Developmental Phonological Disorders

Developmental Phonological Disorders

Foundations of Clinical Practice

Susan Rvachew
Françoise Brosseau-Lapré

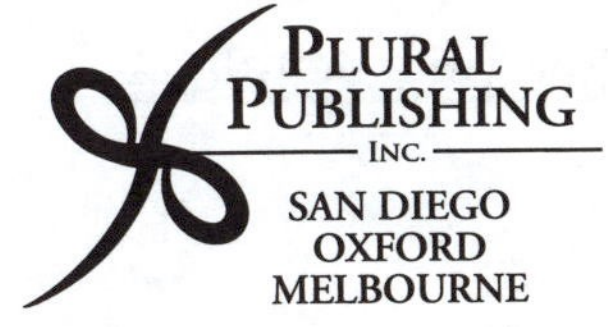

MW

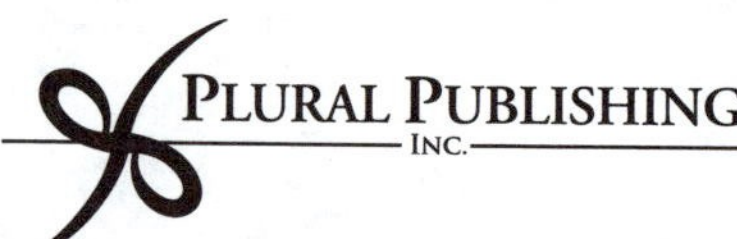

5521 Ruffin Road
San Diego, CA 92123

e-mail: info@pluralpublishing.com
Web site: http://www.pluralpublishing.com

49 Bath Street
Abingdon, Oxfordshire OX14 1EA
United Kingdom

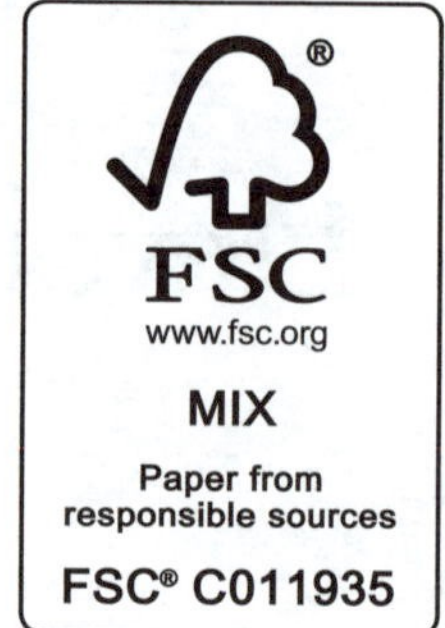

Typeset in 11/13 Palatino by Flanagan's Publishing Services, Inc.
Printed in the United States of America by McNaughton & Gunn

Library of Congress Cataloging-in-Publication Data

Rvachew, Susan.
Developmental phonological disorders : foundations of clinical practice / Susan Rvachew, Francoise Brosseau-Lapre.
p. ; cm.
Includes bibliographical references and index.
ISBN-13: 978-1-59756-377-2 (alk. paper)
ISBN-10: 1-59756-377-3 (alk. paper)
I. Brosseau-Lapré, Françoise. II. Title.
[DNLM: 1. Articulation Disorders—therapy. 2. Child. 3. Language Development. WL 340.2]

618.92'855—dc23

2012005789

4/8/14

Contents

Foreword

Developmental phonological disorders (DPD) are at the center of the profession of speech-language pathology. These disorders have high prevalence in children and frequently accompany other kinds of communicative disorders. A course on DPD is among the first clinical courses in most academic curricula. A sure knowledge of DPD is leverage for understanding other disorders of communication and also for understanding the clinical process itself. The early appearance of the DPD course in a curriculum does not mean it is an easy subject matter. On the contrary, DPD necessarily demands background information from several fields of study, because phonological development, typical or atypical, is a process that draws on a range of knowledge and skills in the developing child. DPD unfolds across several domains of study, including speech perception, speech motor control, phonology and other aspects of linguistics, acoustics, and child development, to name a few. Children are complex, and so is phonological development. The need for cross-disciplinary knowledge is ever-increasing as relevant new information is gathered from fields such as genetics, sociolinguistics, neurolinguistics, and the neurosciences in general. The perspectives in this book are an effective introduction to DPD but also to the larger field of speech-language pathology.

All of the different kinds of knowledge mentioned above are brought to bear on an individual child with a DPD. The way in which the different pieces of knowledge fit together varies from child to child and the enterprising clinician is sensitive to individual differences. Although general patterns can be useful in assessing and treating DPD, ultimately the clinician must recognize the individuality of each child. As the authors note in the introduction to Part I, the development of speech emerges from the interaction of multiple endogenous and exogenous components. To be effective in working with children with DPD, clinicians have to be keen observers, insightful synthesizers, and strategic planners. This sounds like a tall order, and it is. However, Rvachew and Brosseau-Lapré pave the way to fulfilling that order, beginning with comprehensive and insightful summaries of information from the basic sciences such as speech perception, motor control, and phonological development, and then proceeding to detailed accounts of clinical approaches for assessment and treatment, which are enriched by a large number of demonstrations and case studies that illustrate the blending of art and science in clinical practice.

This book welcomes the reader to participate in a productive learning experience that is systematic and rewarding. The first part of the book arms a reader with extensive background information on phonological representation, speech perception, speech motor control, and normal phonological development. The second part builds on the first by moving into clinical assessment, including general issues in assessment of DPD, speech sample analysis, classification of DPD, and treatment planning. The third part elaborates approaches to intervention, with separate chapters on input-oriented approaches, output-oriented approaches, and phonological approaches. The text is complemented by numerous illustrations, case studies, demonstrations, and tables. Well-defined learning objectives are guideposts to the wealth of knowledge that awaits the reader. The information content of this book is considerable, but the authors have artfully organized the material to take readers through the landscape of DPD. Throughout the book, Rvachew and Brosseau-Lapré weave scholarship of the highest caliber with practical wisdom gained through clinical experience and clinical teaching. This book is a generous sharing of expertise. Readers of this book who are new to the profession of speech-language pathology will be well prepared for their first supervised clinical experience in working with a child with DPD. Readers with more experience, even those who have previous coursework in DPD, will find much in this book to warrant close attention and implementation in clinical practice.

Developmental Phonological Disorders: Foundations of Clinical Practice is a book that will have enduring value for individual clinicians and for the profession of speech-language pathology. It is a landmark publication that shows how DPD has matured as a research and clinical specialty. It succeeds in a most difficult undertaking—revealing how complex a subject matter is while showing how that complexity is tractable in the clinic.

Ray D. Kent, PhD
Professor Emeritus of Communicative Disorders
University of Wisconsin-Madison

Acknowledgments

This book is a collaboration between a teacher and a student, both speech-language pathologists, written with the hope that it will serve other teachers and students, including practicing speech-language pathologists who are working to understand the foundations of our clinical practice and maximize outcomes for the children under their care. We wish to thank those who have taught us — beginning with our most important teachers, the children themselves, many of whom appear in the demonstrations and case studies of this book, thanks to the generosity of their parents, who hope that their child's speech data will help other children with developmental phonological disorders. We are grateful to many teachers from our past who helped position us to benefit from the large body of published scholarship and create new research that forms the basis for this book. These individuals include Susan's thesis advisors, Dr. D. G. Jamieson and Dr. E. Slawinski. On a related point we must acknowledge the excellent services offered by the library at McGill University, without which this book could not have been written.

We are indebted to many people who helped us during the writing process by reading and commenting on portions of the book, especially Dr. Ray D. Kent and Dr. Barbara Hodson. Dr. Jon Preston and Dr. Benjamin Munson were also helpful in this regard. We are very happy to share photos and figures provided to us by our very generous colleagues: Dr. Lisa Goffman (Figure 1–5), Dr. Andrea MacLeod (Figure 1–9), Dr. Amy Glaspey (Figure 5–2), Dr. L. D. Shriberg (Figure 7–3), Drs. Edwards, Beckman, Munson, Kurtz, & Windsor (Figure 7–10), and Dr. May (Barbara) Bernhardt (Figure 10–2).

We acknowledge the support of the staff at Plural Publishing throughout the 3-year process with much gratitude. It is with sadness that we note the passing of Dr. Sadanand Singh who, after initiating the project by inviting us to write the book with such enthusiasm and clear vision, was unable to see its completion.

We thank our families whose many sacrifices in support of the writing process are too many to list. Susan expects that Ken and Vivian will stop bringing breakfast in bed upon its publication! Françoise expects Ray, Sophie, and her parents will no longer ask, "Are you done yet?"

Part I

Phonology from a Developmental Perspective

Speech is a quintessential human behavior. The human fetus listens to and learns from speech in the womb and the newborn prefers to listen to the mother's voice above all other auditory inputs. Babies in interaction with their parents engage in heroic efforts to make speechlike sounds, an effort richly rewarded by the emergence of babble by 9 months of age. The use of speech for communication appears shortly thereafter, and by 4 years of age the child is producing meaningful speech in well-formed sentences that are fully intelligible to their communication partners. For some children, the achievement of intelligible speech proves to be an immensely difficult task. The failure to achieve speech that is intelligible enough to serve the social and functional needs of the child in his or her community has immediate and long-term implications that are far from trivial. Learning to help such children is the topic of this book. As with any topic, it cannot be understood fully unless one begins at the beginning. How is it that the typical child learns to produce intelligible speech?

Babble refers to speechlike syllables produced in a rhythmic fashion by normally developing infants between 7 and 11 months of age.

From our perspective, the acquisition of intelligible speech emerges from a perfect marriage of phonetics and phonology. According to old custom, fortuity in marriage requires "something old, something new, something borrowed, and something blue" at the onset. Our approach to the topic has each of these elements. There is certainly no escape from something very old, and that is an ancient debate about the nature of development itself. Throughout the history of human thought, there have been two basic ideas about how developmental change comes about, whether one is talking about concrete structure such as the embryo or abstract knowledge such as grammatical systems. One view founds development on a process of progressive differentiation whereby all the complex structure that will appear during development is present in some prototypical but undifferentiated form in the initial state; the final predetermined form is actualized through a programmed sequence of divisions into finer levels of structure. This view is described as an "inside out" theory because the primary change agent is situated within the organism. This is the model that underlies Jakobson's (1968) view of phonetic development in which infant babble is seen (wrongly, it turns out) as comprising all the sounds of the worlds' languages albeit produced in unstructured form. Jakobson also posited that babbling is followed by a relatively silent interval, after which speech development unfolds by an ordered and universal series of splits yielding major sound classes—consonants versus vowels and then nasals versus orals—followed by further divisions within those classes to produce additional oppositions such as those marking place of articulation. An alternative model views development proceeding via an "outside in" process in which external forces act on the initial state to add complexity in successive steps through a series of generative processes. According to this model of gradual additive complexity the steps are not built into the original state and therefore a predetermined outcome is not assumed. Gould (2002) explains that developmental biology tends to models based on progressive differentiation because of the repeatable and predictable nature of the outcome whereas evolutionary science relies on the notion of additive complexity as an explanation for outcomes that occur only once as a result of a particular, indeed unrepeatable, trajectory of environmental forces. We strongly recommend Gould's essay that traces the central ideas in these alternative models of development back through the history of science to recurring themes in creation myths. Not only is the essay more entertaining and erudite than anything we can accomplish, it shows clearly that both views are so fundamental and long-standing that one would be foolish to treat either with disrespect or claim that one or the other model is simply wrong. We will, however, go so far as to suggest that the preference for models of progressive differentiation in developmental science is based on an illusion of predetermined outcomes. Our experience as parents and as clinicians in pediatric rehabilitation hospitals provides us with an appreciation for the enormous variability in the developmental trajectories that can occur. The well-known challenge of explaining the coexistence of variability and constancy remains. As with the related "nature-nurture" debate, a new synthesis that dissolves the boundaries between "outside in" and "inside out" processes is required (de Waal, 1999; Spencer et al., 2009).

The **"nature-nurture"** debate imposes a false dichotomy between innate factors and environmental influences as explanations for developmental outcomes. Modern science supports an integrated perspective.

Thelen and Smith (1994) sought to achieve this synthesis when they presented the dynamic systems approach as "a biologically valid, but nonreductionist, account of the development of behavior" (p. xviii). This perspective provides "something new" to our approach to developmental phonological disorders (DPD) in relation to the dominant approaches of the past four decades. During this time many different theories of phonology have been introduced to speech-language pathologists (SLPs). As outlined by Ball, Müller, and Rutter (2010) the theories vary greatly in the details of their formal structure and the proposed mechanisms of developmental change. Most theories posit an innately given abstract linguistic structure providing a distinct preformationist flavor to the underlying "inside out" developmental model.

Others draw fairly direct links between speech acquisition and maturation in other domains such as oral-motor or cognitive development, but these alternatives also have difficulty accounting for variable developmental pathways given the linearity of the proposed linkages.

Recently, dynamic systems theory has been applied to the domain of phonological development (e.g., Bybee, 2001), building on connectionist modeling approaches (Munakata & McClelland, 2003) and earlier constructivist accounts of phonological learning (Ferguson & Farwell, 1975). Within a dynamic system, new behaviors emerge from the interactions among multiple components. Those components that arise endogenously, from the so-called biological aspects of the organism's function, and those that arise exogenously from the physical and social environment have equal importance in the developmental process. The multiple components that contribute to the emergence of a new behavior self-organize to meet the demands of a new task in a specific context. A fundamental characteristic of a dynamic system is nonlinearity—gradual and linear changes at a microscopic scale interact to produce new behaviors that emerge as a macroscopic discontinuity. In this book, speech development is viewed as the emergent product of cross-domain knowledge, environmental inputs, and the social and functional needs of the child. Certain concepts from dynamic systems theory will re-occur throughout and therefore they are presented in Table I–1 for easy reference. An example of the application of these concepts to a familiar aspect of cognitive development is discussed next as a means of illustrating some of the core constructs of the theory.

Smith, Thelen, Titzer, and McLin (1999) conducted an in-depth investigation of infant performance in the A-not-B task, a classic paradigm developed by Piaget as a means of testing the infant's achievement of object permanence. The task involves encouraging the infant to search for a desired object that the experimenter hides (in full view of the infant) on repeated trials at a specific location A before hiding the same object at a new but close and similar location B. At the age of 8 months the infant will search again at A when the object is switched to the B location but infants who are 4 months older will search correctly at B when confronted with this task. According to Piaget, sensorimotor exploration of the environment coupled to the mechanisms of assimilation and adaptation

Esther Thelen (1941–2004), a psychologist well known for her studies of rhythmic movement patterns conducted from a dynamic systems theory perspective, is especially recognized for the *embodiment hypothesis*, the notion that cognition is grounded in our perceptions of and actions on the world throughout the life span.

Preformationism is the idea that the form of a living structure pre-exists its development. Philosphically, this idea is opposed to *epigenesis* and both ideas predate the discovery of the genetic code and the molecular basis of developmental biology.

Jean Piaget (1896–1980) was a Swiss developmental psychologist whose theory of cognitive development continues to be influential for its focus on *constructivist (experiential) learning*. Despite the focus on experience with the world as a learning mechanism, cognitive maturation also plays a large role in the theory, mandating a rigid progression through a specific series of stages leading from a sensory-motor understanding of the world toward abstract thought.

Table I–1. *Concepts from Dynamic Systems Theory*

Multicausality	New behaviors arise from the complex interactions among multiple endogenous and exogenous components that have causal equivalence.
Self-organization	The constraints binding the constituent parts spontaneously break, creating instability, and then the constituents reform into a new, stable configuration.
Phase transition	Nonlinear or discontinuous change in the qualitative behavior of the system at the macroscopic level.
Nonlinearity	Linear change at the microscopic scale drives change at the macroscopic scale; gradual change at the microscopic scale can lead to large discontinuities at the macroscopic scale; even small differences at the beginning state can lead to large differences in the outcome.
Heterochronicity	The constituent components in the system change according to their own separate but interacting timetables.
Control parameter	The last of many necessary components to reach some critical level or to be recruited to the task in a given context before the system moves to a new configuration.
Coordinative structure	A functional grouping of components that provides dynamic stability through synergistic coordination of the components within the system.
Dynamic stability	Occurs when the coordinative structure flexibly self-adjusts to the ongoing demands of the task context.
Representational state	A time-dependent state in which an event in the world is re-presented to the nervous system as a particular pattern of neural activation in the absence of the input that specified the original event.

Source: Definitions are adapted from the following sources: Fogel and Thelen (1987); Smith and Thelen (2003); Spencer and Schoner (2003); Stephen, Dixon, and Isenhower (2009); and Thelen and Smith (1994).

are core developmental processes. Despite this focus on the importance of the environment to developmental change, development itself was fixed into an invariant maturational sequence that led the child toward abstract and symbolic knowledge structures that are increasingly distanced from perception and action. Successful search behavior in the A-not-B task was thought to signal the beginnings of detached sensorimotor representations that explained simultaneous advances in multiple domains including object permanence, means-end and imitation skills. The Piagetian view has not held up under the weight of evidence from experiments showing that infant performance in the task is highly context dependent and not at all age-specific: small modifications can result in success for 8-month-olds and failure for 3-year-olds. For example, simply standing the infant up in between the last A trial and the first B trial induces a correct B reach after the switch in hiding location. On the other hand, toddlers will fail the task when objects are hidden in sand, presenting a flat surface with undistinguished hiding locations during trials. These experiments show that performance during the task is not an indicator of maturational change in a knowledge structure that can be abstracted from the details of the task itself. In fact, every feature of the task is critical: the number of A trials in advance of the first B trial, the perceptual salience of the hiding locations, the nature of the hidden object, the length of delay between the hiding and the search, and the infant's posture. These aspects of the task can be manipulated to produce different outcomes in children of different ages. Furthermore, the impact of time and sequencing of events on the way in which the multiple endogenous and exogenous components interact have been precisely modeled for this task (Smith & Thelen, 2003). On any given trial, past experience in the experimental protocol combine with current proprioceptive inputs to account for the strength of the infant's sensory-motor memory for past reaches to A; this sensory-motor memory competes with activation levels for a reach to B that, in younger infants, tend to decay during the delay between the hiding of the object at B and the search. Smith et al. (1999) explain older infants' success in the classic task as a result of improvements in spatial perception that occur as infants gain independence in locomotion as well as refinements in reaching skills that increase flexibility in motor control.

Speech development can also be seen as emerging from the interaction of multiple endogenous and exogenous components, illustrated in Plate 1. Throughout development speech input from the environment is a powerful exogenous component (Plate 1A). We stress the importance of this variable to the development of speech perception skills, speech motor control, and phonological development in Part I of this book. In Part III, the research on environmental contributions to phonological development is used as a guide to the development and selection of therapeutic approaches to the remediation of DPD. Phonological development is dependent on normal auditory and perceptual processing of this input (Plate 1B); we cover the development of speech perception skills in depth in Part I (Chapter 2) and review the literature on the perceptual and phonological processing skills of children with DPD in Part II (Chapter 7). The importance of speech practice—ongoing experience with the phonetic substrate of the sound system of the language from the earliest vocalizations in infancy—is also stressed as a crucial aspect of phonological development (Plate 1D). The development of speech motor control from infancy through adolescence is described in Part I (Chapter 3) and interventions to promote speech motor control are covered in Part III (Chapter 10). Lexical development (Plate 1F) is equally important since, as explained in Chapter 4, phonological knowledge emerges within the lexicon itself; however, the details of lexical development are not covered in detail with the expectation that important aspects of language development that contribute to phonological knowledge will be encountered by the student elsewhere. Crucial aspects of social and cognitive development are also raised repeatedly, although individual chapters are not devoted to these important topics. Within a dynamic system it is often difficult to identify the relevant variables and it is not always

Speech perception refers to the construction of a sound-based representation of speech input, enabling many different kinds of operations on that speech input such as discrimination or identification of sounds and syllables and recognition of spoken words.

The mental **lexicon** organizes information about all the words that a given talker knows, that is, meaning, pronunciation, grammatical inflections, and so forth.

obvious which variable is the control parameter that moves the child into a new mode of functioning. For example, the powerful role of shape perception in lexical learning is surprising and therefore not systematically exploited in speech-language interventions (Smith, Jones, Landau, Gershkoff-Stowe, & Samuelson, 2002). It is hoped that once you are sensitized to the sometimes unexpected nature of these nonlinear relationships, you will be alert to the relevance of learning that will occur outside the context of this text especially as the future is guaranteed to yield many exciting new discoveries in areas such as neurolinguistics and epigenetics.

Infant performance during the A-not-B task is determined in part by their specific history of sensory-motor experiences during the experiment. Similarly, phonology emerges in part from an interweaving of the child's perceptual and motor experiences during the production of speech. However, representational states play a large role in the child's context-dependent behavior during the A-not-B task (Spencer & Schoner, 2003) and are similarly crucial during speech development. The conception of linguistic representations adopted in this book is borrowed from proponents of the multiple representations approach (Beckman & Edwards, 2000; Munson, Edwards, & Beckman, 2005; Pierrehumbert, 2003a, 2003b). Three of several possible levels of representation receive primary emphasis: acoustic-phonetic representations (Plate 1C) are abstracted from the child's experience with speech input and help the child recognize speech sounds even when they are produced by many different talkers in varying contexts; articulatory-phonetic representations (Plate 1E) reflect the child's knowledge of the articulatory characteristics of sounds and allow planning and production of speech output; and phonological representations (Plate 1G) reflect knowledge about the sound system that is generalized across the lexicon and linked to perceptual and articulatory knowledge. These three kinds of representations differ from traditional notions of the phone and phoneme in that they are gradient categories rather than discrete units. Furthermore, they are acquired gradually as dynamic and context specific categories rather than static elements selected from the input in accordance with prespecified options. An organizational scheme for relating linguistic units at the levels of the segmental and prosodic levels of the phonological hierarchy has also been borrowed, in this case from Bernhardt and Stemberger (1998).

Gradient categories are frequency distributions of sounds that vary in their acoustic qualities so that they are not all equivalent exemplars of the category; some are better exemplars of the category than the other and listeners are sensitive to fine acoustic details that account for these differences along the gradient in category goodness.

This brings us to the requirement for "something blue," an element in the wedding ritual that symbolizes fidelity. It has been our goal throughout the writing of this text to remain faithful in every instance to the research evidence. Throughout, we have a particular point of view and have not attempted to present a variety of theoretical perspectives as in a survey text. However, every point made in the text is supported by high quality empirical research. In each chapter, key studies are described in detail and data that may be useful to clinicians and researchers is presented in full. We feel that it is essential for SLPs to understand the research methods that are used to conduct empirical research in phonological development and disorders so that past, current, and future research can be evaluated for its validity and its relevance to practice.

It may seem odd to emphasize the importance of the scientific foundation of the field while invoking a superstition meant to bring luck in a context where there are uncertain outcomes ahead. There is a certain irony but perhaps a hint of felicity too as the model of phonological development that we are supporting here gives an important role to chance as one of many components in a multi-determined system. The child is seen as actively constructing phonological knowledge through his or her own interactions with a complex social and linguistic environment in real time. Certain constraints on what is possible and functional produce an outcome that permits most of us to communicate with each other verbally from an early age. At the same time, chance events account for striking disparities among children in their level of speech and language development that are not usually observed in other developmental domains, even when we restrict our view to those following a normal[1] trajectory. It has been suggested that researchers, looking at variability in phonological development, were "focusing on the wrong properties of linguistic systems" because "the variation that occurs within a species represents the superficial effects of environmental factors in more accessible structures" as opposed to the less accessible but invariant and defining structures of the organism (Dinnsen, 1992; p. 192). In contrast, we prefer Blumberg's (2009) view of archetypal structures when he remarks: "Left to its own devices, nature always takes exception to the rule, undermines the archetype, and reminds us that our ideas about what is natural and what we should do to correct nature's "imperfections" are as sound as a sandcastle battered by a rising tide." (p. 4)

As we are Canadians, we are using the term **speech-language pathologists (SLPs)** throughout this book to denote the professionals who serve individuals with communication disorders with the understanding that the term is meant to be synonymous with equivalent professional titles used in other countries such as *speech therapist* or *speech and language therapist*.

An archetype is the original form of a structure from which all others are copied.

[1]There has been a trend in recent years toward the substitution of the word "typical" for "normal" that has been carried over from casual discourse to scientific writing in a fashion that is imprecise and often inappropriate to the context. The trend appears to date from the appearance of "person-first" style guidelines that promote the use of terms such as "children with language impairment" versus "language-impaired children" to describe research participants. We are in complete agreement with the person-first guidelines and the extension of these guidelines to the description of children in the control groups (American Psychological Association: Public Interest Directorate, 2011). Throughout this book we stress the enormous variability that occurs in developmental trajectories for speech and language development. In fact, we define DPD largely in relation to the distribution of speech accuracy scores within the child population as a whole. We would not describe any particular child as being "normal" or "typical," thus implying that any one child could exemplify the prototypical standard against which other children can be compared. However, the term "normal" in the scientific sense of a distribution of test scores is essential to the definition of DPD, relating to the "normal curve" and defining a range of test scores that captures the performance levels of the majority of children in the population. Children who fall below the range defined by one standard deviation below the mean can be defined as falling within the DPD category, as discussed in greater depth in Part II. Notice that in each use of the term "normal" a specific distribution of numbers is the reference

References

American Psychological Association: Public Interest Directorate. (2011). *Enhancing your interactions with people with disabilities*. Retrieved June 14, 2011, from http://www.apa.org/pi/disability/resources/publications/enhancing.aspx

Ball, M. J., Müller, N., & Rutter, B. (2010). *Phonology for communication disorders*. New York, NY: Psychology Press.

Beckman, M. E., & Edwards, J. (2000). The ontongeny of phonological categories and the primacy of lexical learning in linguistic development. *Child Development, 71*, 240–249.

Bernhardt, B., & Stemberger, J. P. (1998). *Handbook of phonological development from the perspective of constraint-based phonology*. San Diego, CA: Academic Press.

Blumberg, M. S. (2009). *Freaks of nature: What anomolies tell us about development and evolution*. Oxford, UK: Oxford University Press.

Bybee, J. (2001). *Phonology and language use*. Cambridge, UK: Cambridge University Press.

de Waal, F. B. M. (1999). The end of nature versus nurture. *Scientific American, 281*(6), 94–99.

Dinnsen, D. A. (1992). Variation in developing and fully developed phonetic inventories. In C. A. Ferguson, L. Menn, & C. Stoel-Gammon (Eds.), *Phonological development: Models, research and implications* (pp. 191–210). Timonium, MD: York Press.

Ferguson, C., & Farwell, C. B. (1975). Words and sounds in early acquisition. *Language, 51*(2), 419–439.

Fogel, A., & Thelen, E. (1987). Development of early expressive and communicative action: Reinterpreting the evidence from a dynamic systems perspective. *Developmental Psychology, 23*, 746–761.

Gould, S. J. (2002). The narthex of San Marco and the pangenetic paradigm. In S. J. Gould (Ed.), *I have landed: The end of a beginning in natural history* (pp. 271–284). New York, NY: Harmony Books.

Jakobson, R. (1968). *Child language, aphasia, and phonological universals*. A. Keiler, Trans. The Hague: Mouton.

---

and not a whole person or even a population of people. We can expect that every individual will fall at various points along the "normal curve" for different measures of functioning, some of us excelling at language, for example, while failing miserably at swimming and none of us being so bold as to describe ourselves as "typical" exemplars of the human form! We use the term "typical" to describe certain participants of studies where it was the preferred term of the authors of the cited papers. Otherwise, we use the term "normal" to indicate a range of performance levels on a specific measure of developmental functioning for a group of children or to define an individual's performance on a specific measure relative to the range of scores obtained by a normative group of children. Here again, it is important to remember from your statistics classes that a normative reference is not a group of "normal people" but a distribution of numbers obtained from a defined sample of people, usually but not always constructed to represent the population as a whole. In our view, the term "normal" in its scientific sense describes the observed range of "natural imperfections" whereas the term "typical" invokes the prescriptive notion of the "archetype" that we are eschewing in this text.

Munakata, Y., & McClelland, J. L. (2003). Connectionist models of development. *Developmental Science, 6*(4), 413–429.

Munson, B., Edwards, J., & Beckman, M. E. (2005). Phonological knowledge in typical and atypical speech-sound development. *Topics in Language Disorders, 25*(3), 190–206.

Pierrehumbert, J. (2003a). Phonetic diversity, statistical learning, and acquisition of phonology. *Language and Speech, 46*, 115–154.

Pierrehumbert, J. (2003b). Probabilistic Phonology: Discrimation and Robustness. In J. H. a. S. J. R. Bod (Ed.), *Probability theory in linguistics.* Cambridge, MA: MIT Press.

Smith, L. B., Jones, S. S., Landau, B., Gershkoff-Stowe, L., & Samuelson, L. K. (2002). Object name learning provides on-the-job training for attention. *Psychological Science, 13*(1), 13–19.

Smith, L. B., & Thelen, E. (2003). Development as a dynamic system. *Trends in Cognitive Sciences, 7*, 343–348.

Smith, L. B., Thelen, E., Titzer, R., & McLin, D. (1999). Knowing in the context of acting: The task dynamics of the A-not-B error. *Psychological Review, 106*, 235–260.

Spencer, J. P., Blumberg, M. S., McMurray, B., Robinson, S. R., Samuelson, L. K., & Tomblin, J. B. (2009). Short arms and talking eggs: Why we should no longer abide the nativist-empiricist debate. *Child Development Perspectives, 3*(2), 79–87.

Spencer, J. P., & Schoner, G. (2003). Bridging the representational gap in the dynamic systems approach to development. *Developmental Science, 6*(4), 392–412.

Stephen, D. G., Dixon, J. A., & Isenhower, R. W. (2009). Dynamics of representational change: Entropy, action and cognition. *Journal of Experimental Psychology: Human Perception and Performance, 35*, 1811–1832.

Thelen, E., & Smith, L. B. (1994). *A dynamic systems approach to the development of cognition and action*. Cambridge, MA: MIT Press.

Chapter 1

Describing Phonological Knowledge at Multiple Levels of Representation

Types of Phonological Knowledge

1.1.1. List and define four types of phonological knowledge.

1.1.2. Distinguish phonetic encoding from phonological knowledge.

1.1.3. Distinguish segmental and suprasegmental characteristics of speech.

Before turning to the topic of phonological development it is necessary to understand the different types of phonological knowledge and the tools that are used to describe phonological knowledge at these different levels of representation. The ability to use speech sounds to transmit meaning is dependent on multidimensional knowledge of the sound system of the talker's (and the listener's) language (Munson, Edwards, & Beckman, 2005). Four types of phonological knowledge will be introduced briefly. Subsequently, the different tools and units of analysis used to describe each type of phonological knowledge will be covered.

When you greet your friend with, "Nice weather today," it is obvious that *articulatory knowledge* is required to accurately produce the speech sounds in the phrase. You must possess motor plans that are flexible enough to ensure accurate production of each sound across a variety of phonetic and prosodic contexts. You must also be able to execute those plans, precisely coordinating the various articulators involved. Learning to produce speech sounds accurately and consistently also requires finely tuned *perceptual knowledge* of

Articulatory knowledge is encoded in the form of *articulatory-phonetic representations* that support the production of the speech sound categories available for use in speech communication.

Perceptual knowledge is encoded in the form of *acoustic-phonetic representations* that support the perception of speech sound categories that are available for use in speech communication.

Parametric phonetics is concerned with the physical reality of speech sounds.

Phonetic encoding involves the abstraction of phonetic categories from the parametric phonetic space.

Phonological representations reflect knowledge of how speech sounds are contrasted and combined to create meaningful words in the language.

the sound system of the language. The communicative exchange that you have initiated will not be successful unless you and your listener can encode the fine acoustic details of the utterance and are both aware of the many subtle acoustic differences that distinguish sounds such as the "n," the "t," and the "d" in the spoken greeting. Articulatory and perceptual knowledge are both concerned with phonetic levels of representation. Phonetics is concerned with the study of the sounds that are available for use in speech communication from the perspective of their physical production and perception (Ohala, 1999). Phonetic knowledge includes parametric phonetics and phonetic encoding (Pierrehumbert, 2003b). The parametric level of representation involves the physical reality of speech sounds—the production of speech with the vocal apparatus and the transmission of those sounds through the air to the ear of the listener. Phonetic encoding involves the abstraction of phonetic categories from the parametric phonetic space.

Given that you intend to transmit a specific message to your listener you must also have *phonological knowledge* of how speech sounds are contrasted and combined to create meaningful words in the language. In this text we focus on the segmental aspects of phonological knowledge, meaning knowledge of the way in which phonemes such /t/ and /d/ are used to code meaning. Suprasegmental characteristics of speech such as intonation patterns also carry meaning as you would note in the difference between the cheery rendition of "Nice weather today" on a sunny June morning in comparison with the sarcastic version that you might produce if it were –30°C and snowing! *Social-indexical knowledge* of linguistic characteristics that mark membership in different social groups defined by categories such as gender, social class, race, and sexual orientation will also receive little attention in this text but nonetheless constitutes an important aspect of phonological knowledge that has a distinct developmental trajectory and which may be difficult for certain children to acquire. We now turn to the units of analysis and measurement tools that are used to describe phonological knowledge.

Describing Articulatory Knowledge

1.2.1. Derive a phonetic repertoire from a broad transcription of a sample of a child's speech.

1.2.2. List 6 instrumental means of describing articulatory knowledge and evaluate the advantages of these techniques relative to phonetic transcription as a representation of the child's articulatory knowledge of the sound system.

1.2.3. Define motor equivalence.

International Phonetic Alphabet

A standard tool for representing speech is the International Phonetic Alphabet (IPA), developed over one hundred years ago as a set of universal characters to represent speech sounds in terms of articulatory characteristics, specifically voicing and place and manner of articulation (International Phonetic Association, 1999). Each of the universal characters in the alphabet represents a unique phone or speech sound. As shown in Figure 1–1, the consonant symbols represent 11 places of articulation (arranged in the columns of the consonant chart) and 8 manner classes (arranged in the rows of the chart). The consonants might be produced with vocal fold vibration to produce a voiced sound or without vocal fold vibration to produce a voiceless sound. Vowels are represented according to three dimensions. The placement of the primary constriction is described along a continuum from front to back; degree of opening of the vocal tract varies from close to open (in some charts this dimension is referred to as tongue height varying from high to low); finally, the presence or absence of lip rounding during production of the vowel distinguishes pairs of vowels that share characteristics along the other two dimensions.

The **International Phonetic Alphabet (IPA)** was developed over 100 years ago as a set of universal characters to represent speech sounds in terms of articulatory characteristics.

These consonant and vowel symbols can be used by a trained listener to create a *broad transcription* of speech produced by any talker in the world. Care must be taken to represent the speech as the transcriber heard it produced and not as one might expect the utterance to be said. A teacher might introduce the principal by saying [mɪz tʃæn hæz sʌmθɪŋ tu ʃoʊ ʌs] ("Ms. Chan has something to show us") but later during recess describe the class clown to a colleague by mumbling [ʔi ʃɝ ɪz sʌmfn̩] ("He sure is something"). Even adults are unlikely to produce all utterances in accordance with the dictionary pronunciation guide; much variation in pronunciation occurs across and within talkers as a function of sociolinguistic and pragmatic factors.

A **broad transcription** represents the phonetic categories produced by the talker as perceived by the listener.

A narrow transcription is created by using the diacritics to provide additional phonetic detail about the sounds that were produced. Consider for example, the varied articulatory characteristics of the [t] in [tʰek ðə plæstɪk fʊt̚bɑl aʊɾəv ðə bæθt̪ʰʌb] ("Take the plastic football out of the bathtub"). Variations in suprasegmental characteristics can also be represented, for example, [ɪts ə ˈtʰaɪˌgɚ] ("It's a tiger!") in comparison to [ɪz ɪɾə ˌtʰaɪˈgɚː] ("Is it a tiger?").

When creating a **narrow transcription**, the transcriber uses *diacritics* to represent as much phonetic detail as possible about the production of each phonetic category as produced by the talker.

Phonetic transcription has a number of advantages as a means of describing a talker's articulatory knowledge. The primary advantage is that a trained listener can produce a description of a talker's performance quickly and easily with little or no technology. The absence of intrusive technology means that young children's performance can be observed during natural speaking situations ensuring the ecological validity of the results of your observation of the

An advantage of phonetic transcription is the potential to obtain an ecologically valid description of the child's speech.

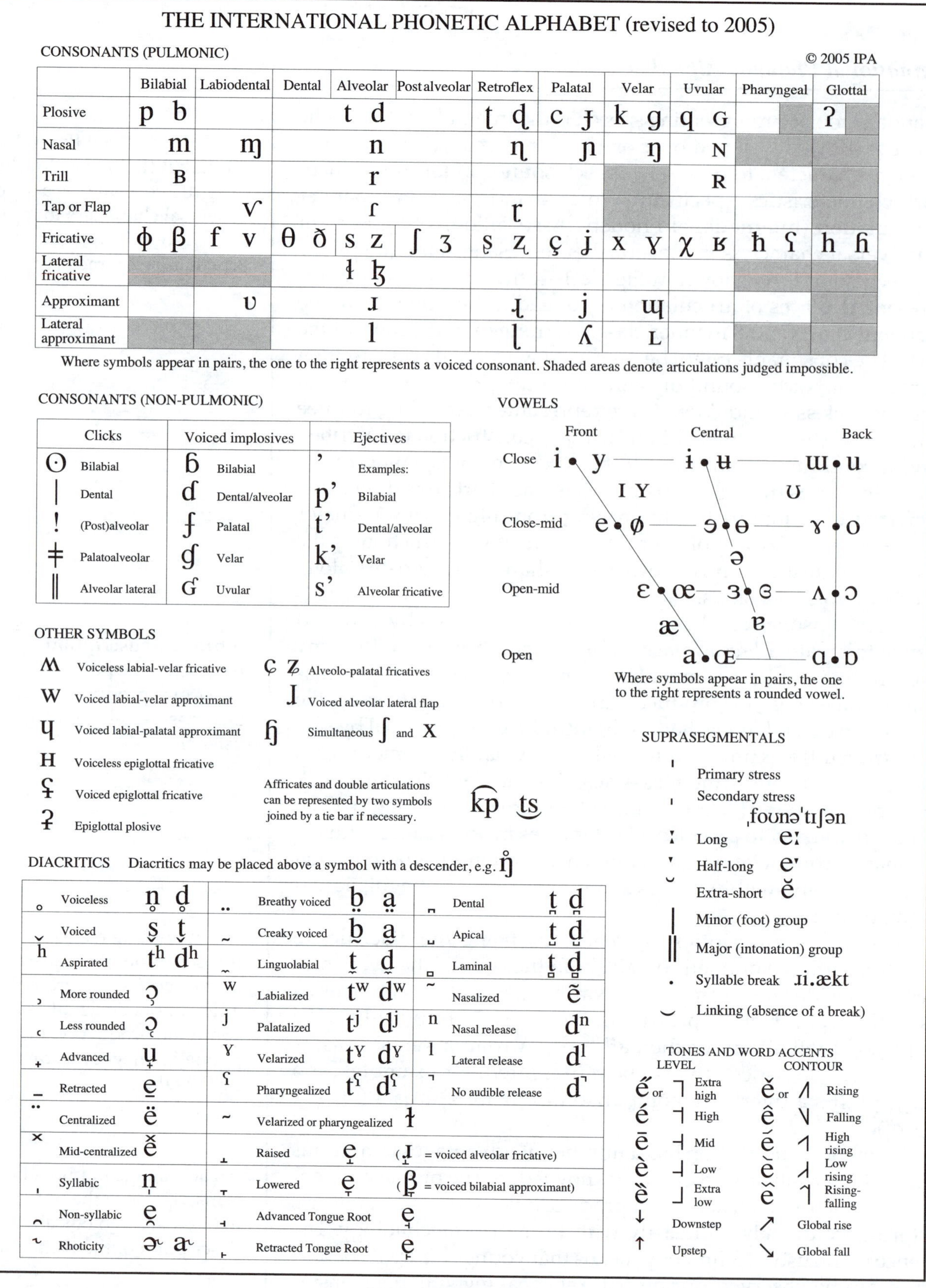

Figure 1–1. *The International Phonetic Alphabet. Source: http://www.langsci.ucl.ac.uk/ipa/ipachart.html. Copyright 2005 by The International Phonetic Association. Reprinted with permission from the International Phonetic Association.*

child's speech performance. With practice, you can learn to derive a phonetic repertoire from the transcription of the child's speech with very little delay, allowing you to provide immediate feedback to the child's parents or teachers about the child's articulatory abilities. As shown in Figure 1–2, a phonetic repertoire is simply an inventory of the phones that the child uses when speaking. The inventory of consonants is organized by place and manner of articulation, mirroring the organization of consonants on the IPA chart in Figure 1–1. Similarly, the vowels are organized in groups to reflect the location of the major constriction (front, central, or back) and listed in order from relatively closed to relatively open. By convention, a phone that occurs only once in the speech sample is shown between parentheses. The phonetic repertoire includes phones even if they are not phonemic in the language that the child is learning. Notice that in Figure 1–2, the English-learning child produced a phone that sounded and looked like a voiced bilabial fricative and thus the symbol [β] appears on the chart even though this sound is not typically used in English. Notice also that the sounds are listed on the chart even if they are not used correctly; thus, [l] is shown in the phonetic repertoire even though it was used at the beginning of the words

A phonetic repertoire is simply an inventory of the phones that the child uses when speaking, usually organized by place and manner of articulation.

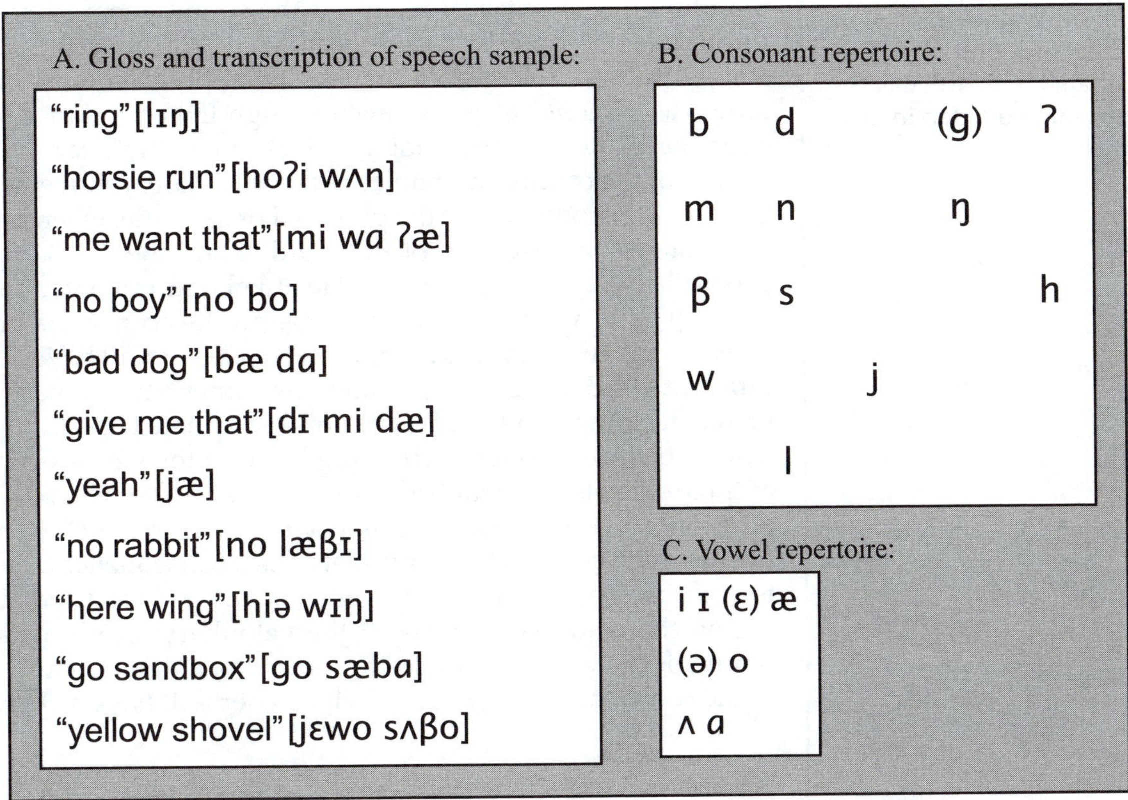

A. Gloss and transcription of speech sample:
"ring" [lɪŋ]
"horsie run" [hoʔi wʌn]
"me want that" [mi wɑ ʔæ]
"no boy" [no bo]
"bad dog" [bæ dɑ]
"give me that" [dɪ mi dæ]
"yeah" [jæ]
"no rabbit" [no læβɪ]
"here wing" [hiə wɪŋ]
"go sandbox" [go sæbɑ]
"yellow shovel" [jɛwo sʌβo]
B. Consonant repertoire:
b d (g) ʔ
m n ŋ
β s h
w j
l
C. Vowel repertoire:
i ɪ (ɛ) æ
(ə) o
ʌ ɑ

Figure 1–2. Example of orthographic gloss and phonetic transcription of a speech sample taken from a hypothetical 18-month old child (A) with the consonant repertoire (B) and the vowel repertoire (C) derived from the sample.

"ring" and "rabbit."[1] The phonetic repertoire can be a very useful tool for identifying children whose speech development is delayed or for describing changes in a child's speech development over time (Dinnsen, Chin, Elbert, & Powell, 1990; Stoel-Gammon, 1985), even when the child is at the prelinguistic stage of speech development as discussed further in Chapters 4 and 5.

Phonetic transcription provides an inaccurate picture of articulation for a number of reasons including biased perception by the transcriber, imposition of discrete categories on a continuous acoustic substrate, and segmentation and linear ordering of phones associated with articulatory gestures that overlap in time and space.

The phonetic transcription and phonetic repertoire shown in Figure 1–2 describe the child's articulatory knowledge at the level of *articulatory-phonetic representations.* For example, the transcription of the child's production of the word "bad" as [bæ] suggests that he represents this word as if it is composed of two phones, an oral plosive produced with an initial closure of the lips and simultaneous vocal fold vibration followed by a vowel produced with a relatively open vocal tract and a constriction placed near the front of the oral cavity. However, this description of the child's speech is a highly abstract representation that remains far removed from his actual articulatory behavior. Phonetic transcription provides an inaccurate picture of articulation for a number of reasons. First, it is a transformation of the sounds that the listener hears, and as will be explained further in this chapter, human speech perception is invariably biased by numerous factors especially past language experience and thus phonetic transcriptions cannot be an accurate rendition of the physical reality of the sound energy transmitted through air or the articulatory gestures that produced that sound energy. Second, the system requires that speech sounds be represented as discrete categories even though the boundaries between one phone category and another are not perfectly clear as a consequence of the continuous nature of the articulatory movements that underly the production of the phones. For example, when transcribing a talker's production of the word "and" the SLP is forced to choose between the open front vowel [æ] and the open-mid front vowel [ɛ] and yet the vowel that was produced may be part way between the two and furthermore, each listener will have a slightly different standard for determining how "open" the vowel has to be before deciding that [ænd] is a more appropriate transcription than [ɛnd]. The transcription further implies that the word is composed of three discrete segments produced in linear order when in fact the articulatory gestures that are associated with the two phones will overlap each other in time and space. As a consequence of anticipatory coarticulation, the vowel might actually be nasalized, depending on the degree of closure of the velopharyngeal port and the timing of the velar gesture as the talker transitions from the vowel to the consonant. Once again, each listener will have a slightly dif-

[1]Throughout this text [w] will appear on such charts as a voiced bilabial approximant although, as noted on the IPA chart it is a voiced bilabial-velar approximant, which recognizes the high-back position of the tongue dorsum that combines with the bilabial constriction during the production of this glide.

ferent standard for determining how much nasality in the vocalic portion of the word they will tolerate before deciding whether [ænd] or [æ̃nd] is the more appropriate transcription. Finally, the IPA implies that there is a one-to-one relationship between articulatory gestures and phonetic categories when in fact the relationship is many-to-one. In order to describe speech at a more purely articulatory level of representation, different analysis tools are required. In the next section, technologies that can be used to visualize articulatory gestures and vocal tract shapes are briefly introduced.

Visual Analysis of Articulation

Visualization of the vocal tract has been accomplished with the use of various forms of x-ray technology for many decades. A well-known example is provided by Delattre and Freeman (1968) who recorded cineradiographic images of articulatory movements during the production of [ɹ] in real time. This study revealed considerable variation in articulatory patterns for the phone with talkers employing 8 different types of tongue shapes involving varying degrees of constriction in the pharyngeal, palatal, and lip regions of the supralaryngeal vocal tract. These findings have been generally confirmed by subsequent studies using magnetic resonance imaging (Alwan & Narayanan, 1997) and ultrasound (Gick & Campbell, 2003) to visualize articulatory movements and vocal tract shapes. Figure 1–3 presents a series of line tracings derived from magnetic resonance images of the vocal tract during [ɹ] production that illustrate the many-to-one relationship between articulatory patterns and phonetic categories (Alwan & Narayanan, 1997).

Visualization of the vocal tract with various technologies reveals considerable variation in articulatory patterns for the production of [ɹ] in real time by different talkers.

Electropalatography (EPG) is a technology that is used to provide information about patterns of tongue contact with the palate during speech production. EPG data is transmitted from a series of electrodes that are embedded in a pseudopalate to a computer that displays the pattern of contacts by electrode over time on the computer monitor. Typically, the pseudopalate is custom made for each user's hard palate (e.g., Reading/WINEPG; McLeod & Singh, 2009), an expensive process that has largely reserved this technology for research purposes. Recently, a system has been developed that reduces the cost of creating the pseudopalate thus improving access to the technology for speech assessment and intervention in regular clinical practice (Logometrix EPG; Schmidt, 2007). EPG has proven useful for the investigation of normal articulatory phenomena such as coarticulation (Gibbon, 1999), as shown in Figure 1–4. EPG has also revealed interesting patterns of atypical articulatory behavior among children with DPD and is proving to be an effective treatment tool for some children as discussed further in Chapters 7 and 10.

Electropalatography (EPG) is a technology that is used to provide information about patterns of tongue contact with the palate during speech production. EPG has proven useful for the investigation of normal articulation development and atypical patterns of articulation. EPG is proving to be an effective treatment tool for some children with DPD.

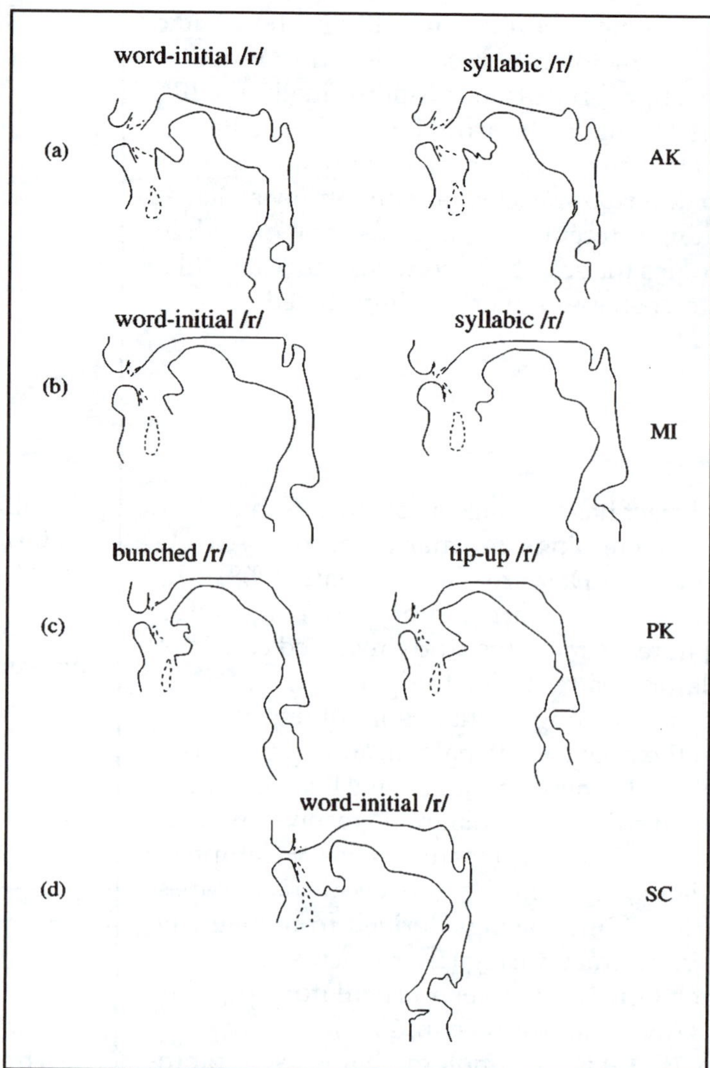

Figure 1–3. *Sagittal profiles of the vocal tract during production of [ɹ] by 4 different adult talkers.* Source: *Alwan, Narayanan and Haker (1997). Toward articulatory-acoustic models for liquid approximants based on MRI and EPG data. Part II. The rhotics.* Journal of the Acoustical Society of America by Acoustical Society of America, 101, *Figure 1, p. 1079. Reproduced with permission from American Institute of Physics for the Acoustical Society of America.*

Kinematic Descriptions of Articulation

Kinematic analyses involve direct measurements of the direction, amplitude, speed, and/or force of movement of specific articulators during speech production.

Kinematic analyses involve direct measurements of the direction, amplitude, speed, and/or force of movement of specific articulators during speech production. A technology used in research applications is the electromagnetic midsagittal articulograph (EMMA), developed to track the locations of transducers that are attached to the tongue, jaw, lips, and teeth along the midsagittal plane and plot

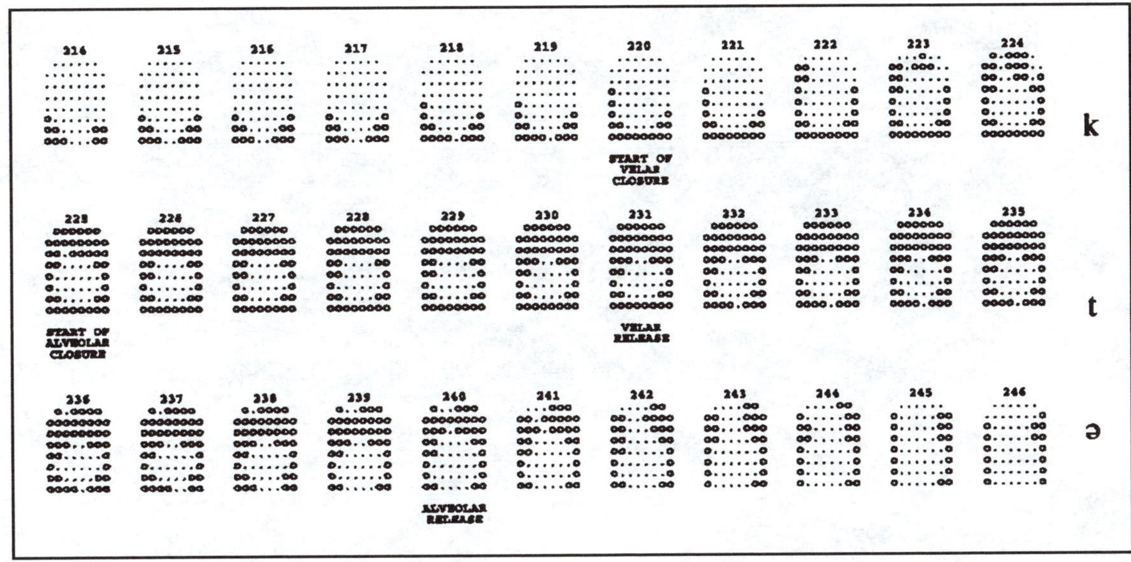

Figure 1–4. *EPG display showing simultaneous tongue tip/blade and tongue body contact with the palate during lingual coarticulation of [kt] during production of the word "tractor" by a 12-year-old girl with normal speech.* Source: *Gibbon, F. E. (1999). Undifferentiated lingual gestures in children with articulation/phonological disorders.* Journal of Speech, Language, and Hearing Research, 42, *Figure 2, p. 386. Reprinted with permission of the American Speech-Hearing-Language Association.*

their trajectories in an anatomically defined coordinate space in real time (Nieto-Castanon, Guenther, Perkell, & Curtin, 2005). EMMA provides data that is comparable to older x-ray microbeam systems (Westbury, Hashi, & Lindstrom, 1998) while being cheaper, safer, and generally more accessible. These techniques have revealed many interesting aspects of adult articulatory behavior including large degrees of intertalker variability (Westbury et al., 1998) and intratalker variability (Nieto-Castanon et al., 2005) in lingual movement patterns during production of [ɹ].

With children, less invasive procedures are used to track the locations of markers placed on the child's face, especially upper and lower lips, as illustrated in Figure 1–5, which shows the apparatus used by Lisa Goffman to study the development of speech motor control in children with typical and atypical speech development. Displays that represent the amplitude of articulator movement over time are produced and velocity of articulator movement can be calculated. Variability in these movement patterns over many repetitions of a given utterance can also be measured, typically using the spatiotemporal index (STI) as shown in Figure 1–6, which presents data from a study by Sadagopan and Smith (2008), who found that movement variability increased with sentence complexity and decreased with age. This is just one of many studies showing interactions among lower levels (e.g., articulatory) and higher levels (e.g., syntactic) of representation.

The **spatiotemporal index (STI)** quantifies variability in oral movements over many repetitions of an utterance (after normalizing for duration and amplitude).

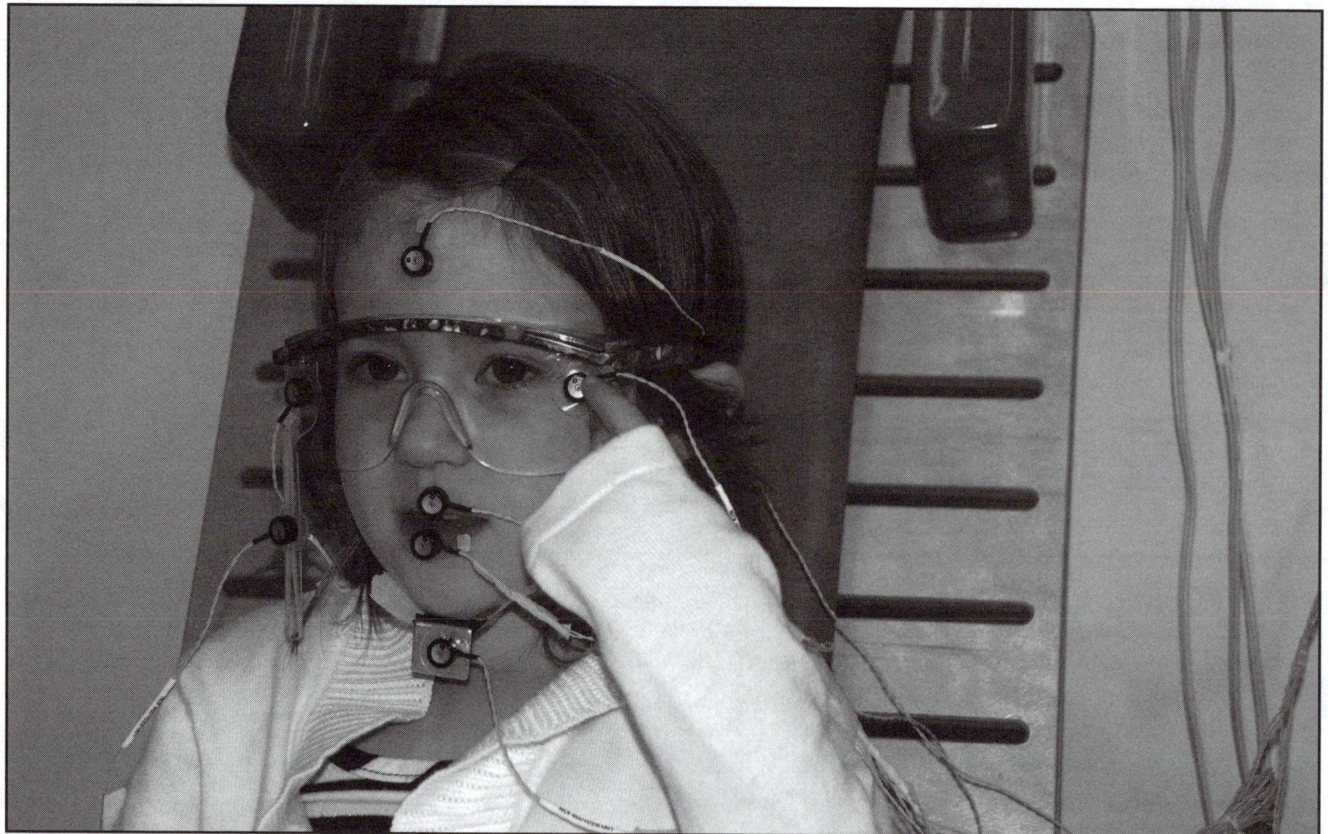

Figure 1–5. *Apparatus for obtaining kinematic measurements of lip and jaw movements. Provided by Dr. Lisa Goffman.*

Pressure transducers can be used to measure the pressure exerted by one articulator against another. For example, Hinton and Arokiasamy (1997) measured interlabial pressure during the production of labial stops in connected speech by normal adult female talkers and found that less than 20% of the maximum available interlabial force was used during these speaking conditions. Dworkin and Culatta (1980) measured tongue strength for three groups of school-age children: children with tongue thrust and open bite but normal speech; children with tongue thrust, open bite, and frontal lisps; and children with normal occlusion and normally developing speech. All three groups of children demonstrated comparable tongue strength when requested to apply maximum tongue strength against resistance.

Motor Equivalence and Articulatory Targets

Studies that utilize the imaging and kinematic technologies described in the previous sections reveal the many-to-one relationship between articulatory gestures and phonetic categories. Every time a consonant described as an alveolar fricative is produced, the

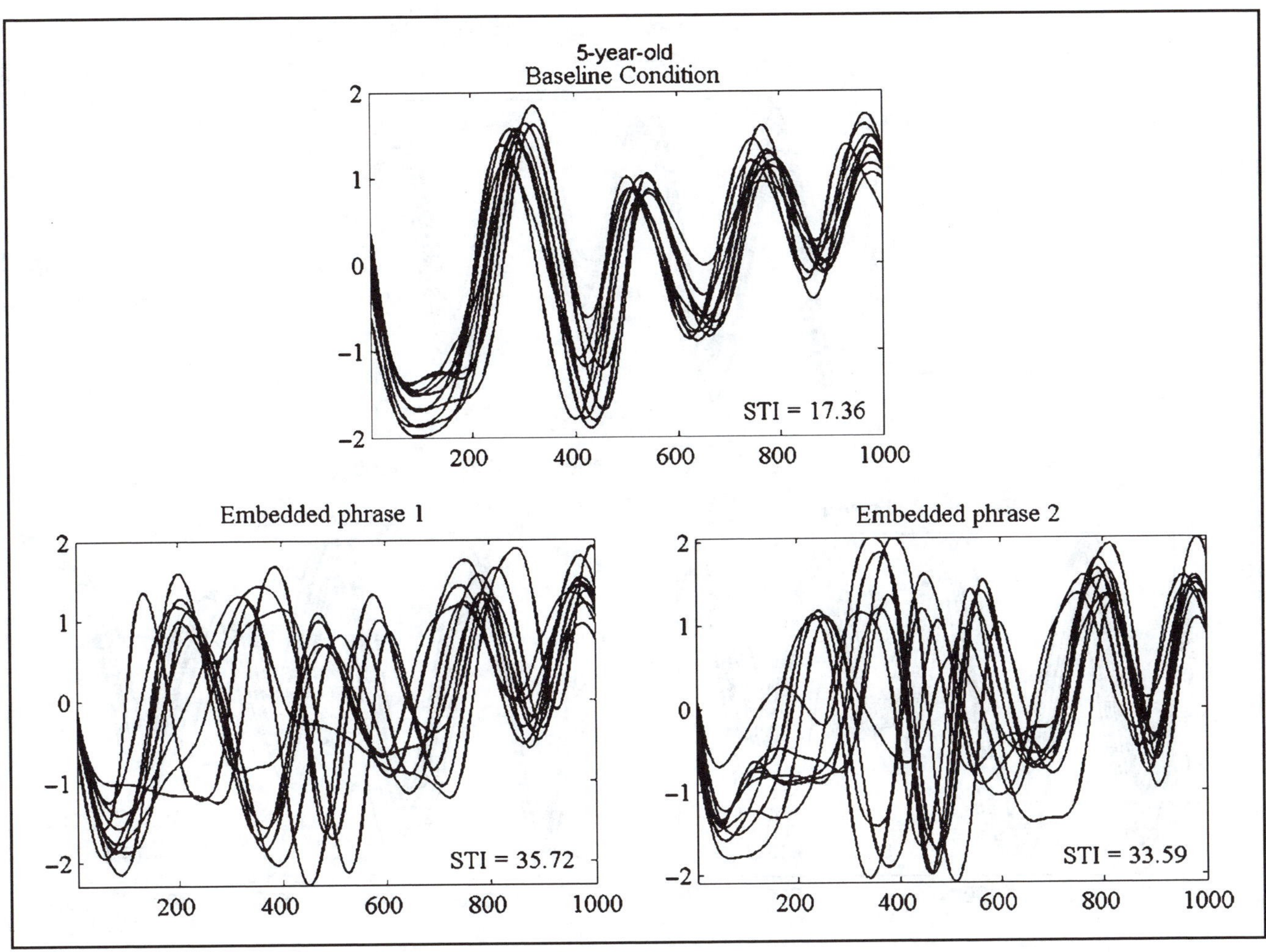

A

Figure 1–6. *Time and amplitude normalized trajectories of lower lip movements of a 5-year-old (**A**) and a 12-year-old (**B**) child while producing the phrase "Buy Bobby a puppy" in the baseline (simple sentence) and embedded (complex sentence) conditions.* Source: *Sadagopan, N., and Smith, A. (2008). Developmental changes in the effects of utterance length and complexity on speech movement variability.* Journal of Speech, Language, and Hearing Research, 51, *Figure 3, p. 1144 (**A**) and Figure 4, p. 1145 (**B**). Reprinted with permission of the American Speech-Hearing-Language Association.* continues

articulatory gestures will be somewhat different. Variations related to coarticulatory effects are well known; for example, the placement of the tongue tip is likely to be more forward when the consonant is produced in the syllable [sti] as compared to [sku]. However, coarticulatory effects due to different phonetic contexts are not the only reason for gestural variability. Some variability reflects the fact that different combinations of articulatory gestures will have the same acoustic effects, a phenomenon called motor equivalence. For example, when producing the [u] vowel it is necessary to create a relatively long cavity in front of the constriction in the oral cavity. Lengthening of the front cavity can be accomplished by moving the tongue dorsum farther back or by protruding the lips further

Motor equivalence refers to the phenomenon whereby different combinations of articulatory gestures produce the same acoustic effects.

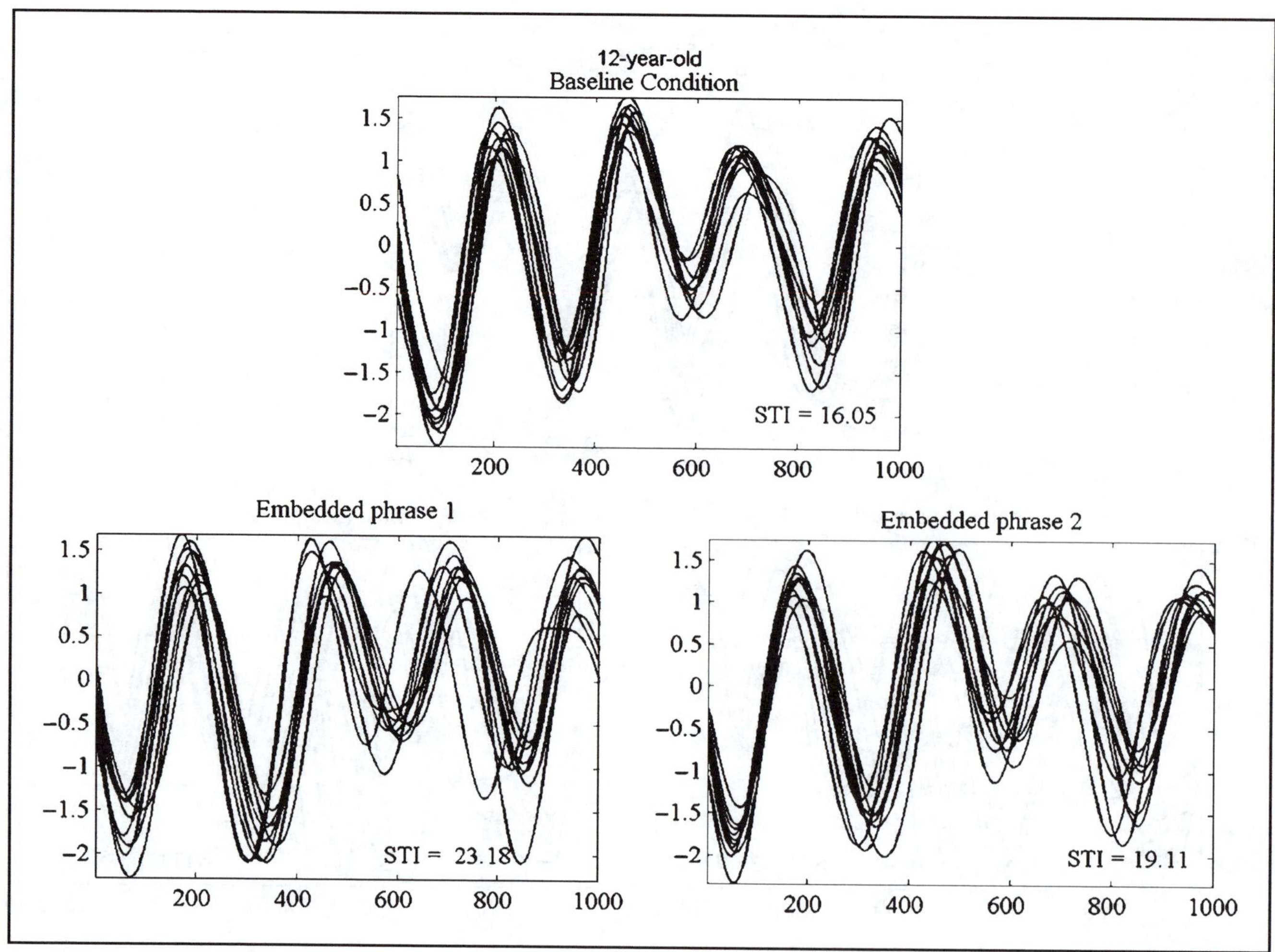

B

Figure 1–6. continued

forward. This phoneme also requires a relatively closed vocal tract which can be accomplished by varying degrees of jaw raising or lip closure. The exact combination of gestures that is produced is thought to reflect the principle of economy of effort within the context of the preceding and following sound sequence. The degree to which the talker manipulates the jaw, the lips, or the tongue when speaking might also vary systematically across language groups (Gick, Wilson, Koch, & Cook, 2004), regardless of phonetic context. There also appear to be speaker-specific preferences even within language groups. Maeda (1990) modeled the vocal tract profiles of two female speakers of French from cineradiographic data and documented patterns of interarticulator compensation during the production of different vowels. Among other findings, their data showed that degree of jaw closure does not relate in a straightforward way to vowel identity along the continuum of vowels described as varying from close to open. Degree of jaw closure can be compensated for by positioning of the tongue dorsum so that a supposedly open vowel could be produced with a more closed jaw posture provided that the tongue dorsum is adjusted to compensate. Furthermore, these adjustments did not simply reflect coarticulatory effects. There were clear intertalker preferences in the use of the jaw to effect differences in vowel quality as shown in Figure 1–7. This figure traces changes in tongue position relative to jaw position during the production of the vowels [a] and [i]. It is clear that the first talker is relying more on tongue dorsum movements than changes in jaw height to produce these vowels. For both speakers, changes in tongue dorsum position were found to be linearly related to jaw height.

These findings about variability in articulatory gestures have implications for the way we think about the goals of speech as a motor task and further highlight the inadequacy of the IPA as a description of what the talker is doing during the act of speaking. As already noted, it cannot be said that the talker's goal, when producing the word "sea" is to produce a linear ordering of phones, first an alveolar fricative and then a close-front unrounded vowel. It is not more accurate to suggest that the talker is attempting to produce an overlapping sequence of articulatory gestures. Rather it

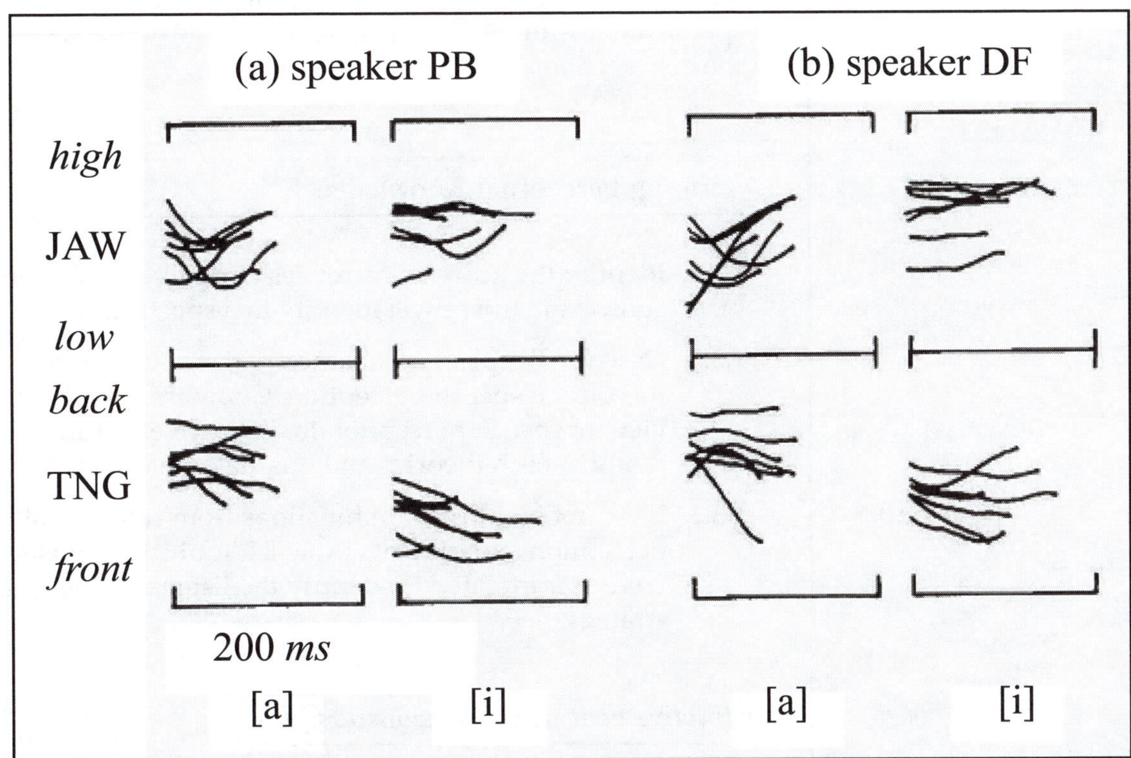

Figure 1–7. *Superimposed temporal patterns of tongue-dorsum and jaw movements during production of the vowels [a] and [i] in different phonetic contexts by two female French-speakers.* Source: *Maeda, S. (1990). Compensatory articulation during speech: Evidence from the analysis and synthesis of vocal-tract shapes using an articulatory model. In W. Hardcastle and A. Marchal (Eds.),* Speech Production and Speech Modelling, *The Netherlands: Kluwer Academic Publishers. Figure 7, p. 145. Copyright © 1990 Springer. Reprinted with permission from Springer Science+Business Media B.V.*

appears that the talker is attempting to shape the vocal tract in such a way as to produce sounds that will be perceived by the listener to be the desired word. Many combinations of articulatory gestures will accomplish the goal and many factors determine the exact solution to the problem at any given time for any given talker.

Summary: Articulatory Knowledge

A phonetic transcription of a talker's speech and an associated phonetic repertoire can provide a snapshot of the individual's phonological knowledge at the level of articulatory-phonetic representations. For example, the phonetic repertoire for the hypothetical toddler shown in Figure 1–2 shows that the child has an established repertoire of labial and alveolar phones but no knowledge of the labiodental and dental places of articulation. It must be remembered that phonetic transcription provides an abstract representation of the child's articulatory knowledge and not a veridical representation of physiological reality. More precise visual tools and kinematic measurements reveal the underlying continuity and nonlinearities in the articulatory movements that comprise speech sounds. A similar tension exists between acoustic-phonetic representations of speech and the underlying raw acoustic information as discussed in the next section.

Describing Perceptual Knowledge

1.3.1. Identify the acoustic correlates of distinctive features to consonant and vowel identity in a spectrogram.

1.3.2. Describe the primary characteristics of exemplar-based theories of speech perception. Compare and contrast this view of speech perception to distinctive feature theory, motor speech theories and quantal-enhancement theory.

1.3.3. Interpret identification functions from categorical perception experiments in which multiple acoustic cues were manipulated to identify the listener's cue weighting strategy.

Distinctive Features and Acoustic Cues

Acoustic cues are hypothesized units of essential acoustic information that define speech sounds in the perceived acoustic waveform.

One approach to the problem of understanding how the listener perceives speech input as a linearly ordered string of speech sounds is tied to the notion that speech must contain acoustic cues that can be associated with natural categories of speech sounds in a reasonably straightforward fashion. Jakobson, Fant, and Halle (1963) declared that acoustic "wave traces contain too much information and that means must be provided for selecting the essential information" (p. 11). They proposed a solution whereby phonemes were minimally contrasted on the basis of bundles of binary features, each of which could be defined by their acoustic attributes. For example, [n] and [t] form a minimal pair of consonants that are similar except for a distinctive difference with respect to the feature [nasal]; specifically, [t] is designated as [−nasal] and [n] as [+nasal] on the basis of the absence and presence (respectively) of a nasal murmur—identifiable on a spectrogram as a series of weak nasal resonances interspersed with marked antiresonances. Their proposed set of distinctive features was supplanted by the more familiar Chomsky and Halle (1968) features that are based on a combination of auditory and articulatory features. Recently, Ladefoged (1999) argued for the utility of describing phoneme classes in terms of features that are defined in acoustic terms. For example, voice was defined as the presence of periodic low-frequency energy, sibilant by the presence of aperiodic high-frequency energy, and sonorant by the presence of periodic energy with well-defined formants (see Ladefoged, 1999, Table 19.3). The acoustic correlates of these features can be observed in Plate 2, which presents an acoustic representation of the phrase "Nice weather today!" in the form of a broad band spectrogram at the top of the figure and a waveform display at the bottom. The waveform shows variations in the amplitude of sound energy over time. The corresponding spectrogram displays changes in the relative concentration of energy at different frequencies over time, with frequency shown on the y-axis, time on the x-axis and relative amplitude of the frequency components represented by the brightness of the colors. The waveform display provides some information about major sound classes. For example, in the word "nice" the highest amplitude peak is associated with the vowel and the lower amplitude peak is associated with the consonant. Similarly in the two syllables of the word "today" the vowels are associated with relatively high amplitude peaks and the consonants are associated with relatively low amplitude peaks. Some temporal information is apparent in the waveform display and relative duration readily differentiates the fricatives [s] and [ð] from the stops [t] and [d]. The spectrogram provides additional indicators of phonetic features. The nasal murmur marked as "a" differentiates [+nasal] from [−nasal] consonants. As marked by the "b," [+sonorant] segments are clearly differentiated from [−sonorant] segments by the presence of periodic energy (regular vertical striations) and well-defined formants (horizontal yellow bars marking concentrations of acoustic energy in a given frequency region). The [+sibilant] fricative [s] is identified by the aperiodic high frequency energy marked as "c" which can be contrasted with the fricative [ð] which is not only [−sibilant] as indicated by the low amplitude, low frequency energy but also [+voice] as indicated by periodic energy shown as vertical striations in the area of the spectrogram marked as "d."

The acoustic correlates of place of articulation are indexed in the Jakobson, Fant, and Halle (1963) feature system by two pairs of

A **distinctive feature** is an acoustic or articulatory parameter whose presence or absence defines a phonetic category in contrast to another phonetic category.

A **waveform display** shows variations in the amplitude of sound energy over time.

A **spectrogram** displays changes in the relative concentration of energy at different frequencies over time, with frequency shown on the y-axis, time on the x-axis, and relative amplitude of the frequency components represented by the intensity of the color scale (may vary in brightness as shown in the color spectrogram in Plate 2 or in darkness as shown in gray scale spectrograms in later figures in this book).

The four corners of the **vowel space** are defined by the extreme values of the acoustic features *grave, diffuse, compact,* and *acute.*

opposed features that describe the distribution of acoustic energy in the spectrum. Consonants and vowels with a *compact* spectrum show energy concentrated in a single central region of the spectrum in contrast to segments that show a more diffuse distribution of energy with additional peaks in the spectrum. The stop [k] is [+compact] in contrast to the stop [t] which is a [−compact] (i.e., diffuse) consonant because it has two prominent energy peaks in the release burst and following aspiration noise (see "d" on Plate 2 marking an area on the spectrogram with energy concentrated at approximately 3300 and 6600 Hz). A second pair of features, grave and acute, serves to contrast spectra with predominantly low frequency energy versus predominantly high frequency energy, respectively. Labial consonants are [+grave] whereas alveolar consonants are [−grave] (i.e., acute). These features also define the four corners of the vowel space, as illustrated in Figure 1–8. The top part of the figure shows the frequency spectra for the corner vowels [u] (close back), [i] (close front), [ɑ] (open back), and [æ] (open front—the IPA chart shows [a] as the vowel in the open front corner of the vowel space but this vowel is not used, at least not phonemically, in Canadian English). The features as defined are difficult to see in these raw acoustic representations but can be observed after some transformation of the data as shown in the bottom part of the figure. The scatter plot shown in Figure 1–8 represents ten productions of each of the four vowels as produced by adult female talkers in the context of single-syllable words such as "shoe," "feet," "pop," and "cat." The first and second formant frequencies (in Hz) were derived from frequency spectra as shown in the top part of the figure and then converted to the Mel scale in order to reflect human perception of pitch (Stevens, Volkmann, & Newman, 1937). Next, each vowel was given a value on the grave-acute dimension by calculating [(Mel1 + Mel2)/2] and a value on the compact-diffuse dimension by calculating [Mel2 – Mel1]. The vowels were then plotted in feature space, which results in four distinct clusters of vowels, with [ɑ] the most compact and [i] the least compact and [u] the most grave, and [æ] the least grave of all the vowels.

The utility of any proposed feature and the associated acoustic cue is not determined by examining the acoustic characteristics of speech however. Rather, it is necessary to investigate the perceptual responses of listeners to speech input that has been structured to highlight the acoustic-phonetic information that is presumed to constitute an acoustic cue to a given distinctive feature.

Categorical Perception

Early speech perception studies presented listeners with naturally produced recordings of syllables or words selected to represent each feature contrast that was of interest to the investigator. Typically, only a single token would be presented of each syllable or

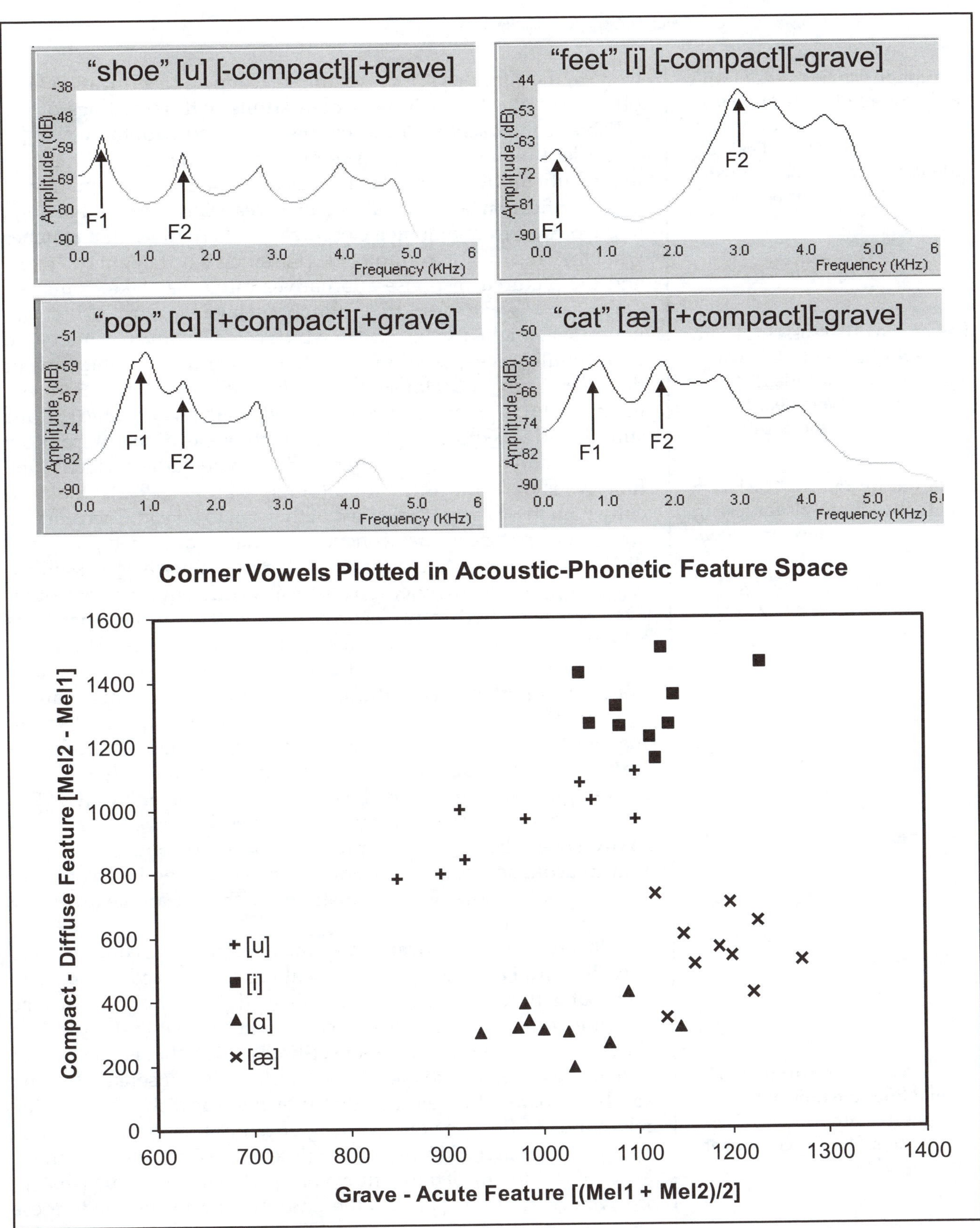

Figure 1–8. *Frequency spectra of the corner vowels [u], [i], [ɑ], and [æ] (top). Acoustic-phonetic characteristics of 10 productions of each of the corner vowels produced by adult female talkers and plotted with respect to the feature dimensions grave versus acute and compact versus diffuse* (bottom).

Perception can be assessed with a closed-set **identification task** in which the listener points to pictures or letters to indicate the identity of the syllable or word that was heard.

Perception can be assessed with a **discrimination task** in which listeners indicate whether pairs of stimuli were heard to the same or different.

The **oddity and ABX tasks** are alternative protocols for testing discrimination.

Voice-onset-time (VOT) quantifies the time of voicing onset relative to the release burst for the consonant.

word in the stimulus set. For example, using an identification task, Miller and Nicely (1955) presented adults with recordings of CV syllables composed of 16 consonants combined with the vowel [ɑ] and asked the listeners to write down what they heard (the task made difficult by the overlay of masking noise). An adaptation of the identification task for children involves asking the child to point to the picture from among a closed-set of alternatives that matches what they heard. For example, the presented word might be "rake" and the pictured response alternatives might be "lake," "make," "rake," and "wake" (Waldman, Singh, & Hayden, 1978). A discrimination task might also be used in which listeners are presented with two stimuli and expected to indicate whether they are the same or different (Graham & House, 1971). Alternative discrimination testing procedures are the oddity task in which the listener hears three stimuli and is required to indicate which one is different from the other two and the ABX task in which the listener judges which of the first two is the same as the third (Singh & Becker, 1972). One difficulty with these early studies is that they fail to take into account the continuous nature of the acoustic cues that underly the presumed distinctive features. As is apparent in Figure 1–8, each vowel spoken within a phonetic category is acoustically different from each other even when plotted in phonetic feature space. Studies that have attempted to predict perceptual responses on the basis of the number of differences in binary features between a pair of stimuli have not lead to perfectly straightforward results; some pairs that are separated by an equal number of features are not equally discriminable and sometimes pairs differentiated by a larger number of features are more difficult to discriminate than pairs differentiated by a single feature (Graham & House, 1971; Miller & Nicely, 1955). The advent of technology to synthesize speech allowed researchers to investigate listeners' perceptual responses to continuous variation in acoustic cues. The major characteristics and outcomes of these types of studies will be illustrated with an example involving voice-onset time.

In a typical categorical perception experiment, a continuum of speech stimuli are created that vary along a single acoustic parameter that is thought to cue a given distinctive feature contrast. The example to follow illustrates perception of the feature [+voice] on the basis of variation in voice-onset-time (VOT), that is, the time of voicing onset relative to the release burst for the consonant. Voicing can begin before the release burst (voicing lead), shortly after the release burst (short lag voicing) or significantly after the release burst, usually accompanied by aspiration (long lag voicing). Although we are used to thinking of the feature [voice] in binary terms such that [p] is [−voice] and [b] is [+voice] the underlying acoustic cue to these categories is continuous in nature. Furthermore, the way in which the continuum of potential VOT values is organized into categories differs by language group as shown in Figure 1–9 for English and French. Understanding how listeners organize continuous varia-

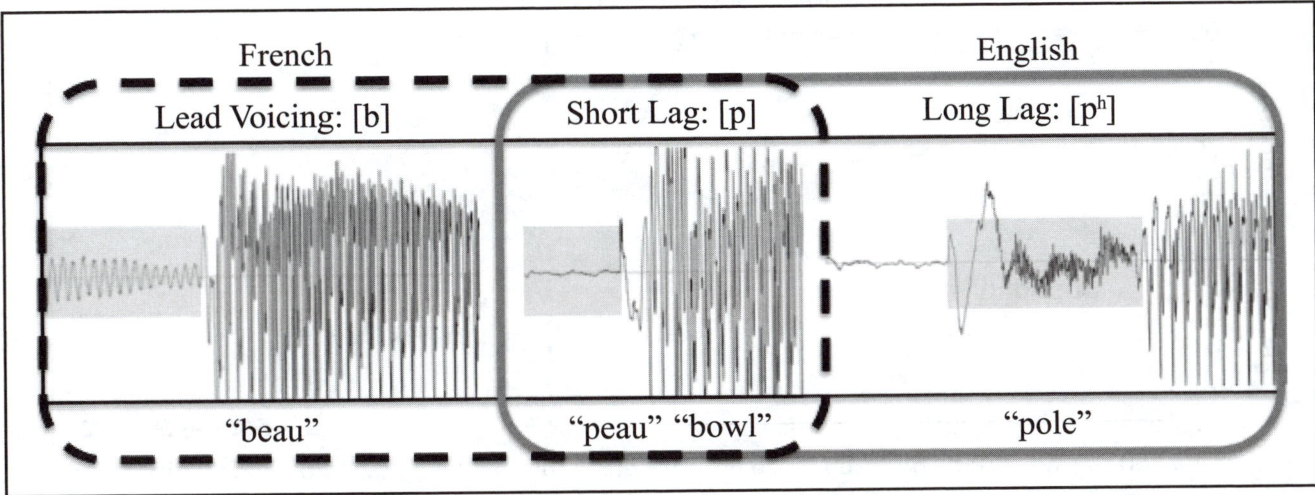

Figure 1–9. *Waveforms showing voicing lead (gray shading marks voicing before release of the stop consonant), short lag voicing (gray shading marks short interval between release of the stop and onset of voicing) and long lag voicing (gray shading marks long interval between release of the stop and onset of voicing). The [b] and [p] categories are realized as voicing lead and short lag voicing in French, whereas the same categories are realized as short lag voicing and long lag voicing in English. Printed with permission from Dr. Andrea MacLeod.*

tions in VOT into phonetic categories requires that the investigator present listeners with speech stimuli in which VOT has been systematically manipulated but all other acoustic characteristics of the stimuli have been held constant across the continuum. Identification and discrimination task responses to VOT continua reveal categorical perception of this feature as illustrated in Figure 1–10.

Figure 1–10 shows identification task performance for one listener who responded to 15 tokens of a VOT continuum in which the first stimulus "to" had a VOT of +80 ms and the fifteenth stimulus "do" had a VOT of 10 ms. VOT was varied in 5-ms steps across the continuum (the middle part of Figure 1–10 shows every second stimulus with the interval between stimulus onset and the onset of voicing shaded to indicate the progressively shorter duration of this interval from stimulus 1 to stimulus 15). The listener's task was to listen to each word, presented in random order with 16 repetitions of each stimulus, and indicate whether the word was 'to' or "do." The identification function plots the number of "to" responses per stimulus. The listener identified all stimuli with a VOT greater than 45 ms as "to" and all stimuli with a VOT less than 30 ms as "do." The category boundary (the point at which 50% of responses are assigned to each response category) is located at approximately 40 ms and the category boundary width is slightly more than 15 ms (marked as the shaded region between approximately 30 and 45 ms where the listener is less than 75% certain about the identity of the stimuli). As perceptual abilities mature the slope of the identification function will become steeper and the width of the category boundary will become narrower, as discussed in greater detail in

The **category boundary** is the point on the *identification function* at which 50% of responses are assigned to each response category. **Category width**, the region marking less than 75% certainty about the identity of the stimuli, narrows with age and experience.

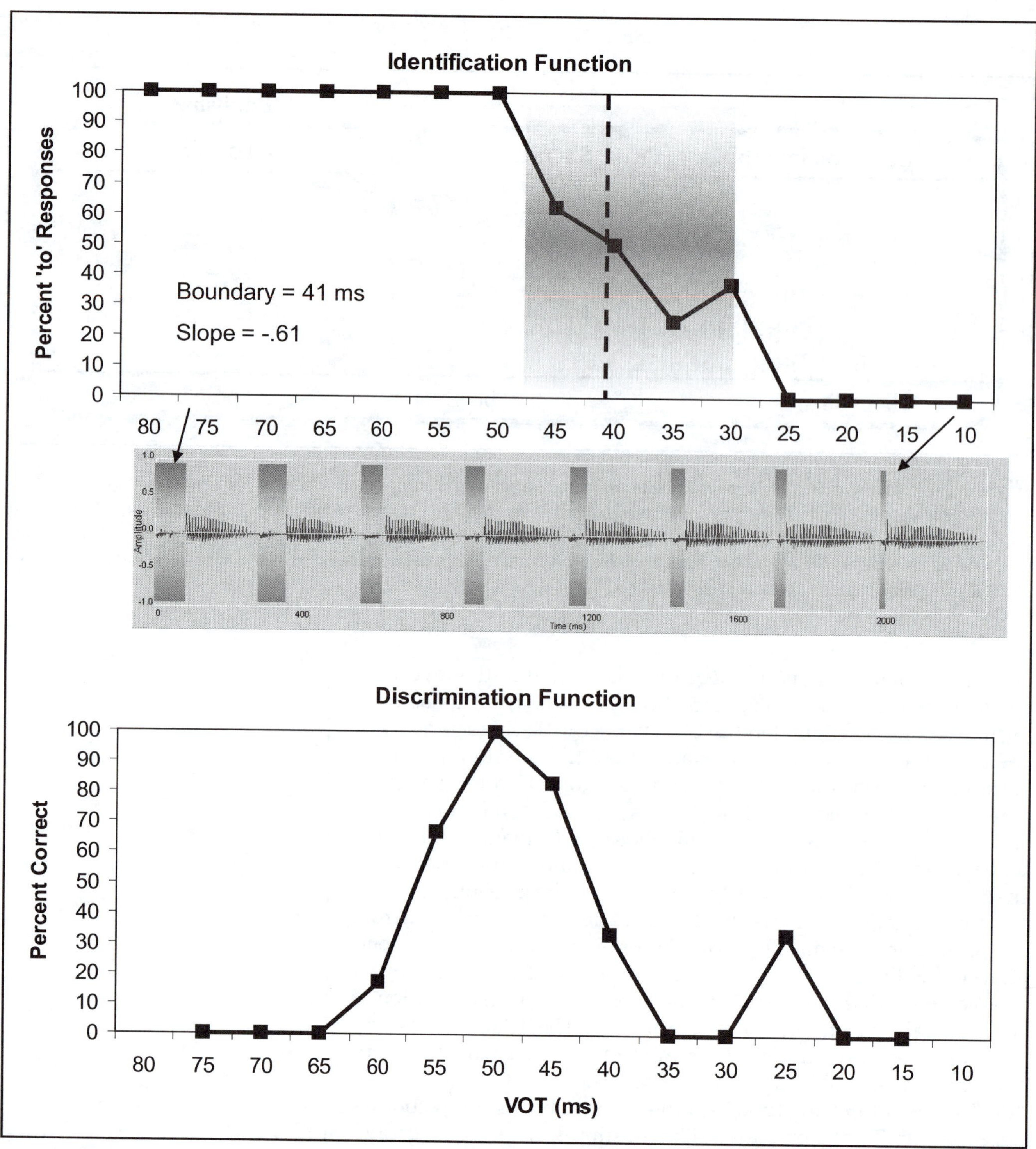

Figure 1–10. *Identification function plotting one English adult listener's responses to a 15 stimulus continuum that varies in 5 ms steps from 80 to 10 ms of voice-onset-time. Dashed vertical bar indicates the category boundary and shading marks the width of the boundary region. The middle part of the figure shows the waveform of every second stimulus with the interval between stimulus onset and voicing onset marked with gray shading to highlight the linear progression of reduced voice-onset-time across the continuum. The lower part of the figure shows the discrimination function for the same listener and stimuli, indicating a marked peak in discrimination accuracy at 50 ms. The discrimination function illustrates categorical perception such that the listener is unable to discriminate a 10-ms difference in VOT when the two stimuli lie clearly within the listener's [t] or [d] categories but is able to discriminate a 10-ms difference in VOT when the stimuli cross into the boundary region between the two phonetic categories.*

Chapter 2. The lower part of the figure shows a discrimination function for the same listener. In this case the listener responded to pairs of stimuli that were always 10 ms different (e.g., 80 ms vs. 70 ms or 35 ms vs. 45 ms, etc.). All possible stimuli were presented equal numbers of times and stimulus order within each pair was counterbalanced so that in half the trials the stimulus with the larger VOT preceded the stimulus with the lower VOT and in the remaining trials the order was reversed. The listener judged whether the two stimuli sounded the "same" or "different" with 16 repetitions of each pair presented in random order. The figure plots the percentage of correct responses with points centered over the VOT value that lies between the pair of stimuli to which the listener responded. A large peak in discrimination performance is apparent at 50 ms VOT indicating that the listener always heard the pair of stimuli contrasting 60 and 40 ms VOT to be different. The most important point that is illustrated by the discrimination function is that perceptual performance is not linearly related to the acoustic differences between the stimuli. The stimulus pair contrasting 80 ms and 70 ms of VOT was consistently heard to be the same as was the stimulus pair contrasting 20 ms versus 10 ms of VOT. However, trials that included a stimulus that fell within the listener's boundary region were heard to be different most of the time even though these pairs also involved a 10 ms difference in VOT. For this specific listener, the discrimination peak is shifted about 10 ms higher than the identification boundary so that it occurs at the edge of the boundary region. Typically, these experiments involve averaging perceptual responses across many listeners who speak the same language, often leading to smoother functions and a very close relationship between the category boundary and the discrimination peak (Abramson & Lisker, 1970).

A defining feature of **categorical perception** is that discrimination performance is not linearly related to acoustic differences between stimuli. Within-category stimuli are difficult to discriminate whereas between-category stimuli are easy to discriminate even when the acoustic difference is constant.

Complexity in Perceptual Encoding

The picture drawn of perceptual encoding thus far is based on the false assumption that phonetic segments are directly recoverable from the acoustic waveform. Looking at the waveform and spectrogram shown in Plate 2 it is tempting to think that our speech perception system need only segment the first word in the spectrogram into the three pieces marked "a," "b," and "c" and then identify the appropriate bundle of features for each segment in order to yield the phonetic representation [nɑɪs]. Discontinuities in the spectrogram readily yield the impression of discrete segments and many of the features seem to be visible in the spectrogram reinforcing the impression that phonetic encoding is a simple process. The first 50 ms appear to indicate that it is [+nasal] (nasal murmer) and [−compact] (diffuse distribution of energy at the point of release of the consonant into the vowel) indexing the location of the segment [n] at the beginning of this word. Having recovered the distinctive

Perceptual encoding is a complex process in that phonetic segments are *not* directly recoverable from the acoustic waveform.

features from the acoustic signal that lead to identification of the segments, the acoustic information itself can be discarded as the language processor proceeds to lexical access. In fact, speech processing is highly complex and the assumption that the features are transparently available in the acoustic signal cannot be supported (Nittrouer, 2002a, 2006). Two categories of problems arise with this simplistic view: those associated with the lack of invariant cues to the identity of features or phonetic segments and those associated with the nonlinearity of acoustic-phonetic information in the acoustic signal.

The **lack of invariant acoustic cues** to the identity of a given phone or phone sequence when produced within and across speakers, language groups, speaking registers, and phonetic contexts complicates perceptual encoding of speech.

The acoustic information that is associated with a given phone or phone sequence varies greatly within and across speakers, language groups, speaking registers, and phonetic contexts. Differences among speakers of different ages can be dramatic as illustrated in Figure 1–11, which plots the extreme corners of the vowel space with respect to the grave-acute and compact-diffuse feature dimensions as estimated from samples of speech recorded from English-learning infants, aged 10 to 18 months of age, and their mothers. The speech samples were recorded as part of a study on cross-linguistic development of vowel production (Rvachew, Alhaidary, Mattock, & Polka, 2008; Rvachew, Mattock, Polka, & Menard, 2006). For this figure, vowels that had the most extreme values of the acute, grave, compact, and diffuse features were selected from all of the vowels that the mother and infant produced during the recording session (20 English-learning infants varying in age between 10 and 18 months and 5 mothers are represented in the figure). For the infant samples, feature values were regressed on age (in days) and used to estimate the corners of the vowel space for an infant aged 10 and 18 months old. In an extensive review of the literature, Vorperian and Kent (2007) linked changes in the acoustic vowel space from infancy through adulthood to anatomical changes in the vocal tract. Undoubtedly, maturation of speech motor control and phonological development also plays a role. The differences in the shape, size and location of the vowel space for infants, children, and adults are so marked that it is clear that some form of speaker normalization is required in order for listeners to hear such acoustically different vowels as being phonetically equivalent. Some success in computer identification of vowels despite differences in talker age and gender has been achieved by researchers who have proposed invariant relationships among the first three formants and between formants and fundamental frequency (e.g., Syrdal & Gopal, 1986), although these talker normalization algorithms do not achieve humanlike levels of identification accuracy.

Speaker normalization is the process by which the listener perceives common phonetic categories produced by talkers with vocal tracts of different sizes.

Even when one examines the vowels from a single age and gender, considerable variation in the acoustic characteristics of specific vowels occurs within and across language groups. Plate 3 shows the feature values of the vowels [i], [u], and [a] as spoken by English, Russian and Swedish mothers in an adult-directed and infant-directed speaking register (Kuhl et al., 1997). Cross-linguistic

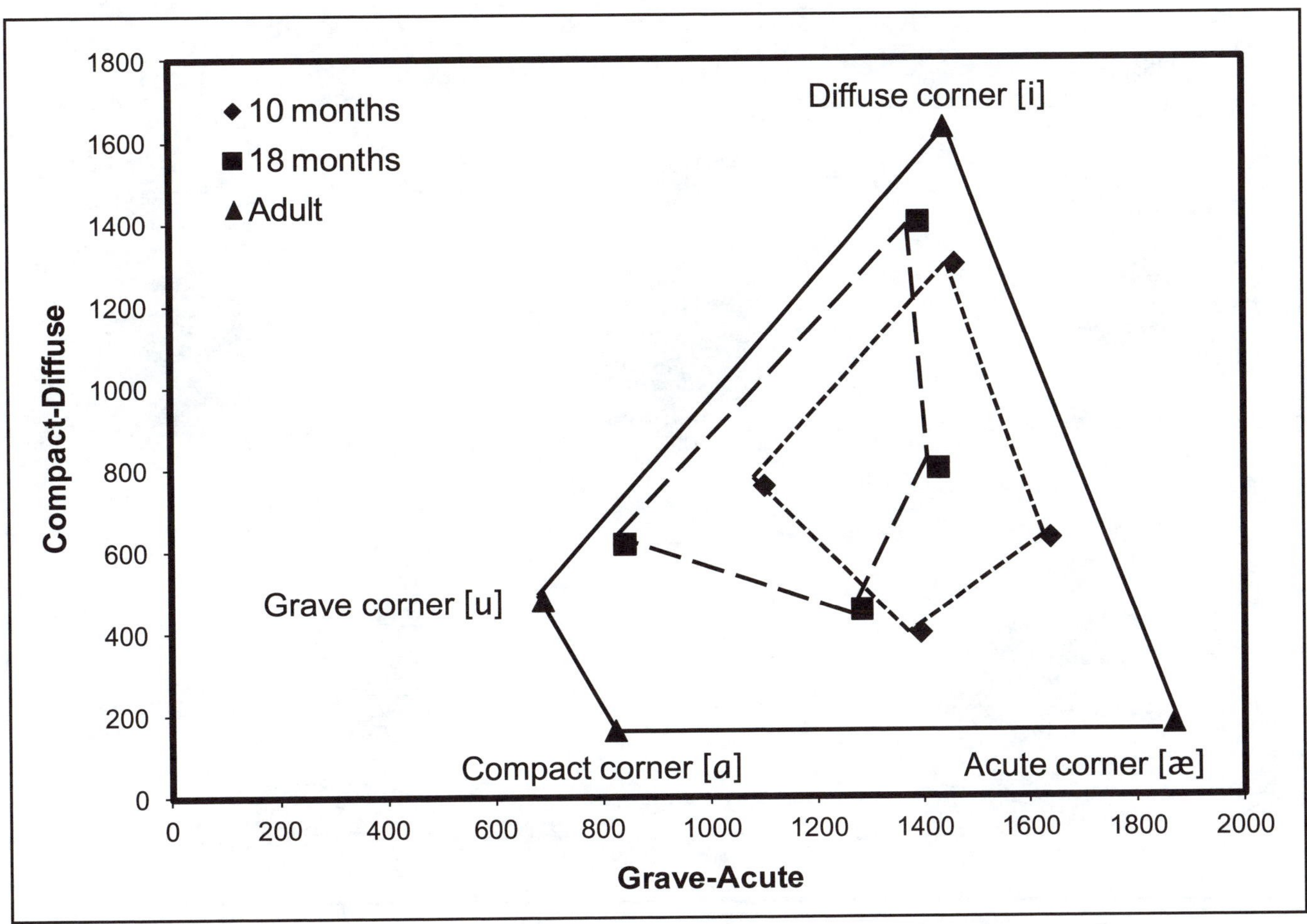

Figure 1–11. *Corners of the vowel space estimated for 10- and 18-month-old infants and their English-speaking mothers, plotted in mels in feature space. For the adult space the most diffuse vowel is [i], the most grave vowel is [u], the most compact vowel is [ɑ], and the most acute vowel is [æ] for these Canadian English speakers. Source: Adapted from Rvachew, S., Mattock, K., Polka, L., and Menard, L. (2006). Developmental and cross-linguistic variation in the infant vowel space: The case of Canadian English and Canadian French.* Journal of the Acoustical Society of America, 120*(4), pp.* 2250–2259.

differences in the locations of the corners of the vowel triangle are apparent. It is also clear that perceptual contrast between the vowel categories was enhanced by the mothers in all three language groups when using the infant-directed speaking register.

Variations introduced by phonetic context are readily apparent when examining cues to consonant place of articulation. Figure 1–12 (top) illustrates the formant frequency transitions associated with the syllables [bɑ], [dɑ], and [gɑ], showing how the direction of these transitions appear to cue the labial, alveolar and velar places of articulation. The syllable [dɑ] has a falling F2 in contrast to the rising F2 in [bɑ] and a relatively flat F3 in contrast to the rising F3 in [gɑ]. However, the spectrogram of the syllables [di] and [du] in the lower part of Figure 1–12 shows that the falling F2 contour is not a reliable cue to [d] identity with the F2 slightly rising in the syllable

Acoustic cues to consonant place of articulation include formant transitions that vary with phonetic context and the spectral characteristics of the release burst which may be less variable with phonetic context.

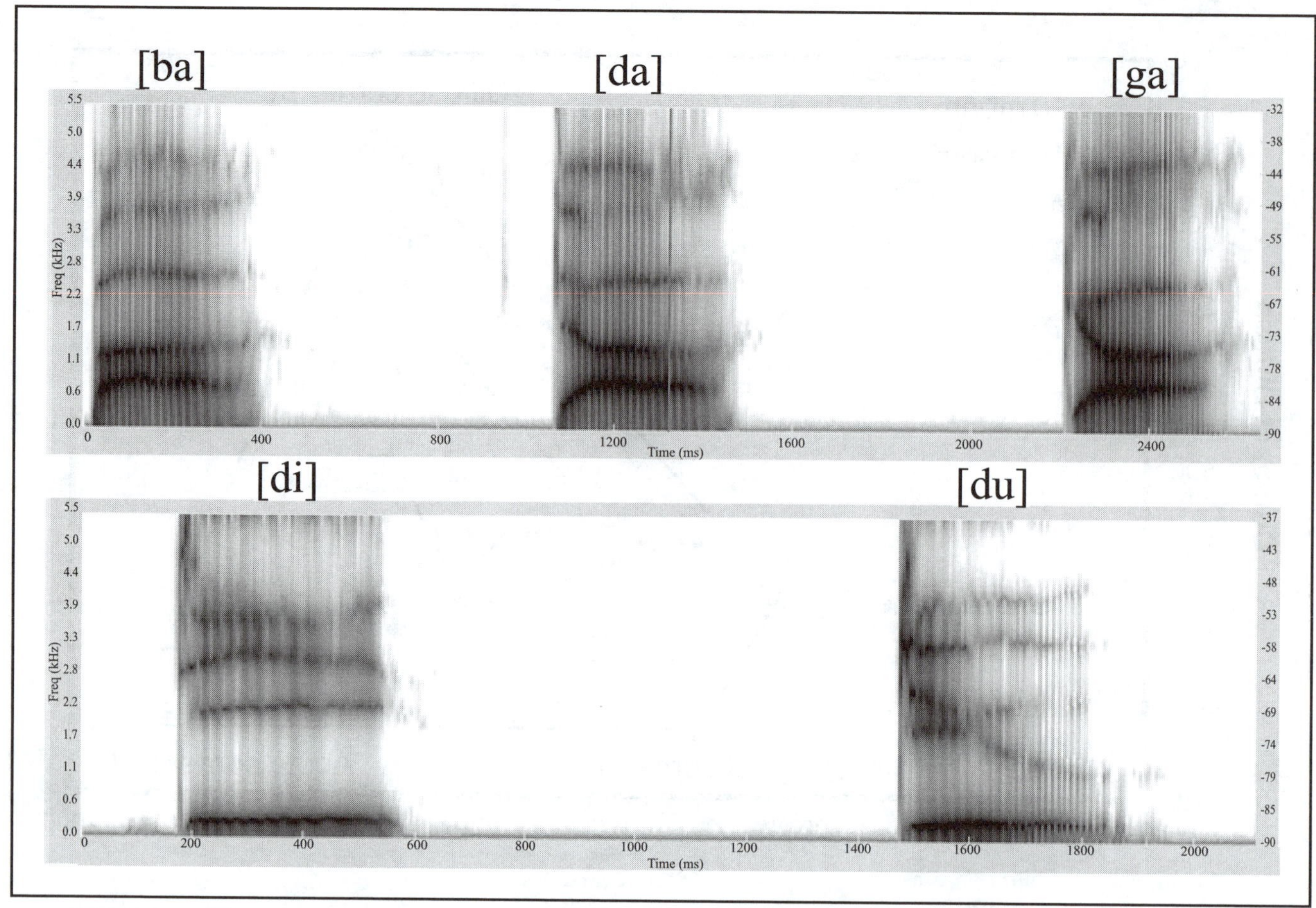

Figure 1–12. *Variations in formant transition contours as a function of phonetic context. The top spectrogram represents the syllables [ba], [da], and [ga], whereas the lower spectrogram represents the syllables [di] and [du], spoken by the same adult male talker.*

[di] and falling in the syllable [du]. Of course, the formant transitions are not the only cues to stop place of articulation. The release bursts also carry information about place features and it has been suggested that context-invariant cues can be derived from the spectral characteristics of the first 25 ms of the syllable onset (Stevens & Blumstein, 1978).

The existence of multiple cues to the identity of features and segments highlights the complexity of the process of phonetic encoding and presents a challenge to the view that speech is perceived by detecting specific acoustic cues. Studies in which multiple acoustic cues are manipulated in a systematic fashion demonstrate that speech perception involves integrating information provided by multiple cues to form a unitary phonetic percept (Repp, 1982). For example, in prevocalic contexts, [voice] judgments are influenced by many different cues including VOT and the "F1 cutback cue." The F1 cutback cue arises because aspiration, associated in English with [−voice] stops, obscures the early part of the F1 transition so that the transition has a higher starting frequency and shorter

Speech perception involves integrating information provided by multiple cues to form a unitary phonetic percept using a language specific organizing strategy.

duration than it does when [+voice] stops are produced at the same place of articulation. The way in which the many cues to [voice] are integrated to influence voicing judgments in speech perception experiments depends on syllable location and place of articulation of the consonant and language background of the listener (Benki, 2003). Place of articulation judgments for stop consonants are also influenced by multiple cues including spectral characteristics of the release burst, starting frequencies of the formant transitions, formant transition trajectories, and even VOT (Benki, 2001). Fricative place of articulation is similarly cued by multiple characteristics of the syllable with characteristics of the noise portion, the formant transitions, and the steady state (vowel) portions of the syllable all playing a role. It is clear that listeners do not simply detect cues and match them up to features in order to identify phonetic segments in the speech input. Each listener must learn a language-specific organizational strategy for integrating spectral and temporal information provided by the input in order to abstract phonetic information from the speech input (Nittrouer, 2002a).

This discussion about multiple cues to feature and segment identity is related to the issue of nonlinearity in the speech signal. The multiple acoustic cues associated with a given feature are not bundled together at discrete time intervals; rather they are spread throughout the utterance so that it is impossible to slice up acoustic waveforms into discrete phonetic segments. Coleman (2003) has demonstrated that temporal smearing of acoustic cues can occur over quite long time intervals that exceed the duration of the words in which a given segment occurs. For example, acoustic differences between utterances such as "utter said again" versus "utter shed again" appear as early as half a second prior to the local differences associated with the fricative noises themselves as a consequence of more anterior productions of the [t] in "utter" spoken before "said" compared to "shed."

The impossibility of mapping directly from the acoustic signal to phonetic segments led to the development of the motor theory of speech perception. This theory has evolved considerably during the past half century but it has remained centered on the claim that the objects of speech perception are articulatory gestures rather than acoustic cues. The underlying premise is that, although the acoustic cues for a given segment may not be invariant, the intended articulatory gestures are and, therefore, it must be the gesture that is perceived. For example, when the listener is presented with syllables containing either the rising F2 or the falling F2 transition depicted in the lower spectrogram of Figure 1–12, the consonant [d] is heard because the "intended gesture" at syllable onset is the same in both syllables. A related assumption is that both the production and the perception of phonetic gestures is controlled by a neural module that has evolved in the human specifically for the task of extricating the overlapping coarticulated gestures that are characteristic of speech production (Liberman & Whalen, 2000). In

According to the **motor theory of speech perception**, the objects of speech perception are articulatory gestures rather than acoustic cues.

the case of the syllables [di] and [du] the formant trajectories are different due to coarticulation of the consonant and vowel gestures but the hypothesized specialized module renders them perceptually equivalent due to recovery of the shared intended gesture at syllable onset. However, it has been shown that many speech perception phenomena thought to be reliant on species-specific knowledge of human vocal tract function can be observed in animals and can be explained by general auditory factors (for review, see Diehl, Lotto, & Holt, 2004). An alternative version of this theory—called the direct realist theory of speech perception—rejects the notion of a specialized module but maintains that the objects of speech perception are articulatory gestures, although in this theory it is the actual rather than intended gestures that are thought to be directly perceived by the listener (Galantucci, Fowler, & Turvey, 2006). The hypothesis that actual vocal tract gestures are the objects of speech perception does not solve the invariance or nonlinearity problems however or provide a satisfactory explanation for the humanlike perceptual responses of animals to speech stimuli.

Neurons discovered in the premotor cortex of the chimpanzee brain that respond when producing goal-directed movements *and* when watching others produce the same goal-directed hand movements are called **mirror neurons**.

The discovery of neurons in the premotor cortex of the monkey brain that respond when producing goal-directed hand movements and while watching others produce the same goal-directed hand movements, or while hearing the consequences of those actions (Kohler et al., 2002), has been claimed as evidence in support of both the motor theory and the direct realist theory of speech perception (Galantucci et al., 2006; Studdert-Kennedy, 2002). Brain-imaging studies reporting activation in premotor cortex during production and perception of speech (e.g., Fidriksson et al., 2009; Pulvermüller et al., 2006) have led to the suggestion that similar "mirror" neurons in the human brain allow for the recovery of articulatory gestures from speech input. However, lesion studies do not support the hypothesis that frontal brain regions play a primary role in speech perception or speech recognition (Hickock, 2008; Lotto, Hickok, & Holt, 2009).

Quantal-enhancement theory is a sophisticated version of a distinctive feature account of speech perception that defines distinctive features in terms of the interaction between articulatory parameters and their acoustic effects.

Quantal-enhancement theory is a sophisticated version of a distinctive feature account of speech perception that defines distinctive features in terms of the interaction between articulatory parameters and their acoustic effects (K. N. Stevens & Keyser, 2009). The central idea is that continuous changes in certain articulatory parameters result in discontinuities in acoustic output such that the acoustic parameters can be described as being quantal, that is, forming discrete categories. For example, closure of the vocal tract from the full-open to the full-closed position is a continuous variable but at a certain degree of closure, turbulence will be produced in the airstream that is associated with a sudden and dramatic increase in the amplitude of noise production that marks the boundary between sonorants and obstruents (i.e., consonants). The linkage of the acoustic cues to specific articulatory states and movements is expected to result in more or less invariant cues to feature identity with a single primary cue for each distinctive feature. Taking into account the fact that the primary cues may be obscured or modified by overlapping articulatory gestures in running speech, it is proposed that secondary cues serve to enhance the perceptual salience of the primary cues. For example, in a phrase such as, "I can't go," the primary cues to the distinctive features that define the [n] and the [t] may be reduced or even completely obscured by the closure and release phases of the [g] articulation; enhancing gestures such as lowering of the velum during the vowel and closing the glottis at the end of the vowel provide acoustic information that cues the presence of the missing segments. This line of research is dependent on studies that involve acoustic analysis of speech and modeling of vocal tract phenomena. The findings provide a valuable picture of the relationship between articulatory events and acoustic consequences and point to important acoustic parameters that inform listeners' perception of speech input. However, studies of the way in which human listeners actually perceive speech raise questions about this view of speech perception, especially from a developmental perspective.

At this point it is necessary to reconsider the foundation of this approach to speech perception, specifically the view that there is "too much information" in the acoustic waveform (Jakobson et al., 1963). The fundamental idea is that listeners pick out the critical acoustic cues to distinctive features and discard the remaining acoustic information as irrelevant. In fact, recent research completely undermines this view of speech processing and leads to the conclusion that humans perceive the "whole" of speech and not just the critical details (Nittrouer, 2006). There are two kinds of studies that challenge the standard view of the importance of acoustic cues to speech perception. In some studies the critical acoustic cues are removed from the speech input, leaving just the "blurry outlines" of the signal. In other studies, the supposedly irrelevant details in the speech input are amplified by increasing rather than controlling variability in these parameters. Some examples of these sorts of studies follow.

Successful perception of stimuli in which the acoustic cues to phoneme identity have been removed, leaving only the "blurry outlines" of speech, challenges the standard view of the importance of acoustic cues to speech perception.

Remez, Rubin, Pisoni, and Carrell (1981) tested adults' perception of time-varying sinusoidal patters that were based on spoken versions of the sentence, "Where were you a year ago?" The sinusoidal patterns that were created contained little of the acoustic information that would be considered critical for recovering the acoustic cues to the distinctive features that make up the phonetic segments in the sentence. Three sinusoids that followed the center frequencies of the formants in the naturally produced sentence were combined but the resulting waveform was significantly different from speech. The three-tone patterns did not reproduce the harmonic structure of speech, thus obliterating acoustic cues to sonorant versus nonsonorant elements as well as cues reliant on the relationship between formants and fundamental frequency and cues to place of articulation based on the spectra of release bursts and formant transitions. In short, the stimuli were designed to capture global amplitude and frequency variations in speech while stripping the signal of local detail. Although listeners typically reported that the stimuli sounded like "science fiction sounds" or some other non-speech stimulus, the majority of subjects were able to transcribe some or all of the sentence when instructed to do so.

Noise vocoding is another transformation of speech that preserves gross temporal cues in speech while removing spectral information and thus eliminating most phonetic details. The stimuli are created by dividing natural recordings of speech into a given number of frequency bands and determining the amplitude envelope of each frequency band; this information is then used to shape a white noise band that has been filtered to match the frequency range of the corresponding speech frequency band. Studies involving this form of speech distortion have become popular because the technique simulates the kind of speech input heard by cochlear implant users. Shannon, Zeng, Kamath, Wygonski, and Ekelid (1995) created stimuli from 2, 3, or 4 frequency bands. They found that adult listeners were able to achieve remarkable recognition performance after 8 to 10 hours of exposure to the vocoded speech. The adult listeners were able to identify consonants and vowels in nonsense syllables and recognize sentences with close to perfect accuracy. Sounds that represented voice and manner contrasts were recognized with only two frequency bands of noise present in the stimuli but recognition of place of articulation did not exceed 60% accuracy even with four noise bands.

These and other studies of the perception of distorted speech indicate that listeners' can perceive speech even when the primary acoustic cues have been removed. The acoustic information that is "left over" after these distortions proves to be useful for perception rather than irrelevant as previously presumed. Another line of research that challenges prior assumptions about aspects of speech that are supposedly irrelevant to linguistic processing investigates the role of indexical information in speech and language processing. Although both linguistic and indexical information are transmitted simultaneously in the speech signal, it was once thought that the indexical properties of speech were filtered out of the speech signal in order to extract the linguistic message (Halle, 1985). However, laboratory research with adults and children demonstrates that fine acoustic details of speech, including those associated with both linguistic and indexical information, are stored in long-term representations of speech (e.g., Nygaard, Sommers, & Pisoni, 1994). When research participants perform word recognition and talker recognition tasks with stimuli that are recorded from multiple talkers and return to the lab a week or more later to perform speech perception tasks with stimuli recorded from these talkers, talker specific details impact on the listeners' future processing of speech (Goldinger, 1996). Furthermore, the highly variable speech input associated with multiple talkers helps children to learn new words (Richtsmeier, Goffman, & Hogan, 2009).

Laboratory research with adults and children demonstrates that fine acoustic details of speech, including those associated with both linguistic and indexical information, are stored in long-term representations of speech.

Exemplar-based (or probabilistic) models of speech perception view these distributions of richly detailed memory traces of experienced words as the key to developing a language-specific strategy for encoding speech input (Johnson, 2007; Pierrehumbert, 2003a, 2003b). Phonetic categories are an emergent property of the distribution of acoustic details across phonetic space. For example, consider the distributions of vowels shown in Plate 3. Learners of all three languages—English, Russian, and Swedish—will have access to a mental map of the vowel space in memory that locates the corners of the vowel triangle within the clusters of vowels that have extreme values along the compact-diffuse and grave-acute feature dimensions. These clusters are located differently for each language and thus perceptual decisions will be different for listeners of each language. A vowel with graveness and diffuseness values of approximately 1000 mels will be readily identifiable as most similar to the other vowels in the cluster labeled /u/ to the English listener. A Russian or Swedish listener, hearing the same vowel, would need other information in order to decide which cluster the vowel is most similar to; the similarity judgment will be facilitated by the storage of increasingly detailed memory traces of words containing these vowels. The decision will also involve information about the probability density of the clusters (in other words an ambiguous vowel is more likely to be assigned to a more frequently occurring vowel category). Nonacoustic information such as visual and articulatory properties of the vowel and nonphonetic information such as semantic or syntactic context can also influence the perceptual similarity judgment. Computer modeling of the process of matching new forms to exemplars of words stored with full acoustic-phonetic detail have shown that many aspects of human perceptual behavior including top-down processing influences, talker normalization, and generalization learning can emerge without building in specific rules for identifying categories or storing prototypes of categories (Beckman & Edwards, 2000; Guenther & Gjaja, 1996; Johnson, 2007). Although the example of phonetic learning that is provided here makes use of the same kinds of acoustic parameters that are thought to be important in the distinctive feature approach, the proposed learning process is markedly different because the acoustic parameters do not themselves point to category membership; rather any given "acoustic cue" is only informative within the context of the full distribution of acoustic and nonacoustic information with which it is associated. Phonetic structure can emerge even when the learner is unaware of the linguistic significance of the input, purely on the basis of the statistical properties of the input, as has been shown in laboratory studies of infant perceptual learning (Maye, Werker, & Gerken, 2002; see Chapter 2 for more details). As mentioned earlier, Rvachew et al. (2006) recorded babbling samples from 20 English-learning infants. We identified the first and second formant frequencies of all 1,424 vowels produced by these infants. We also conducted the same analysis for vowels produced by 3 of the mothers while talking to their infants. Figure 1–13 (top) reveals that the distribution of first formant frequencies is roughly unimodal

Exemplar-based (or probabilistic) models of speech perception view these distributions of richly detailed memory traces of experienced words as the key to developing a language-specific strategy for encoding speech input.

Knowledge of **phonetic structure** can emerge even when the learner is unaware of the linguistic significance of the input, purely on the basis of the statistical properties of the input.

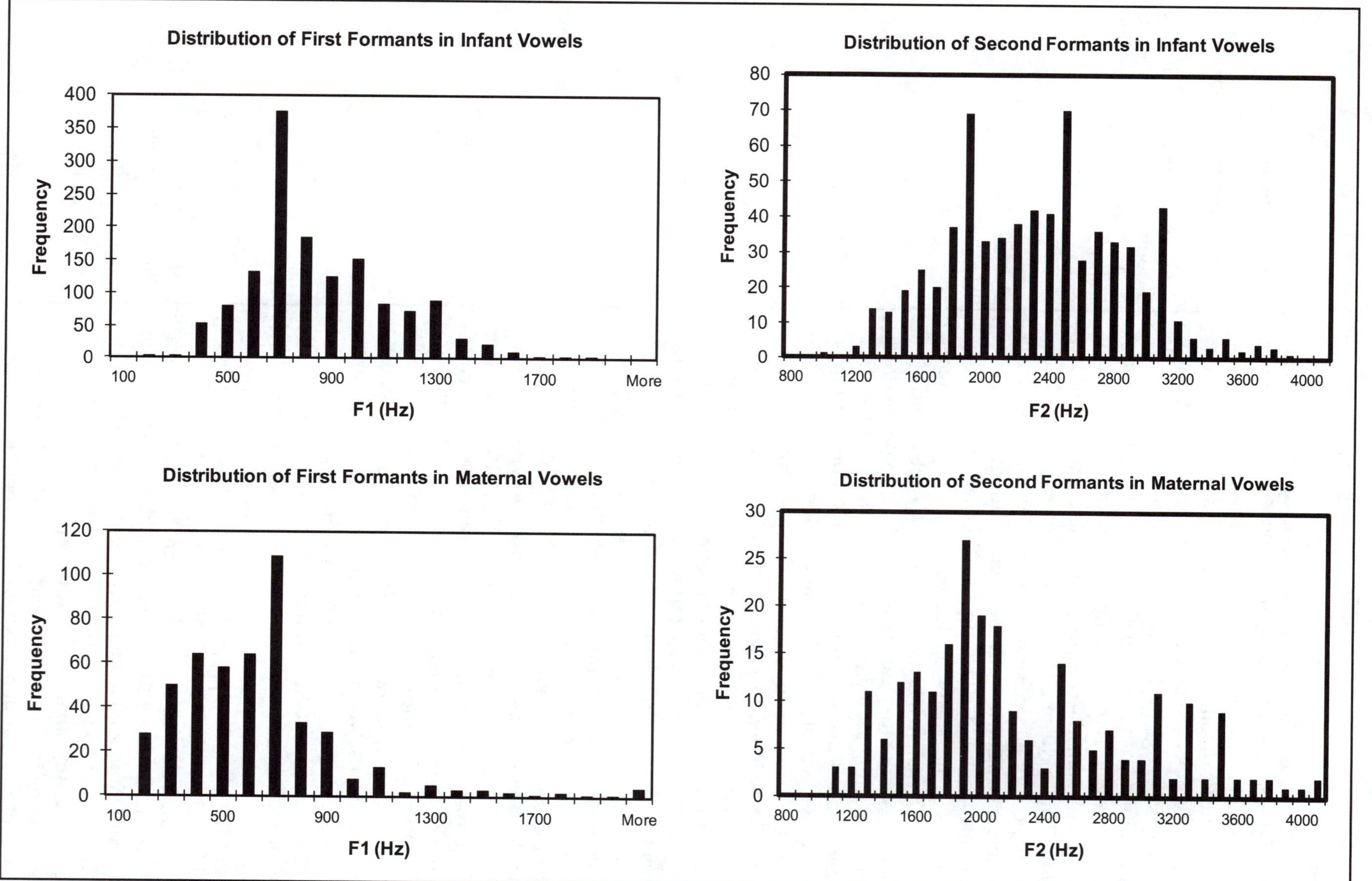

Figure 1–13. *Formant frequencies of vowels produced by 3 English-speaking mothers* (top) *and 20 English-learning infants* (bottom)*: unimodal distribution of first formant frequencies* (left)*; tri-modal distribution of the second formant frequencies for vowels with modal F1 values* (right)*; peaks in the infant F2 distribution correspond to the compact, acute, and diffuse corners of the infants' vowel spaces respectively. Printed with permission from Susan Rvachew.*

with the modal vowel having a frequency of approximately 700 Hz for both maternal and infant vowels although the maternal distribution is somewhat more complex than that produced by the infants. The F1 parameter is associated with the open-close dimension (or vowel height) with more close vowels having lower F1 frequencies and more open vowels having higher F1 frequencies. The finding that 700 Hz is a frequently occurring F1 frequency in the infant sample is not unexpected as it corresponds to the well-known preference of infants for central and mid-open vowels, presumably produced with the vocal tract in a relatively neutral position (Kent & Bauer, 1985; Kent & Murray, 1982). The bottom part of Figure 1-13 shows the distribution of second formant frequencies for vowels that had a first formant near the modal frequency of 700 Hz. This distribution of second formant frequencies is interesting because it does not show an undifferentiated and continuously distributed range of values that would suggest more or less random experimentation with the tongue advancement parameter; rather there is a clear trimodal distribution in the infant distribution. The first peak is associated with extreme values of compactness, the second with extreme values of acuteness, and the third with extreme values of diffuseness in the infant vowel spaces. In Rvachew et al. (2008) we obtained adult listener judgments for the corner vowels in the infants' babble and found that the compact vowels were identified as [ɑ] most often and the acute vowels were identified as [æ] most often; given the relatively high first formant of the most diffuse vowels in the infant spaces these vowels were identified as more central vowels such as [ə], [ɪ], or [ɛ] rather than [i] as would be expected for an adult vowel space. Even though the infant vowel space does not exactly correspond to the more complex adult space shown in the top right corner of Figure 1–13, the trimodal distribution of second formant frequencies across the infant vowel space gives a clear sense of emerging phonetic structure during the prelinguistic period. As the child gains experience with speech input, perceptual knowledge of the vowel system will become gradually more adultlike and incremental restructuring of productive knowledge of the vowel space will also occur, reflecting improvements in both perceptual knowledge and speech motor control. Not only is the process gradual but it is reciprocal, with cross-modal correlations between the child's accumulating perceptual, articulatory and visual experience with speech serving to enhance knowledge of specific phonetic elements.

Assessment of Perceptual Knowledge

Thus far, two approaches to perception testing have been discussed. In one approach, listeners are presented with clearly produced exemplars of specific phonetic categories and asked to discriminate or identify them. This approach assumes that perceptual knowledge is discretely organized: a listener either does or does not have knowledge of the phonetic categories under investigation. As discussed further in Chapters 4 and 7, this approach led to erroneous conclusions about speech perception development and the speech perception skills of children with phonological disorders. Most children and adults can identify such stimuli, especially under ideal listening conditions. Categorical perception tasks are a significant advance because they take into account the continuous nature of the acoustic information that is associated with each phonetic category. Individual differences in perceptual ability can be quantified on the basis of differences in the location or width of the category boundary between two phonetic units. However, even this approach was predicated on the assumption that phonetic units were differentiated on the basis of universal cues that were intrinsically available to the listener. Exemplar-based models assume that the phonetic units are abstracted by each listener from the input. The strategy for processing the input must be discovered anew by each language learner and will reflect the sum total of the individual's language experience. By this view, speech perception assessment must be designed to ask different questions. It is not enough to know whether the listener can discriminate one sound from another sound. We want to know what information the listener is attending to when they make decisions about the identity of speech sounds. We want to know the listener's strategy for weighting the relative importance of different types of information when processing speech. We want to know if the listener's speech processing strategy is flexible enough to allow accurate perception with degraded stimuli or under difficult listening conditions. Some perception testing tasks that allow us to address these kinds of questions were introduced in the previous section. Experiments with vocoded speech and with speech produced by multiple talkers have shown that listener's attend to and store more of the speech signal than previously thought. Two additional types of assessment strategies will be highlighted in this section: experiments that investigate listeners' "cue weighting" strategies and experiments that investigate speech perception performance with "gated speech."

Phonetic structure can emerge even when the learner is unaware of the linguistic significance of the input, purely on the basis of the statistical properties of the input. Therefore, when testing **perception skills**, we want to know which cues are attended and how they are weighted when the listener perceives speech under varied listening conditions.

The first example concerns the fact that many speech contrasts are cued by more than one acoustic difference. For example, the words "shoe" and "Sue" and "seat" and "sheet" are differentiated by steady state spectral cues in the fricative and vocalic portions of the word and by dynamic spectral cues that join these portions of the syllable together. In another example, words such as "pot" and "pod" are differentiated by multiple cues to word final stop consonant voicing category with vowel duration being longer and F1 offset frequency being lower in voiced contexts compared to voiceless contexts. The difference between the words "say" and "stay" also involves the integration of temporal and spectral cues at word onset. Experiments can be designed to determine whether listeners attend more to one cue than another when these cues are manipulated independently, as shown in Figure 1–14. In these experiments two speech continua are created to represent two values of one of the speech cues (e.g., high vs. low F2 onset frequency in shoe/sue, high vs. low F1 offset frequency in pot/pod or low vs. high vowel F1 onset frequency in say/stay); the second cue is varied in equal steps across each continuum to combine with each value of the first cue (e.g., multiple values of fricative centroid in shoe/sue, vowel duration in pot/pod, or stop gap duration in say/stay). Hypothetical data are shown in Figure 1–14 to demonstrate the outcome when one listener weights Cue B more highly than another (Figure 1–14, top comparison) and when a listener places more weight on Cue A than another (Figure 1–14, bottom comparison). This assessment technique has been used to compare listening strategies across different groups of listeners, for example, adults who speak English versus Arabic (Crowther & Mann, 1994), children versus adults with normal speech development (Nittrouer, 2002b), children growing up in poor versus middle-class homes (Nittrouer, 1996), and adults with normal hearing versus those with cochlear implants (Peng, Lu, & Chatterjee, 2009). These studies are important because they show that cue weighting strategies differ remarkably between groups of listeners as a function of language exposure. There are no universal cues to phonetic category identity as once thought. Rather each listener must develop a language-specific strategy for processing all information in the speech input based on language specific distributions of acoustic parameters in the input. These studies also show that speech perception is influenced by both bottom-up (acoustic-phonetic) and top-down (phonological) processes.

Studies show that **cue weighting strategies** differ between groups of listeners as a function of language exposure and that speech perception is influenced by bottom-up (acoustic-phonetic) and top-down (phonological) information and processes.

Studies that employ "gated speech stimuli" are not concerned with the processing of specific acoustic cues. Rather, these studies reveal whether the participants' perceptual representations for speech are detailed enough to support word recognition even when the speech input is degraded. The research strategy is relatively simple: recordings of naturally produced speech are digitized and then progressively larger pieces of the word are removed from the end. The research participant attempts to identify the remainder of the word. Edwards, Fourakis, Beckman, and Fox (1999) gated recordings of words that contrasted word-final consonants that differed in place of articulation (e.g., Pete, peak, peep) as well as a similar word with no word final consonant (e.g. pea). The words were presented to children in a live-voice condition, a recorded whole-word condition and in three different gating conditions: with the portion after the stop burst removed; with the stop burst removed; and with part of the final formant transitions removed. The child's task was to point to one of 4 pictures to identify each word, with the words presented in random order. The children were all approximately 4 years old, 6 with normally developing speech and 6 with

Studies involving the perception of **"gated speech stimuli,"** in which slices are removed from the end of the word before presentation for identification, show that children with DPD have difficulty perceiving speech under conditions of reduced cue redundancy.

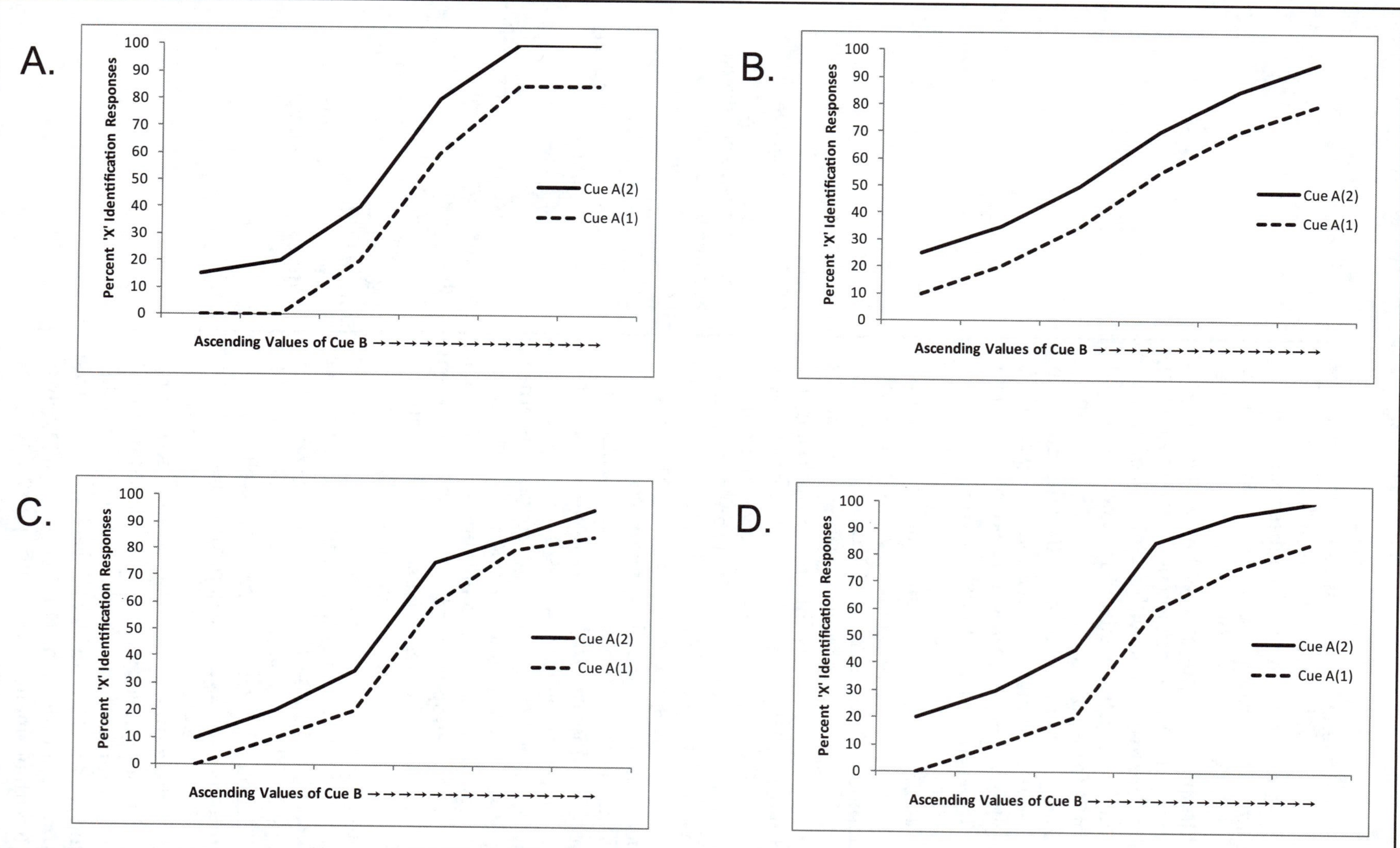

Figure 1–14. Hypothetical data from a cue weighting study illustrating identification functions for continua in which Cue A was manipulated independently of Cue B by creating two separate continua in which values of Cue B were varied in 7 equal steps orthogonally to two different values of Cue A to create stimuli that will be perceived as belonging to one of two different categories X or Y. Subjects are asked to identify the category membership of each stimulus. Identification functions at the top are separated by approximately the same distance but the slopes of the functions in A are much steeper than in B reflecting greater weighting of Cue B by the listeners who provided the identification functions in A compared to B. Identification functions at the bottom are primarily differentiated by the greater distance between the functions in D compared to C indicating that the listeners who provided these functions weighted Cue A more strongly in their listening judgments than did the listeners who provided the identification functions in C.

delayed phonological development. Children in both groups identified words in the live-voice condition equally well and all children had difficulty when the release burst or portions of the formant transitions were removed, as shown in Figure 1–15. Children with delayed phonological development had significantly more difficulty in the mildest gating condition and in the recorded whole-word condition than did children with normally developing speech. The children's stored representations for the test words were not robust enough to support word recognition even with only slightly diminished redundancy of acoustic information in the signal.

Summary: Perceptual Knowledge

Speech perception does begin with the processing of acoustic information from the speech input. Speech research has revealed many acoustic cues that serve as important sources of information to the listener when perceiving speech. However, these cues do not act as automatic pointers to specific distinctive features or phonetic categories. Phonetic categories are an emergent property of the distribution of acoustic information across parametric phonetic space, built up over time as the language learner stores detailed memory traces

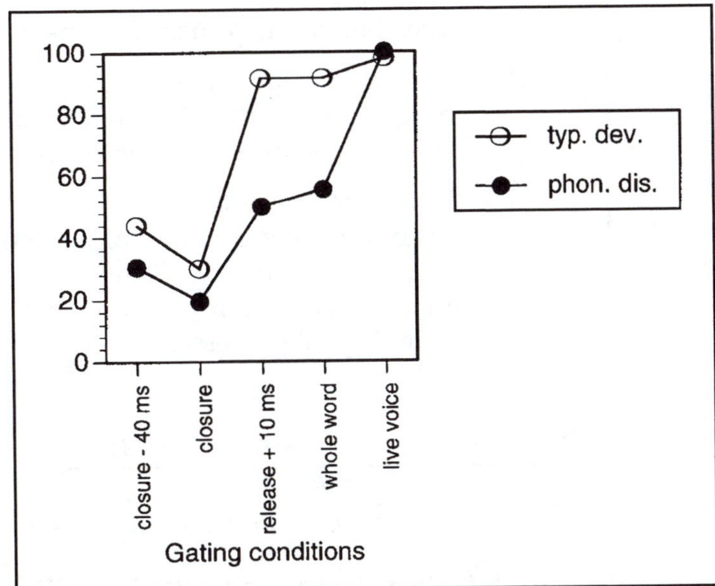

Figure 1–15. *Mean percent correct word identification performance for children with typically developing speech or delayed phonological skills when the words were presented live-voice or under 4 different gating conditions.* Source: Edwards, J., Fourakis, M., Beckman, M. E., and Fox, R. A. (1999). *Characterizing knowledge deficits in phonological disorders.* Journal of Speech, Language, and Hearing Research, 42, *lower left of Figure 2, p. 177. Reprinted with permission of the American Speech-Hearing-Language Association.*

of experienced words. Each language learner must discover a strategy for abstracting phonetic structure from the input that is adapted to the nature of the input that is received. Assessing the language learner's perceptual knowledge requires sophisticated tools that reveal the listener's perceptual strategies for making sense of highly complex and variable input that seems at times to carry "too much information," while being heard in environments that frequently degrade access to that input.

Describing Phonological Knowledge

1.4.1. Complete an independent analysis of a speech sample recorded from a child, deriving a phonemic repertoire and relating it to the child's phonetic repertoire by identifying allophonic rules, neutralization rules, phonotactic constraints, and inventory constraints.

1.4.2. Diagram the prosodic units of utterances at multiple tiers of the phonological hierarchy, from the syllable to the utterance tier, including the linkages between tiers.

1.4.3. Identify the features for each consonant in English and diagram the hierarchical relationships between them, according to the principles of default specification.

1.4.4. From the perspective of multilinear phonology, describe three classes of explanation for word productions by children that mismatch the adult target.

1.4.5. Define "phonological process" and list eight phonological processes that are commonly occurring in the speech of English-speaking children. Given a sample of speech, identify error patterns that correspond to these phonological processes.

Segmental Phonological Knowledge

The Phoneme and the Phonemic Repertoire

Phonological knowledge is often described in terms of **phonemes** which are the smallest segments used to distinguish meaning in the language.

Once the listener has abstracted phonetic units from the spoken input, a more abstract level of phonological knowledge is required in order to derive meaning from the utterance. Phonological knowledge is often described in terms of phonemes, which are the smallest segments used to distinguish meaning in the language. Phonemes are a smaller subset of the phonetic inventory of the language. The relationship between phones and phonemes varies from one language to another as does the relationship between phones and the acoustic-phonetic and articulatory-phonetic substrate of the phones themselves. As alluded to in the previous section, the voicing contrast is realized differently in English and French. As shown in Figure 1–16, French and English both use the phonemes /p/ and /b/ (shown by convention between slashes, to contrast with the phones, shown between square brackets). In French, each phoneme has a single allophone, /p/ is produced as the phone [p] with short lag voicing and /b/ is produced as the phone [b] with lead voicing (MacLeod & Stoel-Gammon, 2009). We can tell that /p/ and /b/ are contrasting phonemes in French because two words that differ by only this sound have different meanings. For example, "peau" means "skin" and "beau" means "beautiful." In English, the /p/ is produced as [pʰ] in prevocalic positions unless preceded by /s/ in which case it is produced as the short lag variant [p]. The two phones [p] and [pʰ] are recognized by English listeners as sounding different but they are functionally equivalent: allophones of the same phoneme /p/. We know that these two phones are allophonic variants of /p/ because they occur in complementary distribution meaning that they always occur in different environments and thus there is no opportunity for the two variants to contrast meaning. A word such as [spʰɪl] would not typically be produced in English; if you were to produce it the listener would hear it as a peculiar-sounding version of the word "spill" rather than a word with some other meaning. On the other hand, the phoneme /b/ is associated with a single phone [b] that is typically produced in English with short lag voicing although lead variants may occur. The short lag

Allophones are different phonetic variants of a single phoneme.

Two phones occur in **complementary distribution** when they always occur in different (nonoverlapping) environments.

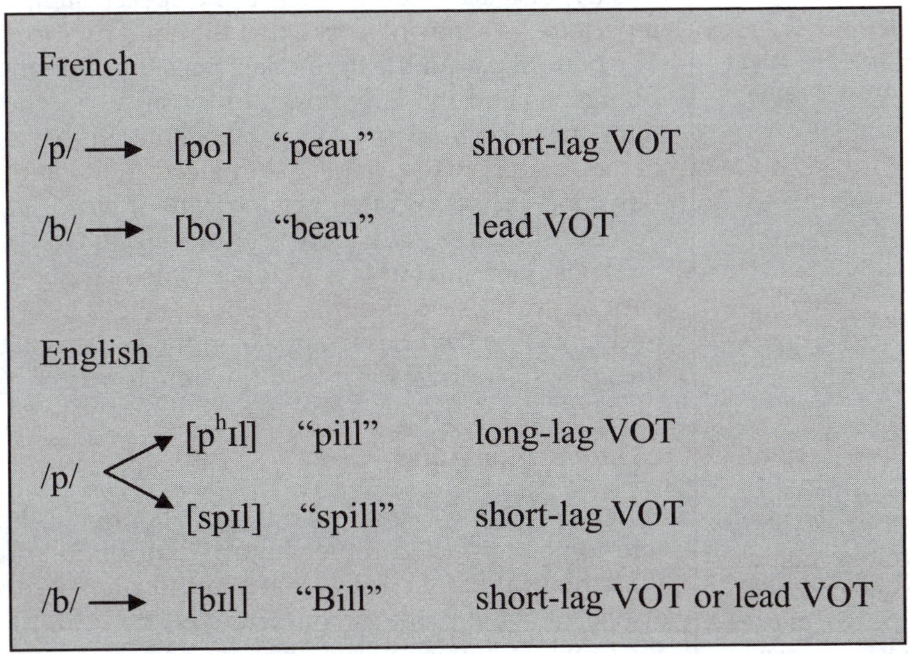

Figure 1–16. *Allophonic variants of the phonemes /p/ and /b/ in word-initial position in French and English.*

Two phones occur in **free variation** when they can occur in the same environment without impacting on the meaning of a word.

and lead variants are in free variation in the word-initial position: either variant is perceived as [b] and [bɪl] will be understood to mean "Bill" whether the [b] is produced with –30 or +10 ms of VOT.

Allophonic Rules

It is important to be able to identify allophonic rules in a speech sample because children sometimes develop phonological systems that are not in accordance with the adult system.

It is important to be able to distinguish allophones and phonemes in a speech sample because children sometimes develop phonological systems that are not in accordance with the adult system. Camarata and Gandour (1984) described an unusual distribution of stop production by a 3½-year-old boy who had a history of chronic otitis media (ear infections), shown in Figure 1–17. The examples of the child's speech that are shown in the table at the top of the figure reveal three stop consonant phones: [b], [d], and [g]. However, [d] and [g] are in complementary distribution: [d] appears only before diffuse vowels ([i], [u]) and [g] appears only before compact vowels ([æ], [ə], [o], [ɑ]). The child's pattern of stop usage appears to reflect assimilation of diffuse consonants with diffuse vowels and compact consonants with compact vowels. Understanding this child's underlying phonological system is critical to the success of the intervention program and thus an accurate description of the phonetic repertoire, the phonemic repertoire and the relationship between them is clinically important.

A **phonemic repertoire** is a list of the phonemes that the talker uses to contrast meaning.

Figure 1–18 provides another example (in this case hypothetical) of a nonstandard pattern of allophonic variants. The figure demonstrates the difference between the phonetic repertoire and the phonemic repertoire. The phonetic repertoire lists each of the phones that this hypothetical toddler uses in the speech sample. The phonemic repertoire lists the phonemes that the child uses to contrast meaning. The bottom part of the figure describes the relationship between the phonemes and the allophones in those cases where there is more than one allophone for a given phoneme. In this example, the phoneme /s/ has two variants, [s] in word-initial and word-final positions and [x] (a voiceless velar fricative) word-internally between vowels. Similarly, /f/ has two variants, [f] in word-initial and word-final positions and [ʍ] (a voiceless labial-velar glide) word-internally between vowels. Notice that [s] and [x] show complementary distribution in that they never appear in the same syllable contexts and thus cannot contrast meaning; the same is true of [f] and [ʍ].

Neutralization Rules

A **neutralization rule** is characterized by multiple realizations of the same phoneme but in this case the two phones are used to contrast meaning in one context but the contrast is neutralized in another context.

When examining a speech sample for allophonic variants it is important to not confuse complementary distribution of two allophones with neutralization rules that may apply to certain phonemes. A neutralization rule is characterized by multiple realizations of the same phoneme but the different phones that are used are not in complementary distribution. In the case of a neutralization rule, the two phones in question are used to contrast meaning in one context

Examples of Stop Production in Different Vowel Contexts

[b]		[d]		[g]	
bee	[bi]	tea	[di]	kite	[gæ]
bath	[bæ]	key	[di]	tie	[gæ]
pan	[bæŋ]	kick	[di]	clown	[gæŋ]
bus	[bə]			train	[gæŋ]
				cup	[gə]
boot	[bu]			duck	[gə]
book	[bu]	two	[du]	goat	[go]
boat	[bo]	cook	[du]	doe	[go]
ball	[bɑ]			car	[gɑ]
				dog	[gɑ]

Relationship Between Stop Phonemes and Phones

/b/ ⟶ [b] diffuse and compact vowel contexts

/d/ ⟶ [d] diffuse vowel contexts

/d/ ⟶ [g] compact vowel contexts

Figure 1–17. *Portion of speech sample* (top) *recorded from a 3½-year-old-boy who experienced chronic otitis media and description of the relationship between phonemes and allophones in his stop consonant system* (bottom). Source: *Camarata, S., and Gandour, J. (1984). On describing idiosyncratic phonologic systems.* Journal of Speech, Language, and Hearing Research, 49, *Table 1, p.* 263. *Adapted with permission of the American Speech-Hearing-Language Association.*

(and thus are clearly separate phonemes) but the phonemic contrast is neutralized in another context. Examine the sample shown in Figure 1–19. In this case, the hypothetical child was asked to produce words that form minimal pairs—words that differ by only one phoneme—so that the pattern is plain to see. Although this is a hypothetical sample, it is not an unusual pattern (e.g., Chiat, 1989);

Two words form a **minimal pair** when they differ by only one phoneme.

Speech Sample Recorded from Hypothetical Toddler

[bæ hoxi i gæs] "black horsie eat grass"

[waɪ si we daʊn hiə ɑ gæxi] "white sheep lay down here all grassy"

[pis gɪ mi sʌm jɛwo he] "please give me some yellow hay"

[wʌn tu fi fo faɪ tɪkən] "one two three four five chicken(s)"

[hɪm hæpi kaʊ muː] "him happy cow moo"

[hæpi kaʊ wæʍi mumuː] "happy cow laughing moo moo"

[bɪ baʊn ɑ dʊri] "big barn all dirty"

[fɑmo kɔʍi ʔəʔə] "farmer coughing– coughing noises"

[ɑ dʌxi hɪm ni bæf] "all dusty, him need bath"

Phonetic Repertoire (Consonants)

p b	t d	k g	ʔ
m	n		
f	s	x	h
ʍ w		j	

Phonemic Repertoire (Consonants)

p b	t d	k g	
m	n		
f	s		h
w		j	

Relationship Between Fricative Phonemes and Phones

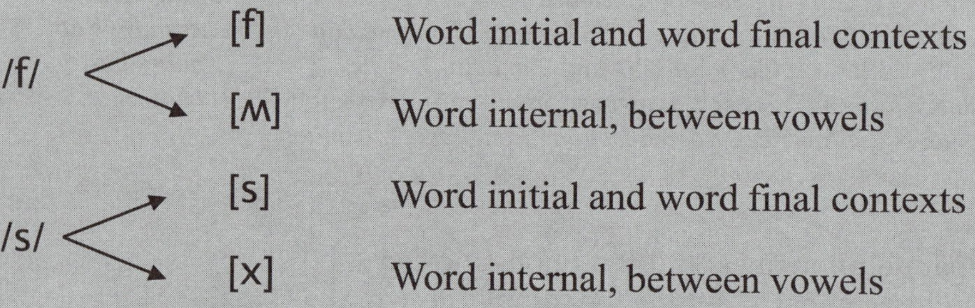

Figure 1–18. *Portion of hypothetical speech sample* (top) *along with phonetic and phonemic consonant repertoires derived from the sample* (middle) *and description of the relationship between phonemes and allophones in the toddler's voiceless fricative system* (bottom).

Speech Sample Recorded from Hypothetical Child

Word-Initial Position	Word-Final Position
[t^{h}u] "Sue"	[pis] "piece"
[t^{h}u] "two"	[pit̚] "Pete"
[t^{h}i] "see"	[pæs] "pass"
[t^{h}i] "tea"	[pæt̚] "pat"
[p^{h}ɑɪ] "fie" (fee, fie, fo, fum…)	[kʌf] "cuff"
[p^{h}ɑɪ] "pie"	[kʌp̚] "cup"
[p^{h}it] "feet"	[kæf] "calf"
[p^{h}it] "Pete"	[kæp̚] "cap"

Realization of the Stop-Fricative Contrast

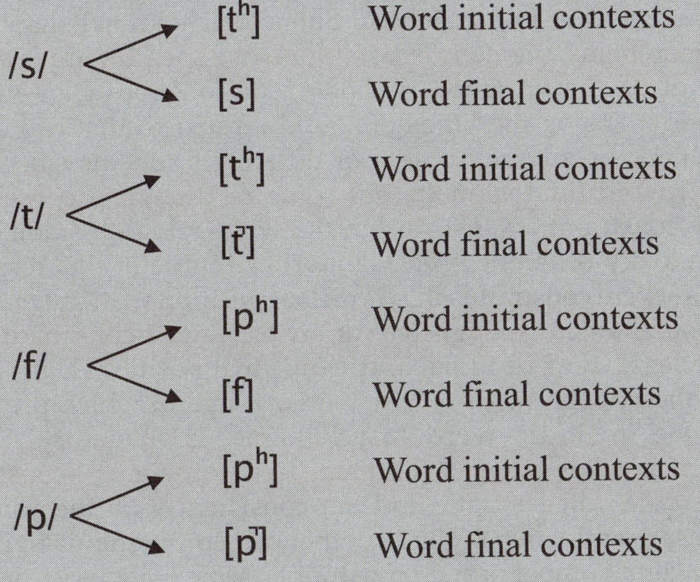

Figure 1–19. *Portion of hypothetical speech sample* (top) *and description of the relationship between phonemes and allophones in the toddler's voiceless fricative system* (bottom), *illustrating neutralization of the /s/-/t/ contrast in the word-initial position.*

even among children with normally developing speech, fricatives may emerge earlier in word- or utterance-final than in word- or utterance-initial position (Kent & Bauer, 1985). The first thing to notice about the sample in Figure 1–19 is that the aspirated and unreleased variants of /t/ appear in complementary distribution: [tʰ] is exclusive to the word-initial position, whereas [t̚] is exclusive to the word-final position. The same pattern applies to the aspirated and unreleased variants of /p/. Therefore, the aspirated and unreleased variants are allophones of their respective stop phonemes. However, /t/ and /s/ and their phonetic variants [t̚] and [s] are not in complementary distribution; on the contrary, both phones occur in the word final position and contrasting use of these phones in minimal pair words signal differences in meaning and thus are clearly different phonemes. Again, the same pattern applies to the /p/ and the /f/ phonemes: [kæf] refers to the baby cow, whereas [kæp̚] refers to headgear. However, no fricative sounds are used in word initial position resulting in a neutralization of the contrasts between /t/ and /s/ and between /p/ and /f/ in this word position. Nonetheless, all four phonemes are clearly present in the child's phonemic repertoire.

Phonotactic Constraints

Phonotactic constraints are restrictions on the kinds of sound sequences that can occur.

Another aspect of segmental phonological knowledge that will be apparent in a phonetic transcription of a speech sample of sufficient length is the presence of phonotactic constraints; in other words, restrictions on the kinds of sound sequences that can occur. English allows a large number of different phonemes in word-initial and word-final contexts but some restrictions do occur such as the constraint against /ŋ/ in the word initial position. English is markedly different from Mandarin Chinese in this respect which has severe constraints in word-final position with only nasal consonants allowed. In English a variety of 2- and 3-consonant sequences are legal in word-initial and word-final positions but /ps/ is proscribed in contrast to French, a language in which pronunciation of the "p" in the word "psychologue" is obligatory. As with the phonemic inventory, a child may have phonotactic constraints that are quite idiosyncratic and not consistent with the adult system. Close examination of the hypothetical sample shown in Figure 1–18 reveals a number of such constraints. Most obvious is complete lack of consonant sequences in word-initial or word-final position. The sample also reveals a constraint against stop consonants in word-final position but nasals and fricatives are used in this position.

Inventory Constraints

Inventory constraints comprise those phonemes or sound classes that are completely absent from the repertoire.

Finally, the child's speech sample should be examined for inventory constraints—phonemes or sound classes that are completely absent from the child's repertoire. Careful organization of the repertoire according the IPA chart will help you to spot missing elements quickly. In the case of the example in Figure 1–18 it is readily apparent that no postalveolar obstruents are used by the child. Furthermore, affricates and liquids are absent from the phonetic and phonemic repertoires. There are many specific phonemes not represented in this sample but it is clearly too short for clinical purposes such as diagnosis or treatment planning. More information about appropriate sampling methods is provided in Chapter 6.

Independent Versus Relational Descriptions of Segmental Phonological Knowledge

The phonetic and phonemic repertoires provide an independent description of the child's knowledge of the sound system at the phonetic and segmental phonological levels of representation. The analysis is predicated on the assumption that the child might develop an underlying phonological system that is different from the adult model. The child's use of speech sounds to convey meaning is considered independently of the adult system. In contrast, a relational analysis describes the child's speech output in relation to the adult versions of the child's intended words.

An **independent analysis** of the child's speech aims to describe the child's phonological knowledge independently of the adult system.

When conducting a relational analysis of a child's speech, the child's production of a given word is compared to the adult model and each phoneme is judged according to the chosen scoring system of which the simplest is a binary correct/incorrect judgment. The traditional basis for a relational description of a child's segmental phonological knowledge is a five-way scoring system however: each phoneme is judged to be correct, an omission, a substitution, a distortion, or an addition in relation to the adult model (Shriberg & Kent, 2003). Typically, this analysis is focused on the consonant targets although it may be applied to the vowels as well. An example of the five-way scoring system as applied to a single word in shown in Figure 1–20. The target word "pussycat" contains four consonants: /p/, /s/, /k/, and /t/. The child's production of the word contained a correct production of /p/, a lateralized distortion of /s/, a substitution of [t] for /k/, omission of /t/, and addition of [w]. When this kind of analysis is applied to a sample of speech that is structured to include all of the phonemes in the language that the child is learning, it is typically used to identify the phonemes that the child has mastered and those that the child has yet to learn.

A **relational analysis** of the child's speech compares the child's production of words to the adult targets or models.

A relational description of this kind can form the basis for a detailed description of a child's phonological knowledge as will be shown in detail in Chapters 5 and 6. This description by itself does not constitute a description of the child's underlying phonological knowledge without further analysis however. It is important not to confuse the goals or the outcome of the two kinds of analysis. Just as a phonetic repertoire and a phonemic repertoire provide very different types of information, a phonemic repertoire is not at all the same thing as a list of the sounds that a child has mastered. Consider again the sample of speech shown in Figure 1–18. The child's phonemic repertoire contains the consonants [b d g m n f s h w j]

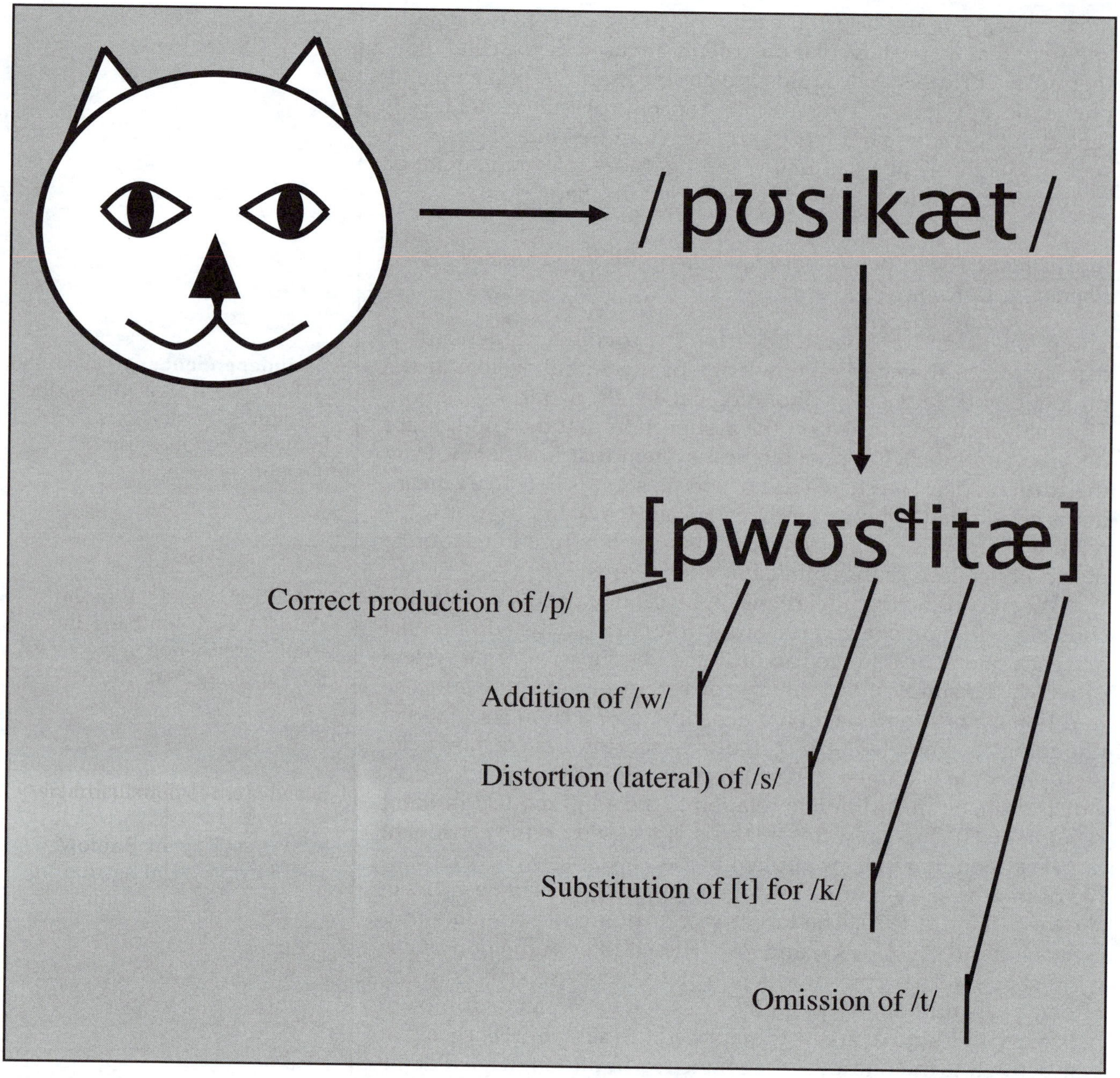

Figure 1–20. *Illustration of the five-way scoring system when conducting a relational analysis of a child's speech production.*

meaning that the child uses these phonemes contrastively. Looking at his use of these phonemes throughout the speech sample it can be seen that only [m n] might be said to be mastered in that they were used correctly in relation to the adult targets (disregarding the grammatical errors).

Covert Contrast

The determination of a child's phonemic repertoire based on a phonetic transcription of the child's speech reflects the sensitivity of the listener to phonemic contrasts in the child's speech. Given that the child's phonological system may be different from that of the adult listener's, it is possible that the child may be producing contrasts that are imperceptible to the adult who is transcribing the child's speech. When this happens the child is said to be producing a covert contrast. Covert contrasts are well documented in normal and atypical speech and are revealed by acoustic analysis of the child's speech output (Baum & McNutt, 1990; Macken & Barton, 1980) or instrumental descriptions of the child's articulatory patterns (Gibbon, 1999). Figure 1–21 illustrates this phenomenon with some data from a child who was one of 62 normally developing 4-year-old children who took part in a study of fricative development. The phonetic transcription of her efforts to produce the phonemes /s/ and /θ/ in word-initial and word-final positions revealed consistent use of [θ] for both phonemes in both word positions suggesting no phonological knowledge of the contrast between the phonemes. An identification test of her ability to identify words such as "sick" and "thick" revealed that she did not have perceptual knowledge of this contrast either, at least when cued by differences in the spectral characteristics of the fricative noise. Acoustic analysis of the spectrum of the noise portion of words targeting /s/ and /θ/ revealed that the centroid of the noise was not significantly higher for target /θ/ noise than for target /s/ noise as would be expected for correct productions of these phonemes (the centroid is the mean frequency of the spectrum, weighted by amplitude). The duration of the target /s/ noise was significantly longer than target /θ/ noise, however, indicating that she was differentiating these phonemes on the basis of noise duration. When describing her phonological knowledge on the basis of a perceptual analysis alone (i.e., phonetic transcription) it appears as if she has no knowledge of this contrast. Acoustic analysis reveals a covert contrast that is not apparent to adult listeners for whom duration is not a primary cue to the identity of these fricatives. This child appears to have both /s/ and /θ/ in her phonemic repertoire with /s/ produced as a relatively long noise with [θ]-like spectral properties and /θ/ produced as a shorter noise with [θ]-like spectral properties. Covert contrasts have been shown to be a positive prognostic indicator in that children with covert knowledge of a phoneme learn it more easily than children who have no knowledge of the same phoneme (Tyler, Edwards, & Saxman, 1990). This example illustrates the importance of a detailed description of a child's phonetic knowledge when attempting to understand the child's phonological knowledge.

Acoustic analysis may reveal **covert contrasts** in the child's speech—productive manipulation of cues to produce phonemic contrasts that are imperceptible to the adult listener.

Multilinear Phonology

Thus far, we have been describing phonological knowledge in terms of the phoneme as if phonemes were sequentially ordered isolated linguistic units. A strictly segmental description of phonological knowledge misses important aspects of the child's underlying phonology.

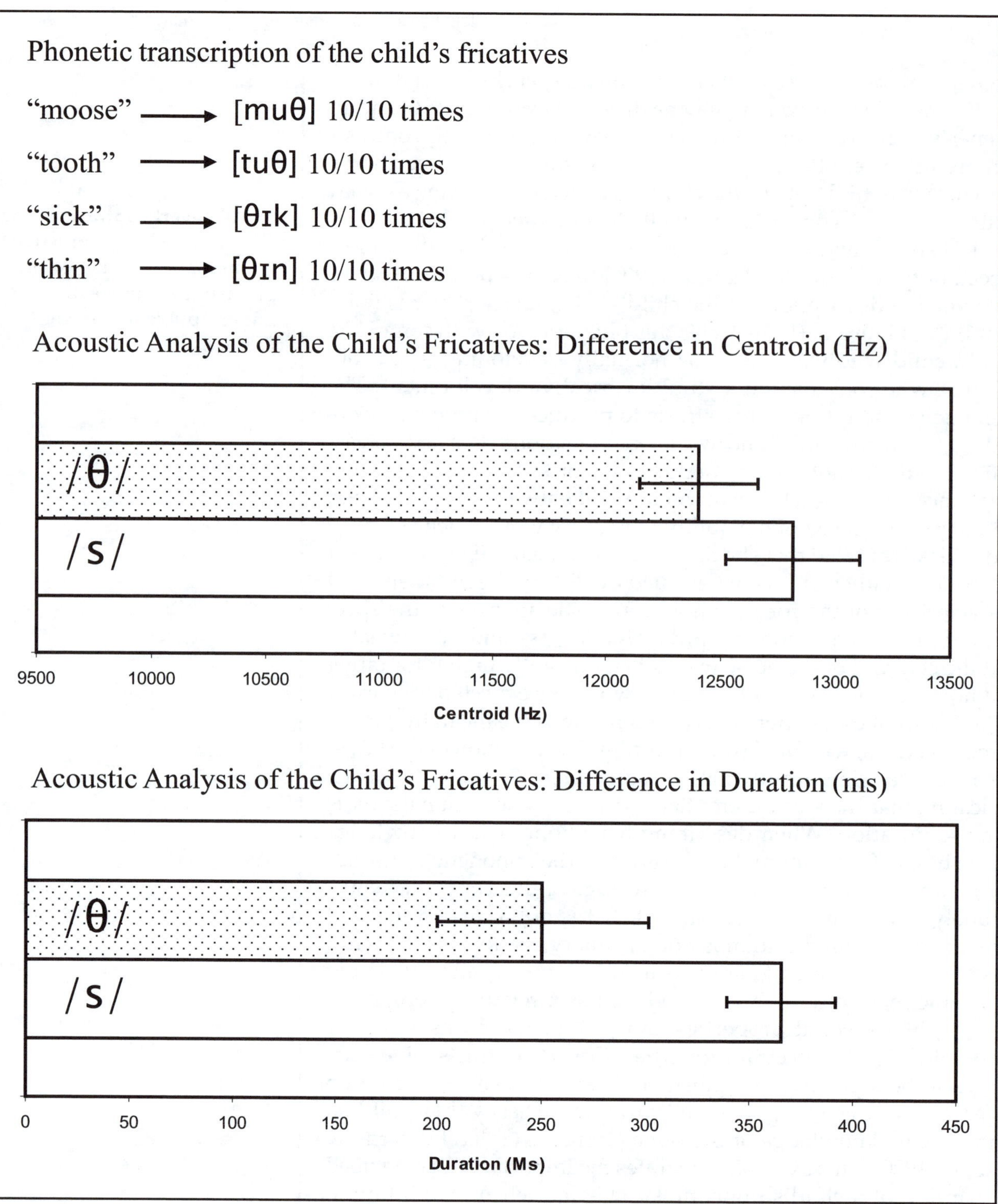

Figure 1–21. *Illustration of a covert contrast in a 5-year-old girl with normally developing speech. As shown by phonetic transcription of her repeated efforts to produce the target phonemes /s/ and /θ/, the child appears to have no contrast between the phonemes as she produces all target fricatives as /θ/ on a consistent basis* (top). *A bar chart showing the mean centroid of her /s/ and /θ/ targets with overlapping error bars indicates no significant difference between these fricatives with respect to their spectral characteristics* (middle). *A bar chart showing the mean duration of her /s/ and /θ/ targets with nonoverlapping error bars indicates that this child differentiates these phonemes on the basis of duration of the fricative noise* (bottom). Source: *Adapted from Ohberg, A. (2006).* Articulatory, perceptual, and phonological determinants of accurate production of /s/. *Unpublished master's thesis, McGill University, Montreal, Quebec. Printed with permission.*

Notice that the description of the sample presented in Figure 1–19 reveals a pattern of contrast neutralization that is applied to two phonemes, /s/ and /f/, that are related to each other. In order to capture this regularity in the child's pattern of phonetic realization of the fricative phonemes it is necessary to describe phonological knowledge at the subphonemic level, with phonemes defined by their features. Another regularity in the application of this neutralization rule involves the location of the phoneme—the contrast between fricatives and stops is retained in word final position but neutralized in word initial position. In order to capture this regularity, it is necessary to describe phonological knowledge at levels that are larger than the phoneme.

Multilinear phonology comprises a set of phonological theories that describe phonological representations in terms of a hierarchical organization of linguistic units.[2] Separate levels of representation are posited for prosodic and segmental constituents. In the next two sections, the prosodic levels of representation are described. Specifically, the levels or tiers in the representational hierarchy that are covered are the utterance, intonational phrase, phonological phrase, prosodic word, foot, syllable, onset and rhyme, and skeletal tiers. The first thing to keep in mind is that these labels, when used in the context of prosodic phonology, do not correspond to their meanings in other contexts. For example, a phonological phrase is not the same thing as a syntactic phrase and a prosodic word is not the same thing is a lexical word. Simply because there is insufficient space to diagram all the tiers for a complete phrase on one page, the initial focus is on the units at and above the level of the syllable. A description of the intrasyllabic units follows once the larger units have been tackled. In the diagrams to appear in the next two sections the segments are represented as phonemes for the sake of

Multilinear phonology comprises a set of phonological theories that describe phonological representations in terms of a hierarchical organization of linguistic units. Separate levels of representation are posited for prosodic and segmental constituents.

[2]There are many different versions of multilinear phonological theory, including nonlinear, autosegmental, metrical, or prosodic phonology. These theories share the multitiered hierarchical organization of phonological units but there is a large degree of variation in the choice of units, their arrangements within the hierarchy, and the terms used to describe them. Even individual theorists have been known to change their minds frequently about what to call units and how best to organize them. Sometimes the differences in terminology reflect individual preferences for the naming of similar units; in other cases the differences in terminology reflect significant theoretical disputes about the nature of the underlying units. For advanced students, an understanding of these theoretical disputes can be valuable. When linguists are able to derive multiple solutions to a particular phonological problem (such as, for example, the best way to represent affricates or liquids) it is a fair bet that developing children will also derive multiple solutions to the same problem. Knowing the range of possible solutions can help the clinician to plan effective interventions, especially for children with unusual underlying phonological systems. Nonetheless, making sense of these many changes in representational architecture and nomenclature is a very difficult task for a beginning student and thus, in this text, a single view is presented. The particular version of nonlinear phonological theory that is presented was selected because it has been presented repeatedly in the clinical literature for over two decades and is associated with an empirically validated assessment tool and treatment approach.

convenience; however, as will be explained in the section that describes the segmental units, phonemes are properly represented as a hierarchical arrangement of features. The feature hierarchy is covered after the prosodic tiers have been described.

The Prosodic Hierarchy

One aspect of **prosody** is the manipulation of duration, pitch, and loudness cues to emphasize certain syllables relative to others, thus creating variations in phrasal stress over the course of an utterance.

The arrangement of phonological units on the tiers of the prosodic hierarchy reflects the impact of prosody on speech perception and speech production (Gerken & McGregor, 1998). One aspect of prosody is the manipulation of duration, pitch, and loudness cues to emphasize certain syllables relative to others, thus creating variations in phrasal stress over the course of an utterance that communicate lexical, syntactic, or pragmatic information. These same aspects of speech can be manipulated in concert with pauses to create boundary cues that signal junctures between words and phrases within utterances. Each language has a characteristic melody or meter which is determined in part by the arrangement of stressed and unstressed syllables. In English, there is a preference for alternation of stressed and unstressed syllables although sequences of two unstressed syllables (but not more) may occur within phrases. English is said to be a stress-timed language in that it is spoken with approximately equal duration between stressed syllables. Certain other languages, such as French, are said to be syllable-timed because the syllables themselves are produced with approximately equal duration.

Utterances, the largest units in the prosodic hierarchy, are bounded by nonhesitation pauses.

The phonological tiers are illustrated for four different utterances (U) in Figure 1–22. You will see that the way in which the constituents are linked between tiers differs from one example to the next as a function of the prosody of the utterance and therefore careful attention to phrasal stress and boundary cues in a child's speech will be important when describing his or her phonological knowledge from the nonlinear perspective. Utterances, which are the largest units in the prosodic hierarchy, are bounded by nonhesitation pauses (Shattuck-Hufnagel & Turk, 1996). Utterances are roughly isomorphic with sentences although sometimes an utterance may contain more than or less than one full sentence. In Figure 1–22, the four examples cover a range of full sentences that might be spoken by a child but varying in length and complexity: Mummy loves me (A); I love elephants (B); After dinner, I had a bath (C); and Daddy is driving the blue car (D).

An **intonational phrase** is defined by a perceptually coherent intonation contour.

In each example, the second tier down from the U is the intonational phrase (IP), defined by a perceptually coherent intonation contour (there appears to be considerable variation in the literature as to the labeling and definition of this tier of the prosodic hierarchy; for further discussion, see Shattuck-Hufnagel & Turk, 1996). The number of IPs at this level will be determined by the boundary cues perceived in the utterance that themselves will be influenced by syntactic and pragmatic factors. For the examples shown in

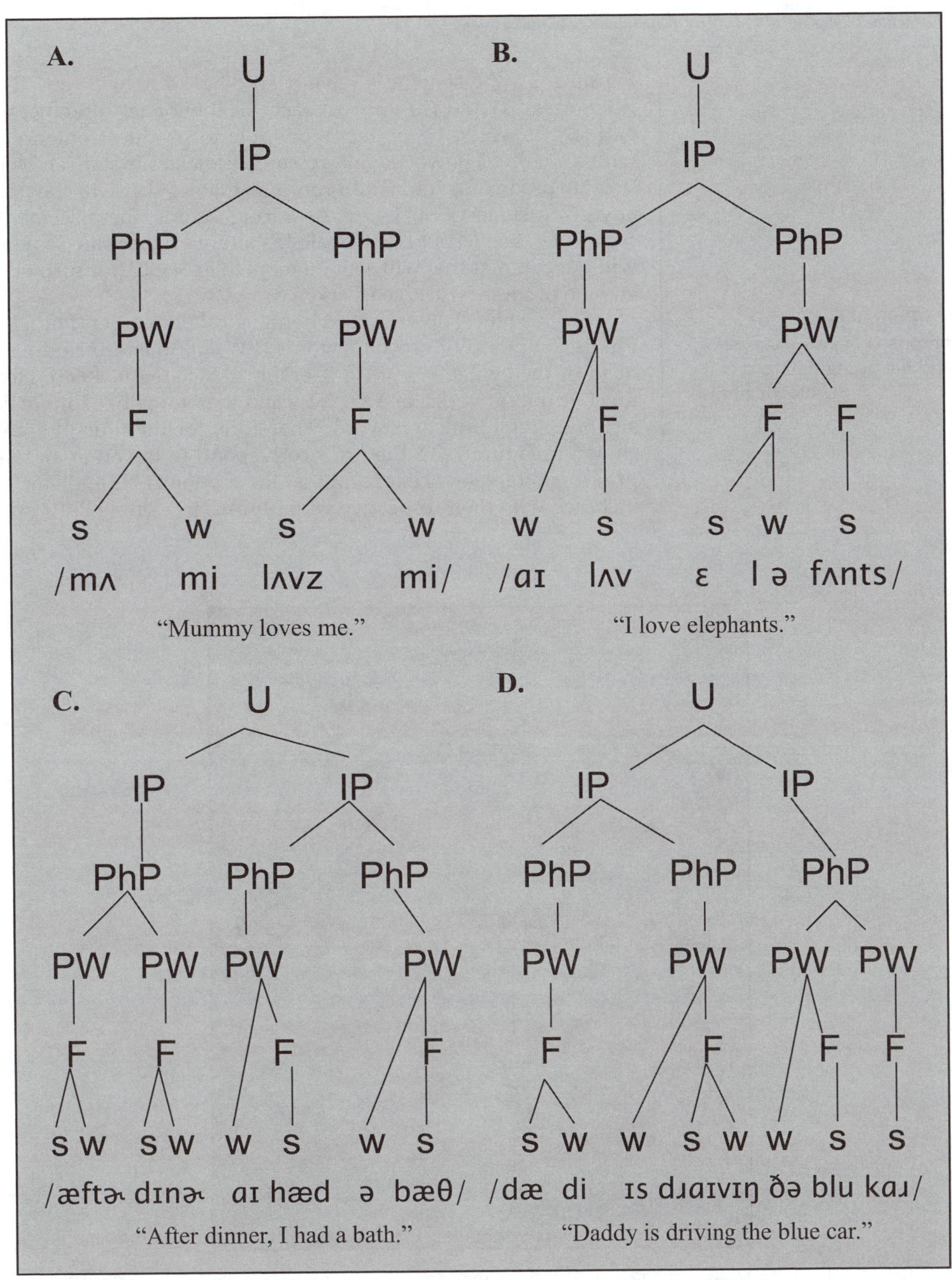

Figure 1–22. *Illustration of the top six tiers of the prosodic hierarchy for four sentences. Specifically, the utterance (U), intonational phrase (IP), phonological phrase (PhP), prosodic word (PW), foot (F), and syllable (s = strong, w=weak) tiers are shown for each sentence.*

Phonological phrases are composed of *prosodic words* up to and including the head of the syntactic phrase.

Figure 1–22, the sentences have been diagramed with one IP for utterances (A) and (B) but two each for the longer utterances (C) and (D). It would be perfectly possible to produce sentence (D) with a single IP, however, and research indicates that it can be difficult to predict the intonation contours that a talker will choose for any given syntactic structure. As a rough guide, the placement of commas in text tend to demarcate IPs although there are sentences without commas that will contain more than one IP (for further discussion of these issues, see Gerken & McGregor, 1998).

The next level down is the Phonological Phrase tier (PhP). Each PhP is composed of prosodic words (PW) up to and including the head of the syntactic phrase (Gerken & McGregor, 1998). Heads must be nouns, verbs, or adjectives and therefore PhPs cannot consist of a single function word. Therefore, for the four utterances shown in Figure 1–22, the PhPs correspond to the noun and verb phrases in the sentences except that the pronouns "I" and "me" are included with their respective verb phrases in a single PhP.

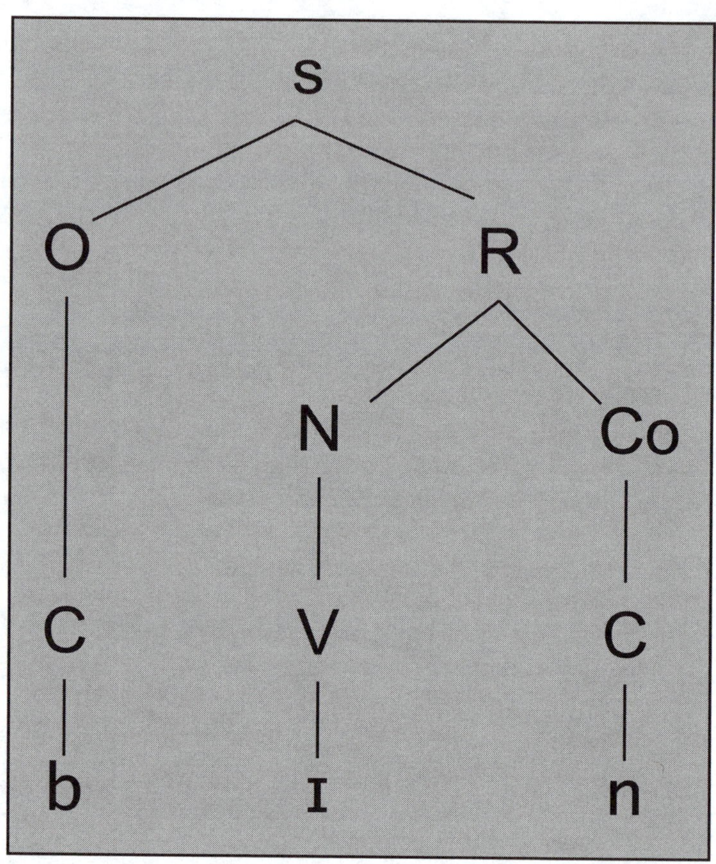

Figure 1–23. *Diagram of syllabic and subsyllable units for a single syllable word "bin." S = strong syllable, O = onset, R = rime, N = nucleus, Co = Coda, C = nonsyllabic timing unit, and V = syllabic timing unit.*

The prosodic word tier captures lexical words and adjacent function words into PW units. Notice that the final PW in utterance (B) is the single lexical word "elephants" but the final PW in utterance (C) contains two lexical words because the function word "a" is included along with the noun "bath." Similarly the verbs in each utterance capture neighboring pronouns or auxiliary verbs.

Each **prosodic word** consists of a lexical word and adjacent function words.

The next tier down identifies the foot (F) units in the utterance, each of which links to a single strong (i.e., stressed) syllable or maximally two syllables, the first of which is strong and the second of which is weak (unstressed). Unless it is monosyllabic, a metrical foot in English must be trochaic which means that it cannot consist of a weak syllable followed by a strong syllable. Most words in English have a trochaic structure (e.g., "Mummy" → ['mʌmi], "driving" → ['dɹɑɪvɪŋ] but some words and many word combinations have an iambic stress pattern (e.g., "a bath" → [ə'bæθ]). Iambic words and word combinations cannot be captured within a single foot because the foot must begin with a strong syllable. Words with more than two syllables cannot be captured within a single foot either (e.g., notice that the word "elephant" → ['ɛləˌfʌnt] in utterance B is composed of two metrical feet).

Each **foot** unit in the utterance links to a single strong (i.e., stressed) syllable or maximally two syllables, which in English must have a trochaic stress pattern, that is, strong syllable followed by a weak syllable.

The lowest level shown in Figure 1–22 is the syllable tier. Notice that each syllable is marked by a symbol indicating its relative stress as being strong (s) or weak (w). In some representations these diagrams will denote the syllable with the Greek letter sigma and indicate syllable strength with a subscript, that is, σ_s and σ_w. The sigma has been omitted here for convenience following Gerken and McGregor. Typical definitions of the syllable demand that each one contain at least a vowel with adjacent consonants when they occur (Gerken & McGregor, 1998).

Each syllable is marked on the **syllable tier** by a symbol indicating its relative stress as being strong or weak, that is, σ_s or σ_w.

The prosodic hierarchy is characterized not only by the arrangement of different linguistic units on these separate tiers but by the nature of the linkages between the tiers. These linkages are governed by the Strict Layering Hypothesis (Shattuck-Hufnagel & Turk, 1996). Simply put, each constituent on any given tier should link to one or more constituents on the next tier down with the set of linkages expected to be both exclusive and exhaustive. In other words, a constituent on a given tier should not link to constituents on any other tier except the immediately lower tier and all of the constituents on the immediately lower tier should be linked up to the immediately higher tier. Exceptions do occur, however, and these exceptions play a role in predicting certain speech and language production phenomena as discussed further in Chapter 4. A common exception occurs in utterances (B), (C), and (D) in the form of "unfooted" syllables. Consider utterance (B) for example: according to the Strict Layering Hypothesis the first PW should be composed exclusively of one or more feet units but, in fact, it links to both a foot from the next tier down and a w-syllable from two tiers down. Furthermore, all syllables on the syllable tier should be exhaustively linked to the foot tier above but the first w-syllable

According to the **Strict Layering Hypothesis**, linkages between tiers are expected to be both exclusive and exhaustive.

(associated with the word "I") bypasses the foot tier and is linked directly to the PW tier. This occurs because the first metrical foot must align with the first stressed syllable which is "love," leaving the syllable "I" in its "unfooted" state, linked directly to the first PW.

Syllables and Intrasyllabic Units

The **hierarchical organization of the syllable** posits that the syllable consists of an obligatory *rime* and an optional *onset* with the rime itself composed of an obligatory *nucleus* with an optional *coda* on the next tier.

Timing units on the **skeletal tier** allocate time for the production of the segments to which they are associated.

The hierarchical organization of the syllable is illustrated for a simple word in Figure 1–23. This structure posits that the syllable consists of an obligatory rime (R) and an optional onset (O) with the rime itself composed of an obligatory nucleus (N) with an optional coda (Co) on the next tier (O'Grady & Dobrovolsky, 1997). The skeletal tier holds timing units that are marked C for nonsyllabic units (roughly equivalent to consonants) and V for syllabic units (roughly equivalent to vowels although sometimes consonants act as syllable nuclei). Described as "enablers" by Bernhardt and Stemberger (1998), the timing units allocate time for the production of the segments to which they are associated but are nonetheless independent of those segments and thus there can be more segments than timing units and vice versa. Examples of single syllable words are shown in Figure 1–24, illustrating complex onsets and codas that contain more than one C unit as well as syllable nuclei with a long vowel or a diphthong necessitating more than one V unit in each

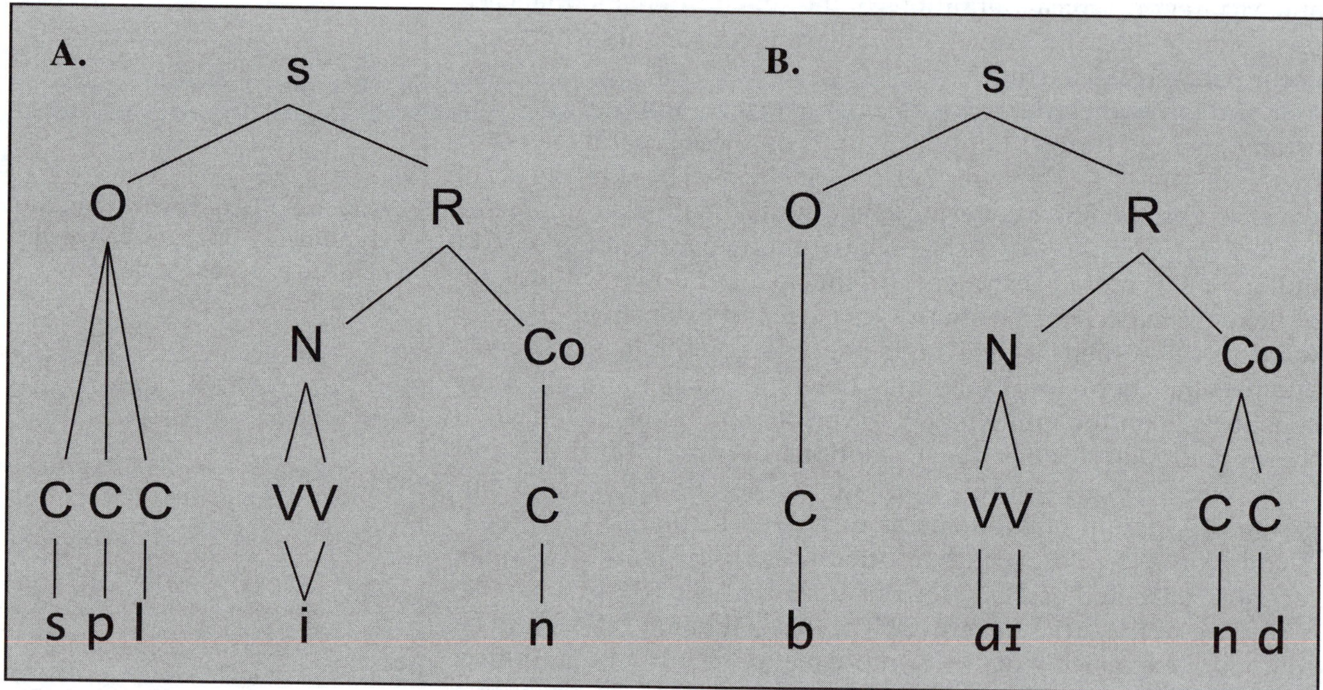

Figure 1–24. *Illustration of the syllabic and subsyllabic units for two words with complex elements: (**A**) "spleen" contains a complex onset and a long vowel; (**B**) "bind" contains a complex coda and a diphthongal vowel.*

case. By some accounts, the inclusion of the /s/ in the onset of the word "spleen" (see Figure 1–24A) would not be permitted because it violates the Sonority Sequencing Principle. In other words, each phoneme from the nucleus toward the edge of the word is expected to be less sonorant that its predecessor, with the sonorancy hierarchy from most to least sonorant being low vowels → high vowels → glides → liquids → nasals → voiced fricatives → voiceless fricatives → voiced stops → voiceless stops (Ball, Müller, & Rutter, 2010). The /s/ stands out as being more sonorant than the /p/ and thus it does not "fit." Different metaphonological solutions to the problem have been proposed that each involve excluding the /s/ from the onset and linking it directly to the syllable tier, in which case it is connected either to the syllable to which the rest of the consonant sequence belongs or to a separate "headless syllable" (for further discussion of these issues, see Bernhardt & Stemberger, 1998). Other researchers have suggested that the tendency to produce words that conform to the Sonority Sequencing Principle has phonetic rather than phonological origins (for further discussion, see Ball et al., 2010). Given that the treatment of this single exception (in English) to the Sonority Sequencing Principle remains controversial, the simplest representation is adopted here: all consonants to the left of the nucleus that form a legal word-initial consonant sequence in accordance with English phonotactic constraints will be placed together in the onset of the syllable; remaining consonants to the right of the nucleus will be placed together in the coda.

According to the **Sonority Sequencing Principle**, each phoneme from the nucleus toward the edge of the word is expected to be less sonorant than its predecessor.

Determining the syllable structure of single syllable words is relatively straightforward. The treatment of word internal consonants in multisyllabic words is complex in some cases. Figure 1–25 illustrates the syllabification of two words that contain word-internal consonant sequences. In part A of the figure, the word "elderly" contains no complex onsets or codas because the sequence /ld/ is not a legal onset in English and therefore the /l/ is placed in the coda of the first syllable and the /d/ in the onset of the second. In part B, the word "extra" contains a four-consonant sequence /kstɹ/. The three consonants to the left of the second nucleous /stɹ/ form a legal word-initial cluster and are therefore placed in the onset of the syllable and the /k/ is placed in the coda of the preceding syllable.

Phonotactic constraints are not the only consideration when determining the syllable structure of words. The syllable, onset-rime, and skeletal tiers are part of the prosodic hierarchy and prosody plays an important role in syllabification. Figure 1–26 illustrates the influence of syllable stress on the placement of word-internal consonants in the onset or coda of the first or second syllable of the word. Two word-internal exemplars of /ʃ/ appear in the phrase "washing machine." The first occurs in the context of a trochaic word "washing," that is, a word with a s-w stress pattern. The second occurs in the context of an iambic word "machine," that is, a word with a w-s stress pattern. In the second word, the /ʃ/ is unambiguously in the onset of the second syllable. In the first word,

Phonotactic constraints and prosody play important roles in the syllabification of words.

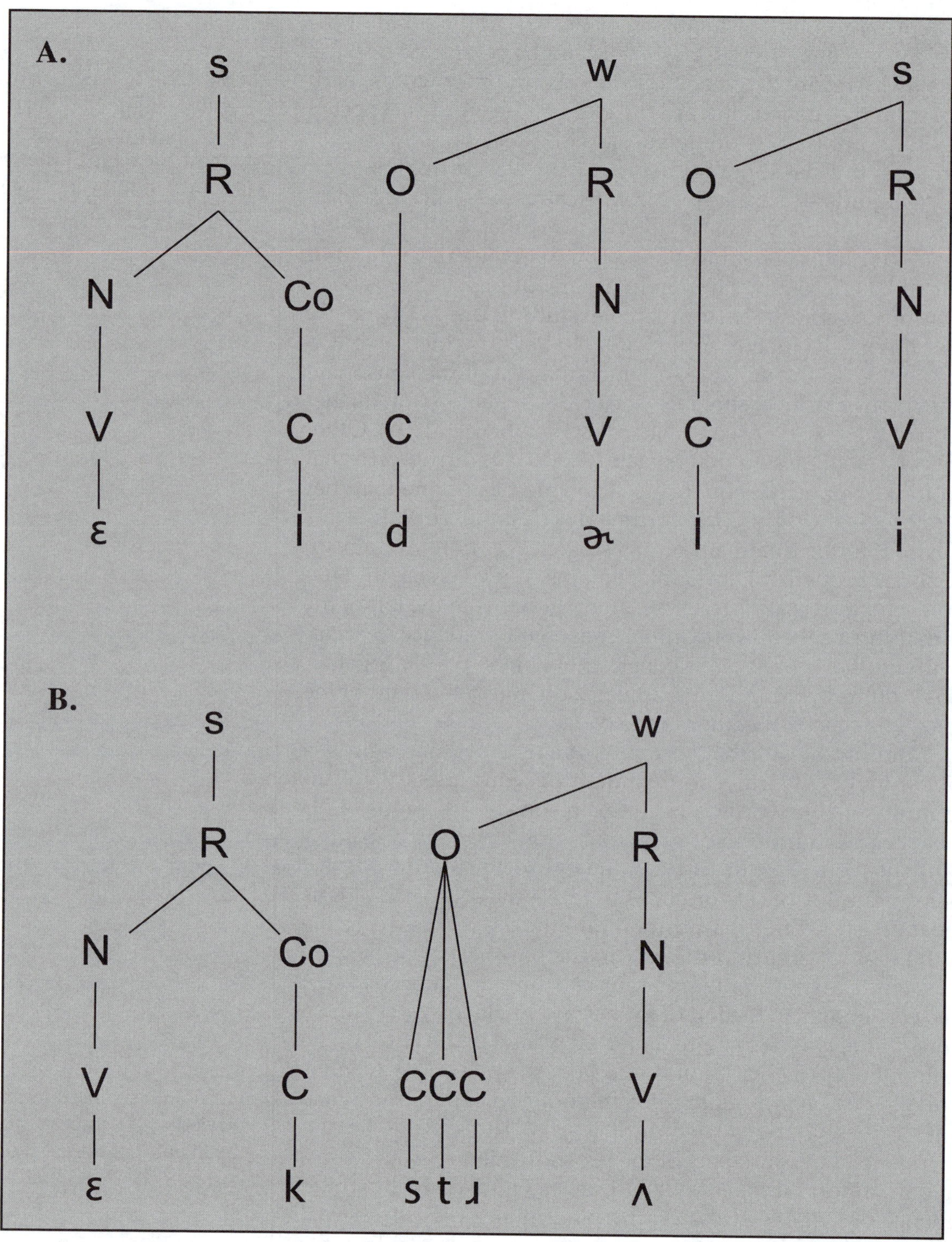

Figure 1–25. *Illustration of the syllabic and subsyllabic units for two words with word-internal consonant sequences: (**A**) "elderly" contains no complex onsets because the consonant sequence does not form a legal English onset; (**B**) "extra" contains a four-consonant sequence that is split to place the legal three-consonant sequence in the onset of the second syllable leaving the /k/ in the coda of the first syllable.*

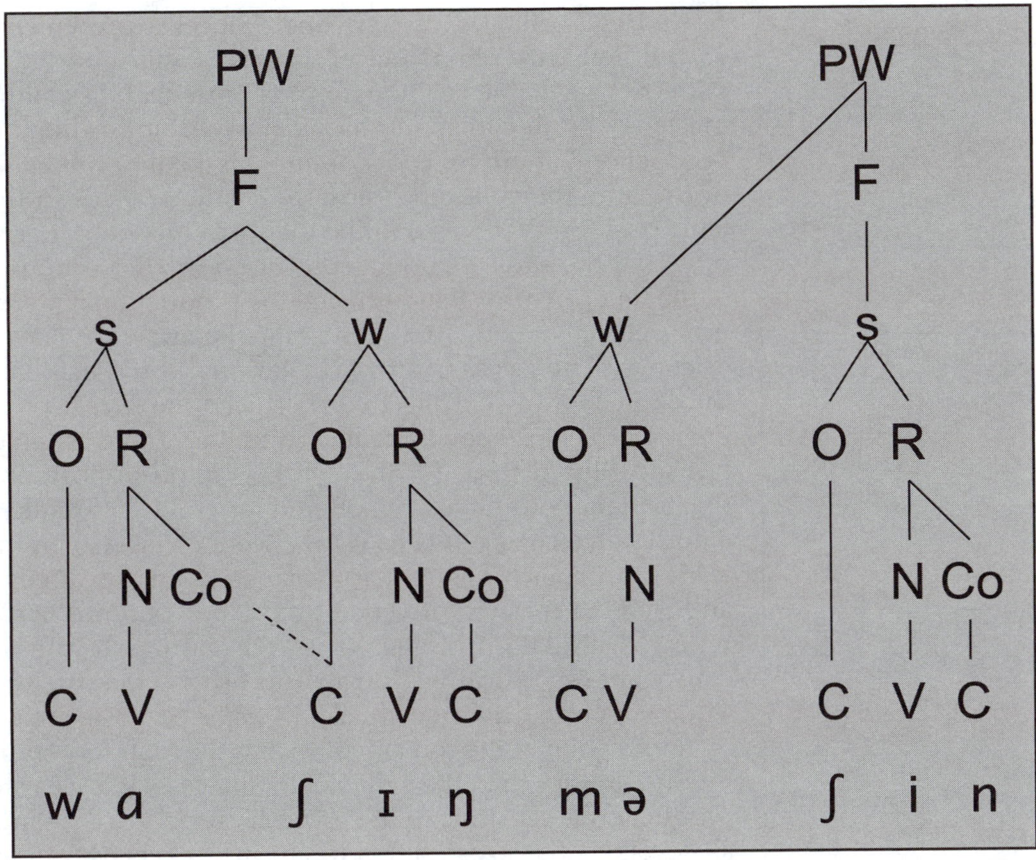

Figure 1–26. *Example of ambisyllabic /ʃ/ in the trochaic word "washing" compared to second /ʃ/ in the word "machine" that is in the onset of the last syllable.*

the /ʃ/ is ambisyllabic meaning that it is in the onset of the second syllable but it is also captured by the rime of the first syllable so that it becomes the coda of the first syllable and the onset of the second syllable simultaneously. The ambisyllabic syllable position has been proposed for languages such as English and German to account for certain phonetic phenomena. Notice that voiceless consonants that occur in the onsets of stressed syllables in English are aspirated whether the onset occurs in a word-initial or word-internal position, e.g., "support" → [sə'pʰɔɝt], "potato" → [pʰə'tʰeɾo], "pecan" → [pʰə'kʰɑn]. However, these same consonants, when produced in the onset of a word-internal unstressed syllable are pronounced differently: /p/ and /k/ will be unaspirated and /t/ will be produced as a flap, for example, "happy" → ['hæpi], "pocket" → ['pʰɑkɪt], "butter" → ['bʌɾɚ]. Ambisyllabicity is a controversial concept that is inconsistent with the common practice of "maximizing onsets" when syllabifying words. However, as has been reported repeatedly in the literature, children treat ambisyllabic consonants as if they there were codas more often than not (Bernhardt & Stemberger, 2002; Kehoe & Lleo, 2002; Marshall & Chiat, 2003; Rvachew

An **ambisyllabic consonant** is positioned in the onset of the second syllable of a trochee but is also captured by the rime of the first strong syllable so that it becomes the coda of the first (strong) syllable and the onset of the second (weak) syllable simultaneously.

& Andrews, 2002). Rvachew and Andrews presented data from 18 children with phonological disorders and reported production patterns by syllable position for phonemes that the children had not mastered. Production patterns in ambisyllabic position mirrored the production pattern for codas about half the time; about one-quarter of the time the children produced a unique error in the ambisyllabic position that was not like their production pattern for onsets or codas; the same error was produced in all positions about 20% of the time; an error that mirrored the production pattern for onsets occurred only about 10% of the time. Examples of one child's productions of voiceless fricatives in various word positions are reproduced in Table 1–1. This child produced the fricatives with a high degree of consistency in coda and ambisyllabic syllable positions but substituted stops for these targets in onset positions. Alternative explanations have been offered for children's tendency to treat ambisyllabic consonants as if they were codas. Given that the pattern is particularly common for velar stops and fricatives, Bernhardt and Stemberger suggested that production patterns in this position reflect assimilation of shared vowel features to the intervocalic consonant (specifically [Dorsal] and [+continuant]). Marshall and Chiat suggested that the children's error patterns are conditioned by the location of the consonant within the foot (foot-initial vs. foot-internal) rather than the syllable. In any case, it is clear that speech production is sensitive to the prosodic structure of words and thus all levels of the prosodic hierarchy must receive attention when describing children's phonological knowledge.

Segmental Tiers

The primary assumption of multilinear phonology is that **the feature is the basic unit of analysis**. Features can be deleted, inserted, and reordered independently of the segments.

Bernhardt and Stemberger (1998) state that the primary assumption of multilinear phonology is that the feature is the basic unit of analysis. Not only are phonemes described as a set of features, but features are ascribed properties formerly thought to be unique to segments—specifically, features can be deleted, inserted, and reordered independently of the segments. This property of features is

Table 1–1. *Examples of Allison's Productions of Voiceless Fricatives by Syllable Position*

Target	Word-Initial Onset	Word-Internal Onset	Ambisyllabic	Word-Internal Coda	Word-Final Coda
/f/	fish [pɪs]	uniform [jubo]	muffin [mʌfɪn]	halftime [ʔæftaim]	giraffe [dəwæf]
/θ/	thumb [dʌm]	panther [pædoɹ]	Cathy [kæfi]	bathtub [bæθtʌb]	mammoth [mainəf]
/s/	sadly [dɑdi]	casino [kətino]	glasses [wæsəs]	police chief [wis tʃif]	yes [jɛs]
/ʃ/	shovel [dʌfəl]	machine [mətin]	washing [wæʃɪŋ]	fishhook [pɪsʔʊk]	rubbish [wʌbɪs]

Source: Adapted from Rvachew, S., and Andrews, E. (2002). The influence of syllable position on children's production of consonants. *Clinical Linguistics and Phonetics*, *16*, Table 5, p. 193. Used with permission of Taylor and Francis Ltd.

made possible by the hierarchical organization of the tiers at the prosodic and segmental levels of the phonological hierarchy. In this section, the feature hierarchy and the features are described, as posited by Bernhardt and colleagues (Bernhardt & Stemberger, 1998; Bernhardt, Stemberger, & Major, 2006; Bernhardt & Stoel-Gammon, 1994).

A diagram of the feature hierarchy for the description of consonants is shown in Figure 1–27. The feature set chosen for this diagram deliberately reflects articulatory dimensions of speech and focuses on the English consonant system although two features specific to vowels are shown as detailed further below. It is recognized that features are discrete categories imposed upon a phonetic substrate that is continuous in nature. The category boundaries are not always agreed upon by linguists, may vary from one language to another, and most certainly vary among individual children. The feature distinctions described here form just one of many possible ways of representing the sound system of English.

The features are organized around three nodes, the Root node, the Laryngeal node, and the Place node. The Root node, situated on the segmental tier, attaches to the timing units on the skeletal tier. Manner features are organized around the Root node: [+sonorant] applies to vowels, glides, liquids, nasals, and the glottals /h/ and [ʔ]; [+consonantal] covers oral stops, fricatives, and affricates; [+nasal]

The **Root node**, situated on the segmental tier, attaches to the timing units on the skeletal tier. Manner features are organized around the Root node.

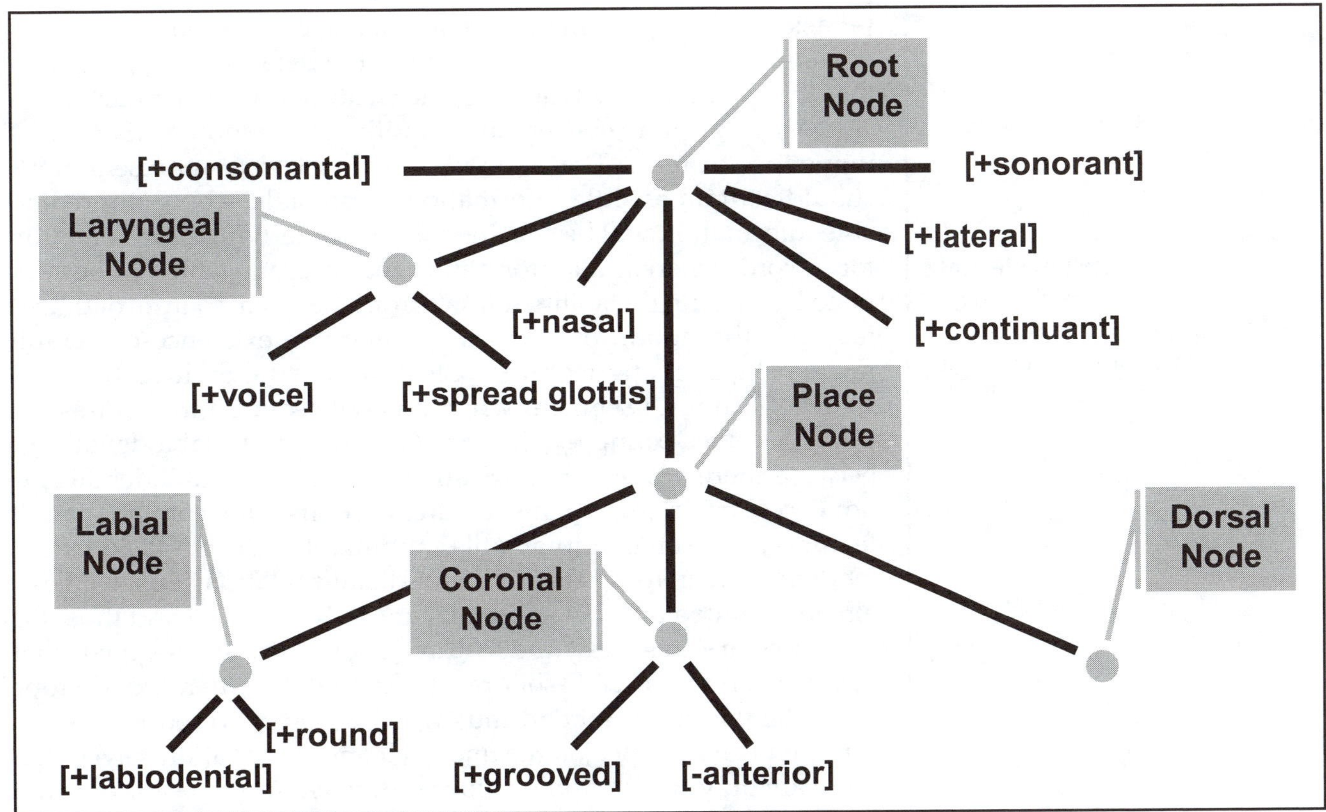

Figure 1–27. Diagram of the feature hierarchy for consonants (see text for details).

applies to the nasal consonants in English but may apply to nasal vowels, as in French or in certain child phonologies; [+continuant] refers to vowels, glides, liquids, and fricatives; and [+lateral] applies to all variants of /l/ and to lateral fricatives. The liquids /ɹ/ and /l/ are specified [+sonorant] and [+consonantal] simultaneously, at least in the onset position.

The nasals and liquids are sometimes called the "sonorant obstruents."

The **Laryngeal node** carries the features [+voice] and [+spread glottis].

The Laryngeal node carries the feature [+voice], which characterizes the sonorants which are voiced by default and the voiced obstruents. The second feature on this node [+spread glottis] is specified when stops are aspirated and applies by default to the voiceless fricatives.

The **Place node** links directly to the Root node and connects to three additional nodes that organize the major place features: *Labial, Coronal,* and *Dorsal.*

The Place node links directly to the Root node and connects to three additional nodes that organize the major place features: Labial, Coronal, and Dorsal, which in turn dominate more specific place features. All consonants produced with the lips are [Labial]. Connecting to the Labial node, [+labiodental] describes /f/ and /v/ and [+round] applies to rounded vowels and /w/. All phonemes produced with the tongue tip or blade are [Coronal] with the postalveolars being specified as [−anterior] and the interdentals being specified as [−grooved] (in contrast to the stridents, which are produced with a central groove in the tongue). The velar consonants are specified as [Dorsal] as are all vowels which are further described with the features [+high] and [+back]. Specifically, the [+back] vowels are /u, ʊ, o, ɔ, ə, ʌ, ɑ, a/, whereas /i, ɪ, e, ɛ, æ/ are [−back]; and the [+high] vowels are /i, ɪ, u, ʊ/, whereas the [−high] vowels are /æ, ɑ, a/. The vowel /ɛ/ is the default vowel, meaning that this vowel occurs when no place features are specified.

Underlying lexical representations should be underspecified in that only unpredictable information need be specified.

An important concept in multilinear phonology is that of underspecification. The basic idea is that lexical representations should contain as little information as possible—only unpredictable information will be specified in the underlying representation for a word, whereas all information that is predictable can be supplied by rule. Predictability follows from the binary nature of (most) features, the notion of markedness and the existence of default relationships among features. A feature may be omitted from the specification for a segment when it is not required for contrastive purposes. For example, /f/ and /v/ are clearly labiodental but because there are no labial fricatives that are not labiodental it is not necessary to specify this feature in English: the combination of features [+consonantal][Labial][+continuant] will be [+labiodental] by default. Regarding the notion of default relationships, we have already pointed out that sonorants are always voiced and thus it is not necessary to specify the feature [+voice] for any segment that has been specified as [+sonorant]. On the other hand, oral stops might be voiced or not and thus when a stop is voiced it is necessary to specify [+voice] in the underlying representation. Given that there are only two possible values of this feature, if [+voice] is not specified for an oral obstruent, then [−voice] is assumed and therefore it is not necessary to specify [−voice] in the underlying lexical representations for words such as "pea" and "pies," for example. The value of the feature that must be specified is usually the marked value of the feature. Markedness reflects sound characteristics such as distribution patterns across world languages and age of acquisition. For example, voiceless obstruents are widespread, being present in all languages, and they appear earlier than voiced obstruents in development, and thus [−voice] is the unmarked or default value of [voice] for obstruents. Given radical underspecification some segments require almost no specification. The glottal stop is specified simply by the Laryngeal node; having no specified place it is predictably [−consonantal]. Specification of the Laryngeal and Place nodes only yields /t/ because the [+consonantal], [−voice], and [Coronal] features are filled in by default. Although /t/ is the maximally underspecified consonant in English, default options for any given feature may vary across languages; even within a language the defaults in child phonologies may not be the same as the defaults in the adult system. Bernhardt and Stemberger (1998) propose default underspecification as a variant of radical underspecification that allows certain redundant or predictable features to be specified because this system seems to provide a more adequate explanation for children's phonological patterns. Table 1–2 shows the specified features for each consonant in English.

Usually only the marked value of a feature is specified. **Markedness** reflects sound characteristics such as distributional patterns across world languages and age of acquisition.

Figure 1–28 diagrams prosodic and segmental tiers for the word "chicken," beginning with the foot tier. This word forms a single trochaic foot being composed of a strong syllable followed by a weak syllable. The word has a CVCVC structure with the second consonant (C2) being ambisyllablic. The affricate in the onset position (C1) consists of two consonants, linked to a single timing unit, that share the features [+consonantal] and [−anterior] as well as the default Laryngeal node feature [−voice]. The first segment is [−continuant] (by default) while the second is [+continuant] (and thus the specification "branching continuant" as indicated in Table 1–2). The following vowel is [+sonorant] by default but is specified with the [+ high] place feature on the Dorsal node. C2 is specified as being [+consonantal] and Dorsal but defaults to [−voice]. The second vowel is the default vowel and thus no place features are specified. The final consonant, C3, is specified as [+nasal]. No place is specified (although the Place node is) and thus the C3 defaults to Coronal place.

Rules in Nonlinear Phonology

Two rules in nonlinear phonology can explain variance in the child's production from the child's underlying representation for a given word: spreading rules and delinking rules. Notice that the child's production might be perfectly consistent with the child's underlying representation while being different from the adult model. In this case, no rule is required to explain the difference—the child's representation is described in terms of the prosodic elements and features that exist underlyingly according to the evidence that is available.

Two rules in nonlinear phonology can explain variance in the child's production from the child's underlying representation for a given word: **spreading rules** and **delinking rules**.

Table 1–2. Default Underspecified Feature Matrix for Adult English Consonant Phonemes

Segment	Root Node	Laryngeal Node	Place Node
/m/	[+consonantal] [+nasal]		[Labial]
/n/	[+consonantal] [+nasal]		
/ŋ/	[+consonantal] [+nasal]		[Dorsal]
/p/	[+consonantal]		[Labial]
/b/	[+consonantal]	[+voice]	[Labial]
/t/	[+consonantal]		
/d/	[+consonantal]	[+voice]	
/k/	[+consonantal]		[Dorsal]
/g/	[+consonantal]	[+voice]	[Dorsal]
/f/	[+consonantal] [+continuant]		[Labial]
/v/	[+consonantal] [+continuant]	[+voice]	[Labial]
/θ/	[+consonantal] [+continuant]		[Coronal]:[−grooved]
/ð/	[+consonantal] [+continuant]	[+voice]	[Coronal]:[−grooved]
/s/	[+consonantal] [+continuant]		
/z/	[+consonantal] [+continuant]	[+voice]	
/ʃ/	[+consonantal] [+continuant]		[Coronal]:[−anterior]
/ʒ/	[+consonantal] [+continuant]	[+voice]	[Coronal]:[−anterior]
/tʃ/	[+consonantal] branching [+continuant]		[Coronal]:[−anterior]
/dʒ/	[+consonantal] branching [+continuant]	[+voice]	[Coronal]:[−anterior]
/w/	[+sonorant]		[Labial]:[+round]
/j/	[+sonorant]		
/h/		[+spread glottis]	
/l/	[+sonorant][+consonantal] [+lateral][a]		
/ɹ/	[+sonorant][+consonantal]		[Coronal]:[−anterior] [Labial]:[+round]

Note. Small changes to these feature specifications appear in Bernhardt and Stemberger (1998) that reflect chronic issues within linguistics about the nature of certain phonemes, e.g., appropriate specification for affricates, the specification of /h/ as [+consonantal] versus defaulting to [−consonantal] and the specification of the liquids as sonorants or consonants (specifications that may depend on syllable position). The exact resolution of these issues is not of primary concern in this book because the feature specifications are not presumed to be universal and these specifications may vary among children.

[a][+lateral] may not be specified for /l/ in English because /l/ and /ɹ/ are differentiated by the features [Coronal][−anterior] and [+round] (in the onset position).

Source: Adapted from Bernhardt, B., and Stoel-Gammon, C. (1994). Nonlinear phonology: Introduction and clinical application. *Journal of Speech and Hearing Research*, 37, Table 1, p. 129. Used with permission of the American Speech-Language and Hearing Association.

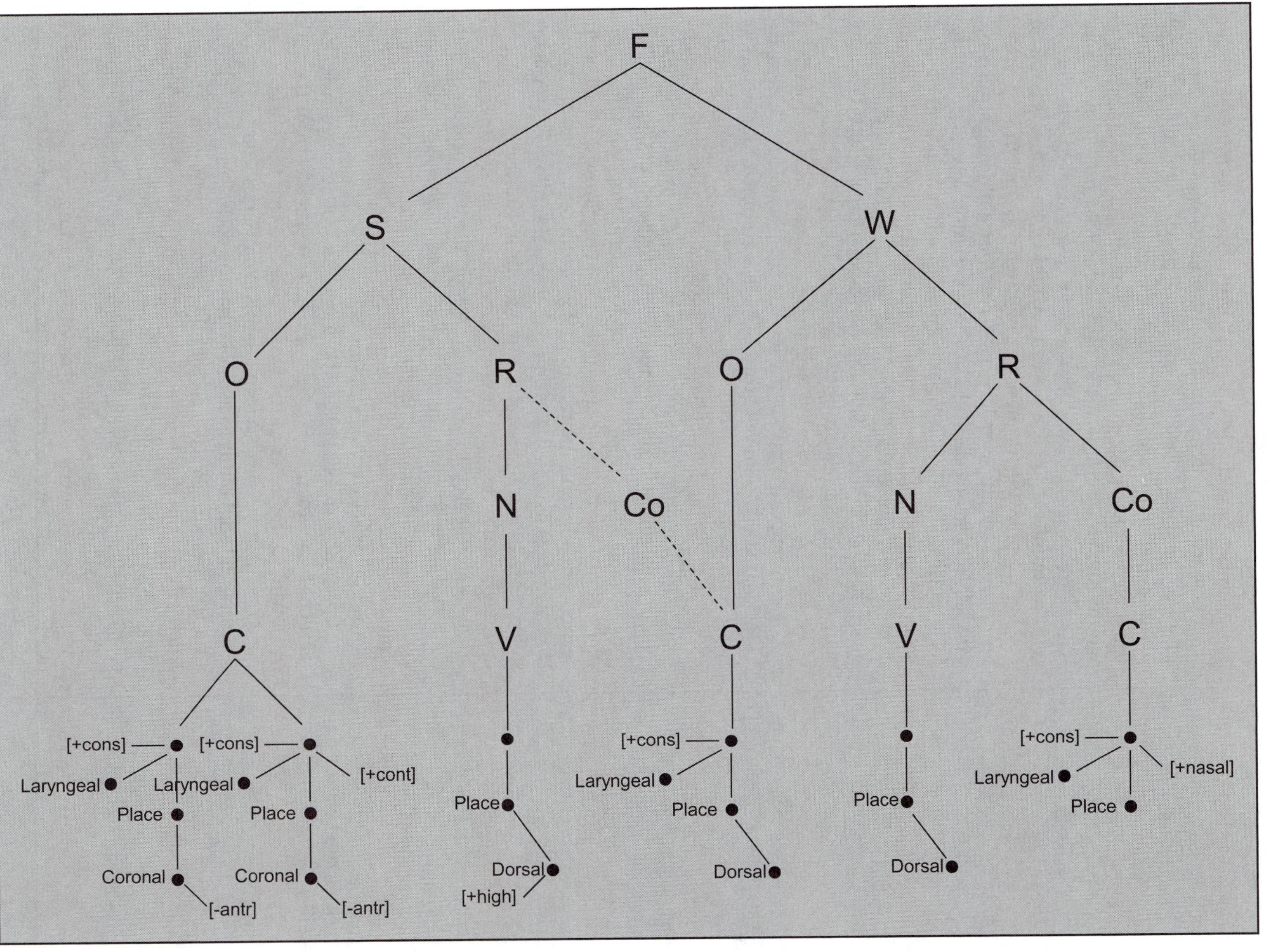

Figure 1–28. *Phonological hierarchy, starting with the foot tier and including specified features, for the word "chicken." Abbreviations are [+cons] for [+consonantal] and [−antr] for [−anterior]. Root node is unlabeled.*

For example, two children who failed to produce final consonants might have quite different underlying phonologies. One child might produce the words "pea," "Pete," and "peed" with an acoustically identical [pi] syllable and fail to discriminate perceptually between the three words. A pervasive pattern of omitting final consonants would further strengthen the hypothesis that the child's phonological system disallows codas. In this case the child's underlying representation for the three words would be the same, lacking any coda at all relevant levels of the hierarchy as shown in part A of Figure 1–29 for the word "peed." Another child might also produce all three words as [pi] but show variation in vowel duration, for example, "Pete" → [pʰi] and "peed" → [pʰiː], indicating some knowledge of the missing coda. Perceptual recognition of the distinction between "pea," "Pete," and "peed" would provide further proof that the child's underlying representation is adultlike but the coda is delinked due a production constraint as diagramed in part B of Figure 1–29. All units lower than the coda are also delinked.

Delinking can occur at any level of the phonological hierarchy.

Delinking can occur at any level of the phonological hierarchy. In the example shown in Figure 1–30, it is assumed that the underlying representation for the word "facecloth" is roughly adultlike except that the final consonant is represented as the default consonant /t/. Delinking of several elements results in the surface form [pestɑʔ], as follows: the [+continuant] feature is delinked from the first segment so that it defaults to an oral stop but with Labial place of articulation preserved; the /k/ target in the onset of the second syllable defaults to Coronal place of articulation after the Dorsal node is delinked; the liquid that should follow is completely unexpressed after the second timing unit in the complex onset is delinked; finally, delinking of the Place node from the final segment leaves a glottal stop by a default. Again, the assumption that the child has some knowledge of the delinked elements requires evidence from multiple sources such as use of the structures in other words or contexts, accurate speech perception responses, and/or acoustic evidence of covert contrasts.

Spreading rules explain the movement of features from one segment to another.

Spreading rules explain the movement of features from one segment to another. In Figure 1–31, Dorsal spreads from the coda consonant to the onset of the word "dog" so that the onset is produced as [g] in the surface form. In this example the coda is retained resulting in [gɑg] but it is possible that the coda could be delinked after the spreading occurs so that the surface form would be [gɑ]. Alternatively, the Place node of the coda might be delinked resulting in [gɑʔ] or Dorsal might be delinked resulting in [gɑd]. The consonant in the onset position is vulnerable to spreading because it is unspecified for Place. It is highly unlikely that a word such as "bog" would be pronounced as [gɑg] due to spreading because the specification of Labial would block spreading of Dorsal from the coda to the Place node of the onset.

It is important to note that spreading is not the only potential explanation for a production such as [gɑg] in place of "dog."

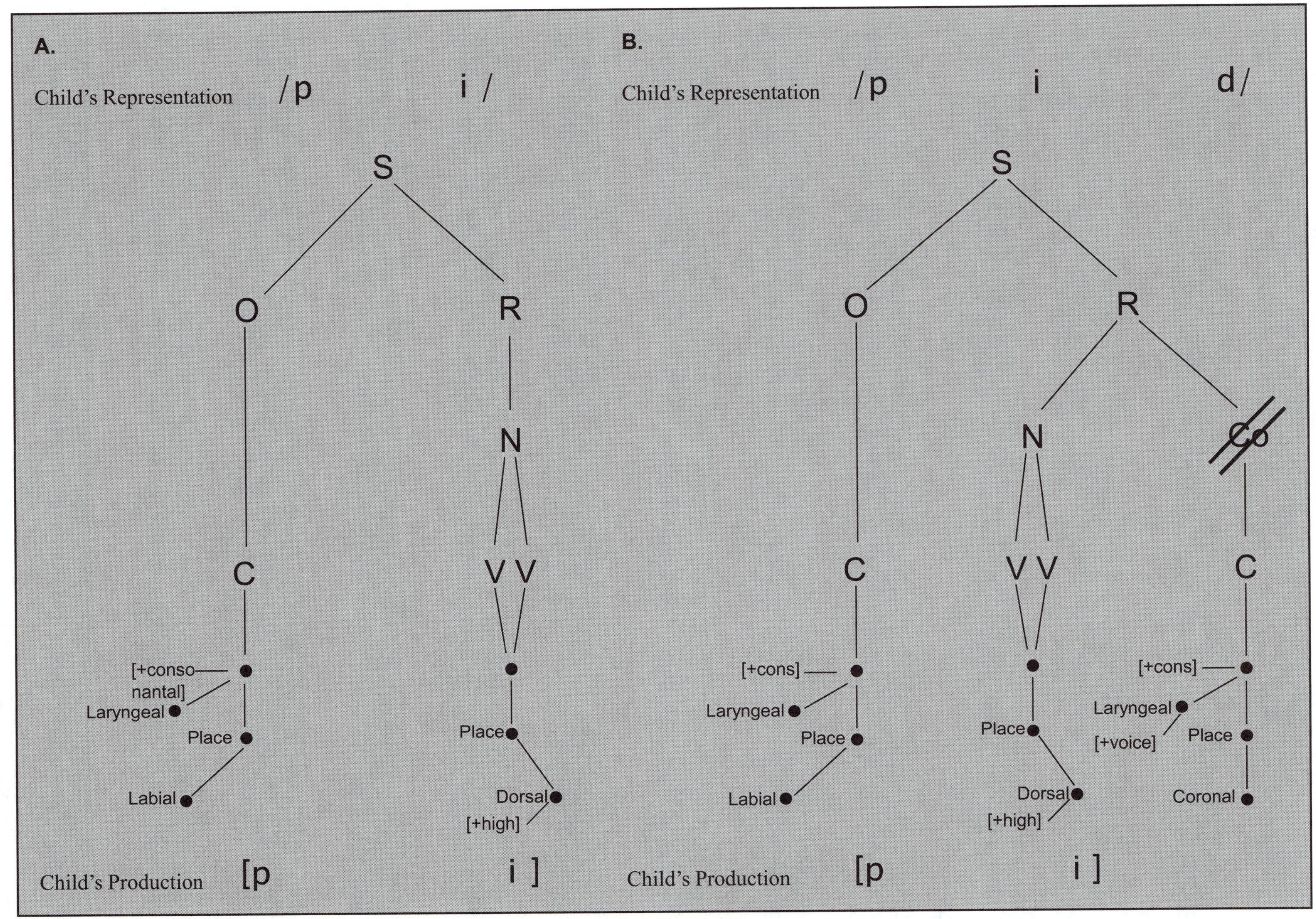

Figure 1–29. *Alternative underlying representations for the word "peed" in children who omit the final consonant.* **A.** *Coda is omitted because it is absent from the underlying representation.* **B.** *Coda is present in the underlying representation but delinked due to production constraints.*

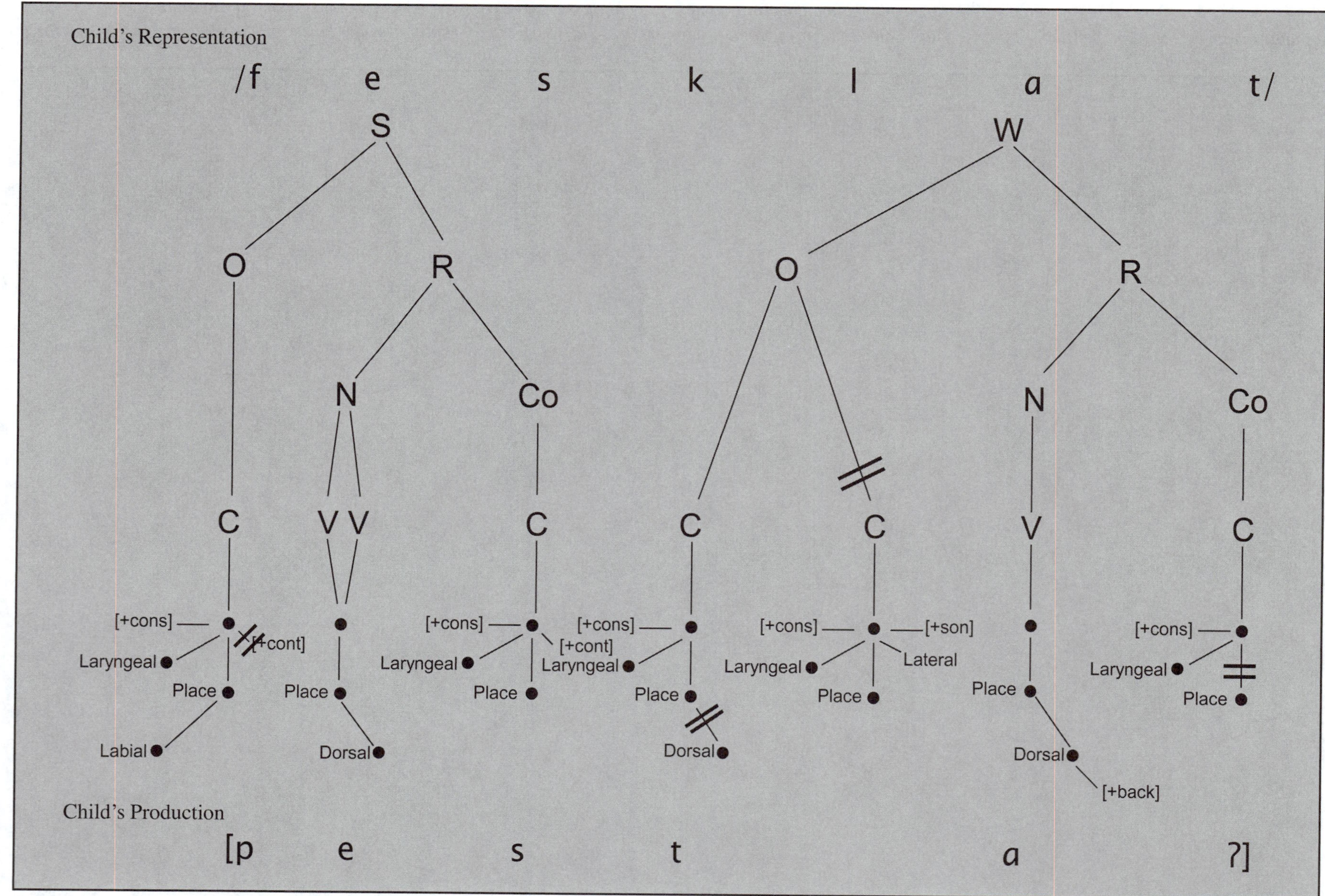

Figure 1–30. *Phonological hierarchy, starting with the syllable tier and including specified features, for the word "facecloth." Delinking of [+continuant] from /f/, [Dorsal] from /k/, the timing unit for /l/ and the Place node from /t/ results in the surface form [pes.taʔ]. Abbreviations are [+cons] for [+consonantal], [+cont] for [+continuant], and [+son] for [+sonorant]. Root node is unlabeled.*

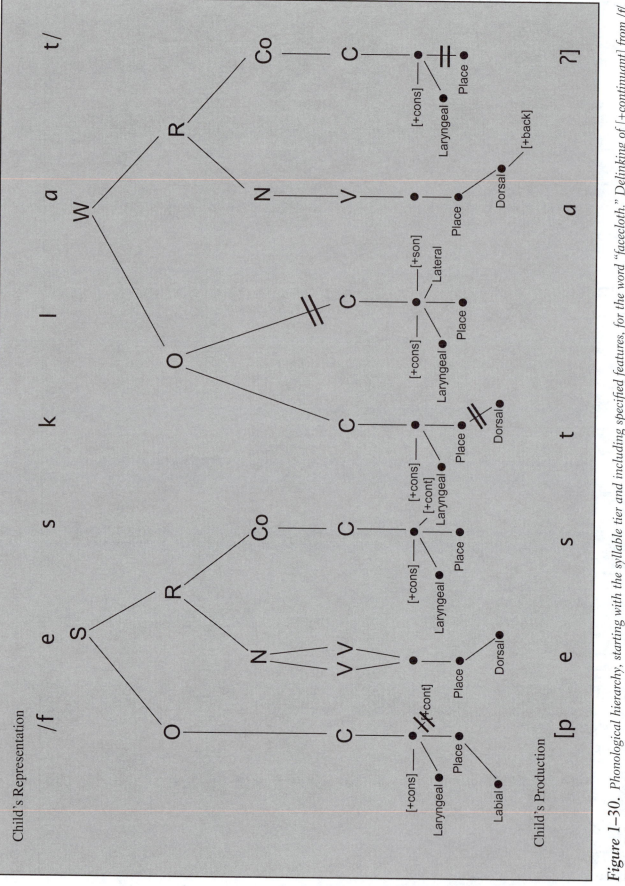

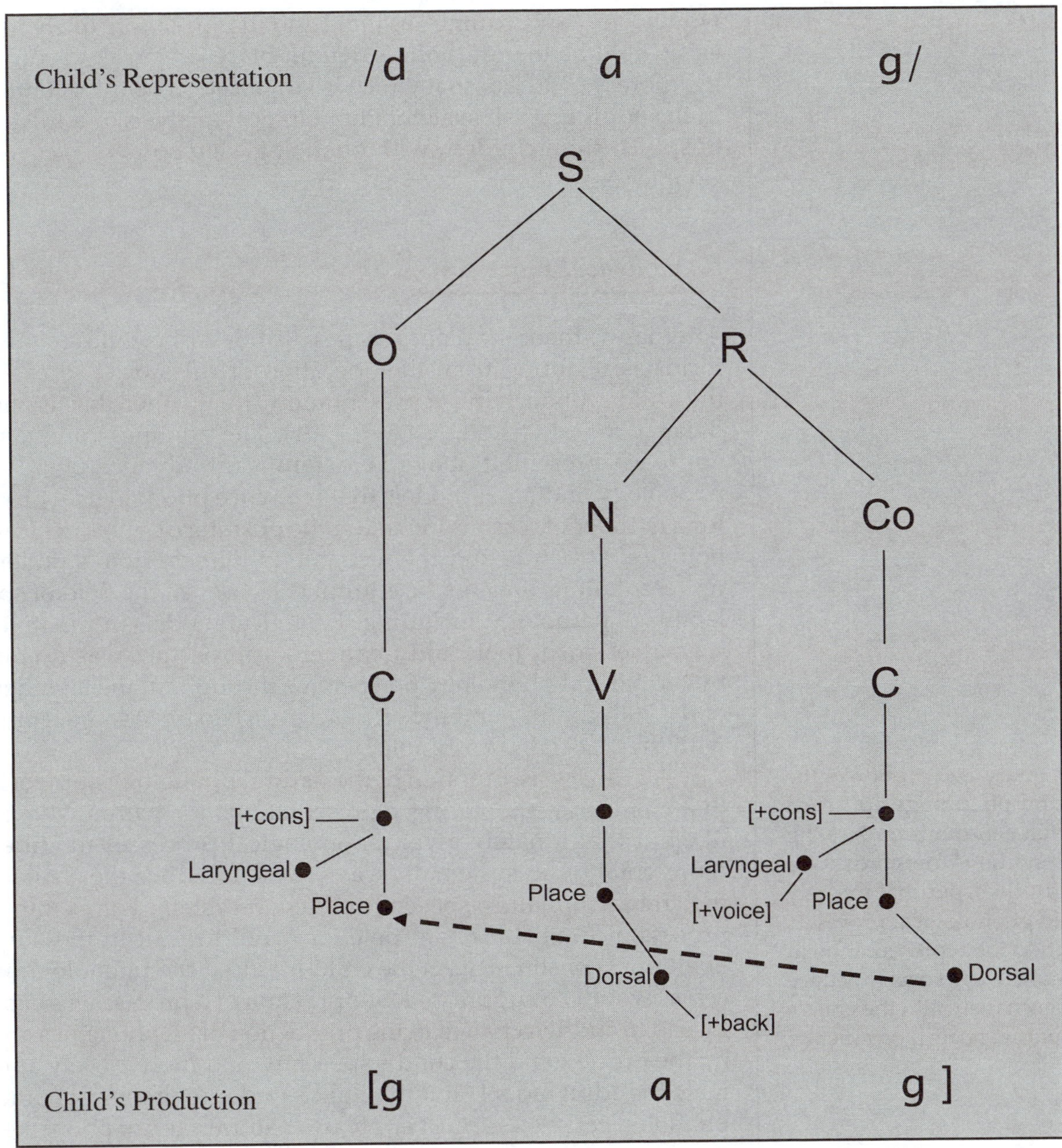

Figure 1–31. *Phonological hierarchy, starting with the syllable tier and including specified features, for the word "dog." Spreading of Dorsal from the coda to the onset results in the surface form [gag]. Abbreviation is [+cons] for [+consonantal]. The Root node is unlabeled.*

Spreading patterns can only be identified after analysis of the child's productions across a range of consonants and words. In this example, it would be necessary to verify that the child produced the /d/ target as expected in other words not containing the Dorsal feature. If the child produced the words "dot" and "dumb" correctly it would seem likely that substitution of [g] for /d/ in the word "dog" results from spreading. However, if the child produced the words "dot" and "dumb" as [gɑk] and [gʌm], a more likely hypothesis would be that the child's default place is Dorsal, in contrast to the more typical Coronal which is supposed to be the default place in the adult English system. Phonological analysis of a full sample of speech from children with phonological disorders is covered in Chapter 6.

Phonological Processes

Alternative theoretical approaches also describe children's surface forms as resulting from the operation of rules or "processes" on the child's underlying representation (for further discussion, see Baker, Croot, McLeod, & Paul, 2001). The nonlinear phonological approach presented above is a significant advance over natural phonology and other models that reference phonological processes for a number of reasons including the positing of a hierarchical phonological structure and the recognition that children's underlying representations may not be adultlike. However, the field of speech-language pathology, including theoretical models, normative data sets, assessment tools and treatment approaches, was dominated by the natural phonology perspective throughout the later decades of the 20th century and thus it is necessary to have some familiarity with the associated terminology.

A primary assumption of the **natural phonology approach** was that children's underlying representations for words were adultlike, but that innately given phonological processes modified the representation in systematic ways so as to reduce the challenge to the child's immature speech production system.

A primary assumption of the natural phonology approach was that children's underlying representations for words were adult-like but that innately given phonological processes modified the representation in systematic ways so as to reduce the challenge to the child's immature speech production system. For example, the process of final consonant deletion would result in the omission of all final consonants. As the child matured the phonological processes would be suppressed. Suppression of a process was expected to lead to sudden change in the production of all phonemes affected by the process and the child's speech would more closely approximate the adult model (and the child's underlying representation). A phonological process must apply to a natural class of phonemes and it must result in a simplification of the target phonemes. Distortions of phonemes (e.g., "shoe" → [ʃˡu]), errors that are specific to a single phoneme (e.g., "think" → [fɪŋk]), and errors that are more complex than the target (e.g., "yak" → [ɹæk]) would not be considered to be phonological processes. Furthermore, phonological process are expected to be "natural" in that they should be commonly occurring in children's speech as well as adult speech and across different languages. For example, final consonant devoicing (e.g., "dog" → [dɑk]) commonly occurs in both child and adult speech and is even obligatory in certain languages.

Table 1–3 lists some phonological processes that are observed frequently in the speech of English-speaking children, as described by Shriberg and Kwiatkowski (1980). The processes included were

Table 1–3. *List of Phonological Processes with Examples of Errors That Count and Do Not Count as Exemplars of the Process*

Exemplar of Process	*Dubious Exemplar*	*Not an Exemplar*
Final Consonant Deletion		
"dog" → [dɑ] "pants" → [pæ]	"far" → [fa] "boat" → [boʔ]	"toast" → [tos] "bottle" → [bɑdo] "car" → [kɑo] "butter" → [bʌɾə]
Velar Fronting		
"sing"→ [sɪn] "cob" → [tɑb] "go" → [do]	"dog" → [dɑd] "cone" → [t̡jon]	"key" → [kji] "coffee" → [pɑfi]
Stopping of Fricatives or Affricates		
"sew"→ [do] "shy" → [taɪ] "chew" → [tu]	"house" → [ʔaʊs]	"zoo" → [ju] "peach" → [pits] "push" → [pʊs] "see" → [tsi]
Palatal Fronting		
"sheet"→ [sit] "chalk" → [tsɑk] "measure" → [mɛzɝ] "jump" → [zʌmp]	"shock" → [pɑk]	"show" → [tʃo] "jello" → [wɛwo] "she" → [θi] or [s̪i] or [ʃ̪i]
Liquid Simplification		
"rat"→ [wæt] "lake" → [jeɪk] "run" → [jʌn] "bar" → [bɑo] "little" → [wɪɾə]	"row" → [ɹ̰oʊ] "rabbit" → [ɹ̬æbɪt]	"bird" → [bʊd]
Unstressed Syllable Deletion		
"about"→ [baʊt] "telephone" → [tɛfon]	"probably" → [prɑbli]	"alligator" → [æʔɪgeə] "button" → [bʌʔn̩]
Cluster Reduction		
"spot"→ [pɑt] "post" → [pos] or [pot] "bread" → [bɛd] "grow" → [woʊ] "steep" → [θip]	"card" → [kɑd]	"swim" → [θwɪm] "broke" → [bwok] "batman" → [bæmæn]

continues

Table 1–3. continued

Exemplar of Process	*Dubious Exemplar*	*Not an Exemplar*
Assimilation		
"dog"→ [gɑg]	"black" → [bwæk]	"down doggie" → [gaʊŋ gɑgi]
"cups" → [pʌps]		
"knife" → [maɪf]		
"lamb" → [næm]		
"boat" → [bop]		
"band" → [bæ̃nd]		
"dress" → [bwɛs]		

chosen specifically because they can be claimed to be natural due to their frequency of occurrence in the speech of normally developing children. There are two idiosyncratic characteristics about the list, however. The first is that processes related to voicing were omitted due to the extreme difficulty that clinicians have with reliable narrow transcription of voicing features. The second is that all types of errors relating to liquids including both those typically considered to be different types of processes and those considered to be distortions were bundled together into a single category called "liquid simplifications," again reflecting the fact that clinicians often have difficulty differentiating the various errors that affect this class of phonemes. Table 1–3 also lists errors that are sometimes mistaken for a given phonological process and some errors that are dubious exemplars of the process in question. Each of the eight processes are discussed in turn.

Final consonant deletion is manifested by complete omission of the coda.

Final consonant deletion is manifested by complete omission of the coda. Omission of one member of a final cluster or substitution of a glottal stop for the final consonant would not be coded as this process. Any cases of omission of liquid consonants in the coda position should be considered in the context of other liquid errors to be sure that they are not another manifestation of liquid simplification. Substitution of a vowel for a final liquid is coded as vocalization or vowelization by some clinical phonologists and as liquid simplification in the Shriberg and Kwiatkowski (1980) coding system. If the only exemplars of final consonant deletion to occur in the child's speech involve liquids it is more prudent to code these errors as liquid simplification.

Velar fronting describes a pattern of substitution of Coronal consonants for Dorsal consonants.

Velar fronting describes a pattern of substitution of Coronal consonants for Dorsal consonants. Some errors involving lingual consonants actually reflect an articulatory pattern called an "undifferentiated lingual gesture" (discussed further in Chapter 7). In this case the child produces these phonemes with a large part of the tongue dorsum and blade in contact with the full palate and alveolar ridge simultaneously. The percept of [k] or [t] depends on the spatial and temporal characteristics of the release, but in fact none of the phones produced in this fashion involve discrete closing gestures such as tongue dorsum to velum or tongue tip to alveolar ridge as one expects for the production of phones characterized by the features Coronal or Dorsal. Phones that sound like [t͡j] or [k͡j] are better described as distortions than phonological processes. Substitution of labials or other front consonants for velars are not properly coded as velar fronting as they are not the typical errors and thus not "natural." Most likely, these other front substitutions can be explained by some other rule or process such as assimilation.

Stopping describes the substitution of a stop for a fricative or an affricate, usually one similar in place of articulation to the target. Other errors for fricative or affricate targets that do not involve substitution of a stop are not coded as stopping. Substitution of an affricate for a fricative (e.g., /s/ → [ts] or /ʒ/ → [dʒ]) is called affrication rather than stopping. Note that this error actually results in a surface form that is more complex than the target and is thus not typically considered to be a natural phonological process.

Stopping describes the substitution of a stop for a fricative or an affricate.

Palatal fronting is coded when a postalveolar fricative or affricate is produced with alveolar place of articulation. Other fronted substitutions would not typically occur and probably should not be coded as palatal fronting. Other errors for postalveolar fricatives such as affrication or distortion do not count as palatal fronting either.

Palatal fronting is coded when a postalveolar fricative or affricate is produced with alveolar place of articulation.

Liquid simplification includes liquid gliding (substitution of glides for liquids in the onset position) and vocalization/vowelization (substitution of vowels for liquids in the coda position). Normally occurring distortions such as labialized or derhotacized variants of [ɹ] would not be coded as phonological processes. These errors are included in the liquid simplification category in the Shriberg and Kwiatkowski (1980) system. It is important to be aware of whether a given normative study of liquid production distinguished between substitution and distortion errors when determining the age at which most children suppressed the process or mastered this category of sounds. Errors on rhotic vowels would not be coded as liquid simplifications.

Liquid simplification includes liquid gliding and vocalization/vowelization.

Unstressed syllable deletion requires that the entire syllable be absent from the target word and must be distinguished from weakening of the unstressed syllable. It does not seem reasonable to say that a child has deleted an unstressed syllable if it is not present in the child's underlying representation and thus local norms for the pronunciation of words should be taken into account (in fact, this is true for all phonological processes). The pronunciation of "probably" as [pɹɑbli] is so pervasive in some dialects that this could be an example where weak syllable deletion would not be a reasonable description of the child's production, especially in the case of a preliterate child.

Unstressed syllable deletion requires that the entire syllable must be absent from the target word and must be distinguished from weakening of the unstressed syllable.

Cluster reduction involves reducing a consonant sequence in an onset or coda to fewer than the required number of segments.

Cluster reduction involves reducing a consonant sequence in an onset or coda to fewer than the required number of segments. The consonant sequence must be contained within the onset or the coda of the same syllable for the sequence to be coded as a cluster. Therefore the production of "Batman" as [bæmæn] should be coded as final consonant deletion rather than cluster reduction because the omitted /t/ is in the coda of the first syllable whereas the /m/ is in the onset of the second syllable. Word-final liquid+obstruent sequences form questionable clusters because the liquid might be considered to be part of the syllable nucleus. Therefore, "card" → [kɑd] could be described as omission of a rhotic vowel rather than cluster reduction. Similarly, syllabic nasals and liquids should not be coded as clusters and therefore "puddle" ([pʌdl̩]) → [pʌd] should be coded as weak syllable deletion rather than cluster reduction.

The identification of all phonological processes requires that the **entire speech sample** be taken into account because processes must apply to a natural class of phonemes and thus one is looking for error patterns rather than isolated instances of sound changes.

The identification of all phonological processes requires that the entire speech sample be taken into account because processes must apply to a natural class of phonemes and thus one is looking for error patterns rather than isolated instances of sound changes such as those shown in Table 1–3. In the case of assimilation errors, it is necessary to show that the particular error occurs in a specific context. Therefore, in the case of regressive velar assimilation, the most commonly occurring assimilation error, it is important to show that appropriate articulation of /d/ and /g/ occurs in other words where there is no opportunity to spread Dorsal to the Coronal segment. In the example of "black" → [bwæk], it is unlikely that this is labial assimilation (as opposed to liquid simplification) unless /l/ was normally produced correctly, for example, "glass" → [glæs]. Other place and manner features are subject to regressive assimilation too and, although less common, progressive assimilation does occur. Assimilation can occur between coda and onset, between coda and vowel and between the two consonants in a complex onset or coda.

Summary: Phonological Knowledge

A full accounting of a child's phonological knowledge requires attention to a number of different phonological constituents and the relations between them. At the very least, the child's use of syllables, onsets, rimes, codas, and features must be described. An inventory of the constituents and combinations of constituents that the child uses at every level of the phonological hierarchy must be provided. Interactions between these levels of the phonological hierarchy must be taken into account, such as the constraint against [−continuant] segments in the coda position as shown in Figure 1–20. Hypotheses about the child's underlying knowledge of phonological constituents relative to productive knowledge of those constituents should be formed and rules proposed to explain discrepancies between underlying knowledge and surface forms. Although this level of description is concerned with abstract knowledge of the sound system of the language, it is clear that careful attention to the child's knowledge of the child's phonetic knowledge in the perceptual and articulatory domains is important to the development of this description. Chapters 5 and 6 provide more information about how to conduct a detailed analysis of a child's phonological knowledge. At this point, familiarity with the basic units of analysis provides an essential foundation for the study of the normal course of phonological development.

References

Abramson, A. S., & Lisker, L. (1970). Discriminability along the voicing continuum: Cross language tests. In *Proceedings of the International Congress of Phonetic Sciences, 6th, Prague, 1967* (pp. 569–573). Prague Academia.

Alwan, A., Narayanan, S., & Haker, K. (1997). Toward articulatory-acoustic models for liquid approximants based on MRI and EPG data. Part II. The rhotics. *Journal of the Acoustical Society of America, 101*, 1078–1089.

Baker, E., Croot, K., McLeod, S., & Paul, R. (2001). Psycholinguistic models of speech development and their application to clinical practice. *Journal of Speech, Language, and Hearing Research, 44*, 685–702.

Ball, M. J., Müller, N., & Rutter, B. (2010). *Phonology for communication disorders*. New York, NY: Psychology Press.

Baum, S. R., & McNutt, J. C. (1990). An acoustic analysis of frontal misarticulation of /s/ in children. *Journal of Phonetics, 18*, 51–63.

Beckman, M. E., & Edwards, J. (2000). The ontongeny of phonological categories and the primacy of lexical learning in linguistic development. *Child Development, 71*, 240–249.

Benki, J. R. (2001). Place of articulation and first formant transition pattern both affect perception of voicing in English. *Journal of Phonetics, 29*, 1–22.

Benki, J. R. (2003). *Perception of VOT and first formant onset by Spanish and English speakers*. Paper presented at the 4th International Symposium on Bilingualism.

Bernhardt, B., & Stemberger, J. P. (1998). *Handbook of phonological development from the perspective of constraint-based phonology*. San Diego, CA: Academic Press.

Bernhardt, B., & Stemberger, J. P. (2002). Intervocalic consonants in the speech of English-speaking Canadian children with phonological disorders. *Clinical Linguistics and Phonetics, 16*, 199–214.

Bernhardt, B., Stemberger, J. P., & Major, E. M. (2006). General and nonlinear phonological intervention perspectives for a child with resistant phonological impairment. *Advances in Speech-Language Pathology, 8*, 190–206.

Bernhardt, B., & Stoel-Gammon, C. (1994). Nonlinear phonology: Introduction and clinical application. *Journal of Speech and Hearing Research, 37*, 123–143.

Camarata, S., & Gandour, J. (1984). On describing idiosyncratic phonologic systems. *Journal of Speech and Hearing Disorders, 49*, 262–266.

Chiat, S. (1989). The relation between prosodic structure, syllabification and segmental realisation: Evidence from a child with fricative stopping. *Clinical Linguistics and Phonetics, 3*, 232–242.

Chomsky, N., & Halle, M. (1968). *The sound pattern of English.* New York, NY: Harper & Row.

Coleman, J. (2003). Discovering the acoustic correlates of phonological contrasts. *Journal of Phonetics, 31,* 351–372.

Crowther, C. S., & Mann, V. A. (1994). Use of vocalic cues to consonant voicing and native language background: The influence of experimental design. *Perception and Psychophysics, 55,* 513–525.

Delattre, P., & Freeman, D. C. (1968). A dialect study of American r's by x-ray motion picture. *Linguistics, 44,* 29–68.

Diehl, R. L., Lotto, A. J., & Holt, L. L. (2004). Speech perception. *Annual Review of Psychology, 55,* 149–179.

Dinnsen, D. A., Chin, S. B., Elbert, M., & Powell, T. W. (1990). Some constraints on functionally disordered phonologies: Phonetic inventories and phonotactics. *Journal of Speech and Hearing Research, 33*(1), 28–37.

Dworkin, J. P., & Culatta, R. A. (1980). Tongue strength: Its relationship to tongue thrusting, open-bite, and articulatory proficiency. *Journal of Speech and Hearing Disorders, 45*(2), 277–282.

Edwards, J., Fourakis, M., Beckman, M. E., & Fox, R. A. (1999). Characterizing knowledge deficits in phonological disorders. *Journal of Speech, Language, and Hearing Research, 42,* 169–186.

Fidriksson, J., Moser, D., Ryalls, J., Bonilha, L., Rorden, C., & Baylis, B. (2009). Modulation of frontal lobe speech areas associated with the production and perception of speech movements. *Journal of Speech, Language, and Hearing Research, 52,* 812–819.

Galantucci, B., Fowler, C. A., & Turvey, M. T. (2006). The motor theory of speech perception. *Psychonomic Bulletin and Review, 13,* 361–377.

Gerken, L., & McGregor, K. (1998). An overview of prosody and its role in normal and disordered child language. *American Journal of Speech-Language Pathology, 7,* 38–48.

Gibbon, F. E. (1999). Undifferentiated lingual gestures in children with articulation/phonological disorders. *Journal of Speech, Language, and Hearing Research, 42,* 382–397.

Gick, B., & Campbell, F. (2003). *Intergestural timing in English /r/.* Paper presented at the 15th International Conference of Phonetic Sciences, Barcelona.

Gick, B., Wilson, I., Koch, K., & Cook, C. (2004). Language-specific articulatory settings: Evidence from inter-utterance rest position. *Phonetica, 61,* 220–233.

Goldinger, S. D. (1996). Words and voices: Episodic traces in spoken word identification and recognition memory. *Journal of Experimental Psychology, Learning, Memory, and Cognition, 22,* 1166–1183.

Graham, L. W., & House, A. S. (1971). Phonological oppositions in children: A perceptual study. *Journal of the Acoustical Society of America, 49*(2B), 559–566.

Guenther, F. H., & Gjaja, M. N. (1996). The perceptual magnet effect as an emergent property of neural map formation. *Journal of the Acoustical Society of America, 100*(2), 1111–1121.

Halle, M. (1985). Speculations about the representation of words in memory. In V. A. Fromkin (Ed.), *Phonetic linguistics* (pp. 101–104): New York, NY: Academic Press.

Hickock, G. (2008). Eight problems for the mirror neuron theory of action understanding in monkeys and humans. *Journal of Cognitive Neuroscience, 21,* 1229–1243.

Hinton, V. A., & Arokiasamy, W. M. C. (1997). Maximum interlabial pressures in normal speakers. *Journal of Speech, Language, and Hearing Research, 40*, 400–404.

International Phonetic Association. (1999). *Handbook of the International Phonetic Association: A guide to the use of the International Phonetic Alphabet*. Cambridge, UK: Cambridge University Press.

Jakobson, R., Fant, C. G. M., & Halle, M. (1963). *Preliminaries to speech analysis: The distinctive features and their correlates* (10th ed.). Cambridge, MA: MIT Press.

Johnson, K. (2007). Decisions and mechanisms in exemplar-based phonology. In M. J. Sole, P. Beddor, & M. Ohala (Eds.), *Experimental approaches to phonology. In honor of John Ohala* (pp. 25–40). Oxford, UK: Oxford University Press.

Kehoe, M. M., & Lleo, C. (2002). Intervocalic consonants in the acquisition of German: Onsets, codas or something else? *Clinical Linguistics and Phonetics, 16*, 169–182.

Kent, R. D., & Bauer, H. R. (1985). Vocalizations of one-year-olds. *Journal of Child Language, 12*, 491–526.

Kent, R. D., & Murray, A. D. (1982). Acoustic features of infant vocalic utterances at 3, 6, and 9 months. *Journal of the Acoustical Society of America, 72*, 353–365.

Kohler, E., Keysers, C., Umiltà, A., Fogassi, L., Gallese, V., & Rizzolatti, G. (2002). Hearing sounds, understanding actions: Action representation in mirror neurons. *Science, 297*, 846–848.

Kuhl, P. K., Andruski, J. E., Chistovich, I. A., Kozhevnikova, E. V., Ryskina, V. L., Stolyarova, E. I., . . . Lacerda, F. (1997). Cross-language analysis of phonetic units in language addressed to infants. *Science, 277*, 684–686.

Ladefoged, P. (1999). Linguistic phonetic descriptions. In W. J. Hardcastle & J. Laver (Eds.), *The handbook of phonetic sciences*. Hoboken, NJ: Blackwell. Blackwell Reference Online. Retrieved July 2, 2010, from http://www.blackwellreference.com/subscriber/tocnode?id=g9780631214786_chunk_g978063121478619.

Liberman, A. M., & Whalen, D. H. (2000). On the relation of speech to language. *Trends in Cognitive Sciences, 4*(5), 187–196.

Lotto, A. J., Hickok, G. S., & Holt, L. L. (2009). Reflections on mirror neurons and speech perception. *Trends in Cognitive Sciences, 13*, 110–114.

Macken, M., & Barton, D. (1980). A longitudinal study of the acquisition of the voicing contrast in American English word initial stops, as measured by voice onset time. *Journal of Child Language, 7*, 41–72.

MacLeod, A. A. N., & Stoel-Gammon, C. (2009). The use of voice onset time by early bilinguals to distinguish homorganic stops in Canadian English and Canadian French. *Applied Psycholinguistics, 30*, 53–77.

Maeda, S. (1990). Compensatory articulation during speech: Evidence from the analysis and synthesis of vocal-tract shapes using an articulatory model. In W. Hardcastle & A. Marchal (Eds.), *Speech production and speech modeling* (pp. 131–149). The Netherlands: Kluwer Academic.

Marshall, C., & Chiat, S. (2003). A foot domain account of prosodically-conditioned substitutions. *Clinical Linguistics and Phonetics, 17*(8), 645–657.

Maye, J., Werker, J. F., & Gerken, L. (2002). Infant sensitivity to distributional information can affect phonetic discrimination. *Cognition, 82*, B101–B111.

McLeod, S., & Singh, S. (2009). *Speech sounds: A pictoral guide to typical and atypical speech*. San Diego, CA: Plural.

Miller, G. A., & Nicely, P. E. (1955). An analysis of perceptual confusions among some English consonants. *Journal of the Acoustical Society of America, 27*, 338–352.

Munson, B., Edwards, J., & Beckman, M. E. (2005). Phonological knowledge in typical and atypical speech-sound development. *Topics in Language Disorders, 25*(3), 190–206.

Nieto-Castanon, A., Guenther, F. H., Perkell, J., & Curtin, H. D. (2005). A modeling investigation of articulatory variability and acoustic stability during American English /r/ production. *Journal of the Acoustical Society of America, 117*(5), 3196–3212.

Nittrouer, S. (1996). The relation between speech perception and phonemic awareness: Evidence from low-SES children and children with chronic otitis media. *Journal of Speech and Hearing Research, 39*, 1059–1070.

Nittrouer, S. (2002a). From ear to cortex: A perspective on what clinicians need to understand about speech perception and language processing. *Language, Speech, and Hearing Services in Schools, 33*, 237–252.

Nittrouer, S. (2002b). Learning to perceive speech: How fricative perception changes and how it stays the same. *Journal of the Acoustical Society of America, 112*(2), 711–719.

Nittrouer, S. (2006). Children hear the forest. *Journal of the Acoustical Society of America, 120*(4), 1799–1802.

Nygaard, L. C., Sommers, M. S., & Pisoni, D. B. (1994). Speech perception as a talker-contingent process. *Psychological Science, 5*(1), 42–46.

O'Grady, W., & Dobrovolsky, M. (1997). *Contemporary linguistics* (3rd ed.). New York, NY: St. Martin's Press.

Ohala, J. J. (1999). The relation between phonetics and phonology. In W. J. Hardcastle & J. Laver (Eds.), *The handbook of the phonetic sciences*. Hoboken, NJ: Blackwell. Blackwell Reference Online. Retrieved July 13, 2009, from http://www.blackwellreference.com/subscriber/tocnode?id=g9780631214786_chunk_g978063121478622.

Ohberg, A. (2006). *Articulatory, perceptual, and phonological determinants of accurate production of /s/.* Unpublished master's thesis, McGill University, Montreal, Quebec.

Peng, S. C., Lu, N., & Chatterjee, M. (2009). Effects of cooperating and conflicting cues on speech intonation recognition by cochlear implant users and normal hearing listeners. *Audiology and Neurotology, 14*(5), 327–337.

Pierrehumbert, J. (2003a). Phonetic diversity, statistical learning, and acquisition of phonology. *Language and Speech, 46*, 115–154.

Pierrehumbert, J. (2003b). Probabilistic phonology: Discrimation and robustness. In R. Bod, J. Hay, & S. Jannedy (Eds.), *Probability theory in linguistics* (pp. 177–228). Cambridge, MA: MIT Press.

Pulvermüller, F., Huss, M., Kherif, F., del Prado Martin, F., Hauk, O., & Shtyrov, Y. (2006). Motor cortex maps articulatory features of speech sounds. *Proceedings of the National Academy of Sciences, 103*, 7865–7870.

Remez, R. E., Rubin, P. E., Pisoni, D. B., & Carrell, T. D. (1981). Speech perception without traditional speech cues. *Science, 212*, 947–949.

Repp, B. H. (1982). Phonetic trading relations and context effects: New experimental evidence for a speech mode of perception. *Psychological Bulletin, 92*, 81–110.

Richtsmeier, P. T., Gerken, L., Goffman, L., & Hogan, T. (2009). Statistical frequency in perception affects children's lexical production. *Cognition, 111*, 372–377.

Rvachew, S., Alhaidary, A., Mattock, K., & Polka, L. (2008). Emergence of the corner vowels in the babble produced by infants exposed to Canadian English or Canadian French. *Journal of Phonetics, 36*, 564–577.

Rvachew, S., & Andrews, E. (2002). The influence of syllable position on children's production of consonants. *Clinical Linguistics and Phonetics, 16*(3), 183–198.

Rvachew, S., Mattock, K., Polka, L., & Menard, L. (2006). Developmental and cross-linguistic variation in the infant vowel space: The case of Canadian English and Canadian French. *Journal of the Acoustical Society of America, 120*(4), 2250–259.

Sadagopan, N., & Smith, A. (2008). Developmental changes in the effects of utterance length and complexity on speech movement variability. *Journal of Speech, Language and Hearing Research, 51*, 1138–1151.

Schmidt, A. M. (2007). Evaluating a new clinical palatometry system. *Advances in Speech-Language Pathology, 9*, 73–81.

Shannon, R. V., Zeng, F.-G., Kamath, V., Wygonski, J., & Ekelid, M. (1995). Speech recognition with primarily temporal clues. *Science, 270*(5234), 303–304.

Shattuck-Hufnagel, S., & Turk, A. E. (1996). A prosody tutorial for investigators of auditory sentence processing. *Journal of Psycholinguistic Research, 25*, 193–247.

Shriberg, L. D., & Kent, R. D. (2003). *Clinical phonetics* (3rd ed.). Boston, MA: Allyn and Bacon.

Shriberg, L. D., & Kwiatkowski, J. (1980). *Natural Process Analysis: A procedure for phonological analysis of continuous speech samples*. New York, NY: MacMillan.

Singh, S., & Becker, G. M. (1972). A comparison of four feature systems using data from three psychophysical methods. *Journal of Speech and Hearing Research, 15*, 821–830.

Stevens, K. N., & Blumstein, S. E. (1978). Invariant cues for place of articulation in stop consonants. *Journal of the Acoustical Society of America, 64*(5), 1358–1368.

Stevens, K. N., & Keyser, S. J. (2009). Quantal theory, enhancement and overlap. *Journal of Phonetics*. doi:10.1016/j.wocn.2008.1010.1004.

Stevens, S. S., Volkmann, E. B., & Newman, J. (1937). The mel scale equates the magnitude of perceived differences in pitch at different frequencies. *Journal of the Acoustical Society of America, 8*, 185.

Stoel-Gammon, C. (1985). Phonetic inventories, 15–24 months: A longitudinal study. *Journal of Speech and Hearing Research, 28*, 505–512.

Studdert-Kennedy, M. (2002). Mirror neurons, vocal imitations, and the evolution of particulate speech. In I. M. S. V. Gallese (Ed.), *Mirror neurons and the evolution of brain and language: Advances in consciousness research* (Vol. 42, pp. 207–227). Amsterdam, Netherlands: John Benjamin.

Syrdal, A. K., & Gopal, H. (1986). A perceptual model of vowel recognition based on the auditory representation of American English vowels. *Journal of the Acoustical Society of America, 79*, 1086–1100.

Tyler, A. A., Edwards, M. L., & Saxman, J. H. (1990). Acoustic validation of phonological knowledge and its relationship to treatment. *Journal of Speech and Hearing Disorders, 55*, 251–798.

Vorperian, H. K., & Kent, R. D. (2007). Vowel acoustic space development in children: A synthesis of acoustic and anatomic data. *Journal of Speech, Language, and Hearing Research, 50*, 1510–1545.

Waldman, F. R., Singh, S., & Hayden, M. E. (1978). A comparison of speech-sound production and discrimination in children with functional articulation disorders. *Language and Speech, 21*, 205–230.

Westbury, J. R., Hashi, M., & Lindstrom, M. J. (1998). Difference among speakers in lingual articulation for American English /ɹ/. *Speech Communication, 26*, 203–226.

Chapter 2

Speech Perception Development

Assessment of Speech Perception Skills in Infancy

2.1.1. Describe two behavioral assessment methods for use during infancy, specifically habituation procedures and the visually reinforced head-turn procedure and indicate the advantages and disadvantages of each approach to determining the infant's speech perception abilities.

2.1.2. Describe the basic characteristics of an ERP experiment designed to investigate the infant's brain responses to a change in stimulus.

2.1.3. Describe the typical outcome of an fMRI experiment.

It is still common to refer to infancy as the "prelinguistic period" despite many decades of research that firmly roots the beginnings of phonological knowledge in the development of the infant's ability to perceive language-specific phonological units during the first year of life. Our understanding of the profound implications of infant speech perception development for language acquisition dates to the seminal study by Eimas, Siqueland, Jusczyk, and Vigorito (1971) in which it was shown that 1- and 4-month-old infants perceive the VOT contrast [b] versus [p] in a categorical fashion. At the time, the results of this and similar studies were interpreted within the framework of a "detector model" in which phonetic elements were identified via species-specific innate feature detectors; it was believed that exposure to specific phonetic input enhanced the sensitivity of these detectors and that lack of such experience within a critical period resulted in a loss of sensitivity (Eimas, 1975). This model of the speech perception process has since been proven

Peter D. Eimas (1934–2005) conducted ground breaking studies using the high-amplitude sucking technique to demonstrate categorical perception of speech sound contrasts in infants as young as one month of age.

to be untenable; however, the remarkable abilities demonstrated by infants continue to fascinate and the method used to assess the infants' speech perception abilities has stood the test of time.

The **high-amplitude sucking procedure** is one of many procedures for detecting discrimination responses in groups of infants that involve habituating the infant to one stimulus before introducing a contrasting stimulus.

Eimas et al. (1971) used the high-amplitude sucking procedure, a technique that continues to be in common use for testing speech perception in the youngest infants. With this procedure, specific speech input is provided to the infant contingent on a criterion rate of nonnutritative sucking resulting in an initial increase in the infant's sucking rate followed by a decline as the infant habituates to the stimulus; subsequent to habituation, a new stimulus is introduced and an increase in the infant's sucking rate is interpreted as evidence that the infant discriminates the new stimulus from the initial input. A related procedure, the visual habituation task, in which the auditory input is provided contingent upon the infant's looking at a visually interesting pattern, is used with older infants. A variation on this procedure, the sequential preferential looking task, provides an index of the infant's preference for listening to one or another stimulus. All habituation procedures provide evidence of discrimination for groups of infants, however, as the rates of sucking (or looking) are compared for groups of infants who experienced a change in stimulus relative to a group of infants who experienced no change after the habituation criterion was reached. A large body of literature on speech discrimination during the latter half of the first year has involved the visually reinforced head-turn procedure, in which the infant receives visual reinforcement for turning to look at the reinforcement display when the sound input changes from one phonetic category to another. An advantage of this procedure is that multiple trials can be administered to an individual infant and thus the researcher can determine whether each individual infant in the study was able to discriminate the test contrast. The use of these behavioral measures has provided a detailed picture of the course of speech perception development during the first years of life (Polka, Jusczyk, & Rvachew, 1995; Polka, Rvachew, & Mattock, 2007).

With the **visually reinforced head-turn procedure**, the infant receives visual reinforcement for turning to look at the reinforcement display when the sound input changes from one phonetic category to another.

As attention has turned to understanding the mechanisms that underlie the development of speech perception during infancy, neurophysiological techniques have become prominent in this field of research. The recording of event-related potentials (ERPs) is particularly common due to the relative ease of application of this procedure with infants and young children (Cheour, Korpilahti, Martynova, & Lang, 2001; Dehaene-Lambertz & Gliga, 2004; Mills & Neville, 1997). ERPs are patterns of electrical activity, measured from the brain through the skull and scalp, in response to a specific event, which in this context is carefully controlled speech input. ERPs can be elicited by unattended stimuli, and thus the technique does not require the attention and cooperation required by behavioral assessment methods. Brain activity is recorded at frequencies that reflect both sensory and cognitive processing of the auditory input.

Event-related potentials (ERPs) are patterns of electrical activity, measured from the brain through the skull and scalp, in response to a specific event such as carefully controlled speech input. Brain activity is recorded at frequencies that reflect both sensory and cognitive processing of the auditory input.

Electrophysiological studies of speech perception often exploit a particular pattern of brain activity called the mismatch negativity (MMN) which reflects the suppression of neuronal response to a repeated stimulus followed by renewed activity caused by the response of other neurons when a change in stimulus is introduced, as shown in Plate 4. This experimental design is referred to as the oddball paradigm; typically the repeated stimulus is called the standard whereas the infrequently presented stimulus is termed the deviant. The standard stimuli do not have to be acoustically identical; indeed, it is by observing the degree of suppression that is induced when similarities and differences among the standards are varied at acoustic, phonetic, phonemic, prosodic, or indexical levels that the researcher can trace the emergence of perceptual representations in the developing brain.

Another noninvasive procedure for studying the neurophysiology of speech perception is functional magnetic resonance imaging (fMRI) which measures changes in blood flow related to neural activity. This procedure is more commonly used with adults but studies with infants and young children are appearing with increasing frequency in the literature (Dehaene-Lambertz, 2004). Typical experimental paradigms involve alternating a rest phase or control condition with the experimental condition in which the stimulus of interest is presented either for passive listening or active response on the part of the participant. In contrast to ERPs, fMRI has poor temporal resolution but good spatial resolution which permits identification of brain regions that contribute to the cognitive processes engaged by the stimuli and tasks presented during the course of the experiment. Subsequent to data processing, brain maps are produced that show regions of the brain in which changes in blood flow were statistically correlated with the pattern of stimulus presentations during the experiment.

Functional magnetic resonance imaging (fMRI) measures changes in blood flow related to neural activity, permitting identification of brain regions that contribute to the cognitive processes engaged by the stimuli and tasks presented during the course of the experiment.

In this chapter, speech perception development is described as illuminated by behavioral and neurophysiological studies. The development of speech perception skills for phonetic, prosodic, and phonemic elements are described first for the infant period. A review of changes in speech perception during late and middle childhood follows. In the third and final section of the chapter, factors that contribute to the course of speech perception development are discussed, including environmental influences, biological constraints, and learning mechanisms.

Speech Perception Development in Infancy

2.2.1. Describe two important transitions in speech perception development that occur during the infant period.

2.2.2. Initially, the remarkable speech perception abilities of the neonate were taken as evidence of innate feature detectors for the perception of phonemes with the role of the input being restricted to maintenance of language-specific categories. Identify and describe six types of research evidence that invalidate the feature detector model and support the view that the child is actively learning language-specific phonetic categories from the input.

2.2.3. Interpret toddler mispronunciation detection performance as shown in Figure 2–10, in relation to the outcome of the habituation experiments summarized in Table 2–1.

Phonetic Perception in Early Infancy

Infants demonstrate **language-general phonetic perception** during the first 6 months of life, as they are able to discriminate a wide range of phonetic contrasts, including those that are used in the infant's ambient language environment and those that are not.

During the first 6 months of life, infants are able to discriminate a wide range of phonetic contrasts, including those that are used in the infant's ambient language environment and those that are not. Behavioral studies have revealed discrimination of both prevoiced and long lag voicing contrasts among stop consonants (Eimas et al., 1971; Streeter, 1976). Manner distinctions have been discriminated successfully by infants in this age range when presented with stops versus glides (Hillenbrand, Minifie, & Edwards, 1979), stops versus nasals, affricates versus fricatives, (Tsao, Liu, & Kuhl, 2006) and [ɹ] versus [l] within the liquid class (Eimas, 1975). Sensitivity to place of articulation has been observed for stops (Jusczyk & Thompson, 1978; Moffitt, 1971), glides (Eimas & Miller, 1980; Jusczyk, Copan, & Thompson, 1978), and fricatives (Levitt, Jusczyk, Murray, & Carden, 1988). Very young infants are able to discriminate oral vowel contrasts as well as contrasts between nasal and oral vowels (Trehub, 1973, 1976). Most of this research has involved the presentation of single CV syllables but some studies have demonstrated the perception of stop consonants in the initial and medial position of two syllable nonsense words (Jusczyk & Thompson, 1978), in the coda position of CVC syllables and in complex onsets, specifically [sta] versus [ska] (Eimas & Miller, 1991). However, young infants failed to discriminate stop consonants embedded in the 3-syllable nonsense words [atapa] versus [ataba] (Trehub, 1974).

ERP studies have confirmed **categorical perception** of phonetic contrasts in early infancy.

ERP studies have confirmed categorical perception of phonetic contrasts in early infancy. Dehaene-Lambert and Baillet (1998) presented 3-month-old infants with three types of trials consisting of repeated sequences of four stimuli from a voiced place-of-articulation continuum ([ba] vs. [da]): during control trials the four stimuli were identical; during within-category trials the fourth stimulus was acoustically different from the preceding three but within the same phonetic category; during across-category trials the fourth stimulus was both acoustically and phonetically different from the preceding three stimuli with the acoustic difference equal in magnitude to that presented in within-category trials. The mismatch response was larger for across-category trials than for within-category trials; furthermore, the topography of the brain activation pattern was distinct for the processing of phonetic differences relative to that observed for the processing of acoustic differences. The authors concluded that 3-month-old infants already possess a dedicated neuronal network for phonetic processing that involves the temporal cortices.

The visually reinforced head-turn paradigm has been used to explore equivalence classification by infants in the 6 to 9 months age range, providing evidence that infants can attend to phonetic categories while ignoring variation in irrelevant parameters. Hillenbrand (1984) trained infants to respond to a change from [ma] to [na] produced by a single male talker, and then introduced new stimuli with changes in vowel and talker in successive stages of the experiment so that the infants learned to categorize [ma, mi, mu] versus [na, ni, nu]. Hillenbrand (1983) used the same procedure to teach infants to categorize CV syllables on the basis of nasal [m, n, ŋ] or oral [b, d, g] onset. Kuhl (1979) found that infants could discriminate vowel categories despite irrelevant variation in pitch contours and talkers. Neonates, within days of birth, have demonstrated discrimination of [pa]—[ta] stimuli despite irrelevant talker variation as indexed by MMN responses in an ERP study (Dehaene-Lambertz & Pena, 2001).

Equivalence classification by 6- to 9-month-old infants shows that infants of this age can attend to phonetic categories while ignoring irrelevant parameters.

These reports of remarkable speech perception performance by neonates have been used to support a view of phonology whereby knowledge of all possible phoneme contrasts is innately given and the linguistic environment serves to select from a finite pool of discrete categories. This theoretical perspective has led clinicians to discount the role of individual differences in speech perception learning as a causal factor in phonological disorders. Consequently, speech perception interventions fell into disfavor in the latter half of the 20th century. This is a misleading interpretation of the infants' performance in these experiments however.

The first misconception is that the infant has knowledge of discrete phonetic categories. In fact, speech perception is influenced by fine-grained acoustic details and the way that those acoustic details are distributed within and between phonetic categories. For example, variations in perceptual salience play a role in the perception of contrasts within the vowel class. Polka and Bohn (2003) described robust and predictable perceptual asymmetries in the discrimination of vowel contrasts that is evident in both infants and adults. Recall that the visually reinforced head-turn procedure involves presenting the infants with a stream of stimuli from one phone category (the background or standard stimulus) and reinforcing the infant for responding to a change to a new phone category (the foreground or target stimulus) during test trials. An infant is judged to have succeeded at the task if a criterion proportion of correct responses is observed, counting both anticipatory looking at the reinforcement box during change trials and refraining from responding during no-change trials. For almost every vowel contrast tested, infants were more likely to respond to changes in one

The now-discredited **feature detection model** of speech perception suggested that the infant perceives discrete phonetic categories at birth. In fact, speech perception is influenced by fine-grained acoustic details and the way that those acoustic details are distributed within and between phonetic categories.

direction than the other. For example, when 6-month-old English-learning infants were presented with [y] as the background vowel, over 75% responded to a change to [u] (with the [y]—[u] vowel tokens representing a German vowel contrast); in contrast, virtually no English-learning infants of the same age succeeded at the task when [u] was the background stimulus and [y] was the target (Polka & Werker, 1994). Further research with the sequential preferential listening procedure showed that 4-month-old infants' listening preferences parallel directional asymmetries for speech discrimination. Young infants preferred to listen to [u] in contrast to [y], regardless of whether their home environment exposed them to French, a language in which [y] is phonemic, or English, which does not include [y] in the phonemic inventory. Altogether, the directional asymmetries across a range of studies reveal the special status of vowels that are on the periphery of the vowel space as opposed to the interior of the vowel space, as plotted in F1-F2 acoustic parameter space (Figure 2–1). Polka and Bohn (2011) propose that the peripheral vowels [i], [u], and [a] are "natural referent vowels [that] support and guide the development of vowel perception by attracting infant attention and providing stable perceptual forms for the language

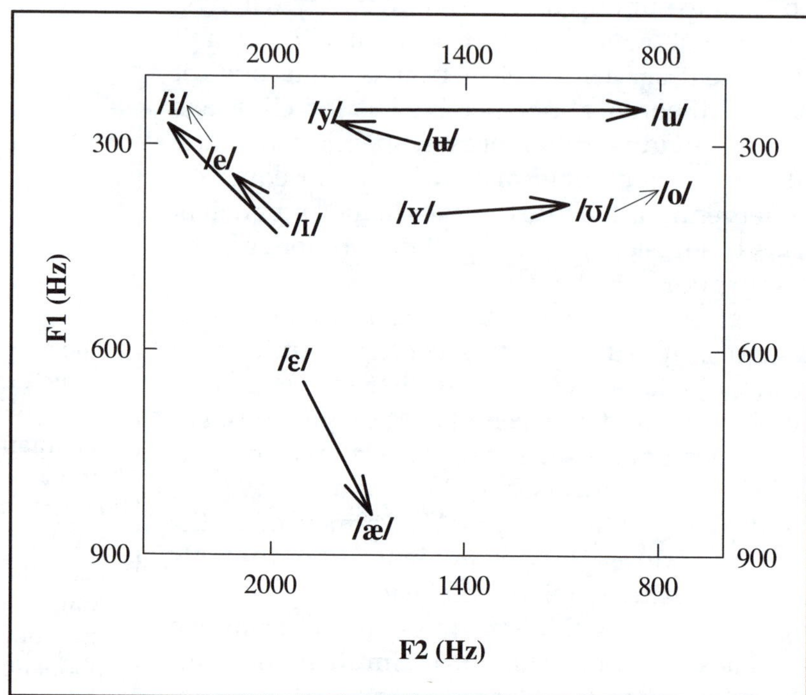

Figure 2–1. *Plot of F1/F2 frequencies for contrasts showing asymmetries in infant vowel discrimination. Arrows point to the reference vowels for the contrast; vowel changes in this direction were easier to discriminate. Formant frequency values are approximate. From Polka and Bohn (2003). Asymmetries in vowel perception.* Speech Communication, 41, *Figure 1a, p. 223. Reproduced with permission of Elsevier BV.*

learner" (p. 474). These vowels are characterized by extreme degrees of formant convergence relative to other vowels that enhances perceptual salience and facilitates talker normalization. The natural referent vowels provide the infant with a universal minimal vowel set that can be used as anchor points for the discovery of other vowels in the native language inventory. Note that these vowels are "natural" not because they are innately given phonetic categories but because of the perceptual salience of their acoustic characteristics. Knowledge of these anchor vowels facilitates the perceptual learning of the other vowels in the learner's vowel system. Research with infants learning one language and with infants learning multiple languages simultaneously provides further evidence that perceptual development involves active learning from the acoustic-phonetic input rather than a passive process of selecting from innately given categories (Mattock, Polka, Rvachew, & Krehm, 2010; McMurray & Aslin, 2005; McMurray, Tanenhaus, & Aslin, 2002). In fact, infants' sensitivity to within-category acoustic variation helps them to discover phonetic categories from the input. We discuss the powerful statistical learning mechanism that underlies this developmental process later in this chapter.

The **natural referent vowels** [i], [u], and [a] provide the infant with a universal minimal vowel set that can be used as anchor points for the discovery of other vowels in the native language inventory. Note that these vowels are "natural" not because they are innately given phonetic categories but because of the perceptual salience of their acoustic characteristics.

Although infants have been observed to discriminate many native and nonnative phonetic contrasts it is not true that they can perceive any potential contrast from all the world's languages. Lasky, Syrdal-Lasky, and Klein (1975) assessed perception of voicing contrasts by 4- to 6-month-old infants living in monolingual Spanish-speaking environments. Three voicing contrasts were targeted in bilabial stop + [a] syllables: –60 versus –20 ms VOT, which is phonemic in Thai but not Spanish or English; –20 versus +20 ms VOT which is phonemic in Thai and Spanish but not English; and +20 versus +60 ms VOT which is phonemic in English but not Thai or Spanish. Spanish-learning infants discriminated stimuli that crossed the Thai boundary (–20 vs. –60 ms), and the English boundary (+20 vs. +60 ms); they were unable to discriminate stimuli that crossed the Spanish boundary (–20 vs. +20 ms), however. The authors conclude that this result is inconsistent with Eimas' (1975) hypothesis of innate feature detectors since this view of perceptual development posits that specific input is required to maintain perception of native language contrasts whereas a mechanism to explain the induction of the ability to perceive a native language contrast is required in the case of Spanish.

Although infants have been observed to discriminate many native and nonnative phonetic contrasts it is not true that they can perceive any potential contrast from all the world's languages. Certain **voicing contrasts** are difficult for infants to perceive, for example.

A further challenge to the notion of feature detectors came from Eilers and Minifie's (1975) finding that 4-month-old infants were unable to perceive the [sa] versus [za] contrast although other infants of the same age discriminated [sa] versus [va] and [sa] versus [ʃa] (Figure 2–2). These researchers suggested that infant perception of VOT in stop consonants is accomplished by attending to the F1 cutback cue rather than VOT itself. Levitt et al. (1988) showed that 2-month-old infants can discriminate CV syllables on the basis of formant frequency transitions appropriate to [fa] and [θa] even if the fricative noise portion of the syllables is spectrally identical.

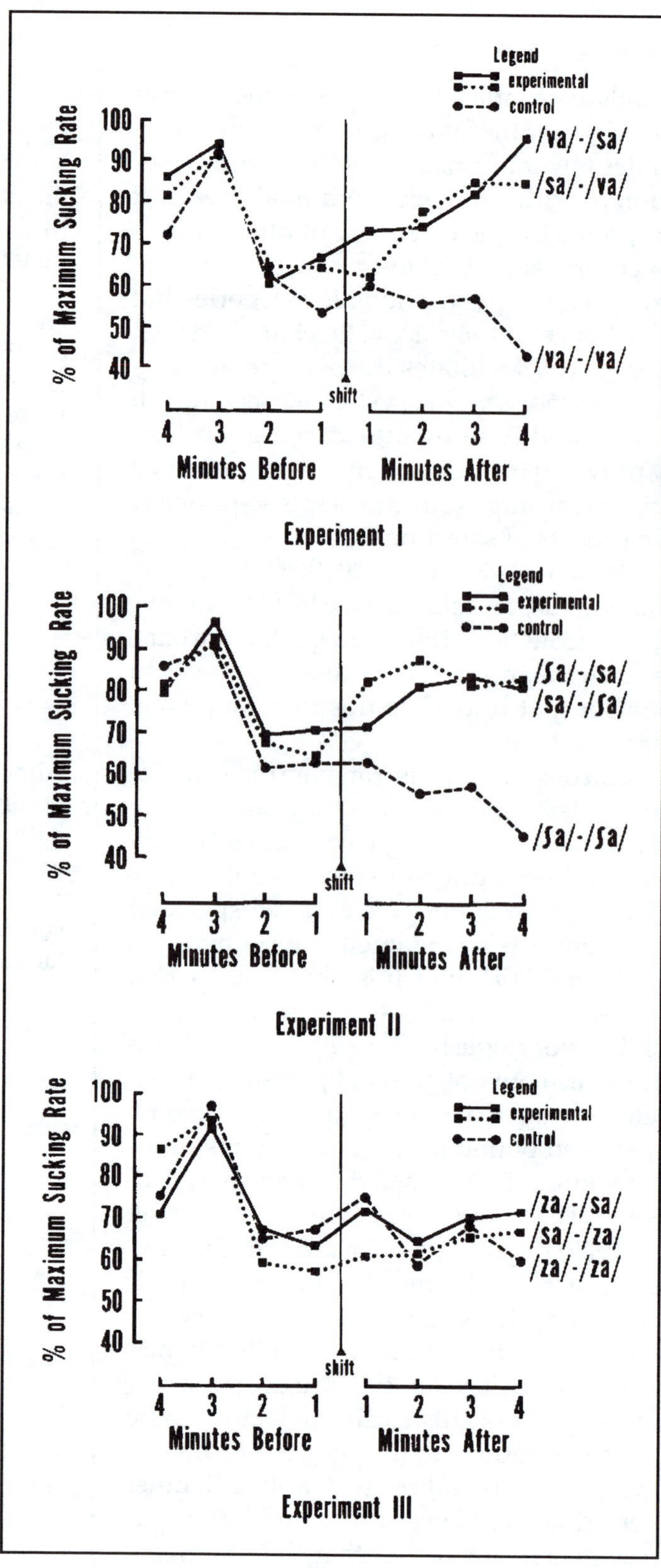

Figure 2–2. *Mean sucking rates expressed as a percentage of the maximum prehabituation sucking level for four minutes before and four minutes after the sound change in the experimental conditions compared to no sound change in the control condition. From Eilers and Minifie (1975). Fricative discrimination in early infancy.* Journal of Speech, Language, and Hearing Research, *Figure 1 (Experiment I, p. 163), Figure 2 (Experiment II, p. 164), and Figure 3 (Experiment III, p. 165). Reprinted by permission of the American Speech-Hearing-Language Association.*

Nittrouer (2001) attempted to determine if infants place greater weight on formant transition cues than spectral or temporal cues at the syllable onset when discriminating fricative place and stop VOT contrasts. She was unable to answer the question because infant performance with unmodified natural speech recordings of syllables such as [su] versus [ʃu] and [tɑ] versus [dɑ] was so unreliable, in a study employing the visually reinforced head-turn procedure with 6- to 14-month-old infants. Although 65% of the infants succeeded with a vowel contrast (e.g., [sɑ] versus [su]) fewer than half the infants met criterion for discrimination of the fricative or the VOT contrast. Nittrouer reminds us that, in studies employing the high amplitude sucking procedure or the visually reinforced head-turn procedure, it is common for half the infants tested to fail the procedure due to "fussiness." The data from these infants are routinely discarded under the assumption that the infants would have performed just like the successful infants if they had not been feeling fussy on the day of testing.[1] However, Nittrouer tested the same infants on multiple contrasts over multiple occasions and was able to show that infant performance was systematically associated with specific contrasts rather than being determined by random factors. She concluded that the results challenge the hypothesis of innate phonetic categories. Certainly the results reveal variable performance across phonetic categories and individual differences across infants that may have implications for later phonological development.

Individual differences in infant perceptual performance may also have implications for the identification of different sub-types of developmental phonological disorders and the underlying causal factors. Dyslexia is a neurodevelopmental reading disability that has genetic correlates that overlap with developmental phonological disorders as discussed further in Chapter 7. The MMN procedure has been used to study responses to a short versus long vowel contrast that is phonemic in Finnish (specifically, "ka" vs. "kaa" syllables). In these studies infants who were at-risk for reading disability due to family history of dyslexia were compared to infants with no genetic risk for dyslexia. MMN responses to these syllables were significantly different in newborns and 6-month-old infants when the stimuli were presented at a slow rate (Leppanen, Pihko, Eklund, & Lyytinen, 1999; Pihko, 1999).

Individual differences in perceptual performance may have implications for later phonological development. Some neurodevelopmental disorders such as **dyslexia** are associated with speech perception deficits in infancy.

To summarize, certain perceptual abilities appear to be in place early in infancy independent of specific language input. At least some infants are capable of discriminating a wide variety of phonetic contrasts even when the contrasts tested are not phonemic in the language that the infant is hearing in the ambient input. ERP studies confirm that perception of these contrasts is categorical in nature. Behavioral and ERP studies show that infants are capable

[1]Exclusion rates for electrophysiological studies of infant speech perception ability are similarly high.

of equivalence classification of highly variable stimuli that share a common phone or feature. Phonetic perception in early infancy is not entirely unconstrained, however. The corner vowels [i], [u], and [a] are particularly salient to infants and appear to act as natural referent vowels in vowel perception tasks. Certain contrasts appear to be easier to perceive than others, such as the long lag voicing contrast in comparison to the short lag voicing contrast, or vowel contrasts in comparison to fricative contrasts. Individual differences in perceptual performance are observed even for easy contrasts, however, and when infants are successful with the perception of a contrast it is likely that they are not integrating across the same acoustic cues as adult listeners. Learning a language-specific strategy for perceiving speech is a gradual process that involves the mapping of distributions of continuous acoustic parameters to discrete phonetic categories. An important part of this process is achieved before the end of the first year of life as discussed next.

Environmental Influences on Phonetic Perception in Infancy

A gradual shift from language-general to **language-specific phonetic perception** occurs between 6 and 12 months of age.

Early evidence of a **shift to language-specific perceptual processing** of language input is a progressive decline in sensitivity to nonnative vowels beginning around 6 months of age. Declining sensitivity to nonnative consonants occurs toward the end of the first year.

In the previous section, cross-linguistic studies of very young infants revealed universal aspects of early speech perception abilities. Cross-linguistic studies also reveal the influence of the language environment on infant speech perception, with a gradual shift from language-general to language-specific perception occurring for the phonetic aspects of speech between 6- and 12-months of age. The most dramatic and frequently reported change during the second half of the first year is a loss of sensitivity to nonnative phonetic contrasts.

Early evidence of a shift to language specific perceptual processing of language input is a progressive decline in sensitivity to nonnative vowels with 6-month-old infants typically being unable to discriminate nonnative vowel contrasts. This has been shown for perception of a German vowel contrast [y]-[u] by German- and Canadian English-learning infants (Polka & Werker, 1994), for a Catalan contrast [e]-[ɛ] by Spanish- and Catalan-learning infants (Bosch & Sebastián-Gallés, 2003), and for a Swedish contrast [y]-[i] by Swedish and American English-learning infants (Kuhl, Williams, Lacerda, Stevens, & Lindblom, 1992). Kuhl et al. observed a "perceptual magnet effect" for the perception of native-language vowels in their study: infant responses suggested that the perceptual distance between the prototype of a native language vowel category and acoustically similar variants was less than the perceptual distance between the prototype of a nonnative vowel and acoustically similar variants despite constant acoustic distances in the native and nonnative test conditions. The shift to language-specific perception occurs at a later age for consonants than for vowels. In a series of studies involving both cross-sectional and longitudinal designs, Werker and colleagues (Werker, Gilbert, Humphrey,

& Tees, 1981; Werker & Lalonde, 1988; Werker & Tees, 1983, 1984) demonstrated that discrimination of two nonnative consonant contrasts by English-learning infants declined to negligible levels by approximately 10 months of age (specifically, the Hindi retroflex versus dental alveolar stop contrast and the Salish uvular versus velar fricative contrast), whereas infants learning these languages perceived these contrasts without difficulty when tested between 10 and 12 months of age.

Maintenance of native-language contrasts is not the only process that has been observed during infancy. Learning of voicing contrasts involves a more complex process in languages such as Spanish and French where the boundary between voiced and voiceless stops is approximately 0 ms VOT. Recall that Lasky et al. (1975) found that 4- to 6-month-old Spanish-learning infants discriminated the English long lag voicing contrast rather than the Spanish short lag voicing contrast. Eilers, Gavin, and Wilson (1979) found that 6- to 8-month-old Spanish-learning infants discriminated both the Spanish and the English voicing contrast. A similar developmental pattern was observed for French-learning infants in a study in which deceleration in heartbeat upon presentation of a category change was taken as evidence of discrimination (Hoonhorst et al., 2009). As shown in Figure 2–3, the 4-month-old infants responded to stimulus pairs that crossed boundaries at −30 ms and +30 ms VOT whereas 8-month-old infants were responsive to the stimulus

For some phonetic categories, environmental input results in **shifts in the perceptual category boundary to a language-specific location**. For example, French- and Spanish-learning infants shift perceptual sensitivity from the long lag to the short lag voicing contrast.

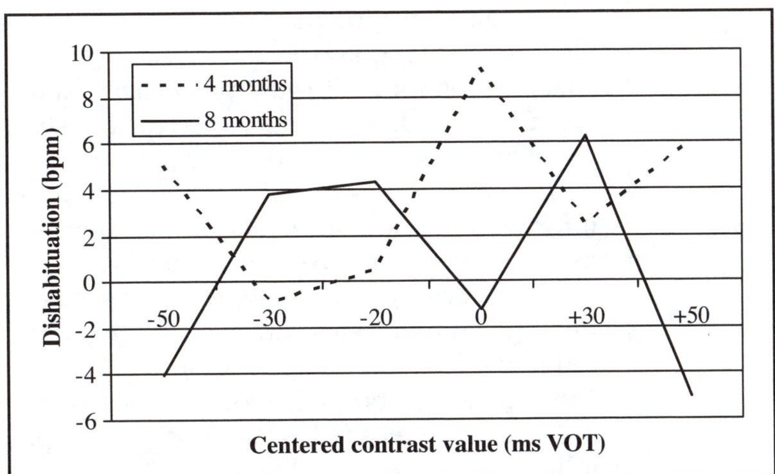

Figure 2–3. *Dishabituation scores (expressed in heart beats per minute) for French-learning infants listening to six pairs of stimuli that differed by 20 ms VOT centered on −50, −30, −20, 0, +30, and +50 ms VOT. The 4-month-olds show dishabituation peaks at the language-general boundaries of -30 and +30 ms VOT. The 8-month-olds show a peak at the French-language boundary of 0 ms VOT. Reprinted from* Journal of Experimental Child Psychology, 104, *Hoonhorst et al., French native speakers in the making: From language-general to language-specific voicing boundaries, Figure 4, p. 361, Copyright 2009, with permission from Elsevier.*

pair that crossed the boundary at 0 ms VOT. Therefore, in Spanish- and French-learning infants, the category boundary for voiced and voiceless stops shifts from approximately +30 ms to approximately 0 ms between 6 and 8 months of age.

Language experience also results in **facilitation of perceptual performance** with heightened sensitivity to native language phonetic contrasts.

Another process involving native-language contrasts is that of facilitation. Language-specific perception of liquids also emerges late in the first year, with Japanese-learning and English-learning infants both demonstrating discrimination of [ɹa] versus [la] at 6 months of age (Kuhl et al., 2006). Between 6 and 12 months, significant attenuation of discrimination was observed for Japanese infants while significant facilitation was observed for English-learning infants. Facilitation was also observed in a study of affricate versus fricative perception by Mandarin- and English-learning infants. Mandarin and English both contrast an affricate with a fricative but at slightly different places of articulation (palatal, [tɕ^{h}] vs. [ɕ], in Mandarin; postalveolar, [tʃ] vs. [ʃ], in English). Both contrasts are cued by differences in rise time and fricative duration. Adult speakers of English and Mandarin can discriminate both contrasts but achieve better performance with the native contrast suggesting that the cues are weighted differently across the two languages. Mandarin and English learning infants were able to discriminate the Mandarin contrast at 7 and at 11 months of age but performance improved with age for the Mandarin group and declined with age for the English group. In contrast, performance improved with age for perception of the English contrast by English-learning infants. This study highlights the point that perceptual learning in infancy is not just about the placement of boundaries between phone categories. The language-learner must also learn the precise acoustic specification for the prototype of each phonetic category.

Other studies have explored the questions of what kind of language input is required to shape perception of a given phonetic contrast. These studies reveal that exposure to the underlying acoustic information is not sufficient to maintain phonetic perception. For example, Pegg and Werker (1997) investigated discrimination by English-learning infants of voiceless aspirated [t^{h}], voiced unaspirated [d̥], and voiceless unaspirated [t$^{=}$] in CV syllables. In English, [t^{h}] is the long lag allophone of /t/ that occurs in words such as "top," [d̥] is the short lag allophone of /d/ that occurs in words such as "dog," whereas [t$^{=}$] is the short lag allophone of /t/ that occurs following /s/ in words such as "stop." The naturally recorded exemplars of [d̥a] and [t$^{=}$a] had similar VOT (approximately 6 ms) but [t$^{=}$a] had a lower starting frequency for the second formant transition; [t^{h}a] began with longer VOT (over 20 ms) than the other two phones but had a lower starting frequency for the second formant transition, similar to [t$^{=}$a]. They found that 6- to 8-month-old infants were able to discriminate the subtle difference between [t$^{=}$a] and [d̥a], whereas 10- to 12-month-old English-learning infants were not when tested with the visually reinforced head-turn procedure. Both younger and older infants could discriminate [t^{h}a] from [d̥a] however. This study demonstrates that passive exposure to relevant acoustic input is insufficient to maintain discrimination of a phonetic contrast. Indeed, the study calls into question the notion of maintenance as an explanation for infant perception of native-language contrasts. Rather, one sees a strategic shift in perceptual sensitivity: younger infants attend to differences based on acoustic differences alone whereas older infants attend to differences that reflect the distribution of acoustic cues in the input.

Passive exposure to relevant acoustic cues is insufficient to maintain **discrimination of a phonetic contrast**. Younger infants attend to differences based on acoustic differences alone whereas older infants attend to differences that reflect the distribution of acoustic cues in the input.

Perhaps more surprising than the loss of sensitivity to phones that occur in the input is the finding of continued perception of some contrasts in the absence of phonetic input. For example, Best, McRoberts, and Sithole (1988) demonstrated that adults and 14-month-old infants from English-speaking backgrounds can discriminate Zulu click contrasts even though these sounds are not used phonemically or allophonically in English. They concluded that perception of these contrasts is maintained because the phones are not assimilated by the listener into any of the native language phonological categories. In contrast, perception of the Salish velar versus uvular ejective contrast is lost before 12 months of age because these phonemes are assimilated by the English listener into the voiceless velar stop category, albeit as unusual sounding exemplars of the English /k/ (Best, McRoberts, LaFleur, & Silver-Isenstadt, 1995). Therefore, changes in speech perception during the first year of life reflect linguistic processes in which the functional significance of the phonetic input plays a role in shaping speech perception development.

Increasingly, ERP procedures are being used to investigate the processes that underlie the apparent loss of perceptual ability for nonnative phonetic contrasts that occurs during the first year of life. Cheour et al. (1998) examined MMN responses in an oddball paradigm to two deviant vowels, [ö] and [õ], in relation to the standard vowel, [e]. The standard vowel is phonemic in both Finnish and Estonian as is the deviant [ö]; the second deviant [õ] is phonemic only in Estonian, however. The participants were Finish-learning infants tested at age 6 months and again at age 12 months and Estonian-learning infants tested once at 12 months of age. The results, illustrated in Figure 2–4, show that the MMN response at 6 months reflects the acoustic properties of the vowels: the Finnish infants show a larger MMN in response to [e] versus [õ] than [e] versus [ö] because the acoustic difference between the standard and the deviant is larger in the case of the Estonian contrast compared to the Finnish contrast. When retested at 12 months however, the Finnish infants show a MMN for the Finnish contrast that is larger than that observed for the Estonian contrast at 6 or 12 months of age. The Estonian infants tested at 12 months of age show the reverse pattern with a comparatively larger MMN for the Estonian contrast. This study demonstrates that, in parallel with changes in behavioral performance, linguistic input enhances MMN amplitude for native-language contrasts and attenuates MMN amplitude for

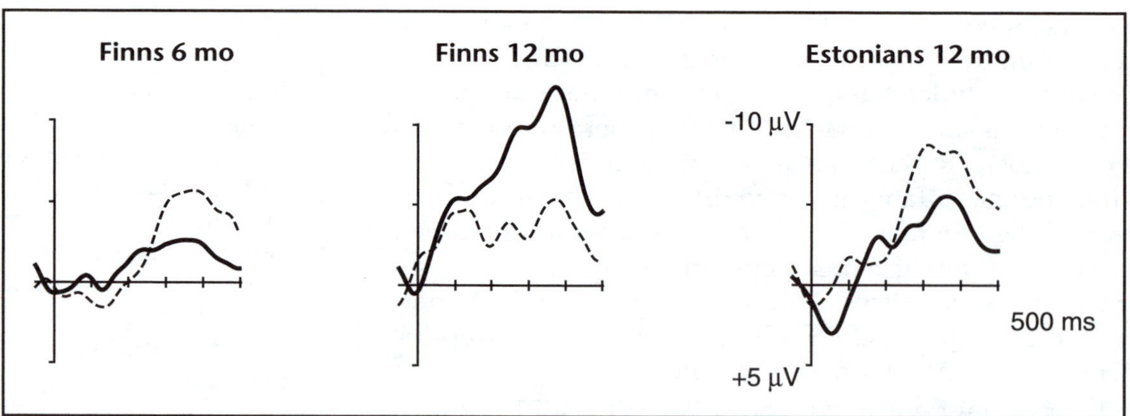

Figure 2–4. *MMN amplitude at the central Cz electrode, displayed as the grand-average, deviant-standard difference waveform, averaged across nine infants, for Finnish-learning infants aged 6 and 12 months and Estonian-learning infants aged 12 months. The solid line represents the difference in MMN amplitude for the standard [e]—deviant [ö], a vowel shared by Finnish and Estonian. The dashed line represents the difference in MMN amplitude for the standard [e]—deviant [õ], an Estonian vowel. From Cheour et al. (1998). Development of language-specific phoneme representation in the infant brain. Reprinted by permission from Macmillan Publishers Ltd:* Nature Neuroscience, 1, *Figure 2, p. 352, copyright 1998.*

ERP studies show that brain responses to nonnative phonetic contrasts are attenuated but not lost. Perceptual performance at younger ages reflects **acoustic differences between stimuli** whereas ERP responses later in infancy reflect linguistic differences in phonetic category membership.

nonnative contrasts. In contrast to behavioral studies, however, the neurophysiological evidence indicates that at some level discrimination of nonnative phonetic contrasts is retained throughout the first year, as evidenced by significant if attenuated MMN responses to nonnative contrasts for both younger and older infants. Perceptual performance at younger and older ages may reflect different aspects of the stimulus: the topography and amplitude of the MMN response early in life reflects acoustic differences between stimuli whereas changes in the topography and amplitude of the MMN response later in infancy reflect linguistic differences in phonetic category membership. A longitudinal ERP study of the emergence of the voicing contrast in English-learning infants confirms these developmental patterns for native and nonnative phones and reveals considerable individual differences among infants in the time course of the shift from language-general to language-specific processing (Rivera-Gaxiola, Silva-Pereyra, & Kuhl, 2005). These findings have implications for the assessment of children with speech and language disorders: clearly, it is not enough to know whether a child can discriminate a phoneme contrast on the basis of its acoustic characteristics; rather it is necessary to be sure that the child is aware of the functional significance of the contrast and can identify members of the two categories on the basis of language-specific acoustic cues.

Speech perception development has been described as an "innately guided learning process" (Jusczyk & Bertoncini, 1988). The process is innately guided in the sense that there are inherent constraints on the types of input that influence the learning of perceptual categories, with the special status of the peripheral vowels as natural referents for the learning of native-language vowel contrasts being one example. Clearly, the process also involves learning: the initial universalist view, whereby the phonetic categories were innately given at birth but that linguistic input was required to maintain perception of language-specific categories, is not tenable. The infant must learn language-specific strategies for weighting the acoustic cues that define the prototypes of the phonetic categories that exist in the native language and shift the category boundaries to language specific locations. Neurophysiological studies demonstrate that perception of acoustic differences between nonnative phones is never completely lost; rather, the infant appears to acquire a qualitatively new strategy for discriminating speech sounds that reflects the functional significance of any given phone in relation to other phones in the language being learned. These new studies that highlight the role of learning in the acquisition of language-specific speech perception in early life have important implications for the treatment of developmental phonological disorders. This new perspective raises the possibility that slow learning or mislearning of perceptual categories during the first year of life contributes to delayed speech development. These studies highlight the importance of the specific acoustic characteristics of the input to which the infant is exposed and provide guidance for the development of interventions to ensure that children acquire the perceptual knowledge that is the foundation of phonological development.

These studies have also shifted the attention of researchers to the study of the learning mechanisms that account for the infant's extraordinary perceptual learning in early life. Jusczyk and Bertoncini believed that speech is an especially salient signal for infants: in essence, infants arrive in the world prepared to listen to, remember and learn from speech input. They believed that the properties of speech that make it "special" are related to its rhythm or prosody. In the next section, infant perception of phonological units at prosodic levels of the phonological hierarchy are considered.

Perception of Prosodic Units in Infancy

The phonetic content of speech is delivered in the context of fluent connected speech which has a language-specific prosodic structure. Recall from Chapter 1 that prosody involves the manipulation of duration, pitch, and loudness cues to create variations in phrasal stress over the course of an utterance which, together with boundary cues, signal junctures between phonological words, phrases, and utterances. A significant amount of prosodic information reaches the infant even before birth since transmission of sound from the external environment to the fetus occurs in a nonlinear pattern with some intrauterine amplification of frequencies below 400 Hz, attenuation of frequencies between 400 and 12500 Hz and a gradual reversal of the attenuation for higher frequency sounds (Lecanuet et al., 1998).

A significant amount of **prosodic information** reaches the infant even before birth.

Shortly after birth, **infants prefer to listen to their native language** compared to a foreign language with different rhythmic qualities.

Shortly after birth, infants prefer to listen to their native language compared to a foreign language with different rhythmic qualities (Moon, Cooper, & Fifer, 1993; comparing English and Spanish). More recent research shows that fetal responses to novel language input can be obtained using heart rate measures, demonstrating that infants are learning about the ambient language prior to birth (Kisilevsky et al., 2009; comparing English and Mandarin). Further evidence of fetal learning comes from DeCasper and Spence (1986) who asked mothers to read a specific passage daily during the final 6 weeks of pregnancy. At birth the familiar passage was found to be more reinforcing to the infant, in comparison to a novel passage, even though both passages were read by a stranger. The role of prosody in the shaping of infant listening preferences was examined by Mehler et al. (1988) in a series of studies involving 2-day-old French-learning and 2-month-old English-learning infants. They found that newborns can discriminate their native language from a foreign language and demonstrated that this ability is based on the prosodic characteristics of the speech input because it is retained even after low-pass filtering of the stimuli which strips away the phonetic content while leaving the prosodic pattern of the language input intact.

In a subsequent series of studies Nazzi, Bertoncini, and Mehler (1998) directly assessed the hypothesis that newborn infants are sensitive to the rhythmic properties of language input by presenting infants with pairs of foreign language samples that systematically contrasted different rhythmic classes, low-pass filtered in every case. Sentences were recorded in Japanese (a mora-timed language), Italian and Spanish (syllable-timed languages), and Dutch and English (stress-timed languages). The rhythmic hypothesis was confirmed in that French-learning newborn infants were observed to discriminate foreign languages from different rhythmic classes but not from within the same rhythmic class. Research with 5-month-old infants revealed a similar pattern of language discrimination ability (Nazzi, Jusczyk, & Johnson, 2000). In this study, older infants retained the ability to discriminate two languages from different rhythmic classes. They were also able to discriminate languages from the same rhythmic class but only as long as one sample in the pair represented the native language.

Infant attention to the rhythmic qualities of the language input leads to the acquisition of language specific strategies for the segmentation of prosodic units such as phonological phrases and words from the language input. The **prosodic bootstrapping hypothesis** posits that the infant's access to these prosodic units facilitates acquisition of phonetic, lexical and syntactic knowledge.

Infant attention to the rhythmic qualities of the language input leads to the acquisition of language specific strategies for the segmentation of prosodic units such as phonological phrases and words from the language input. The prosodic bootstrapping hypothesis posits that the infant's access to these prosodic units facilitates acquisition of phonetic, lexical, and syntactic knowledge (Nazzi & Ramus, 2003). There is some evidence that infants learn to segment larger prosodic units earlier and then progress to smaller units within the prosodic hierarchy (Johnson & Seidl, 2008). Typical studies of clause segmentation present infants with the same phonetic and lexical content embedded in passages that vary the placement of clause boundaries. For example, Soderstrom, Nelson, and Jusczyk (2005) familiarized 6-month-old English learning infants with passages containing clause-coincident (e.g., "eat leafy") and clause-straddling (e.g., ("eat. Leafy") word sequences. The head-turn preference procedure revealed that infants preferred to listen to passages that contained familiar phrases spoken with the same prosodic contour that was presented during the familiarization phase indicating that they were sensitive to the clause boundary cues (long pause between the words, longer duration of the vowel in the word preceding the boundary, and a pitch peak on the word following the boundary). Johnson and Seidl (2008) found that Dutch-learning infants weighted pause duration more strongly than pitch changes in their detection of clause boundaries in this same task, reflecting their experience with the narrower pitch range of Dutch compared to English.

Investigations of infant perceptual sensitivity to smaller units indicates that a limited ability to discriminate stress patterns in prosodic words is available at birth (Ooijen, Bertoncini, Sansavini, & Mehler, 1997; Sansavini, Bertoncini, & Giovanelli, 1997). Phonetic complexity interacts with the prosodic characteristics of the speech input to determine infant performance, however. For example, 1-month-old infants can discriminate [maɹana] from [malana] if the middle syllable has exaggerated stress cues characteristic of infant-directed speech. The same phonetic sequence with equal stressed syllables or less exaggerated stress on the middle syllable cannot be discriminated by such young infants (Karzon, 1985). Similarly, a bias in listening preference for trochaic versus iambic stress patterns can be observed in infants learning stress-timed languages, but this bias is observed at earlier ages when the stimuli are phonetically simple (Höhle, Bijeljac-Babic, Herold, Weissenborn, & Nazzi, 2009) than when the stimuli are phonetically complex (Jusczyk, Cutler, & Redanz, 1993).

A bias in **listening preference for trochaic versus iambic stress patterns** can be observed in infants learning stress-timed languages, but this bias is observed at earlier ages when the stimuli are phonetically simple than when the stimuli are phonetically complex.

Electrophysiological responses to nonsense words with different stress patterns show that the trochaic stress bias is shaped by language input in the first four months of life (Friederici, Friedrich, & Christophe, 2007). As shown in Figure 2–5, significant mismatch responses are obtained with the oddball paradigm when German-learning infants hear an iambic deviant stimulus within a stream of trochaic syllables but the reverse pattern is obtained for French-learning infants. The trochaic bias emerges for infants learning stress-timed languages in behavioral responses between 6 and 9 months of age (Höhle et al., 2009; Jusczyk et al., 1993). Interestingly, 6-month-old French-learning infants do not show a listening preference for either strong-weak or weak-strong stress patterns although they are able to discriminate trochaic and iambic words (Höhle et al., 2009).

Emergence of a language-specific strategy for processing the rhythmic structure of the native language plays a role in the infant's developing ability to segment words from the continuous stream of speech input. Word segmentation is a very difficult problem because words do not contain any obvious boundaries such as pauses between them and adults produce only a small percentage

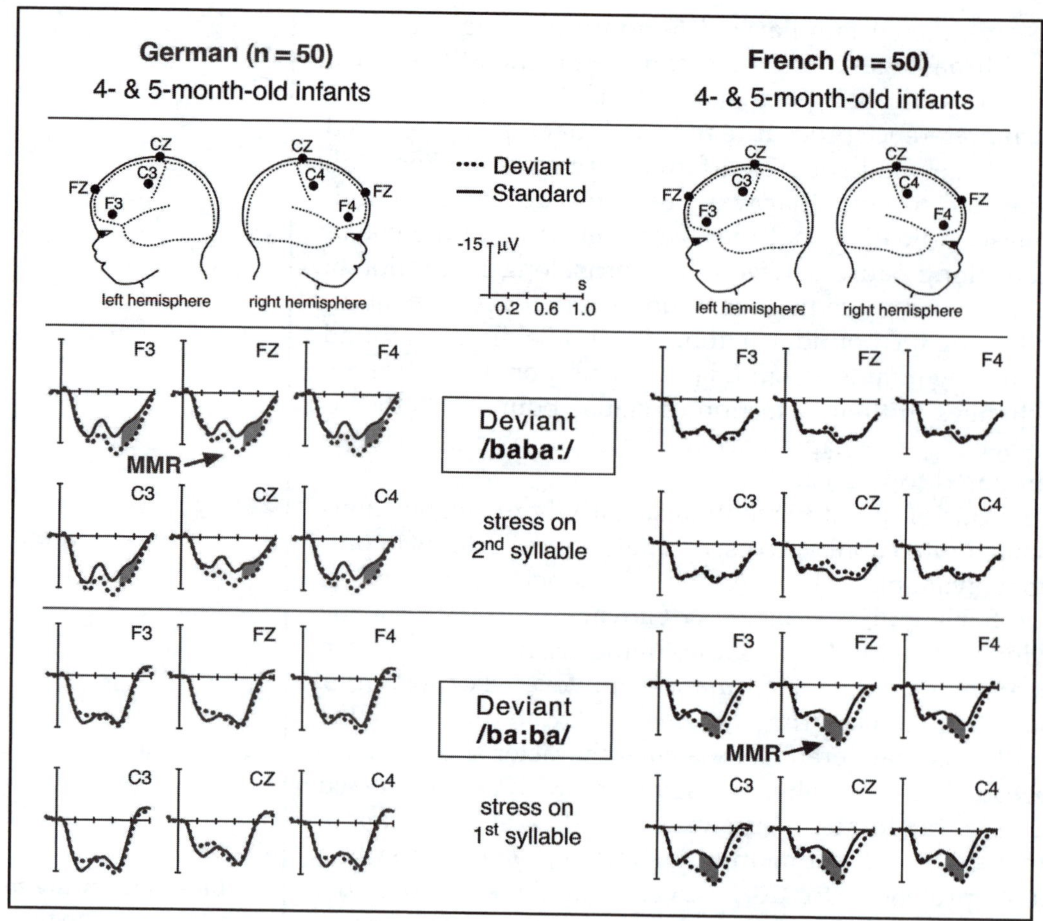

Figure 2–5. *Mismatch responses recorded from German-learning infants in response to trochaic deviant stimuli presented in a stream of iambic nonsense words (left) and from French-learning infants to iambic deviant stimuli presented in a stream of trochaic nonsense words (right), in an ERP study involving 4- and 5-month-old infants. From Friederici et al. (2007). Brain responses in 4-month-old infants are already language specific.* Current Biology, 17(14), *Figure 2, p. 1210. Reproduced with permission of Cell Press.*

of words in isolation when speaking to babies (Gerken, 2009). Cues to word boundaries include phonotactic sequences (e.g., certain phone sequences occur more frequently within words than between them), allophonic details (e.g., aspirated stops are more like to occur in an onset than a coda), and syntactic regularities (e.g., a noun is likely to follow a function morpheme such as "the" or "a"). It is difficult to see how the infant might learn these cues without knowing what the words are however. Attention to the prosodic structure of the language provides the infant an initial segmentation strategy and helps to explain how infants acquire some word segmentation abilities prior to the acquisition of a lexicon. Word boundaries are likely to coincide with the clause boundaries that attract infant attention at birth and, in English, stressed syllables are a reliable cue to word onsets.

In a series of 15 experiments, Jusczyk, Houston, and Newsome (1999) explored infants' ability to segment words with a trochaic or iambic stress pattern from continuous speech. The infants were 7.5 months old from English-speaking homes. The head turn preference procedure was used to assess the infants' preference for stimuli that were identical to or similar to the familiarization stimuli, presented as lists of isolated words or as passages, alternating conditions from experiment to experiment. The words used in the experiments were sometimes single syllable words such as "king" or "tar" and other times bisyllable words such as "kingdom" or "guitar." Sometimes the infants were tested for recognition of syllable sequences that crossed word boundaries such as "tar is." The infants learned to recognized bisyllabic trochaic words, whether presented in passages or as isolated words, and they did not confuse single syllables such as "king" with bisyllables such as "kingdom." On the other hand, their pattern of listening preferences suggested that they did not learn to segment iambic words and confused single syllables such as "tar" with bisyllables such as "guitar." Furthermore, infants at this age appeared to segment fluent speech into trochaic feet (e.g., "tar is") rather than iambic words ("guitar"). Further study revealed that 10.5-month-old infants were able to segment words with an iambic stress pattern from fluent speech and no longer missegmented words on the basis of the trochaic foot.

The implication of Jusczyk et al.'s (1999) findings is that the English-learning infant's initial strategy for segmenting words from fluent speech is based on a trochaic word template. This initial strategy provides the infant with a basis for learning other word boundary cues, culminating in the infant's ability to segment words with an iambic stress pattern toward the end of the first year. Infants show improving knowledge of language specific word boundary cues including phonotactic constraints (Mattys & Jusczyk, 2001) and allophonic regularities (Jusczyk, Hohne, & Bauman, 1999) between 9 and 12 months of age.

The English-learning infant's initial reliance on a **trochaic word template** provides a basis for learning language-specific word boundary cues linked to phonotactic constraints and allophonic regularities before the end of the first year.

To summarize, infants are attentive to the rhythmic characteristics of the ambient language at if not before birth as indexed by an ability to discriminate the native language from foreign languages from a different rhythmic class. Clause boundaries appear to help infants recognize previously heard language input and aid in the learning of other metrical properties of the native language. Between 4 and 9 months of age listening preferences for language specific word stress patterns emerge, forming a foundation for the discovery of a variety of word boundary cues that allow effective application of language specific word segmentation strategies before the end of the first year. Throughout this period interaction between phonetic and prosodic processing occurs such that prosody aids in the processing of phonetic information and phonetic knowledge enhances the infant's ability to segment fluent speech into prosodic units. In Chapter 4 we show that this interaction between phonetic and prosodic processing continues to be important for phonological learning later in life. We stress the importance of attending to interactions between these levels of phonological knowledge in assessment and treatment planning in Part II and Part III of this book.

During the first year the infant has accomplished a qualitative shift from language-general to language-specific processing of phonetic and prosodic elements and is now aware of phonetic contrasts, allophonic variation, rhythmic patterns, and phonotactic regularities that are characteristic of the ambient language. During the second year the infant must make a second qualitative shift, from phonetic to phonemic knowledge of the sound system of the language being learned.

Phonemic Perception and Word Learning in Infancy

One could argue that the perceptual knowledge learned by the infant in the first year is linguistic in nature in that it is language-specific and is not a simple reflection of the acoustic characteristics of the units that are perceived. Perceptual sensitivity to phonetic contrasts is enhanced for those contrasts that are phonemic in the language being learned and attenuated for those contrasts that are not phonemic even when the language provides allophonic exposure to the underlying phonetic content. The perceptual distance between phones is determined by the functional significance of the phonetic elements in the language being learned by the infant (Kuhl et al., 1992). These phonetic perception skills cannot be said to be phonemic, however, until the infant uses this knowledge in the identification and discrimination of meaningful words.

Phonemic perception skills emerge when the infant employs phonetic perceptual abilities in the identification and discrimination of meaningful words.

In an early study on the shift from phonetic to phonemic perception, Russian-learning toddlers were taught nonsense word labels for novel objects and then asked to act upon the objects in various ways when they were presented in triads such as [bɑk], [mɑk], and [zub] (Shvachkin, 1948/1973). The results suggested that, in the early stages of word learning, words are represented globally at a whole-word level; ability to represent words on the basis of minimal phonemic contrasts emerged gradually over the second year of life. In a replication of this general finding with English-learning infants, Garnica (1973) showed that there is not a universal order of contrast emergence in phonemic perception although there were common findings. Both researchers found that a word shape contrast emerged very early, specifically the presence versus absence of a consonant in the onset (e.g., [bos] vs. [os]). Subsequently the children demonstrated the ability to perceive sonorant versus stop contrasts at the phonemic level (e.g., [bɑk]

In the early stages of word learning, **words are represented globally** at a whole-word level.

vs. [mɑk]). A voicing contrast was the last to emerge in both language groups.

More recent methods of assessing word learning in infants require less physical ability and cooperation from the infant and provide sophisticated controls for potential confounds such as experimenter bias (Werker, Cohen, Lloyd, Casasola, & Stager, 1998). Specifically, the switch task is a modification of the visual habituation procedure used with younger infants. Videos or still photos of interesting objects and recordings of nonsense words produced with an infant-directed speaking register are prepared. The toddler is shown, in alternating trials, two word-object combinations (e.g., object A/[lɪf] and object B/[nim]) until a predetermined reduction in looking time to the visual stimuli is observed. After the habituation criterion has been met, two test trials are presented, one in which an object is presented with the expected word (e.g., same trial: object A/[lɪf]) and one in which the expected object-name pairing is switched (e.g., switch trial: object B/[lɪf]). Finally, a third object and a novel word (object C/[pok]) is presented to ensure that the child remained engaged with the procedure throughout the duration of the task. During the test phase of the experiment, greater looking at the visual stimulus during the switch trial as compared to the same trial is the index of successful word learning.

The **switch task** is an ingenious modification of the visual habituation procedure that tests the infant's ability to learn the association between novel word forms and novel objects.

Stager and Werker (1997) pioneered the use of the switch procedure to study the emergence of word learning in infants aged 8 through 14 months of age. Infants aged approximately 14 months are able to succeed at this task with phonetically different object names but 8- to 12-month-old infants do not appear to notice the switch even though infants in this age range are clearly able to process the phonetic differences between the novel words. Although 14-month-old infants are able to map novel words to objects when the words are phonetically different (object A/[lɪf] and object B/[nim]) they are unable to succeed at this task when the nonsense words are minimal pairs (object A/[bɪ] and object B/[dɪ]). Furthermore, 14-month-old infants failed to notice the switch when habituated to a single object word pairing (e.g., object A/[bɪ]) and tested with both same (e.g., object A/[bɪ]) and switch (e.g., object A/[dɪ]) trials whereas 8-month-old infants succeeded at this task. Toddlers were clearly able to discriminate the words as shown by their performance in the standard visual habituation paradigm (i.e., [bɪ] paired with checkerboard pattern during habituation and [dɪ] paired with the same checkerboard pattern during test); nonetheless, they seemed unable to attend to the fine phonetic detail in words and map those words to meaning at the same time. Subsequent studies determined that word learning ability in the switch task emerges after 14 months of age and before 20 months of age (Werker, Fennell, Corcoran, & Stager, 2002). Individual variability is observed during this age range such that some 14-month-olds are able to map minimal pair nonsense words to novel objects but some 17-month-olds cannot; in fact, the toddler's

Most 14-month-old toddlers succeed at the switch task and learn new word-object pairings **when the words are phonetically different** but not when the new words are minimal pairs.

vocabulary size provides a better predictor of word learning ability than age during this period. These findings have been confirmed by ERP in subsequent investigations (Mills et al., 2004). A summary of these findings is shown in Table 2–1.

A related but different line of research has investigated toddlers' awareness of mispronunciations of familiar words using a preferential looking task. Swingley and Aslin (2000) presented 18- to 23-month-old toddlers with pictures of two familiar objects (e.g., apple, baby) followed by a recorded request which may contain either a correct or a mispronounced version of one of the words (e.g., Where's the apple? Can you find it?; *or* Where's the opple? Can you find it?). Looking times to the target picture (in this example, the apple) were compared for conditions in which the target was correctly pronounced versus incorrectly pronounced, as shown in Figure 2–6 (Swingley, 2008). Infants throughout the age range tested demonstrated longer looking times in the correctly pronounced target condition (although looking times to the target were significantly above chance in the incorrectly pronounced condition). These results indicate that older toddlers' perceptual representations are sufficiently detailed to allow for some differentiation of misarticulated

The **preferential looking task** shows that older toddlers' perceptual representations are sufficiently detailed to allow for some differentiation of misarticulated words from their correctly pronounced targets.

Table 2–1. *Summary of Results of Selected Studies Employing the "Switch Task" to Investigate Early Word Learning Abilities*

Study	*Child Characteristics*	*Stimulus A*	*Stimulus B*	*Significant Recovery on Switch*
1	8-month-olds	[lɪf]	[nim]	no
	14-month-olds	[lɪf]	[nim]	yes
	14-month-olds	[bɪ]	[dɪ]	no
2	14-month-olds	[bɪ]	[dɪ]	no
	17-month-olds	[bɪ]	[dɪ]	yes
	20-month-olds	[bɪ]	[dɪ]	yes
	Comprehension ≥200 words	[bɪ]	[dɪ]	yes
	Comprehension <200 words	[bɪ]	[dɪ]	no
	Production ≥25 words	[bɪ]	[dɪ]	yes
	Production <25 words	[bɪ]	[dɪ]	no
3	14-month-olds	[bɪn]	[dɪn]	no

Sources: Above data are from: Study 1. Stager, C.L., & Werker, J. F. (1997). Infants listen for more phonetic detail in speech perception than in word-learning tasks. *Nature*, 388(6640), 381–382. Study 2. Werker, J. F., Fennell, C.T., Corcoran, K.M., & Stager, C. L. (2002). Infants' ability to learn phonetically similar words: Effects of age and vocabulary size. *Infancy*, 3(1), 1–30. Study 3. Pater, J., Stager, C. L., & Werker, J. F. (2004). The perceptual acquisition of phonological contrasts. *Language*, 80, 384–402.

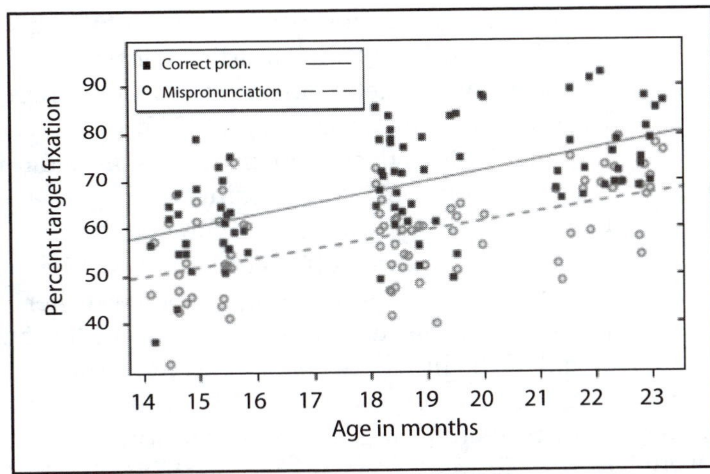

Figure 2–6. *Using a preferential looking task to assess children's detection of mispronunciations. This figure shows the outcome of several studies in the form of percent target fixations when the word was pronounced correctly (e.g.,* "dog," squares) *versus incorrectly (e.g., "tog,"* circles). *The lines drawn through the plot show a linear regression of fixation percentage on age for correct pronunciations* (solid line) *and mispronunciations* (dashed line). *From Swingley (2008). The roots of the early vocabulary in infants' learning from speech.* Current Directions in Psychological Science, *by American Psychological Society, 17, Figure 2, p. 310. Reproduced with permission of Blackwell Publishing, Inc.*

words from their correctly pronounced targets. Fennell and Werker (2003) have confirmed that toddlers as young as 14 months of age are sensitive to mispronunciations of familiar words when tested in the switch task. At the same time, they are not completely sure which acoustic-phonetic differences are phonemically significant. In fact, even nonphonetic differences such as changes in talker or intonation can make it difficult for infants to recognize recently learned words. Stabilization of the child's perceptual knowledge of acoustic-phonetic representations for words requires a lot of experience with variable input in meaningful contexts. We return to this important point in Chapter 9 when we cover perceptual interventions for the remediation of developmental phonological disorders.

Infant responses to speech discrimination tasks and toddler responses to word learning tasks give the impression of a marked discontinuity as the infant negotiates the shift from phonetic to phonemic perception of speech. On the other hand, continuity from the first to the second year of life is indicated by correlations between infant speech perception performance and language development during the second year. Recall that individual differences in speech perception development are observed during early infancy. Not only do large numbers of infants fail to complete the speech perception tasks, not all infants who complete the task will show clear evidence of the ability to discriminate a given contrast (e.g., Polka & Werker, 1994). ERP studies confirm individual variation in the course of phonetic development in the first year. In a longitudinal study, Rivera-Gaxiola et al. (2005) traced changes in the P150-250,[2] believed to reflect acoustic processing, and the N250-550, believed to reflect phonetic processing, in response to native and nonnative VOT contrasts. The results showed that some infants had shifted to the more mature pattern of strong N250-550 responses to the native contrast at 7 months of age, whereas others did not make this shift until 11 months of age. Tsao, Huei-Mei, and Kuhl (2004) investigated the link between speech perception at age 6 months and language development at 13, 16, and 24 months of age. The number of trials required to reach criterion for perception of a vowel contrast in the first year was significantly (and negatively) correlated with various measures of vocabulary and grammatical performance throughout the second year of life. Behavioral measures of word learning by toddlers are also associated with language test performance in preschoolers (Bernhardt, Kemp, & Werker, 2007; Hohle, van de Vijver, & Weissenborn, 2006). Höhle et al. (2006) suggested that infant responding to mispronounced words during the preferential looking task may indicate a generalized problem with information processing on the part of children with poor language skills or a specific problem with unstable phonological representations for familiar words. In the next section, the path toward the achievement of stable adultlike perceptual representations for words is described.

Speech perception performance by infants during the first year of life is correlated with word learning performance and measures of language ability during the second year of life.

Speech Perception Development in Childhood

2.3.1. Identify 5 changes in speech perception performance that occur during childhood.

2.3.2. Distinguish between a word identification task designed to measure speech perception skills and a matching task designed to measure phonological awareness skills in terms of the procedures and stimuli used and in terms of the underlying knowledge that is tapped by the tasks.

[2]ERP waveforms in response to a stimulus take the form of a characteristic series of positive and negative peaks that occur at characteristic time intervals in relation to stimulus onset. ERP components are labeled according to the polarity of voltage deflection (N; negative, and P; positive) and their characteristic latency in ms. An N200 is a negative peak (valley) occurring approximately 200 ms after stimulus onset. ERP components measured from the infant brain may be broader and less well defined than those recorded from the adult brain and thus the component in this case is described with a range such as the P150 to 250. These peaks can also be labeled to reflect their relative latency so that P1 is the earliest positive peak and P2 is the next to occur and so on. This labeling system recognizes individual differences in the latency of these peaks especially as a function of age.

2.3.3. Describe the major milestones along the path toward the achievement of phonemic awareness.

Development of Perceptual Representations for Words

At the end of the infant period, the toddler has perceptual awareness of the phone categories and rhythmic structures that are characteristic of the native language and is able to use this knowledge to extract word forms from the speech input and associate those words with specific referents. However, perceptual knowledge at this age is far from mature as will be shown in this section that focuses on the achievement of adultlike speech perception skills in English-speaking children. A number of different research paradigms have been used to study the child's knowledge of the precise acoustic-phonetic characteristics of the phonemes in the native-language sound system. One method involves assessing children's ability to detect mispronunciations of words although with older children a forced-choice picture pointing task is used rather than the visual preference task that is used with infants and toddlers.

Vance, Rosen, and Coleman (2009) developed a test in which correct and incorrect versions of target words were recorded from an adult female talker of standard British English. The words were carefully selected to be in the productive vocabulary repertoires of 2- to 4-year-old children. The child was shown a picture of two boys on a computer screen and told that one boy said things right while the other got them a little bit wrong. The child's task was to select one or the other boy to indicate whether each presented word was pronounced correctly or not. The 30 test items were presented in quiet conditions and with background noise of multitalker babble with a signal to noise ratio of +2 dB. The simulated articulation errors included confusions of voicing or place or manner of articulation, targeting consonants with the exception of one vowel error. A test of speech discrimination ability using an ABX task and CVC nonsense words was also administered to each child in quiet and in noise. Speech perception performance on these four tasks was shown to improve significantly with age although there was considerable intrasubject variability at each age level, as shown in Figure 2–7. The ABX task was more difficult than the mispronunciation detection task. Some children attained perfect scores when tested in quiet conditions but ceiling effects were not observed for performance in noise. Age-corrected composite scores on these measures of speech perception ability were correlated with standardized scores on a test of receptive vocabulary skills.

The **ability to detect mispronunciations of words** continues to mature throughout childhood, when tested in quiet and noisy conditions. As in infancy, this perceptual ability is correlated with language skills in childhood.

Even studies employing undegraded adult-produced speech, presented in quiet conditions, have found that mispronunciation detection improves with age and is significantly correlated with other aspects of language development such as vocabulary size and especially phonological awareness (Claessen, Heath, Fletcher,

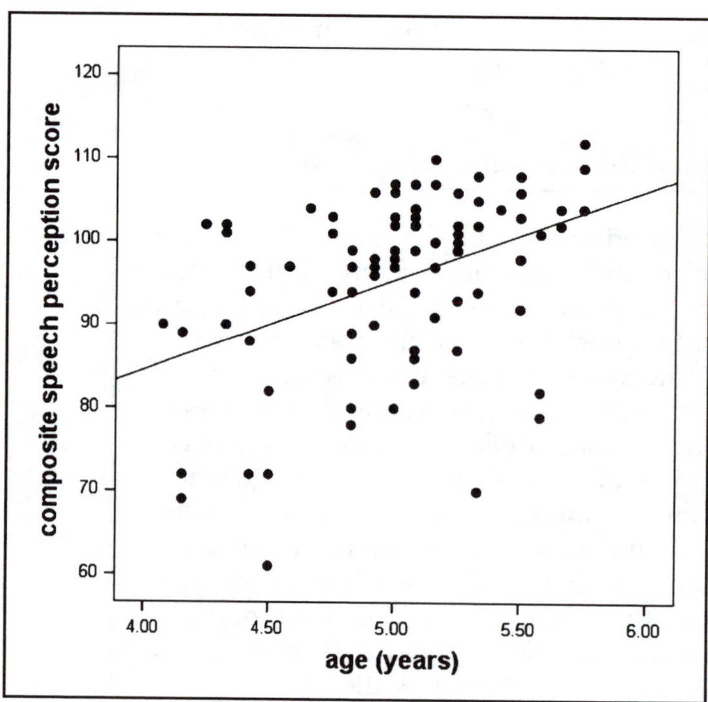

Figure 2–7. Children's composite speech perception scores as a function of age reflecting mispronunciation detection in quiet, mispronunciation detection in noise and ABX discrimination performance. From Vance et al. (2009). Assessing speech perception in young children and relationships with language skills. International Journal of Audiology *by British Society of Audiology, 48(10), Figure 1, p. 713. Reproduced with permission of Taylor & Francis Inc.*

Hogben, & Leitao, 2009; McNeill & Hesketh, 2010). McNeill and Hesketh also reported that it is easier for children to detect mispronunciations that impact the prosodic structure of the target words, that is, when the errors are deletions or transpositions; mispronunciations of individual segments, both vowels and consonants, were more difficult for the children to perceive. In fact, the three most difficult items on their test involved vowel substitutions.

Another method for studying speech perception development involves the presentation of words from synthetically produced speech sound continua for identification from the child so that developmental changes in the location and width of the category boundary can be described (see Chapter 1 for details of this method). In general, these studies reveal that the locations of category boundaries are roughly appropriate in very early childhood but the achievement of a sharply sloped identification function with a narrow boundary width is a protracted process (Burnham, Earnshaw, & Clark, 1991). Zlatin and Koenigsknetcht (1975) investigated identification of the minimal pairs bees/peas, bear/pear, dime/time, and goat/coat in 2-year-olds, 6-year-olds, and adults. With respect to boundary location, no significant differences were observed except that 2-year-olds shifted their perception from /g/ to /k/ at a significantly later lag point than 6-year-olds or adults. The 2-year-old group also demonstrated significantly wider boundary widths for all four continua in comparison with adults and for the labial continua in comparison with the 6-year-olds. The 6-year-old group demonstrated similar boundary widths to the adult group except for the velar continuum. Krause (1982) investigated perceptual knowledge of a cue to postvocalic voicing, specifically vowel duration in the words bip/bib, pot/pod, and back/bag. In this study, differences in boundary location and slope of the identification function were compared for 3-year-olds, 6-year-olds, and adults, with both variables changing progressively with age and not being mature at age 6 years. Specifically, adult listeners shifted their responses from the voiceless to the voiced category at shorter vowel durations and demonstrated steeper slopes in their identification functions.

Hazan and Barrett (2000) used this same method to study the development of perceptual ability for the contrasts /g/-/k/, /d/-/g/, /s/-/z/, and /s/-/ʃ/ in word-initial position between 6 and 12 years of age, in a study involving 84 children. Age effects for boundary location were not observed but a strong effect of age was observed for the slope (gradient) of the identification function, as shown in Figure 2–8. Between-subjects variation within age groups was greatest for the youngest children and still greater than that observed in adults at age 12 years, especially for the fricative contrasts.

When word identification skills are assessed using **synthetic speech continua** that systematically vary specific acoustic cues, developmental changes are observed in the *width of the category boundary* and the *steepness of the identification function* through late childhood.

Taken together these studies show that children are able to identify clear exemplars of words that contrast phonemes that differ by a single phonetic feature as early as age 2 years; however, the ability to assign words with ambiguous acoustic cues to discrete phoneme categories does not reach maturity until very late childhood. Two additional research paradigms have explored the reasons for late maturation of speech perception abilities: those involving the presentation of stimuli with degraded acoustic information and those involving trading relations among competing cues to phoneme identity.

One method of degrading the acoustic information available in recorded words is to "gate" the speech stimuli by removing progressively larger chunks from the ends of the words, as described when discussing the study conducted by Edwards et al. (1999) in Chapter 1 (see Figure 1–15 and related discussion). This research team used these same gated stimuli to assess the development of word final consonant discrimination among 120 children approximately 3, 5, and 7 years of age, in comparison with adult performance on this word identification task (Edwards, Fox, & Rogers, 2002). When listening to ungated recordings of the words tap/tack and cap/cat, 3-year-old children performed significantly worse than older children or adults who achieved similar performance.

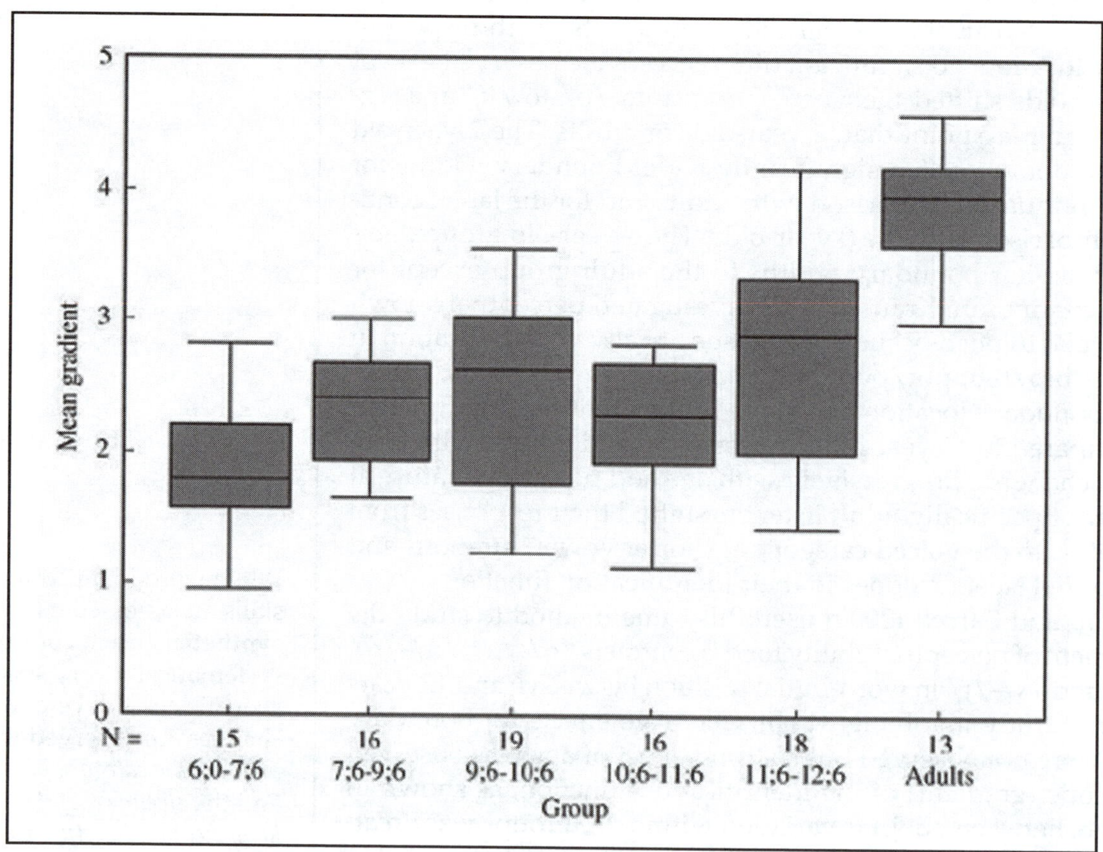

Figure 2–8. *Mean gradients (slopes) of the identification functions by age averaged across the functions obtained for synthetic speech continua contrasting goat/coat, date/gate, sue/zoo, and sue/shoe. From Hazan and Barrett (2000). The development of phonemic categorization in children aged 6–12.* Journal of Phonetic, 8, *Figure 3, p. 388 (A) and Figure 2, p. 387 (B). Reproduced with permission of Academic Press.*

When the words were presented with the final 20 or 40 ms excised from the words significant differences were apparent between all age groups. On average, older children's representations were more detailed at the acoustic-phonetic level than younger children's but still not sufficiently well specified to permit adultlike performance on this task.

Many studies have found that children require a **higher signal-to-noise ratio** to achieve the same perceptual performance as adults even for very simple detection and discrimination tasks.

Another strategy for degrading the speech input is to present it in the context of background noise. Many studies have found that children require a higher signal-to-noise ratio to achieve the same perceptual performance as adults even for very simple detection and discrimination tasks (Elliott, Longinotti, Clifton, & Meyer, 1981; Fallon, Trehub, & Schneider, 2000; Maillart, Schelstraete, & Hupet, 2004; Nozza, 1988). Furthermore, the poorer performance of children relative to adults for speech discrimination in noise tasks can be attributed to perceptual rather than nonsensory factors (i.e., cognitive, memory, attention factors associated with task complexity). These findings have implications for classroom acoustics and the use of amplification during speech therapy as discussed further in Chapter 9.

Linguistic factors also play a role in speech perception performance under conditions of stimulus degradation (Eisenberg, Shannon, Martinez, Wygonski, & Boothroyd, 2000). In this study 5-year-old children demonstrated significantly poorer speech recognition accuracy for vocoded speech in comparison to 12-year-olds and adults (see Chapter 1 for a description of vocoded speech). However, the performance difference between younger and older children was much greater for sentence recognition than for recognition of kindergarten level single words; the older children appeared to be more adept at using linguistic context to support speech recognition when spectral cues in the input were reduced.

Morrongiello, Robson, and Best (1984) assessed 5-year-olds' perception of trading relations between temporal and spectral cues to the say/stay contrast using synthetic speech continua. In one continuum, the starting frequency of the first formant was lower than in the other continuum (appropriate for the word "stay") and the duration of the silent interval between the fricative noise and the onset of the vowel was varied systematically in both continua. Both adult and child listeners showed a trading relationship for these two acoustic cues such that stimuli from the continua were heard as "stay" with shorter silent intervals if the stimulus also contained the lower F1 onset cue. The effect was not as great for child listeners as for adult listeners however suggesting that children weighted the temporal cue more highly than the spectral cue when identifying the s-cluster than did adults.

Nittrouer (2002b) has investigated children's weighting strategies for multiple acoustic cues extensively, especially in the context of fricative contrasts. Recall from Chapter 1 that the contrast between /s/ and /ʃ/ is cued by differences in the centroid of the fricative noise as well as the starting frequency of the F1 transition. Children and adults identified stimuli from two continua in which one contained formant transitions appropriate for /s/ and the other contained formant transitions appropriate for /ʃ/. Both continua varied the centroid (center pole) frequency of the fricative noise in equal steps. The results for 3-, 5-, and 7-year-old children compared to adults are shown in Figure 2–9. In this figure the slope of the identification functions indicates the relative weight that the listener assigns to the frequency of the fricative noise when identifying the stimuli; the separation between the identification functions for stimuli with /s/ or /ʃ/-transitions indicates the weight assigned to the formant transitions when assigning stimuli to phonetic categories. The children's responses in this study represent a developmental increase in the weight assigned to the spectrum of the fricative noise and a developmental decrease in the weight assigned to the formant transitions. In this study, the performance of the children was still not adultlike at 7 years of age (Nittrouer & Miller, 1997).

Developmental changes in **weighting strategies** for multiple acoustic cues to phoneme identity are important factors that impact children's perceptual performance.

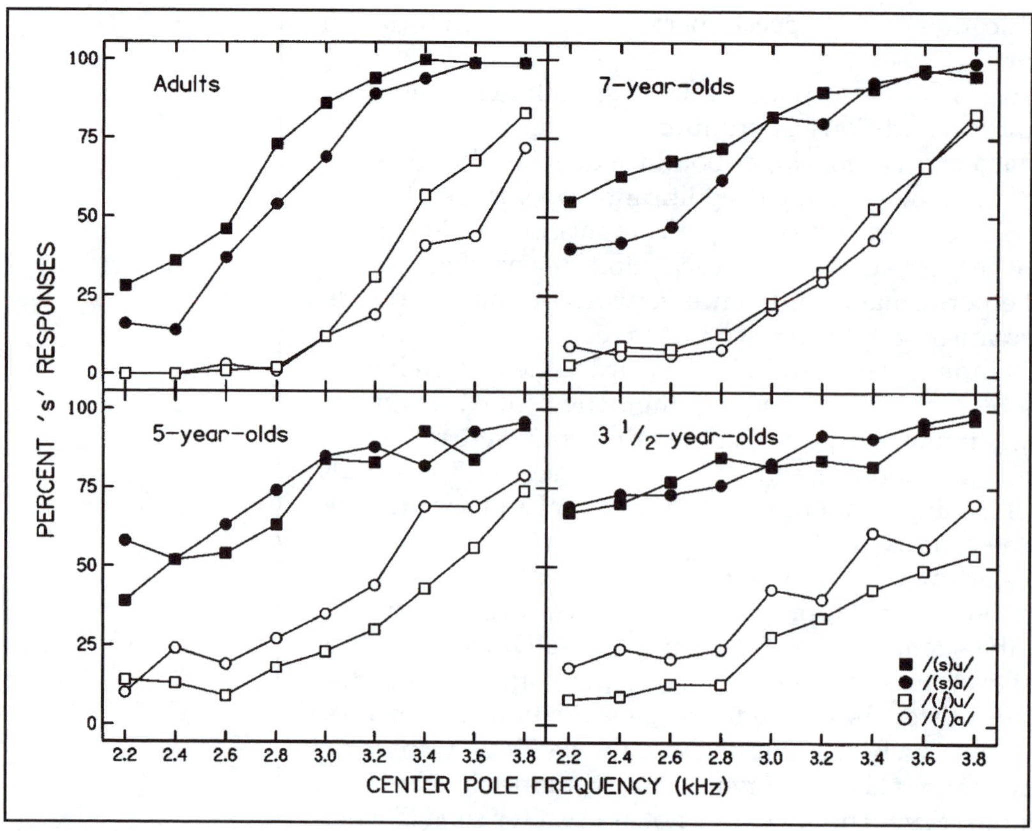

Figure 2–9. *Child and adult identification functions for synthetic continua with 9 step variation of the fricative noise spectrum and dichotomous variation of the formant transitions. From Nittrouer (2002b). Learning to perceive speech: How fricative perception changes and how it stays the same.* Journal of the Acoustical Society of America *by Acoustical Society of America, 112(2), Figure 1, p. 713. Reproduced with permission of American Institute of Physics for the Acoustical Society of America.*

These two studies do not indicate that there is a general tendency on the part of children to weight formant transition more heavily than other acoustic cues in speech input. Rather, the weighting strategy that is learned is contrast- (and language-) specific. When children and adults were tested for their relative weighting of noise spectrum versus formant transition cues to the /f/ - /θ/ contrast it was found that children aged 4 to 8 years and adults all weighted the formant transitions more than the noise spectrum (Nittrouer, 2002b). Indeed there was very little developmental change in responses to the /f/ - /θ/ contrast. Nittrouer concludes that, "As children gain experience with their native language, it is proposed, perceptual attention (i.e., weight) gradually shifts to take advantage of the properties of the acoustic signal that are most informative regarding phonetic structure" (p. 718).

In summary, assessment of speech perception skills in childhood confirms that most young children are able to perceive well produced words contrasting a variety of phonemic contrasts when presented in quiet conditions with a good signal-to-noise ratio. Nonetheless, speech perception follows a protracted course of gradual refinement throughout childhood and is still not adultlike at age 12 years. Children's cumulative experience with language allows them to encode increasingly detailed acoustic-phonetic representations for words and learn a flexible strategy for weighting temporal and spectral information so as to derive phonological structure from the language input (Nittrouer, 2002a). Eventually, the child is able to recognized words with a high degree of accuracy even when they are ambiguous or degraded exemplars of the target items or when the speech is presented in a noisy environment.

Development of Segmented Phonological Representations for Words

Tests of word recognition employing minimal pair words, such as those discussed in the previous section, provide a measure of the child's phonemic perception skills because they tap the listener's knowledge of the way that acoustic-phonetic information is organized to contrast meaning in the language. When the child indicates that [biːd] and [biːd̥] represent an object that can be threaded, whereas [bitʰ] and [bit̚] represent a red vegetable, she demonstrates knowledge of the phonemes /d/ and /t/. When the child rejects [t͡su] and [s̪u] and [ɬu] as correctly pronounced exemplars of the word "Sue" he reveals the specificity of his perceptual representation for the phoneme /s/. Performance on these kinds of tasks does not reveal the underlying structure of the child's phonological representations in the lexicon, however. It is not clear that the underlying representations are segmented at the level of the phoneme itself and it cannot be determined if the child's lexicon is organized at the level of the phoneme either. Although it seems obvious to literate adults that the word "bead" is composed of three sounds /b/, /i/, and /d/, as explained in Chapter 1, there are no segments in the acoustic input and it is possible to perform speech perception tasks by comparing whole word input to whole word representations. Awareness of subsyllabic units—onsets, rimes, phonemes—emerges developmentally from the organization of the lexicon as the child's store of perceptual representations grows in size (Beckman & Edwards, 2000; Ferguson & Farwell, 1975; Metsala & Walley, 1998).

Phonological awareness of subsyllabic units—onsets, rimes, phonemes—emerges developmentally from the organization of the lexicon as the child's store of perceptual representations grows in size.

In clinical practice the tests that tap this level of phonological representation are measures of phonological awareness. There are many different types of phonological awareness tests, varying along three dimensions. First, the tests require more or less conscious awareness of linguistic units on the part of the child. Tests that tap conscious awareness are called measures of metaphonological or explicit awareness, whereas those that tap less conscious awareness are measures of epiphonological or implicit awareness (Gombert, 1992; Savage, Blair, & Rvachew, 2006). For example, a task in which the child indicates that the words "map" and "men" go together whereas "map" and "toad" do not is a measure of implicit phonological awareness of onsets. A task in which the child is asked to "say the word sunshine without sun" taps explicit knowledge of syllables. As shown in these examples, phonological awareness tests also vary in terms of the phonological units that they target. Finally, the cognitive difficulty of the tasks varies considerably with tasks that provide picture support and employ real word stimuli reducing the memory load and complexity relative to those that ask children to manipulate subsyllabic units in nonsense words. Phonological awareness tests are not measures of speech perception ability per se, but performance on these measures of phonological processing is closely related to the child's speech perception abilities (Joanisse, Manis, Keating, & Seidenberg, 2000; Lyytinen et al., 2004; Rvachew & Grawburg, 2006) and thus the development of phonological awareness skills is discussed briefly here.

There are many kinds of **phonological awareness tests** that vary along three dimensions: *explicitness of the level of awareness* tapped by the task; the *phonological unit* that must be accessed during the task; and the *cognitive demands* required while performing the task.

Implicit awareness of **larger phonological units** has been observed in some 2- and 3-year-old children.

Implicit awareness of larger phonological units—words, syllables, and rimes—has been demonstrated by some 2- and 3-year-old children (Chaney, 1992; Lonigan, Burgess, Anthony, & Barker, 1998). For example, Lonigan et al. presented preschoolers with three kinds of cognitively complex tasks: oddity, elision, and blending. The rime oddity task involved presenting the children with sets of three pictured words and asking them to select the word that did not sound the same as the other two. The elision task involved deletion of a specific element from a word (with picture support for some items); for example, "Say *sunshine* without saying *shine*" or "Say *carpet* without saying *pet*." Children were also presented with parts of words and asked to blend them together into one word. One-quarter of the 2-year-old children in the sample performed at above chance levels on the rime oddity task but alliteration oddity (i.e., matching words with the same onset) was not achieved by a significant proportion of the sample until age 4 or 5. Among middle-class children, 43% were able to complete the word level elision items with picture support (i.e., sunshine) at age 2 years but few were able to succeed with the syllable level items (i.e., carpet). Between 75 and 100% of middle-class children were responding at above chance levels on all of the test tasks by the age of 5 years. Considerably fewer children from lower income homes were successful with these tasks at all age levels.

Implicit awareness of phonemes is not typically seen in children younger than 5 years of age.

Implicit awareness of phonemes, even when situated in the onset or coda position of CVC words, is not typically seen in children younger than 5 years of age (Lonigan et al., 1998). Byrne and Fielding-Barnsley (1993) found that kindergarten students continued to make word similarity judgments based on global similarity more easily than on the basis of individual phonemes. In this study, a phoneme identity test was administered in which the child had to match one of two items to the target on the basis of shared first sound. Two versions of the test were constructed, one in which the foils (incorrect items) were closely matched to the target in global similarity and another in which they were not. Global similarity was calculated on a phoneme by phoneme basis to reflect the overlap in distinctive features. For example, in the matched version of the test the response alternatives corresponding to the target *pot* were *peach* and *duck* whereas the response alternatives in the unmatched version were *peach* and *leg*. Test scores were significantly better in the unmatched than matched condition. Carroll and Snowling (2001) also found that kindergarten-age children found it more difficult to reject phonetically similar foil items, in comparison to semantically similar or unrelated foils, in rime and onset matching tasks. Taken together these studies suggest that even at age 5 years, children's judgments about word similarity are influenced by global similarity at the word level, suggesting that implicit awareness of individual phonemes in words remains somewhat unstable.

Kindergarten-age children do not appear to have explicit awareness of phonemes as measured by elision or deletion tasks, with most children succeeding on few if any items requiring elision of a phoneme throughout the kindergarten year (Chiappe, Siegel, & Gottardo, 2002; Lonigan et al., 1998; Rosner & Simon, 1971). By third grade many children can perform elision tasks at the phoneme level, even those that require elision of a phoneme from a complex onset or coda (McBride-Chang, 1995; Rosner & Simon, 1971).

By third grade many children can perform **explicit elision tasks** at the phoneme level.

Many studies suggest that children's implicit and explicit knowledge of phonological units becomes stable for larger units before smaller units. However, this does not mean that the emergence of awareness of larger versus smaller units occurs during discrete stages of development. Furthermore, the developmental order in which these skills develop is influenced by the type of representations that are accessed in the context of the task in which the child is engaged. Savage, Blair, and Rvachew (2006) assessed implicit and explicit knowledge of heads, rimes, onsets and codas by 4- to 6-year-old children. Two tasks were employed, a matching task, in which the child responded "same" or "different" to indicate whether two words shared a given element, and a common unit task, in which the child pronounced the common element. Items were controlled to be identical sets of CVC word pairs across both tasks. The results, as shown for nonreaders in Figure 2–10, revealed the expected finding for implicit awareness: on the matching task more correct responses were obtained for awareness of the larger units compared to smaller units. The pattern of results was somewhat different for explicit awareness: on the common unit task the best results were obtained for onsets; surprisingly, the children were essentially unable to pronounce common rimes when presented with items such as "pin" and "fin." The results for children

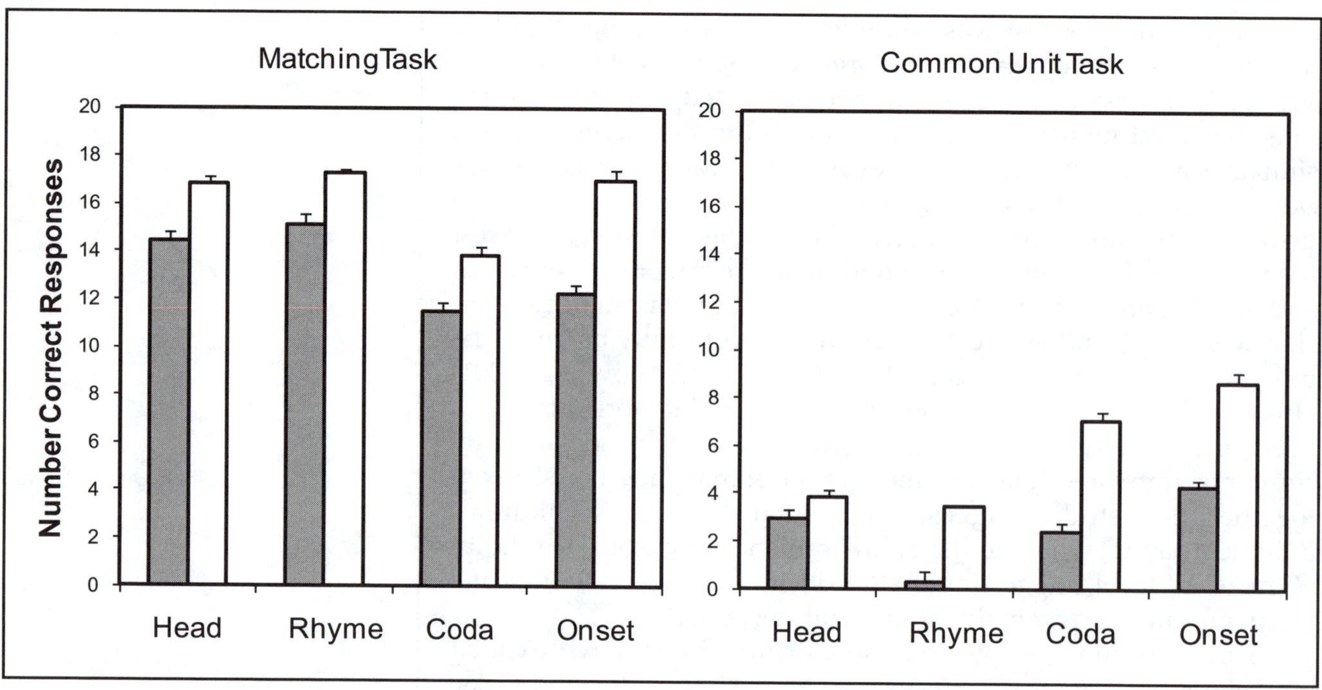

Figure 2–10. *Number of correct responses by 4- to 6-year-old children on tests of implicit (matching task) and explicit (common unit task) phonological awareness for four phonological units: Head (e.g., heart, harp), Rime (e.g., heart, cart), Coda (e.g., heart, boot) and Onset (e.g., heart, horse). Adapted from Savage, Blair, and Rvachew (2006). Rimes are not necessarily favored by prereaders: Evidence from meta- and epilinguistic phonological tasks.* Journal of Experimental Child Psychology, *94, pp. 183–205. Reproduced with permission of Academic Press.*

who had some reading ability showed strong awareness of onsets on both tasks. It seems probable that these two tasks differentially require access to acoustic-phonetic and articulatory-phonetic representations in addition to phonological knowledge of the words presented to the children. Common rimes appear to have strong perceptual salience for young children in the matching task; on the other hand, it is easier for them pronounce the first sound of two words sharing a common onset. Overall, the research evidence supports Anthony and Lonigan's (2004) conclusion that phonological awareness "develops from sensitivity to words to sensitivity to phonemes . . . in a quasi-parallel progression rather than a temporally discrete, sequential progression" (p. 52).

Interventions that target **phonological awareness as a crucial prereading skill** that emerges during the preschool period have become important parts of speech-language pathology practice.

Phonological awareness is a crucial prereading skill that emerges during the preschool period. Interventions that target phonological awareness to prevent delayed acquisition of reading and screening to identify children who have poor phonological awareness and are thus at risk for reading disability have become important parts of speech-language pathology practice. It can be seen from this brief review that assessment tools and intervention tasks must be carefully designed to be valid and developmentally appropriate.

Mechanisms That Underly Speech Perception Development

2.4.1. Define experience expectancy and explain how this concept relates to speech perception development in the human infant.

2.4.2. Describe Hickok and Poeppel's model for the processing of spoken language input by the adult brain.

2.4.3. Describe the relationship between the language environment and developmental changes in brain responses to linguistic stimuli.

2.4.4. Define statistical learning.

Thus far, we have described the course of speech perception development through infancy and childhood, as summarized in Figure 2–11. It can be seen that the child's achievement of mature speech perception abilities involves the successful negotiation of several important challenges. First, the child must develop a language-specific strategy for processing speech input, learning to attend selectively to acoustic information that is functionally relevant in the language being learned. Once on the way to acquiring perceptual knowledge of the phonetic system of the native language, the toddler must learn to use this knowledge to map words to referents, gradually acquiring implicit knowledge of the individual phonemes that make up words. After school entry the child learns to access this phonological knowledge explicitly for the purpose of learning to read. In the final section of this chapter we discuss some of the environmental factors, biological mechanisms, and cognitive processes that are involved in the acquisition of mature perceptual knowledge of the native language phonological system.

Experience Expectancy and Environmental Factors

Two distinct processes are thought to mediate the effect of experience on brain development (Greenough, Black, & Wallace, 1987). Experience-expectant plasticity is characteristic of early development. This mechanism involves two phases: initially, spontaneous activation of neurons leads to an oversupply of synaptic connections in anticipation of certain species-specific experiences; later, these experiences serve to prune the connections, shaping the structure through selective survival of those connections that are optimally responsive to the particular experiences that are provided. This mechanism has evolved in the organism to take advantage of the stimuli that are reliably present in the environment and the range of experiences that are normally encountered by the developing organism.

Experience-expectant plasticity shapes neural structure through selective survival of synaptic connections that are optimally responsive to stimuli that are reliably present in the environment and experiences that are normally encountered by the developing organism.

Age	Milestone	Stage
Birth	Discriminate native from foreign language	Language-general phonetic perception
1–2 mos	Discriminate lead and long-lag VOT contrasts in stop consonants	
2–4 mos	Discriminate many native and non-native vowel and consonant contrasts	
4 months	Discriminate some but not all fricative contrasts	
4–6 mos	Listening bias for words with trochaic stress pattern (English-learning infants)	
6 months	Segment clauses in continuous speech	
6–9 mos	Equivalence classification of phones belonging to a major sound class	
6–8 mos	Marked decline in perception of non-native vowel contrasts	Language-specific phonetic perception
7 months	Segment words with trochaic stress pattern (English-learning infants)	
8 months	Language specific shift in VOT boundary (e.g., French- and Spanish-learning infants)	
9 months	Segment words based on phonotactic cues	
10 months	Marked decline in perception of non-native consonants	
11 months	Segment words with iambic stress pattern (English-learning infants)	
14 months	Fast-mapping of phonetically dissimilar words in switch task	
17 months	Fast-mapping of phonetically dissimilar words in switch task	Phonemic perception
24 months	Adult-like VOT boundaries for bilabial and alveolar but not velar stops in word identification task	
3 years	Implicit awareness of words and syllables	Implicit phonological awareness
4 years	Implicit awareness of rimes	
5 years	Implicit awareness of onsets and codas	
6 years	Adult-like VOT category boundaries for bilabial and alveolar but not velar stops	Explicit phonological awareness
9 years	Explicit awareness of phonemes	
12 years	Slopes of identification functions and variability of perceptual performance still not adult-like	

Figure 2–11. *Milestones in the development of speech perception, word recognition and phonological awareness skills.*

Experience-dependent plasticity is characteristic of later development and involves the formation of new synapses in response to experiences that may be unique to the individual.

Experience-dependent plasticity involves the formation of new synapses in response to experiences that may be unique to the individual.

Experience expectancy in species-specific perceptual development was studied in depth by Gottlieb (2002) in the context of duckling acquisition of selective sensitivity to the maternal call. This research reveals many important aspects of environmental input that are relevant to the study of infant speech perception. In the wild, ducklings become responsive to the maternal call shortly after hatching, with certain species-specific acoustic characteristics of the maternal call capturing the ducklings' attention: repetition rate in the case of mallard ducklings and a descending frequency glide in the case of wood ducklings. Laboratory studies demonstrated that successful imprinting to the maternal call is dependent on a highly specific sequence of experiences during and after the embryonic stage of development. Wood ducklings must hear the vocalizations of their siblings as embryos (i.e., embryonic contact calls) with self-vocalizations and maternal calls during this period being ineffective. Sibling calls must contain a range of acoustic characteristics that includes the specific features of the maternal call. The optimal input appears to be a range of inputs that sensitize the duckling to a critical acoustic feature (e.g., repetition rate or frequency glide) rather than the specific form of the maternal call itself. In the absence of appropriate input during the embryonic stage the duckling would remain open to imprinting to a variety of calls including that of the chicken after hatching! Furthermore, the timing of the input was found to be critical as exposure to embryonic contact calls after hatching did not restore the perceptual selectivity lost due to deprivation during the embryonic stage. Introduction of premature visual stimulation was found to interfere with the effect of embryonic exposure to sibling calls on learning the maternal call. Finally, imprinting to the maternal call requires tactile contact with siblings as normally experienced during social rearing. To summarize, learning from the input was highly dependent on who provided the input, the specific form of the input, the social context in which the input was provided, and the timing and sequencing of the input with respect to other developmental events. These factors can be considered in the context of human infant listening preferences and perceptual learning in the neonatal period.

Experience-dependent perceptual learning is highly dependent on who provides the input, the specific form of the input, the social context in which the input is provided, and the timing and sequencing of the input with respect to other developmental events.

Vouloumanos and Werker (2007) demonstrated that neonates, 1 to 4 days old, prefer to listen to speech when presented with a choice of single words spoken by a human in an infant-directed register versus a nonspeech analogue of the words (sine-wave analogues of speech created as described in Chapter 1). Although the nonspeech stimuli retained the temporal and spectral characteristics of natural speech they had a completely unnatural source and were not as attractive to the infants as nonsense words produced by an adult female talker. The neonate's preference for speech in comparison to other auditory stimuli at birth cannot be assumed to be experience-independent because the fetus receives and learns from speech input, showing a preference for the maternal voice, the maternal language, and passages read by the mother during the last month of pregnancy (DeCasper & Fifer, 1980; DeCasper & Spence, 1986; Kisilevsky et al., 2009; Moon et al., 1993). Quite probably the newborn's preference for human speech input results from experience-expectant processes.

Infants prefer to listen to speech over other auditory inputs and to infant-directed over adult-directed speech, a listening preference that is probably driven by the melodic contour of infant-directed speech.

Infant listening preferences are driven by the form as well as the source of the input. Infants show a preference for infant-directed speech over adult-directed speech throughout the first year of life, regardless of whether the speech is produced by a female or male talker (Cooper & Aslin, 1990). In comparison to adult-directed speech, so-called motherese has a number of distinctive characteristics including prosodic repetition across utterances, longer pauses between utterances and overall shorter duration of individual utterances. Within utterances, the talker will use a higher overall pitch and wider pitch excursions and greater overall amplitude modulation. Fernald and Kuhl (1987) demonstrated that 4- to 6-month-old infants are specifically attracted to the fundamental frequency contours in the speech input rather than the amplitude modulation or the temporal pattern. However, younger infants prefer to listen to speech that contains the full range of spectral information in contrast to low-pass filtered speech, raising the question of whether selective attention to the pitch contour in motherese requires experience with the full range of acoustic qualities that contribute to exaggerated prosody (Panneton Cooper & Aslin, 1994; also see ERP study by Sambeth, Ruohio, Alku, Fellman, & Huotilainen, 2008).

Infant-directed speech may serve to **exaggerate certain phonetic contrasts**. In particular, the point vowels are produced with more extreme acoustic features in infant-directed than in adult-directed speech.

In addition to being characterized by a melodic pattern that is especially attractive to the infant listener, infant-directed speech serves to exaggerate phonetic contrast. Although the effect of the infant-directed register on consonants is somewhat ambiguous (e.g., see Englund, 2005), phonetic contrast for vowel categories is enhanced in motherese (Kuhl et al., 1997; Werker et al., 2007). For example, the point vowels are produced with more extreme acoustic features in infant-directed than in adult-directed speech (see Plate 3, reprinted from Kuhl et al., 1997). Furthermore, it has been shown that this stretching of the vowel space is specific to infant-directed speech as it does not occur in speech directed to pets even though pet-directed speech shares the prosodic characteristics of the infant-directed speaking register (Burnham, Kitamura, & Vollmer-Conner, 2002). The important role of the infant-directed speaking register in speech perception learning was demonstrated by Liu, Kuhl, and Tsao (2003). They found that the size of the maternal vowel space while talking to her infant was correlated with the infant's ability to discriminate a native language phonetic contrast. This research team also explored the importance of the social context in which the speech input is provided to the infant (Kuhl, Tsao, & Liu, 2003). In this study, exposure to Mandarin was used to maintain English-learning infants' sensitivity to a Mandarin phonetic contrast. Some infants interacted with a female Mandarin talker who used infant-directed speech during naturalistic play sessions, whereas others were exposed to Mandarin input provided via videorecordings. Perception of a Mandarin consonant contrast was assessed when the infants were 10 to 12 months old, revealing maintenance of the ability to perceive the contrast only in those infants who were exposed to it in the context of human interactions. Exposure to audiovisual recordings of Mandarin speech input was not sufficient to maintain the infants' perception of a nonnative contrast; in fact, perception declined to levels similar to that observed in other American infants who had no exposure to Mandarin. ERP studies confirm the important role of the infant-directed speaking register in modulating infant attention to linguistic content, thus facilitating speech perception development and language learning (Zangl & Mills, 2007).

The importance of the infant's early preference for speech input is highlighted by cases where this experience-expectant process is lacking. Autistic children tend to show listening preferences that are not the same as those observed in normally developing infants. For example, they prefer to listen to superimposed voices over their mother's voice alone and nonspeech analogues over infant-directed natural speech input (for review, see Kuhl, Coffey-Corina, Padden, & Dawson, 2005). The degree of preference for nonspeech over speech input was correlated with severity of the autism symptoms on a measure of social communication abilities. High functioning autistic children showed normal MMN responses to phonetic contrasts but components of the evoked potentials related to attention were atypical. Children with the most marked preference for nonspeech input and the most severe autistic symptoms however showed abnormal MMN responses to a [ba]—[wa] contrast indicating difficulties with phonetic perception as well as attention.

Studies of hearing-impaired children suggest that early experience with speech plays a role in the human tendency to attend to speech signals. Houston, Pisoni, Kirk, Ying, and Miyamoto (2003) used the visual habituation procedure to assess responses to speech by normal-hearing infants and children who had received cochlear implants. During the habituation phase a speech stimulus (e.g., "hop hop hop") was alternated with silence in blocks of trials until the habituation criterion was met at which point the test trials were introduced. The test trials consisted of either the familiar stimulus (e.g. "hop hop hop") or a novel stimulus (e.g., prolonged "ah"). Difference in looking time to sound versus silent trials during the habituation phase indexed attention to speech, whereas difference in looking time to the familiar versus novel stimulus during the test phase indexed speech discrimination. Both 6- and 9-month-old normal-hearing infants showed significant attention to speech in comparison to silence whereas this difference in looking time was not statistically significant even 6 months after implantation for the hearing-impaired children. Only the infant who received a cochlear implant at the youngest age (6 months) showed a trend toward longer looking times during speech trials versus silent trials, a trend which emerged during the period 6 to 15 months postimplantation. On the other hand, infants with cochlear implants did show reliably longer looking times to novel versus familiar stimuli during the test phase of the experiment, indicating the emergence of gross speech discrimination abilities. The authors concluded that early auditory deprivation disrupts active attention to speech input that in turn may impact on the acquisition of language-specific speech perception skills, word segmentation strategies, and auditory-visual and auditory-motor integration abilities.

Early auditory deprivation disrupts active attention to speech input that in turn may impact on the acquisition of language-specific speech perception skills, word segmentation strategies, and auditory-visual and auditory-motor integration abilities.

Another means of investigating attention to auditory stimuli is the distraction masker technique. A distraction masker is an extraneous noise that does not share any frequency components with the target signal and thus it causes informational masking rather than energetic masking of the signal. Werner and Bargones (1991) demonstrated that adult detection of lower frequency pure-tones was not affected by the presence of high frequency noise; infants on the other hand had significant difficulty with tone detection in the presence of a distraction masker reflecting their poorer selective attention skills. Polka, Rvachew, and Molnar (2008) replicated this result for speech input, finding that normal-hearing infants have significant difficulty discriminating [bu] versus [gu] in the presence of high-frequency bird calls whereas this contrast was easy for the infants to perceive under quiet conditions. Interestingly, infants with a past history of otitis media had no more or less difficulty than infants with no such history under distracting conditions; however, their performance in quiet was similar to their performance in noise, suggesting that they had generalized difficulties with attention to speech. Subsequent studies investigated environmental stimuli that help the infant cope with distraction (Versele, Polka, & Panneton, 2008). Access to a dynamic image of the talker's face and presentation of the speech stimuli in an infant-directed style appears to help some infants recover their attention to the target syllables in the presence of a distraction masker whereas visual input with adult-directed speech does not reduce the distraction effect. Infant-directed speech without the visual face input also benefits infant selective attention to speech in the presence of a distraction masker.

Infant-directed speech may help infants attend to speech in a distracting environment and process speech when there is background noise.

Language learning in natural environments takes place in the presence of considerable background noise. Typically this background noise consists of multiple talkers which provides both informational and energetic masking because the target speech input is masked at the auditory periphery by the overlapping frequency components of the background speech. Furthermore, the infant must sort out the multiple sources of the speech to focus on the specific input stream that is being addressed to the infant, a task that depends on many cognitive and perceptual processes (Newman, 2009). Mothers accentuate the prosodic characteristics of infant-directed speech in noisy environments when talking to children as old as 2 years (Newman, 2003). Newman and Hussain (2009) reported that 4.5-month-old infants preferred infant-directed to adult-directed speech in a noisy environment whereas they listened equally long to passages read in either speaking register in quiet conditions. Further research is required to determine if the infant-directed register helps infants to learn from speech input when presented in a noisy environment.

To summarize, the infant is born with a strong interest in speech as an important species-specific signal. Very quickly the infant develops a preference for the mother's voice and the exaggerated prosodic characteristics of the infant-directed speaking register. Infant-directed speech also serves to highlight certain phonetic contrasts and the learning of those contrasts is enhanced when such input is provided in natural social learning interactions. Auditory deprivation early in life and certain neurodevelopmental disorders interfere with the experience-expectant processes that lead to a heightened attention to speech input and appear in turn to delay the acquisition of speech perception and language skills. For those infants who listen to speech however, the input is an important driver of speech perception development. We now turn to the impact of speech input on brain development in relation to the acquisition of language-specific speech perception skills.

Biological Mechanisms

The infant can learn from the speech input only if the input is received through a properly functioning auditory system. The basic structure of the auditory system is established during embryonic development. Moore and Linthicum (2007) describe subsequent development as occurring in three sharply delimited stages. The first stage occurs during the second prenatal trimester and is marked by maturation of the cochlea and myelination of the intracochlear portion of the auditory nerve. The perinatal stage, lasting through the sixth postnatal month, sees rapid maturation of the brainstem pathway. The final stage is protracted with gradual myelination of the auditory cortex progressing through 12 years of age. Progressive myelination throughout the auditory system enhances conduction speed and synchronicity, contributing to maturation of auditory brainstem and cortical evoked potentials. However, the relationship between structure and function in auditory system development is reciprocal; not only does maturation of the auditory system enable transmission of sound energy, sound input itself plays a role in auditory system development specifically with respect to dendritic growth, synaptic remodeling, and the progression of myelination. These authors speculate that auditory deprivation during the different phases of auditory system maturation will have distinct impacts on speech perception and language development. In particular, they speculated that auditory deprivation during the perinatal period

The **cochlea matures during the second trimester** and maturation of the brainstem pathway follows through the sixth postnatal month. Gradual mylenation of the auditory cortex is a protracted process lasting through 12 years of age.

would lead to difficulties with sound discrimination and attention to speech. Sound deprivation at later ages should affect development of auditory cortex, manifested in delayed latencies or atypical topography of the components of auditory evoked emissions and resulting in difficulties with word learning and recognition. Eggermont and Ponton (2003) described the maturation of auditory evoked potentials in children who have cochlear implants. They reported that the positive components of cortical auditory evoked potentials resume maturation after cochlear implantation with a delay that reflects the duration of deafness, accounting for the restoration of open set word recognition in quiet conditions. On the other hand, certain negative components do not emerge even many years after receiving the cochlear implant; their research suggests that maturation of the superficial layers of auditory cortex requires auditory input during a critical period in early childhood. Altered maturation of the upper layers of auditory cortex in children with cochlear implants is associated with poor speech recognition in noise.

According to the **dual-stream model of cortical organization for speech processing** the initial stages of speech perception involve bilateral processing of speech to derive acoustic-phonetic and phonological representations. Subsequent processing diverges into a *ventral stream* that maps sound to meaning and a *dorsal stream* that maps sound to articulatory-based representations.

Cortical organization for the processing of spoken language input goes well beyond the auditory cortex of course. Hickok and Poeppel (Hickok & Peoppel, 2004, 2007) have proposed a dual stream model for the adult brain that is illustrated in Figure 2–12. Mapping of sound to meaning occurs via the left-dominant ventral stream that allows for flexible and parallel processing at multiple levels of representation in broadly distributed neural networks. Initial sensory processing of the spectral and temporal characteristics of the sound input occurs bilaterally in dorsal superior temporal gyrus followed by access to phonological representations in middle to posterior portions of the superior temporal sulcus. Hickok and Peoppel (2007) propose that segment level information, occurring on a fast time scale, and prosodic level information, occurring on a slower time scale, must be analyzed separately and then integrated before accessing phonological representations for words. Furthermore, they propose that the right hemisphere is specialized for long-term integration whereas short-term integration occurs bilaterally. This view contrasts with an alternative hypothesis that the left hemisphere processes rapid temporal cues, whereas the right hemisphere is specialized for the processing of spectral cues in speech (Zatorre, Berlin, & Penhune, 2002). Subsequent to phonological processing, projections through posterior inferior temporal lobe (specifically portions of the middle temporal and the inferior temporal gyrus) link phonological representations to widely distributed semantic representations. Mapping of phonological representations to articulatory representations occurs via the strongly left-lateralized dorsal stream. This stream includes an area at the parietotemporal boundary in the sylvian fissure that serves as a sensorimotor interface for mapping between auditory and articulatory representations of speech that themselves are located in the frontal lobe, specifically parts of premotor cortex and Broca's area, that subserve articulation and phonological short-term memory.

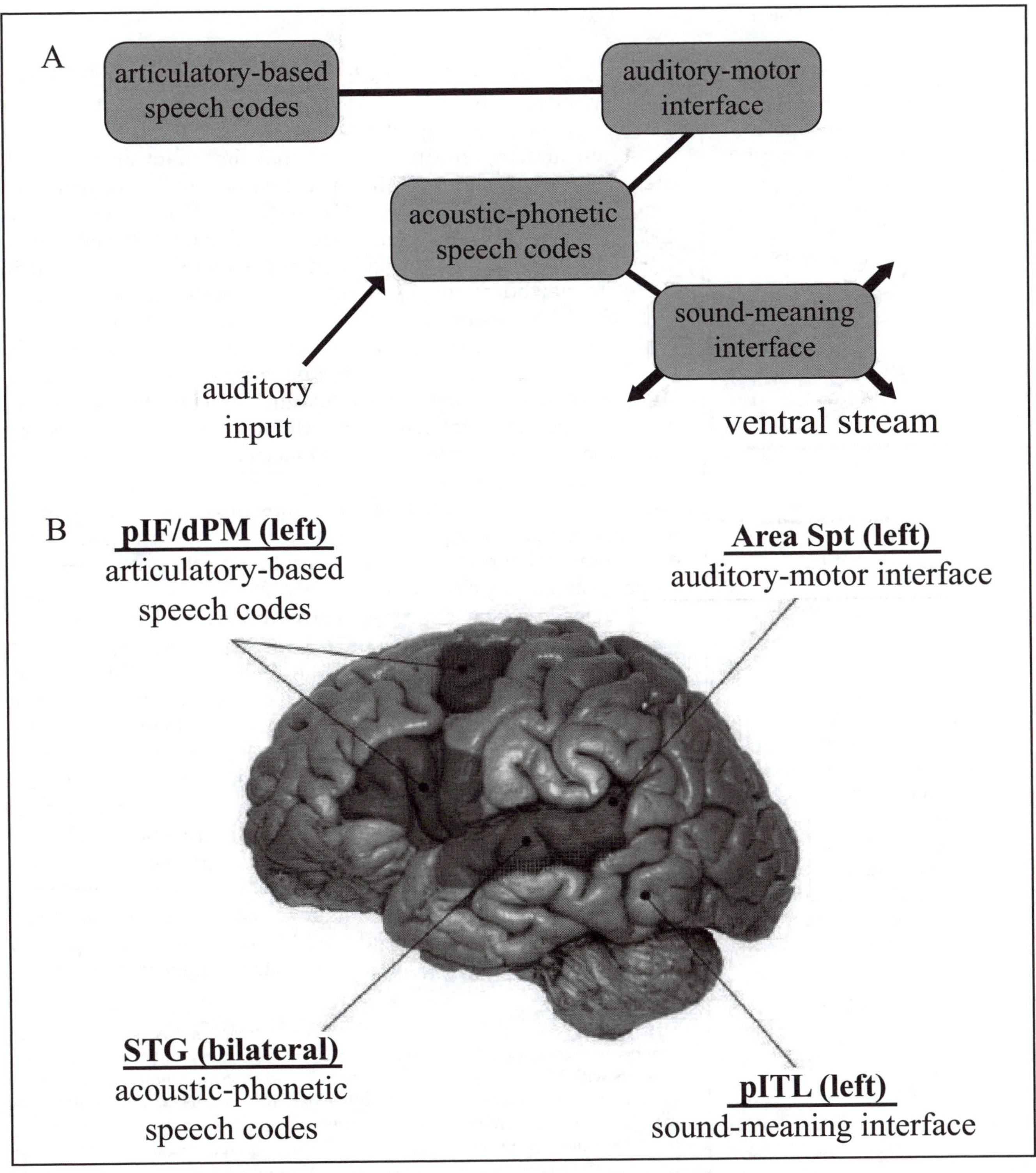

Figure 2–12. *Dual-stream model of cortical organization for speech processing.* **A.** *Initial stages of speech perception involve bilateral processing of speech to derive acoustic-phonetic and phonological representations. Subsequent processing diverges into a ventral stream that maps sound to meaning and a dorsal stream that maps sound to articulatory-based representations.* **B.** *General locations of model components shown on a lateral view of the brain. Abbreviations: pIF, posterior Inferior Frontal; dPM, dorsal Premotor Cortex; Spt, parietotemporal boundary area in the Sylvian fissure; STG, Superior Temporal Gyrus (the stippled area on STG is the Superior Temporal Sulcus); pITL, posterior Inferior Temporal Lobe. From Hickok and Poeppel (2004). Dorsal and ventral streams: a framework for understanding aspects of the functional anatomy of language.* Cognition, *92, Figure 1, p. 71. Reproduced with permission of Elsevier BV.*

Hickok and Peoppel (2007) assign speech perception to the dorsal pathway and speech recognition to the ventral pathway although initial sensory and phonological processing is shared by these streams.[3]

Brain-imaging studies suggest that the infant brain is well prepared for speech processing at the earliest stages of language acquisition.

Brain imaging studies suggest that the infant brain is well prepared for speech processing at the earliest stages of language acquisition (Dehaene-Lambertz, Hertz-Pannier, Dubois, & Dehaene, 2008; Dehaene-Lambertz, Pannier-Hertz, & Dubois, 2006; Friederici, 2006; Paterson, Heim, Thomas Friedman, Choudhury, & Benasich, 2006). In newborns and 3-month-olds, left-dominant increases in cerebral blood flow over temporal regions were observed in response to speech input in comparison to silence. In 3-month-olds, left dominant ERP responses have been observed for both tones and CV syllables. At the same age, right dominant ERP responses have been observed for sentences with normal pitch contours and phrase boundaries versus sentences that lacked these prosodic cues. Overall, these studies indicate engagement of superior temporal, inferior parietal and frontal brain regions in very young infants in response to varying types of speech input that suggest significant developmental continuity in the neural networks associated with speech and language processing.

Neurophysiological changes associated with the **shift to language-specific processing of speech** include increasingly focal and left-lateralized responses to the between-category stimulus change, reflecting integration of auditory representations with higher cognitive networks.

Other studies have traced changes in brain function as the infant navigates the shift from language general to language specific perception of phonetic contrasts. For example, Minagawa-Kawai, Mori, Naoi, and Kojima (2007) used near-infrared spectroscopy to describe the neurophysiological changes that are associated with the acquisition of a vowel duration contrast by Japanese-learning infants aged between 3 and 28 months of age. Infants listened passively to repetitions of a two-syllable word ([mama]) in which the last word in the sequence differed from the previous repetitions ([mama:]). On different days, infants were exposed to a within-category and a between-category change in vowel duration but with absolute difference in duration held constant. The results revealed marked developmental remodeling of the amplitude, within-hemisphere topography and laterality of ERP responses. In infants younger than 6 months

[3]Hickok and Poeppel (2007) distinguish speech perception and speech recognition because these skills "double dissociate" in adult stroke patients (specifically, patients with Wernicke's aphasia may show good discrimination of syllables but poor word comprehension whereas other patients with lesions in frontal areas may have impaired syllable discrimination but good word comprehension). By their definitions, a speech perception task involves perceptual operations on sublexical units but a speech recognition task requires the listener to link the stimulus with representations in the mental lexicon. Speech perception and speech recognition are seen as aspects of speech processing, a term used to cover any task involving aurally presented speech. It is not clear that the boundaries between these levels of processing can be drawn so distinctly in the infant and young child when the linkages between acoustic-phonetic, phonological, and semantic representations are in the early stages of development. Furthermore, Hickok and Poeppel (2004) point out that the extent to which each pathway is employed in any given task depends upon the exact task requirements and the specific strategies that the individual listener uses during task completion.

of age, diffuse and bilateral ERP responses were observed to both within- and between-category changes in vowel duration. The shift from language-general to language-specific processing of the phonetic contrast was indicated by greater amplitude of responses to the between-category change compared to within-category change at 6 months although the ERP responses were not left-lateralized at this young age. The shift from phonetic to phonemic processing was indexed by a temporary loss of phoneme specific responding at 10 months of age followed by recovery of specific responses to the between-category change at 13 months with emerging left-dominance. In infants aged 25 months or older, increasingly focal and left-lateralized responses to the between-category change were observed, a pattern of ERP response that was very similar to that observed in Japanese-speaking adult listeners. The authors speculate that early processing of speech relies primarily on auditory mechanisms and that the observed qualitative shifts in neurophysiological responses reflect an integration of auditory representations with higher cognitive networks. The focus and specificity of neural responses observed in the oldest infants, as shown in Figure 2–13, reflects the acquisition of stable neural representations that can be resistant to change even with intensive exposure to second language input (Kuhl et al., 2008; Zhang et al., 2009).

Developmental changes in functional lateralization for word recognition have been described for monolingual English-learning (Mills, Coffey-Corina, & Neville, 1997) and Spanish-English bilingual toddlers (Conboy & Mills, 2006). In both studies, ERPs were recorded from 13- and 20-month-olds while they listened to familiar and unfamiliar single words. Analysis of the results focused on the P100, thought to index sensory processing of the speech input, and the N200 and N375, thought to index higher level word recognition processes. Maturation of these components is reflected in reductions in the latency of the peak. Changes in lateralization of the amplitudes and focalization of ERP responses index increasing specialization of specific brain areas for speech and language processing. The P100 shows greater left lateralization to known words for monolingual children with higher percentile rankings on vocabulary measures. Among bilingual children, the P100 is more left lateralized for known words in the dominant language for children with greater total conceptual vocabulary size. The negative components are more right lateralized during the early stages of word learning and become more symmetrical with increasing word familiarity. Developmental changes in these negative components are linked to absolute vocabulary size and age rather than relative language skill within a given age group. Overall, studies of monolingual and bilingual children demonstrate that brain maturation for language processing, especially as reflected by the negative ERP components, reflects the child's language experience rather than general brain maturation processes.

Studies of **monolingual and bilingual children** demonstrate that brain maturation for language processing, especially as reflected by the negative ERP components, reflects the child's language experience rather than general brain maturation processes.

To summarize, studies employing diverse imaging technologies to describe brain responses to multiple forms of auditory

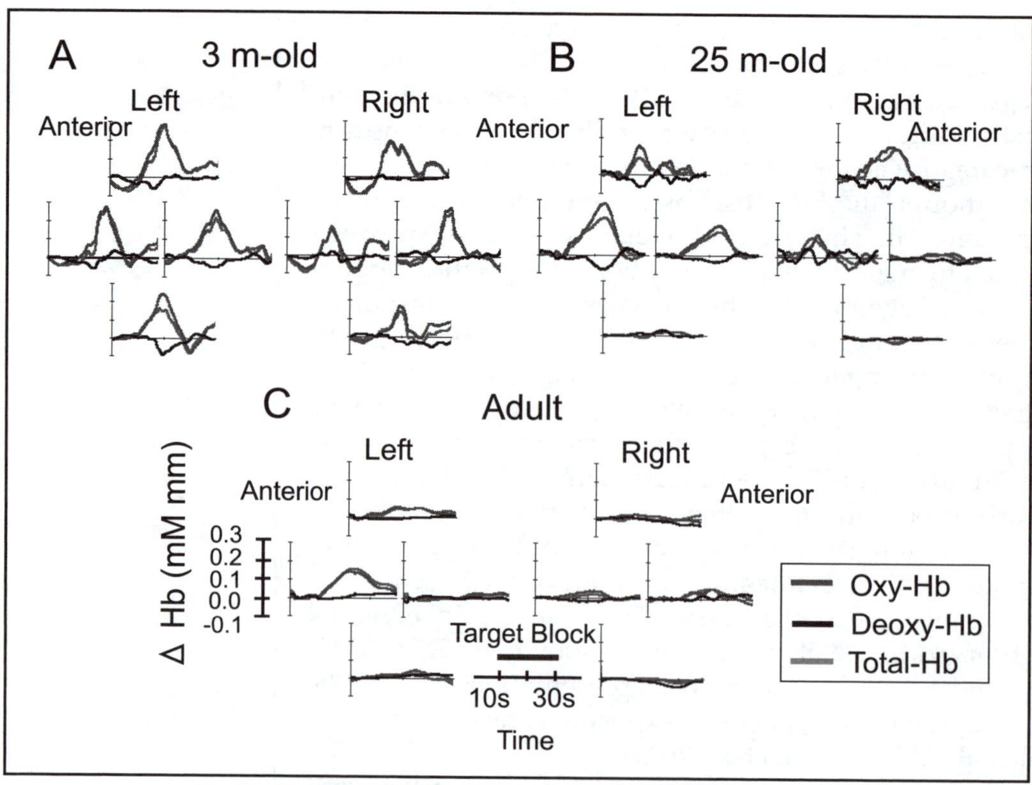

Figure 2–13. *Near infrared spectroscopy responses from 8 channels placed over the temporal areas of the right and left hemispheres from 3 of 6 groups of subjects in a study of the acquisition of a Japanese vowel duration contrast. Automatic change detection responses to [mama:] in contrast to [mama] regardless of whether the change was phonemic were observed in all age groups but the topography of the responses varied with age: (**A**) responses from 3-month-olds were bilateral and broadly distributed; (**B**) responses from older infants were less broadly distributed with left-dominance emerging; and (**C**) responses from adults were focal and left-lateralized. From Minagawa-Kawai et al. (2007). Neural attunement processes in infants during the acquisition of a language-specific phonemic contrast.* Journal of Neuroscience: The Official Journal of the Society for Neuroscience *by Society for Neuroscience, 27(2), Figure 3, p. 318. Copyright 2007. Reproduced with permission of Society for Neuroscience.*

input provide converging evidence of structural and functional specialization for speech processing in the infant brain at the earliest stages of language learning. Early processing of speech input reflects resolution of auditory rather than phonological properties of speech. Maturation of the P1 (P100 in the infant brain) correlates with relative indices of language development, suggesting that individual differences in early sensory processing may explain some part of variation in rate of language learning. Reciprocal relationships between maturation of brain function and language learning are clearly evident however. The latency and topography of ERP responses to within-category and between-category phonetic contrasts undergo qualitative shifts as the infant progresses from language-general to language-specific processing of speech and from phonetic to phonemic processing of language. Different neurophysiological responses to familiar and unfamiliar words are observed within the same bilingual infant in the dominant versus nondominant language. It is clear that specific aspects of the infant's experience with language input are driving developmental reorganization of certain ERP components. In general these developmental changes are characterized by greater neural efficiency, reflected in earlier latencies, greater amplitudes, increasing focalization and stronger left-dominance of brain responses to language-specific and familiar speech input. Some of the cognitive-linguistic learning processes that are associated with these neurophysiological changes are considered in the next section.

Cognitive Learning Processes

The first year of life is marked by a qualitative shift in the mode of speech perception: initially the infant perceives speech via language-general psychoacoustic mechanisms; gradually the infant's perceptual behavior becomes attuned to a set of language-specific phonetic categories. The process by which the ambient language shapes the infant's perceptual representations is dependent at least in part on a statistical learning mechanism that is sensitive to the distribution of acoustic cues in the speech input. For example, the top part of Figure 1–13 illustrates the distribution of first and second formant frequencies of vowels in the speech produced by mothers while speaking to their infants. A useful statistical learning mechanism must be sensitive to the clustering that is apparent in the distribution of F2 values, with modal F2s occurring at 1900, 2500, and 3100 Hz, as well as correlations among acoustic parameters such as the relationship between this particular distribution of F2 values and the modal value of F1 that occurs at 700 Hz. Given the facts of early perceptual learning, the mechanism must also be able to function with data that is acquired incrementally, without prior knowledge of the number of categories present in the system and without supervision, that is, explicit information about the category membership of each incoming exemplar. A number of computational models have been developed that meet these requirements and successfully learn phonetic categories given reasonably realistic distributions of abstracted acoustic cues to certain phonetic contrasts (e.g., for VOT, see McMurray, Aslin, & Toscano, 2009). Other researchers have modeled the implementation of statistical learning in the brain, simulating the perceptual magnet effect when presenting self-organizing networks with formant frequency information (Guenther & Gjaja, 1996) or synthetic vowels preprocessed with a model of the auditory periphery (Salminen, Tiitinen, & May, 2009).

A **statistical learning** mechanism allows the child to acquire knowledge of linguistic structure by tracking the distribution of acoustic-phonetic cues in the language input.

The existence of statistical learning has been demonstrated in behavioral studies with infants, employing natural or artificial distributions of speech and nonspeech stimuli. For example, Maye, Weiss, and Aslin (2008) created multiple continua of stimuli representing the Hindi contrast between prevoiced and voiceless unaspirated stops, specifically the dental [da] versus [ta] and the velar [ga] versus [ka], as produced by a male talker and digitally altered to vary in voice-onset-time between −100 and +21 ms VOT. English-learning infants, aged 8 months, were assigned to one of three different familiarization conditions: one group heard all of the VOTs but distributed in bimodal fashion to represent prevoiced and voiceless categories; another group heard all of the VOTs but distributed in a unimodal fashion to represent a single category; a control group heard a repeating sequence of tones (Figure 2–14A). After the familiarization phase all of the infants were tested for their ability to discriminate between stimuli with −50 versus +7 ms VOT, using a visual habituation procedure. Some infants were exposed during familiarization to the dental continua and others to the velar continua. In the bimodal condition, some infants were tested with the contrast that they were not exposed to during familiarization; this testing condition measured generalization of learning from one place of articulation to another. The results, as shown in Figure 2–14B, indicate that even brief laboratory exposure to a bimodal distribution of VOTs facilitated perception of a nonnative VOT contrast. Furthermore, this facilitation effect was shown to generalize from one place of articulation to another. This is one of several studies showing that the way in which acoustic cues are distributed in speech influences infants' extraction of phonetic categories from language input (e.g., Anderson, Morgan, & White, 2003; Maye, Werker, & Gerken, 2002).

The way in which **acoustic cues** are distributed in speech influences infants' extraction of phonetic categories from language input early in infancy and impacts on word learning later in the infant period.

The statistical distribution of acoustic cues in the ambient language environment also impacts on word learning later in the infant period. Mattock, Polka, Rvachew and Krehm (2010) used the switch task to investigate word learning by 17-month-old infants who were monolingual learners of English or French or simultaneous French-English bilinguals. The task was structured to teach the infants to pair the words "bowce" and "gowce" to novel objects. Although the phonemes /b/ and /g/ are phonemic in both English and French, the phonetic implementation is not identical. For all groups, word learning was best when the distribution of phonetic cues in the experimental input matched their environmental input. For example, bilingual infants could learn the task when both French and English versions of the words were presented. French monolingual infants could learn the new words only when presented with French input; they were unable to succeed with bilingual or monolingual English input that provided very subtle differences in the distribution of VOT cues relative to their experience with stop VOT in the ambient language environment.

The statistical learning mechanism allows the infant to discover word boundaries by tracking **transitional probabilities** between sequences of phones or syllables in the speech input.

Further to the topic of word learning, the statistical learning mechanism allows the infant to discover word boundaries by tracking transitional probabilities between sequences of phones or syllables in the speech input. Pelucchi, Hay, and Saffran (2009) demonstrated this by exposing English-learning infants to Italian sentences and testing their ability to segment words from this input using a preferential looking procedure (the experimental design

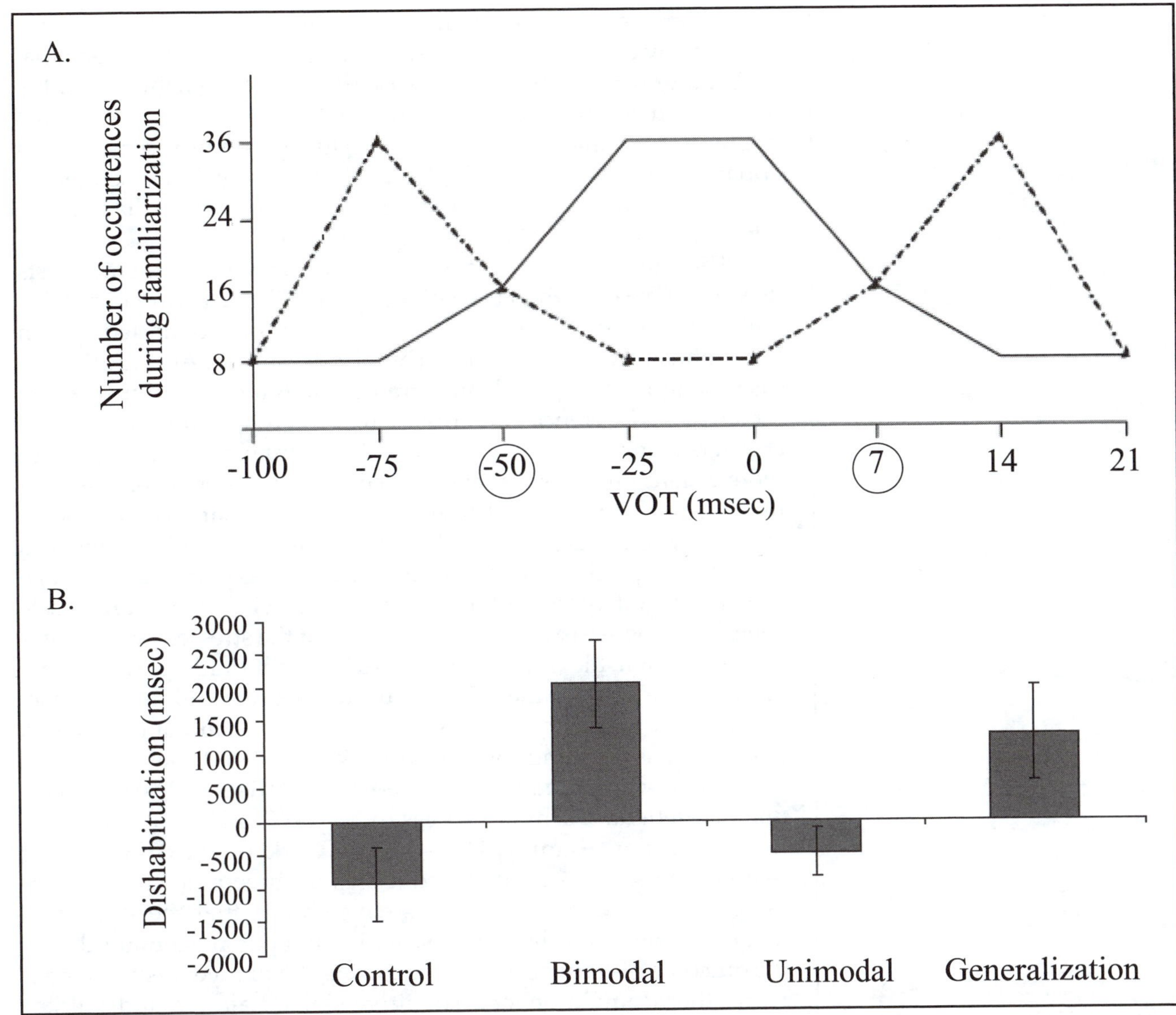

Figure 2–14. *Demonstration of statistical learning by 8-month-old English-learning infants.* **A.** *Presentation frequency by VOT during the familiarization phase in the bimodal condition* (dotted line) *and unimodal condition* (solid line). *Test stimuli are circled.* **B.** *Mean dishabituation (average looking time for two change trials minus average for final two habituation trials) by condition, collapsed across velar and dental places of articulation. Error bars indicate 1 standard error. From Maye, J., Weiss, D. J., and Aslin, R. N. (2008). Statistical phonetic learning in infants: facilitation and feature generalization.* Developmental Science *by European Society for Developmental Psychology,* 11(1), *Figure 2, p. 125 and Figure 3, p. 127. Reproduced with permission of Blackwell Publishing Ltd.*

was similar to that implemented by Jusczyk, Newsome, and Houston to study the emergence of segmentation abilities for words with trochaic and iambic stress patterns, as described earlier in this chapter). The four trochaic target words in the familiarization passages (*fuga, melo, bici,* and *casa*) were presented with equal frequency but the transitional probability of the syllable sequences varied. The transitional probability of the syllables in the words *fuga* and *melo* was 1.00 for each word because the constituent syllables did not occur in any other words. However, for *bici* and *casa*, the transitional probability was lower at .33 because the stressed syllables *bi* and *ca* occurred in combination with other syllables to form other words within the familiarization passages. During the test phase it was apparent that words with high transitional probability sequences were easier for the 8-month-old infants to recognize than words with lower transitional probability sequences.

The importance of the statistical learning mechanism manifests itself most clearly when transitional probability cues are in conflict with other potential cues to word boundaries in connected speech (e.g., Johnson & Jusczyk, 2001; Thiessen & Saffran, 2003). Although Jusczyk and colleagues demonstrated that 6-month-old infants are sensitive to differences in stress pattern as reported earlier in this chapter, Thiessen and Saffran found that infants of this age were more reliant on statistical cues to word boundaries when learning to recognize new words. These results suggest that it is the infant's sensitivity to statistical cues that leads English-learning infants to discover the predominance of the trochaic stress pattern. By the age of 9 months, infants were apt to treat stressed syllables as word onsets even when the statistical cues indicated that the stressed syllable was the second syllable of an iambic word. It is not until approximately 11 months of age that the infant is able to integrate both types of cue, allowing more consistent recognition of trochaic and iambic words in the English-learning context (Jusczyk et al., 1999).

Other studies have confirmed that statistical learning is a domain-general learning process, not specifically tied to linguistic stimuli. For example, Dawson and Gerken (2009) found that 4-month-olds could abstract sequences of three-note chords from musical input. Other researchers have shown that the shift from language-general to language-specific phonetic perception that is the outcome of statistical learning during the first year is associated with other domain general cognitive skills. Lalonde and Werker (1995) demonstrated that the decline in perceptual ability for nonnative consonant contrasts is correlated with visual categorization skills and success on the A-not-B task (traditionally thought to index object permanence but known to be associated with executive functions). In a similar study, Conboy, Sommerville, and Kuhl (2008) found that perception of a nonnative voicing contrast was negatively associated with performance on tasks involving inhibitory cognitive control. In contrast, perceptual performance for native language phonemic contrasts was not associated with domain-general cognitive skills or use of communicative gestures but was positively correlated with vocabulary size. The relationship between cognitive control and language development has been studied in preschool and school-age children in relation to family socioeconomic status as well as home and school environment variables (Noble, McCandliss, & Farah, 2007; Noble, Norman, & Farah, 2005; Stevens, Lauinger, & Neville, 2009). These studies raise the question of the nature of the relationship among these variables—it cannot be assumed that cognitive control or other executive functions are causally related to language development. In fact, Noble et al. suggest that high SES families are able to provide home and school environments that support superior language development that in turn drives performance on measures of executive function.

In this chapter, speech perception development, with a focus on the infant period, has been presented as the foundation of phonological development. Four critical events in this developmental trajectory have been highlighted: (1) the shift from language general to language specific phonetic perception, occurring during the first year of life; (2) the emergence of phonemic perception coincident with word learning in the second year of life; (3) the gradual acquisition of implicit phonological awareness skills throughout the preschool period; and (4) the learning of explicit phonological awareness skills during the early school years. These developments are supported by experience expectant and experience dependent processes that, in normal development, take advantage of an exquisite match between the ambient language environment and a neurophysiological substrate that is perfectly adapted for learning from linguistic input at if not before the infant's birth. The next chapter also focuses on the early stages of speech development, in this case describing the development of speech production abilities.

References

Anderson, J. L., Morgan, J. L., & White, K. S. (2003). A statistical basis for speech sound discrimination. *Language and Speech, 46*, 155–182.

Anthony, J. L., & Lonigan, C. J. (2004). The nature of phonological awareness: Converging evidence from four studies of preschool and early grade school children. *Journal of Educational Psychology, 96*(1), 43–55.

Beckman, M. E., & Edwards, J. (2000). The ontongeny of phonological categories and the primacy of lexical learning in linguistic development. *Child Development, 71*, 240–249.

Bernhardt, B., Kemp, N., & Werker, J. F. (2007). Early word-object associations and later language development. *First Language, 27*(4), 315–328.

Best, C. T., McRoberts, G. W., LaFleur, R., & Silver-Isenstadt, J. (1995). Divergent developmental patterns for infants perception of two non-native consonant contrasts. *Infant Behavior and Development, 18*, 339–350.

Best, C. T., McRoberts, G. W., & Sithole, N. N. (1988). The phonological basis of perceptual loss for non-native contrasts: maintenance of discrimination among Zulu clicks by English-speaking adults and infants. *Journal of Experimental Psychology: Human Perception and Performance, 14*, 345–360.

Bosch, L., & Sebastián-Gallés, N. (2003). Simultaneous bilingualism and the perception of a language-specific vowel contrast in the first year of life. *Language and Speech, 46*, 217–243.

Burnham, D., Earnshaw, L. J., & Clark, J. E. (1991). Development of categorical identification of native and non-native bilabial stops: infants, children and adults. *Journal of Child Language, 18*, 231–260.

Burnham, D., Kitamura, C., & Vollmer-Conner, U. (2002). What's new, pussycat? On talking to babies and animals. *Science, 296*(5572), 1435.

Byrne, B., & Fielding-Barnsley, R. (1993). Recognition of phoneme invariance by beginning readers: Confounding effects of global similarity. *Reading and Writing, 6*, 315–324.

Carroll, J. M., & Snowling, M. J. (2001). The effects of global similarity between stimuli on children's judgment of rime and alliteration. *Applied Psycholinguistics, 22*(3), 327–342.

Chaney, C. (1992). Language development, metalinguistic skills, and print knowledge in 3-year-old children. *Applied Psycholinguistics, 13*, 485–514.

Cheour, M., Ceponiene, R., Lehtokoski, A., Luuk, A., Allik, J., Alho, K., & Näätänen, R. (1998). Development of language-specific phoneme representation in the infant brain. *Nature Neuroscience, 1*, 351–353.

Cheour, M., Korpilahti, P., Martynova, O., & Lang, O.-H. (2001). Mismatch negativity and late discriminative negativity in investigating speech perception and learning in children and infants. *Audiology and Neurotology, 6*, 2–11.

Chiappe, P., Siegel, L. S., & Gottardo, A. (2002). Reading-related skills of kindergartners from diverse linguistic backgrounds. *Applied Psycholinguistics, 23*(1), 95–116.

Claessen, M., Heath, S. M., Fletcher, J., Hogben, J., & Leitao, S. (2009). Quality of phonological representations: A window into the lexicon. *International Journal of Language and Communication Disorders, 44*(2), 121–144.

Conboy, B. T., & Mills, D. L. (2006). Two languages, one developing brain: Event-related potentials to words in bilingual toddlers. *Developmental Science, 9*(1), F1–F12.

Conboy, B. T., Sommerville, J. A., & Kuhl, P. K. (2008). Cognitive control factors in speech perception at 11 months. *Developmental Psychology, 44*(5), 1505–1512.

Cooper, R. P., & Aslin, R. N. (1990). Preference for infant-directed speech in the first month after birth. *Child Development, 61*(5), 1584–1595.

Dawson, C., & Gerken, L. (2009). From domain-generality to domain-sensitivity: 4-month-olds learn an abstract repetition rule in music that 7-month-old do not. *Cognition, 111*, 378–382.

DeCasper, A. J., & Fifer, W. P. (1980). Of human bonding: Newborns prefer their mothers' voices. *Science, 208*, 1174–1176.

DeCasper, A. J., & Spence, M. J. (1986). Prenatal maternal speech influences newborns' perception of speech sounds. *Infant Behavior and Development, 9*(2), 133–150.

Dehaene-Lambertz, G. (2004). Bases cérébrales de l'acquisition du langage: apport de la neuro-imagerie. *Neuropsychiatrie de l'enfance et de l'adolescence, 52*, 452–459.

Dehaene-Lambertz, G., & Baillet, S. (1998). A phonological representation in the infant brain. *NeuroReport, 9*(8), 1885–1888.

Dehaene-Lambertz, G., & Gliga, T. (2004). Common neural basis for phoneme processing in infants and adults. *Journal of Cognitive Neuroscience, 16*(8), 1375–1387.

Dehaene-Lambertz, G., Hertz-Pannier, L., Dubois, J., & Dehaene, S. (2008). How does early brain organization promote language acquisition in humans. *European Review, 16*(4), 399–411.

Dehaene-Lambertz, G., Pannier-Hertz, L., & Dubois, J. (2006). Nature and nurture in language acquisition: anatomical and functional brain-imaging studies in infants. *Trends in Neurosciences, 29*(7), 367–373.

Dehaene-Lambertz, G., & Pena, M. (2001). Electrophysiological evidence for automatic phonetic processing in neonates. *NeuroReport, 12*(14), 3155–3158.

Edwards, J., Fourakis, M., Beckman, M. E., & Fox, R. A. (1999). Characterizing knowledge deficits in phonological disorders. *Journal of Speech, Language, and Hearing Research, 42*, 169–186.

Edwards, J., Fox, R. A., & Rogers, C. L. (2002). Final consonant discrimination in children: Effects of phonological disorder, vocabulary size, and articulatory accuracy. *Journal of Speech, Language, and Hearing Research, 45*, 231–242.

Eggermont, J., & Ponton, C. W. (2003). Auditory-evoked potential studies of cortical maturation in normal hearing and implanted children: Correlations with changes in structure and speech perception. *Acta Otolaryngology, 2003*, 123.

Eilers, R. E., Gavin, W., & Wilson, W. R. (1979). Linguistic experience and phonetic perception in infancy: A cross-linguistic study. *Child Development, 50*, 14–18.

Eilers, R. E., & Minifie, F. D. (1975). Fricative discrimination in early infancy. *Journal of Speech and Hearing Research, 18*, 158–167.

Eimas, P. D. (1975). Auditory and phonetic coding of the cues for speech: Discrimination of the [r-l] distinction by young infants. *Perception and Psychophysics, 18*(5), 341–347.

Eimas, P. D., & Miller, J. (1980). Contextual effects in infant speech perception. *Science, 209*, 1140–1141.

Eimas, P. D., & Miller, J. L. (1991). A constraint on the discrimination of speech by young infants. *Language and Speech, 34*, 251–263.

Eimas, P. D., Siqueland, E. R., Jusczyk, P. W., & Vigorito, J. (1971). Speech perception in infants. *Science, New Series, 171*(3968), 303–306.

Eisenberg, L. S., Shannon, R. V., Martinez, A. S., Wygonski, J., & Boothroyd, A. (2000). Speech recognition with reduced spectral cues as a function of age. *Journal of the Acoustical Society of America, 107*(5), 2704–2710.

Elliott, L. L., Longinotti, C., Clifton, L., & Meyer, D. (1981). Detection and identification thresholds for consonant-vowel syllables. *Perception and Psychophysics, 30*, 411–416.

Englund, K. T. (2005). Voice onset time in infant directed speech over the first six months. *First Language, 25*(2), 219–234.

Fallon, M., Trehub, S. E., & Schneider, B. A. (2000). Children's perception of speech in multitalker babble. *Journal of the Acoustical Society of America, 108*(6), 3023–3029.

Fennell, C. T., & Werker, J. F. (2003). Early word learners' ability to access phonetic detail in well-known words. *Language and Speech, 46*, 245–264.

Ferguson, C., & Farwell, C. B. (1975). Words and sounds in early acquisition. *Language, 51*(2), 419–439.

Fernald, A., & Kuhl, P. K. (1987). Acoustic determinants of infant preference for motherese. *Infant Behavior and Development, 10*(3), 279–293.

Friederici, A. D. (2006). The neural basis of language development and its impairment. *Neuron, 52*(6), 941–952.

Friederici, A. D., Friedrich, M., & Christophe, A. (2007). Brain responses in 4-month-old infants are already language specific. *Current Biology, 17*(14), 1208–1211.

Garnica, O. K. (1973). The development of phonemic speech perception. In T. E. Moore (Ed.), *Cognitive development and the acquisition of language* (pp. 215–222). New York, NY: Academic Press.

Gerken, L. (2009). *Language development*. San Diego, CA: Plural Publishing.

Gombert, J. E. (1992). *Meta-linguistic development*. London, UK: Harvester.

Gottlieb, G. (2002). On the epigenetic evolution of species-specific perception: The developmental manifold concept. *Cognitive Development, 17*, 1287–1300.

Greenough, W. T., Black, J. E., & Wallace, C. S. (1987). Experience and brain development. *Child Development, 58*, 539–559.

Guenther, F. H., & Gjaja, M. N. (1996). The perceptual magnet effect as an emergent property of neural map formation. *Journal of the Acoustical Society of America, 100*(2), 1111–1121.

Hazan, V., & Barrett, S. (2000). The development of phonemic categorization in children aged 6-12. *Journal of Phonetics, 28*, 377–396.

Hickok, G., & Peoppel, D. (2004). Dorsal and ventral streams: a framework for understanding aspects of the functional anatomy of language. *Cognition, 92*, 67–99.

Hickok, G., & Poeppel, D. (2007). The cortical organization of speech processing. *Nature Reviews: Neuroscience, 8*, 393–402.

Hillenbrand, J. (1983). Perceptual organization of speech sounds by infants. *Journal of Speech and Hearing Research, 26*(2), 268–282.

Hillenbrand, J. (1984). Speech perception by infants: Categorization based on nasal consonant place of articulation. *Journal of the Acoustical Society of America, 75*(5), 1613–1622.

Hillenbrand, J., Minifie, F. D., & Edwards, T. J. (1979). Tempo of spectrum change as a cue in speech-sound discrimination by infants. *Journal of Speech and Hearing Research, 22*(1), 147–165.

Höhle, B., Bijeljac-Babic, R., Herold, B., Weissenborn, J., & Nazzi, T. (2009). Language specific prosodic preferences during the first half year of life: Evidence from German and French infants. *Infant Behavior and Development, 32*(3), 262–274.

Hohle, B., van de Vijver, R., & Weissenborn, J. (2006). Word processing at 19 months and its relation to language performance at 30 months: A retrospective analysis of data from German learning children. *Advances in Speech-Language Pathology, 8*, 356–363.

Hoonhorst, I., Colin, C., Markessis, E., Radeau, M., Deltrenre, P., & Serniclaes, W. (2009). French native speakers in the making: From language-general to language-specific voicing boundaries. *Journal of Experimental Child Psychology, 104*, 353–366.

Houston, D. M., Pisoni, D., Kirk, K. I., Ying, A., & Miyamoto, R. T. (2003). Speech perception skills of deaf infants following cochlear implantation: A first report. *International Journal of Pediatric Otorhinolaryngology, 67*, 479–495.

Joanisse, M. F., Manis, F. R., Keating, P., & Seidenberg, M. S. (2000). Language deficits in dyslexic children: Speech perception, phonology, and morphology. *Journal of Experimental Child Psychology, 77*, 30–60.

Johnson, E. K., & Jusczyk, P. W. (2001). Word segmentation by 8-month-olds: When speech cues count more than statistics. *Journal of Memory and Language, 44*(4), 548–567.

Johnson, E. K., & Seidl, A. (2008). Clause segmentation by 6-month-old infants: A crosslinguistic perspective. *Infancy, 13*(5), 440–455.

Jusczyk, P. W., & Bertoncini, J. (1988). Viewing the development of speech perception as an innately guided learning process. *Language and Speech, 31*(3), 217–238.

Jusczyk, P. W., Copan, H., & Thompson, E. (1978). Perception by 2-month-old infants of glide contrasts in multisyllabic utterances. *Perception and Psychophysics, 24*, 515–520.

Jusczyk, P. W., Cutler, A., & Redanz, N. (1993). Infants' preference for the predominant stress patterns of English words. *Child Development, 64*, 675–687.

Jusczyk, P. W., Hohne, E. A., & Bauman, A. (1999). Infants' sensitivity to allophonic cues for word segmentation. *Perception and Psychophysics, 61*(8), 1465–1476.

Jusczyk, P. W., Houston, D. M., & Newsome, M. (1999). The beginnings of word segmentation in English-learning infants. *Cognitive Psychology, 39*(3–4), 159–207.

Jusczyk, P. W., & Thompson, E. (1978). Perception of a phonetic contrast in multisyllabic utterances by 2-month-old infants. *Perception and Psychophysics, 23*(2), 105–109.

Karzon, R. G. (1985). Discrimination of polysyllabic sequences by one- to four-month-old infants. *Journal of Experimental Child Psychology, 39*(2), 326–342.

Kisilevsky, B. S., Hains, S. M. J., Brown, C. A., Lee, C. T., Cowperthwaite, B., Stutzman, S. S., . . . Wang, Z. (2009). Fetal sensitivity to properties of maternal speech and language. *Infant Behavior and Development, 32*(1), 59–71.

Krause, S. E. (1982). Vowel duration as a perceptual cue to postvocalic consonant voicing in young children and adults. *Journal of the Acoustical Society of America, 71*(4), 990–995.

Kuhl, P. K. (1979). Speech perception in early infancy: Perceptual constancy for spectrally dissimilar vowel categories. *Journal of the Acoustical Society of America, 66*(6), 1668–1679.

Kuhl, P. K., Andruski, J. E., Chistovich, I. A., Kozhevnikova, E. V., Ryskina, V. L., Stolyarova, E. I., . . . Lacerda, F. (1997). Cross-language analysis of phonetic units in language addressed to infants. *Science, 277*, 684–686.

Kuhl, P. K., Coffey-Corina, S., Padden, D., & Dawson, G. (2005). Links between social and linguistic processing of speech in preschool children with autism: Behavioral and electrophysiological measures. *Developmental Science, 8*(1), F1–F12.

Kuhl, P. K., Conboy, B. T., Coffey-Corina, S., Padden, D., Rivera-Gaxiola, M., & Nelson, T. (2008). Phonetic learning as a pathway to language: New data and native language magnet theory expanded (NLM-e). *Philosophical Transactions of the Royal Society, 363*, 979–1000.

Kuhl, P. K., Stevens, E., Hayashi, A., Deguchi, T., Kiritani, S., & Iverson, P. (2006). Infants show a facilitation effect for native language phonetic perception between 6 and 12 months. *Developmental Science, 9*(2), F13–F21.

Kuhl, P. K., Tsao, F., & Liu, H. (2003). Foreign-language experience in infancy: Effects of short-term exposure and social interaction on phonetic learning. *Proceedings of the National Academy of Sciences, 100*(15), 9096–9101).

Kuhl, P. K., Williams, K. A., Lacerda, F., Stevens, K. N., & Lindblom, B. (1992). Linguistic experience alters phonetic perception in infants by 6 months of age. *Science, 255*(606–608).

Lalonde, C. E., & Werker, J. F. (1995). Cognitive influences on cross-language speech perception in infancy. *Infant Behavior and Development, 18*, 459–475.

Lasky, R., Syrdal-Lasky, A., & Klein, R. E. (1975). VOT discrimination by four to six and a half month old infants from Spanish environments. *Journal of Experimental Child Psychology, 20*, 215–225.

Lecanuet, J.-P., Gautheron, B., Locatelli, A., Schaal, B., Jacquet, A.-Y., & Busnel, M.-C. (1998). What sounds reach fetuses: Biological and non-biological modeling of the transmission of pure tones. *Developmental Psychobiology, 33*(3), 203–219.

Leppanen, P. H. T., Pihko, E., Eklund, K. M., & Lyytinen, H. (1999). Cortical responses of infants with and without a genetic risk for dyslexia: II. Group effects. *NeuroReport, 10*, 969–973.

Levitt, A., Jusczyk, P. W., Murray, J., & Carden, G. (1988). Context effects in two-month-old infants' perception of labiodental/interdental fricative contrasts. *Journal of Experimental Psychology: Human Perception and Performance, 14*(3), 361–368.

Liu, H.-M., Kuhl, P. K., & Tsao, F.-M. (2003). An association between mothers' speech clarity and infants' speech discrimination skills. *Developmental Science, 6*(3), F1–F10.

Lonigan, C. J., Burgess, S. R., Anthony, J. L., & Barker, T. A. (1998). Development of phonological sensitivity in 2- to 5-year-old children. *Journal of Educational Psychology, 90*(2), 294–311.

Lyytinen, H., Aro, M., Eklund, K., Erskine, J., Guttorm, T., Laakso, M., . . . Torppa, M. (2004). The development of children at familial risk for dyslexia: Birth to early school age. *Annals of Dyslexia, 54*(2), 184–220.

Maillart, C., Schelstraete, M.-A., & Hupet, M. (2004). Phonological representations in children with SLI: A study of French. *Journal of Speech, Language, and Hearing Research, 47*, 187–198.

Mattock, K., Polka, L., Rvachew, S., & Krehm, M. (2010). The first steps in word learning are easier when the shoes fit: Comparing monlingual and bilingual infants. *Developmental Science, 13*, 229–243.

Mattys, S. L., & Jusczyk, P. W. (2001). Phonotactic cues for segmentation of fluent speech by infants. *Cognition, 78*(2), 91–121.

Maye, J., Weiss, D. J., & Aslin, R. N. (2008). Statistical phonetic learning in infants: Facilitation and feature generalization. *Developmental Science, 11*(1), 122–134.

Maye, J., Werker, J. F., & Gerken, L. (2002). Infant sensitivity to distributional information can affect phonetic discrimination. *Cognition, 82*, B101–B111.

McBride-Chang, C. (1995). What is phonological awareness? *Journal of Educational Psychology, 87*, 179–192.

McMurray, B., & Aslin, R. N. (2005). Infants are sensitive to within-category variation in speech perception. *Cognition, 95*, B15–B26.

McMurray, B., Aslin, R. N., & Toscano, J. C. (2009). Statistical learning of phonetic categories: Insights from a computational approach. *Developmental Science, 12*(3), 369–378.

McMurray, B., Tanenhaus, M. K., & Aslin, R. N. (2002). Gradient effects of within-category phonetic variation on lexical access. *Cognition, 86*, B33–B42.

McNeill, B. C., & Hesketh, A. (2010). Developmental complexity of the stimuli included in mispronunciation detection tasks. *International Journal of Language and Communication Disorders, 45*(1), 72–82.

Mehler, J., Jusczyk, P., Lambertz, G., Halsted, N., Bertoncini, J., & Amiel-Tison, C. (1988). A precursor of language acquisition in young infants. *Cognition, 29*(2), 143–178.

Metsala, J. L., & Walley, A. C. (1998). Spoken vocabulary growth and the segmental restructuring of lexical representations: Precursors to phonemic awareness and early reading ability. In J. L. Metsala & L. C. Ehri (Eds.), *Word recognition in beginning literacy* (pp. 89–120). Mahwah, NJ: Erlbaum.

Mills, D. L., Coffey-Corina, S., & Neville, H. J. (1997). Language comprehension and cerebral specialization from 13 to 20 months. *Developmental Neuropsychology, 13*(3), 397–445.

Mills, D. L., & Neville, H. (1997). Electrophysiological studies of language and language impairment. *Seminars in Pediatric Neurology, 4*(2), 125–134.

Mills, D. L., Prat, C., Zangl, R., Stager, C. L., Neville, H. J., & Werker, J. F. (2004). Language experience and the organization of brain activity to phonetically similar words: ERP evidence from 14- and 20-month-olds. *Journal of Cognitive Neuroscience, 16*, 1452–1464.

Minagawa-Kawai, Y., Mori, K., Naoi, N., & Kojima, S. (2007). Neural attunement processes in infants during the acquisition of a language-specific phonemic contrast. *Journal of Neuroscience, 27*(2), 315–321.

Moffitt, A. R. (1971). Consonant cue perception by twenty-to-twenty-four-week-old infants. *Child Development, 42*, 717–741.

Moon, C., Cooper, R. P., & Fifer, W. P. (1993). Two-day-olds prefer their native language. *Infant Behavior and Development, 16*(4), 495–500.

Moore, J. K., & Linthicum Jr., F. H. (2007). The human auditory system: A timeline of development. *International Journal of Audiology, 46*, 460–478.

Morrongiello, B. A., Robson, R., & Best, C. T. (1984). Trading relations in the perception of speech by 5-year-old children. *Journal of Experimental Child Psychology, 37*, 231–250.

Nazzi, T., Bertoncini, J., & Mehler, J. (1998). Language discrimination by newborns: Toward an understanding of the role of rhythm. *Journal of Experimental Psychology: Human Perception and Performance, 24*(3), 756–766.

Nazzi, T., Jusczyk, P. W., & Johnson, E. K. (2000). Language discrimination by English-learning 5-month-olds: Effects of rhythm and familiarity. *Journal of Memory and Language, 43*(1), 1–19.

Nazzi, T., & Ramus, F. (2003). Perception and acquisition of linguistic rhythm by infants. *Speech Communication, 41*, 233–243.

Newman, R. S. (2003). Prosodic differences in mothers' speech to toddlers in quiet and noisy environments. *Applied Psycholinguistics, 24*, 539–560.

Newman, R. S. (2009). Infants' listening in multitalker environments: Effect of the number of background talkers. *Attention, Perception, and Psychophysics, 71*(4), 822–836.

Newman, R. S., & Hussain, I. (2009). Changes in preference for infant-directed speech in low and moderate noise by 4.5- to 13-month-olds. *Infancy, 10*(1), 61–76.

Nittrouer, S. (2001). Challenging the notion of innate phonetic boundaries. *Journal of the Acoustical Society of America, 110*(3), 1598–1605.

Nittrouer, S. (2002a). From ear to cortex: A perspective on what clinicians need to understand about speech perception and language processing. *Language, Speech, and Hearing Services in Schools, 33*, 237–252.

Nittrouer, S. (2002b). Learning to perceive speech: How fricative perception changes and how it stays the same. *Journal of the Acoustical Society of America, 112*(2), 711–719.

Nittrouer, S., & Miller, M. E. (1997). Developmental weighting shifts for noise components of fricative-vowel syllables. *Journal of the Acoustical Society of America, 102*(1), 572–580.

Noble, K. G., McCandliss, B. D., & Farah, M. J. (2007). Socioeconomic gradients predict individual differences in neurocognitive abilities. *Developmental Science, 10*(4), 464–480.

Noble, K. G., Norman, M. F., & Farah, M. J. (2005). Neurocognitive correlates of socioeconomic status in kindergarten children. *Developmental Science, 8*(1), 74–87.

Nozza, R. J. (1988). Auditory deficit in infants with otitis media with effusion: More than a "mild" hearing loss. In D. J. Lim (Ed.), *Recent advances in otitis media* (pp. 376–379). Toronto, Canada: B.C. Decker.

Ooijen, B. v., Bertoncini, J., Sansavini, A., & Mehler, J. (1997). Do weak syllables count for newborns? *Journal of the Acoustical Society of America, 102*(6), 3735–3741.

Panneton Cooper, R., & Aslin, R. N. (1994). Developmental differences in infant attention to the spectral properties of infant-directed speech. *Child Development, 65*, 1663–1677.

Paterson, S. J., Heim, S., Thomas Friedman, J., Choudhury, N., & Benasich, A. A. (2006). Development of structure and function in the infant brain: Implications for cognition, language and social behaviour. *Neuroscience and Biobehavioral Reviews, 30*(8), 1087–1105.

Pegg, J. E., & Werker, J. F. (1997). Adult and infant perception of two English phones. *Journal of the Acoustical Society of America, 102*(6), 3742–3753.

Pelucchi, B., Hay, J. F., & Saffran, J. R. (2009). Statistical learning in a natural language by 8-month-old infants. *Child Development, 80*(3), 674–685.

Pihko, E., Leppanen, P. H. T., Eklund, K. M., Cheour, M., Guttorm, T. K., and Lyytinen, H. (1999). Cortical responses of infants with and without a genetic risk for dyslexia: I. Age effects. *NeuroReport, 10*, 901–905.

Polka, L., & Bohn, O. (2003). Asymmetries in vowel perception. *Speech Communication, 41*, 221–231.

Polka, L., & Bohn, O. (2011). Natural referent vowel (NRV) framework: An emerging view of early phonetic development. *Journal of Phonetics, 39*, 467–478.

Polka, L., Jusczyk, P. W., & Rvachew, S. (1995). Methods for studying speech perception in infants and children. In W. Strange (Ed.), *Speech perception and linguistic experience: Issues in cross-language research* (pp. 49–89). Timomium, MD: York.

Polka, L., Rvachew, S., & Mattock, K. (2007). Experiential influences on speech perception and speech production in infancy. In E. Hoff & M. Shatz (Eds.), *Blackwell handbook of language development* (pp. 153–172). Hoboken, NJ: Blackwell.

Polka, L., Rvachew, S., & Molnar, M. (2008). Speech perception by 6- to 8-month-olds in the presence of distracting sounds. *Infancy, 13*, 421–439.

Polka, L., & Werker, J. F. (1994). Developmental changes in perception of nonnative vowel contrasts. *Journal of Experimental Psychology: Human Perception and Performance, 20*(2), 421–435.

Rivera-Gaxiola, M., Silva-Pereyra, J., & Kuhl, P. K. (2005). Brain potentials to native and non-native speech contrasts in 7- and 11-month-old American infants. *Developmental Science, 8*, 162–172.

Rosner, J., & Simon, D. P. (1971). The auditory analysis test: An initial report. *Journal of Learning Disabilities, 4*, 384–392.

Rvachew, S., & Grawburg, M. (2006). Correlates of phonological awareness in preschoolers with speech sound disorders. *Journal of Speech, Language, and Hearing Research, 49*, 74–87.

Salminen, N. H., Tiitinen, H., & May, P. J. C. (2009). Modeling the categorical perception of speech sounds: A step toward biological plausibility. *Cognitive, Affective, and Behavioral Neuroscience, 9*(3), 304–313.

Sambeth, A., Ruohio, K., Alku, P., Fellman, V., & Huotilainen, M. (2008). Sleeping newborns extract prosody from continuous speech. *Clinical Neurophysiology, 119*(2), 332–341.

Sansavini, A., Bertoncini, J., & Giovanelli, G. (1997). Newborns can discriminate the rhythm of multisyllabic stressed words. *Developmental Psychology, 33*(1), 3–11.

Savage, R., Blair, R., & Rvachew, S. (2006). Rimes are not necessarily favored by prereaders: Evidence from meta- and epilinguistic phonological tasks. *Journal of Experimental Child Psychology, 94*, 183–205.

Shvachkin, N. K. (1948/1973). The development of phonemic speech perception in early childhood. In C. Ferguson & D. Slobin (Eds.), *Studies of child language development*. New York, NY: Holt, Rinehart & Winston. (Original work published in 1948).

Soderstrom, M., Nelson, D. G. K., & Jusczyk, P. W. (2005). Six-month-olds recognize clauses embedded in different passages of fluent speech. *Infant Behavior and Development, 28*(1), 87–94.

Stager, C. L., & Werker, J. F. (1997). Infants listen for more phonetic detail in speech perception than in word-learning tasks. *Nature, 388*(6640), 381–382.

Stevens, C., Lauinger, B., & Neville, H. (2009). Differences in neural mechanisms of selective attention in children from different socioeconomic backgrounds: An event-related brain potential study. *Developmental Science, 12*(4), 634–646.

Streeter, L. A. (1976). Language perception of 2-month-old infants shows effects of both innate mechanisms and experience. *Nature, 259*, 39–41.

Swingley, D. (2008). The roots of the early vocabulary in infants' learning from speech. *Current Directions in Psychological Science, 17*(5), 308–312.

Swingley, D., & Aslin, R. N. (2000). Spoken word recognition and lexical representation in very young children. *Cognition, 76*(2), 147–166.

Thiessen, E. D., & Saffran, J. R. (2003). When cues collide: Use of stress and statistical cues to word boundaries by 7- to 9-month-old infants. *Developmental Psychology, 39*(39), 706–716.

Trehub, S. E. (1973). Infants' sensitivity to vowel and tonal contrasts. *Developmental Psychology, 1973*, 91–96.

Trehub, S. E. (1974). *Auditory-linguistic sensitivity in infants* (Doctoral dissertation, McGill University, 1973). *Dissertation Abstracts International, 34*, 6254B.

Trehub, S. E. (1976). The discrimination of foreign speech contrasts by infants and adults. *Child Development, 47*(2), 466–472.

Tsao, F., Huei-Mei, L., & Kuhl, P. K. (2004). Speech perception in infancy predicts language development in the second year of life: A longitudinal study. *Child Development, 75*(4), 1067–1084.

Tsao, F., Liu, H., & Kuhl, P. K. (2006). Perception of native and non-native affricate-fricative contrasts: Cross-language tests on adults and infants. *Journal of the Acoustical Society of America, 120*, 2285–2294.

Vance, M., Rosen, S., & Coleman, M. (2009). Assessing speech perception in young children and relationships with language skills. *International Journal of Audiology, 48*(10), 708–717.

Versele, J., Polka, L., & Panneton, R. (2008). *Effects of voice quality and face information on infants' speech perception in noise.* Presented at the XVth

International Conference on Infant Studies. Vancouver, BC, Canada, March 2008.

Vouloumanos, A., & Werker, J. F. (2007). Listening to language at birth: Evidence for a bias for speech in neonates. *Developmental Science, 10*(2), 159–164.

Werker, J. F., Cohen, L. B., Lloyd, V. L., Casasola, M., & Stager, C. L. (1998). Acquisition of word-object associations by 14-month-old infants. *Developmental Psychology, 34*(6), 1289–1309.

Werker, J. F., Fennell, C. T., Corcoran, K. M., & Stager, C. L. (2002). Infants' ability to learn phonetically similar words: Effects of age and vocabulary size. *Infancy, 3*(1), 1–30.

Werker, J. F., Gilbert, J. H., Humphrey, K., & Tees, R. C. (1981). Developmental aspects of cross-language speech perception. *Child Development, 52*(1), 349–355.

Werker, J. F., & Lalonde, C. E. (1988). Cross-language speech perception: Initial capabilities and developmental change. *Developmental Psychology, 24*(5), 672–683.

Werker, J. F., Pons, F., Dietrich, C., Kajikawa, S., Fais, L., & Amano, S. (2007). Infant-directed speech supports phonetic category learning in English and Japanese. *Cognition, 103*(1), 147–162.

Werker, J. F., & Tees, R. C. (1983). Developmental changes across childhood in the perception of non-native speech sounds. *Canadian Journal of Psychology, 37*(2), 278–286.

Werker, J. F., & Tees, R. C. (1984). Cross-language speech perception: Evidence for perceptual reorganization during the first year of life. *Infant Behavior and Development, 7*(1), 49–63.

Werner, L. A., & Bargones, J. Y. (1991). Sources of auditory masking in infants: Distraction effects. *Perception and Psychophysics, 50*(5), 405–412.

Zangl, R., & Mills, D. L. (2007). Increased brain activity to infant-directed speech in 6- and 13-month-old infants. *Infancy, 11*(1), 31–62.

Zatorre, R. J., Berlin, P., & Penhune, V. B. (2002). Structure and function of auditory cortex: Music and speech. *Trends in Cognitive Sciences, 6*, 37–46.

Zhang, Y., Kuhl, P. K., Imada, T., Iverson, P., Pruitt, J., Stevens, E. B., . . . Nemoto, I .(2009). Neural signatures of phonetic learning in adulthood: A magnetoencephalography study. *NeuroImage, 46*(1), 226–240.

Zlatin, M. A., & Koenigsknecht, R. A. (1975). Development of the voicing contrast: perception of stop consonants. *Journal of Speech and Hearing Research, 18*(3), 541–553.

Chapter 3

Development of Speech Motor Control

As described in Chapter 2, the infant's speech perception abilities are so extraordinary that learning from the ambient language environment begins prior to birth. In contrast, the infant is born with limited oral motor control and a restricted repertoire of vocalizations. Speech production is a complex motor act that requires the coordination of respiratory, laryngeal, and articulatory subsystems involving over 100 muscles belonging to 5 different structural-functional classes (Kent, 2004). At birth, even features of the infant's cry reflect discoordination of the respiratory and laryngeal subsystems (Grau, Robb, & Cacace, 1995). It will be 6 or 7 months before the infant integrates control of these subsystems sufficiently to permit the emergence of speechlike babble (Oller, 2000). More than 16 years will pass before the child achieves adultlike stability and speed of articulatory movement patterns (Walsh & Smith, 2002). In the first part of this chapter, we trace this developmental trajectory with respect to four specific speech elements: (1) syllables and multisyllabic utterances, (2) vowels, (3) voice-onset time, and (4) pitch contours across an utterance, focusing in these sections on English-learning infants and children. This chapter describes the achievement of speech motor control, as revealed by kinematic and acoustic studies of speech movements.[1] Subsequent to this description of speech development from infancy through adolescence, theories of speech motor control are introduced. In the third and final section of the chapter, mechanisms that contribute to the achievement of speech motor control are discussed, emphasizing the dynamic interplay among structure and function and the causal equivalence of intrinsic and extrinsic factors.

Speech production is a complex motor act that requires the coordination of respiratory, laryngeal, and articulatory subsystems involving over 100 muscles belonging to 5 different structural-functional classes.

[1] Normative data on the achievement of specific phones, derived from studies involving phonetic transcription of speech behavior, are reserved for Chapter 4.

Acoustic and Kinematic Studies of Speech Development

3.1.1. Describe the 5 stages of infant vocal development including acoustic definitions of the characteristic utterance types at each stage.

3.1.2. Distinguish the muscle activation patterns for chewing versus speech and describe the development of these muscle activation patterns during the infant period.

3.1.3. Define differentiation, integration, and refinement and describe how these processes contribute to the development of inter-articulator coordination throughout childhood.

3.1.4. Define dynamic stability and describe how this concept relates to the achievement of higher order gestural goals during speech production.

3.1.5. List six developmental changes in the production of vowels that occur during infancy and childhood.

3.1.6. Describe the acquisition of the voicing contrast in English speech production in relation to the development of perceptual knowledge of this contrast.

Syllables and Multisyllabic Utterances

Infraphonological Description of Infant Speech

Significant advances in the effort to understand the course of infant speech development occurred in the 1970s when researchers moved beyond descriptive metrics that related infant vocalizations to adult linguistic categories. Earlier research that relied on phonetic transcription yielded a number of false conclusions about the nature of early speech development, chief among them a universalist bias that minimized individual differences in early speech development, and a tendency to view babble as a reflexive behavior that was sharply discontinuous with the later emergence of meaningful speech (Irwin, 1947; Jakobson, 1971, as cited in Oller, 2000; Locke, 1983). Guided by new theoretical perspectives and aided by new technical tools, researchers generated detailed descriptions of infant vocal behavior that incorporated, for a given vocalization, the behavioral and social context in which it was embedded, its acoustic characteristics across multiple dimensions, and the associated phonatory and articulatory movements (Koopmans-van Beinum & van der Stelt, 1986; Oller, 1980; Stark, 1980; Stark, Rose, & Benson, 1978). The promise of this approach was fully realized when Oller developed an infraphonological framework for interpreting this descriptive data in relation to an operational definition of the *canonical syllable* (see Oller, 1980 in which the priniciples are refered to as metaphonological; and Oller, 2000, for a full discussion of the infraphonological framework in relation to infrastructural schemes in the sciences). Oller (2000, pp. 12–13) explains that "the [infraphonological] principles indicate the limits on how acoustic features (durations, frequencies, amplitudes, and resonance characteristics) can be implemented in speechlike sounds and on how articulation and phonation must be performed to meet the requirements of well-formedness. Adults and infants can produce sounds that are not well formed with their vocal tracts by violating the infraphonological principles but such vocalizations are not considered to be canonical representations of speech forms."

The **infraphonological framework** relates infant vocalizations to an operational definition of the *canonical syllable* that takes acoustic, articulatory, and phonatory parameters of well-formedness into account.

Although Oller stresses that canonical syllables are recognizable to most human listeners on an intuitive basis as being speechlike whereas noncanonical vocalizations can be subjectively rejected as "not speechlike," a precise and objective definition of the canonical syllable was developed that takes into account a range of phonatory and articulatory characteristics operationalized in acoustic terms. Classification begins with the identification of an utterance which is defined as a vocalization that is produced on a single breath group, typically bounded by an inspiration, silence, or speech produced by the communication partner. Vocalizations that are vegetative or reflexive in nature are excluded from further analysis (grunts, laughs, cries, and other discomfort sounds, cf. Stark et al., 1978). In order to be judged as syllabic, the vocalization must include at least one articulatory gesture that corresponds to a transition from a relatively closed to a relatively open vocal tract (or less commonly in infant speech, a transition from a relatively open to a relatively closed vocal tract); a series of these opening and closing gestures produces what is commonly referred to as *babble,* inducing the percept of an alternating sequence of consonantal and vocalic segments. Yells and whispers are eliminated from the canonical category on the basis of amplitude parameters of the waveform envelope that correspond to loudness characteristics that are readily identified by ear; specifically, the amplitude of the syllable nucleus and margin must differ by at least 10 dB and the intensity range within the syllable must not exceed 30 dB. Resonance characteristics play an important role in the classification of infant vocalizations with the nuclei of canonical syllables expected to be fully resonant as exhibited by substantial energy in the higher frequency ranges. Phonation must also be normal with regularly spaced harmonics in the narrowband spectrogram. Timing characteristics are crucial. The overall duration of a single syllable within an utterance must be between 100 and 500 ms. The formant transitions corresponding to the vocal tract opening gesture must also be of appropriate duration, between 25 and 120 ms. Typically, multiple syllables in a sequence are of roughly similar duration although there is no specific criterion for

An **utterance** is defined as a vocalization that is produced on a single breath group, typically bounded by an inspiration, silence, or speech produced by the communication partner.

rhythmicity in the production of canonical babble beyond the limits on individual syllable duration.

A **canonical syllable (CS)** contains a formant transition with duration between 25 and 100 ms in a syllable no longer than 500 ms produced with higher frequency energy components indicating full oral resonance.

With an operational definition of the well-formed or canonical syllable (CS) in hand it is possible to interpret acoustic descriptions of human vocalizations using a scheme that can be applied equally well to infant or adult vocalizations while not assuming that the infant has the same vocal tract structure, motor control capabilities, articulatory goals, or internalized linguistic categories as the adult talker. The application of this scheme revealed a path toward the achievement of speechlike vocalizations that passes through five stages, marked not by the appearance of unique categories of vocalization but rather by differences in the relative frequency of particular utterance types. Although several stage models have been proposed (Koopmans-van Beinum & van der Stelt, 1986; Oller, 1980; Roug, Landberg, & Lundberg, 1989; Stark, 1980), there are many similarities among them; Oller's (2000) model is elaborated in the next section.

Stages in Infant Speech Development

During the **phonation stage** in the first month or two of life the primary nonreflexive, nondistress vocalization is the *quasiresonant vowel.*

During the *phonation stage* in the first month or two of life the primary nonreflexive, nondistress vocalization is the quasiresonant vowel. Quasiresonant vowels (QRVs) are typically a short utterance, produced with the vocal tract in a more or less resting position. The primary difference between QRVs and CSs is the absence in QRVs of clear upper frequency resonances and obvious formant transitions that would accompany deliberate shaping of the vocal tract to produce a specific vowel or syllable. They sound nasal in quality although they may or may not be produced with the velum lowered. QRVs share many similarities with CSs, however; they are produced with normal phonation and duration and may occur in rhythmic sequences, as shown in Figure 3–1A. Thelen (1991) notes that the QRV, from the dynamic systems perspective, might be considered to be a "stable attractor," a natural result of phonating on expiration while the infant is in a relaxed state. Oller (2000) remarks that QRVs may be the first sound that the infant produces with "contextual freedom" meaning that there is no obvious endogenous or exogenous stimulus. Although nearly all nonreflexive, nondistress vocalizations that are produced during the first 6 to 8 weeks are QRVs, these utterances do not disappear in later stages; on the contrary they occur at high frequencies throughout the first 6 months and are even heard in adulthood (e.g., as filler words such as "um," "hmm").

The **primitive articulation** stage occurs between 1 and 4 months of age and is characterized by an increased frequency of vocalizations in which phonation is interrupted by closures in the back of the vocal tract.

The *primitive articulation* stage emerges next with a peak in the frequency of vocalizations called Goos between 1 and 4 months of age. The term Goo refers to a category of highly variable vocalizations in which phonation is interrupted by a kind of undifferentiated vocal tract closing gesture that is produced in the back of the oral cavity. It is common for an infant to produce a series of Goos during a face-to-face interaction with an adult communication part-

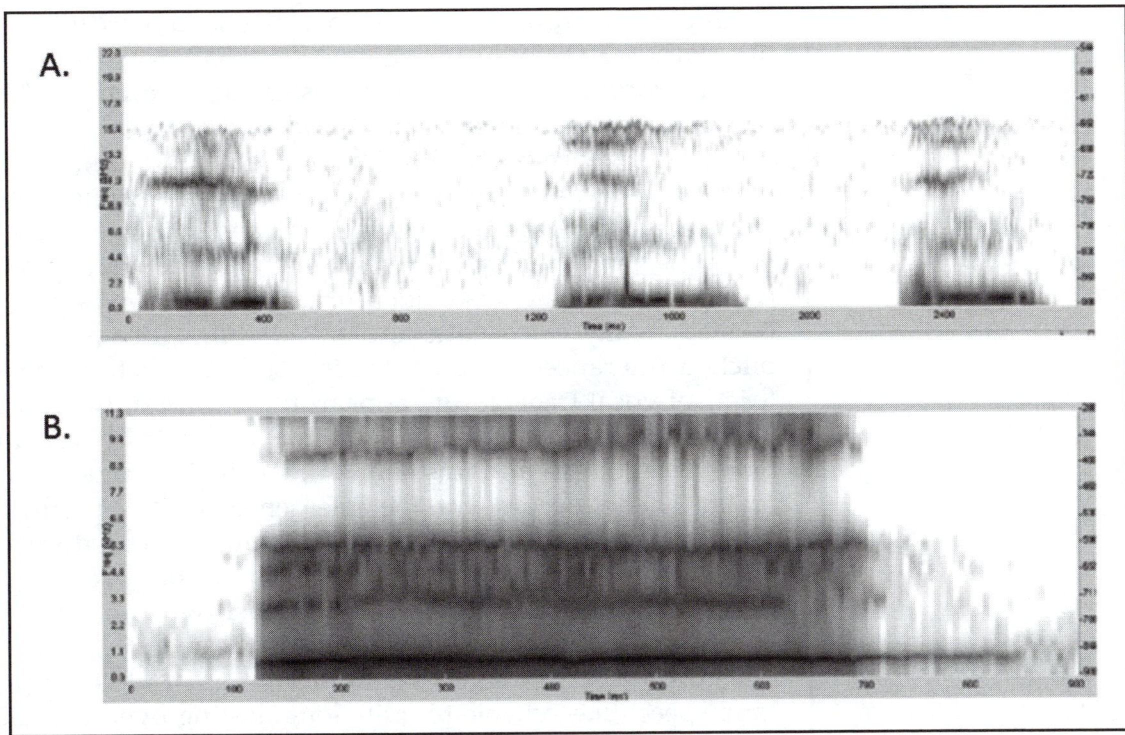

Figure 3–1. *Spectrograms of infant vocalizations contrasting utterances produced with quasiresonance (**A**) versus full resonance (**B**). The series of 3 quasiresonant nuclei are separated by inspirations and are characterized by a primary energy bar below 1200 Hz. The single fully resonant nucleus, perceived as the vowel [e], is produced with strong energy throughout the frequency range shown and the first four formants are clearly visible. Printed with permission from Susan Rvachew.*

ner and the variable nature of the vocalization from one turn to the next during the interaction can be striking. The closing gestures may be complete or partial, resulting in varying degrees of friction during the consonantal element. The degree of vocal tract opening during the nucleus of the vocalization can also vary; neutral positioning resulting in QRVs is typical but open mouth postures leading to a fully resonant vowel occasionally occur; at times the infant may shape the vocal tract for a fully resonant vowel but fail to phonate resulting in a silent opening gesture. The QRV may precede or follow the closure of the vocal tract. Duration and pitch contours are also highly variable.

Dynamic systems theory predicts that phase transitions will be marked by periods of extreme variability and indeed the instability of Goo production soon gives way to the dynamic stability of the *expansion* stage during which the infant gains control over the production of a broad variety of vocalization types. This stage, lasting from approximately 3 or 4 through 6 or 7 months, is characterized by three important advances in speech production ability: (1) systematic exploration of many parameters of speech, leading to (2) an explosion in the diversity of vocalization categories that are

During the **expansion stage**, between approximately 4 and 7 months, the infant produces a broad variety of vocalization types suggesting systematic exploration of many parameters of speech.

produced, including (3) one category that has a particularly speechlike character, the fully resonant vowel (FRV). Stark referred to the infant's vocal behavior during this stage as "speech play" because particular vocalizations are produced "over and over again," with their reoccurrence suggesting "that the infant has some control over the oral gestures involved or that he is experimenting with them" (Stark et al., 1978, p. 44). Experimentation with the loudness parameter appears in the form of whispering and yelling. Exploration of laryngeal parameters is evident in the production of growls, low pitched creaky voiced utterances, and abundant squealing, high-pitched utterances often containing sudden pitch changes. New forms of vocal tract closure appear in the form of the raspberry, a loud trill-like sound produced with the tongue or lips or quite commonly the tongue and lips simultaneously. Experimentation with oral resonance occurs with the emergence of FRVs, produced with an open vocal tract that is typically positioned to produce a central or mid-front vowel. In contrast to the QRV, these vowels are produced with full resonance so that at least two and often three or more formants are clearly measurable in the spectrogram, as shown in Figure 3–1B. Durations vary from short as would be appropriate for a speechlike syllable to quite long, lasting over a second. One FRV may be produced on a single breath group or a series may be produced, interrupted by glottal closures.

Marginal babbling is composed of consonants and vowels but does not meet the criteria for canonical babbling as a result of unusual timing, loudness, phonatory, or resonance characteristics.

Another category of vocalization that emerges during the expansion stage is the marginal syllable. These primitive syllables are perceived as being composed of consonants and vowels but fail to meet the criteria for canonical syllables as described above. Given that the requirements for well-formedness in the syllable are multifaceted, there are many ways in which a syllable can be marginal: the "hallmark of marginal babbling is its variability" (Oller, 2000, p. 177). Marginal syllables are often created by combining other expansion stage vocalizations. As shown in Figure 3–2, they may sound "not speechlike" as a result of unusual timing, loudness, or resonance parameters. Very commonly, atypical phonatory characteristics lead to a marginal syllable even when a consonantal closure is combined with a fully resonant vowel; Figure 3–3 shows narrowband spectrograms of marginal syllables illustrating departures from normal laryngeal function rarely observed in adult speech. The extreme variability in the form of these vocalizations echoes an earlier primitive form, the Goo, while distinguishing them from other expansion stage utterances as well as canonical syllables. Repetition typifies speech play in the expansion stage and canonical babble at later ages. An infant may "practice" squealing, endearingly at first and then annoyingly, for days at a time before switching to growling. In contrast, marginal syllables seem to be different every time and their sporadic occurrence lends them an almost accidental quality.

The emergence of *canonical babbling* is an unmistakable milestone in the life of the infant, easily identified by parents and other

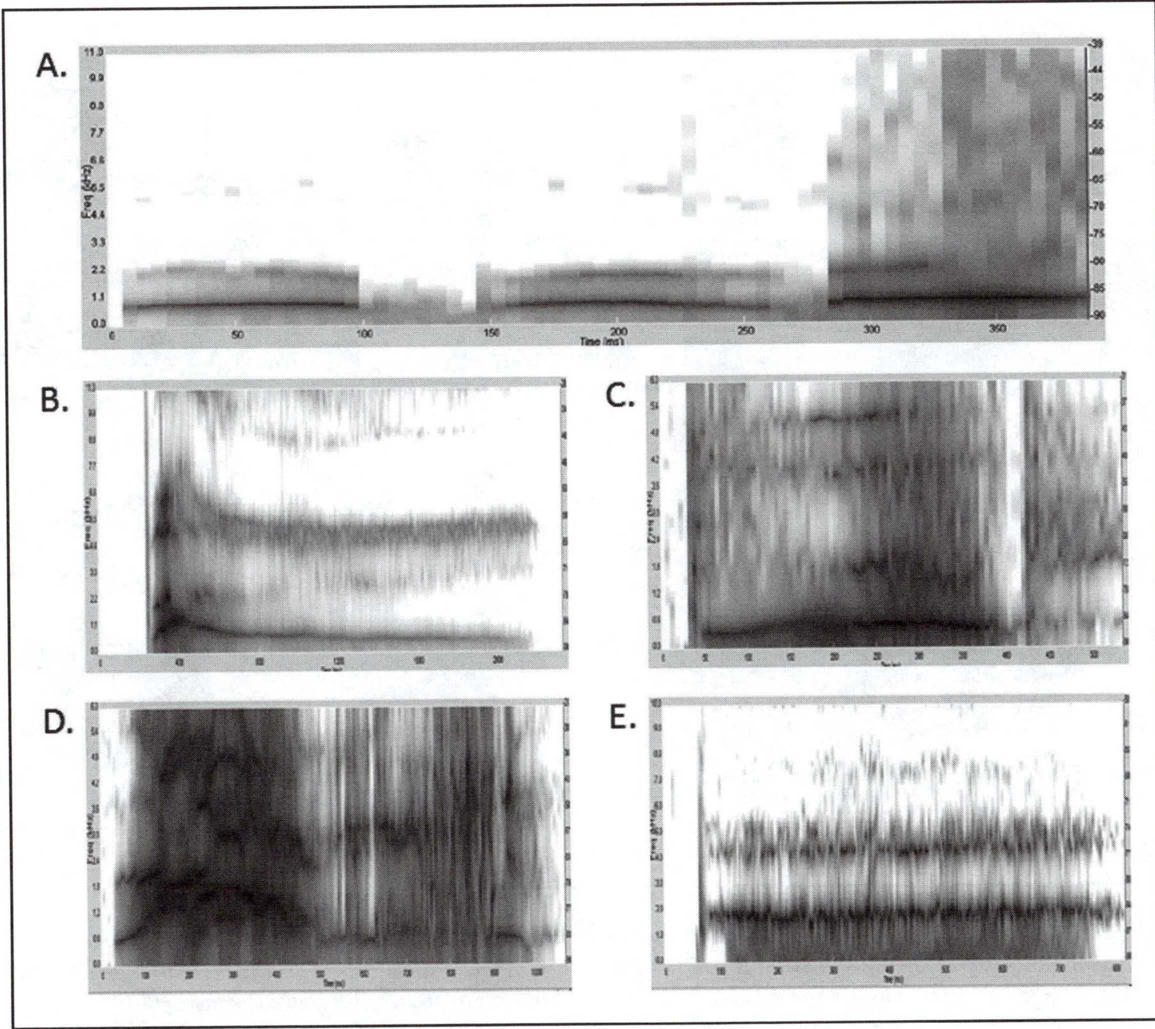

Figure 3–2. *Spectrograms of infant vocalizations categorized as marginal syllables.* **A.** *Utterance produced with minimal vocal tract movement excepting small movements of tongue tip, perceived as [ɖədəɖə] and classed as marginal due to short syllable durations and/or short formant transitions and quasiresonant nuclei given lack of energy above 2 kHz.* **B.** *In contrast, this syllable [bae:] is too long with a duration of 1915 ms.* **C.** *The duration of the transition from the consonant release into the steady-state portion of the vowel is approximately 190 ms giving the perception of an off-glide transition from the initial consonant into the vowel, [bwʊp].* **D.** *This utterance is produced with excessive loudness, explaining the lack of steady formants in the vocalic portion, with [jaʀ] being a rough approximation of the sound of this utterance.* **E.** *A long syllable, [bʌ̤:], produced with low amplitude and extreme breathiness. Printed with permission from Susan Rvachew.*

untrained observers when it occurs, on average at 7 months but always by 11 months in normally developing infants (Eilers & Oller, 1994; Oller, Eilers, & Basinger, 2001). Indeed, these well-formed utterances sound so much like speech that they may be taken for meaningful speech communication. The first author vividly recalls observing a 9-month-old infant repeatedly say "da" while banging a ball, prompting his mother to exclaim "See, he just said truck!" while finding a truck that was hidden behind the baby and

Canonical babbling emerges at 7 months on average and no later than 11 months in normally developing infants.

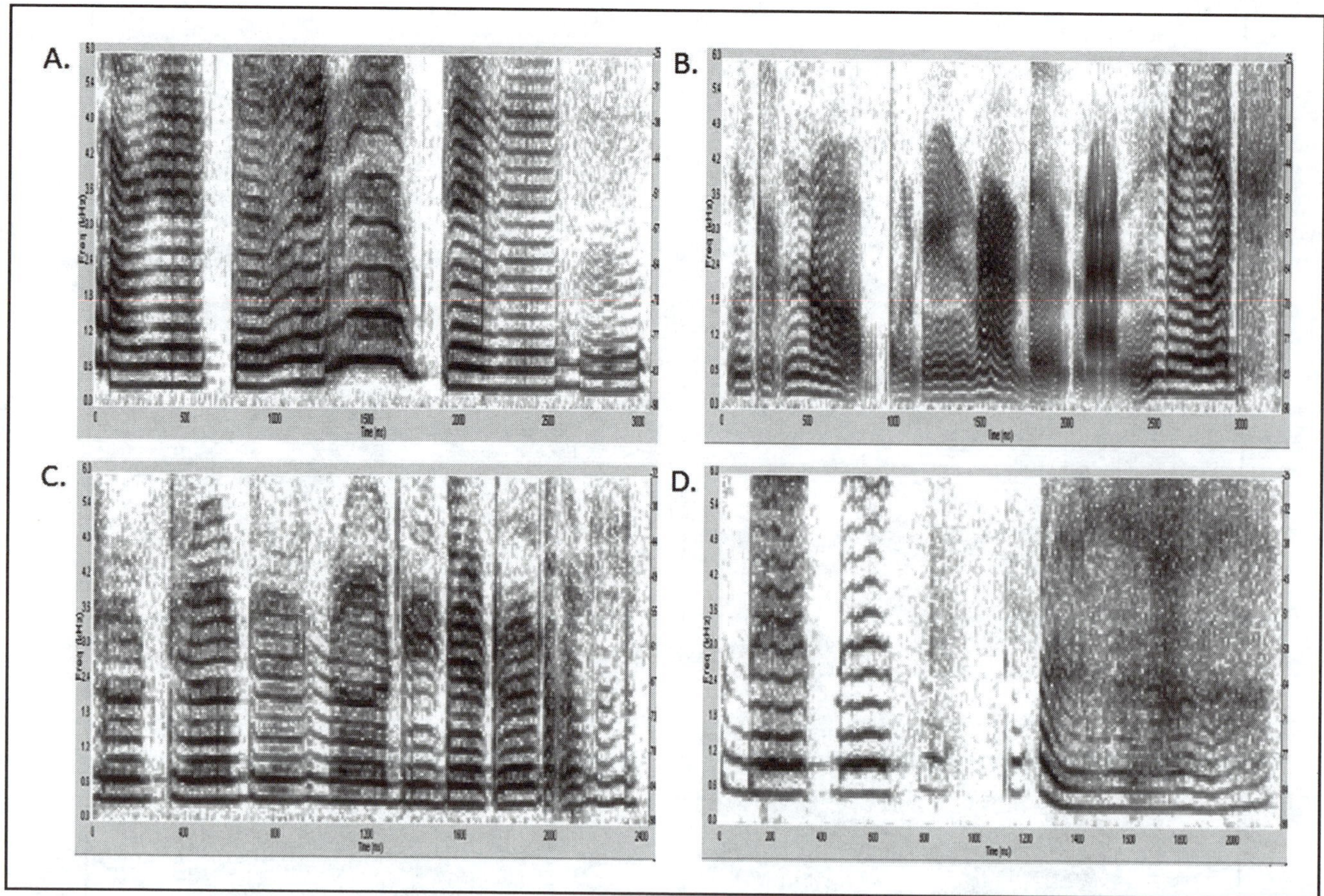

Figure 3–3. *Narrowband spectrograms of infant vocalizations classed as marginal due to unusual phonatory characteristics despite being composed of CV and CVC syllables.* **A.** *An F0 shift or pitch break is visible as a sudden change from harmonics spaced at 400 Hz intervals to harmonics spaced at 800 Hz intervals at approximately 1200 ms; the last syllable in the utterance is also marginal due to quasiresonance and harmonic doubling.* **B.** *The ripples in the harmonics are characteristic of tremor, perceived as a vibrato sound.* **C.** *Harmonic doubling is apparent in syllables 3 and 4 as a parallel series of harmonics interleaved with the original harmonics and associated with mild harshness in the voice.* **D.** *The sudden change in the harmonic structure in the final syllable, blurring the harmonics throughout the frequency range is associated with a rough and breathy voice quality. From Rvachew, Creighton, Feldman, & Sauve (2002). Acoustic-phonetic description of infant speech samples: coding reliability and related methodological issues.* Acoustics Research Letters Online *by American Institute of Physics, 3(1), Table 2, p. 26 and Mm. 2. Reproduced with permission of American Institute of Physics.*

substituting it for the ball. This incident explained the unusually large reported vocabulary size but also foretold rapid acquisition of expressive language skills for this child, unsurprisingly as early referential use of language is associated with repeated use of specific consonants in babble (McCune & Vihman, 2001). As described earlier in this section, the speechlike character of the vocalizations that emerge during the canonical stage is attributed to how well the syllables are formed, consisting of a clear syllable margin resulting from closure of the oral vocal tract, smoothly changing but rapid formant transitions corresponding to the vocal tract opening gesture, combined with a fully resonant vowel that is produced with

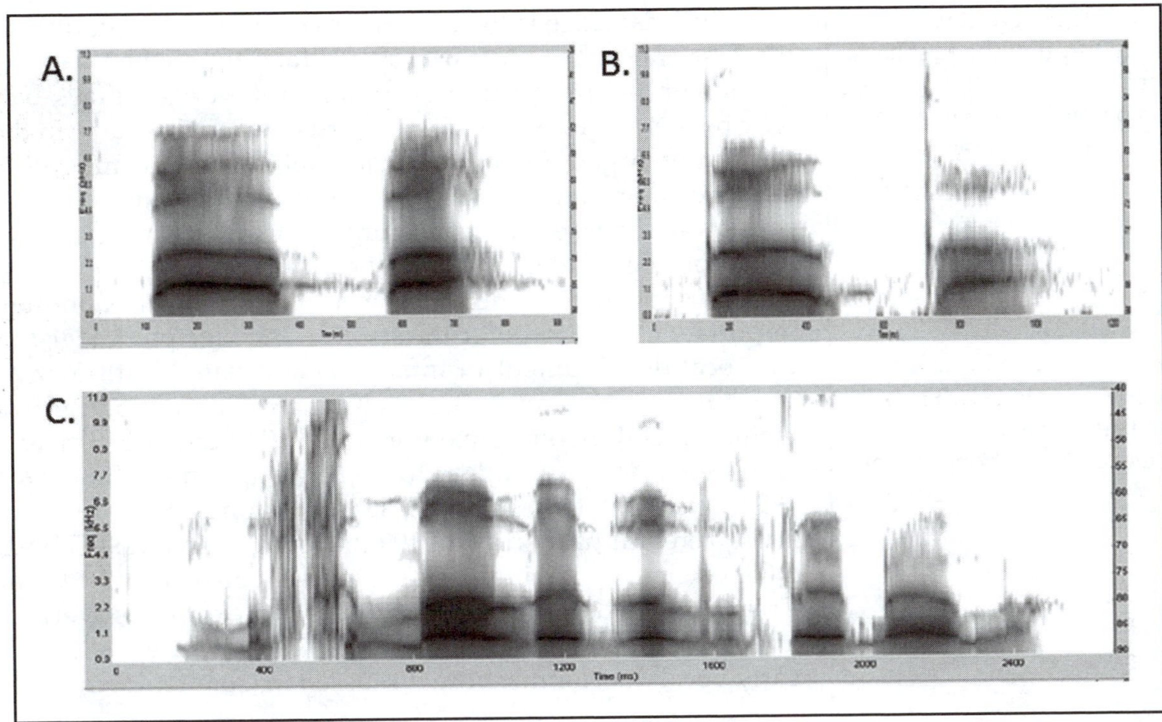

Figure 3–4. *Broadband spectrograms of canonical utterances produced by a 14-month-old Arabic-learning infant.* A. *Reduplicated babble,* [bæbæ]. B. *Reduplicated babble,* [dædʌ]. C. *Variegated babble,* [nʊθɬɪnælʌdɛðɪnænʌ]. *Printed with permission from Abdulsalam Alhaidary.*

normal phonation and a relatively short duration (see examples in Figure 3–4). Reduplication of these vocalizations is not obligatory. First, variegated syllable sequences—in which there is variation in the consonantal and/or vocalic elements within a sequence—occur contemporaneously with reduplicated babble (Mitchell & Kent, 1990; Smith, Brown-Sweeney, & Stoel-Gammon, 1989). Second, single syllables may be classified as canonical and in fact multisyllabic utterances remain relatively rare even at one year of age (Kent & Bauer, 1985). Nonetheless, periods of practice with long sequences of syllables, produced with increasingly regular timing as the infant ages, is a defining feature of the canonical babbling stage.

Although CSs are speechlike in form there is no expectation that they be communicative in function. In fact, infants are very happy to vocalize when they are alone, during so-called crib monologues or when the parent is ignoring the baby and conversing with another adult, apparently for self-stimulation (Locke, 1989). The canonical babbling stage coincides with beginning receptive language skills and overlaps with the emergence of intentional communication; babbled utterances do not immediately serve the communicative needs of the child, however, as often the infant will resort to nonverbal gestures or more primitive forms of vocalization to demand attention or comment on the environment (McCune, Vihman, Roug-Hellichus, Bordenave Delery, & Gogate, 1996).

Although canonical syllables are speechlike in form there is no expectation that they be communicative in function.

The **integrative stage** lasts roughly through the first half of the second year of life, a time when babbling co-exists with the production of meaningful words.

The final stage is the *integrative* stage, lasting roughly through the first half of the second year of life, a time when babbling co-exists with the production of meaningful words. In fact, babbling may be literally integrated with words during this stage in the production of jargon, utterances that combine nonmeaningful babble with meaningful words. Gibberish is also produced, utterances that consist of sequences of nonmeaningful syllables produced with prosodic contours that mimic those heard in meaningful phrases.

Atypical vocal development in infancy is associated with many types of primary and secondary developmental phonological disorder.

Identification of delayed onset of canonical babbling is an important clinical skill for the speech-language pathologist. Atypical vocal development in infancy is associated with many types of primary and secondary developmental phonological disorder including childhood apraxia of speech (Velleman & Strand, 1994) and speech delay secondary to hearing impairment (Eilers & Oller, 1994), cleft palate (Chapman, Hardin-Jopnes, Schulte, & Halter, 2001), cerebral palsy (Levin, 1999), Down syndrome (Cobo-Lewis, Oller, Lynch, & Levine, 1996), very low birth weight (Rvachew, Creighton, Feldman, & Sauve, 2005), and extreme poverty (Oller, Eilers, Basinger, Steffens, & Urbano, 1995). Strategies to facilitate early vocal development are discussed in Chapters 9 and 10.

Development of Mandibular Control During Babbling

Moore and colleagues conducted a series of electromyographic studies of the development of coordinated muscle activity during chewing, silent jaw oscillation, babbling, and speech in infants aged 9 through 22 months (Moore & Ruark, 1996; Steeve & Moore, 2009; Steeve, Moore, Green, Reilly, & Ruark McMurtrey, 2008) in comparison to the adult pattern of muscle activity for chewing, jaw oscillation and speech (Moore, 1993; Moore, Smith, & Ringel, 1988), in each case focusing on mandibular (lower jaw) movements. Interpretation of these data is facilitated by understanding the primary features of the adult pattern for these behaviors as illustrated in Figure 3–5. Muscle activation patterns that are characteristic for chewing are shown in Figure 3–5A: activity of the three jaw elevator muscles (masseter, temporalis, and medial pterygoid) is reciprocally organized in time with the activation of the anterior belly of the digastric muscle which acts to depress the mandible. Rhythmic and reciprocal activation of antagonist muscle groups (i.e., muscles that raise the jaw versus the muscle that lowers the jaw) is well known to be the dominant pattern for chewing. Surface similarities in the rhythmicity of the alternating pattern of jaw raising and lowering in chewing and speech have led to the proposal that specialized neural mechanisms that support alimentary behaviors are exploited in the production of babble (Lund & Kolta, 2006; MacNeilage, 1998). However, the organization of muscle activation patterns during speech differs markedly from that observed during chewing, as shown in Figure 3–5B: over and above the minimal activation of the masseter and temporalis muscles, the striking pattern observed in this

In the adult, rhythmic and *reciprocal activation of antagonist muscle groups* is the dominant pattern for **chewing**, a coordinative organization that optimizes occlusal force generation.

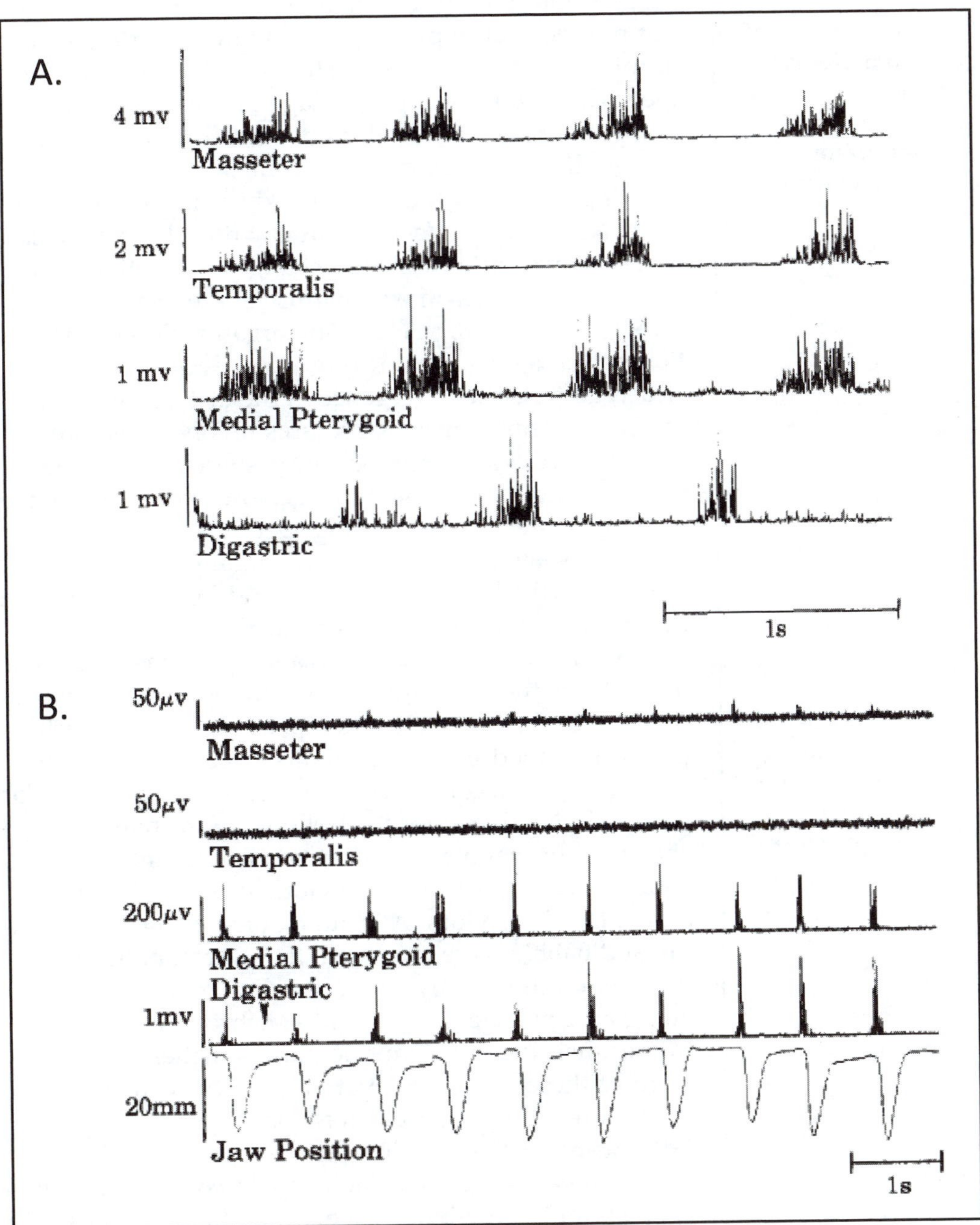

Figure 3–5. *Electromyographic records of activity from the right masseter, temporalis, medial pterygoid, and anterior belly of the digastrics muscles, recorded from adults during* (**A**) *chewing and* (**B**) *repetitions of the syllable [a] from a closed jaw position. Vertical jaw displacement is also shown in* (**B**). *From* Moore et al. *(1988). Task specific organization of activity in human jaw muscles.* Journal of Speech, Language, and Hearing Research, 31, *Figure 2, p. 674; Figure 3, p. 775; Figure 5, p. 677. Reprinted with permission of the* American Speech-Hearing-Language Association.

In the adult, **coactivation of antagonist muscles** is the predominant pattern during speech, optimizing jaw stability as a dynamic support for rapid articulatory movements.

figure is the highly correlated activation of the medial pterygoid and the anterior belly of the digastrics muscle. Coactivation of antagonist muscles is the predominant pattern during speech, including simple repetitive vowels as shown in the figure, and in connected speech as when reading a passage (Moore, 1993; Moore et al., 1988). The pattern of mandibular coordination during voluntary silent jaw oscillations was distinct from the patterns observed during chewing and from those observed during speech, contributing to the conclusion that "activity in jaw muscles can be coordinated in several ways, either through changes in relative timing of activity, or through changes in which muscles are recruited for a given task" (Moore et al., 1988, p. 676). The organization of the muscle activation patterns observed during nonspeech and speech movements clearly reflects the divergence in the task requirements rather than the isomorphism in the structures involved. Moore posits that the coordinative organization of the system during chewing is specialized to optimize occlusal force generation. In contrast, coactivation of antagonistic muscles during speech results in mechanical stiffening of the system, optimizing jaw stability as a dynamic support for the rapid articulatory movements and frequent changes in direction that are required for speech production.

In young infants, **coordinative organization of muscle activation patterns** is poorly specified during speech and nonspeech tasks.

A study of the muscle activation patterns for chewing and babble in 9-month-old infants demonstrated that the coordinative organization of this system across speech and nonspeech tasks is quite poorly specified in young infants (Steeve et al., 2008). The degree of coupling (i.e., correlated muscle activity) was low for all muscle groups indicating poor underlying coordinative organization for chewing and babble, a finding not consistent with the notion that babbling emerges from a previously established infrastructure for alimentary behaviors. Although some differences between chewing and babble were observed, the overall pattern of muscle activity was roughly similar with coupling greater among agonist than antagonist muscle groups and synchrony also greater among the former than the latter muscle pairs. Further study of the development of these muscle activation patterns during infancy suggests gradual refinement and differentiation with age (Moore & Ruark, 1996; Steeve & Moore, 2009; Steeve et al., 2008). These small sample studies revealed gradual increases in coupling and synchrony for agonists and reductions in synchrony for antagonists during chewing between 9 and 22 months of age. These findings correspond to emergence of the expected pattern of reciprocal activity of muscle groups that raise the jaw versus those that lower the jaw while chewing. During the production of CV syllables, coupling and synchrony of both agonist and antagonist muscle pairs increased during this same period. Gradual stabilization of the typical pattern of coactivation of antagonist muscle groups for speech was more advanced for these simple syllables relative to reduplicated and variegated babble, however.

The research findings reviewed here have important clinical implications. Some approaches to speech therapy assume that speech requires stabilization of earlier appearing nonspeech behaviors but these studies clearly disconfirm this hypothesis. Rather, speech and nonspeech oral behaviors involve distinct coordinative structures that develop along divergent but parallel paths. For this reason we advise against the use of nonspeech oral motor exercises in speech therapy in Chapter 10 while describing procedures for facilitating vocal play and the development of early speech behaviors in functional contexts.

Speech and nonspeech oral behaviors involve distinct coordinative structures that develop along divergent but parallel paths.

Organization of Supralaryngeal Articulatory Gestures in Meaningful Speech

Toward the end of the second year of life the child has achieved sufficient control of the respiratory, laryngeal, and supralaryngeal articulatory systems to produce speech in single syllable babbles and reduplicated and variegated multisyllable babbles. The child is also producing a growing number of meaningful words, either singly or in combination with babble or other words to produce jargon and short phrases. Precise spatial and temporal organization of articulatory gestures is required for consistent production of all these types of speech. Complexity is added in the case of meaningful speech by the need to integrate the gestural coordination challenge with increasing linguistic processing demands. The development of interarticulator coordination within and across syllables during the early stages of language development has been studied using kinematic and acoustic analysis methods as described in Chapter 1. Although the methods vary, the primary conclusions are corroborated across studies. Certain key studies are reviewed to highlight the critical findings about early developments in speech motor control.

Kinematic studies of toddler's lip and jaw movements during the second year of life reveal considerable continuity between babble and speech, a finding that supports the conclusions of the electromyography studies discussed in the previous section. Nip, Green, and Marx (2009) recorded the speed of lower lip and jaw movements using infrared light-emitting markers and a specialized camera system as described in Chapter 1 (see Figure 1–5). The speed of these movements was investigated for silent spontaneous jaw movements, babbles, and meaningful words produced by 24 infants recorded every 3 months between 9 and 21 months of age. Silent jaw movements decreased, while meaningful words increased in frequency during the period of study. The speed of opening and closing movements for both jaw and lower lip increased with age, although most of the increase occurred between 9 and 15 months with a plateau observed thereafter. Articulator movement speeds for babble and words were not significantly different from each

Kinematic studies of toddlers' lip and jaw movements during the second year of life reveal considerable continuity between babble and speech.

other but both were significantly faster than articulator speeds for silent voluntary jaw movements.

Kinematic and acoustic studies of interarticulator coordination in children reveal three primary developmental processes: **differentiation**, **integration**, and **refinement**.

Kinematic and acoustic studies of interarticulator coordination in children reveal three primary developmental processes: differentiation, integration, and refinement. Early in development, differentiation is particularly important as the young child gains independent control of the multiple components of a given task. Instantiation of a new coordinative structure may also involve the integration of a new behavior into a previously established motor behavior. Once the child has achieved a coordinative structure that resembles the mature form, interarticulator coordination undergoes gradual refinements in speed, precision, and stability. All three processes were observed by Green, Moore, Higashikawa, and Steeve (2000) when they studied the coordination of upper and lower lip and jaw movements during the production of disyllables by infants, toddlers and children. Extent of articulator movement is plotted against time for the syllable "baba" as produced by a 1-year-old infant, a 2-year-old toddler, a 6-year-old child, and an adult talker in Figure 3–6.

In 1-year-old infants, the jaw is making the primary contribution to oral closure during speech, suggesting that motor control is achieved for the jaw before other articulators.

Adult production of "baba," as shown in Figure 3–6 (upper left), is characterized by closely correlated rising and falling trajectories of all three articulators, a pattern referred to as high interarticulator coupling. In the adult, the lower lip and the jaw both make a significant contribution to the achievement of vocal tract closure at the syllable onsets, whereas the contribution of the upper lip is minimal. This pattern contrasts markedly with the pattern observed in the one-year-old infants: Figure 3–6 (lower right) indicates that the jaw is making the primary contribution to oral closure and the lip movements are not in phase with the jaw trajectory. Overall, the kinematic patterns observed in infants suggests that motor control is achieved for the jaw before other articulators, reinforcing the impression obtained across many studies employing kinematic, electromyographic, and acoustic measures (Green, Moore, & Reilly, 2002; Moore & Ruark, 1996; Nip et al., 2009; Nittrouer, 1993; Steeve et al., 2008). Nonetheless, these same studies demonstrate that jaw movements are clearly imprecise in infancy. For example, Green et al. (2000) report many instances of poor mandibular force control resulting in excessive compression of the lips during articulation of these labial syllables by their one-year-old participants.

Improvement in inter-articulator coordination during the second year of life is characterized by **integration** of lip movements into the previously established jaw movement trajectory.

By age two as shown in Figure 3–6 (lower left), upper and lower lip movements showed a single undifferentiated rising and falling trajectory that spanned the entire disyllabic utterance. During this period the relative contribution of the jaw to the oral closing gesture decreased and the contribution of both lips increased. Improvement in interarticulator coordination during the second year of life is therefore characterized by integration of lip movements into the previously established jaw movement trajectory. The tight spatial and temporal coupling of upper and lower lip movements observed in the 2-year-olds is described as an example of "motor overflow,"

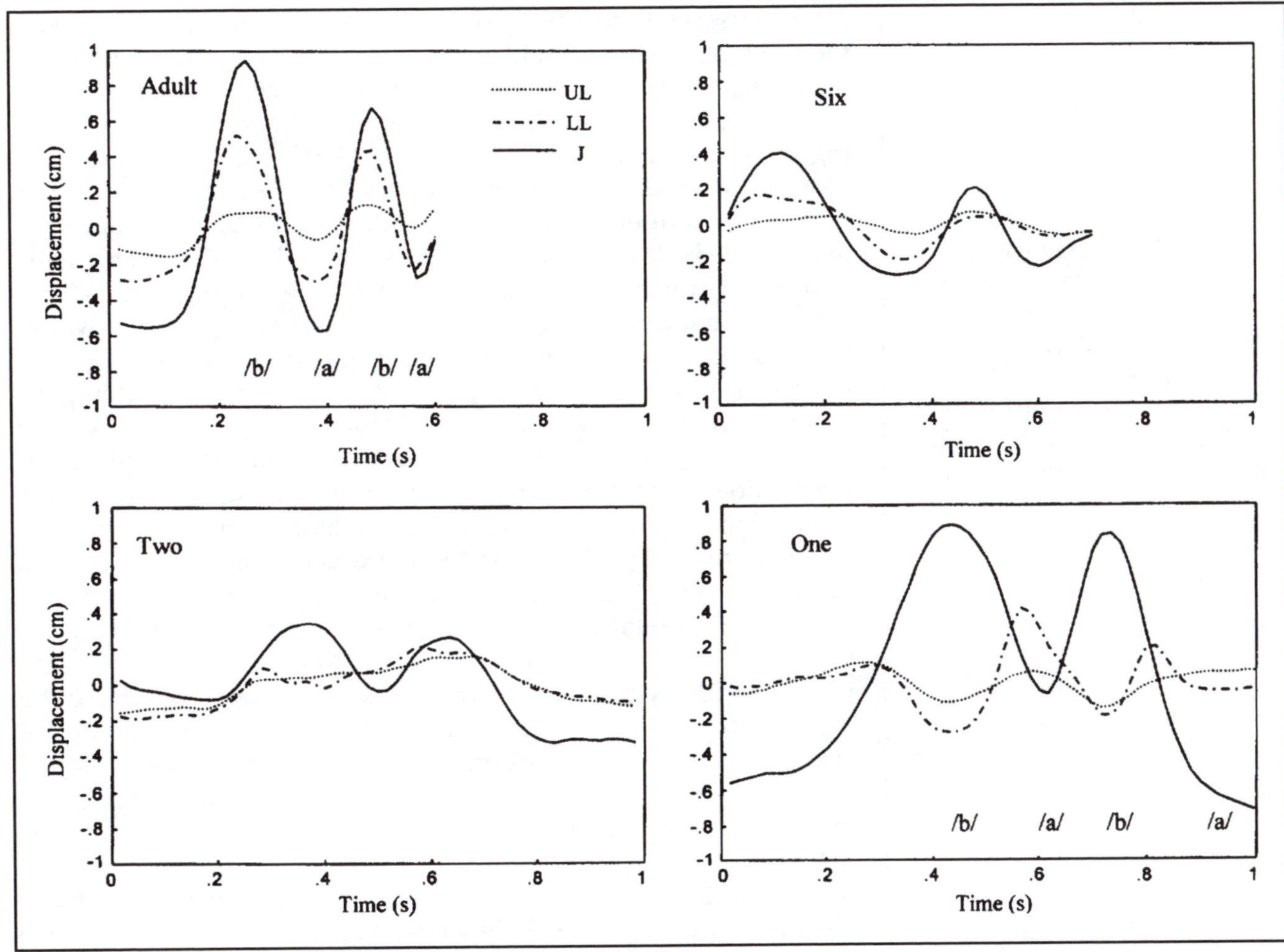

Figure 3–6. *Kinematic tracings from upper lip (UL), lower lip (LL), and jaw (J) during production of the disyllable "baba" by an adult, 6-year-old, 2-year-old, and 1-year-old talker. Jaw movement was subtracted from lower lip movement to get the lower lip tracing. The upper lip tracing has been inverted. Each signal is centered about its mean. From Green et al. (2000). The physiologic development of speech motor control: Lip and jaw coordination.* Journal of Speech, Language, and Hearing Research, 43, *Figure 4, p. 246. Reprinted with permission of the American Speech-Hearing-Language Association.*

a common feature of immature movements observed across multiple motor domains. A noticeable change in the movement pattern between 2 and 6 years is the differentiation of the upper and lower lip movements resulting in a coordinative structure that is similar to the adult pattern, as illustrated in Figure 3–6 (upper right). In this figure it can be seen that the lower lip trajectory is roughly synchronized with the jaw and no longer tightly coupled with the lower lip. At age 6, the lower lip and jaw jointly make the primary contribution to oral closure while the lower lip makes only a minimal contribution. Changes between age 6 and adulthood reflect an ongoing process of refinement in movement control and coordination.

Differentiation of the upper and lower lip movements occurs between 2 and 6 years of age.

Changes between age 6 years and adulthood reflect an ongoing process of **refinement** in movement control and coordination.

Kinematic studies of the development of interarticulator coordination have focused on the jaw and lips because these articulators can be observed directly. Efforts to understand the coordination of tongue movements with jaw and lip articulation have been based on acoustic analyses. A number of studies have traced the achievement of gestural coordination within and across syllables during the production of disyllables with iambic and trochaic stress patterns (Goodell & Studdert-Kennedy, 1993; Nittrouer, 1993; Nittrouer, Studdert-Kennedy, & McGowan, 1989; Nittrouer, Studdert-Kennedy, & Neely, 1996). These studies show that intersyllabic gestural organization is achieved earlier in development than intrasyllabic organization with levels of intersyllabic gestural overlap in the unstressed syllable being adultlike at age 3 years. Overall, the results of these two studies do not support the general hypothesis that children's early interarticulator coordination is characterized by excessive gestural overlap that subsequently declines with maturation; rather, the observed effects and changes with age were highly specific to the segments and syllable structures involved. In other words, the degree of overlap was adultlike in some cases, declined with age in others and increased with age in others. The unifying interpretative framework invokes again the developmental processes of integration, differentiation, and refinement. For example, the toddlers gradually learn to execute temporal overlap of the spatially separable consonant and vowel gestures in [bɑ] and [bi] syllables but to delay execution of the vowel in the context of lingual onsets. Goodell and Studdert-Kennedy conclude that the differences observed in the youngest toddlers "reflect the children's difficulties in timing both the precise duration of a gesture and its onset or offset with respect to other gestures . . . [and the need to learn] to differentiate, and to bring under independent control, the several gestures that compose the sequence of syllables in an utterance" (p. 724).

Acoustic analysis of iambs and trochees shows that intersyllabic **gestural organization** is achieved earlier in development than intrasyllabic organization with levels of intersyllabic gestural overlap in the unstressed syllable being adultlike at age 3 years.

Age-related refinements in the production of prosodic patterns have also been investigated in kinematic studies. Goffman and Malin (1999) compared child and adult productions of the nonsense words ['pʌpəp], [pə'pʌp], ['fʌfəf], and [fə'fʌf] in the context of the carrier phrase "It's Sam's ______," using acoustic and kinematic measures. Some of the kinematic data from this study are shown in Figure 3–7, illustrating differences in performance for child and adult subjects across iambic and trochaic words. The children (aged 3;10 to 4;2) produced longer movements than adults but all participants produced final syllable lengthening in both iambic and trochaic contexts. Children and adults produced iambs and trochees with distinct movement patterns. However, the children produced trochees as if they had a strong-strong stress pattern, suggestive of unmodulated syllables in babble, and unlike the modulated strong-weak pattern observed in the adults, as shown on the left side of Figure 3–7. Both child and adult talkers modulated the weak-strong syllable sequence in the iambs as shown on the right side of Figure 3–7. Interestingly, stability in reproducing the movement pattern was greater for the iambic words than the trochaic words for both adults and children, reflecting the precision that is required to

Kinematic studies show greater stability of movement patterns during production of iambic words than trochaic words for both adults and children, reflecting the precision that is required to achieve the target form that is more distinctive in comparison to an unmodulated movement pattern.

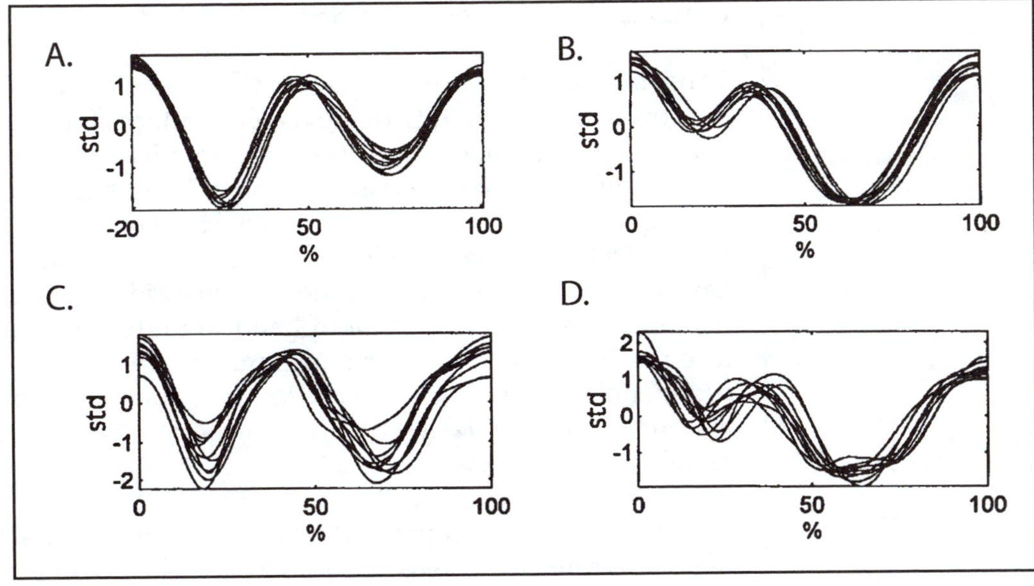

Figure 3–7. *Time and amplitude normalized kinematic tracings of displacement of the lower lip during productions of the nonsense words ['pʌpəp]* (left) *and [pə'pʌp]* (right)*, recorded from an adult* (top) *and child* (bottom)*. The corresponding spatiotemporal indexes for the repeat productions shown are:* (**A**) *adult trochee STI = 8.56,* (**B**) *adult iamb STI = 8.99,* (**C**) *child trochee STI = 18.15, and* (**D**) *child iamb STI = 14.24. Adapted from Goffman & Malin (1999). Metrical effects on speech movements in children and adults.* Journal of Speech, Language, and Hearing Research, 42, *Figure 5, p. 1009. Used with permission of the American Speech-Hearing-Language Association.*

achieve the target form that is more distinctive in comparison to an unmodulated movement pattern.

Walsh and Smith (2002) and Smith and Zelaznick (2004) described the achievement of speech motor control for even longer phrases in a cross-sectional kinematic study spanning the age range 4 through 22 years. The trajectory of upper lip, lower lip, and jaw movements were recorded during production of the phrases "Buy Bobby a puppy" and "Mommy bakes pot pies." Duration, displacement, velocity, and spatiotemporal index measures were calculated separately for male and female participants in each age group. Consistency and speed increased and interarticulator coupling improved over the full age range studied with the oldest group of children (16-year-olds) still not showing fully adultlike levels of speech motor control. The results suggested that the children achieved near adultlike consistency for jaw movements before lip movements. They also found that the children achieved near adultlike speaking rates at the expense of temporal consistency in their speech production. A developmental increase in synergy of lower lip and jaw movements was also observed across the age range. The protracted developmental course observed in these studies could not be attributed simply to maturation of craniofacial structures since there were no sex differences in the results obtained from adolescent participants.

Kinematic studies of lip and jaw movement patterns during phrase production show that consistency, speech, and interarticulator coupling continue to improve through at least 16 years of age.

Gestural Goals in Connected Speech

Thus far, we have reviewed studies showing developmental improvements in stability of movement patterns for a single articulator (e.g., the jaw) and increases in interarticulator coupling (e.g., synergy of lower lip with jaw trajectory). These studies might leave the impression that the developmental challenge is to achieve control of each of these individual structures. Smith and colleagues have conducted a series of studies aimed at identifying the unit of planning in speech motor control and to understanding the interface between speech motor and linguistic planning in language production. Smith (2006) concluded that speech motor control is hierarchically organized with planning occurring at multiple levels of the hierarchy at once.

Smith and Zelaznik (2004) examined the lower levels of the hierarchy when they compared relative stability in the achievement of lip aperture size versus lip and jaw coupling over repeated productions of "Buy Bobby a puppy." Lip aperture is described as a higher order synergy whereas coupling of the upper or lower lip movements with the jaw trajectory are considered to be lower order synergies. Lip aperture (the size of the opening between the lips) is the dynamically controlled target—in other words, the motor goal—whereas maintaining lip-to- jaw synergy provides the means to achieve the goal. Stability in the achievement of lip aperture and of lip-to-jaw synergy both improved with age but stability was always greater for the higher level synergy, whereas variability was greater for the lower level synergy. Stability in the higher level synergy can be achieved despite variability in the lower level synergy because of a phenomenon called "motor equivalence," a term meaning (in this context) that multiple combinations of motor movements can achieve the same vocal tract constriction (Perkell et al., 2000). This behavior is also an example of dynamic stability, "that is, an overall task orientation and resistance to minor perturbations" (Fogel & Thelen, 1987, p. 749). Wohlert and Smith (2002) reported that electromyography recordings from the upper lip show that neural commands to the upper lip muscles are significantly more variable in 7- and 12-year-old children than in young adults. However, it appears that children are able to compensate for minor perturbations to the movement trajectories of specific articulators that result from these variable muscle activations to achieve relatively stable higher order goals.

Motor equivalence means that multiple combinations of motor movements can achieve the same vocal tract constriction.

Children are able to compensate for minor perturbations to the movement trajectories of specific articulators that result from variable muscle activations to achieve relatively stable higher order goals thus demonstrating **dynamic stability**.

Smith and Zelaznik (2004) demonstrated that the unit of planning goes beyond the activation of a specific muscle or the movement of a given articulator. Goffman and Smith (1999) suggest that the goal of speech production is to produce perceptually distinguishable linguistic units, including units as small as the segment. In their kinematic study, lip and jaw trajectories were recorded from 4- and 7-year-old children and young adults as they produced the words *man, ban, pan, fan,* and *van* at the end of a carrier phrase. These words were chosen because they appear to represent a common motor plan or template but with contrasts differing only in the presence or absence of a single gesture or the setting of a single parameter: specifically, lowering the velum differentiates [m] from [b]; laryngeal vibration distinguishes [p] from [b]; degree of vocal tract closure contrasts [p] and [f]. As would be expected given the preceding discussion, the children were more variable than adults in the basic movement parameters that described their labial closing and opening gestures (displacement, velocity, duration). Nonetheless, a statistical pattern sorting algorithm was able to discern 5 distinct movement patterns in the child data at significantly better than chance levels, identifying the five segments from normalized velocity profiles with as much accuracy as was observed for the adult kinematic tracings. They concluded that "the crucial result is that segmental specificity does not appear to be emerging as a consequence of developmental changes in standard movement components" (p. 657). Rather, higher level goals, such as achieving specific segmental outcomes that will be perceived as intended by the listener, have input to the motor system and allow the child to achieve dynamic stability in the achievement of those goals long before adultlike motor control of the individual components has been attained.

Further studies have investigated the response of the motor system to more complex linguistic input. Sadagopan and Smith (2008) examined duration and stability of lower lip movements for the phrase "Buy Bobby a puppy" when said alone or when embedded in one of two longer more complex utterances, specifically "They asked us to buy Bobby a puppy this week" and "You buy Bobby a puppy now if he wants one" (see examples in Chapter 1, Figure 1–6). The talkers were children aged 5 through 16 years and young adults. The spatiotemporal index and duration of the target phrase "Buy Bobby a puppy" was plotted as a percentage of the adult value in the three conditions. Children at all ages showed reduced stability when the phrase was embedded in a longer more complex utterance in contrast to the adults who were able to produce the phrase with equal stability in all conditions. Children younger than 12 produced the phrase at a slower rate in the embedded conditions compared to the baseline condition. Interestingly, adults and older children produce the phrase at a faster rate in the embedded conditions relative to baseline, an effect not observed in the younger children. The authors speculate that adults and older children are planning their utterances in longer chunks than the younger children. The results further suggest that children aged 12 and older are showing evidence of a shift to more mature motor planning strategies; however, even 16-year-olds show reduced stability of movement patterns in response to increased linguistic processing loads.

Adults and older children plan their **utterances in longer chunks** than the younger children.

Vowels

Development of the Vowel Space in Infancy

According to **frame/content theory**, the developing infant gradually differentiates tongue movements from the jaw allowing for the production of different consonants and vowels (content) via modulation of cyclical mandibular movements (frame) hypothesized to have evolved from chewing.

In the previous section we described developmental changes in the syllabic organization of speech. Not surprisingly, the relevant studies had a strong focus on the jaw as the critical articulator since mandibular oscillation is proposed as the basic movement underlying the production of syllables, with elevation of the jaw resulting in consonants and lowering of the jaw resulting in vowels (MacNeilage & Davis, 2000). According to the "frame/content" theory, the first few years of speech development are dominated by the "frame"; in other words, mandibular oscillations lead to predictable patterns of apparent consonant-vowel co-occurrences that reflect a lack of independence of the tongue from the jaw. Specifically, labial closures of the vocal tract should be paired with central vowels because the tongue is simply carried passively by the jaw in its central resting position during the biphasic oscillation of the mandible for the production of babble or early words. Similarly, vocal tract closures involving the blade of the tongue (i.e., alveolar consonants) should be paired with front vowels, whereas vocal tract closures involving the tongue dorsum (i.e., velar consonants) should be paired with back vowels because in each instance the tongue position is static during the opening and closing phases of the jaw. According to the theory, gradual differentiation of the frame results in superposition of "content." A gradual reduction of frame dominance and the emergence of specific content would be revealed by combinations of segments that are less constrained by the biomechanical factors that were sole drivers of the frame in the early stage of speech development. Efforts to support the theory are almost exclusively based on phonetic transcription studies (e.g., Davis & MacNeilage, 1995) that are not discussed here due to the many shortcomings of this technique as an adequate tool for description of infant speech movements. However, it is clear that any effort to trace the acquisition of speech motor control in early childhood cannot ignore the tongue! Unfortunately, kinematic studies of jaw trajectories are relatively straightforward whereas kinematic techniques for visualizing tongue movements (e.g., EMMA and ultrasound, as described in Chapter 1) are not readily applied to infants and young children and thus direct study of the early development of tongue control is difficult. Acoustic studies of the development of vowel production do provide a window on the acquisition of lingual control, however, notwithstanding complications introduced by the ever-changing size and shape of the vocal tract, as discussed further in later sections of this chapter.

Studies of infant vowel production often describe the vowel space as a whole simply because it is not possible to ask the infant to produce a specific vowel. All of the infant's vocalizations are recorded and fully resonant vowels produced with normal phonation and relatively stable formants are selected for spectral analysis. Once the vowels have been plotted on the F1 and F2 axes the center and corners of the vowel space can be identified and the area of the vowel space can be described. Kent and Murray reported that the vowel space increased in size between 3 and 9 months of age, especially in the F1 dimension as shown in Figure 3–8. In this cross-sectional study, the center of the vowel space remained static with the "average vowel" having an F1, F2, and F3 of approximately 1, 3, and 5 kHz for 3-, 6-, and 9-month-olds respectively, values that would be expected for the infant vocal tract in the neutral or "schwa" position. Overall, the acoustic characteristics of the vowels produced by these young infants were consistent with mid-front and central articulations.

An infant's **vowel space** is identified by plotting the F1 and F2 frequencies of all the vowels produced during a given sampling interval.

Rvachew and colleagues have described changes in the mean and standard deviation of the F1 and F2 frequencies for three different groups of normally developing English-learning infants between 8 and 18 months of age in one longitudinal and two cross-sectional studies. Rvachew, Mattock, Polka, and Ménard (2006) observed a significant decline in mean second formant frequencies but not mean first formant frequencies over this age range in their English-learning sample. In all three studies English-learning infants were observed to increase the standard deviation of observed F2 frequencies but not F1 frequencies (Rvachew et al., 2005; Rvachew et al., 2006; Rvachew, Slawinski, Williams, & Green, 1996). The effect of increasing the range and variance of F2 frequencies is to expand the vowel space into the diffuse and grave corners (Rvachew, et al., 2006), resulting in a gradual increase in the number of vowels that are perceived by adults to be [i] or [u] as opposed to more central vowels (Polka, Rvachew, & Mattock, 2007). Ishizuka, Mugitani, Kato, and Amano (2007) demonstrated that this rapid expansion of the vowel space in the first 18 to 24 months of life also results in the development of more distinct (i.e., less overlapping) specific vowel categories.

Cross-linguistic studies of infant vowel production show universal expansion of the vowel space in the first 18 to 24 months of life that results in the development of more distinct (i.e., less overlapping) specific vowel categories.

Taken together, these studies give the impression that the first year of life is marked by changes in the tongue height parameter, indexed by an expansion of the vowel space along the F1 dimension, whereas the second year of life is characterized by changes in the tongue advancement parameter, indexed by an expansion of the vowel space along the F2 dimension. Especially when interpreted in view of the kinematic studies discussed earlier in this chapter, the notion of "frame dominance" may be supported for the earliest stages of speech development. It is not clear that the child's productive output is dominated by the mandibular frame throughout the canonical babbling, integrative and first word stages as predicted however (e.g., MacNeilage & Davis, 2000). Sussman examined CV coarticulation in two longitudinal case studies using locus equations which are essentially linear regression equations that relate second formant frequencies at two time points in the syllable: release of the consonant and midpoint of the vowel (Sussman, Duder, Dalston, &

The first year of life is marked by changes in the tongue height parameter, indexed by an expansion of the vowel space along the F1 dimension, whereas the second year of life is characterized by changes in the tongue advancement parameter, indexed by an expansion of the vowel space along the F2 dimension.

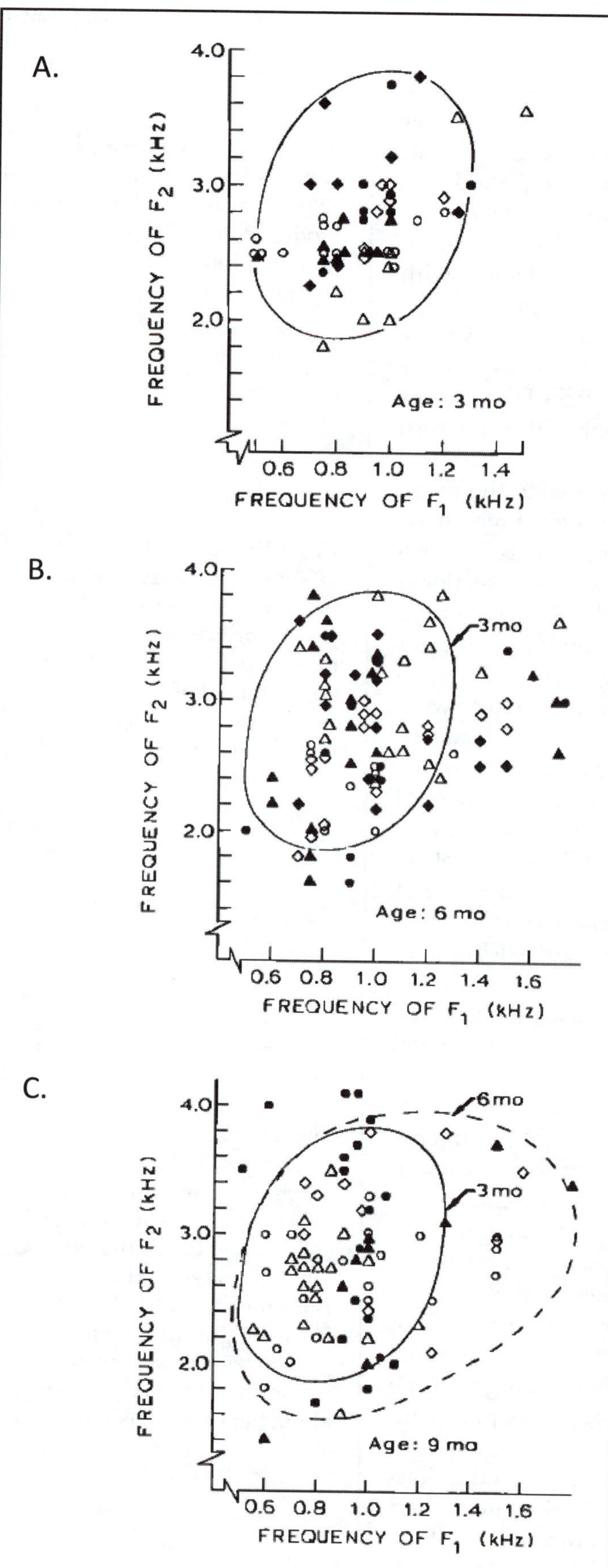

Figure 3–8. *F1-F2 plots of vowels produced by infants recorded at 3 months (***A***), 6 months (***B***) and 9 months (***C***) of age. Each symbol represents a different infant in a given age group. Lines are drawn to enclose approximately 100% of the vowels at each age. From Kent & Murray (1982). Acoustic features of infant vocalic utterances at 3, 6, and 9 months.* Journal of the Acoustical Society of America *by Acoustical Society of America, 72, Figures 8, 9, and 10, p. 357. Reproduced with permission of American Institute of Physics for the Acoustical Society of America.*

Caciatore, 1999; Sussman, Minifie, Buder, Stoel-Gammon, & Smith, 1996). These children achieved adultlike values of the slopes of the locus equations in labial, alveolar and velar consonant contexts between 7 and 12 months of age for babble and real words. Thus, it appears that children are motivated to modulate the mandibular frame and impose specific segmental content during the first year of life.

Goldfield (2000) addressed the question of whether infants are actively exploring the F1-F2 vowel space by examining vowel production in single syllable utterances versus multivowel sequences recorded from 6-month-old infants. The vowel space was larger for single vowels than for vowels produced within multivowel sequences. Changes in F1 and F2 frequencies within a multivowel sequence suggested that the infants were actively and systematically varying the height or anterior-posterior position of the tongue within the sequence of vowels. We conclude the section on infant vowel production on this note in order to emphasize the point that development during this period is not solely driven by biomechanical constraints on vocal output. The infant's role in actively seeking to explore the possibilities of the developing vocal tract and map productive output to the perceptual phonetic categories that are being learned in the first year of life must not be forgotten.

Vowel Production in Childhood

Descriptions of the acoustic vowel space provide information about vowel development across the lifespan. In an extensive review of this literature, Vorperian and Kent (2007) reported that the center of the F1-F2 plot declines to lower values of F1 and F2 between age 4 years and adulthood. Furthermore, the area of the acoustic vowel space declines over this period for both males and females. Both of these changes are predicted by reductions in the length of the vocal tract. These kinds of normative data are of clinical value because vowel space area is associated with speech intelligibility. Although the overall area of the vowel space is expected to decline with age, an unusually small space at a given age can explain poor speech intelligibility (Higgins & Hodge, 2001; Hodge, 1999). For example, Liu, Tsao, and Kuhl (2005) recorded words containing the point vowels from young adults with dysarthria secondary to cerebral palsy and from young adults with normal speech and plotted their acoustic vowel spaces as shown in Figure 3–9. On average the talkers with dysarthria evidenced a smaller vowel space area in comparison to the normal talkers; naïve listeners were able to identify 56% of the words spoken by the talkers with dysarthria and 97% of the words spoken by the talkers with normal speech. Furthermore, vowel space area was significantly correlated with speech intelligibility (r = .86).

Mean F1 and F2 at the center and overall area of the vowel space declines between age 4 years and adulthood, reflecting **reductions in the length of the vocal tract**.

Among young adults with *dysarthria*, **vowel space area** is correlated with speech intelligibility.

Investigation of the acoustic characteristics of specific vowels is possible with older children and adults. Means and standard

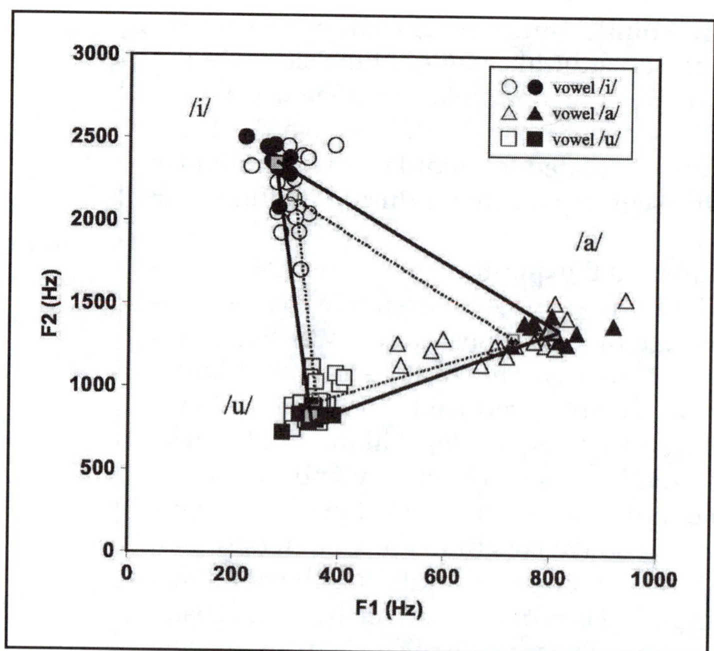

Figure 3–9. Vowel space of Mandarin talkers with normal speech (filled markers) or dysarthria secondary to cerebral palsy (open markers). Each marker represents the mean F1-F2 coordinate of the vowels /i/, /a/, and /u/ as produced by a single talker. From Liu et al (2005). The effect of reduced vowel working space on speech intelligibility in Mandarin-speaking young adults with cerebral palsy. Journal of the Acoustical Society of America by Acoustical Society of America, 117(6), Figure 1, p. 3883. Reproduced with permission of American Institute of Physics for the Acoustical Society of America.

deviations of the F1, F2, and F3 values for a broad range of vowels as produced by children and adults speaking North American English are provided by Peterson and Barney (1952), Hillenbrand, Getty, Clark, and Wheeler (1995), Lee, Potamianos, and Narayanan (1999), and Assman and Katz (2000), collectively covering the age range from 3 years to adults. Lee et al. sampled the broadest range with samples of child talkers recorded at each age from 5 through 18 years as well as a group of adults. For clinical purposes these data are useful because they provide a foundation for the application of spectral analysis to the treatment of speech sound disorders, as demonstrated in Chapter 10. From the research perspective, these investigations provide information about factors that influence the course of speech development. All studies show a downward trajectory in formant frequencies with age as well as differences between male and female talkers that can be predicted by growth in the vocal tract and larynx. Other age trends, such as a reduction in duration magnitude and variability, and a corresponding reduction in within-subject formant and spectral envelope variability, most likely reflect maturation of speech motor control, with adultlike levels of variability achieved at approximately 14 years of age (Lee

Age-related reductions in duration magnitude and variability, and a corresponding reduction in within-subject formant and spectral envelope variability, most likely reflect maturation of speech motor control, with adultlike levels of variability achieved at approximately 14 years of age.

et al., 1999). Despite the greater variability at younger ages, even children as young as three accomplish adultlike within-vowel formant trajectories leading to a high degree of listener identification accuracy (Assman & Katz, 2000). Some findings appear to reflect sociolinguistic phenomena, such as a significant difference in F1 for male and female children and a decline in F1 after age 18 for adult females that could not be explained by biomechanical factors (Lee et al., 1999). In a reanalysis of Lee et al.'s data, Whiteside (2001) found that adult women produced more distinct vowels especially on the periphery of the vowel space, when compared to adult men and to 18-year-old males and females. This greater distinctiveness of vowel production is associated with a broader range of F1 and F2 values, similar to what is seen for women in the infant-directed versus adult-directed speech context as described in Chapter 1 (e.g., see Plate 3). Both Hillenbrand et al. and Lee et al. were surprised to find that vowel durations were longer for female adult talkers than for male talkers even though Hillenbrand et al. recorded single words, whereas Lee et al. (1999) recorded words in the context of a carrier phrase. Hillenbrand documented an interesting pattern of *overshoot* across a variety of parameters. Specifically, vowel duration, formant frequencies, fundamental frequency, spectral envelope measures, and the associated variabilities all declined with age, reaching their minimum values at approximately age 14 years; interestingly, all of these values subsequently increased to finally converge on the adult values at a later age.

Even children as young as 3 accomplish adultlike within-vowel formant trajectories leading to a high degree of listener identification accuracy.

In comparison to younger women and adult men, adult women produce more distinct vowels, associated with a broader range of F1 and F2 frequencies and longer durations.

When F1-F2 coordinates, measured at the midpoint of the vowel, are plotted for specific vowels, a considerable amount of overlap between adjacent vowel categories is observed in the speech of adult male, adult female and child talkers, as illustrated in Figure 3–10 (Hillenbrand et al., 1995). Despite all of this overlap in what is assumed to be the primary cue to vowel identity, listeners were able to identify these vowels with surprising accuracy; specifically these vowels as produced by women, men and children were heard as intended 96, 95, and 93% of the time, respectively; confusions were most common for [ɔ]-[ɑ], [æ]-[ɛ], and [ɛ]-[ɪ]. Further investigation revealed that the identity of these vowels is determined not just by the achievement of a static vocal tract configuration; rather, the duration of the vowel and dynamic changes in the formants throughout the production of the syllable nucleus play a role. Assman and Katz (2000) demonstrated that these dynamic, time-varying cues to vowel identity are especially important for disambiguating vowels that are close or overlapping in the F1-F2 space; for example, the formant trajectories move in opposite directions during the production of [e] and [ɛ] when produced by English speakers. It is possible that these time varying cues are particularly salient in the speech of children in comparison to the static spectral cues which may be less salient when fundamental frequency is high. The importance of these time-varying cues to segment identity (for consonants and vowels) is just one reason that syllables are preferred over isolated segments when presenting stimuli in speech perception or speech

Dynamic, time-varying cues to vowel identity are especially important for disambiguating vowels that are close or overlapping in the F1-F2 space.

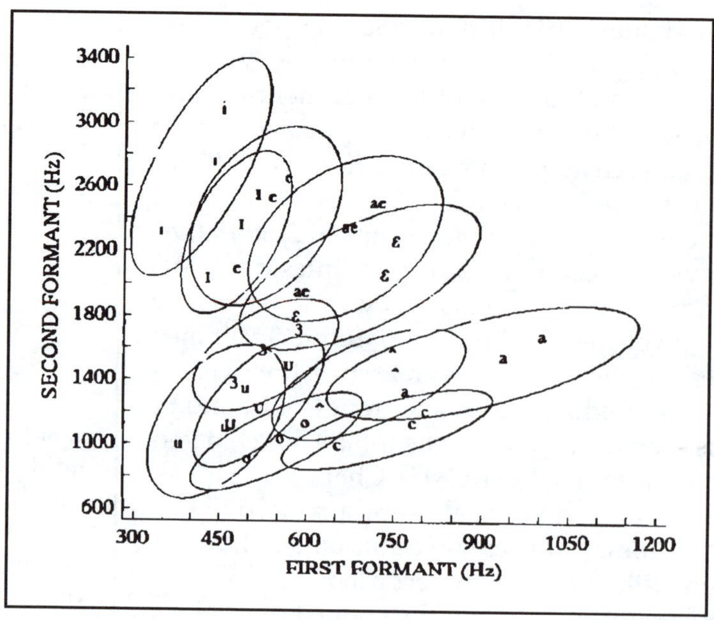

Figure 3–10. *Average values of F1 and F2 for men, women, and child talkers shown inside ellipses encompassing all of the vowels produced in each vowel category. "ae" = [æ], "c" = [ɔ], and "3" = [ɝ]. From Hillenbrand (1995). Acoustic characteristics of American English vowels.* Journal of the Acoustical Society of America *by Acoustical Society of America, 97(5), Figure 3, p. 3103. Reproduced with permission of American Institute of Physics for the Acoustical Society of America.*

production intervention tasks, a point that is discussed further in Chapters 9 and 10.

Manipulation of vowel duration is important, not only for distinguishing vowel categories such as [i] versus [ɪ], but also for cuing final consonant voicing, for example, [bæt] versus [bæːd]. Buder and Stoel-Gammon (2002) studied the development of children's ability to manipulate these two types of vowel duration differences in a cross-linguistic study that included Swedish and American toddlers aged 24 and 30 months. In Swedish and in English the tense-lax vowel pair [i] versus [ɪ] is produced with a qualitative difference such that the tense vowel is more "close" and a quantitative difference such that the tense vowel is longer in duration. However, the qualitative cue is weighted more highly in English whereas the quantitative cue is weighted more highly in Swedish, a language that contains 9 pairs of vowels contrasted by duration. With respect to the difference in vowel duration that occurs before voiced and voiceless final consonants, this generally unmarked pattern must be suppressed in Swedish to enhance the salience of the extensive system of phonemically contrastive short-long vowel pairs. Buder and Stoel-Gammon found that the quantitative difference in vowel duration between [i] and [ɪ] emerged earlier in Swedish toddlers compared to English toddlers, illustrating the interaction of phonetic and phonological factors in speech development.

Krause (1982a) studied the development of the vowel duration cue to final stop consonant voicing in 3- and 6-year-old children and adults. Significant differences in vowel duration before voiced and voiceless stops were observed for all three age groups. No significant age effect was observed in the voiceless stop context. However, vowels before voiced stops became progressively shorter with age suggesting that the contrast was exaggerated in the speech of the youngest children. Furthermore, variability of production over repeated trials declined with age. These findings for productive use of this cue mirror Krause's (1982b) findings for perception of word final voiced and voiceless stops, as reported in Chapter 2: these same children were observed to require larger differences in vowel duration to identify the voiced stop category and the slopes of their identification functions were shallower in comparison to those obtained from adults, indicating more variable responding to the stimuli close to the category boundary.

Voice Onset Time

Although vowel duration is the most salient cue to the voicing contrast in the postvocalic position, manipulation of voice onset time (VOT) is essential to the production of voicing in the prevocalic position. Manipulation of the VOT cue requires that the child learn to produce the appropriate laryngeal gestures in order to modulate airflow and subglottal pressure and to coordinate the timing of laryngeal and supralaryngeal articulatory gestures in a manner appropriate to the particular voicing category (Koenig, 2000). Macken and Barton (1980) conducted a longitudinal investigation of the acquisition of the stop consonant voicing contrast by recording four English-learning toddlers at biweekly intervals between approximately 16 and 26 months of age. The samples of speech were recorded during semistructured play sessions involving toys selected to prompt production of the stops at labial, alveolar and velar place of articulation. Average VOTs by voicing category were plotted to show how these values evolved between 16 and 26 months of age for each child and place of articulation. The results are shown for one child and one phoneme pair in Figure 3–11; the pattern of results shown in this figure reveals a multistage process toward the acquisition of the voicing contrast that is characteristic of the general findings across infants and phonemes. Recall from Chapter 2 that language general perception of the short lag versus long lag voicing contrast is present at birth and that the shift to language specific perceptual processing of this contrast occurs between 6 and 8 months of age. However, phonemic perception of the voicing contrast is reportedly quite late developing, appearing during the latter half of the second year. Turning now to productive acquisi-

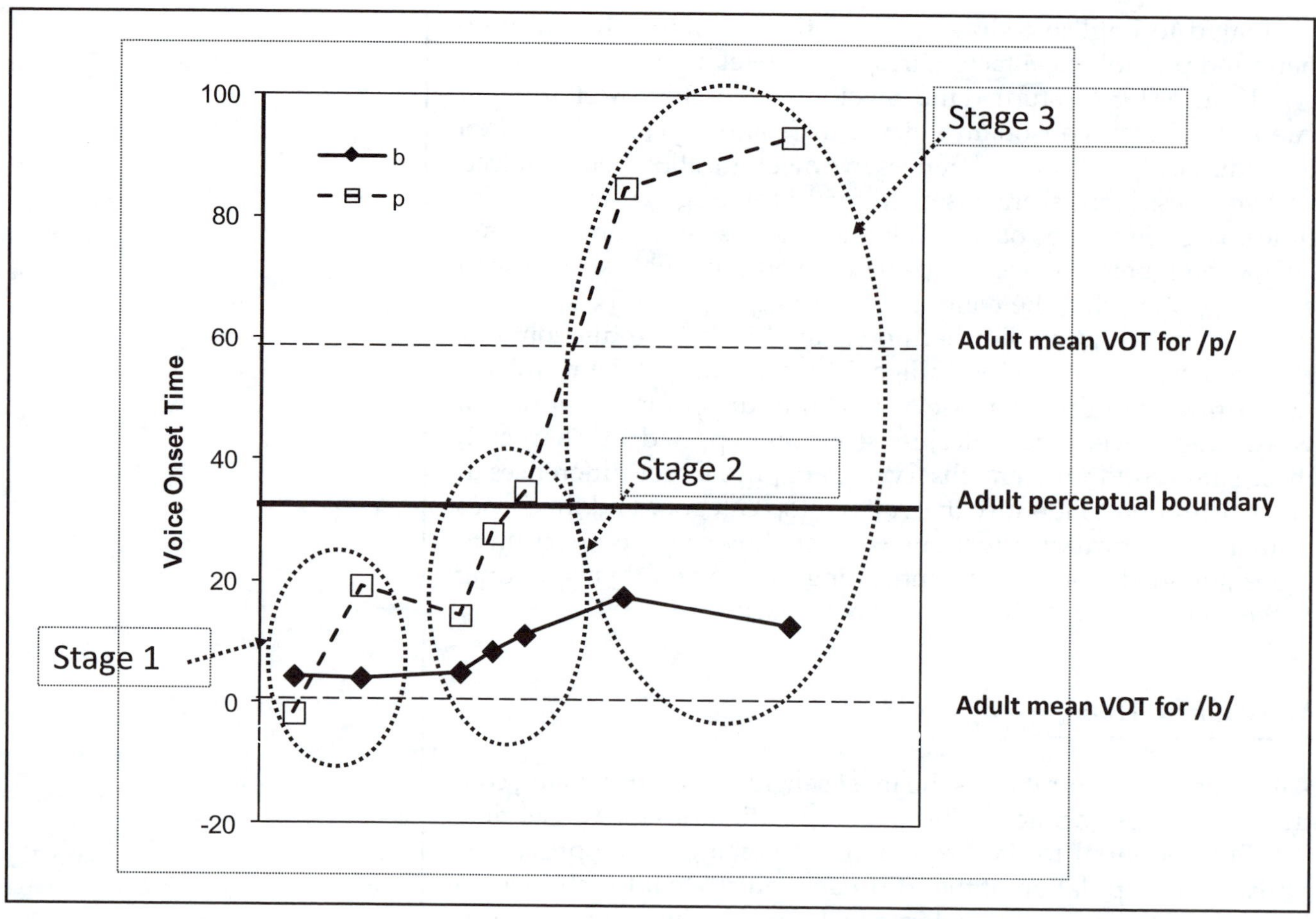

Figure 3–11. *Mean voice onset time values (in ms) for target /p/ and /b/ in word initial position as produced by a female toddler at multiple sampling intervals between 16 and 26 months of age plotted from left to right. Three stages in the acquisition of the voicing contrast are marked by ellipses: Stage 1, no contrast; Stage 2, covert contrast; Stage 3, overshoot. Adapted from Macken and Barton (1980). A longitudinal study of the acquisition of the voicing contrast in American English word initial stops, as measured by voice onset time.* Journal of Child Language, *7, Table 6, p. 63 and Figure 5, p. 66.*

Acoustic analysis of toddlers' production of voiced and voiceless stops reveals three stages toward acquisition of the **voicing contrast**: no contrast, covert contrast, and overshoot.

tion of the contrast, Figure 3–11 shows that the initial stage involves production of a short lag (i.e., voiceless unaspirated) stop for both voiced and voiceless targets. This finding has been replicated in many studies for children speaking varied languages (e.g., Eilers, Oller, & Benito-Garcia, 1984, Spanish; MacLeod, Rvachew, & Polka, 2009, French). Lowenstein and Nittrouer (2008) describe this stage as being consistent with the "everything moves at once" principle that is common to early undifferentiated movements of the articulators; the subsequent development of long lag or voicing lead productions requires that the laryngeal gestures be differentiated from the supralaryngeal articulatory gestures. During the second stage, the VOT for voiceless targets diverges from that for voiced targets so that a covert contrast is now present in the child's speech; the difference in VOT is not perceptually apparent to the adult listener but the voiceless targets are produced with measurably longer VOT than the voiced targets. During the third stage, the mean VOT for voiceless targets lengthens considerably so that it surpasses the boundary for adult identification of voiceless stops in relation to voiced stops. Not only is the contrast now perceptible to adult listeners, but the child's production of the contrast appears to reflect a pattern of overshoot as has been described for other speech targets in childhood.

Zlatin and Koenigsknecht (1976) reported VOT values for the production of word initial stops in relation to the participants' own perceptual category boundaries in a study that compared 2-year-olds, 6-year-olds, and adults. For the voiced stop categories, the use of voicing lead increased with age. When producing voiceless stop targets, mean lag times were similar across age groups but varied with place of articulation as velar stops showed the longest voicing lags. Adults produced discrete distributions of VOTs for voiced and voiceless targets at all places of articulation whereas VOT distributions were overlapping for both 2-year-olds and 6-year-olds, as shown in Figure 3–12. More than 90% of the children's productions for voiced targets fell within the child's perceptual category for the voiced target even at age two years. Voiceless targets were much more variable in relation to the toddler's own perceptual categories however with poor accuracy for all places of articulation observed at this age. At age 6, performance was adultlike for labial and alveolar targets but not yet for the velar target. Figure 3–12 illustrates that the increase in VOT values falling within the /k/ perceptual category reflects both increasing stability in production and a narrowing in the width of the perceptual boundary between /g/ and /k/. These data reinforce Macken and Barton's conclusions; acquisition of the voicing contrast in production involves a gradual process of differentiation, refinement and stabilization. Perceptual and productive mastery of the contrast occurs over a protracted time period with the impression of a reciprocal relationship between the two domains although perceptual development leads productive acquisition in time.

Productive acquisition of the voicing contrast between 2 and 6 years of age includes declining overlap between categories and greater correspondence with perceptual categories.

In English-speaking children, the voiced category is acquired in production before the voiceless category and labial and alveolar targets are mastered earlier than velar targets.

Perceptual and productive mastery of the voicing contrast occurs over a protracted time period with the impression of a reciprocal relationship between the two domains although perceptual development leads productive acquisition in time.

Fundamental Frequency Contours

Laryngeal control is important not only for the production of segments but also for the manipulation of the suprasegmental aspects of speech. As discussed in Chapters 1 and 2, variations in fundamental frequency, duration, and amplitude create contrasting patterns of phrasal stress over the course of an utterance; manipulation of these same acoustic parameters serves to mark the boundaries between phonological words and phrases. Therefore, imprecise control of fundamental frequency (F0) can be expected to impair the child's ability to communicate lexical, syntactic, and pragmatic information that depends on prosodic information that is conveyed at many levels of the phonological hierarchy. In fact, inappropriate manipulation of fundamental frequency contours is a known correlate of motor speech disorders that has been shown to impair speech intelligibility (Laures & Weismer, 1999). A detailed review of

Imprecise control of fundamental frequency can be expected to impair the child's ability to communicate lexical, syntactic, and pragmatic information that depends on prosodic information that is conveyed at many levels of the phonological hierarchy.

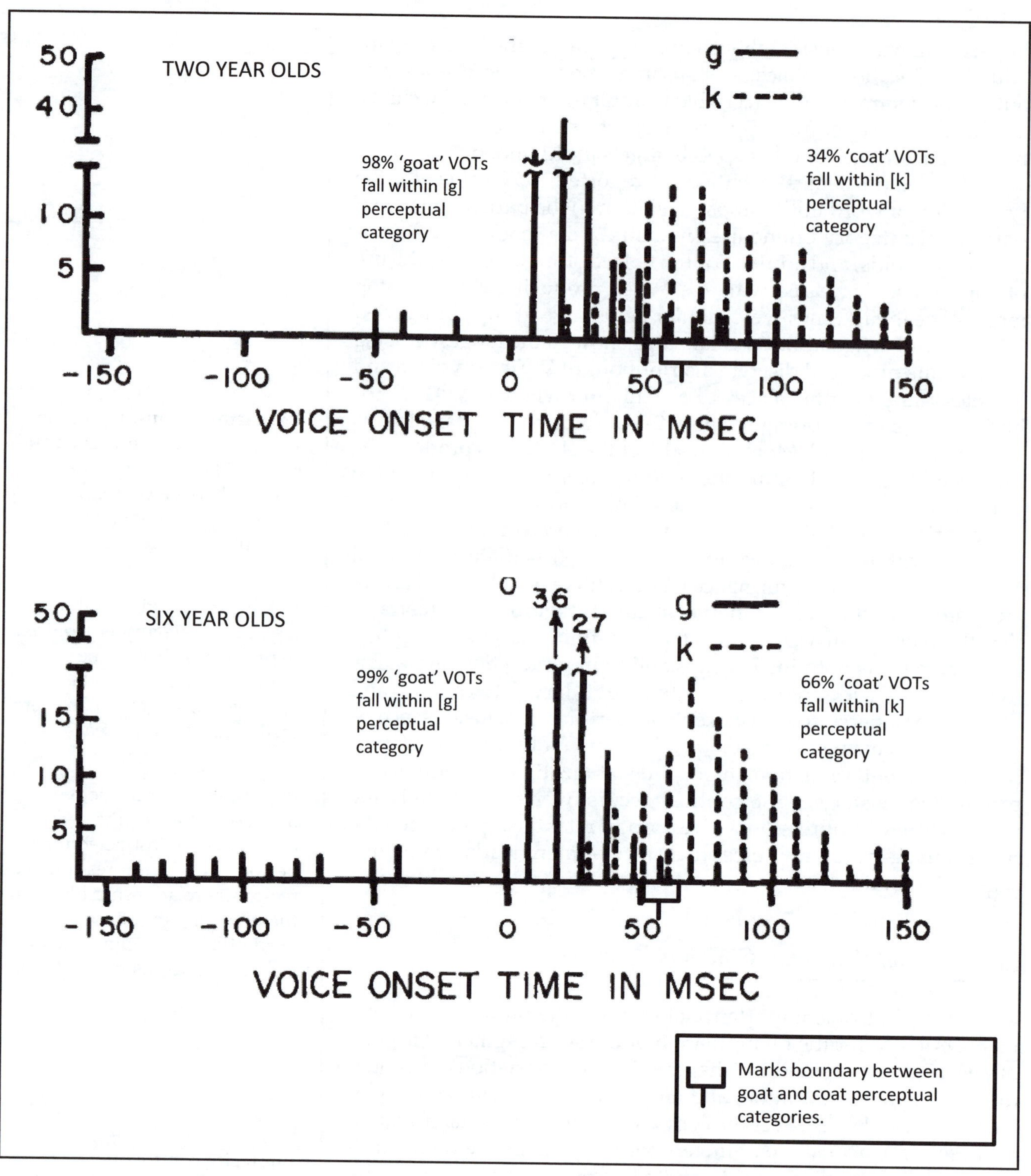

Figure 3–12. *Distributions of voice onset time values (in ms) for target /g/ and /k/ as produced in the words "goat" and "coat" by ten 2-year-old children (top) and ten 6-year-old children (bottom) in relation to their perceptual categories for this phonemic contrast. Adapted from Zlatin and Koenigsknecht (1976). Development of the voicing contrast: A comparison of voice onset time in stop perception and production.* Journal of Speech, Language, and Hearing Research, 19, *Figure 2, p.* 98 *and Figure* 3, *p.* 99. *Used with permission of the American Speech-Hearing-Language Association.*

the literature on the development of fundamental frequency control and its relation to the acquisition of prosody is not undertaken here; the reader is referred to sources such as Snow and Balog (2002). However, a brief review follows that focuses on lexical stress and the production of phrase boundaries.

Detectable and deliberate manipulation of F0 requires a relatively stable background level of F0 in the child's speech. However, continuous declines in mean F0 are observed throughout childhood with the average between infancy and adulthood being approximately 1 octave for females and 2 octaves for males (Vorperian & Kent, 2007). Furthermore, between utterance variability in F0 also changes with maturation, with significant declines observed in childhood but variability increasing again following puberty (Lee et al., 1999). The child's use of F0 to create contrasting lexical and phrasal stress patterns must be adjusted to cope with these developmental changes in level and variance in mean F0.

In order to produce lexical tone contrasts (for example the falling tone associated with trochees and the rising tone associated with iambs) the child must learn to control variation in F0 within an utterance. The research evidence regarding the age at which this kind of control emerges is contradictory. A predominance of falling tones has been reported for early infant utterances that has been attributed to physiological factors such as falling subglottal pressure at the end of a breath group (e.g., Kent & Murray, 1982). Furthermore, changes in between- and within-utterance variability have been tied to linguistic milestones, enhancing the impression that early F0 contours are constrained by physiological factors, whereas later emerging control of F0 is motivated by linguistic factors (Amano, Nakatani, & Kondo, 2006). On the other hand, Davis, MacNeilage, Matyear, and Powell (2000) reported that English-learning prelinguistic infants produced both falling and rising contours in babbled disyllables with no apparent trochaic bias. Numerous studies have reported cross-linguistic differences in the frequency of rising and falling tones in babbled disyllables with continuity in the proportion of usage of these patterns into the first word stage (e.g., for French vs. Japanese, Hallé, De Boysson-Bardies, & Vihman, 1991; for English vs. French, Whalen, Levitt, Hsiao, & Smorodinsky, 1995). Therefore, some researchers conclude that the control of F0 for the production of lexical tone emerges during the integrative stage of early vocal development.

Some of the confusion in this literature may reflect the fact that the rhythmic qualities of speech that the infant is sensitive to are signaled by multiple acoustic correlates. In order to reproduce the prosodic contours that occur in the input, the child must learn to manipulate these cues in conjunction with each other in order to reproduce adultlike lexical tone contrasts. Kehoe, Stoel-Gammon, and Buder (1995) studied acquisition of lexical stress in toddlers aged 18 to 30 months and found that about 30% of the stress patterns produced were perceived by adults to be inaccurate even

Speech development between 18 and 30 months involves improved stability in the use of individual parameters (F0, duration, amplitude) and increased correlation of these parameters within stressed syllables for the production of lexical stress contrasts.

though the acoustic analyses demonstrated that the infants were manipulating F0, duration, and amplitude to mark stressed syllables. The results suggested that development involves improved stability in the use of individual parameters (F0, duration, amplitude) and increased correlation of these parameters within stressed syllables with maturation. Their review of the literature further suggests that sampling procedures will have a significant effect on results, with children's ability to control F0 likely to be better for familiar words and in spontaneous speech than for imitation tasks and for nonsense words.

In early speech development, lexical and utterance boundaries are often confounded; with increased linguistic sophistication the child will have a growing need to manipulate lexical tone and phrase and utterance boundaries independently. Phrase final syllables are typically marked by a steep decrement in F0 as well as other cues such as increased duration and a pause at the phrase juncture. The phrase final syllable may or may not coincide with an utterance juncture. Snow and Balog (2002) reviewed studies in which accent range (degree of pitch change) was taken as an indication of boundary marking. By comparing accent range in stressed and unstressed syllables across single and two-syllable words they were able to conclude that children were using F0 contours to signal grammatical boundaries during the single word stage. Control of utterance internal phrase boundaries is more difficult and may involve a protracted developmental course, however. Katz, Beach, Jenouri, and Verma (1996) found that 5- and 7-year-old children were able to manipulate duration but not F0 to mark phrase boundaries for utterances such as "pink, and green and white" versus "pink and green, and white." Large differences in research procedure in studies of young children compared to older children make it difficult to trace the emergence of these boundary marking cues because children's performance on these structured tasks may not reflect their knowledge as well as the spontaneous language sampling that typically is used with younger children.

Summary of Studies of Speech Development

We have traced the development of speech motor control from birth through to adulthood with respect to four speech behaviors: syllabic organization, vowel production, voice onset time contrasts, and fundamental frequency contours. Certain processes were common to the acquisition of all these behaviors. The general time course of events was also shared—in each case the early emergence of an adultlike coordinative infrastructure was followed by a protracted period of refinement. The earliest stages of speech development are marked by active and deliberate exploration of the possibilities of the vocal tract, culminating in the coordination of the multiple speech subsystems for the production of canonical syllables.

The infant's production of reduplicated and variegated babble at approximately 7 months of age marks the emergence of syllabic organization in speech. Initially, alternating sequences of consonants and vowels during syllable production are accomplished largely through jaw oscillation. Although the jaw makes the primary contribution to early syllabic organization, jaw movements are far from mature at this young age; in fact, muscle activation patterns for mandibular control are loosely specified for chewing and for speech in 9-month-old infants.

An adultlike coordinative infrastructure for speech emerges gradually over the next 24 months. A key event is the establishment of mandibular control, reflected in decreased synchrony of muscle activation among antagonist muscle groups during chewing and increased synchrony among antagonist muscle groups during speech. Integration of lip movements into the increasingly stable jaw movement pattern during syllable production also occurs during this period. Furthermore, tongue movements gradually become differentiated from the jaw as evident by the achievement of adultlike locus equations by 12 months of age and steady expansion of the vowel space along the F1 and F2 dimensions during the first 18 months of life. Adultlike formant frequency trajectories leading to perceptually accurate vowel production and mature patterns of intersyllabic coarticulation by age 36 months reflect continued differentiation of tongue from jaw as well as tongue blade from tongue dorsum. Differentiation of laryngeal and supralaryngeal gestures is also observed with the emergence of the long lag voicing category and increasingly stable use of F0 contours to mark lexical tone and utterance final prosodic boundaries.

Although the overall coordinative infrastructure for speech resembles the adult form in early childhood, children's articulatory movements are characterized by smaller displacements, longer durations, lower velocities, and greater variability than those observed in young adults. Gradual refinement toward adult values for displacement, duration, velocity, and variability continues past the age of 16 years with the process being far from linear however. Nonlinearity is evident not only in the pace of change with age but differences in rate of change across different articulators and subsystems. For example, kinematic studies of lip and jaw movements during sentence production show that children achieve 60% of adult values for displacement by age 12 with steady increases thereafter; in contrast, 90% of adult duration values are achieved by age 12 and then a plateau is observed between 12 and 16 years. Overshoot has been observed for vowel formant frequencies, vowel durations, spectral envelopes, and fundamental frequencies with children exceeding adult values in early adolescence and returning to the adult target in later adolescence. During the toddler period the same phenomenon was observed for stop VOTs. Variability is observed to be less for higher order coordinative goals (i.e., lip aperture) than for lower order coordinative structure (i.e., lower lip and jaw synergy). Variability increases with linguistic complexity as late as age 16 years. Increased levels of variability throughout childhood may provide flexibility to the system that allows for adaptation to ongoing developments in other domains including vocal tract structure, neurophysiological function, cognitive load, and linguistic knowledge.

Walsh and Smith (2002) concluded that "At present, there is not a widely accepted, comprehensive model for the acquisition of speech motor processes. Such a model would specify the factors contributing to speech motor development as the child matures and the time course of acquisition of various components of speech motor performance" (p. 1127). In the next section we describe some influential theories of speech motor control. Although these theories have largely dealt with adult speech motor processes, they provide a basis for identifying factors that potentially contribute to the acquisition of speech motor control and for considering the strength of the current evidence for the role of these factors.

Theories of Speech Motor Control

3.2.1. Distinguish between the following psycholinguistic processes: lexical access, phonological encoding, motor planning, motor programming, and motor execution.

3.2.2. Describe how a child might learn to produce an iambic utterance such as [pə'pʌp] (see Figure 3–7) from the perspective of Schema Theory (see text and Figures 3–13 and 3–14).

3.2.3. Identify two primary weaknesses with Schema Theory as an explanation for the development of speech motor control.

3.2.4. Define and differentiate: internal forward model, feed-forward command, and internal inverse model.

3.2.5. Describe the DIVA model and each of its components as shown in Figure 3–15.

3.2.6. Describe the probable roles of unsupervised, supervised, and reinforcement learning in the development of internal models for speech motor control during early speech acquisition.

Psycholinguistic Models of Speech Production

In Chapter 1 we indicated that articulatory knowledge at multiple levels of the phonological hierarchy would be required in order to greet your friend with the phrase "Nice weather today!" A number of different psycholinguistic models propose a multistage process for accessing and implementing this knowledge, with the stages typically being phonological encoding, motor planning, motor programming and finally execution of the utterance (Baker, Croot, McLeod, & Paul, 2001). Naturally the process must begin, as illustrated in Plate 5, with conceptual preparation of the message to be transmitted, a stage that is followed by selection of lexical items and other information that is important to the construction of the form of the message. There is considerable disagreement among theorists about how information is stored in the lexicon and the amount of phonological detail that is contained within lexical entries (Dell, 1988; Levelt, Roelofs, & Meyer, 1999; Shattuck-Hufnagel, 1999). These debates are well beyond the scope of this chapter and deal with details that may be independent of the motor planning, programming, and execution stages of the process in any case. Therefore, we simply point out that the phonological representations in the lexicon do not provide enough information to directly guide speech production. If phonological representations are structured in a manner similar to that described in Chapter 1, the default feature specifications will not provide enough information to guide production of the segments. Furthermore, as pointed out earlier, one of the characteristics of mature speech production is the ability to plan utterances in relatively long chunks, probably at the level of the phonological phrase. The metrical frame for a phonological phrase is often not the same as the concatenated metrical frames for the individual words that make up the phrase. Therefore, during phonological encoding it may be necessary to resyllabify the constituent morphemes to integrate the phonological, morphological, syntactic, and intonational characteristics of the phonological phrase by constructing an utterance-specific metrical frame. Segments are then selected and fit into the slots in the frame. The output of this stage is an abstract but utterance-specific representation of the phonological phrase that specifies segmental and metrical information. A highly simplified representation of a metrical frame with filled segment slots is illustrated in Plate 5.

This utterance-specific abstract representation serves as input to the motor planning stage of the process. Many models propose that the talker selects or constructs a plan for the production of syllable-sized units. In Levelt's model (e.g., Levelt et al., 1999), motor plans for a few hundred frequently used syllables are accessed from a syllabary in the form of gestural scores, as described by Browman and Goldstein (1989), whereas motor plans for infrequent syllables must be constructed online. The gestural score for each syllable outlines a spatiotemporal pattern of articulator specific gestures that is abstract but context specific. Browman and Goldstein graphically represented these plans in the manner shown in Plate 5, with constriction degree and constriction placement parameters specified for the velum, tongue body (TB), tongue tip (TT), lips, and glottis. In this example the first syllable to be articulated is [naɪs]. Production

Psycholinguistic models propose a multistage process for accessing and implementing phonological knowledge to produce an utterance.

Conceptual preparation of the message to be transmitted is followed by *selection of lexical items* and other information that is important to the construction of the form of the message.

Subsequent to lexical access, **phonological encoding** serves to integrate the phonological, morphological, syntactic, and intonational characteristics of the phonological phrase by constructing an utterance specific *metrical frame* into which segments are inserted.

Many models propose that the talker selects or constructs a plan for the production of syllable-sized units during the **motor planning stage**.

The **gestural score** for each syllable outlines a spatiotemporal pattern of articulator-specific gestures that is abstract but context specific.

of the syllable begins with the velum open and the tongue tip on the alveolar ridge; therefore the parameters are shown as constriction degree WIDE for the velum and CLOSED for the tongue tip which is placed on the ALVEOLAR RIDGE (ALV). The tongue body gestures for the diphthong—starting as NARROW PHARYNGEAL (NAR PHGL) and ending with WIDE PALATAL (WIDE PAL)—overlap with the tongue tip, velar, and glottal gestures for the consonants at the beginning and end of the syllable. For the final consonant, the parameters for the tongue tip are CRITICAL (CRIT) for constriction degree and ALVEOLAR RIDGE for constriction placement. The glottis constriction degree is WIDE as this is a voiceless fricative. Browman and Goldstein propose that these invariantly specified gestures result in variable speech output when the gestural score is stretched or shrunk in space and time in accordance with the metrical frame and to accommodate different speaking styles (see also Saltzman & Munhall, 1989). For example, in formal speaking situations or when reading a list of words, the individual articulatory gestures may have greater extent but less overlap resulting in reduced coarticulation. Rapid connected speech will lead to overlapping gestures that are reduced in time and space resulting in common processes such as segment deletions and assimilations. The motor plan or gestural score provides a basis for motor programming, the stage at which commands are generated to specify the patterns of muscle activity that are required to produce the desired direction, force, range, and speed of movement of the individual muscles. Execution of the program results in articulation of the syllable.

Browman and Goldstein proposed a theory in which invariantly specified gestures are the basic units of phonology; these gestures result in variable speech output when the gestural score is stretched or shrunk in space and time in accordance with the metrical frame.

The motor plan or gestural score provides a basis for **motor programming**, the stage at which commands are generated to specify the patterns of muscle activity that are required to produce the desired direction, force, range, and speed of movement of the individual muscles.

Execution of the program results in articulation of the syllable.

The "box-and-arrow" illustration in Plate 5 is presented as a kind of metaphor for speech production that serves to identify some of the processes that might be involved while not explaining how any of these processes actually work at a neurophysiological or biomechanical level. We turn now to two theories of the motor planning and programming processes that have been developed with sufficient detail to allow for testing through behavioral experiments and computational modeling.

Motor Schema Theory

Motor Schema Theory was introduced in 1975 by Richard A. Schmidt as a new theory of discrete motor learning that had the potential to solve the *storage problem* (how does the learner store so many discrete motor plans) and the *novelty problem* (how does the learner learn a new motor plan).

Closed-loop control occurs when performance is compared to an internalized target trajectory or goal and errors are corrected online in response to error messages as they occur.

Open-loop control involves execution of a preprogrammed movement without recourse to feedback.

Motor Schema Theory was introduced by Schmidt (1975) as a solution to two persistent problems in theories of speech motor control: the storage problem and the novelty problem. At the time, theorists posited either closed-loop or open-loop control mechanisms: closed-loop control occurs when performance is compared to an internalized target trajectory or goal and errors are corrected online in response to error messages as they occur; open-loop control involves execution of a preprogrammed movement without recourse to feedback. Early closed-and open-loop models of speech motor control assumed storage of information that was unique to each discrete task, defined by Schmidt as a task lasting less than

5 seconds from recognizable onset to offset. Given that speech production was estimated to involve more than 100,000 discrete allophones (taking into account phonetic context) Schmidt felt that the storage problem would be insurmountable without modifications to the earlier theories. Schmidt was also trying to explain how the learner added new programs or adapted old programs to new circumstances, a particularly acute problem in the developmental context.

Schmidt's (1975; 2003) innovation was the notion of the generalized motor program (GMP) that specifies the broad outlines of a movement while providing for adaptation to variable task demands through the scaling of a rate parameter and a force parameter. Schmidt proposed that appropriate setting of the parameters is accomplished by reference to a learned set of relationships among the target, the initial conditions, and prior experience with production of a general class of movement patterns, as outlined in Figure 3–13. These relationships include two schemata: a recall schema and a recognition schema. The recall schema specifies the relationship between the parameters for a given GMP and the outcomes that

A **generalized motor program (GMP)** specifies the broad outlines of a movement while providing for adaptation to variable task demands through the scaling of a *rate parameter* and a *force parameter*.

Appropriate setting of the parameters is accomplished by reference to a learned set of relationships among the target, the initial conditions, and prior experience with production of a general class of movement patterns.

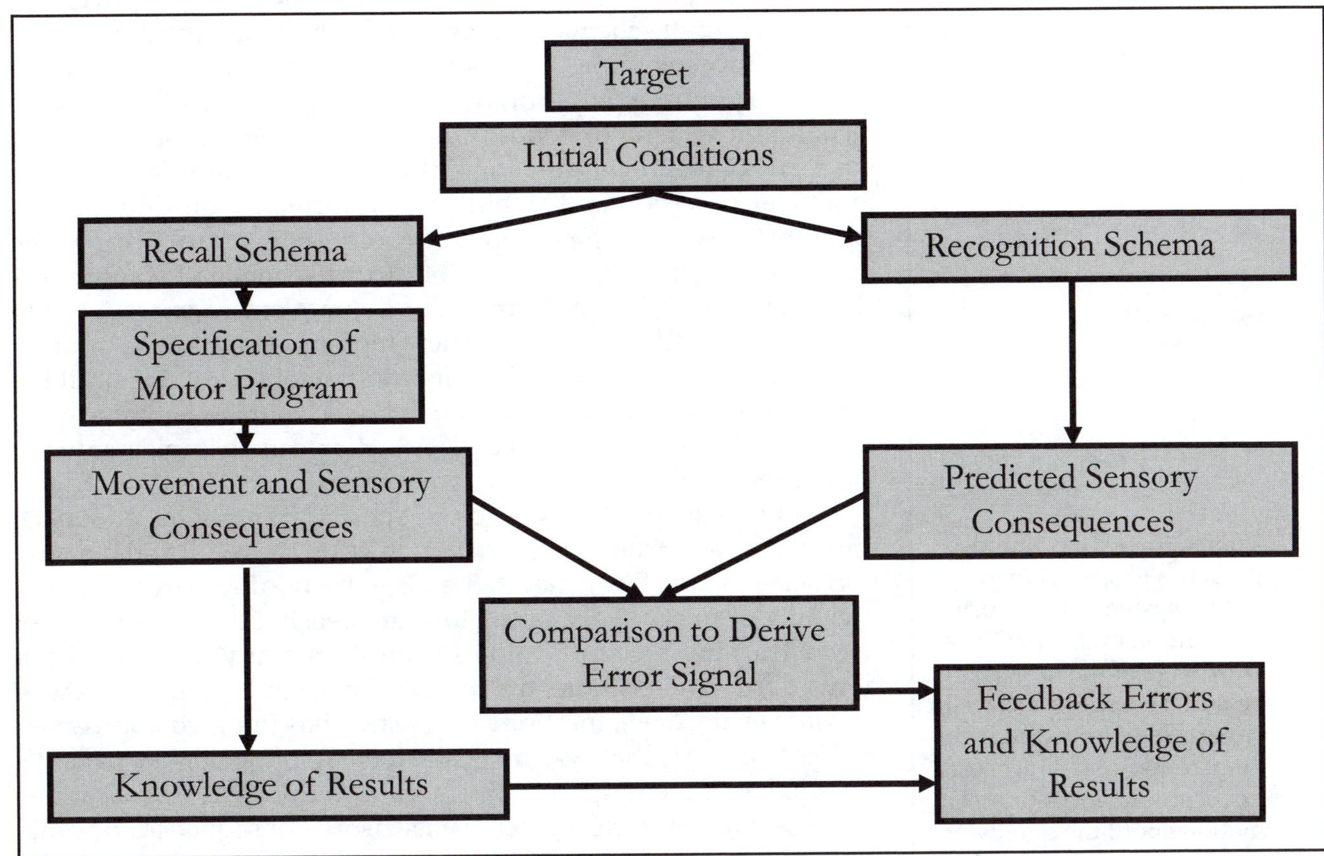

Figure 3–13. *Fundamental relationships involved in the acquisition, maintenance, and performance of a motor skill. Adapted from Kent and Lybolt (1982). Motor schema as a basis for motor learning.* General Principles of Therapy, *Table 1, p. 14. Used with permission of Thieme Medical Publishers, Inc.*

The **recall schema** specifies the relationship between the parameters for a given GMP and the outcomes that will be achieved.

will be achieved, allowing the talker to choose parameters for a given speaking situation either by repeating previously practiced parameter settings or by interpolating between known settings. Presumably the notion of an adaptable generalized motor plan reduces the storage load while the ability to select new parameters on the basis of past experience solves at least part of the novelty problem. Recall of the GMP for a given task and selection of the parameters in accordance with the initial conditions leads to specification of a motor program for execution of the movement. During production of the movement the talker will experience the sensory consequences of the articulatory movements involved (somatosensory, proprioceptive, auditory) and may determine if the desired target was achieved (knowledge of results). Based on past experience with feedback during similar movements, a recognition schema predicts the sensory consequences that should occur upon execution of the motor program. The error signal that is derived from comparison of the expected sensory consequences with the actual sensory consequences is integrated with knowledge of results to refine the schemata. Specifically, new information about the relationship between the outcome of the movement, the initial conditions and the parameters that were used to execute the movement allows the recall schema to more accurately define the parameters in the future; the same information, combined with knowledge of the sensory consequences of the movement as executed, allows the recognition schema to better predict the sensory consequences of the correct movement; updating of the schemata in this way leads to greater precision and stability of performance on future trials. Note that this is an open-loop model of motor control because the feedback results in updating of the stored schemata for future trials rather than online adjustment of the movement in response to error. The disadvantage is that a new motor plan cannot be brought online in response to changing environmental conditions until the current program has run its course; the advantage is that a well-learned motor program for a discrete action can be implemented in the absence of peripheral sensory feedback.

Based on past experience with feedback during similar movements, a **recognition schema** predicts the sensory consequences that should occur upon execution of the motor program.

Motor schema theory leads to specific hypotheses about the impact of practice and feedback variables on the recall and recognition schema and has generated a large body of research in many domains of motor learning including speech. Some principles of motor learning for application in speech therapy that have been derived from these studies are reviewed in Chapter 10. As reviewed by Maas et al. (2008), this body of research has founded approaches to speech therapy that systematically focus attention on the patient's knowledge of the target and the initial conditions as well as access to knowledge of performance (i.e., sensory consequences or other information about the quality of the movement) and knowledge of results (i.e, accuracy of the outcome with respect to the target or goal of the movement).

Schema theory has founded approaches to speech therapy that systematically focus attention on the patient's knowledge of the target and the initial conditions as well as access to **knowledge of performance** (i.e., sensory consequences or other information about the quality of the movement) and **knowledge of results** (i.e., accuracy of the outcome with respect to the target or goal of the movement).

Typical studies in this field involve teaching participants to perform a simple movement pattern with visual feedback. For example, Wulf, Schmidt, and Deubel (1993) presented young adults with normal motor skills a visual pattern on a screen; after removing the visual image of the pattern, the participants would try to reproduce it by pushing a horizontal lever; subsequent to the attempt, visual feedback indicated whether the movement matched the spatiotemporal characteristics of the model. Participants were trained with 3 different versions of the pattern and then tested with a fourth version for which they had received no prior practice. Feedback was provided for training patterns but not the test pattern. Figure 3–14 provides examples of patterns representing two different GMPs, one that was taught with variations in the rate parameter (Figure 3–14A) and another that was taught with variations in the force parameter (Figure 3–14B). Learning was assessed by determining if the movements produced during test trials were consistent with the modeled rate or force parameter and by observing whether the global movement trajectory was consistent with the GMP, as illustrated in Figure 3–14C. Although this experiment seems far removed from speech, some researchers have applied similar research techniques to patients with speech disorders. For example, Clark and Robin (1998) conducted a very similar experiment with elderly adults except that the participants were required to reproduce a visual pattern by moving their jaw. After training in the production of the jaw movement at variable rates, participants with apraxia of speech, conduction aphasia, or normal speech were tested for their ability to match the same general movement pattern modeled at an untrained rate. Some patients showed difficulty learning the GMP, whereas others had difficulty with parameterization but no particular pattern served to differentiate the diagnostic groups from each other.

You can see from Figure 3–14 how each of the GMPs specifies the relative timing and force of the muscle contractions that must be produced by the effectors in order to reproduce a pattern of movements that belongs to the same general class. Changing the rate or the force parameter alters the absolute amplitude of the trajectories in the spatial and temporal domains but does not change the fundamental relationships among these parameters within the GMP. Understanding the difference between the GMP and the parameters in these movement trajectories is potentially important because the training conditions that promote learning of a new GMP versus generalization of learning across new parameterizations within a GMP are reportedly different. Despite empirical validation of some of the principles of motor learning that are associated with this theory, there are significant conceptual problems with this theoretical perspective. Application of the principles of learning requires that one be able to clearly identify discrete motor tasks that collectively represent a single GMP. Operationalizing these fundamental constructs can prove to be problematic in the domain of functional motor skills such as picking up your coffee cup or saying the word "nice."

Understanding the difference between the GMP and the parameters in these movement trajectories is potentially important because the training conditions that promote learning of a new GMP versus generalization of learning across new parameterizations within a GMP are reportedly different; however, operationalizing these fundamental constructs can prove to be problematic in the domain of functional motor skills.

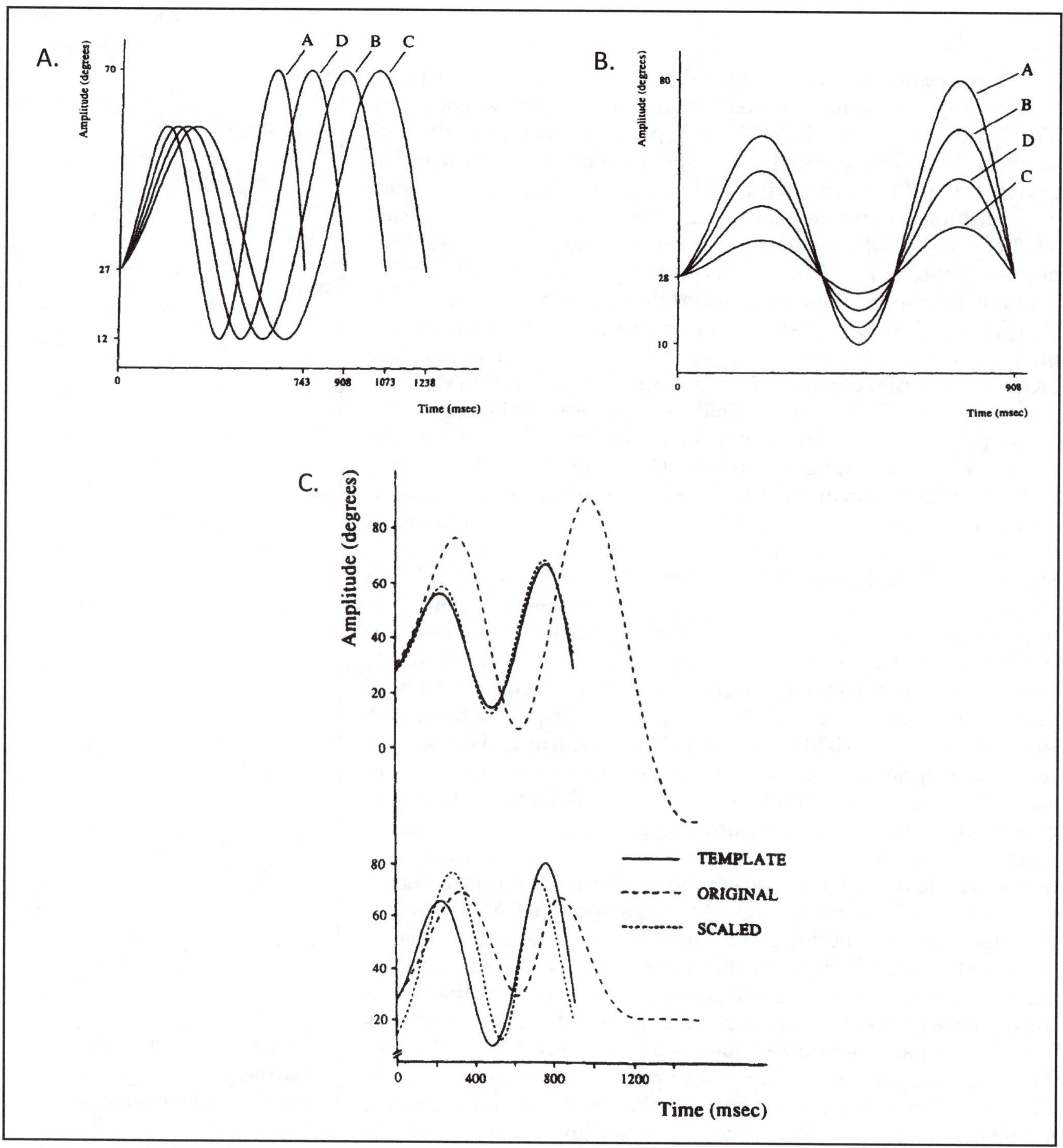

Figure 3–14. *Visual representations of spatiotemporal patterns provided as models for the production of arm movements while pushing a horizontal lever in a study to examine differential learning of gross motor plans (GMPs) versus parameters: (**A**) one GMP modeled to vary rate; (**B**) another GMP modeled to vary force (patterns marked A, B, and C were taught with feedback and then the participant's ability to match the pattern marked D was tested without feedback; and (**C**) test movement trajectories were scaled and then compared to the model to determine if the movement was consistent with the GMP (the scaled trajectory fits the GMP in the upper part of the example but does not in the lower part). From Wulf, Schmidt, & Deubel. Reduced feedback frequency enhances generalized motor program learning but not parameterization learning. Copyright © 1993 by the American Psychological Association. Reproduced with permission.* Journal of Experimental Psychology: Learning, Memory, and Cognition, 19*(5), Figure 1, p. 1136, Figure 5, p. 1143, Figure 2, p. 1138. The use of APA information does not imply endorsement by APA.*

The experimental tasks thus far are constrained so that the participants make a simple extension-flexion-extension-flexion sequence of movements around a single joint that bears little relationship to functional movements using the same effectors. No syllables can be spoken with a simple movement of the jaw—coordination with multiple supralaryngeal articulators as well as the laryngeal and respiratory systems will be necessary. Reaching for one's coffee cup also requires coordination of multiple components, with reaching and grasping components overlapping in time and space. The planning and execution of this action is typically successful despite the sudden appearance of obstacles such as your orange juice order or your partner's reading glasses. Consider that you can articulate "Nice weather today" while chewing your toast, reaching for the coffee, and avoiding the orange juice and you can see that the complexities abound! Under these real-world conditions it has proved quite impossible to isolate discrete units of action that can be grouped into generalized classes that are controlled by a single GMP.

One challenge to the validity of schema theory is that the notion of a generalized motor plan with scalable rate or force parameters has not proven useful for the grouping of functional movement patterns.

The first difficulty is that the notion of uniform scaling of rate and force parameters has not held up under scrutiny. For example, Marteniuk, Leavitt, MacKenzie, and Athenes (1990) observed young adults reaching for and grasping progressively larger objects and found that speed increased with object size; however, the duration of the accelerating part of the movement was constant with object size whereas the time from peak deceleration to object contact was linearly related to object size reflecting the greater precision required to grasp small objects. In this case it can be seen that the relative timing of the two phases of the action is not held constant and thus even this simple but functional task does not fit with the notion of a generalized motor plan. Schmidt (2003) summarizes examples in which the assumption of invariant patterns of relative force within a class of presumably similar movements does not hold (rather devastatingly for a theory of movement, this includes actions that are affected by gravity such as walking with or without a pack). Despite the inherent challenge of identifying GMPs on the basis of scalable rate and force parameters, these concepts have been applied to speech therapy. Maas et al. (2008, p. 280) suggested that "the syllables 'tie' and 'sigh,' while sharing the same articulator, might involve different GMPs because they differ in relative movement amplitude (full closure vs. narrow constriction) [thus predicting transfer of training] across place of articulation (same GMP) but not across manner of articulation (different GMPs)." It is difficult to imagine how any two syllables with different phonetic content could be considered to differ by any scalable rate or force factor; even syllables with the same phonetic content fit uneasily into the concept of a GMP because it is well known that linear changes in speaking rate do not result in uniform kinematic effects on speech production, either within or across talkers (Adams & Weismer, 1993). Recall also Goffman and Smith's (1999) study in which the kinematic patterns (velocity templates) of the words *man, ban, pan, fan,* and *van* were found to form 5 unique patterns rather than clusters of related words differing only in the setting of a specific parameter.

A second challenge to the validity of schema theory is the lack of a mechanism within the theory to explain motor equivalence.

Another serious problem is the lack of a mechanism within the theory to explain motor equivalence, a phenomenon elegantly exemplified by studies in which an articulator is perturbed unexpectedly during speech. Abbs and Gracco (1983) recorded EMG activity from facial muscles including the upper and lower lip muscles of young adults while they produced utterances that included intervocalic labial consonants. On some trials a downward load was placed on the bottom lip during the labial closing gesture. Subjectively, the talkers were not bothered by the perturbation and listeners could not discern any distortion in the resulting speech output. The EMG data reveal that compensatory movements of the lower and upper lip occurred from the first perturbed trial. The movements of the upper and lower lips and the corresponding muscles were varied rather than stereotypical but the joint activity of these effectors covaried in a predictable fashion to achieve labial closure despite these unpredictable perturbations to the planned lower lip trajectory. In other words, the higher-order goal was achieved despite variability in upper and lower lip movements, foreshadowing Smith and Zelaznik's (2004) finding that children achieve greater stability for lip aperture size than for lower order synergies during sentence production. The results suggest the dynamic interplay of two different sensorimotor processes that independently affect the upper and lower lip. Compensatory increases in lower lip muscles reflect closed-loop feedback processes, in other words a direct corrective response to the error induced by the perturbation. Increases in upper lip muscle activation that contribute to labial closure cannot be due to feedback since the upper lip is not the site of the perturbation or the source of the error feedback. Upper lip compensatory actions are attributed to a feed-forward mechanism. Feed-forward processes are predictive rather than reactive: the system monitors peripheral sensory events and predicts the likely outcome relative to the expected target, allowing for continuous and proactive adjustments throughout the system to achieve the motor goal. From the dynamic systems perspective, this experiment presents an example of a coordinative structure in which a complex organization of interacting components achieves a specific goal via the "temporary marshaling of many degrees of freedom into a task-specific, functional unit" (Kelso, Tuller, Vatikiotis-Bateson, & Fowler, 1984; p. 828). Within a coordinative structure, there is no need to control each component independently; rather, the components are "soft-assembled" (rather than hardwired) to cooperate together to achieve the higher order goal. Kelso et al. (1984) demonstrated the task-specificity of coordinative structures for speech by conducting perturbation experiments similar to the one described above, comparing local and remote reactions to perturbations of

When articulators are unpredictably perturbed during speech, the dynamic interplay of closed-loop feedback processes and open-loop feed-forward processes permits achievement of the higher order motor goal.

Feed-forward processes are predictive rather than reactive: the system monitors peripheral sensory events and predicts the likely outcome relative to the expected target, allowing for continuous and proactive adjustments throughout the system to achieve the motor goal.

the lower jaw during production of the syllables [bæb] and [bæz]. The researchers observed compensatory responses of the lower lip during production of both syllables when the lower jaw was displaced during the closing phase of the articulatory gesture; compensatory responses were observed in the upper lip only during [bæb] production whereas compensatory responses were observed in the tongue only during [bæz] production. These authors suggest that these compensatory responses of the coordinative structure for the production of a given phoneme, observed under peculiar laboratory conditions, are actually fundamental to our understanding of normal speech production; the widely and rapidly varying phonetic conditions under which any phoneme is articulated during language production requires flexible and task specific adaptations by the articulators. We now turn to models of speech motor control that incorporate sufficient dynamic flexibility to account for motor equivalence and other fundamental characteristics of speech production and speech development.

A **coordinative structure** is a functional grouping of components that is soft-assembled to achieve a specific task by adapting in a dynamic and flexible manner to varying inputs without requiring independent control of each individual component.

Auditory Feedback Based Models of Speech Motor Control

In the previous section we introduced an open-loop model of speech motor control in which feedback was used to learn a motor program that would achieve a specific target given a particular set of initial conditions. The model failed to explain how motor plans might be altered online to adapt to changing environmental conditions and did not allow for the many-to-one relationship between motor plans and a specific target (i.e., motor equivalence). Current theories of motor control incorporate several of the earlier concepts, especially retaining the notion of the motor program and highlighting the importance of predicting the sensory consequences of implementing the program. However, the adaptability of the motor program is enhanced by reference to an *internal model*: a neural system that simulates the behavior of a sensorimotor system in relation to the external environment (Wolpert & Kawato, 1998).

An **internal model** is a neural system that simulates the behavior of a sensorimotor system in relation to the external environment.

An internal model is analogous to a mental map or mental image (Gabbard, 2009) and thus we begin by considering an example in which a mental map of the self in relation to the environment plays a role in the solution to an everyday planning problem. It is important for most of us to be able to find our way from the bed to the bathroom even when the lights are out. After moving into a new apartment some trial and error learning with the lights on will be required to learn the task while becoming familiar with a new floor plan and a novel placement of your furniture. With time you will learn to predict the sensory consequences of a successful negotiation of the path from the bed to the bathroom, 6 steps to the bedroom door, over the lintel and then a small left-turn, two steps across the hall, and you're there. You may have to learn more than one trajectory—if you have left your shoes in front of the easy chair to the left you will have to make a little detour around them at the second step from the bed. Every time that you traverse one of these alternative trajectories you receive multiple kinds of sensory feedback so that eventually you can predict the sensory feedback that you will receive once you have embarked on one or the other path. Now you are ready to make the trip in the middle of the night with the lights off. You select the unobstructed trajectory because you remember that your shoes are in the closet. You lack visual feedback from the environment but you can generate this internally as a consequence of your prior experience. However, if you have forgotten that you left a stepstool just outside the room and slightly to the right of the door frame you will receive somatosensory feedback—ouch!—on step 7 letting you know that you have selected the wrong environmental context and therefore you have to adjust your trajectory. Alternatively, if you remember before you reach the bedroom door—Watch out for the stepstool!—you should be able to visualize the altered environmental context and select a new trajectory on the basis of internal rather than direct feedback, subsequently achieving your target, perhaps with an expected brush-up against the left doorframe but avoiding an injury to your right toes.

An **internal forward model** predicts the future state of the sensorimotor system given its current state and the motor plan that has been implemented, taking context into account.

This example allows us to introduce several new concepts while highlighting the fact that there are actually different kinds of internal models involved in the process. First, an *internal forward model* predicts the future state of the sensorimotor system given its current state and the motor plan that has been implemented, taking context into account, in essence modeling the causal relationship between actions and their consequences (Wolpert & Flanagan, 2001). The forward model allows for smooth execution of locomotion from the bed to the bathroom even though visual feedback is lacking and certain sensory feedback is slow to arrive due to delays in neural transmission of sensory signals. For example, in the unobstructed example, you do not have to stop at the lintel and think, "Ok, I've made it to the bedroom door, now I have to adjust my trajectory 45° to the left"; you can plan this adjustment in advance because you can predict arrival at the lintel when you implement the plan for achieving the intermediate target. In the obstructed example, bumping into the stepstool created a *prediction error* that indicates an unexpected environmental context; the prediction error signaled the need to select a different motor plan better suited to the actual context. The motor plan, sometimes called a *feed-forward command*, is generated by an *internal inverse model* that is able to determine the correct motor plan given knowledge of the current state and the desired state of the system (in essence reversing the forward model that predicts the end state given the current state and the motor plan). Generating the new motor plan at the obstructed doorway requires a transformation of aggregate sensory information and internal feedback into motor commands that will achieve the desired trajectory and end state (Wolpert, Ghahramani, & Flanagan, 2001).

A **feed-forward command** is the motor plan generated by the *internal inverse model.*

The **internal inverse model** is able to determine the correct motor plan given knowledge of the current state and the desired state of the system.

Let us now consider these concepts in the context of syllable production. In the example above, movements were planned to transport oneself toward a visually defined target along a trajectory formulated in terms of spatial coordinates. In speech, the movements of multiple articulators must be coordinated in time and space to achieve targets that are defined in auditory-perceptual terms along trajectories that are formulated in acoustic-phonetic space (Gracco & Abbs, 1986; Perkell et al., 2000). Just as the doorway provides some latitude as to the precision of one's path out of the room, auditory-perceptual targets are not absolute values of particular acoustic cues; rather these targets are multidimensional regions in acoustic-phonetic space, bounded by the distribution of cue values that are provided in the input (McMurray, Aslin, & Toscano, 2009) and shaped by principles of articulatory coherence (Schwartz, Basirat, Ménard, & Sato, 2010).

In speech, the movements of multiple articulators must be coordinated in time and space to achieve targets that are defined in auditory-perceptual terms along trajectories that are formulated in acoustic-phonetic space.

Auditory-perceptual targets are not absolute values of particular acoustic cues; rather these targets are multidimensional regions in acoustic-phonetic space, bounded by the distribution of cue values that are provided in the input and shaped by principles of articulatory coherence.

For example one might wish to produce a pattern of formant frequency changes similar to those shown in the top middle portion of Figure 1–12: a rising F1, falling F2, and rising F3 with the resulting steady states being roughly equally spaced and the listener's percept being [da]; starting with the jaw almost but not closed and the lips in a neutral position this can be accomplished by moving the tongue tip from the alveolar ridge to the lower incisors in coordination with a small jaw lowering gesture and appropriate airflow and laryngeal parameters. Patterns of muscle activation across the appropriate groups of muscles will produce stabilization of certain articulators as well as specific movements of other articulators with characteristic amplitudes, velocities and movement trajectories; these lower level synergies will combine to create a higher level synergy, specifically a change in vocal tract shape that produces the desired acoustic output that is perceived by the listener to be the syllable [da]. Production of these muscle activation patterns will result in several kinds of sensorimotor consequences with each type of feedback having its own characteristic neural transmission time with proprioceptive feedback from muscles and joints being faster than auditory and somatosensory feedback (Schmidt, 1975). The internal forward model will map the relationships between the sensory feedback associated with execution of the motor commands required to produce a specific vocal tract shape and the resulting acoustic output. The internal inverse model translates between the auditory-perceptual goals and the requisite vocal tract shapes and the motor commands required to achieve those vocal tract shapes given the current state of the articulators and relevant contextual information (Perkell et al., 1997). Normally, an adult can produce a syllable or a sequence of syllables without auditory feedback because the forward model allows one to predict the sensory consequences of executing a given motor plan; being able to predict the state of the vocal tract at the offset of the first syllable allows one to guide the articulators through the first syllable with the aid of internal feedback and to plan the articulation of the subsequent

Normally an adult can produce a syllable or a sequence of syllables without auditory feedback because the forward model allows one to predict the sensory consequences of executing a given motor plan.

syllable, accounting in part for co-articulatory effects as previously described (Goodell & Studdert-Kennedy, 1993; Guenther, 1995). When an unexpected event occurs, such as the perturbation to the bottom lip that was provided in the experiments conducted by Abbs and Gracco (1983), both direct feedback and the forward model play a role in achieving the desired outcome. Sensory feedback from the lower lip produces a prediction error that signals a need for compensatory responses but the correction is applied synergistically to the entire system in order to achieve the ultimate goal: the desired auditory-perceptual outcome. Recently, Lackner and Tuller (2008) described "this adaptive flexibility as a dynamic system that evolves in response to the altered actor-environment interaction in a given goal-directed task . . . Adaptive behavior is thus a property of a system that includes the actor, the environment, and the task or goal" (p. 100). Keeping the complexity of this system in mind will be important as we consider the implications for treatment in Chapter 10. In the next section, we describe an auditory feedback model of speech motor control in detail. The advantage of this model—the DIVA model—is that the functional task of speech production is viewed as the achievement of acoustic goals that will be perceived by the listener as a particular string of phonemes.

DIVA Model

The **DIVA (Directions into Velocities of Articulators) model** is a computational model of segmental speech production.

The DIVA (Directions into Velocities of Articulators) model is a computational model of segmental speech production that is designed to be neurologically plausible (Guenther & Vladusich, 2009; Guenther, 1995, 2003, 2006; Guenther, Ghosh, & Tourville, 2006; Guenther, Hampson, & Johnson, 1998; Perkell et al., 2000). The model uses a feedback control system to develop an internal model of the relationship between acoustic signals and vocal tract shapes. The model uses an inverse kinematic model to plan movement trajectories in acoustic space that will achieve the desired auditory-perceptual goals and to transform the acoustic trajectories into feed-forward commands that are specified in terms of velocity and position of articulators. The components of the model in relation to hypothesized neural correlates are described below, with reference to Figure 3–15. We begin by focusing on mature speech production.

Production of speech begins with activation of a unit in the **Speech Sound Map** which typically corresponds to a syllable.

Production of speech begins with activation of a unit in the Speech Sound Map which typically corresponds to a syllable although a unit in the speech sound map might be associated with a single segment or a short sequence of syllables. fMRI studies of adults engaged in nonword reading supports the hypothesis that the ventral premotor cortex (vPMC) is involved in syllable level processing (Peeva et al., 2010). Activation of the units corresponding to the target syllable in the Speech Sound Map leads to signals that encode the requisite motor commands (Feed-Forward Control System) and the sensory expectations associated with executing those motor commands (Feedback Control System). Inhibitory pro-

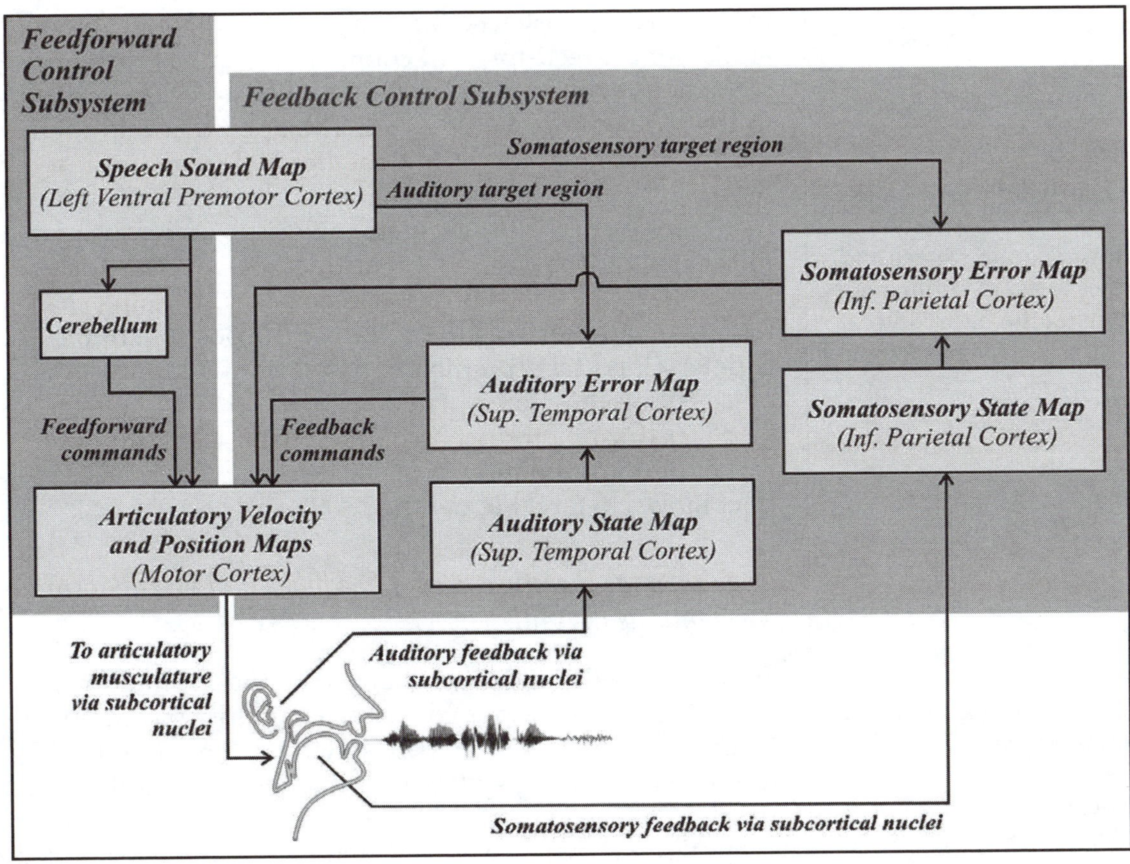

Figure 3–15. Schematic of the components of the DIVA model (see text for details). From Guenther, Ghosh, & Tourville (2006). Neural modeling and imaging of the cortical interactions underlying syllable production. Brain and Language *by Academic Press, 96, Figure 1, p. 282. Reproduced with permission of Academic Press.*

jections from the Speech Sound Map in vPMC to the Auditory Error Map, hypothesized to reside in the superior temporal gyrus, allow for the coding of prediction errors in the event that auditory feedback during production of the syllable (encoded in the Auditory State Map) does not match sensory expectations. Similarly, learned tactile and proprioceptive correlates of the syllable are encoded in the Somatosensory Error Map, hypothesized to be located in the supramarginal gyrus, allowing for the coding of mismatches to somatosensory feedback received in the Somatosensory State Map in the inferior parietal cortex. These error signals are transmitted through the cerebellum to generate corrective feedback commands that impact on the velocity and position of articulators and serve to tune the forward model. It is expected that prediction errors are rare in mature speech, however, and thus feed-forward control plays the major role in adult speech production.

Feed-forward commands from the Speech Sound Map in vPMC to primary motor cortex have two routes, direct projections from vPMC (the motor plan) and projections through the cerebellum that provide state information from the forward model and

The **feedback control system** involves inhibitory projections from the Speech Sound Map to the Auditory and Somatosensory Error Maps allowing for the coding of prediction errors in the Auditory and Somatosensory State Maps in the event that sensory feedback during syllable production does not meet expectations.

It is proposed that error signals are transmitted through the cerebellum to generate corrective feedback commands that impact on the velocity and position of articulators and serve to tune the forward model.

from actual sensory feedback. In the computational model the generation of the feed-forward commands requires a number of transformations or mappings on the route from the Speech Sound Map to the Articulatory Synthesizer. The Speech Sound Map activates multidimensional target regions defined in an auditory and orosensory planning space. Movements in auditory planning space are then transformed into articulator velocities (in essence a motor plan for achieving the desired vocal tract shape). The forward model tracks the vocal tract's position in auditory planning space without relying on auditory feedback; rather the position of the vocal tract is determined by a prediction based on the known consequences of executing the motor plan combined with actual somatosensory feedback during production of the syllable. This information allows for continuous updating of the feed-forward command as the vocal tract moves to target (Guenther, 2003).

The forward model tracks the vocal tract's position in auditory planning space and generates forward commands for achieving the desired vocal tract shape.

Experimental Investigations of Feedback and Feed-Forward Mechanisms in Adult Speech

Tourville, Reilly, and Guenther (2008) induced auditory feedback control of speech production in the laboratory by altering the acoustic characteristics of the talker's own speech while feeding it back to the talker during syllable production. The adult subjects were required to read CVC words that contained the vowel /ɛ/; each subject's own speech was captured by microphone and fed back to the talker over headphones in real time; on randomly selected trials the first formant of the vowel was shifted up or down while they produced the word so that the subjects heard themselves produce a vowel that was slightly more like /æ/ (upward shift) or slightly more like /ɪ/ (downward shift) than the intended vowel /ɛ/; feedback of their own speech was unperturbed on 30% of trials. Talkers compensated during the perturbed trials by adjusting their articulatory output to produce an F1 shift in the direction opposite to the feedback perturbation. These compensatory responses occurred within the utterance that was affected by the shifted feedback, 75 to 150 ms after the onset of the perturbation, reflecting neural delays in delivery of the perturbed feedback. A simulation of this experiment with the DIVA computational model exactly replicated the behavioral effect and supported the hypothesis that the compensation involves the interaction of feedback control and feed-forward processes. Furthermore, imaging of neural responses during perturbed feedback in comparison to normal feedback trials revealed increased activation of bilateral superior temporal cortex with projections to right ventral premotor cortex. The authors interpreted the imaging results as reflecting the activation of the Auditory Error Map in temporal cortex followed by the transmission of corrective commands to frontal areas that generate compensatory articulatory commands.

Auditory feedback control of speech production is studied in the laboratory by altering the acoustic characteristics of the talker's own speech while feeding it back to the talker during syllable production.

Imaging of neural responses during perturbed auditory feedback in comparison to normal feedback trials revealed increased activation of bilateral superior temporal cortex with projections to right ventral premotor cortex.

Guenther and Vladusich (2009) describe a similar experiment in which a small stiff balloon, placed between the molars, was inflated on random trials during production of VCV syllables in order to perturb somatosensory feedback during consonant production. In this case, neural activation increased in bilateral supramarginal gyrus during perturbed trials relative to trials with normal feedback; furthermore, the role of right ventral premotor cortex in the generation of compensatory responses during feedback control was confirmed.

Imaging of neural responses during perturbed somatosensory feedback resulted in increased *activation in bilateral supramarginal gyrus.*

The Tourville et al. study described above involving intermittent perturbation of the talker's F1 was a variation on a seminal study conducted by Houde and Jordan (1998) that demonstrated speech adaptation to altered auditory feedback, applied continuously as the talkers produced many hundreds of trials. The experiment has been repeated in various forms by other researchers (Purcell & Munhall, 2006; Shiller, Sato, Gracco, & Baum, 2009; Villacorta, Perkell, & Guenther, 2007), confirming in every case significant although incomplete compensation indexed by a shift in self-produced speech to counter the perturbation during the period of altered feedback, as well as adaptation indexed by persistence of the effect when feedback was blocked by masking noise and when normal feedback was resumed. Other effects that have been observed include generalization of the adaptation effect to new vowels (Houde & Jordan, 2002) and shifts in perceptual boundaries after adaptation (Shiller et al., 2009). Houde and Jordan (2002) further observed the compensation effect during baseline responses when their adult subjects returned to the lab one month after the initial experiment to repeat the procedure using the same apparatus but without altered feedback. This finding confirms that the subjects learned context specific internal models that they re-activated when they returned to the experimental environment, a phenomenon observed in prism experiments and other studies of visuomotor adaptations (Imamizu & Kawato, 2009).

Compensation and negative aftereffects with exposure to altered auditory, somatosensory, and visual feedback indicate that adults develop context-specific internal models that are specifically adapted to these laboratory conditions.

Speech adaptation has also been observed in studies in which altered somatosensory feedback was induced with a thick artificial palate that changed the shape of the alveolar ridge (Aasland, Baum, & McFarland, 2006; Baum & McFarland, 1997). These experiments involved an hour of practice in the production of utterances containing the fricative /s/ with the artificial palate in place. The results also revealed compensation during altered sensory feedback and adaptation as indexed by negative aftereffects (i.e., target overshoot) subsequent to removal of the artificial palate. In experiments involving auditory and/or somatosensory perturbations of feedback during speech, prediction errors occur when sensory feedback does not match the expected sensory consequences of executing the motor plan for the target phoneme; these prediction errors lead to a new forward model that is adapted to the altered sensorimotor mapping in the experimental context. Adaptation studies in other domains have implicated the cerebellum in the development of both forward and inverse internal models (Imamizu & Kawato, 2009; Ito, 2008; Wolpert, Miall, & Kawato, 1998).

Development of Internal Models

In **unsupervised learning,** the environment provides inputs that are not specified as desired targets or as reinforcements or punishments for desired responses.

Supervised learning involves specification of a target, either from the external environment or from an internal representation; repeated attempts to reproduce the target lead to errors that gradually tune the internal model so that an accurate match between the target input and the output of the motor command can be reliably achieved.

In **reinforcement learning,** the environment may or may not provide a target input, but does provide reinforcement or punishment to indicate whether a given behavior is desirable or not.

These experimental manipulations demonstrate that feedback plays a role in the development of internal models and these models are tractable to some degree throughout the lifespan. In normal development, the internal models that guide speech production are developed in infancy as a consequence of three kinds of learning mechanisms. Computational modelers refer to these mechanisms as unsupervised, supervised, and reinforcement learning (Wolpert et al., 2001). In unsupervised learning, the environment provides inputs that are not specified as desired targets or as reinforcements or punishments for desired responses. The well-known Hebbian learning rule, whereby the strength of a connection is increased when there is a coincidence of firing of a pre- and postsynaptic neuron, is a simple form of unsupervised learning. Supervised learning involves specification of a target, either from the external environment or from an internal representation; repeated attempts to reproduce the target lead to errors that gradually tune the internal model so that an accurate match between the target input and the output of the motor command can be reliably achieved. In reinforcement learning, the environment may or may not provide a target input, but does provide reinforcement or punishment to indicate whether a given behavior is desirable or not. Wolpert et al. (2001) suggest that Purkinje cells in the cerebellum play a role in supervised learning and that dopaminergic systems in the basal ganglia are implicated in reinforcement learning.

The DIVA computational model is a developmental or adaptive model in which the mappings between auditory targets, vocal tract shapes, and articulatory movements are learned by applying unsupervised and then supervised learning rules sequentially during training (Guenther, 1995; Guenther & Vladusich, 2009). Initially, during a "babbling" stage, random articulator movements are induced that lead the model to learn the mapping between directions in orosensory space and articulator movements. The result is a learned inverse kinematic mapping that links changes in vocal tract configuration to the associated movements in a task-related grouping of articulators (i.e., a coordinative structure). Linkage of vocal tract configurations to speech sounds also occurs during this stage via Hebbian learning: when babbling results in output that corresponds to a language specific acoustic-phonetic representation as perceived by the speech recognition system, a unit in the Speech Sound Map is activated. Over time the model learns all the vocal tract configurations that will result in a given speech sound output, with enhanced precision in dimensions that are critical for production of the target but increased variability in dimensions that do not have much impact on the resulting acoustic-phonetic output. Subsequently, in an "imitation" stage, a specific acoustic target is presented leading to activation of the corresponding unit in the Speech Sound Map which in turn triggers readout of a feed-forward command. Initially, execution of the feed-forward command will result in auditory errors, leading the feedback system to generate corrective commands specified in articulatory terms. The transformation of auditory errors into corrective articulatory commands is enabled by the learning that took place during the babbling phase. Successive trials of supervised learning leads to a progressive reduction of errors and tuning of the inverse model so that eventually the feed-forward command can be executed without error and without recourse to feedback control. Supervised learning in computational models is entirely dependent on the feedback of errors in relation to an externally or internally specified target. Other theorists have pointed to the importance of the social context and communicative partner which provide reinforcement for the production of native-language speech units and information about the function of specific speech responses in natural learning situations (Howard & Messum, 2011; Kröger, Kopp, & Lowit, 2010).

Factors That Contribute to the Development of Speech Motor Control

3.3.1. From the perspective of the DIVA model, describe how the infant adapts to developmental changes in the structure of the vocal tract during the acquisition of speech motor control.

3.3.2. Identify two types of evidence for the importance of the auditory environment for the development of speech motor control. Describe two roles of auditory input in the development of speech motor control.

3.3.3. Suggest two roles for the social environment in early speech production learning and provide research evidence to support these hypotheses.

The DIVA model provides us with a framework for identifying potential factors that may impact on the child's path toward the achievement of mature speech motor control. Clearly maturation of biomechanical and neurophysiological structures associated with speech production will be an important factor. However, the child's access to and ability to process both auditory and somatosensory feedback will be critical determinants of speech development given the central role of feedback in the development of internal models. Cognitive, social, or other factors that impact on the child's access to learning opportunities through exploration and imitation will also serve to support or hinder speech development. Literature related to development in these areas is covered in the final section of this chapter.

Maturation of Biomechanical and Neurophysiological Structures

Maturation of the Vocal Tract

Descriptions of developmental change in the dimensions of the infant vocal tract have been improved by the advent of magnetic resonance imaging. The impact of these morphological changes on the possible acoustic output of the infant vocal tract has been explored using sophisticated modeling and speech synthesis techniques. Studies using MRI confirm the long-standing impression that vocal tract development does not involve a simple linear increase in vocal tract length (Fitch & Giedd, 1999). Although vocal tract length is strongly correlated with an individual's height, increases in vocal tract length are slower than increases in body height early in development. Growth of the pharyngeal cavity is disproportionately large relative to oral cavity growth throughout development: during childhood, pharyngeal cavity length increases by 22%, whereas increases in oral cavity length average only 12%; between puberty and adulthood, the pharyngeal cavity lengthens again by 25% in comparison with a 5% increase in oral cavity length. This disproportionate growth in the size of the pharyngeal cavity is significantly greater in adolescence than in childhood and in males than in females although significant sex differences are not observed prior to puberty.

Growth of the pharyngeal cavity is disproportionately large relative to oral cavity growth throughout development.

The newborn vocal tract is significantly different from the adult structure as illustrated in Figure 3–16 (Vorperian, Kent, Gentry, & Yandell, 1999). The high larynx position and engagement of the velum with the epiglottis obligates nasal breathing and encourages quasiresonant vocalizations early in life. The short length of the vocal cavity accounts for the high natural resonating frequency of the infant tract relative to the adult tract. The forward position of the tongue in a relatively small oral cavity along with the fat deposits in the cheeks (i.e., "sucking pads") restrict the motion of the tongue and the variety of vowels that are produced in the earliest stage of speech production.

The newborn vocal tract is significantly different from the adult structure.

Major developmental changes in vocal tract structure that begin approximately 3 months after birth include the descent of the larynx which is associated with the disengagement of the epiglottis from the velopharynx, lengthening of the pharyngeal cavity, and a sharper angle between the oral and pharyngeal cavities (Kent & Vorperian, 1995). The shape of the vocal tract approximates the adult model at age 6 years although continued changes occur through puberty (Crelin, 1987). Vorperian, Kent, Gentry, and Yandell (1999) described the growth of the supralaryngeal vocal tract in one infant who received repeated MRI scans between birth and 30 months of age. They found that changes in the size of various vocal tract structures were generally coordinated, even during growth spurts that occurred between 1 and 4 months of age and again between 12 and

Major developmental changes in vocal tract structure begin approximately 3 months after birth.

The shape of the vocal tract approximates the adult model at age 6 years although continued changes occur through puberty.

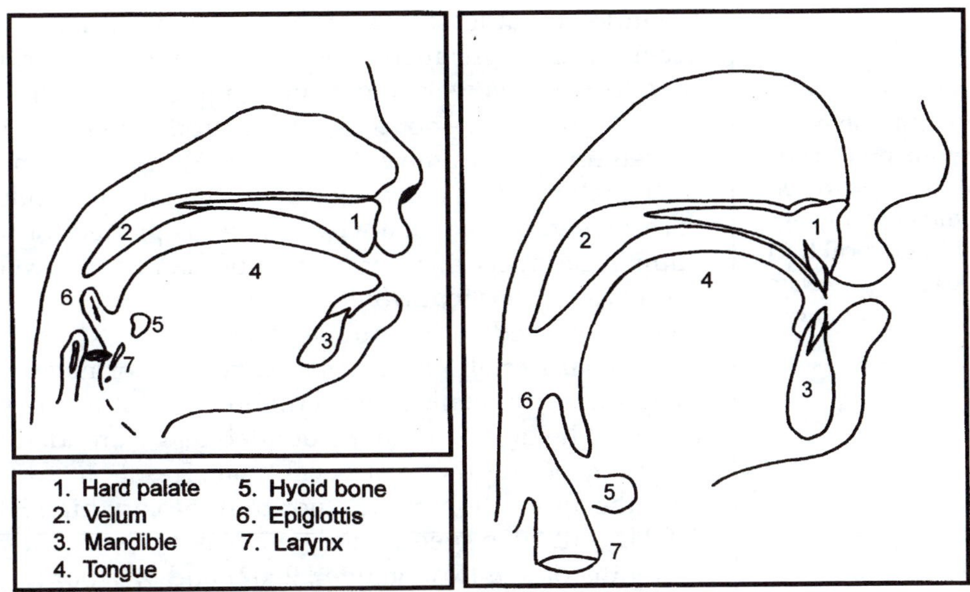

Figure 3–16. Line drawings of the infant and adult vocal tracts (see text for details). Reprinted from International Journal of Pediatric Otorhinolaryngology, 49, *Vorperian, H. K., Kent, R. D., Gentry, L. R., & Yandell, B. S. (1999). Magnetic resonance imaging procedures to study the concurrent anatomic development of vocal tract structures: Preliminary results. Figure 1, p. 198, Copyright 1999, used with permission from Elsevier.*

15 months of age. Their data showed that most of the increase in vocal tract length could be explained by the descent of the larynx and tongue but lengthening of the hard palate and increases in lip thickness also played a significant role. The data for this subject indicated that laryngeal descent was the most important factor during the first year, whereas descent of the tongue and lengthening of the hard palate made a greater contribution to vocal tract growth during the second year of life.

The model of speech motor control presented in the previous section rests on the assumption that the infant can produce speech sounds that are perceptually equivalent to adult-produced phonetic categories and that the infant recognizes this equivalency. The plausibility of this hypothesis has been enhanced by the application of the Variable Linear Articulatory Model (VLAM) to synthesize vowels that would be produced by vocal tracts having the dimensions observed for different age groups (Ménard, Davis, Boë, & Roy, 2009; Ménard, Schwartz, & Boë, 2002, 2004). Ménard and her colleagues asked adults to identify vowels synthesized for vocal tracts sizes and fundamental frequencies representing a 4-week-old infant, 2-, 4-, 8-, and 12-year-old children, a 16-year-old adolescent, and a 21-year-old adult male. They found that perceptually acceptable point vowels ([i], [u], [a]) could be produced by all vocal tracts, including the newborn configuration. Even the nonpoint vowels synthesized for the infant vocal tract configuration were accurately identified by at least 50% of the listeners. Although identification accuracy and agreement was considerably less for infant vowels than for adult vowels, the results indicated that the infant's vocal tract anatomy does not prevent the production of the full range of vowels used in the ambient language. At the same time, infant vocal tract anatomy does at least partly explain infant production preferences: when the maximal vowel space is plotted for the infant and adult vocal tracts, a larger portion of the infant vowel space corresponds to vowels that would be perceived to be low or front vowels when compared to the adult vowel space.

The infant's vocal tract anatomy does not prevent the production of the full range of vowels used in the ambient language although infant vocal tract anatomy does partly explain infant production preferences.

Ménard et al. (2002) also examined normalization of vowel categories across talkers with different vocal tracts. Acoustic cues to vowel height, place, and roundedness were identified that are valid for the full range of vocal tract sizes. Some difficulties arise with the application of the algorithms at very high F0 values (e.g., 450 Hz) but F0 in speechlike utterances rarely exceeds 400 Hz after 6 months of age (Rothganger, 2002) and we found that the F0 of vowels in the context of canonical syllables averaged 307 Hz for the 10- to 18-month-old infants described in Rvachew et al. (2006). Therefore, the infant can potentially perceive equivalency between its own vowel productions and those of adult models using the same normalization algorithms for speechlike vocalizations produced by talkers of all ages. It is important to note, however, that while it is possible for the infant to produce vowels that are perceptually equivalent to adult vowel categories, in many cases the infant would need to employ different articulatory gestures than the adult to achieve the same perceptual outcome. Modeling with VLAM showed that articulatory parameters that produced a given vowel for an infant vocal tract resulted in an acoustic output that was perceived as a different vowel when implemented for the vocal tract of an older child. Therefore, "as growth occurs, reaching a perceptual vocalic target involves the gradual adaptation of articulatory positions to produce the appropriate ranges of articulatory strategies related to the acoustic goal" (Ménard et al., 2009, p. 1283). Callan, Kent, Guenther, and Vorperian (2000) demonstrated that the DIVA model can simulate the retuning of internal models to accommodate morphological changes in the vocal tract from childhood through adulthood. The key feature of the model that permits adaptation of articulatory-perceptual relationships throughout development is the positing of auditory-perceptual targets (as opposed to gestural targets) to plan articulation.

Although it is possible for the infant to produce vowels that are perceptually equivalent to adult vowel categories, in many cases the infant would need to employ different articulatory gestures than the adult to achieve the same perceptual outcome.

Retuning of internal models to accommodate morphological changes in the vocal tract from childhood through adulthood can be simulated with an auditory feedback model in which auditory-perceptual targets are used to plan articulation.

Vocal tract morphology is influenced by growth in bony and skeletal structures as emphasized above but muscles also play a role in the structure and function of the speech system. The muscles involved in speech can be grouped into 5 structural-functional classes, specifically, as described by Kent (2004, p. 496): "(a) joint-related muscles (the muscles of the jaw, such as the masseter and the digastrics), (b) sphincteric muscles (the orbicularis oris muscle of the lips and the constrictor muscles of the pharynx and velopharynx), (c) a muscular hydrostat (the intrinsic muscles of the tongue), (d) muscles specialized for vibration and airway valving (the intrinsic muscles of the larynx), and (e) the muscles that inflate and deflate the lungs (respiratory muscles)." These muscles contain diverse fiber types so that the microscopic anatomy and mechanical properties of the component tissues are unique in relation to other muscles in the body, limb muscles in particular, as speech muscles are specialized for the precise coordination of complex movement sequences at a rapid rate.

The muscles of speech articulation contain diverse fiber types so that the microscopic anatomy and mechanical properties of the component tissues are unique in relation to other muscles in the body, limb muscles in particular, as speech muscles are specialized for the precise coordination of complex movement sequences at a rapid rate.

The development of the oral-facial musculature is influenced by structural changes; for example, the decent of the larynx leads to the vertical orientation of the posterior third of the tongue which in turn contributes to the development of the intrinsic muscles of the tongue. The relationship between structure and function is reciprocal however with oral function playing a major role in the reshaping of the oral cavity and this reshaping itself facilitating new functions (Moss & Salentijn, 1969). This is not to say that vocal tract structure determines function of the articulators or limits vocal output. Crelin (1987) recounts how surprised he was to find his infant grandson making vowel sounds that seemed impossible given the similarity of infant vocal tract morphology to that of the chimpanzee; further investigation revealed that infants and toddlers functionally reconfigure the tract during vocalization to create a variety of fully resonant vowels well before the structural modifications thought to promote human speech production are in place.

The relationship between structure and function is reciprocal; oral function plays a major role in the reshaping of the oral cavity and this reshaping itself facilitates new functions.

Maturation of Neurophysiological Structures

The finding that the production of the full range of vowels can be produced with the newborn vocal tract structure does not mean that the infant has the functional capacity to produce the full range of adult phonetic categories. Another constraint on the infant's speech production capability is maturation of the neurophysiological system that drives the function of the articulatory, laryngeal, and respiratory systems. In this review we focus on the maturation of connectivity between anterior (e.g., posterior ventral premotor cortex, inferior frontal gyrus, or Broca's area) and posterior (e.g., superior temporal gyrus) speech processing regions that are hypothesized to be important for auditory feedback control of speech and the development of internal models (Guenther & Vladusich, 2009). Paus et al. (1999) described structural changes in white matter density in corticospinal and frontotemporal pathways, as derived from MRI scans of normally developing children aged 4 to 17 years. They observed maturational changes that were bilateral for the corticospinal pathways but predominantly left lateralized for the frontotemporal pathways. They noted that the long-term and age-related increases in white matter density in the arcuate fasciculus parallels

Long-term maturational increases in white matter density in the arcuate fasciculus parallels the protracted period of motor development in children and may reflect the importance of feedback between auditory and motor brain regions in speech development throughout childhood.

the protracted period of motor development in children and may reflect the importance of feedback between auditory and motor brain regions in speech development throughout childhood.

Another technique for examining the maturation of these pathways is to examine developmental fluctuations in spontaneous low-frequency fMRI signals (Fransson et al., 2007). Resting state functional connectivity MRI identifies interactions between regional activations while the subject is at rest, that is, not performing any specific task (Fair et al., 2009). Resting state potentials in adults reveal 10 intrinsic networks including strongly lateralized frontotemporal and frontopareital networks and cerebellar networks. Fransson et al. (2007) investigated resting state potentials in preterm infants at term-equivalent age while they were sleeping. They found 5 networks in the infant brain but they did not correspond to resting state networks that have been observed in the adult brain; three of the networks were associated with well-known functional architectures in the infant brain that are involved with visual, auditory, and sensorimotor processing. A striking difference with adult networks was the nonlateralized and cross-hemisphere connectivity of the infant networks. In other words, networks in the adult brain connect functionally related areas along the anterior-posterior direction within a hemisphere whereas networks in the infant brain connect homologous brain regions across hemispheres. Although considerable reorganization of these networks occurs in the first 6 months (Homae et al., 2010), developmental changes occur throughout childhood. Fair et al. (2009) investigated resting state potentials in children aged 8 through 13 years relative to adults and found that networks in children reflected anatomical proximity so that, for example, regions within the frontal lobe were correlated at younger ages but gradually became segregated and then integrated with other regions to form the frontotemporal and frontoparietal networks seen in the adult brain. They attribute these developmental changes to the interaction of "general experiential environment and processing demands . . . with maturational changes of the neural substrate" (p. 8).

In Chapter 3 we reviewed studies confirming that the infant brain is prepared for the processing of spoken language; in particular, increases in cerebral blood flow over left temporal regions have been observed in response to speech input to newborns. The discovery of "mirror neurons" in the monkey brain (see Chapter 1 for discussion) led to interest in the response to speech input of areas of the human brain thought to be homologous to the mirror neuron system (specifically BA44 of Broca's area). Recent studies have attempted to trace the emergence of correlated activity between superior temporal gyrus and Broca's area in infancy. Imada et al. (2006) used magnetoencephalography to record brain responses to pure tones, harmonic chords, and speech syllables in newborns, 6-month-olds, and 12-month-old infants, using a mismatch negativity paradigm. Infants at every age showed activation in superior temporal gyrus in response to all stimuli. Coupling of inferior frontal activation to superior temporal activation occurred only for speech stimuli and only in 6- and 12-month-old infants. They conclude that "speech motor areas are not activated by the perception of speech initially, but require experience to bind perception and action in early speech development" (p. 961).

MEG studies of infant brain responses to speech and nonspeech stimuli suggest that experience is required to bind perception and action as indicated by coupling of inferior frontal and superior temporal activation in response to speech stimuli starting at 6 months along with canonical babbling.

Access to Sensory Feedback

Auditory Input

The DIVA model emphasizes the role of speech input in the formation of auditory-perceptual targets for speech output as well as the importance of auditory feedback of the infant's own speech for the achievement of speech motor control. This model leads to the prediction that the speech environment will influence the characteristics of the infant's speech output from the beginning of the canonical babbling stage. Natural tests of the hypothesis involve variations in the amount of speech input as occurs in the case of hearing impairment and variations in the phonetic content in speech input as occurs across linguistic environments.

Significant hearing impairment dramatically reduces the infant's access to auditory feedback at a critical stage of speech development. Infants with normal hearing and infants with hearing impairment produce similar vocalizations for the first few months but prelinguistic vocal development begins to diverge well before the end of the first year. Koopmans-van Beinum, Clement, and van den Dikkenberg-Pot (2001) observed that vocalizations involving the coordination of the phonatory and articulatory systems were produced less frequently by deaf infants when compared to hearing infants. They concluded that "the development of the separate systems seems to be physiologically and neurologically governed," but "auditory perception and feedback are a prerequisite for the coordination of the movements in the two systems together" (p. 69).

Children with sensorineural hearing impairment demonstrate delayed onset of the canonical babbling stage, a limited range of consonants in the phonetic repertoire and a developmental reduction in the size of the vowel space (Carney, 1996; Eilers & Oller, 1994; Kent, Osberger, Netsell, and Hustedde, 1987; Oller & Eilers, 1988; Stoel-Gammon & Otomo, 1986). The complete lack of overlap in the age of onset for canonical babble among infants with normal hearing and congenital hearing loss, as shown in Figure 3–17, lead to the suggestion that earlier identification of hearing impairment could be accomplished by asking parents about their infant's speech behavior (Oller et al., 2001). The importance of auditory feedback for normal phonetic development is further highlighted by studies of children who have received cochlear implants. Increases in vowel diversity, consonant repertoire, and the emergence of canonical

Children with **sensorineural hearing impairment** demonstrate delayed onset of the canonical babbling stage, a limited range of consonants in the phonetic repertoire, and a developmental reduction in the size of the vowel space.

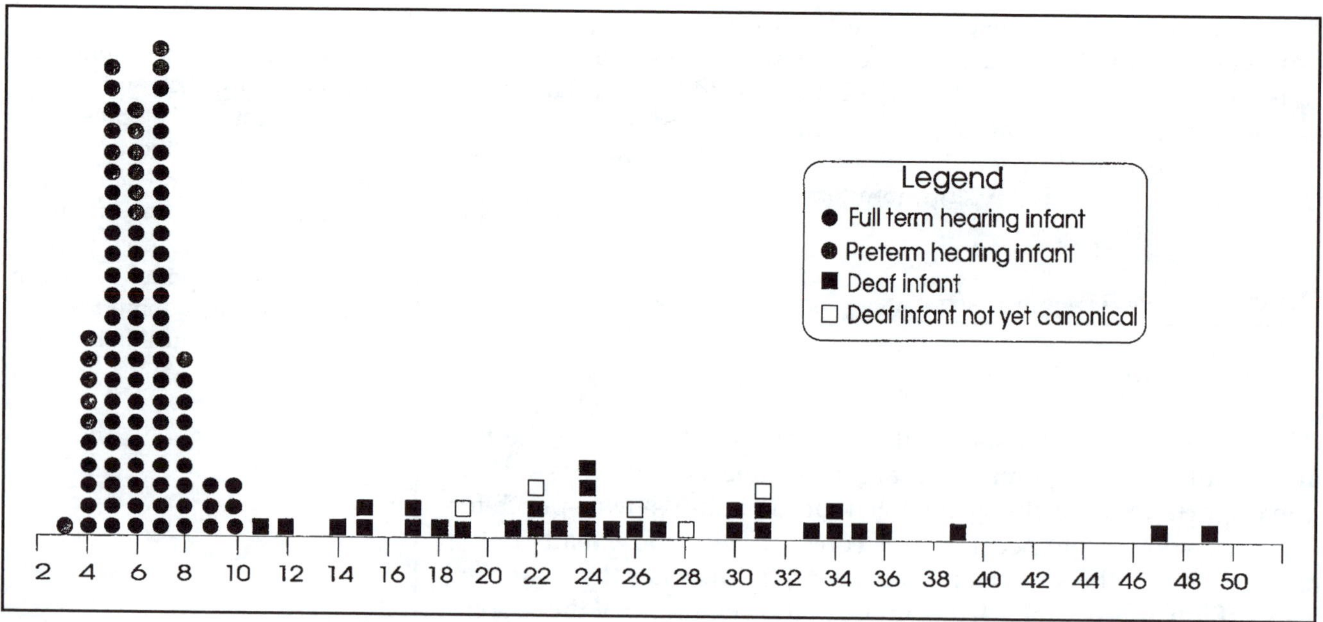

Figure 3–17. Histogram showing age of onset of canonical babbling by infant and age (in months). From Eilers & Oller (1994). Infant vocalizations and the early diagnosis of severe hearing impairment. Journal of Pediatrics *by American Academy of Pediatrics, 124(2), Figure 1, p. 201. Reproduced with permission of Mosby, Inc.*

babble shortly after implant activation have been reported in a number of case studies (Ertmer, 2001; Ertmer & Mellon, 2001; Ertmer et al., 2002).

Even subtle and transient hearing loss, such as that associated with otitis media, has an impact on prelinguistic phonetic development. Rvachew, Slawinski, Williams, and Green (1999) found that infants with early-onset otitis media showed an average 3-month delay in the onset of canonical babble, relative to children who had no ear infections during the first 6 months of life. Relative to the infants with later-onset otitis media, the early-onset group produced fewer canonical babbles throughout the period 6 to 18 months of age, and produced more quasiresonant vowels and more marginal syllables containing a quasiresonant nucleus. Furthermore, these infants were more likely to produce a restricted range of vowels and they did not demonstrate the age-related increase in the range of second formant frequencies that was observed in the later-onset group, as illustrated for two representative infants in Figure 3–18.

Restriction in the vowel space has also been observed in the babble produced by infants with early-onset otitis media with effusion.

Investigations into the "babbling drift hypothesis" also demonstrate that the auditory environment shapes the infant's vocal output, suggesting that supervised learning mechanisms come into play once the infant makes the transition to language-specific perceptual processing of speech input. Cross-linguistic investigations of infant vocal behavior have yielded confusing results because studies employing phonetic transcription tend to obscure individual differences within and across linguistic groups. Investigations that

Investigations into the **babbling drift hypothesis** also demonstrate that the auditory environment shapes the infant's vocal output, suggesting that supervised learning mechanisms come into play once the infant makes the transition to language-specific perceptual processing of speech input.

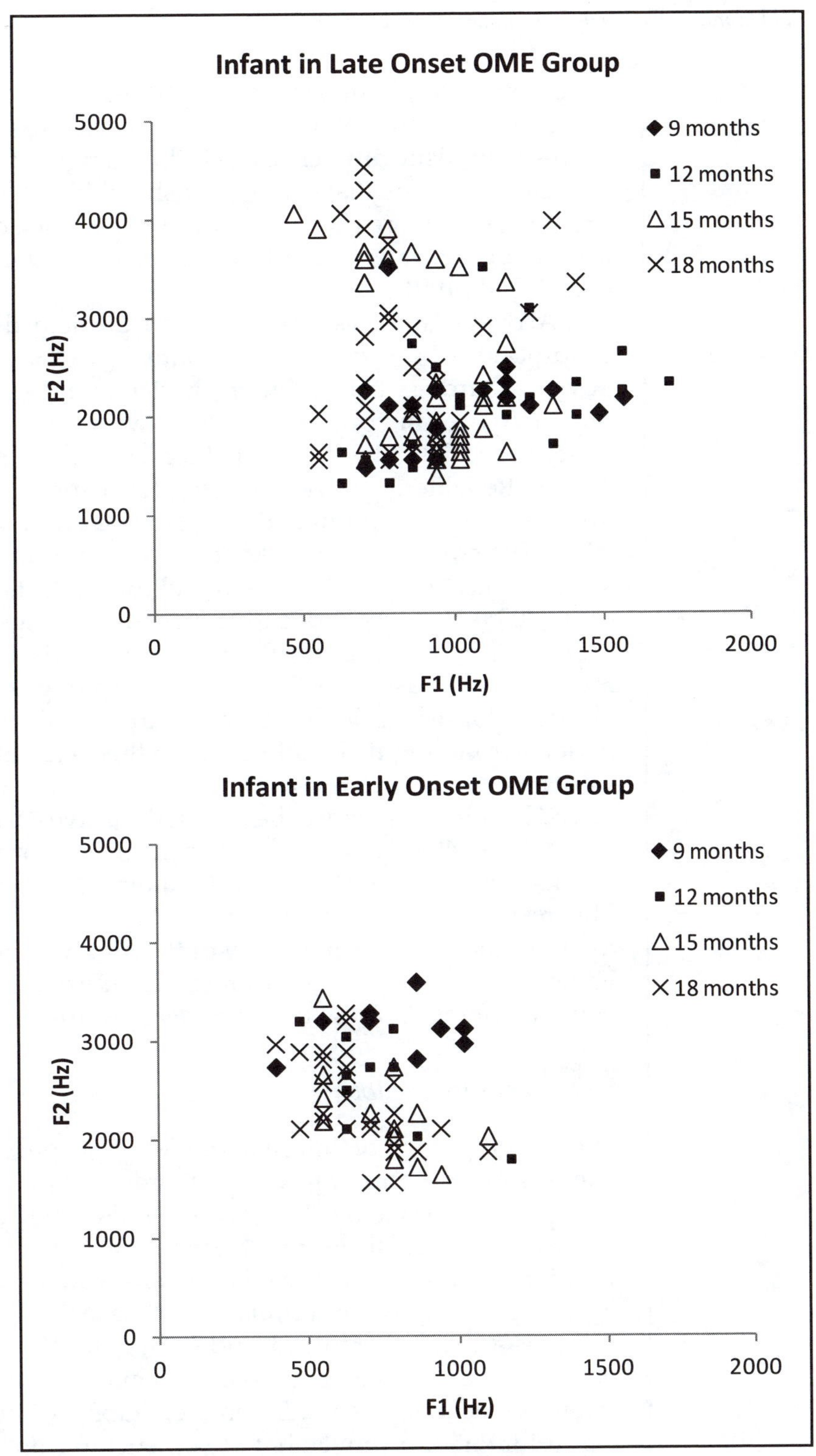

Figure 3–18. *F1-F2 plots showing expansion of the vowel space with age for one infant who did not have otitis media with effusion during the first 6 months of life (top) in comparison with a restricted vowel space throughout the 6- through 18-month period for a second infant who had early onset otitis media with effusion. Adapted from Rvachew et al. (1996). Formant frequencies of vowels produced by infants with and without early onset otitis media.* Canadian Acoustics, 24, *Figure 2. Used with permission from Canadian Acoustical Association.*

have combined phonetic and acoustic analyses to describe the prosodic characteristics of infant speech have led to reports of a variety of cross-linguistic differences including longer utterances in French and more closed syllables in English babbling (Levitt & Aydelott Utman, 1992), more rising F0 contours in French compared to English babble (Whalen, Levitt, & Wang, 1991) and Japanese babble (Hallé et al., 1991).

Acoustic analysis has also been used to describe the vowels produced by infants in the context of canonical syllables. De Boysson-Bardies, Halle, Sagart, and Durand (1989) found striking differences in vowel formants between samples collected from 10-month-old babies learning French, English, Cantonese, and Arabic. Reliable differences in long-term spectra were also found for these language groups (de Boysson-Bardies, Sagart, & Durand, 1984). The cross-linguistic variation in long-term spectra for infant samples was attributed to the vowel formants, however. Rvachew et al. (2006) observed a decline in mean F1 alongside a stable F2 in the vowels of infants aged 10 through 18 months learning Canadian French; in contrast, a decline in mean F2 alongside a stable F1 was observed for infants learning Canadian English over the same time period. Cross-linguistic differences in the shape of the vowel space were associated with a greater frequency of vowels that were perceived by adult listeners to be /u/ in the grave corner of the English infants' vowel spaces in comparison to this corner of the French infants' vowel spaces (Rvachew, Alhaidary, Mattock, & Polka, 2008). This result was observed throughout the age range and appeared to reflect the greater complexity of the high vowel inventory in the French input and mirrored differences in listening preferences for younger infants in these two language groups.

Somatosensory Feedback

The development of internal models for speech motor control requires somatosensory feedback in order to link information about vocal tract shapes to the motor commands that produced them and the resultant acoustic output. A small number of studies have provided information about developmental changes in response to tactile and proprioceptive stimulation of the articulators.

Barlow, Finan, Bradford, and Andreatta (1993) investigated the perioral reflex in infants, school-age children and adults, induced through mechanical stimulation (i.e, "taps") on the outer lip during voluntary lip movements (e.g., sucking on a pacifier in the case of the infants). This brain-stem mediated reflexive response is recorded as electromyographic (EMG) activity in the lip muscles. The latency of the response was observed to decline with age during the first seven months of life but increased again for children aged 4 to 6 years before declining again to approach adult values by age 12 years. Another interesting developmental effect was an age-related increase in the specificity of the response: for infants, the response was observed in obicularis inferior and superior, both ipsilateral and contralateral to the point of stimulation; in adults the response was restricted to one side and strongest for obicularis inferior where the stimulation was applied.

The maturation of a number of other oral reflexes has been studied. Koehler and Hölker (2004) tapped the chin and recorded responses in the masseter muscles. Finan and Smith (2005) assessed the jaw stretch reflex by inducing a rapid downward displacement of the mandible and measuring responses in the jaw closing muscles. Wood and Smith (1992) examined cutaneous reflex responses by providing light sensory stimulation to the midline of the anterior palate, midpalate, tongue tip and lateral margin of the tongue. Responses were recorded as EMG activity in the masseter muscles and jaw closing force at the molars. In these studies developmental changes in latencies and amplitudes of the EMG responses were nonlinear; reflex patterns are significantly more mature in 8- to 10-year-old children relative to preschoolers, whereas latencies of EMG responses decline in the elderly relative to young adults. Wood and Smith also included a small sample of children with speech sound disorders and found a significantly reduced frequency of EMG responses to sensory stimulation in this group.

Other methods for studying somatosensory function include the measurement of vibrotactile thresholds (Andreatta & Barlow, 2009; Fucci, 1972; Fucci, Petrosino, Underwood, & Kendal, 1992), two-point discrimination thresholds (McNutt, 1977; Ringel & Ewanowski, 1965) and oral stereognosis (i.e., oral form discrimination/identification; Locke, 1969; McNutt, 1977; Ringel, House, Burk, Dolinsky, & Scott, 1970). Typically, these studies involve adult subjects or small samples of children with speech disorders (these papers are reviewed in Chapter 7). Investigations of the maturation of these sensory functions during infancy, childhood, and adolescence have not been undertaken and the relationship of oral sensory acuity to speech development has not been systematically explored. Overall, a review of the literature suggests a curious lack of interest in the role of somatosensory feedback in speech development, especially when compared to the rich history of studies on the impact of auditory deprivation and variations in speech input on speech production.

Systematic investigations of oral sensory maturation and the relation of oral sensory acuity to speech development are sparse in the scientific literature.

Speech Motor Adaptation in Childhood

Recall that adults are able to adapt to perturbations in auditory feedback or auditory and sensory feedback during speech production after relatively brief periods of speech practice in the laboratory. Speech motor adaptation is thought to reflect the development of new forward models that map motor commands to the altered sensory outcomes. Some studies have examined this process in children.

In a pioneering adaptation of Houde and Jordan's (1998) procedure to the production of fricatives (/s/ and /ʃ/) by children,

Shiller and colleagues demonstrated that 9- to 11-year-old children are capable of speech motor adaptation under conditions of perturbed auditory feedback. The amount of compensation observed in the children's speech under the perturbed condition was as great for the children as it was for the adults (Shiller, Gracco, & Rvachew, 2010). However, the children did not change their perception of the contrast as a result of participation in the experiment whereas the adults adapted both their production and their perception following perturbed auditory feedback (see also Shiller et al., 2009). In a follow-up study, 5- to 6-year-old children produced the word "head" under conditions of perturbed auditory feedback. The results also revealed that children are capable of speech motor adaptation, but in this study there were differences in the child responses relative to the adult control group. The degree of compensation was not as great among the children and their articulatory manipulations were less likely to result in a vowel that was perceived to be /ɛ/ by adult listeners under conditions of first formant shifting.

A common procedure for investigating speech motor adaptation involves the use of a bite block which, when fixed between the molars during speech, serves to increase the size of the jaw opening while decreasing the contribution of the jaw to the achievement of articulatory goals. Although some studies have yielded uninterpretable results due to measurement problems, at least two studies have shown that children as young as 4 years of age can adapt to this perturbation and produce acceptable point vowels in the bite block condition (Baum & Katz, 1988; Smith & McLean-Muse, 1987). Furthermore, the children demonstrated compensation from the first trial just as adults did, suggesting mature use of internal models to adapt to the perturbation despite the higher levels of variability in speech output observed in the children's responses in both perturbed and normal speaking conditions.

Use of a lip tube to ensure a wider lip opening during production of /u/ produces a more difficult perturbation of the articulators than does the bite block because it alters the geometry of the vocal tract (Ménard, Perrier, Aubin, Savariaux, & Thibeault, 2008). Under these conditions it is not enough to exaggerate the articulatory gestures used for production of /u/ under normal conditions; rather, one must position the articulators for production of another phonemic category, specifically /o/. Under these conditions neither adults nor 4-year-olds fully compensate. Ménard et al. observed some qualitative differences in the response of 4-year-olds to this perturbation relative to adult subjects. First, the children did not show evidence of learning over the 20-trial experiment; although they achieved some productions that were perceptually accurate in a trial-and-error manner they did not progress gradually toward increased rates of accuracy in a manner similar to the adults. Second, the children did not benefit from articulatory instructions that prompted them to begin by producing the /o/ sound whereas adults were more likely to achieve compensation when they were provided with this facilitative context. The authors explain the performance of the 4-year-old children in terms of "immature internal models."

Studies of adaptation in other domains have also suggested qualitative differences in performance for younger versus older children. For example, children are able to adapt to a visuomotor distortion that forces them to shift their reaching movements in space (King, Kagerer, Contreras-Vidal, & Clark, 2009). Furthermore, they generalize this adaptation to the auditory domain when asked to reach to auditory targets after the experimental distortion of the sensory environment has been removed. In this study, children in all age groups from 5 through 10 years demonstrated adaptation, after-effects and generalization from the visual to the auditory domain. However, the authors note in their review of several studies of this nature, that younger children require more trials than older children to learn the adaptation and that their reaching movements are significantly more jerky, suggesting that they are more reliant on feedback control even in the baseline condition before the sensory distortion was introduced.

In some studies, children appear to adapt to perturbations of sensory feedback in multiple domains suggesting mature internal models but they may be more reliant on feedback control during motor movements than adults even under normal conditions without sensory distortion.

Gabbard (2009) suggests that children's ability to learn from motor imagery (i.e., internal rehearsal of movements without overt motor output) also illuminates the process of developing motor programs and internal models for action-perception relationships. Gabbard directly links motor imagery to the notion of the forward model, claiming that a motor image "reflects an internal action representation or internal model of volitional movements [that] is therefore a conscious equivalent to a prediction for that action and is involved in the prediction of the consequences of one's actions" (p. 235). Gabbard reviewed the literature on motor imagery performance in tasks such as visually guided pointing by children, both those who were developing normally and those who had developmental coordination disorder. These studies suggested that the ability to effectively create and use motor imagery emerges between 5 and 7 years in normally developing children although considerable refinement occurs between adolescence and adulthood.

The ability to effectively create and use motor imagery emerges between 5 and 7 years in normally developing children although considerable refinement occurs between adolescence and adulthood.

Social and Cognitive Influences

Finally, we must consider the role of learning and the social and cognitive mechanisms that support the process of acquiring internal models for speech production. The DIVA model posits a two stage learning process in which unsupervised learning with random practice precedes supervised or imitation learning during babbling. Supervised learning occurs when the learner attempts to achieve a specific target and error signals representing discrepancies in the match between target and actual output are used to tune the internal model. The target may be internalized (in the form of an acoustic-phonetic representation for a syllable for example) or it may be provided externally by an adult communication partner as a model to imitate. It seems reasonable to suggest that supervised learning begins to play a role at approximately 6 months of age in the human infant because the shift from language-general to language-specific perception of vowels occurs at this age, suggesting that the infant is acquiring internalized targets to guide speech production learning. Furthermore, canonical babbling is emerging and the repetitive production of speechlike syllables gives the appearance of active efforts to achieve specific speech goals. Imitation of vowels has been suggested for even younger infants however as will be described below.

From the traditional Piagetian perspective the infant has very limited capacity for representation or imitation during the first year of life (Anisfeld, 1984). More recent research demonstrates that infants are fully capable of representing and remembering objects and representing and imitating actions at much earlier ages than once believed possible (Meltzoff, 1999; Meltzoff & Moore, 1998; L. B. Smith, Thelen, Titzer, & McLin, 1999). Reports of infants imitating oral gestures at and shortly after birth (e.g., Meltzoff, 1977) have been difficult to replicate with the exception of one specific gesture (tongue protrusion) and are thus open to multiple interpretations (Jones, 2009). It appears that the development of imitative ability is dependent on sensorimotor experience (Catmur, Walsh, & Heyes, 2009). Nonetheless, delayed imitation skills have been convincingly documented in infants during the first year (e.g., Meltzoff, 1988), confirming that representational abilities and imitation skills emerge very early in life.

Imitation appears to play a role in the development of vowel production ability at least by 20 weeks of age and possibly as early as 12 weeks of age.

With respect to vocal learning, Kuhl and Meltzoff (1996) investigated the role of imitation in the development of vowel production ability in infants aged 12, 16, and 20 weeks. Infants were presented with audiovisual recordings of one of three different vowels ([i], [u], or [a]) for 5 minutes while seated in an infant seat in a sound booth with no human intervention during the procedure. The vowels were produced slowly and clearly by a female talker once every 5 seconds. The experiment was repeated on three separate days and the infant's vocalizations during the silent intervals between vowel presentations were submitted to acoustic and perceptual analyses. These analyses confirmed that the infants were capable at all three ages of producing vowels that were perceived as being [i]-like, [u]-like, or [a]-like (as determined via perceptual analyses) and that differentiation between these three broad categories increased with age (as determined via acoustic analyses). Biological constraints were clear in the raw data in that [a] was produced much more often than front or high back vowels. Nonetheless, the effect of the environmental input and the infants' efforts to match that input was suggested in their vocal output by 20 weeks of age if not before. Kuhl and Meltzoff link the infants' ability to match their vocal output to the speech input provided in this experiment to their capacity for multimodal integration, further exemplified in 4- to 5-month-olds by the ability to recognize facial gestures that correspond to the acoustic form of the vowels [i] or [u] (Kuhl & Meltzoff, 1984; Patterson & Werker, 1999).

Twin studies have shown that individual differences in imitation ability are explained more by shared environment than genetic factors (McEwen et al., 2007), suggesting that the quality of social interactions between infants and their caregivers plays a large role in the infant's propensity to imitate. As discussed in Chapter 2 in relation to the powerful statistical learning mechanism, infants do not attend to all stimuli available to them in the environment; social mediation from parents serves to structure the input and focus the child's attention on important information. We have already noted that the shift to language-specific patterns of phonetic perception requires a human teacher (Kuhl, Tsao, & Liu, 2003). The same may be true for language specific shifts in speech production. Cross-linguistic differences in infant vowel production have been observed in infants as young as 8 months of age (Lee, Davis, & MacNeilage, 2010; Rvachew et al., 2008), differences that may be more readily explained by the phonetic characteristics of infant-directed than adult-directed speech. For example, English-learning infants produce more [u] vowels than French- or Korean-learning infants. However, Lee et al. (2010) compared the phonetic characteristics of infant-directed versus adult-directed speech of English and Korean speaking mothers and found that high back vowels were more prevalent only in the infant-directed context.

The effect of the adult conversation partner on infant vocal output has been directly examined in a number of laboratory based experiments. Bloom (1988) conducted a series of studies in which the experimenter produced specific speech inputs in face-to-face interactions with 3-month-old infants with the type and timing of the input experimentally controlled. Infants were randomly assigned to receive either speech or nonspeech input in a contingent or noncontingent fashion (Figure 3–19). Speech input consisted of phrases such as "hello baby" produced in an infant-directed register whereas nonspeech input consisted of vocalizations such as clicks "tsk, tsk." In the contingent condition, the input was provided contingent upon the infant vocalizing. In the noncontingent condition, the experimenter listened to a recording of another infant and presented vocal input to the infant in front of her in response to the recorded vocalizations (this is called a "yoked condition" because the experimenter is yoked to another infant). Infant vocalizations were coded as syllabic (roughly equivalent to fully resonant) or vocalic (roughly equivalent to quasiresonant) and the outcome measure was the amount of increase in these vocalization types over the baseline condition in which the experimenter provided no speech input to the infant. Percent increase in syllabic-type utterances was greatest when the infants were provided with speech input but the effect was enhanced when the verbal input was provided in a contingent manner (Bloom, 1988; Bloom, Russell, & Wassenberg, 1987). Henning and Striano (2011) provide further evidence that the

Contingent speech input to 3-month-old infants increased the frequency and quality of the infant's vocal output.

	Contingent Input	Noncontingent Input
Speech	Large increase in syllabic vocalizations	Moderate increase in syllabic and vocalic vocalizations
Nonspeech	Large increase in vocalic vocalizations	Large increase in vocalic vocalizations

Figure 3–19. *Outcome of a study in which infants received either speech (e.g., "hello baby") or nonspeech (e.g., "tsk, tsk") input in a contingent or non-contingent temporal pattern. Pattern of increase in syllabic (i.e., fully resonant) and vocalic (i.e., quasiresonant) vocalizations from baseline in the four experimental conditions is shown, summarizing from Bloom (1988). Copyright © 2011 Kathleen Bloom. Printed with permission.*

timing of maternal input plays an important role in early infant development.

The impact of maternal social interaction on the vocal output of older infants has also been examined. Goldstein, King, and West (2003) observed 8-month-old's vocalizations while interacting with their mothers during a baseline period compared to a social interaction period. During the social interaction phase of the experiment mothers smiled at and touched their infants according to a scheduled determined by their own infant's vocalizations or another infant's vocalizations. Once again, contingent social responses increased the quality of the infant's vocal output, in this case resulting in a higher frequency of fully resonant and canonical utterances. Using a similar technique, Goldstein and Schwade (2008) asked mothers to respond verbally as well as nonverbally to their 9-month-old infants according to a contingent or noncontingent schedule. In this study, some mothers were instructed to respond with vowels and others were instructed to respond with words. Replicating previous research, quality of infant vocalizations in the noncontingent conditions did not change between the baseline and social interaction phases of the study whereas there were marked changes for infants in the contingent conditions. Infants whose mothers produced vowels increased their production of vowels and infants whose mothers produced words increased their production of CV syllables. There was no evidence that these infants were imitating the phonetic content in their mother's words, however.

Contingent social responses increased the frequency and quality of vocalizations produced by 8-month-old infants.

Howard and Messum (2011) present a model of early speech acquisition that highlights a third learning mechanism, specifically a form of reinforcement learning that depends upon adult mirroring of infant speech production output. In their model the infant learns the correspondence between his or her speech output and native language speech sound categories when the caregiver either mimics or reformulates the infant's utterances. The results of their computational model that learns to babble and pronounce real words after receiving such inputs from a human interlocutor are impressive and consistent with findings in bird song research that show the importance of adult responses to juvenile vocalizations in the learning of species- and dialect- specific vocalizations (Goldstein, Schwade, Menyhart, & DeVoogd, 2011). Nonetheless, it seems likely that this learning mechanism operates in parallel with supervised learning in which the infant actively attempts to achieve internalized targets.

Taken together these studies suggest at least two important roles for the social environment in speech production learning. First, adult mediators focus the child's attention on what to learn, providing information that is essential to the learning of internalized perceptual targets and reinforcing speech output that approximates native language phonetic categories. Second, adult responses motivate the child to practice speech even when not providing explicit models for imitation or specific reinforcement for a given response. Issues related to practice are explored further in Chapter 10. However, one study that examined the effect of practice on variability will be discussed here because of its explicit relevance to speech motor control. Walsh, Smith, and Weber-Fox (2006) observed lip aperture stability and lower lip/jaw synergy in children and adults as they repeated the nonwords "mab," "mabshibe," "mabfaishabe," "mabshaytiedoib," and "mabteebeebee" in the context of a short sentence. Figure 3–20 shows the familiar pattern of enhanced stability for the higher order synergy (lip aperture) in comparison to the lower order synergy (lower lip/jaw synergy). The children increased stability in lip aperture synergy with practice, whereas adults did not, apparently due to a ceiling effect for the adult group. In fact, for the most difficult nonword the children achieved stability that was equivalent to the adult normalized stability index for lip aperture after practice. Reductions in variability of the lower lip/jaw synergy were not observed with practice for children or adults during this experiment.

Research suggests two important roles for the social environment in speech production learning: adult mediators focus the child's attention on what to learn and adult social responses motivate the child to practice.

Children increased stability in lip aperture after practicing the production of difficult nonwords even though reductions in variability in lower lip/jaw synergy were not observed with practice.

Walsh et al.'s experiment highlights the importance of higher order goals in the achievement of speech motor control. The authors point out that developmental change in the variability of motor movements is often attributed to maturational events in the central nervous system that reduce "neural noise." Although "neural noise" undoubtedly plays an important role in the development of speech perception and speech production skills, it is clear that the child's active participation in learning the sound system of the language is a crucial driver of linguistic development. Maturation of

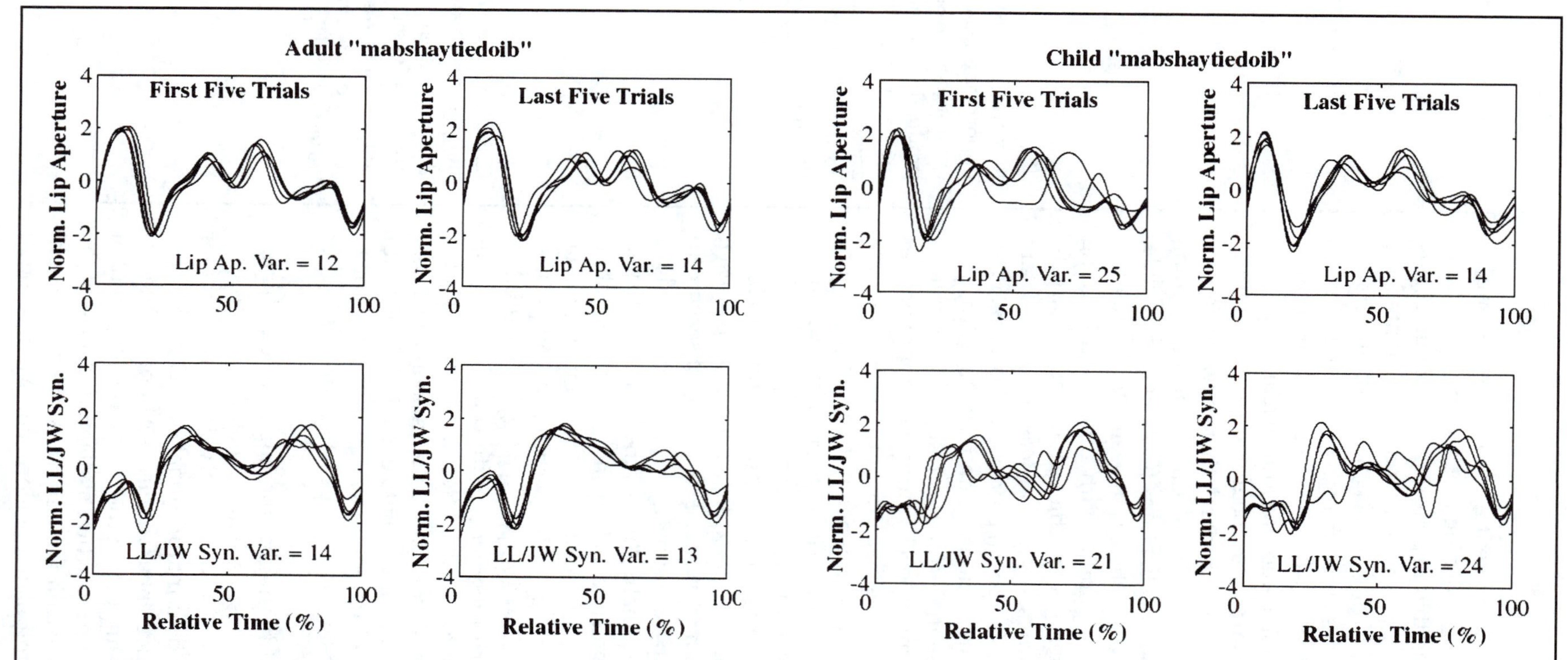

Figure 3–20. *Normalized lip aperture trajectories* (top row) *in comparison to changes in normalized lower lip/jaw synergy* (bottom row) *during repeated productions of the nonword "mabshaytiedoib" in the context of a short sentence. Improvement in stability of lip aperture trajectory (i.e., the higher order gestural goal) is shown from the first 5 to the last 5 repetitions for children (but not adults) who approach adultlike performance with practice. Neither adults nor children show a change in the lower order lower-lip/jaw synergy with practice. Adapted from Walsh, Smith, & Weber-Fox (2006). Short-term plasticity in children's speech motor systems.* Developmental Psychobiology *by International Society for Developmental Psychobiology, 48, Figure 3, p. 666, and Figure 4, p. 667. Reproduced with permission of John Wiley & Sons, Inc.*

articulatory and neurophysiological structures and developmental changes in sensory feedback systems are not the key explanatory factors in speech development. Rather, the child begins very early in life to practice achieving specific acoustic-phonetic targets, providing opportunities for auditory and somatosensory feedback to tune internal models that support the acquisition of motor programs for the production of language-specific speech sounds. Therefore, speech motor development is intimately connected to phonological development, the topic of the next chapter.

References

Aasland, W. A., Baum, S. R., & McFarland, D. H. (2006). Electropalatographic, acoustic, and perceptual data on adaptation to a palatal perturbation. *Journal of the Acoustical Society of America, 119*(4), 2372–2381.

Abbs, J. H., & Gracco, V. L. (1983). Sensorimotor actions in the control of multi-movement speech gestures. *Trends in Neurosciences, 6*, 391–395.

Adams, S. G., & Weismer, G. (1993). Speaking rate and speech movement velocity profiles. *Journal of Speech and Hearing Research, 36*(1), 41.

Amano, S., Nakatani, T., & Kondo, T. (2006). Fundamental frequency of infants' and parents' utterances in longitudinal recordings. *Journal of the Acoustical Society of America, 119*(3), 1636–1647.

Andreatta, R. D., & Barlow, S. M. (2009). Somatosensory gating is dependent on the rate of force recruitment in the human orofacial system. *Journal of Speech, Language, and Hearing Research, 52*, 1566–1578.

Anisfeld, M. (1984). *Language development from birth to three*. Hillsdale, NJ: Lawrence Erlbaum Associates.

Assmann, P. F., & Katz, W. F. (2000). Time-varying spectral change in the vowels of children and adults. *Journal of the Acoustical Society of America, 108*(4), 1856–1866.

Baker, E., Croot, K., McLeod, S., & Paul, R. (2001). Psycholinguistic models of speech development and their application to clinical practice. *Journal of Speech, Language, and Hearing Research, 44*, 685–702.

Barlow, S. M., Finan, D. S., Bradford, P. T., & Andreatta, R. D. (1993). Transitional properties of the mechanically evoked perioral reflex from infancy through adulthood. *Brain Research, 623*(2), 181–188.

Baum, S. R., & Katz, W. F. (1988). Acoustic analysis of compensatory articulation in children. *Journal of the Acoustical Society of America, 84*(5), 1662–1668.

Baum, S. R., & McFarland, D. (1997). The development of speech adaptation to an artificial palate. *Journal of the Acoustical Society of America, 102*, 2353–2359.

Bloom, K. (1988). Quality of adult vocalizations affects the quality of infant vocalizations. *Journal of Child Language, 15*(3), 469–480.

Bloom, K, Russell, A, & Wassenberg, K (1987). Turn taking affects the quality of infant vocalizations. *Journal of Child Language, 14*(2), 211–227.

Browman, C., & Goldstein, L. M. (1989). Articulatory gestures as phonological units. *Phonology, 6*, 201–251.

Buder, E. H., & Stoel-Gammon, C. (2002). American and Swedish children's acquisition of vowel duration: Effects of vowel identity and final stop voicing. *Journal of the Acoustical Society of America, 111*(4), 1854–1864.

Callan, D. E., Kent, R. D., Guenther, F. H., & Vorperian, H. K. (2000). An auditory-feedback-based neural network model of speech production that is robust to developmental changes in the size and shape of the articulatory system. *Journal of Speech, Language, and Hearing Research, 43*, 721–738.

Carney, A. E. (1996). Audition and the development of oral communication competency. In F. Bess (Ed.), *Amplification for children with auditory deficits*. Nashville, TN: Bill Wilkerson Center Press.

Catmur, C., Walsh, V., & Heyes, C. (2009). Associative sequence learning: the role of experience in the development of imitation and the mirror system. *Philosophical Transactions of the Royal Society B: Biological Sciences, 364*, 2369–2380.

Chapman, K. L., Hardin-Jopnes, M., Schulte, J., & Halter, K. A. (2001). Vocal development of 9-month-old babies with cleft palate. *Journal of Speech, Language, and Hearing Research, 44*, 1268–1283.

Clark, H. M., & Robin, D. A. (1998). Generalized motor programme and parameterization accuracy in apraxia of speech and conduction aphasia. *Aphasiology, 12*(7), 699–713.

Cobo-Lewis, A. B., Oller, D. K., Lynch, M. P., & Levine, S. L. (1996). Relations of motor and vocal milestones in typically developing infants and infants with Down syndrome. *American Journal on Mental Retardation, 100*, 456–467.

Crelin, E. S. (1987). *The human vocal tract: Anatomy, function, development and evolution*. New York, NY: Vantage Press.

Davis, B. L., & MacNeilage, P. F. (1995). The articulatory basis of babbling. *Journal of Speech and Hearing Research, 38*, 1199–1211.

Davis, B. L., MacNeilage, P. F., Matyear, C. L., & Powell, J. K. (2000). Prosodic correlates of stress in babbling: An acoustical study. *Child Development, 71*(5), 1258–1270.

De Boysson-Bardies, B., Halle, P., Sagart, L. & Durand, C. (1989). A cross-linguistic investigation of vowel formants in babbling. *Journal of Child Language, 16*, 1–17.

De Boysson-Bardies, B., Sagart, L., & Durant, C. (1984). Discernible differences in the babbling of infants according to target language. *Journal of Child Language, 11*(1), 1–15.

Dell, G. S. (1988). The retrieval of phonological forms in production: Tests of prediction from a connectionist model. *Journal of Memory and Language, 27*, 124–142.

Eilers, R. E., & Oller, D. (1994). Infant vocalizations and the early diagnosis of severe hearing impairment. *Journal of Pediatrics, 124*(2), 199–203.

Eilers, R. E., Oller, D. K., & Benito-Garcia, C. R. (1984). The acquisition of the voicing contrasts in Spanish and English learning infants and children: A longitudinal study. *Journal of Child Language, 11*, 313–336.

Ertmer, D. J. (2001). Emergence of a vowel system in a young cochlear implant recipient. *Journal of Speech, Language, and Hearing Research, 44*, 803–813.

Ertmer, D. J., & Mellon, J. A. (2001). Beginning to talk at 20 months: Early vocal development in a young cochlear implant recipient. *Journal of Speech, Language, and Hearing Research, 44*, 192–206.

Ertmer, D. J., Young, N., Grohne, K., Mellon, J. A., Johnson, C., Corbett, K., & Saindon, K. (2002). Vocal development in young children with cochlear implants: Profiles and implications for intervention. *Language, Speech, and Hearing Services in Schools, 33*, 184–195.

Fair, D. A., Cohen, A. L., Power, J. D., Dosenbach, N. U. F., Church, J. A., Miezin, F. M., . . . Peterson, S. E. (2009). Functional brain networks develop from a "local to distributed" organization. *PLoS Computational Biology, 5*, e1000381. doi:1000310.1001371/journal.pcbi.1000381

Finan, D. S., & Smith, A. (2005). Jaw stretch reflexes in children. *Experimental Brain Research, 164*(1), 58–66.

Fitch, W. T., & Giedd, J. (1999). Morphology and development of the human vocal tract: A study using magnetic resonance imaging. *Journal of the Acoustical Society of America, 106*(3), 1511–1522.

Fogel, A., & Thelen, E. (1987). Development of early expressive and communicative action: Reinterpreting the evidence from a dynamic systems perspective. *Developmental Psychology, 23*, 746–761.

Fransson, P., Skiöld, B., Horsch, S., Nordell, A., Blennow, M., Lagercrantz, H., & Aden, U. (2007). Resting-state networks in the infant brain. *Proceedings of the National Academy of Sciences, 104*, 15531–15536.

Fucci, D. (1972). Oral vibrotactile sensation: an evaluation of normal and defective speakers. *Journal of Speech and Hearing Research, 15*, 179–184.

Fucci, D., Petrosino, L., Underwood, G., & Kendal, C. (1992). Differences in lingual vibrotactile threshold shifts during magitude-estimation scaling between normal-speaking children and children with articulation problems. *Perceptual and Motor Skills, 75*, 495–504.

Gabbard, C. (2009). Studying action representation in children via motor imagery. *Brain and Cognition, 71*, 234–239.

Goffman, L (1999). Prosodic influences on speech production in children with specific language impairment and speech deficits: Kinematic, acoustic, and transcription evidence. *Journal of Speech, Language, and Hearing Research, 42*, 1499–1517.

Goffman, L., & Malin, C. (1999). Metrical effects on speech movements in children and adults. *Journal of Speech, Language, and Hearing Research, 42*, 1003–1015.

Goffman, L., & Smith, A. (1999). Developmental and phonetic differentiation of speech movement patterns. *Journal of Experimental Psychology: Human Perception and Performance, 25*(3), 649–660.

Goldfield, E. C. (2000). Exploration of vocal tract properties during serial production of vowels by full term and preterm infants. *Infant Behavior and Development, 23*, 421–439.

Goldstein, M. H., King, A. P., & West, M. J. (2003). Social interaction shapes babbling: Testing parallels between birdsong and speech. *Proceedings of the National Academy of Sciences, 100*(13), 8030–8035.

Goldstein, M. H., & Schwade, J. H. (2008). Social feedback to infants' babbling facilitates rapid phonological learning. *Psychological Science, 19*, 515–523.

Goldstein, M. H., Schwade, J. H., Menyhart, O., & DeVoogd, T. J. (2011). *From birds to words: Social interactions at small timescales yield big effects on the development of vocal communication*. Paper presented at the 2011 Biennial Meeting of the Society for Research in Child Development, Montréal, Québec, Canada.

Goodell, E. W., & Studdert-Kennedy, M. (1993). Acoustic evidence for the development of gestural coordination in the speech of 2-year-olds: A longitudinal study. *Journal of Speech and Hearing Research, 36*, 707–727.

Gracco, V. L., & Abbs, J. H. (1986). Variant and invariant characteristics of speech movements. *Experimental Brain Research, 65*, 156–166.

Grau, S. M., Robb, M. P., & Cacace, A. T. (1995). Acoustic correlates of inspiratory phonation during infant cry. *Journal of Speech ahd Hearing Research, 38*, 373–381.

Green, J. R., Moore, C. A., Higashikawa, M., & Steeve, R. W. (2000). The physiologic development of speech motor control: Lip and jaw coordination. *Journal of Speech, Language, and Hearing Research, 43*(1), 239–255.

Green, J. R., Moore, C. A., & Reilly, K. J. (2002). The sequential development of jaw and lip control for speech. *Journal of Speech, Language, and Hearing Research, 45*(1), 66–79.

Guenther, F. H. (1995). Speech sound acquisition, coarticulation, and rate effects in a neural network model of speech production. *Psychological Review, 102*(3), 594–621.

Guenther, F. H. (2003). Neural control of speech movements. In A. Meyer & N. Schiller (Eds.), *Phonetics and phonology in language comprehension and production: Differences and similarities* (pp. 209–239). Berlin, Germany: Mouton de Gruyter.

Guenther, F. H. (2006). Cortical interactions underlying the production of speech sounds. *Journal of Communication Disorders, 39*, 350–365.

Guenther, F. H., Ghosh, S. S., & Tourville, J. A. (2006). Neural modeling and imaging of the cortical interactions underlying syllable production. *Brain and Language, 96*, 280–301.

Guenther, F. H., Hampson, M., & Johnson, D. (1998). A theoretical investigation of reference frames for the planning of speech movements. *Psychological Review, 105*(4), 611–633.

Guenther, F. H., & Vladusich, T. (2009). A neural theory of speech acquisition and production. *Journal of Neurolinguistics.* doi:10.1016/j.jneuroling.2009.08.006

Hallé, P. A., De Boysson-Bardies, B., & Vihman, M. M. (1991). Beginnings of prosodic organization: Intonation and duration patterns of disyllables produced by Japanese and French infants. *Language and Speech, 34*, 299–318.

Henning, A., & Striano, T. (2011). Infant and maternal sensitivity to interpersonal timing. *Child Development, 82*(3), 916–931.

Higgins, C. M., & Hodge, M. (2001). F2/F1 vowel quadrilateral area in young children with and without dysarthria. *Canadian Acoustics, 29*, 66–68.

Hillenbrand, J., Getty, L. A., Clark, M. J., & Wheeler, K. (1995). Acoustic characteristics of American English vowels. *Journal of the Acoustical Society of America, 97*(5), 3099–3111.

Hodge, M. (1999). Relationship between F2/F1 vowel quadrilateral area and speech intelligibility in a child with progressive dysarthria. *Canadian Acoustics, 27*, 84–85.

Homae, F., Watanabe, H., Otobe, T., Nakano, T., Go, T., Konishi, Y., & Taga, G. (2010). Development of global cortical networks in early infancy. *Journal of Neuroscience, 30*(14), 4877–4882.

Houde, J. F., & Jordan, M. I. (1998). Sensorimotor adaptation in speech production. *Science, 279*(5354), 1213–1216.

Houde, J. F., & Jordan, M. I. (2002). Sensorimotor adaptation of speech I: Compensation and adaptation. *Journal of Speech, Language, and Hearing Research, 45*(2), 295–310.

Howard, I. S., & Messum, P. (2011). Modeling the development of pronunciation in infant speech acquisition. *Motor Control, 15*, 85–117.

Imada, T., Zhang, Y., Cheour, M., Taulu, S., Ahonen, A., & P. K., Kuhl. (2006). Infant speech perception activates Broca's area: A developmental magnetoencephalography study. *NeuroReport, 17*, 957–962.

Imamizu, H., & Kawato, M. (2009). Brain mechanisms for predictive control by switching internal models: Implications for higher-order cognitive functions. *Psychological Research, 73*, 527–544.

Irwin, O. C. (1947). Infant speech: Consonant sounds according to manner of articulation. *Journal of Speech Disorders, 12*, 402–404.

Ishizuka, K., Mugitani, R., Kato, H., & Amano, S. (2007). Longitudinal developmental changes in spectral peaks of vowels produced by Japanese infants. *Journal of the Acoustical Society of America, 121*, 2272–2282.

Ito, M. (2008). Control of mental activities by internal models in the cerebellum. *Nature Reviews: Neuroscience, 9*, 304–313.

Jakobson, R. (1971). Why "Mama" and "Papa"? In A. Bar-Adon & W. F. Leopold (Eds.), *Child language: A book of readings* (pp. 21–217). Englewood Cliffs, NJ: Prentice-Hall.

Jones, S. S. (2009). The development of imitation in infancy. *Philosophical Transactions of the Royal Society B: Biological Sciences, 364*, 2325–2335.

Katz, W. F., Beach, C. M., Jenouri, K., & Verma, S. (1996). Duration and fundamental frequency correlates of phrase boundaries in productions by children and adults. *Journal of the Acoustical Society of America, 99*(5), 3179–3191.

Kehoe, M. M., Stoel-Gammon, C., & Buder, E. H. (1995). Acoustic correlates of stress in young children's speech. *Journal of Speech and Hearing Research, 38*, 338–350.

Kelso, J. A. S., Tuller, B., Vatikiotis-Bateson, E., & Fowler, C. A. (1984). Functionally specific articulatory cooperation following jaw perturbations during speech: Evidence for coordinative structures. *Journal of Experimental Psychology: Human Perception and Performance, 10*, 812–832.

Kent, R. D. (2004). The uniqueness of speech among motor systems. *Clinical Linguistics and Phonetics, 18*, 495–505.

Kent, R. D., & Bauer, H. R. (1985). Vocalizations of one-year-olds. *Journal of Child Language, 12*, 491–526.

Kent, R. D., & Lybolt, J. T. (1982). Motor schema as a basis for motor learning. In W. H. Perkins (Ed.), *General principles of therapy*. New York, NY: Thieme-Stratton.

Kent, R. D., & Murray, A. D. (1982). Acoustic features of infant vocalic utterances at 3, 6, and 9 months. *Journal of the Acoustical Society of America, 72*, 353–365.

King, B. R., Kagerer, F. A., Contreras-Vidal, J. L., & Clark, J. E. (2009). Evidence for multisensory spatial-to-motor transformations in aiming movements in children. *Journal of Neurophysiology, 101*, 315–322.

Koehler, J., & Hölker, C. (2004). Masseter reflex in childhood and adolescence. *Pediatric Neurology, 30*(5), 320–323.

Koenig, L. L. (2000). Laryngeal factors in voiceless consonant production in men, women, and 5-year-olds. *Journal of Speech, Language, and Hearing Research, 43*, 1211–1228.

Koopmans-van Beinum, F. J. , & van der Stelt, J. M. (1986). Early stages in the development of speech movements. In B. Lindblom & R. Zetterstrom (Eds.), *Precursors of early speech* (pp. 37–50). New York, NY: Stockton Press.

Koopmans-van Beinum, F. J., Clement, C. J., & van den Dikkenberg-Pot, I. (2001). Babbling and the lack of auditory speech perception: A matter of coordination? *Developmental Science, 4*(1), 61–70.

Krause, S. E. (1982a). Developmental use of vowel duration as a cue to postvocalic stop consonant voicing. *Journal of Speech and Hearing Research, 25*, 388–393.

Krause, S. E. (1982b). Vowel duration as a perceptual cue to postvocalic consonant voicing in young children and adults. *Journal of the Acoustical Society of America, 71*(4), 990–995.

Kröger, B. J., Kopp, S., & Lowit, A. (2010). A model for production, perception, and acquisition of actions in face-to-face communication. *Cognitive Processing, 11*, 187–205.

Kuhl, P. K, & Meltzoff, A. N. (1984). The bimodal representation of speech in infants. *Infant Behavior and Development, 7*, 361–381.

Kuhl, P. K., & Meltzoff, A. N. (1996). Infant vocalizations in response to speech: Vocal imitation and developmental change. *Journal of the Acoustical Society of America, 100*, 2425–2438.

Kuhl, P. K., Tsao, F., & Liu, H. (2003). Foreign-language experience in infancy: Effects of short-term exposure and social interaction on phonetic learning. *Proceedings of the National Academy of Sciences, 100*(15), 9096–9101.

Lackner, J. R., & Tuller, B. K. (2008). Dynamical systems and internal models. In A. Fuchs & V. K. Jirsa (Eds.), *Coordination: Neural, behavioral and social dynamics* (pp. 93–103). Berlin, Germany: Springer-Verlag. DOI: 10.1007/978-3-540-74479-5

Laures, J. S., & Weismer, G. (1999). The effects of a flattened fundamental frequency on intelligibility at the sentence level. *Journal of Speech, Language, and Hearing Research, 42*(5), 1148–1156.

Lee, S., Potamianos, A., & Narayanan, S. (1999). Acoustics of children's speech: Developmental changes of temporal and spectral parameters. *Journal of the Acoustical Society of America, 105*(3), 1455–1468.

Lee, S. S., Davis, B. L., & MacNeilage, P. (2010). Universal production patterns and ambient language influences in babbling: A cross-linguistic study of Korean- and English-learning infants. *Journal of Child Language, 37*, 293–318.

Levelt, W. J. M., Roelofs, A., & Meyer, A. S. (1999). A theory of lexical access in speech production. *Behavioral and Brain Sciences, 22*, 1–75.

Levin, K. (1999). Babbling in infants with cerebral palsy. *Clinical Linguistics and Phonetics, 13*(4), 249–267.

Levitt, A. G., & Aydelott Utman, J. G. (1992). From babbling towards the sound systems of English and French: A longitudinal two-case study. *Journal of Child Language, 19*, 19–49.

Liu, H., Tsao, F., & Kuhl, P. K. (2005). The effect of reduced vowel working space on speech intelligibility in Mandarin-speaking young adults with cerebral palsy. *Journal of the Acoustical Society of America, 117*(6), 3879–3889.

Locke, J. L. (1969). Short-term auditory memory, oral perception, and experimental sound learning. *Journal of Speech and Hearing Research, 12*, 185–192.

Locke, J. L. (1983). *Phonological acquisition and change.* New York, NY: Academic Press.

Locke, J. L. (1989). Babbling and early speech: Continuity and individual differences. *First Language, 9*, 191–206.

Lowenstein, J. H., & Nittrouer, S. (2008). Patterns of acquisition of native voice onset time in English-learning children. *Journal of the Acoustical Society of America, 124*(2), 1180–1191.

Lund, J. P., & Kolta, A. (2006). Brainstem circuits that control mastication: Do they have anything to say during speech? *Journal of Communication Disorders, 39*, 381–390.

Maas, E., Robin, D. A., Austermann Hula, S. N., Freedman, S. E., Wulf, G., Ballard, K. J., & Schmidt, R. A. (2008). Principles of motor learning in treatment of motor speech disorders. *American Journal of Speech-Language Pathology, 17*, 277–298.

Macken, M., & Barton, D. (1980). A longitudinal study of the acquisition of the voicing contrast in American English word initial stops, as measured by voice onset time. *Journal of Child Language, 7*, 41–72.

MacLeod, A., Rvachew, S, & Polka, L. (2009). Language background influences the emergence of voice onset time in production and perception. *Journal of the Acoustical Society of America, 125*, 2778.

MacNeilage, P. F. (1998). The frame/content theory of evolution of speech production. *Behavioral and Brain Sciences, 21*, 499–511.

MacNeilage, P. F., & Davis, B. L. (2000). On the origin of internal structure structure of word forms. *Science, 288*, 527–531.

Marteniuk, R. G., Leavitt, J. L., MacKenzie, C. L., & Athenes, S. (1990). Functional relationships between grasp and transport components in a prehension task. *Human Movement Science, 9*(2), 149–176.

McCune, L., & Vihman, M. M. (2001). Early phonetic and lexical development: A productivity approach. *Journal of Speech, Language, and Hearing Research, 44*, 670–684.

McCune, L., Vihman, M. M., Roug-Hellichus, L., Bordenave Delery, D., & Gogate, L. (1996). Grunt communication in human infants (*homo sapiens*). *Journal of Comparative Psychology, 110*, 27–37.

McEwen, F., Happé, F., Bolton, P., Rijsdijk, F., Ronald, A., Dworzynski, K., & Plomin, R. (2007). Origins of individual differences in imitation: Links with language, pretend play, and socially insightful behavior in two-year-old twins. *Child Development, 78*(2), 474–492.

McMurray, B., Aslin, R. N., & Toscano, J. C. (2009). Statistical learning of phonetic categories: Insights from a computational approach. *Developmental Science, 12*(3), 369–378.

McNutt, J. C. (1977). Oral sensory and motor behaviors of children with /s/ or /r/ misarticulations. *Journal of Speech and Hearing Research, 20*, 694–704.

Meltzoff, A. N. (1977). Imitation of facial and manual gestures by human neonates. *Science, 198*, 75–78.

Meltzoff, A. N. (1988). Infant imitation and memory: Nine-month-olds in immediate and deferred tests. *Child Development, 59*, 217–225.

Meltzoff, A. N. (1999). Origins of theory of mind, cognition and communication. *Journal of Communication Disorders, 32*, 251–269.

Meltzoff, A. N., & Moore, M. K. (1998). Object representation, identity, and the paradox of early permanence: Steps toward a new framework. *Infant Behavior and Development, 21*, 201–235.

Ménard, L., Davis, B. L., Boë, L., & Roy, J. (2009). Producing American English vowels during vocal tract growth: A perceptual categorization study of synthesized vowels. *Journal of Speech, Language, and Hearing Research, 52*, 1268–1285.

Ménard, L., Perrier, P., Aubin, J., Savariaux, C., & Thibeault, M. (2008). Compensation strategies for a lip-tube perturbation of French [u]: An acoustic and perceptual study of 4-year-old children. *Journal of the Acoustical Society of America, 106*, 381–393.

Ménard, L., Schwartz, J., & Boë, L. (2002). Auditory normalization of French vowels synthesized by an articulatory model simulating growth from birth to adulthood. *Journal of the Acoustical Society of America, 111*(4), 1892–1905.

Ménard, L., Schwartz, J., & Boë, L. (2004). Role of vocal tract morphology in speech development: Perceptual targets and sensorimotor maps for synthesized vowels from birth to adulthood. *Journal of Speech, Language, and Hearing Research, 47*, 1059–1080.

Mitchell, P. R., & Kent, R. D. (1990). Phonetic variation in multisyllable babbling. *Journal of Child Language, 17*, 247–265.

Moore, C. A. (1993). Symmetry of mandibular muscle activity as an index of coordinative strategy. *Journal of Speech and Hearing Research, 36*, 1145–1157.

Moore, C. A., & Ruark, J. L. (1996). Does speech emerge from earlier appearing oral motor behaviors? *Journal of Speech and Hearing Research, 39*(5), 1034–1047.

Moore, C. A., Smith, A., & Ringel, R. L. (1988). Task specific organization of activity in human jaw muscles. *Journal of Speech and Hearing Research, 31*, 670–680.

Moss, M. L., & Salentijn, L. (1969). The primary role of functional matrices in facial growth. *American Journal of Orthodontics, 55*, 474–490.

Nip, I. S. B., Green, J. R., & Marx, D. B. (2009). Early speech motor development: Cognitive and linguistic considerations. *Journal of Communication Disorders, 42*, 286–298.

Nittrouer, S. (1993). The emergence of mature gestural patterns is not uniform: Evidence from an acoustic study. *Journal of Speech and Hearing Research, 36*, 959–972.

Nittrouer, S., Studdert-Kennedy, M., & McGowan, R. S. (1989). The emergence of phonetic segments: Evidence from the spectral structure of fricative-vowel syllables spoken by children and adults. *Journal of Speech and Hearing Research, 32*(1), 120–132.

Nittrouer, S., Studdert-Kennedy, M., & Neely, S. T. (1996). How children learn to organize their speech gestures: Further evidence from fricative-vowel syllables. *Journal of Speech and Hearing Research, 39*, 379–389.

Oller, D. K. (1980). The emergence of the sounds of speech in infancy. In G. H. Yeni-Komshian, J. Kavanagh & C. A. Ferguson (Eds.), *Child phonology* (Vol. I: Production, pp. 93–112). New York, NY: Academic Press.

Oller, D. K. (2000). *The emergence of the speech capacity*. Mahwah, NJ: Lawrence Erlbaum.

Oller, D. K., Eilers, R. E., & Basinger, D. (2001). Intuitive identification of infant vocal sounds by parents. *Developmental Science, 4*(1), 49–60.

Oller, D. K., Eilers, R. E., Basinger, D., Steffens, M. L., & Urbano, R. (1995). Extreme poverty and the development of precursors to the speech capacity. *First Language, 15*, 167–288.

Patterson, M. L., & Werker, J. F. (1999). Matching phonetic information in lips and voice is robust in 4.5-month-old infants. *Infant Behavior and Development, 22*(2), 237–247.

Paus, T., Zijdenbos, A., Worsley, K., Collins, D. L., Blumenthal, J., Giedd, J. N., . . . Evans, A. C. (1999). Structural maturation of neural pathways in children and adolescents: In vivo study. *Science, 283*, 908–911.

Peeva, M. G., Guenther, F. H., Tourville, J. A., Nieto-Castanon, A., Anton, J., Nazarian, B., & Alario, F. X. (2010). Distinct representations of phonemes, syllables, and supra-syllabic sequences in the speech production network. *NeuroImage, 50*(2), 626–638.

Perkell, J., Guenther, F. H., Lane, H., Matthies, M. L., Perrier, P., Vick, J., . . . Zandipour, M. (2000). A theory of speech motor control and supporting data from speakers with normal hearing and with profound hearing loss. *Journal of Phonetics, 28*, 233–272.

Perkell, J., Matthies, M., Lane, H., Guenther, F. H., Wilhelms-Tricarico, R., Wozniak, J., & Guiod, P. (1997). Speech motor control: Acoustic goals, saturation effects, auditory feedback and internal models. *Speech Communication, 22*, 227–250.

Peterson, G. E., & Barney, H. L. (1952). Control methods used in a study of the vowels. *Journal of the Acoustical Society of America, 24*(2), 175–184.

Polka, L., Rvachew, S., & Mattock, K. (2007). Experiential influences on speech perception and speech production in infancy. In E. Hoff & M. Shatz (Eds.), *Blackwell handbook of language development* (pp. 153–172). Hoboken, NJ: Blackwell.

Purcell, D. W., & Munhall, K. G. (2006). Adaptive control of vowel formant frequency: evidence from real-time formant manipulation. *Journal of the Acoustical Society of America, 120*(2), 966–977.

Ringel, R. L., & Ewanowski, S. J. (1965). Oral perception: 1. Two-point discrimination. *Journal of Speech and Hearing Research, 8*(4), 389–398.

Ringel, R. L., House, A. S., Burk, K. W., Dolinsky, J. P., & Scott, C. M. (1970). Some relations between orosensory discrimination and articulatory aspects of speech production. *Journal of Speech and Hearing Disorders, 35*, 3–11.

Rothganger, H. (2002). Analysis of the sounds of the child in the first year of age and a comparison to the language. *Early Human Development, 75*, 55–69.

Roug, L., Landberg, I., & Lundberg, L.-J. (1989). Phonetic development in early infancy: A study of four Swedish children during the first eighteen months of life. *Journal of Child Language, 16*, 19–40.

Rvachew, S., Alhaidary, A., Mattock, K., & Polka, L. (2008). Emergence of the corner vowels in the babble produced by infants exposed to Canadian English or Canadian French. *Journal of Phonetics, 36*, 564–577.

Rvachew, S., Creighton, D., Feldman, N., & Sauve, R. (2002). Acoustic-phonetic description of infant speech samples: Coding reliability and related methodological issues. *Acoustics Research Letters Online, 3*(1), 24–28.

Rvachew, S., Creighton, D., Feldman, N., & Sauve, R. (2005). Vocal development of infants with very low birth weight. *Clinical Linguistics and Phonetics, 19*(4), 275–294.

Rvachew, S., Mattock, K., Polka, L., & Ménard, L. (2006). Developmental and cross-linguistic variation in the infant vowel space: The case of Canadian English and Canadian French. *Journal of the Acoustical Society of America, 120*(4), 2250–2259.

Rvachew, S., Slawinski, E. B., Williams, M., & Green, C. L. (1996). Formant frequencies of vowels produced by infants with and without early onset otitis media. *Canadian Acoustics, 24*, 19–28.

Rvachew, S., Slawinski, E.B., Williams, M., & Green, C.L. (1999). The impact of early onset otitis media on babbling and early language development. *Journal of the Acoustical Society of America, 105*, 467–475.

Sadagopan, N., & Smith, A. (2008). Developmental changes in the effects of utterance length and complexity on speech movement variability. *Journal of Speech, Language, and Hearing Research, 51*, 1138–1151.

Saltzman, E., & Munhall, K. G. (1989). A dynamical approach to gestural patterning in speech production. *Ecological Psychology, 1*, 333–382.

Schmidt, R. A. (1975). A schema theory of discrete motor skill learning. *Psychological Review, 82*(4), 225–260.

Schmidt, R. A. (2003). Motor schema theory after 27 years: Reflections and implications for a new theory. *Research Quarterly for Exercise and Sport, 74*(4), 366–375.

Schwartz, J., Basirat, A., Ménard, L., & Sato, M. (2010). The perception-for-action-control theory (PACT): A perceptuo-motor theory of speech perception. *Journal of Neurolinguistics.* doi:10.1016/j.jneuroling.2009.12.004

Shattuck-Hufnagel, S. (1999). The role of word structure in segmental serial ordering. *Cognition, 42*(1–3), 213–259.

Shiller, D. M., Gracco, V. L., & Rvachew, S. (2010). Auditory-motor adaptation learning during speech production in 9-11-year-old children. *PLoS ONE, 5*, e12975. doi:12910.11371/journal.pone.0012975

Shiller, D. M., Sato, M., Gracco, V. L., & Baum, S. R. (2009). Perceptual recalibration of speech sounds following speech motor learning. *Journal of the Acoustical Society of America, 125*(2), 1103–1113.

Smith, A. (2006). Speech motor development: Integrating muscles, movements and linguistic units. *Journal of Communication Disorders, 39*, 331–349.

Smith, A., & Zelaznik, H. N. (2004). Development of functional synergies for speech motor coordination in childhood and adolescence. *Developmental Psychobiology, 45*(1), 22–33.

Smith, B. L., Brown-Sweeney, S., & Stoel-Gammon, C. (1989). A quantitative analysis of reduplicated and variegated babbling. *First Language, 9*, 175–190.

Smith, B. L., & McLean-Muse, A. (1987). Effects of rate and bite block manipulations on kinematic characteristics of children's speech. *Journal of the Acoustical Society of America, 81*(3), 747–754.

Smith, L. B., Thelen, E., Titzer, R., & McLin, D. (1999). Knowing in the context of acting: The task dynamics of the A-Not-B error. *Psychological Review, 106*, 235–260.

Snow, D., & Balog, H. L. (2002). Do children produce the melody before the words? A review of developmental intonation research. *Lingua, 112*(12), 1025–1058.

Stark, R. E. (1980). Stages of speech development in the first year of life. In G. H. Yeni-Komshian, J. Kavanagh, & C. A. Ferguson (Eds.), *Child phonology* (Vol. I: Production, pp. 73–92). New York, NY: Academic Press.

Stark, R. E., Rose, S. N., & Benson, P. J. (1978). Classification of infant vocalization. *British Journal of Disorders of Communication, 13*, 41–47.

Steeve, R. W., & Moore, C. A. (2009). Mandibular motor control during the early development of speech and nonspeech behaviors. *Journal of Speech, Language, and Hearing Research, 52*, 1530–1554.

Steeve, R. W., Moore, C. A., Green, J. R., Reilly, K. J., & Ruark McMurtrey, J. L. (2008). Babbling, chewing and sucking: Oromandibular coordination at 9-months. *Journal of Speech, Language, and Hearing Research, 51*, 1390–1404.

Sussman, H. M., Duder, C., Dalston, E., & Caciatore, A. (1999). An acoustic analysis of the development of CV coarticulation: A case study. *Journal of Speech, Language, and Hearing Research, 42*(5), 1080–1096.

Sussman, H. M., Minifie, F. D., Buder, E. H., Stoel-Gammon, C., & Smith, J. (1996). Consonant-vowel interdependencies in babbling and early words: Preliminary examination of a locus equation approach. *Journal of Speech, Language, and Hearing Research, 39*, 424–433.

Thelen, E. (1991). Motor aspects of emergent speech: A dynamic approach. In D. M. Rumbaugh, N. A. Krasnegor, R. L. Schiefelbusch, & M. Studdert-Kennedy (Eds.), *Biological and behavioral determinants of language development* (pp. 339–362). Hillsdale, NJ: Erlbaum.

Tourville, J. A., Reilly, K. J., & Guenther, F. H. (2008). Neural mechanisms underlying auditory feedback control of speech. *NeuroImage, 39*, 1429–1443.

Velleman, S. L., & Strand, K. (1994). Developmental verbal dyspraxia. In J. E. Bankson & N.W. Bernthal, (Eds.), *Phonology: Characteristics, assessment, and intervention* (pp. 110–139). New York, NY: Theime.

Villacorta, V. M., Perkell, J. S., & Guenther, F. H. (2007). Sensorymotor adaptation to feedback perturbations of vowel acoustics and its relation to perception. *Journal of the Acoustical Society of America, 122,* 2306–2319.

Vorperian, H. K., & Kent, R. D. (2007). Vowel acoustic space development in children: A synthesis of acoustic and anatomic data. *Journal of Speech, Language, and Hearing Research, 50,* 1510–1545.

Vorperian, H. K., Kent, R. D., Gentry, L. R., & Yandell, B. S. (1999). Magentic resonance imaging procedures to study the concurrent anatomic development of vocal tract structures: Preliminary results. *International Journal of Pediatric Otorhinolaryngology, 49,* 197–206.

Walsh, B., & Smith, A. (2002). Articulatory movements in adolescents: Evidence for protracted development of speech motor control processes. *Journal of Speech, Language, and Hearing Research, 45,* 1119–1133.

Walsh, B., Smith, A., & Weber-Fox, C. (2006). Short-term plasticity in children's speech motor systems. *Developmental Psychobiology, 48,* 660–674.

Whalen, D. H., Levitt, A. G., Hsiao, P., & Smorodinsky, I. (1995). Intrinsic F0 of vowels in the babbling of 6-, 9-, and 12-month-old French and English-learning infants. *Journal of the Acoustical Society of America, 97,* 2533–2539.

Whalen, D. H., Levitt, A. G., & Wang, Q. (1991). Intonational differences between the reduplicative babbling of French- and English-learning infants. *Journal of Child Language, 18,* 501–516.

Whiteside, S. P. (2001). Sex-specific fundamental and formant frequency patterns in a cross-sectional study. *Journal of the Acoustical Society of America, 110*(1), 464–478.

Wohlert, A. B., & Smith, A. (2002). Developmental change in variability of lip muscle activity during speech. *Journal of Speech, Language, and Hearing Research, 45,* 1077–1087.

Wolpert, D. M., & Flanagan, J. R. (2001). Motor prediction. *Current Biology, 11*(18), R729–R732.

Wolpert, D. M., Ghahramani, Z., & Flanagan, J. R. (2001). Perspectives and problems in motor learning. *Trends in Cognitive Sciences, 5*(11), 487–494.

Wolpert, D. M., & Kawato, M. (1998). Multiple paired forward and inverse models for motor control. *Neural Networks, 11*(7–8), 1317–1329.

Wolpert, D. M., Miall, R. C., & Kawato, M. (1998). Internal models in the cerebellum. *Trends in Cognitive Sciences, 2*(9), 338–347.

Wood, J. L., & Smith, A. (1992). Cutaneous oral-motor reflexes of children with normal and disordered speech. *Developmental Medicine and Child Neurology, 34*(9), 797–812.

Wulf, G., Schmidt, R. A., & Deubel, H. (1993). Reduced feedback frequency enhances generalized motor program learning but not parameterization learning. *Journal of Experimental Psychology: Learning, Memory, and Cognition, 19*(5), 1134–1150.

Zlatin, M. A., & Koenigsknecht, R. A. (1976). Development of the voicing contrast: A comparison of voice onset time in stop perception and production. *Journal of Speech and Hearing Research, 19*(1), 78–92.

Chapter 4

Phonological Development

Normal Phonological Development

In Chapter 3 we emphasized the importance of higher order goals to the child's acquisition of speech motor control. The child talks for the purpose of creating acoustic products that will be perceived by the listener as the child intended. This communicative process works when linguistic knowledge is shared between talker and listener. If the child's phonological system is not congruent with the listener's, the child's speech will be difficult to understand in many instances; as the child's phonological knowledge gradually expands and progressively restructures to match the adult system, the child's speech will become more intelligible. The phonological knowledge that is central to the child's efforts to produce intelligible speech is necessarily described from the listener's perspective. In this chapter we describe the development of phonological knowledge as ascertained by the human listener. Studies involving phonetic transcription and phonological analysis of child speech samples are described, covering a variety of units of analysis and theoretical perspectives, as described in Chapter 1.

Communication works when linguistic knowledge is shared between talker and listener. If the child's phonological system is not congruent with the listener's, the child's speech will be difficult to understand.

In the first section we focus on studies that describe the acquisition of specific phonological units. These studies may have the goal of tracing the steps through which the child passes toward the acquisition of a specific phonological unit or they may attempt to determine the age at which most children acquire a given phonological unit. Sander (1972) outlined some general milestones toward the acquisition of a "speech sound": (1) first appearance of the sound in the repertoire; (2) first correct use of the sound in meaningful words; (3) correct use of the sound more often than not; (4) correct use of the sound most or all of the time, which, for

Mastery of a "speech sound" includes correct use of the sound most or all of the time and not using the sound inappropriately in place of other sounds.

mastery, should include (5) not using the sound inappropriately in place of other sounds. It can be seen that different analysis strategies are required at different stages of development. Early in development an independent analysis of the phones that appear in the child's repertoire will be most appropriate. Later in development a relational analysis of the child's use of phonemes will be required to trace the child's gradual achievement of mastery of a given sound. Additional analyses are required to determine the child's system of underlying phonemic contrasts in addition to counting correct usages of specific sounds in target word positions. Subsequent to Sander's classic paper, other theoretical perspectives have focused attention on features and prosodic structures as important units in addition to phones and phonemes. Normative data are provided first for infants and toddlers and then for older children, in each case at multiple levels of the phonological hierarchy. Brief discussion of the clinical application of these normative data is presented (although clinical assessment of children is covered in greater depth in Chapter 5).

Subsequent to consideration of normative data, theoretical perspectives on phonological development are discussed with an emphasis on the implications for explaining individual differences in phonological development. Studies that explore individual differences and variables that impact on phonological performance and learning are covered in the final section of the chapter.

Emerging Phonological Knowledge in Infants and Toddlers

4.1.1. List three strategies that children use in early language development that result in idiosyncratic productions of word forms.

4.1.2. List three factors that motivate selection and avoidance of words with certain phones or word shapes in early language development.

4.1.3. Explain why traditional forms of phonological analysis are not applicable during early speech/language development.

4.1.4. Describe the profile of a "typical 24-month-old."

4.1.5. Analyze a speech sample recorded from a 2-year-old child and determine if it is consistent with the profile of a "typical 24-month-old."

Charles A. Ferguson (1921–1998) is renowned for many achievements in diverse areas of applied linguistics including bilingualism, sociolinguistics, and this path-breaking research on the early stages of phonological acquisition.

Ferguson and Farwell (1975, Table 7, p. 795) described the acquisition of word-initial consonants in the early words of a small group of infants, observed weekly for 10 months from the time of their first words at approximately 12 months of age. This classic study of the "first 50-word stage" revealed several important principles and phenomena in early phonological acquisition. Although admitting that any attempt to identify autonomous units of analysis in child speech by abstracting from adult language would be a "hazardous past-time," the authors chose to observe the emergence of words and word-initial consonants over time. Words were defined loosely as having a recognizable form and consistent referent without requiring an adult equivalent. Phone classes were identified by grouping phones that were used in the onsets of the same word and by linking words that were produced with the same groups of initial consonants. The authors traced the evolution of the phone classes and their contrastive function over time and discovered several aspects of early phonological acquisition that were unexpected given previous approaches and reports. One set of phone trees from this paper is reproduced in Figure 4–1.

The expansion of the phonetic repertoire, with the rapid increase in the sheer number of different phones in use, is the prominent developmental process in the early period of phonological development. It can be seen in Figure 4–1 that the child's words form only two phone classes at time I, one involving alveolar closure and the other alternating a glottal fricative with an empty onset. Labial and velar places of articulation emerge soon thereafter and then palatal fricatives and affricates appear soon after that. Toward the end of the period of observation increased complexity takes the form of differentiation within phone classes. In T's case for example a single phone class comprised of voiced and voiceless fricatives and affricates at multiple places of articulation splits to form three differentiated phone classes.

Rapid expansion of the phonetic repertoire is a prominent developmental process in the early period of phonological development.

One important finding that is immediately apparent in the depiction of phone classes is the extreme variability of early word productions. This variability is indicated in Figure 4–1 by the phones enclosed in rectangles, reflecting the production of multiple variants of a single word in a recording session (reportedly as many as eight for some cases described in this study). This extreme variability in the production of word forms led them to focus on the word as the phonological unit that appeared to function as the basic contrastive unit at this early period of phonological development. This sense of a word-based phonology revealed itself in at least two ways. First, there were many instances of words in which the phonetic features of the target word occurred but they were not bundled to form the expected phonemes or organized to produce the prosodic structure of the adult target either. One example provided was [gutçɪ] and [gutʃɪdi] as alternative productions of the word "shoe" by one child in the study. A more extreme example is given in Figure 4–2 in the form of 10 different attempts at the word "pen" produced in a single session: neither the CVC structure nor the three phonemes in the target form are consistently matched but attempts at nasality, bilabial closure, alveolar closure, and voicelessness reoccur across attempts. It can be seen that it is quite impossible to analyze many of these utterances in relation to the phonological units in the adult form except that the child appears to be attempting to match some of the segmental features.

Extreme variability in the production of word forms by toddlers supports the hypothesis of a **word-based phonology** whereby the word is the basic contrastive unit during early phonological development.

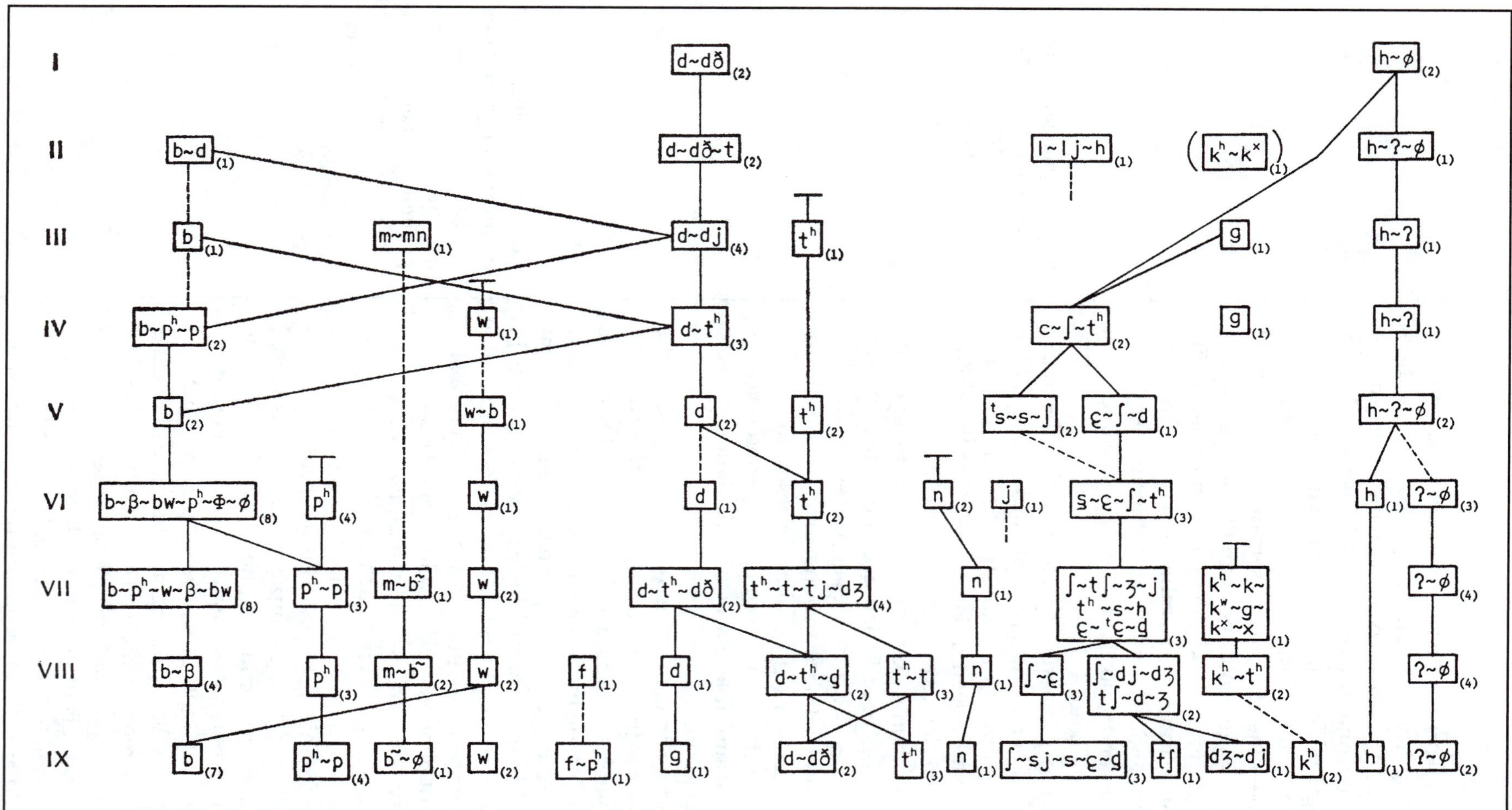

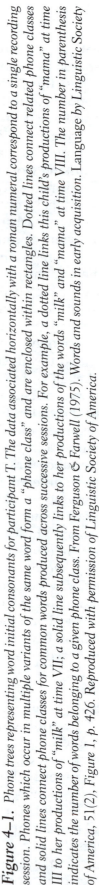

Figure 4–1. *Phone trees representing word initial consonants for participant T. The data associated horizontally with a roman numeral correspond to a single recording session. Phones which occur in multiple variants of the same word form a "phone class" and are enclosed within rectangles. Dotted lines connect related phone classes and solid lines connect phone classes for common words produced across successive sessions. For example, a dotted line links this child's productions of "mama" at time III to her productions of "milk" at time VII; a solid line subsequently links to her productions of the words "milk" and "mama" at time VIII. The number in parenthesis indicates the number of words belonging to a given phone class. From Ferguson & Farwell (1975). Words and sounds in early acquisition.* Language *by Linguistic Society of America, 51(2), Figure 1, p. 426. Reproduced with permission of Linguistic Society of America.*

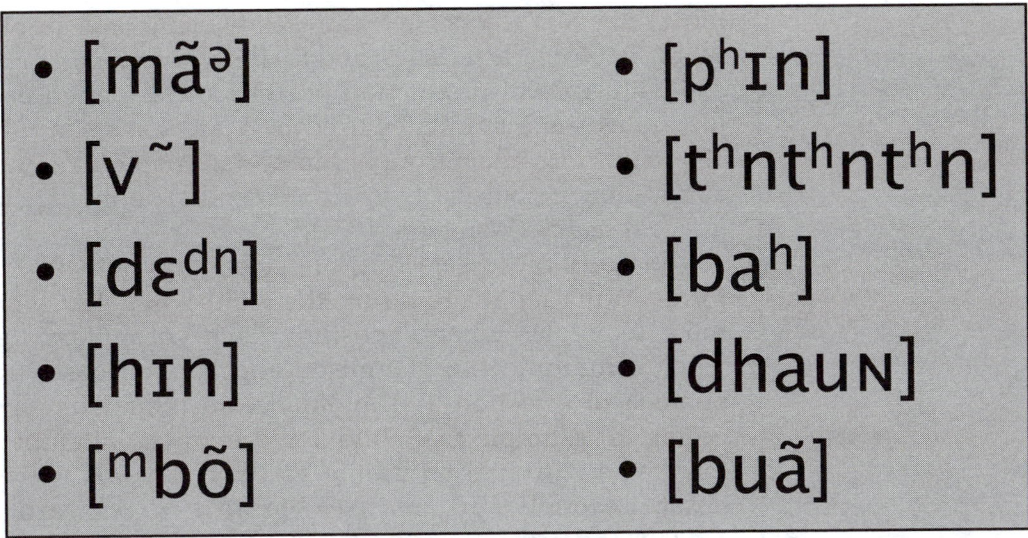

Figure 4–2. *Ten different attempts at the word "pen" recorded from a 15-month-old girl in a 30-minute period, providing evidence for a word-based phonology. Adapted from Ferguson & Farwell (1975).* Words and sounds in early acquisition. Language *by Linguistic Society of America, 51(2), Footnote 8, p. 423. Reproduced with permission of Linguistic Society of America.*

The second form of evidence for an early word-based phonology was revealed by the way in which the toddlers used phone classes to contrast meaning. Child T (see Figure 4–1) produced target /m/ and /n/ in an unconventional fashion throughout the observation period but nonetheless some order was apparent. From time III onward, there was a group of words, with initial /m/ or /n/ target consonants, that were typically produced with an initial [m] except for one session in which [m ~ n] were in free variation for this word set. At time VI, a pair of words with target /n/ onsets ("no," "nose") emerged that were consistently produced with word initial [n]. Although no minimal pairs directly contrasted the phonemes /m/ versus /n/, it appeared that the child contrasted groups of words with the phone classes [m ~ n] versus [n].

The children in this study also provided examples of "progressive idioms," a well-known phenomenon in which the child initially produces a word in an adultlike fashion but later productions of the word are more consistent with the child's constrained phonological system. By some accounts, progressive idioms reflect the emergence of a rule-based phonological system that operates at the level of phonemic segments. This is not necessarily the case, however, as many descriptions of children's early word forms show the child adapting adult forms to preferred word-based templates (also referred to as schema). Vihman (Vihman, 2006; Vihman & Croft, 2007) has argued that toddlers select "production-friendly" templates from the language input and then adapt other words to the developing system of preferred templates. The templates reflect: (1) constraints imposed by the developing speech production mechanism; (2) the

A **progressive idiom** is the precocious production of a word in an adultlike fashion that is later supplanted by a less accurate version more consistent with the child's constrained phonological system.

Young children adapt their word productions to **word-based templates** that reflect mechanism constraints, salience of the input, and individual child-related factors.

most salient or accessible features of the language input, especially word shape characteristics; and (3) individual factors related to the child's history of production practice and experience. Figure 4–3 illustrates some templates used by Waterson's son when he was 18 months old, taken from her important paper demonstrating the application of nonsegmental (i.e., prosodic) phonology to child language research (Waterson, 1971).

In addition to selecting preferred templates from accessible forms in the language input, the child will select words that fit those templates when choosing which vocabulary items to use when communicating. Ferguson and Farwell observed the phenomena of selection and avoidance in their language samples, noting for example that child T did not even attempt any words that begin with [p^h] until time VI when 4 words with target /p/ onsets suddenly appeared (see Figure 4–1). Schwartz and Leonard (1982) documented selection and avoidance in a systematically controlled experiment in which 12 normally developing toddlers were taught to associate nonsense words with unfamiliar referents in 10 biweekly sessions beginning when they were 12 to 15 months of age. The nonsense words were constructed so that half represented phones and word shapes that were IN the child's repertoire, whereas the remainder represented phones and word shapes that were not previously used by the child. IN words were produced imitatively and nonimitatively in greater numbers during the earlier sessions in comparison with OUT words. Phonetic accuracy was

- Stop Structure
  - [beːbeː] *biscuit*
  - [bæbu] *Bobby*
  - [bæbu] *bucket*
- Nasal Structure
  - [ɲẽ ɲẽ] *finger*
  - [ɲeːɲeː] *window*
  - [ɲeɲe] *another*
- Sibilant Structure
  - [ɪʃ] *fish*
  - [ʊʃ] *vest*
  - [byʃ] *brush*

Figure 4–3. *Examples of word templates (or schema) in early phonological development (18-month-old boy). Adapted from Waterson (1971). Child phonology: A prosodic view.* Journal of Linguistics, 7, *pp.* 179–211.

better for IN words than for OUT words, but phonetic accuracy did not differ between imitative and nonimitative productions. They observed a gradual relaxation of selection constraints as the child's vocabulary grew. Subsequent studies established that selection and avoidance of words based on phonetic characteristics applies to the child's productive vocabulary and not to the child's receptive vocabulary (Kay-Raining Bird & Chapman, 1998; Schwartz, Leonard, Loeb, & Swanson, 1987).

Selection and avoidance of words based on phonetic characteristics applies to the child's productive vocabulary and not to the child's receptive vocabulary.

Idiosyncratic patterns of selection and avoidance were one source of individual variation among children in Ferguson and Farwell's sample. As illustrated in Figure 4–1, Child T's preference for words containing sibilants was unique but each child had particular favorite sounds. Individual differences also reflected each child's efforts to approximate adult targets while avoiding homonymy so as to communicate most effectively. In fact, Ferguson and Farwell mentioned that children did not simply avoid "difficult sounds"; rather, children employed novel strategies for preserving lexical contrast and in some cases this meant avoiding relatively "easy sounds" such as [p]. Ingram (1975) documented children's creativity in maintaining lexical contrast, describing novel word productions such as "plane" → [me] which served to avoid overlap with "play" → [pe]. Ferguson and Farwell noted individual differences in the use of strategies such as idiosyncratic patterns of sound avoidance or novel phonological patterns, however. Overall approach to the linguistic challenges of the first 50-word stage varied among children, with some privileging lexical expansion within phone classes or templates and others focusing on phonological differentiation and lexical contrast at the expense of lexical expansion.

Children do not simply avoid "difficult sounds"; rather, children employ novel and creative strategies for preserving **lexical contrast.**

Ferguson and Farwell (1975) conclude their paper by stating "that a phonic core of remembered lexical items and articulations which produce them is the foundation of an individual's phonology, and remains so throughout his entire linguistic lifetime" (p. 437). Over time the child abstracts phonological generalizations from the "phonic core" but in the early stages "traditional forms of phonological analysis are not strictly applicable" (p. 429). We now turn to normative data based on analysis strategies that are appropriate for this age group.

"A phonic core of remembered lexical items and articulations which produce them is the foundation of an individual's phonology, and remains so throughout his entire linguistic lifetime" (Ferguson & Farwell, 1975).

Normative Data: Phonetic Repertoires

In Chapter 1 we demonstrated the procedure for deriving a repertoire of phones used by a young child, based on a broad transcription of the child's speech. In combination with a repertoire of the word or syllable shapes produced by a child, this procedure has become the standard for describing early speech development for clinical and research applications (Stoel-Gammon, 2001). One advantage of the procedure for children with emerging phonological systems is that it can be used when children are still in the integrative stage when babble and meaningful words coexist and when

Deriving the child's **phonetic repertoire** from a transcription of the child's vocal output is an appropriate procedure for describing phonological development when children are in the *integrative stage* when babble and meaningful words co-exist.

meaningful words may be difficult for the listener to reliably associate with adult equivalents. Furthermore, this procedure does not assume adultlike underlying representations and is thus appropriate for the description of a word-based phonology.

The most frequent utterance produced by one-year-old infants consists of a **single vowel**.

Kent and Bauer (1985) described the vocalizations of one-year-old infants using this technique, yielding the following observations: (1) the most frequent utterance observed was a single vowel; (2) central and front vowels were preferred over back and low vowels but [i] and [u] were rarely produced; (3) in CV syllables the preferred consonant was the voiced bilabial stop; (4) consonant and vowel harmony were frequent; and (5) fricatives were most likely to occur in syllable-final position and outnumbered stops in this position. Frequency of occurrence of consonants in CV syllables by place, manner, and voicing category is shown in Table 4–1. Notice

Table 4–1. *Frequency of Occurrence of Word Shapes and of Consonant Features in CV Syllables by Place, Manner, and Voicing Category*

Phonological Unit	*Frequency of Occurrence*
Syllable Shapes	
V	60%
CV	19%
CVCV	8%
VCV	7%
Manner of Articulation	
Stops	74%
Nasals	10%
Fricatives	11%
Glides	5%
Place of Articulation	
Labial	62%
Apical (Alveolar)	18%
Palatal	3%
Velar	10%
Pharyngeal, Glottal	7%
Voicing Category	
Voiced	75%

Note: C = consonant and V = vowel.

Source: Adapted from Kent and Bauer (1985). Vocalizations of one-year-olds. *Journal of Child Language, 12,* 491–526.

that 75% of consonants were classified as voiced (including 85% of all stops) whereas acoustic analysis studies as described in Chapter 3 indicate that children's stops at this age tend to be produced as voiceless unaspirated phones (i.e., [p˚] rather than [pʰ] or [b]) regardless of whether the adult target is a voiced or voiceless phoneme. Phonetic repertoires are based on broad transcriptions of the child speech and, as pointed out at the beginning of this chapter, phonological development is described here from the listener's perspective and native speakers of English will tend to perceive these phones as belonging to the voiced category.

Stoel-Gammon (1985) described the phonetic repertoires of 34 infants followed longitudinally at 3-month intervals between 9 and 24 months of age. Inventories were derived from samples that included both babble and meaningful words as long as they were spontaneous utterances. The children's samples were counted in the data only if the child produced a minimum of 10 meaningful words during a one-hour recording session which meant that many of the children were 18 months old and had a parent-reported vocabulary size of over 30 words at the time when their data was first included in the calculation of inventory sizes. Mean inventory size was larger in word-initial position than word-final position throughout the age range studied. Specifically, the word-initial inventory size was 3.4, 6.3, 6.7, and 9.5 phones at 15, 18, 21, and 24 months, respectively. In contrast, the mean word-final inventory size was 0.6, 2.8, 3.6, and 5.7 at the four observation points. Another interesting finding was that inventory size was positively correlated with age of onset of meaningful speech, with those children who achieved the 10 word per session milestone at the earliest age demonstrating the largest inventories throughout the study. The preference for labial and alveolar stops reported by Kent and Bauer (1985) was replicated in this study. Stoel-Gammon reported that only half the children preferred fricatives in word-final position, however. On the other hand the liquid [ɹ] did tend to appear in word-final position before the word-initial position. Non-English phones occurred only sporadically. In contrast to Ferguson and Farwell (1975), who emphasized individual differences between the children in their study, Stoel-Gammon found that the order of emergence of phones in the children's speech was "highly regular" across the children. She speculates that this is because the children were older and had larger vocabulary sizes than the infants described in Ferguson and Farwell's study.

Consonant inventory size increases between 18 and 24 months and tends to be larger in word-initial than word-final position. Inventory size is correlated with the age of onset of meaningful speech.

Labial and alveolar stops are preferred in the consonant inventories of 1- and 2-year-old toddlers.

Selby, Robb, and Gilbert (2000) followed four children longitudinally from 15 to 36 months of age and derived vowel repertoires from free speech samples using acoustic analyses to support phonetic transcription of the vowels in the children's speech, including all speech-like utterances regardless of whether the utterance had a known or clearly intended referent or meaning. A vowel phone was credited to a child if it appeared at least twice during a one hour recording session. The vowels that appeared in the inventories of at

The **vowel inventory** also increases in size with age. The corner vowels emerge between 15 and 18 months and the full vowel inventory is in place by 36 months.

least 3 of the 4 children increased with age as follows: at 15 months, [ɑ,ɪ,ʊ,ʌ]; at 18 months, [ɑ,i,u,ʊ,ʌ,ɔ,æ]; at 21 months, [ɑ,i,ɪ,ɛ,u,o,ʌ,ɔ]; at 24 months, [ɑ,i,ɪ,ɛ,e,u,o,ɔ,æ]; and at 36 months, [ɑ,i,ɪ,ɛ,e,u,ʊ,o,ʌ,ɔ,æ,ɝ]. The change from 15 to 18 months appears to reflect the expansion of the vowel space that was described in acoustic terms in Chapter 3. Specifically, the infant begins with a small repertoire of central vowels but expansion of the vowel space leads to the emergence of the corner vowels. Subsequent to the anchoring of the space with the establishment of the vowels ([i,u,æ]), further refinement involves the emergence of the full repertoire of central vowels including the rhotic vowels by 36 months of age.

A normative standard for the phonetic repertoire of a child aged 24 months is presented in Table 4–2.

Stoel-Gammon (1987) recommended a normative standard for the phonetic repertoire of a child aged 24 months as presented in Table 4–2. The standard was derived from her longitudinal study in which children were recorded twice for 30 minutes. The first 100 fully or partially intelligible words were included in the analysis. No word was included more than twice and second tokens of a word were included only in those cases where the second token differed from the first. Note that this profile of the typical 2-year-old is based on the repertoire of phones and word shapes. Therefore, the expectation for a cluster or two in word-initial position does not mean that the child is expected to produce the clusters correctly in accordance with the adult target. If the child produces the word "play" as [pwe] and the word "spot" as [θpɑt] these productions would meet the standard. Similarly, the expectations for the number of phones in word-initial and word-final positions only refers to the number of phones observed in the broad transcription regardless of the adult target. In other words, requirements 1 through 4 on Table 4–2 are based on an independent analysis of the child's speech, as defined in Chapter 1. The fifth requirement, however, is based on a relational analysis in which each consonant is compared to the adult target with the expectation being that 70% of consonants will be correctly produced. The profile presented in Table 4–2 is also consistent with more recent data based on picture-naming

Table 4–2. *Expectations for the Typical 24-Month-Old*

1. Word shapes: CV, CVC, CVCV, and CVCVC.
2. Consonant clusters: a few in word-initial position and maybe one or two in word-final position.
3. Initial consonants: 9–10, including exemplars from the classes of stops, nasals, fricatives, and glides.
4. Final consonants: 5–6, mostly stops but including a representative of the nasal, fricative, and liquid classes.
5. Percent match to consonants in the adult target word: 70% correct.

Source: Adapted from Stoel-Gammon (1987). Phonological skills of two-year olds. *Language, Speech, and Hearing Services in Schools, 18,* pp. 327–328. Used with permission of the American Speech-Language and Hearing Association.

data collected from toddlers speaking British English (McIntosh & Dodd, 2008)

Normative Data: Whole Word Measures

Describing a young child's phonological development in terms of a repertoire of phones and word shapes is more appropriate than standard phonological analyses that are used for adult speech because it avoids the assumption that the child has adultlike underlying representations with full knowledge of linearly ordered phonological units at all levels of the phonological hierarchy. Nonetheless, this analysis strategy maintains focus on individual segments and gives the impression that the child's goal is to expand the number of phones available for use in speech production, and furthermore, that the expanding repertoire of phones drives increases in the complexity in the child's word forms. Ingram and Ingram (2001) suggest that this view is inconsistent with the data and recall Ferguson and Farwell's (1975) emphasis on the word as the primary phonological unit in early linguistic development. As described earlier, many aspects of early phonological systems appear to be subservient to the child's need to expand the lexicon while maintaining lexical contrast. Ingram and Ingram (2001) proposed, "that the goal of phonological acquisition is to achieve word productions that will be in close proximity to and eventually match the adult target vocabulary" (p. 274). Ingram (2002) introduced a series of whole word measures that allow us to determine how successful a child is at achieving proximity to adult targets at the whole word level. As the child develops it is expected that his or her word productions will increase in complexity, consistency, and overall proximity to adult targets. The measures were designed to track these changes and are referred to as Phonological Mean Length of Utterance (pMLU), Proportion of Whole Word Proximity (PWP), Proportion of Whole Word Correctness (PWC), and Proportion of Whole Word Variability (PWV).

Whole word measures allow us to determine how successful a child is at achieving **proximity** to adult targets at the whole word level.

Application of these measures begins with the recording of a free speech sample from a child (sampling issues and techniques are discussed in Chapters 5 and 6). The analysis begins with broad transcription of 25 to 50 words, selected in accordance with the Sample Size rule. Given that these are measures designed for very young children or children in the early stages of phonological development, it is very likely that this will include all words in the sample. If the child produces more than 50 words during the recording session, however, a procedure for selecting words that cover the full session (every second or third word, for example) should be adopted. Application of the Lexical Class rule leads to the exclusion of "child words" such as "mama" and "tata," because only common nouns, verbs, prepositions, adjectives, and adverbs that would be used in normal adult conversation are to be counted in the analysis. Further to the issue of word selection, words that would normally be spelled as a compound word ("cowboy") are counted as a single word, whereas apparent compounds that are spelled

When conducting the whole word analysis, the **Sample Size rule** requires selection of 25 to 50 words from a recording of the child's language output.

Application of the **Lexical Class rule** leads to the exclusion of 'child words' such as "mama" and "tata," as only common nouns, verbs, prepositions, adjectives, and adverbs that would be used in normal adult conversation are to be counted in the whole word analysis.

The **Variability rule** excludes all but one production of each unique lexical item for calculation of the pMLU, PWP, and PWC.

The **Phonological Mean Length of Utterance (pMLU)** is arrived at by summing points for each consonant and vowel that is produced correctly in the correct position within the word, subtracting points for additions, and dividing by the number of words.

Proportion of Whole Word Proximity (PWP) is calculated as the pMLU for the child's production divided by the pMLU for the adult target, averaged for the sample.

as two words ("teddy bear") are counted as two words (Compound Word rule).

The Variability rule excludes all but one production of each unique lexical item for calculation of the pMLU, PWP and PWC. All productions of each lexical item are taken into account when calculating PWV as described in detail below.

Calculation of the pMLU requires application of two rules, the Production rule and the Consonants Correct rule. First, according to the Production rule a point is awarded for each consonant and vowel contained within the word with syllabic consonants counting as a single point. Second, according to the Consonants Correct rule an additional point is added for each consonant that was produced correctly. Subsequently, Taelman, Durieux, and Gillis (2005) suggested some refinements to these procedures. They added points for correct consonants only if they occurred in the correct position in the word and points were deducted for additions to a word (essentially consonants adjacent to an added consonant were considered to be incorrect). Some scoring examples are shown in Table 4–3. The pMLU is arrived at by calculating the average number of points for all of the words selected for analysis from the child's speech sample. This table also includes the PWP for each word which is calculated as the points for the child's production divided by the points for the adult target. As shown in Table 4–3, words produced with two syllables tend to receive more points than single syllables words and complex words with many syllables and segments receive the most points of all. The number of points awarded is moderated by the correctness factor however so that the single syllable word "bus" receives more points than the complex target "rooster" that is not

Table 4–3. Examples of Scoring Phonological Mean Length of Utterance

Target Gloss	*Target Transcription*	*Child Transcription*	*Production Rule*	*Consonants Correct Rule*	*PWP[a] for the Word*
bus	[bʌs]	[bʌs]	3 points	2 points	5/5 = 1.00
potato	[pətero]	[tero]	4 points	2 points	6/9 = .66
tunnel	[tʌnl]	[tʌno][b]	4 points	2 point	6/7 = .86
rooster	[ɹustɹ][b]	[wurə]	4 points	0 points	4/9 = .44
cat	[kæt]	[tæk]	3 points	0 points	3/5 = .60
off	[ɑf]	[fɑf]	2 points	1 point	3/3 = 1.00
face	[feɪs]	[feɪst]	3 points	1 point	4/5 = .80
helicopter	[hɛlɪkɑptɹ][b]	[hɛldɪkɹɑptɹ]	9 points	4 points	13/15 = .87

[a]PWP = Proportion of Whole Word Proximity.

[b]Our preference would be to transcribe the last phoneme in these words as the vowel [ɚ] but Ingram (2002) counts these unstressed syllables as syllabic consonants that receive a point according to the Consonants Correct Rule.

produced with any correct consonants. It is further shown that correctly produced words, as in the "bus" example, will receive a PWP of 1.00. The "potato" example shows the impact of omitting the initial weak syllable but the use of the flap in [teɾo] is not penalized as this is perfectly acceptable in the adult input. The examples "tunnel," "rooster," and "helicopter" illustrate the awarding of points for syllabic consonants. The "cat" example illustrates application of Taelman et al.'s Positional rule where no points are awarded for correct consonants that appear in the wrong position or order within the word. The final three examples in the table, "off," "face," and "helicopter," show a limitation on the Production rule: specifically, the number of points given cannot exceed the number of segments in the adult target. Furthermore, in "face" the final [s] is coded as incorrect due to the addition of [t] at the end of the word; similarly, in "helicopter" the [l] and [k] phones are coded as incorrect due to adjacent additions. However, the coding of "off" follows Ingram's original suggestion to simply ignore additions as in this case there is no adjacent consonant to penalize with an error.

Of the remaining whole word measures, the PWC is the most straightforward: simply count the words that were produced correctly and divide by the total number of words selected for analysis. The PWV is more complicated to calculate. In this case, the number of different forms of a word are divided by the number of productions of that word, yielding a number that varies from 0 (no variability) to 1.00 (maximum variability). For example, given multiple productions of the target "bus," the productions [bʌs, bʌs, bʌs] would receive a score of 0 as would [bʌt, bʌt, bʌt], that is, 0 different forms divided by three productions; however, [bʌts, bʌts, bʌs] represents two different forms and would receive a score of .66 whereas [bʌ, bʌt, bʌts] represents three different forms and would receive a score of 1.00 indicating maximum variability for this word in a sample.

The **Proportion of Whole Word Correctness (PWC)** is calculated as the total number of words produced correctly divided by the total number of words selected for analysis.

Proportion of Whole Word Variability reflects the number of unique word forms produced for each word in the sample.

These measures have only recently been proposed and no large scale normative studies have been conducted. However, a few small sample studies, focused on cross-linguistic comparisons or bilingual language development, have been published (Bunta, Davidovich, & Ingram, 2006; Bunta, Fabiano-Smith, Goldstein, & Ingram, 2009; Burrows & Goldstein, 2010; MacLeod, Laukys, & Rvachew, 2011; Saaristo-Helin & Savinainen-Makkonen, 2006). A small amount of English data can be extracted from some of these early papers, as shown in Table 4–4. The table suggests generally greater proximity to adult targets with age although the trend is not monotonic, possibly reflecting differences in coding rules as MacLeod et al. applied the rules that deducted points for additions or errors in segment order. Clearly larger scale cross-sectional or longitudinal studies employing standardized methods for sample collection and scoring are required. Nonetheless, the measure shows great promise as a tool for describing early phonological development at the whole word level and for tracking change as a consequence of intervention with young children.

Proportion of Whole Word Proximity generally increases with age.

Table 4–4. *Mean (Standard Deviation) of Phonological Mean Length of Utterance (pMLU), Proportion Whole-Word Proximity (PWP), and Proportion Whole-Word Correctness (PWC) Data from Selected Published Samples*

Sample	Age (mos)	N	Child pMLU	PWP	PWC
[a]English and other languages	11 to 22	5	3.18 (nr)	.64 (nr)	.12 (nr)
[b]English Monolingual	19	8	3.29 (.52)	.67 (.06)	.15 (.09)
[b]English-French Bilingual	19	11	3.14 (.78)	.66 (.14)	.12 (.09)
[b]English-French Bilingual	25	9	3.90 (.60)	.74 (.04)	.30 (.11)
[b]English Monolingual	36	11	4.70 (.52)	.84 (.06)	.44 (.13)
[b]English-French Bilingual	36	10	4.29 (.51)	.80 (.50)	.44 (.22)
[c]English Monolingual	40	8	6.24 (.33)	.92 (.05)	nr
[b]English-French Bilingual	43	7	4.74 (.21)	.91 (.05)	.66 (.17)
[c]English-Spanish Bilingual	43	8	5.85 (.52)	.86 (.07)	nr

Note: nr = not reported.
[a]Ingram (2002).
[b]MacLeod, Laukys, and Rvachew (2011).
[c]Bunta, Fabiano-Smith, Goldstein, and Ingram (2009).

Clinical Application of Normative Data with Infants and Toddlers

The kinds of measures and descriptive tools that have been described thus far have a number of clinical uses including determining whether a child is eligible for service, diagnosing speech delay or disorder, determining type of speech delay, scheduling the most efficient intensity of service and choosing the most appropriate service delivery model, identifying the most effective approach to intervention, selecting treatment goals, documenting progress toward the achievement of those goals, and deciding when to terminate the treatment program. Upon initial referral of the child for service, however, the speech-language pathologist's typical first task is to determine the child's status in comparison to normally developing age peers. Application of the available normative data to this task in the case of young children is relatively straightforward because the data collection methods used in the scientific literature largely mirror normal clinical practice with this population; in other words, free speech samples, using the mother as a partner in the data collection process is the standard procedure in both contexts. Issues of reliability of the measures do arise, however, because the content of free speech samples are not replicable and the duration of the samples when recorded from young children tends to be short. Morris reported that 20 minute samples recorded from 18- to 22-month-old toddlers yield good test-retest reliability for number of final consonants and word shapes but that number of initial consonants differed across test sessions by an average of one consonant. Taelman et al. (2005) determined that Ingram's suggested sample size of at least 25 words was insufficient if the child's pMLU exceeded 4.5 although we would argue that these whole word measures are not appropriate for children with language ages much beyond 24 or 30 months and complex phonological systems in any case. Fortunately, clinical practice with younger children often allows for multiple observations before a definitive diagnosis is made so that the reliability of one's observations can be established.

Recording and analyzing speech samples from toddlers for comparison to normative data requires samples of sufficient duration. Multiple observations of the child to ensure adequate numbers of utterances for analysis increases confidence in the reliability and validity of the measures.

An example of a speech sample recorded from a 24-month-old monolingual English speaking child is shown in Table 4–5. The table also indicates the pMLU for the adult target and the child's production and the resulting PWP for the first production (i.e., token) of each word (i.e., type). The sample was collected for a study on the development of voice onset time in monolingual and bilingual English- and French-learning toddlers. Although the samples involved unstructured conversation between the child, the mother and the experimenter, materials were provided that targeted voiced and voiceless stops at labial, alveolar and velar place of articulation. The sample contains 50 unique word types and 91 tokens. This sample can be examined for conformity with Stoel-Gammon's (1987) profile of a typical 2-year-old as presented in Table 4–2. In this case no more than two tokens of each word are considered in the analysis which reduced the sample to 61 usable words. The first criterion with respect to word shapes is clearly met with CV ([to], [no]), CVC ([gʌk], [pɪk]), CVCV ([gɑgi], [tetə]), and CVCVC ([tʃɪkɪn], [kɑlɪn]) represented. The child also has a well-developed repertoire of word-initial consonants that includes nasals [m, n], stops [p,b,t,d,k,g], fricatives [(s), h], affricates [tʃ], and glides [w, j], exceeding the requirement for at least 9 different phones in this word position. With respect to the final position, the 7 (to 9) phones present in the sample represent the nasal [n], stop [t,k,g], fricative [(f),s,(ʃ)], affricate [(tʃ)], and liquid [ɹ] sound classes. Clusters are observed in the word-initial [kɹ, (gɹ)] and word-final [ntʃ, (ps), (ts)] positions. Some additional structures, notably the liquid [l] and the clusters [(mb), (ts)] can be seen in ambisyllabic position. The child also produces a range of vowels: [ɑ,i,ɪ,ɛ,e,(u),ʊ,o,ʌ,æ,ɚ,ɝ]. Percent consonants correct for this sample is only 59%, however. Valid comparison to Stoel-Gammon's (1987) standard would require a second recording session and an increase in the size of the sample to 100 usable tokens.

The PWP can also be calculated, based on the first production of each of 39 words meeting the Lexical Class rule, yielding a score of .75. Considering the first token of each type, 18% of words are produced correctly. Overall this child's phonological development appears to be meeting expectations although the percent consonants correct is low, possibly due to the pattern of regressive velar assimilation observed on the words "duck," "dog," and "doggie." This is a phonological process that may occur in the speech of young children as discussed later in the chapter.

Table 4–5. *Speech Sample Recorded from 24-Month-Old English-Speaking Child with Phonological Mean Length of Utterance (pMLU) for the Adult (A) and Child (C) Productions and the Proportion of the Whole-Word Proximity (PWP) Indicated for the First Production of Each Codable Word*

Gloss	Transcription of Child Productions	$pMLU_C/pMLU_A$ = PWP
duck	[gʌk][4] [dʌk][1] [gɑk][2]	4/5 = 0.80
Ernie	[ɚni][1]	5/5 = 1.00
chicken	[tʃɪkɪn][1]	7/7 = 1.00
doggy	[gɑgi][1] [gʌki][1]	5/6 = 0.83
woof	[wʊf]	Excluded
phone	[to][1] [woʊ][1] [dʒo][1]	2/5 = 0.40
hello	[hɛwo][2] [hɑwo][1] [ʌwo][1]	5/6 = 0.83
no	[no][5] [næ][1] [o][1] [do][1] [nɑ][1]	3/3 = 1.00
oink	[oɹnɪtʃ][2]	Excluded
pig	[pɪk][2]	4/5 = 0.80
again	[ʌjɪ][1]	3/6 = 0.50
horse	[hɑɹs][3] [hos][1] [hɑɹʃ][1]	7/7 = 1.00
cat	[kæt][1]	5/5 = 1.00
turtle	[tetʌ]	6/7 = 0.86
crayon	[kɹen][1] [kejən][1]	7/10 = 0.70
yes	[jɛs][1]	5/5 = 1.00
Tara	[taɹʌ][1]	6/6 = 1.00
belly button	[ʌbʌtən][1]	8/13 = 0.62
boots	[bot][1]	5/7 = 0.71
call	[kɑ][1]	3/5 = 0.60
number	[nɛmbɚ][1]	9/9 = 1.00
Ashley	[ɛʃ][1]	3/6 = 0.50
umbrella	[bəwæ][1]	5/11 = 0.46
tell	[tʌ][2] [te][1]	3/5 = 0.60
coming	[kʌmɪn][4] [kʌmɪnk][1]	7/8 = .88
you	[dju][1]	2/3 = 0.66
quack	[kɹæk][1] [kjæk][1] [kɑt][1] [gæ][1]	Excluded
ducky	[dɑgi][1]	5/6 = 0.83
lamb	[næ][1]	2/5 = 0.40
doctor	[dɑtə][1]	6/9 = 0.67

Table 4–5. continued

Gloss	*Transcription of Child Productions*	$pMLU_C/pMLU_A$ = PWP
all right	[ɑɹaɪt][1]	6/8 = 0.75
tea	[tɛ][1]	3/3 = 1.00
pizza	[pitsə][1]	7/8 = 0.88
spaghetti	[dɛdi][1]	5/11 = .46
pickle	[peɪko][1]	6/7 = .86
chips	[tʃɪps][1]	7/7 = 1.00
yogurt	[oɚt][2]	5/9 = 0.56
Grover	[gɹovɚ][1]	9/9 = 1.00
calling	[kɑlɪn][1]	7/8 = 0.88
hungry	[hʌdi][1]	5/10 = 0.50
moo	[mu][1]	Excluded
daddy	[dædi][1]	Excluded
dog	[gɑg][2]	4/5 = 0.80
okay	[ʌkeɪ][1]	4/4 = 1.00
car	[kʌ][1]	3/5 = 0.60
quacks	[gæts][1]	5/9 = 0.56
swimming	[sʌmi][1]	6/10 = 0.60
house	[haʊs][1]	5/5 = 1.00
there	[eɹ][1]	3/5 = 0.60
her	[miɹ][1] [dʌ][1]	2/4 = 0.50

Note: Raw data from one participant enrolled in the study reported in MacLeod, Laukys, and Rvachew (2011). Superscripts indicate number of times the token was observed.

Normative Data: Preschool and School-Age Children

4.2.1. Describe, for children approximately 2, 3, and 4 years of age, the percentage of a child's speech that should be intelligible to a stranger.

4.2.2. Operationalize the constructs "customary production" and "mastery" for different sampling conditions.

4.2.3. Interpret age-of-acquisition charts presented in multiple formats (in particular, see Figure 4–5 versus Table 4–8).

4.2.4. Define developmental versus nondevelopmental errors and typical versus atypical errors and give examples.

4.2.5. List the phonological processes that should be suppressed by 36 months of age. List phonological processes that might still be present with noticeable frequency at 52 months of age.

4.2.6. Compare and contrast two explanations for deletion and/or weakening of weak syllables.

4.2.7. Describe six common types of cluster realization from a nonlinear phonology perspective.

4.2.8. Analyze a speech sample recorded from a preschool-age child and determine if it is consistent with the published normative data for a child of the same age.

Whole Word Accuracy and Connected Speech Measures

Ingram (2002) introduced whole word measures with the assumption that the child is attempting to produce words that match the adult targets. One measure, percentage of whole word correctness, shows that during the first 2 years, no more than 15% of the words produced by the toddlers are correct in relation to the adult target. Table 4–5 shows that gradual improvements to 66% whole words correct occur during the preschool period. Schmitt, Howard, and Schmitt (1983) described the development of whole word accuracy in a cross-sectional study of children aged 3 to 7. In this study, samples of conversational speech, approximately 100 words in length, were recorded from the children. Every word was considered in the analysis and thus the results cannot be compared with the whole word measures reported in Table 4–5 where the analyses excluded many words due to the application of the Lexical Class rule and the correctness judgments were applied to phonetic transcriptions of the children's speech in relation to transcriptions of the adult target. In the Schmitt et al. study, speech-language pathologists listened to the recorded samples one sentence at a time and identified the number of correctly and incorrectly articulated words. Acceptable colloquialisms and contractions were agreed upon by the investigators prior to coding (e.g., "runnin/running," "dunno/don't know," "em/them," "an/and," etc.). The results as shown in Figure 4–4 indicate improvement in percent words correct scores and reductions in between subject variability with age. The 3-year-old group obtained significantly lower scores than all other groups and the children aged 5 to 7 obtained higher scores than all younger age groups.

Percent words correct increases from approximately 68% to 95% between 3 and 7 years of age.

As children produce increasing numbers of words correctly their speech becomes easier for listeners to understand. Coplan and Gleason (1988) investigated age-related changes in intelligibility by asking the parents of young children who were awaiting services in a pediatric emergency department this question: "How clear is

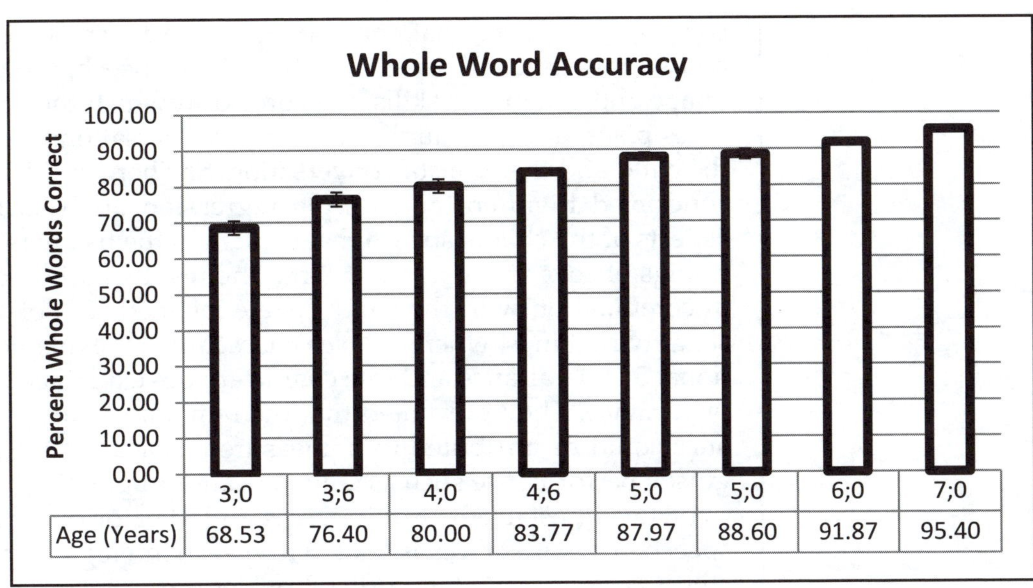

Figure 4–4. *Mean percent whole word accuracy scores obtained from conversational speech samples* (n = *30 children per age group). Standard deviations corresponding to each mean score (shown under the age indicator) are 10.28, 10.72, 10.32, 5.46, 6.04, 7.75, 4.90, and 2.10 for the 3;6, 3;6, 4;0, 4;6, 5;0, 5;6, 6;0 and 7;0-year-old groups respectively. Adapted from Schmitt, Howard, & Schmitt (1983). Conversational speech sampling in the assessment of articulation proficiency.* Language, Speech, and Hearing Services in Schools, 14, *Table 1, p. 211.*

your child's speech? That is, how much of your child's speech can a stranger understand?" Four response alternatives were provided: (1) less than half, (2) about half, (3) three-quarters, and (4) all or almost all. Responses were obtained from parents of 263 children aged 1 to 5. Using a 90th percentile criterion they found that children aged 22 months were 50% intelligible, children aged 37 months were 75% intelligible and children aged 47 months were 100% intelligible. The use of this question and these age cutoffs as a screening tool was validated with a new sample of 151 children, all of whom had been referred due to concerns regarding the child's development. Full speech and language assessment results were used as the criterion measure against which passing or failing the intelligibility screen was validated. Sensitivity, specificity, positive predictive value, and negative predictive value were each found to be .95. Furthermore, the children whose speech was reportedly difficult to understand were frequently found to have difficulties in other areas of development, especially language development, but cognitive and learning disabilities, autism, and hearing impairment were also diagnosed among this subgroup.

An excellent screen for speech delay is the parent's response to this question: "How clear is your child's speech? That is, how much of your child's speech can a stranger understand?" Expected responses (to pass) are "about half" by 22 months, "three-quarters" by 37 months, and "all or almost all" by 47 months.

Shriberg and Kwiatkowski (1982) investigated the relationship between intelligibility and subjective judgments of "severity of involvement" and measures of Percent Consonants Correct (PCC). Listeners reported that speech intelligibility was the primary determinant of their severity ratings. Intelligibility is a multidimensional

Percent Consonants Correct (PCC) is an indicator of the severity of speech impairment that is related to speech intelligibility.

construct, however, that encompasses speech errors, voice quality and suprasegmental aspects of the child's speech, the child's language and pragmatic skills, the context in which the conversation takes place, and the familiarity of the conversational partner with the child and the topic of conversation. Shriberg and Kwiatkowski conducted hierarchical multiple regression analysis to identify aspects of the child's speech that explained the listeners' subjective ratings of severity of involvement. The results indicated that PCC in combination with the child's age explained 73% of variance in severity rankings, whereas voice characteristics explained an additional 5% of variance and rate characteristics explained another 3% of variance. They presumed that the remaining unexplained variance could be attributed to unmeasured aspects of the child's linguistic performance such as language and pragmatic abilities.

Having established that PCC is an indicator of the severity of speech impairment that is related to speech intelligibility, follow-up studies established standardized procedures for deriving the PCC and provided reference data for multiple forms of this metric (Austin & Shriberg, 1997; Shriberg, Austin, Lewis, McSweeny, & Wilson, 1997). The procedures for calculating two forms of the PCC are shown in Table 4-6. Both are based on a narrow transcription of a conversational speech sample that yields a minimum of 100 unique word types. The PCC is derived by counting addition, omission, substitution, and distortion errors as incorrect, with certain exceptions as described in Table 4–6. The PCC-R measure is derived in a similar manner except that distortion errors are scored as correct. Reference data are provided for these two measures for groups of males and females for age categories spanning from 3 to 17 in Table 4–7. The individuals who provided data for this table might have been control group subjects in various studies or children who were treated for speech delay and subsequently achieved normal levels of speaking ability. Their samples were included in the reference data for "normal or normalized speech acquisition" if they met expectations for percentage of intelligible words and their speech was free from errors that were deemed age-inappropriate or atypical. Table 4–7 shows that PCC and PCC-R increase between 3 and 7 years of age with very little change thereafter. Neither measure reaches perfect accuracy for male or female talkers although the female groups achieve scores of at least 98% by age 9.

The **PCC** is derived by counting addition, omission, substitution, and distortion errors as incorrect. The **PCC-R** measure is derived in a similar manner except that distortion errors are scored as correct.

Segmental Norms

The reference data for PCC and PCC-R presented in Table 4–7 show that children achieve adult levels of consonant accuracy in conversation between 7 and 9 years of age. Studies that have sought to determine the age at which specific consonants are mastered have used a different approach, relying on single-word picture naming procedures that ensure elicitation of each English consonant

Table 4–6. *Procedures for Deriving Percent Consonants Correct and Percent Consonants Correct-Revised*

Sampling Rules
1. Record a conversational speech sample containing at least 100 word types.
2. Transcribe the sample, providing both an orthographic (i.e., gloss) and a narrow phonetic transcription.
3. Score only fully intelligible words.
4. Consider only intended consonants in the analysis, excluding intended vowels.
5. Additions of consonants before a vowel are not counted as an error.
6. Postvocalic stressed /ɹ/ is a consonant (e.g., "fair" [feɪɹ]) whereas vocalic /ɝ/ and /ɚ/ are vowels (e.g, "furrier" [fɝiɚ]).
7. Do not score consonants in successive repetitions of a syllable, e.g., ba-ballon, score only first /b/.
8. Do not score consonants in third or successive repetitions of a word unless articulation changes.
Scoring Rules for Percent Consonants Correct (PCC)
1. Score consonants as "incorrect" unless heard as correct (questionable cases are scored as "incorrect").
2. Dialectical variants are glossed as intended in the child's dialect.
3. Fast and casual speech variants are scored as correct, e.g., "dunno"/"don't know" is acceptable.
4. Allophones are scored as correct, e.g., flap in "water" → [wɑɾɚ] is correct.
5. Additions to a target consonant are scored as incorrect.
6. Deletion/omission and substitution errors are scored as incorrect, including voicing errors.
7. Omission of /h/ and substitution of /n/ for /ŋ/ are scored as incorrect in stressed syllables only.
8. Deletion/omission and substitution errors are scored as incorrect, including voicing errors.
9. Distortions of a target consonant, no matter how subtle, are scored as incorrect.
Scoring Rules for Percent Consonants Correct—Revised (PCC-R)
1. Scoring rules 1 through 8 above for PCC apply.
2. Distortion errors are scored as correct.

Source: Adapted from Shriberg and Kwiatkowski (1982). Phonological Disorders III: A procedure for assessing severity of involvement. *Journal of Speech and Hearing Disorders, 47*, Appendix A (p. 267) and Shriberg, L. D., Austin, D., Lewis, B. A., McSweeny, J. L., & Wilson, D. L. (1997). The Speech Disorders Classification System (SDCS): Extensions and lifespan reference data. *Journal of Speech, Language, and Hearing Research, 40*(4), p. 726.

in initial and final and sometimes medial word positions. Clinical application of the normative information that is derived from these studies is not completely straightforward and is dependent on a detailed understanding of the methods that were used to collect and summarize the data. Two popular data sets obtained from North American samples are presented here along with sufficient information to permit accurate interpretation of the tables and charts.

Table 4–7. *Lifespan Reference Data for Percent Consonants Correct (PCC) and Percent Consonants Correct—Revised (PCC-R) for Males and Females by Age Category © 1997 D. Austin and L. D. Shriberg*

	Males				*Females*			
Age Category	PCC		PCC-R		PCC		PCC-R	
Yr;Mos	M	SD	M	SD	M	SD	M	SD
3;00–3;11	79.4	7.9	92.8	4.2	80.9	7.7	94.3	4.3
4;00–4;11	80.2	7.9	93.0	4.2	80.3	7.7	94.1	4.3
5;00–5;11	86.9	7.9	92.9	4.4	87.3	7.6	95.3	4.4
6;00–6;11	90.9	4.3	94.1	3.0	91.6	4.6	95.0	3.0
7;00–7;11	95.7	4.3	96.9	3.0	95.8	4.6	97.2	3.0
8;00–8;11	95.6	4.3	97.5	3.0	95.0	4.6	96.9	3.0
9;0–11;11	96.6	3.5	97.1	3.5	98.2	1.6	98.4	1.5
12;00–17;11	97.5	2.6	98.0	2.3	98.9	1.0	99.2	0.8

Note: The table reports derived rather than actual *SD* for each subsample because these are most appropriate for deriving *z*-scores.

Source: Adapted from Austin and Shriberg (1997). Lifespan reference data for ten measures of articulation competence using the speech disorders classification system (SDSC): Waisman Center on Mental Retardation and Human Development, University of Wisconsin-Madison. Used with permission.

The age of "**customary production**" is the age at which the child produces the sound correctly more often than not.

Sander (1972) created a chart to illustrate the ages at which specific consonants are acquired, pooling data from two previously published large sample studies, specifically Templin's 1957 study of normally developing children aged 3 and older and Wellman, Case, Mengert, and Bradbury's 1931 study that included 2-year-olds. In order to interpret the chart it is necessary, first of all, to distinguish between concepts that apply to individual children versus analyses that are conducted at the group level. The original studies elicited no more than two tokens of each consonant in each of the initial, medial, and final positions of words. The child's performance provides a snapshot of his or her progression along the continuum from not being able to produce the sound at all to complete mastery of the phoneme. One must decide, somewhat arbitrarily, what level of performance corresponds to acquisition of each target phoneme. Sander reasoned that mastery could be defined as perfect performance, which would be accurate articulation of a given consonant in initial, medial, and final word position. Sander felt that this was too stringent a standard for the assignment of acquisition ages to phonemes. He suggested that a more reasonable definition of acquisition would be "customary production," which means producing the sound correctly more often than not, operationalized in this context as "correct production of the consonant in two out of three word positions."

Sander (1972) further distinguished between the average age of acquisition and the normal age limit. The average (or median) age of acquisition is represented by the placement of the left edge of the bars on Figure 4–5, indicating the age at which 50% of children produced the consonant correctly in at least two of three word positions. Average ages provide some sense of the order in which phonemes are typically acquired, information that can be useful for planning therapy as discussed in Chapter 8. The normal limit is represented by the right edge of each bar which indicates the age at which 90% of children produced the consonant correctly in at least two of three word positions. Sander suggested that concern about a child's speech development would be warranted if the child had not achieved customary production of a given consonant at the 90th percentile age indicated on the chart. The length of the bar illustrates the variability among children in the age of acquisition for each phoneme. It can be seen, as a general rule, that variability is less for earlier developing sounds and considerably greater for later developing sounds. The greatest variability was observed for acquisition of /s/, with 50% of children achieving customary production by age 3 but the normal limit occurring at age 8. Some anomalies on the chart reflect the particularities of the data collection and scoring methods employed; for example, the late acquisition of /t/ reflects Templin's requirement that medial /t/ in "skating" and "outing" be produced as a voiceless stop rather than a voiced flap.

The Sander normative chart (Figure 4–5) distinguishes between the average age of acquisition (left-hand edge of the bars) when 50% of children achieved customary production and the normal limit (right-hand edge of the bars) when 90% of the children achieved customary production.

More recent normative data on the acquisition of specific consonants in English were collected by Smit, Hand, Freilinger, Bernthal, and Bird (1990). Children were recruited to represent the age groups 3;0, 3;6, 4;0, 4;6, 5;0, 5;6, 6;0, 7;0, 8;0, and 9;0, with the total sample size being 997. All children were monolingual speakers of Midwestern American English with the sample matched to the demographic characteristics of Iowa and Nebraska at the time of the study with respect to variables such as gender, parental education and population density. Children who were receiving speech therapy were included in a proportion equivalent to the proportions of children receiving such services in the states from which the samples were drawn. A photo-naming task was used to elicit all English consonants except /ʒ/ and word-final /ð/ in single word utterances. Most targets were elicited in word-initial and word-final position but /ɹ,l/ were also elicited in intervocalic position and syllabic forms. Word-initial consonant clusters were elicited in addition to singleton consonants. The number of words used to elicit each target consonant per word position varied from one to four. The percentage of acceptable responses was aggregated across words and children by target and age group. Smit et al. observed the trajectory of improvement in consonant articulation and identified the age at which 90% acceptable articulation was achieved for the target phoneme, yielding the table recreated as Table 4–8.

The **Iowa-Nebraska norms** report the age at which 90% production of a phoneme was achieved, aggregated across all items and children. For some phonemes, marked gender differences were observed.

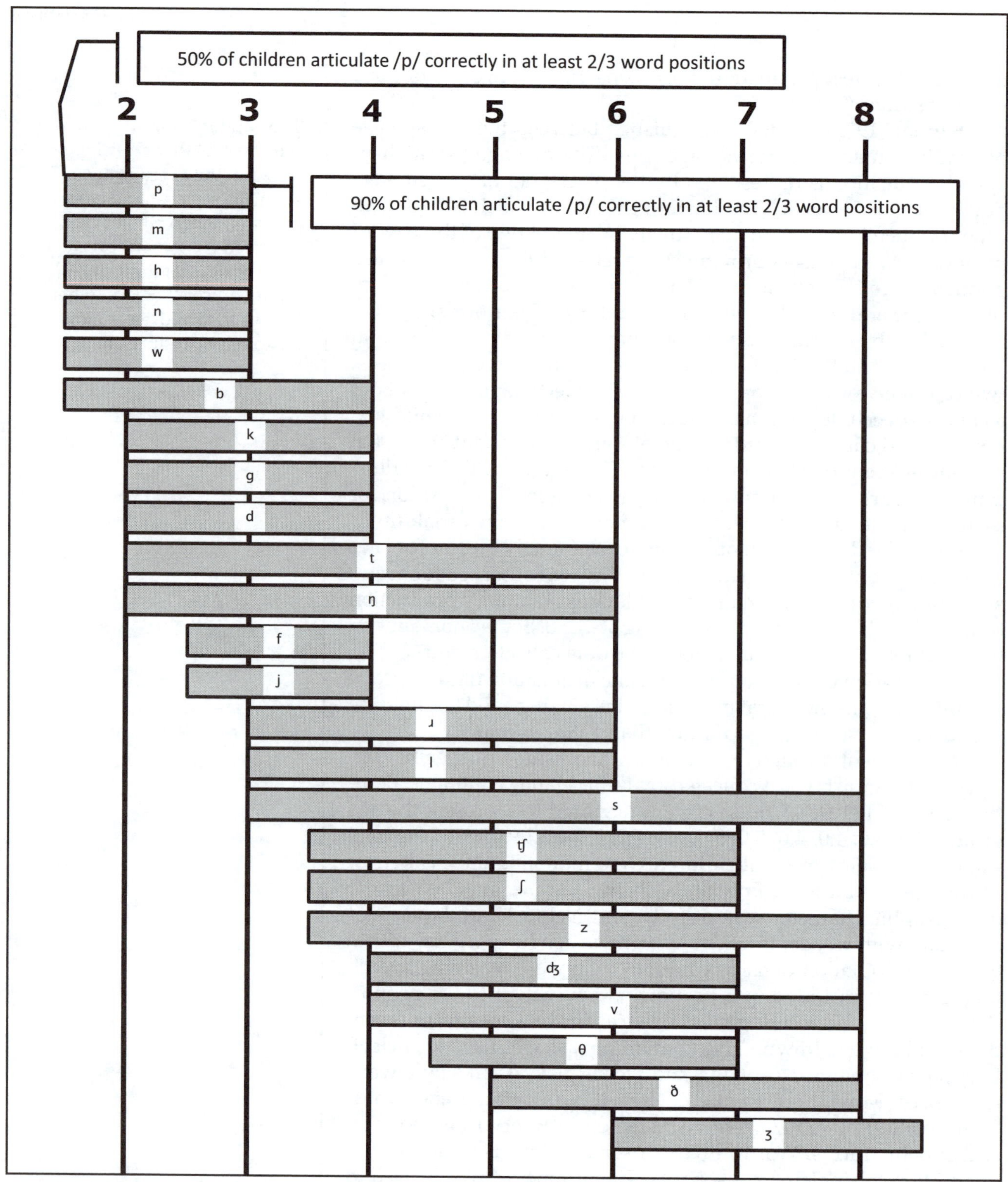

Figure 4–5. *Ages (in years) at which 50%* (left edge of bar) *and 90%* (right edge of bar) *of children achieve customary production of English consonants, when customary production is defined as correct articulation of the consonant in two out of three word positions on a task in which the child has two opportunities to produce each consonant in the initial, medial, and final word positions with small exceptions to take into account phonotactic constraints. Adapted from Sander (1972). When are speech sounds learned?* Journal of Speech and Hearing Disorders, 37, *Figure 1, p. 62. Used with permission of the American Speech-Hearing-Language Association.*

Table 4–8. *Recommended Ages (years;months) of Acquisition by Phoneme or Cluster, Based on 90% Level of Acceptable Articulation*

Phoneme	Females	Males	Phoneme	Females	Males
/m/	3;0	3;0	/ʃ/	6;0	7;0
/n/	3;6	3;0	/tʃ/	6;0	7;0
/-ŋ/	7;0–9;0	7;0–9;0	/dʒ/	6;0	7;0
/h-/	3;0	3;0	/l/ /l-/	5;0	6;0
/w-/	3;0	3;0	/-l/	6;0	7;0
/j-/	4;0	5;0	/ɹ/ /ɹ-/	8;0	8;0
/p/	3;0	3;0	/-ɚ/	8;0	8;0
/b/	3;0	3;0	/tw kw/	4;0	5;6
/t/	4;0	3;6	/sp st sk/	7;0–9;0	7;0–9;0
/d/	3;0	3;6	/sm sn/	7;0–9;0	7;0–9;0
/k/	3;6	3;6	/sw/	7;0–9;0	7;0–9;0
/g/	3;6	4;0	/sl/	7;0–9;0	7;0–9;0
/f/ /f-/	3;6	3;6	/pl bl kl gl fl/	5;6	6;0
/-f/	5;6	5;6	/pr br tr dr kr gr fr/	8;0	8;0
/v/	5;6	5;6	/θɹ/	9;0	9;0
/θ/	6;0	8;0	/skw/	7;0–9;0	7;0–9;0
/ð-/	4;6	7;0	/spl/	7;0–9;0	7;0–9;0
/s/	7;0–9;0	7;0–9;0	/spɹ stɹ skɹ/	7;0–9;0	7;0–9;0
/z/	7;0–9;0	7;0–9;0			

Source: Adapted from Smit et al. (1990). The Iowa Articulation Norms Project and its Nebraska replication. *Journal of Speech and Hearing Disorders*, 55, Table 7, p. 795. Used with permission of the American Speech-Language and Hearing Association.

For example, Figure 4–6 shows the percent acceptable responses for target /ʃ/ aggregated across all participants and plotted by age group. It can be seen that the 90% correct criterion is reached for girls at age 6;0 and for boys at age 7;0. Smit et al. pointed out that their findings are quite similar to those illustrated in Sander's chart with a few notable exceptions: /t/ and /v/ were acquired 2 years earlier in the Smit et al. study, whereas /ŋ/ and /ɹ/ were acquired 2 years later in comparison to the 90th percentile age shown on the Sander chart. The discrepancies for /t/ and /ŋ/ appear to reflect differences in scoring criteria for determining acceptable variants of these phonemes. The authors had no explanation for the discrepant

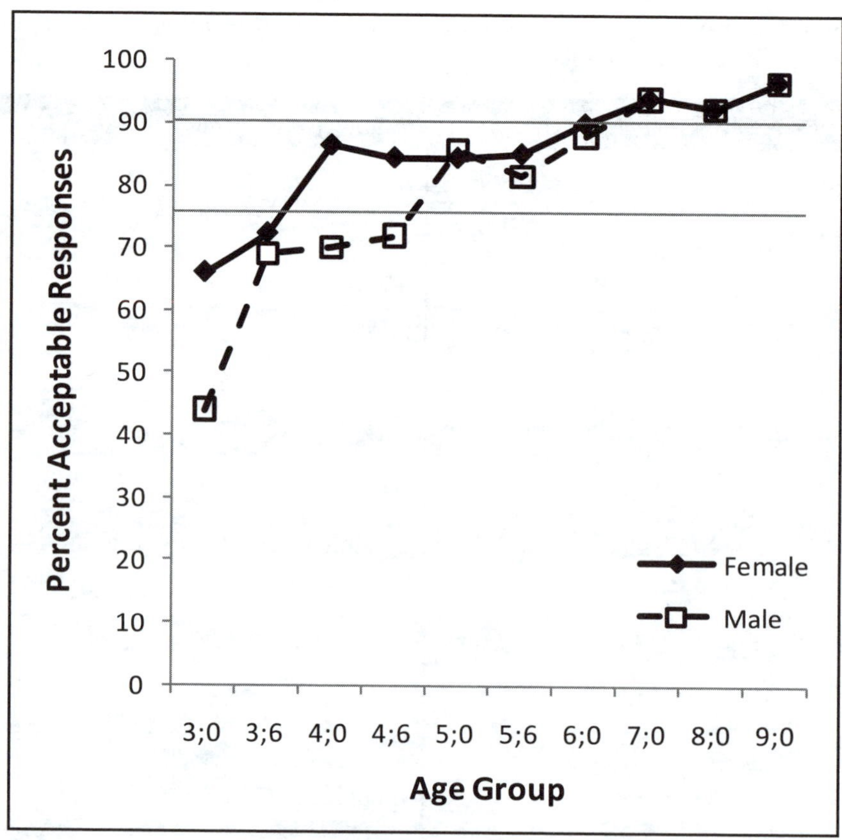

Figure 4–6. *Percent acceptable responses for target /ʃ/ responses by gender and age group (years;months). Adapted from Smit et al. (1990). The Iowa articulation norms project and its Nebraska replication.* Journal of Speech and Hearing Disorders, 55, *Table 4, pp. 786–787 and Figure 14, p. 791.*

findings for /v/ and /ɹ/. Smit's findings are also generally discrepant with those of Prather, Hedrick, and Kern (1975) who reported earlier ages of acquisition for many phonemes in relation to all of the normative studies discussed here. They sampled only the initial and final word positions in their study. These discrepancies across studies reflect the impact of methodological differences as discussed by Edwards and Beckman (2008). Characteristics of the word stimuli such as length in syllables and phonotactic probability of the segment sequences have a significant impact on children's production accuracy. Elicitation, scoring, and transcription procedures also have an important impact on outcomes.

Cross-sectional studies of phoneme acquisition suggest a gradual developmental trajectory with age but rare longitudinal studies suggest that at least some phonemes may be acquired suddenly and rapidly.

Figure 4–6 gives the impression that the developmental course for acquisition of the /ʃ/ phoneme is protracted with girls, as a group, showing 75% acceptable productions at age 3 and 90% acceptable productions at age 6. Cross-sectional data do not illuminate the developmental process for individual children however. Consider the acquisition of /ɹ/ which is one of the few phonemes to have been studied in both cross-sectional and longitudinal studies. Smit's data indicate that boys and girls demonstrated 25% acceptable productions of prevocalic /ɹ/ at age 3;0 and 92% acceptable productions of this allophone at age 8;0. Hoffman, Schuckers, and Daniloff (1980) described 8 preschooler's productions of /ɹ/, /ɝ/ and /ɚ/, measured three times at 4-week intervals. The children, selected because they were normally developing but had not mastered the liquids at study onset, were required to imitate many sentences containing 22 instances each of /ɹ/, /ɝ/ and /ɚ/. Five children showed rapid improvements in production accuracy, whereas three children continued to show almost no gain throughout the course of the study. In general acquisition of /ɚ/ lagged behind the other two allophones. It was not clear what variable or variables triggered sudden emergence of /ɹ/ in these cases but it was interesting to note that no child showed a pattern of slow and gradual improvement that paralleled the developmental pattern that is observed in the aggregate data derived from large group cross-sectional studies. Therefore, Figure 4–6 most likely reflects increasing numbers of children, with advancing age, mastering /ʃ/ rather quickly. However, more longitudinal research with normally developing children is required in order to determine the time course of development by phoneme for individual children.

Smit et al. (1990) also observed the variability in age of acquisition for the sibilants /s, z/ that is seen on the Templin chart. Although the percentage of acceptable productions exceeded 75% at age 3;6, the 90% criterion was not achieved until age 9;0 in their sample, as shown in Figure 4–7. The developmental trajectory for /z/ and for the /s/ clusters was similar to that shown for /s/ in Figure 4–7, with near mastery observed at approximately age 7;0 but performance hovering at or below 90% as late as age 9;0. This particular case, in which the acquisition age for the coronal sibilants is difficult to establish, highlights the fact that there are other variables to consider when judging whether a child's speech performance is within normal limits. One important consideration is the nature of the child's error for a given phoneme.

The acquisition age for the coronal sibilants is difficult to establish, with near mastery observed between 7 and 9 years of age.

Smit (1993a) reported the frequency of different errors by target phoneme and described how this data could be used to identify error types along two dimensions: a child's error for any given consonant can be considered to be developmental or nondevelopmental and typical or atypical. Developmental errors are likely to self-correct whereas nondevelopmental errors are likely to persist unless speech therapy is provided. Typical errors are types of substitutions, omissions or distortions that occur more than 5% of the time in young children's speech whereas atypical errors are rare at any age. For example, Figure 4–8 plots the frequency of occurrence of 4 types of errors for word-final /s/ as a function of age. The error category "null," meaning omission of word-final /s/, is quite frequent with 15% occurrence at age 2;0 but is not seen at all after the age of 3;0. Although it is risky to assume that a pattern observed in cross-sectional data can be generalized to development in an individual, it is likely that a very young child with this error pattern will spontaneously "outgrow" it. Dental distortion of /s/ is another error that is very common, occurring with greater than

Developmental errors are likely to self-correct whereas **nondevelopmental errors** are likely to persist unless speech therapy is provided.

Typical errors are types of substitutions, omissions or distortions that occur more than 5% of the time in young children's speech whereas **atypical errors** are rare at any age.

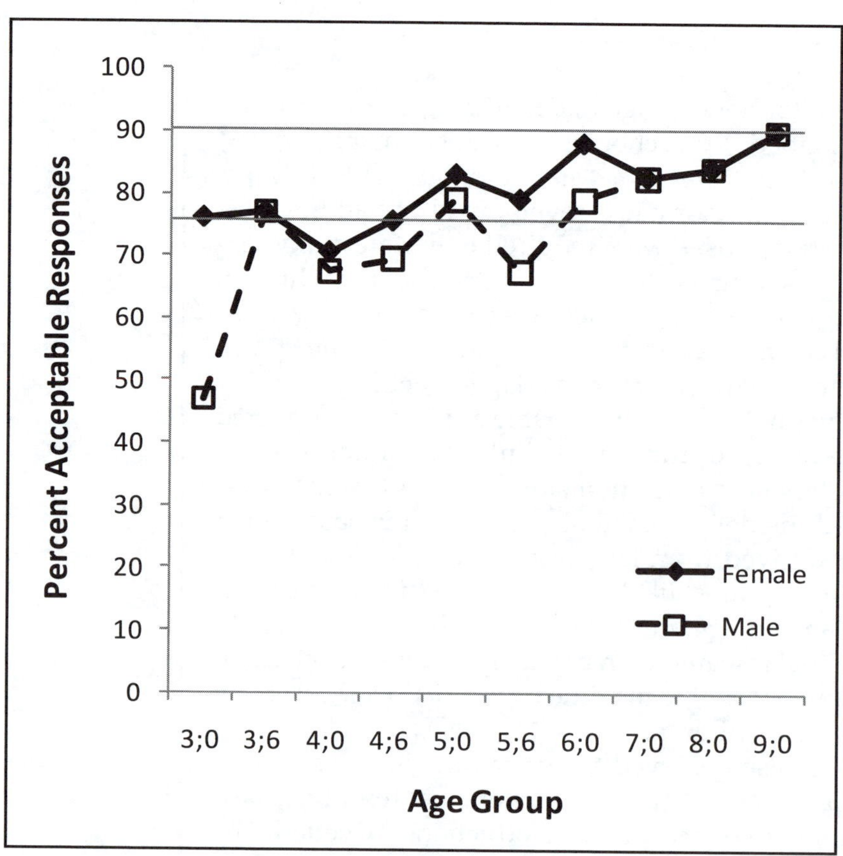

Figure 4–7. *Percent acceptable responses for target /s/ responses by gender and age group (years;months). Adapted from Smit et al. (1990). The Iowa articulation norms project and its Nebraska replication.* Journal of Speech and Hearing Disorders, 55, *Table 4, pp. 786–787 and Figure 10, p. 790.*

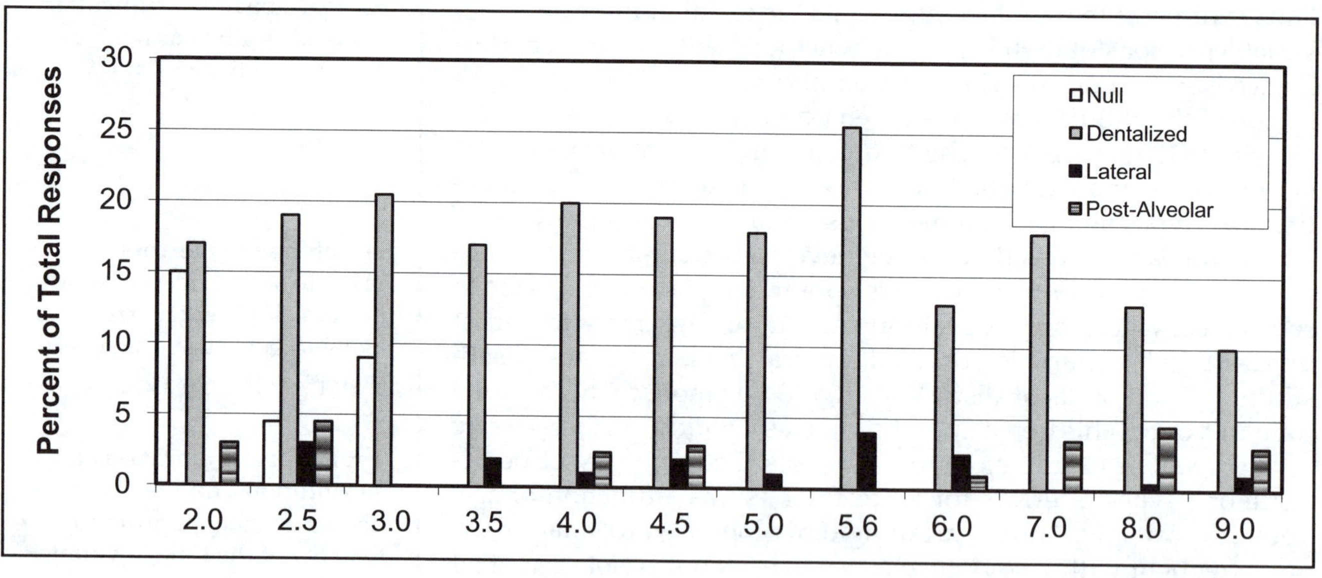

Figure 4–8. *Frequency distribution of common error types for word-final /s/ by age group (in years). Adapted from Smit (1993a). Phonological error distributions in the Iowa-Nebraska Articulation Norms Project: Consonant singletons.* Journal of Speech and Hearing Research, 36, *Figure 3, p. 543. Used with permission of the American Speech-Hearing-Language Association.*

15% frequency before 7 years of age and falling to 10% occurrence at age 9;0. Smit states that there is no reason to believe that this error will self-correct if it persists past this age. Postalveolar distortions of /s/ are atypical throughout the age range studied but the frequency declines with age suggesting that this error may be classified as "atypical developmental" in children younger than age 9;0. Lateral distortions on the other hand are atypical at every age and there is no evidence that this rare distortion self-corrects; indeed, even with intensive speech therapy this can be a difficult error to correct in some cases.

As a second example of different types of errors, Figure 4–9 shows the error distributions for word-initial /ɹ/. In this figure it can be seen that substitution of [w] for /ɹ/ is the most common error type across a broad age range; therefore, it is clearly typical and developmental in preschool-age children. The derhotacized distortion is much less common but occurs with greater than 5% frequency in 2- and 3-year-olds and thus is categorized as a typical error. This error also appears to decline to negligible levels by the age of 8;0. In contrast, labialized and labialized-derhotacized distortions are observed with very low frequency throughout the age range and thus are atypical and probably nondevelopmental errors in a child of any age. Table 4–9 lists some of the typical and atypical errors observed for each consonant in Smit (1993a). More discussion about the use of this kind of information for diagnostic decisions and treatment planning occurs throughout Part II.

Substitution of [w] for /ɹ/ is the most common error type across a broad age range for this phoneme target; therefore, it is clearly typical and developmental in preschool-age children.

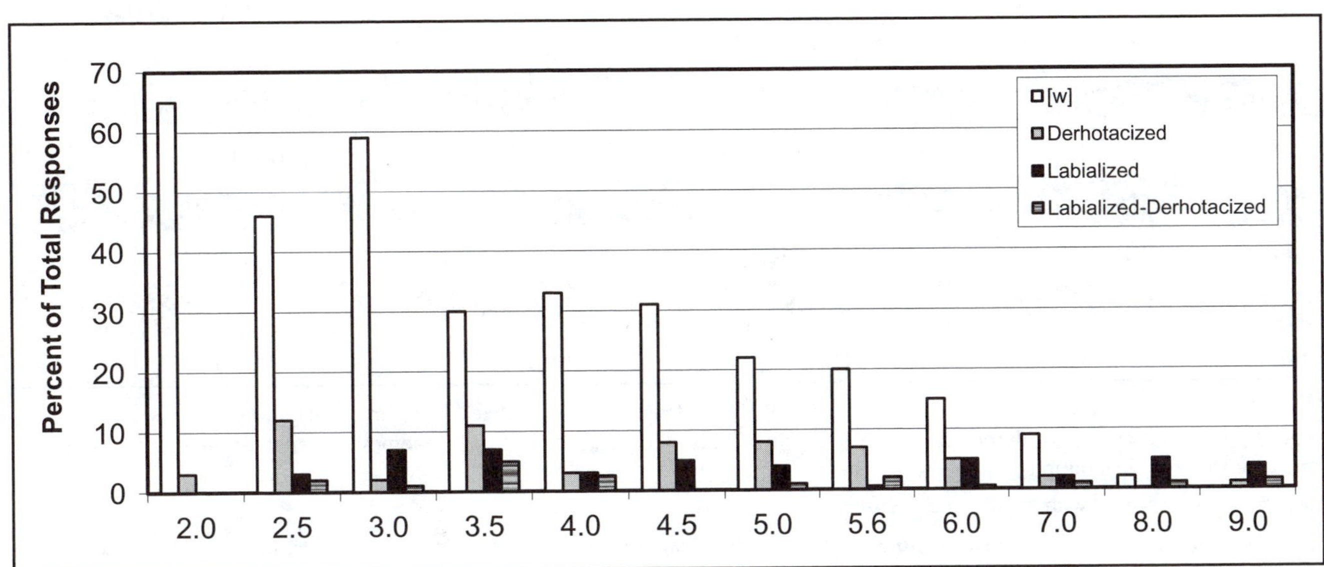

Figure 4–9. *Frequency distribution of common error types for word-initial /ɹ/ by age group (in years). Adapted from Smit (1993a). Phonological error distributions in the Iowa-Nebraska Articulation Norms Project: Consonant singletons.* Journal of Speech and Hearing Research, 36, *Figure 1, p. 537. Used with permission of the American Speech-Hearing-Language Association.*

Table 4–9. Selected Typical[a] and Atypical[b] Errors by Phoneme

Phoneme	Word Initial Position		Word Final Position	
	Typical Errors	Atypical Errors	Typical Errors	Atypical Errors
/m/		[m͊]		[m͊], Ø
/n/		[n͊]		[n͊], Ø
/-ŋ/			[n], [ŋg], [ŋk]	Ø, [n͊], [ŋ͊]
/h-/		Ø, [ʔ]		
/w-/		Ø, [ɹ]		
/j-/	Ø, [w]	[n], [l]		
/p/	[b]	Ø, [h], [t]	Ø	[f], [t]
/b/		[p]	Ø, [p]	
/t/		[k], [ts]	Ø	[k], [d], [tə]
/d/			Ø, [t]	[ʔ]
/k/	[t], [g]	[k̡]		[t], [g], [k̡], Ø
/g/	[d]	[k]	[k]	[ʔ], [t], [d], Ø
/f/	[p], [b]	[h], [w], [ɸ]	Ø, [s], [v]	[p], [b]
/v/	[b], [f]	[β], [w]	[b], [f]	[β], [ɸ]
/θ/	[f], [s], [t], [d]	Ø	[s], [f]	
/ð-/	[d]	[v], [z]		
/s/	[s̪̯], [t], [d]	[s̪̯], [s̡]	[s̪̯], Ø	[s̪̯], [s̡], [ts], [z]
/z/	[d], [z̪]	Ø, [z̪], [z̡], [j]	[z̪], Ø	[d], [s̪̯], [s̡], [z̪], [z̡], [t]
/ʃ/	[s], [t], [d]	[ʃ̪], [ʃ̯], [s̡], [tʃ]	[s], Ø	[ʃ̪], [ʃ̯], [tʃ]
/tʃ/	[t], [d], [ts], [tʃ], [ʃ]	[ʃ̪], [ʃ̯], [tʃ̪]	[ts], [ʃ]	Ø, [t], [ʃ̪], [ʃ̯]
/dʒ/	[d]	[dz], [dz̪̯], [dʒ̯], [tʃ]	[tʃ], [dz]	[dʒ̪], [dʒ̯]
/l/	[w], Ø	[n], [ɹ]	Rounded V, Ø	Unrounded V
/ɹ/	[w], [ɹ̬]	[ɹ̫], Ø	Rounded V, Ø	Unrounded V

Note: The Ø symbol denotes omission of the consonant; V denotes vowel; Denasalized (e.g., [m͊]), palatalized (e.g., [s̡]), dentalized (e.g., [z̪]), lateralized (e.g., [s̪̯],, derhotacized (e.g., [ɹ̬]), and labialized (e.g., [ɹ̫]) variants of phonemes are denoted with standard diacritics for transcribing clinical samples.

[a]Typical errors occurred with greater than 5% frequency at at least one age interval.

[b]Atypical errors occurred occasionally (1 to 4%) or rarely (less than 1%). Only notable atypical variants, for example, those that reoccurred occasionally or rarely across more than one age interval are mentioned here.

Source: Adapted from Smit, A. B. (1993a). Phonological error distributions in the Iowa-Nebraska Articulation Norms Project: Consonant singletons. *Journal of Speech and Hearing Research*, *36*, Tables 2–6 (pp. 536–541).

Thus far, we have focused on consonant production but some researchers have described the accuracy of vowel production as a function of age. Pollock and Berni (2003) administered a photo-naming task to normally developing children aged 18 through 83 months who spoke a range of dialects including Informal Standard English, Southern White Vernacular English, and African American Vernacular English. The photographs elicited 140 words targeting nonrhotic vowels, specifically 11 monophthongs and 3 diphthongs. Responses were scored to take acceptable dialectical variations into account. Accuracy improved with age but was close to ceiling by 36 months. Results are reported separately for a younger group (less than 36 months) and an older group (36 months of older). The percentage of children who achieved at least 85% accuracy was 76% and 96% for the younger and older groups, respectively, whereas the percentage of children who achieved at least 95% accuracy was 35% and 96% for the younger and older groups respectively. Vowel accuracy can also be coded from conversational speech samples, yielding the Percent Vowels Correct (PVC; which includes substitution, addition and distortion errors for nonrhotic and rhotic vowels) or the Percent Vowels Correct—Revised (PVC-R; substitution and addition errors only). Austin and Shriberg (1997) reported that their Normal or Normalized Speech reference sample achieved mean scores of 94.4 (SD = 2.4) and 97.9 (SD = 1.8) for these two measures, respectively. These two data sets give the impression that noticeable vowel errors, even at very low frequencies in the child's speech, are nondevelopmental and possibly atypical past the age of 36 months, especially when they affect nonrhotic vowels.

Accuracy of vowel production improves with age but mastery is achieved by most children by 36 months. Noticeable vowel errors, even at very low frequencies in the child's speech, are nondevelopmental and possibly atypical past the age of 36 months, especially when they affect nonrhotic vowels.

Normative Data for Phonological Processes

Many of the consonant error types shown in Table 4–9 correspond to natural phonological processes such as velar fronting, prevocalic voicing, stopping of fricatives, and final consonant deletion. These patterns did not apply with the consistency that one might expect; in other words the frequency of the error types that corresponded to the processes varied considerably across phonemes and word positions. Smit (1993a) noted that prevocalic voicing applied to stop consonants but not fricatives. Stopping occurred with greater frequency for /f v ð z/ than for /θ s ʃ/; this process was also much more common in word-initial than word-final position. In fact, the fricatives /θ ð/ do not appear to be treated as if they belong to the same natural sound class by children given the strong preference for [d] in place of /ð/ but [f] in place of /θ/. Fronting of velars and palatals was observed almost exclusively in word-initial position. Final consonant deletion did not apply uniformly, being much less likely for targets /k g tʃ dʒ/ in comparison to other obstruents. This study was not designed to examine phonological process use specifically, however. Other researchers have described young children's phonological performance with respect to phonological processes

Although error types revealed in normative studies often correspond to **natural phonological processes**, these errors do not always apply with the consistency across phonemes and word positions that is expected from this theoretical perspective.

rather than on a phoneme-specific basis. We now turn to phonological process norms.

Haelsig and Madison report normative data for children aged 3 to 5 years, collected using a test called Phonological Process Analysis (Weiner, 1979) which uses a picture naming procedure to elicit responses. The test probes 4 syllable structure processes with 50 items, 5 harmony processes with 38 items, and 7 substitution processes with 54 items. The percentage of responses that indicated the presence of each syllable structure process, harmony process, and substitution process is shown in Figure 4–10. Statistical analyses revealed that, overall, there was no significant difference between the performance of the 3;0 and 3;6-year-old groups or between the 4;6- and 5-year-old groups. However, there was a significant reduction in the use of phonological processes after the age of 3;6. Some processes were rarely observed in any age group included in the study, specifically: velar assimilation, prevocalic voicing, gliding of fricatives, affrication, and denasalization. Stopping of fricatives and fronting occurred with noticeable frequency at age 3;0 but their use declined to very low levels before age 4;0. Other processes were relatively common (i.e., occurred with greater than 20% frequency) among the 3;0 and 3;6 age groups but were suppressed thereafter, being close to absent before the age of 5;0: glottal replacement, gliding or vocalization of liquids, and labial assimilation. One process was still in use with 20% or greater frequency in the oldest age groups, namely weak syllable deletion. Haelsig and Madison suggest that cluster reduction is expected through age 5;0 but in fact the frequency of this process falls dramatically after age 3;6, as shown in Figure 4–10.

Phonological process use declines markedly after age 3;6.

The Hodson Assessment of Phonological Patterns (Hodson, 2004) employs an object naming task to probe children's productions of stridents, velars, liquids, nasals, and glides in single and multisyllabic words. Responses are scored to reveal the use of four syllable/word structure patterns: syllable reduction, consonant sequence reduction, prevocalic singleton deletion, and postvocalic singleton deletion. A second class of error patterns, called phoneme class deficiencies, includes omissions of a phoneme or a substitution of one phoneme class for another. For example, within the velar class, "duck" → [dʌ] or [dʌt] would be coded as a phoneme class deficiency but "duck" → [dʌg] would not. Coding of stridents is somewhat unusual in their studies in that stopping is described as "stridency deletion" whereas interdental and lateral distortions are not as long as stridency is maintained.[1] Porter and Hodson (2001) used this tool to describe the use of these phonological patterns in

[1]Ball, Müller, and Rutter (2010) disagree with the division of the fricatives into strident [f v s z ʃ ʒ] versus nonstrident [θ ð] classes, arguing persuasively that sibilant [s z ʃ ʒ] versus nonsibilant [f v θ ð] is a more appropriate natural class division. The reader is referred to their detailed discussion of Hodson's proposed phonological pattern of "stridency deletion."

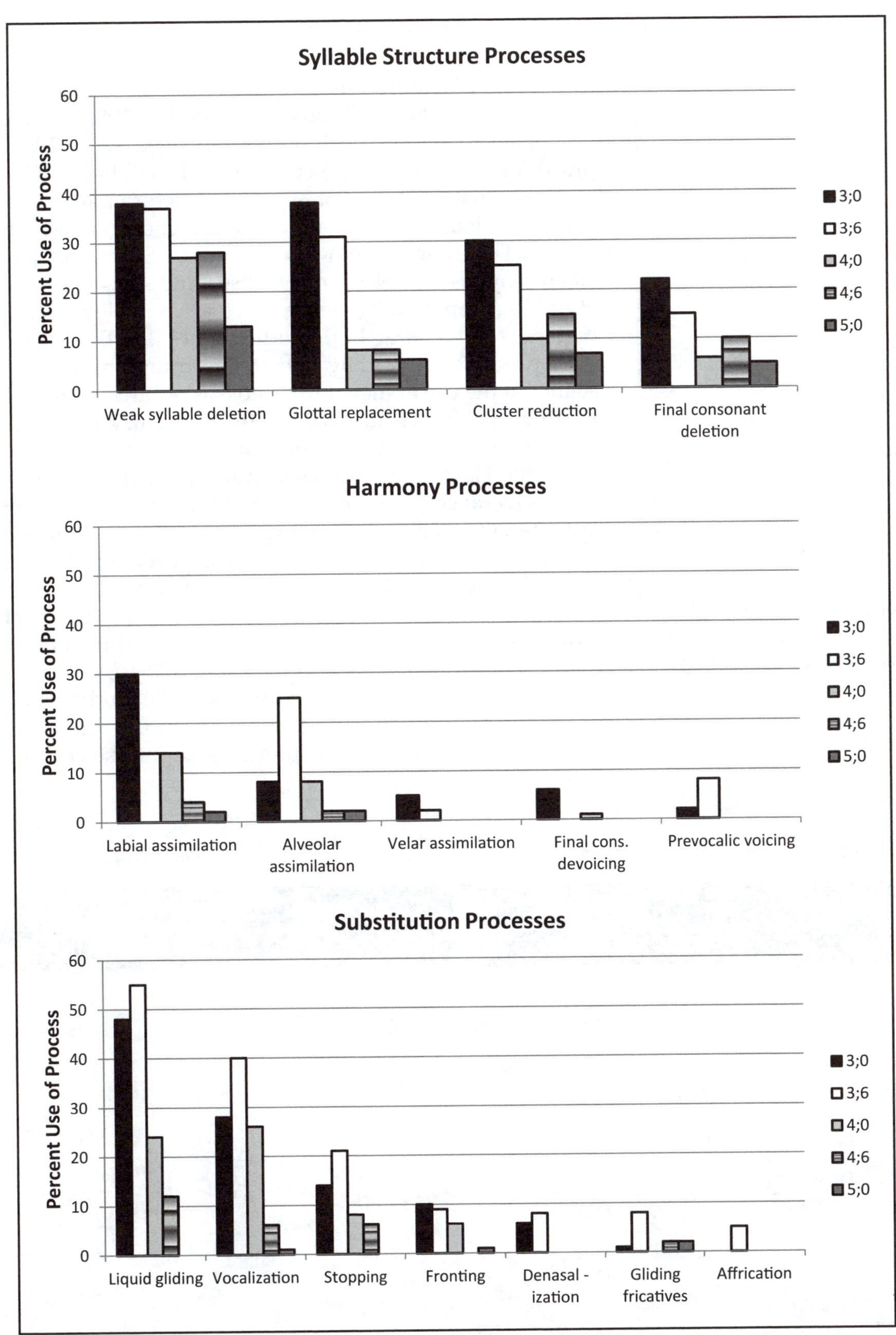

Figure 4–10. *Frequency distribution of syllable structure processes* (top), *harmony processes* (middle) *and substitution processes* (bottom) *by age group (years;months). Adapted from Haelsig and Madison (1986). A study of phonological processes exhibited by 3-, 4-, and 5-year-old children.* Language, Speech, and Hearing Services in Schools, 17, *Tables 1–5, pp. 109–113.*

a sample of 520 children aged 3;0 to 7;0. An earlier prototype of this test was used by Preisser, Hodson, and Paden (1988) to describe the same patterns in the speech of toddlers aged 1;6 to 2;5. The data from these two studies are summarized in Table 4–10, showing the percent use of the syllable/word structure patterns and phoneme class deficiencies for toddlers, preschoolers and school-age children. The coding scheme used in these studies is different from that employed by Haelsig and Madison and, thus, the data sets are not easily compared. However, there are notable similarities and differences. In general, both studies show that the use of phonological processes is typically restricted to young children with sharp declines in the use of these error patterns occurring throughout the second and third years. Overall, the frequency of occurrence of the patterns appears to be somewhat less in the Hodson studies than in the Haelsig and Madison study. Nonetheless, both studies lead to several common conclusions. Cluster reduction (consonant sequence deficiencies) can be expected in 3-year-olds but should fall below the 20% threshold in older children. Strident and velar class deficiencies decline rapidly between year 2 and 3 mirroring the data for stopping of fricatives and fronting in the Haelsig and Madison study. Both studies show continuing difficulties with the liquid class through age 4 years, however. These findings are also consistent with the results of a large sample study conducted in the United Kingdom (Dodd, Holm, Hua, & Crosbie, 2003) which showed stopping and fronting processes suppressed before the end

Strident and velar class deficiencies (i.e., stopping and fronting) decline rapidly between 2 and 3 years of age.

Table 4–10. *Percent Occurrence of Phonological Deviations by Syllable/Word Structure or Phoneme Class and Age Group*

	Age Group							
Deviation	1;6–1;9	1;10–2;1	2;2–2;5	3;0	4;0	5;0	6;0	7;0
Syllable Structures								
Consonant sequences	93.0	76.0	51.0	18.9	6.2	3.1	0.9	0.7
Syllables	43.0	10.0	3.0	2.3	0.8	0.6	0.2	0.0
Postvocalic singletons	45.0	13.0	4.0	2.8	0.6	0.4	0.2	0.0
Prevocalic singletons	14.0	7.0	3.0	1.2	0.3	0.1	0.0	0.0
Phoneme Classes								
Stridents	56.0	41.0	23.0	12.0	5.1	1.7	0.3	0.4
Velars	45.0	23.0	14.0	10.3	3.0	2.3	0.2	0.2
Liquids	91.0	75.0	64.0	29.9	20.5	12.2	4.1	2.6
Nasals/Glides	49.0	23.0	11.0	5.9	1.9	0.8	0.1	0.0

Source: Adapted from Preisser, Hodson, and Paden (1988). Developmental phonology: 18–29 months. *Journal of Speech and Hearing Disorders*, 53, Table 2 (p. 127) and adapted from Porter and Hodson (2001). Clinical forum. Collaborating to obtain phonological acquisition data for local schools. *Language, Speech, and Hearing Services in Schools*, 32, Table 2 (p. 169).

of the third year, cluster reduction largely resolved by age 4;0, and gliding of liquids persisting through to age 6;0.

All normative studies discussed thus far combined data for fronting of velars and fronting of palatals in the same category. Lowe, Knutson, and Monson (1985) reported percent occurrence of fronting for these two sound classes separately in children aged 31 through 54 months. Fronting of velars occurred with 23% frequency versus 17% frequency for fronting of palatals among the children aged 31 to 36 months. The frequency of occurrence fell below 10% for both processes by 42 months of age and to 3% for both processes by 54 months of age.

The findings for gliding of liquids should be discussed in relation to the normative data provided by Smit et al. (1990) and Smit (1993a). Liquid gliding fell below the 20% threshold at age 4;6 in Haelsig and Madison and at age 5;0 in Porter and Hodson. Dodd et al. reported that more than 10% of children used this process at least 5 times through age 5;11 in their sample. Smit et al. suggested that the recommended age of acquisition for the phoneme /l/ should be approximately 6 years and for the phoneme /ɹ/ should be 8 years. The discrepancy between age 4;0 and 6;0 for suppression of liquid gliding and age 6;0 to 8;0 for mastery of /l/ and /ɹ/ has two sources. First, Smit and colleagues use a very stringent standard, requiring 90% correct production for determining the age of acquisition, whereas the "expected age" for occurrence of a phonological process is typically set at a threshold of at least 20% occurrence of the process. Secondly, distortions are not counted as a phonological process but they are coded as an error in the traditional phoneme-level normative studies. In other words, at age 6 or 7 years, liquid gliding is no longer expected but /ɹ/ distortions may still be age-appropriate (depending upon the type of distortion).

Gliding of liquids should be suppressed between 4 and 5 with rare instances through 6 years of age. Distortion of /ɹ/ may persist for several years past this point, however.

One advantage of the phonological approach in comparison to the segmental approach to describing children's phonological development is the attention to both syllable structure and phoneme class error patterns. The high frequency of weak syllable deletion and cluster reduction in 3-year-olds and the persistence of these processes at age 4 years (in the Haelsig and Madison study) points to the necessity of describing children's acquisition of phonological units from the perspective of prosodic or multilinear phonology. In the next section we focus on the prosodic tiers of the phonological hierarchy.

Acquisition of Prosodic Units

Phonological process analysis as described in the preceding section revealed error patterns that altered the syllable structure or overall shape of the target word as well as harmony patterns that involve spreading of features from one segment to another. However, the underlying theoretical approach from which this analysis strategy is derived did not recognize the multilinear or multitiered organization of phonological units across the prosodic and segmental tiers of the phonological hierarchy. In this section we show that the multiple types of error patterns that occur during the production of complex word forms are more adequately described from the multilinear perspective. We begin by considering larger units at relatively high levels of the phonological hierarchy, specifically interactions between the foot and syllable tier.

Young children tend to omit **weak syllables** but not all weak syllables are equally vulnerable to deletion.

In the previous section normative studies indicated that young children tend to omit weak syllables. In this section we show that not all weak syllables are equally vulnerable to deletion. Recall from Chapter 1 that the foot must be composed of a single stressed syllable or a stressed syllable followed by a weak syllable. When prosodic words are combined to form phonological phrases there are instances where weak syllables become "unfooted" as illustrated in Figure 1–22. Gerken investigated toddlers' productions of "footed" and "unfooted" weak syllables in sentences. The toddlers were asked to imitate sentences that had one of two structures, each containing the article "the" as a weak syllable. In one case, the article was linked to the foot tier but in the other the article "the" bypassed the foot tier and linked directly to the prosodic word (PW) tier. Take for example the sentence pair [[TOM]$_{PW}$ [PUSHED the]$_{PW}$ [ZEbra]$_{PW}$] versus [[TOM]$_{PW}$ [PUSHes]$_{PW}$ [the ZEbra]$_{PW}$]. In the sentence "Tom pushed the zebra," the first foot unit aligns with the STRESSED-unstressed syllable pair "PUSHED the" and, thus, in this case the article "the" is captured by a foot unit, satisfying all of the constraints associated with the Strict Layering Hypothesis as explained in Chapter 1. In the sentence "Tom pushes the zebra," the article "the" is unfooted because the first foot unit aligns with the syllable pair "PUSHes" and the second foot unit is forced to align with the stressed-unstressed syllable pair "ZEbra" leaving the article "the" to link directly to the PW tier, violating the exhaustivity constraint. Toddlers aged 25 to 27 months were significantly more likely to preserve the article when imitating sentences in which the article linked to the foot than when imitating sentences in which the article linked directly to the prosodic word, as shown in Figure 4–11. Gerken proposed that children's sentence productions conformed to a trochaic metrical foot production template. In another experiment, however, it was found that preservation of the weak syllable at the beginning of the word "Michelle" was equally likely in the sentences "[Tom]$_{PW}$ [PUSHED]$_{PW}$ [miCHELE]$_{PW}$" versus "[Tom]$_{PW}$ [PUSHes]$_{PW}$ [miCHELE]$_{PW}$." In these sentences the weak syllable of interest is part of a lexical word, specifically "[miCHELE]$_{PW}$." In the first member of the sentence pair, the weak syllable in "Michelle" cannot join with the prosodic word "pushed" to form a two-syllable foot and thus the weak syllable [mɪ] is vulnerable to deletion in both sentences. Gerken concluded that the toddlers structured their sentences into metrical feet that were organized within prosodic words; a prosody-syntax constraint for prosodic words to contain a single

In sentence repetition experiments, English-speaking children's omission or preservation of weak syllables conformed to a **trochaic metrical foot production template**.

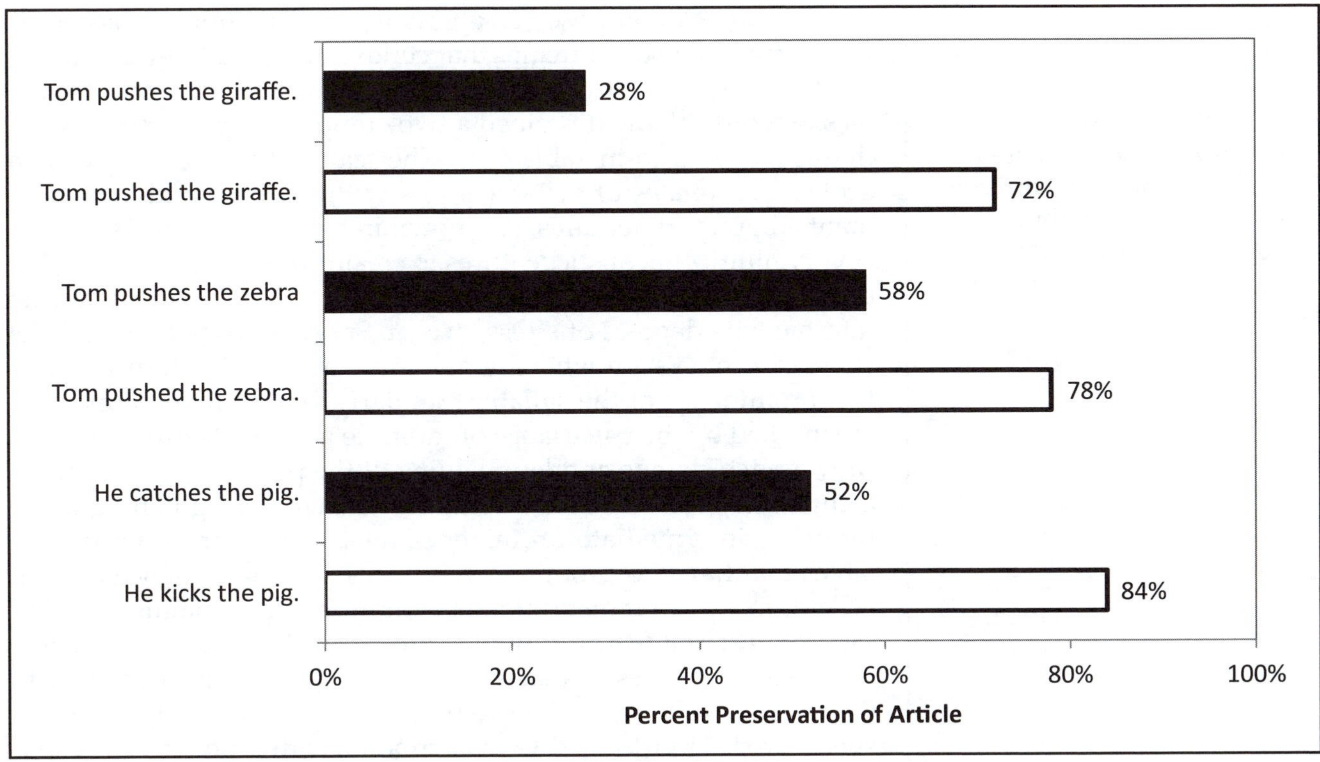

Figure 4–11. *Percent preservation of article by toddlers when imitating sentences with a footed "the"* (open bars) *versus sentences with an unfooted "the"* (closed bars). *Adapted from Gerken (1996). Prosodic structure in young children's language production.* Language, 72, *Table 1, p.* 689.

lexical word outranked the exhaustivity constraint, thus explaining the pattern of weak syllable deletions in both experiments.

Klein (1981) studied toddler's strategies for producing multisyllabic words in single word utterances in a study in which toys and books were used to encourage the production of words up to 5 syllables long by 5 children aged 20 to 25 months. Although three of the children displayed a strong tendency to delete syllables (e.g., "giraffe" → [w{s], "alligater" → [{gejə]), two of the children employed a variety of strategies that served to maintain all of the syllables in a word. These strategies include reduplication (e.g., "tiger" → [taɪtaɪ]), assimilation (e.g., "pocketbook" → [bababʊk]), and neutralization (e.g., "stroller" → [dɔhʌ], "Tina" → [dijʌ], "turtle" → [dɛʔu]). The data also revealed that children will delete weak syllables that are not predicted by the trochaic template hypothesis described above (e.g., "Betty" → [be]). Another syllable weakening pattern that requires explanation is the use of "filler syllables" such as [n̩], [lə], [ɹɪ] or any other phonetic sequence that is substituted routinely for weak syllables in the child's speech (for further discussion, see Echols, 1993; also see sample of speech from a child who used filler syllables extensively in Demonstration 11–2).

Toddlers employ multiple strategies for the production of multisyllabic words, including **reduplication**, **assimilation**, **neutralization,** and **filler syllables,** as well as **weak syllable deletion**. Not all strategies conform to the trochaic metrical foot hypothesis.

The **two-component prominence scale** is based on the known acoustic correlates of syllable stress within words and suprasegmental boundary features.

Snow (1998) proposed an alternative explanation that accounts for the full range of strategies that children use in the production of multisyllabic words by focusing on the relative prominence of syllables in words. Snow described a two-component prominence scale that is reproduced in Table 4–11. The scale is based on the known acoustic correlates of syllable stress within words and suprasegmental boundary features. As shown in Table 4–11, talkers tend to covary multiple acoustic features to create stressed/accented syllables but these features can be manipulated independently to create intermediate degrees of stress/accent. Snow proposed a four-level stress/accent system whereby points are awarded to indicate relative prominence of the syllable. Similarly, phrase final boundaries are marked by the covariance of multiple acoustic features, specifically a pitch change and lengthening of the phrase final syllable in comparison to word final boundaries in which lengthening alone produces intermediate prominence relative to word internal syllables that have no prominence features. The prominence of each syllable in a word is determined by multiplying the points awarded for stress/accent features by the points awarded for boundary features, yielding a result that will vary from 1 to 8, in parallel with the range of vowel durations in English. Snow recorded samples of speech from 11 girls aged 12 to 20 months with productive vocabularies ranging from 30 to 70 words. At least half of the 20 utterances analyzed from each sample were multiword utterances. The syllables in the adult target were coded according to the prominence scale and the transcription of the child's utterances was examined

Table 4–11. *Two Component Prominence Scale*

Points	*Description*	*Prominence Features*	*Example*
Four Levels of the Stress Accent System			
4	Nuclear accent	Pitch change/lengthening on nucleus	it's a *TI*ger
3	Other accent	Pitch change/lengthening elsewhere	the *tiger* can JUMP
2	Tertiary stress	Added length and/or loudness	it's a *hip*oPOtamus
1	Unstressed	No prominence features	it's a *gi*RAFFE
Three Levels of the Boundary System			
2	Phrase-final	Pitch change/lengthening at phrase boundary	it's a *giRAFFE*
1.5	Word-final	Lengthening at word boundary	the tig*er* can JUMP
1	Non-final	No prominence features	it's an E*le*phant

Note: The italicized syllable is the example syllable for the stress or boundary level described in corresponding row. Capital letters mark the syllable with the greatest prominence, that is, nuclear accent in the phrase.

Source: Adapted from Snow, D. (1998). A prominence account of syllable reduction in early speech development: the child's prosodic phonology of tiger and giraffe. *Journal of Speech, Language, and Hearing Research, 41,* pp. 1174–1175. Used with permission of the American Speech-Language and Hearing Association.

for instances of syllable reduction. In the following examples taken from Snow's data, the prominence values are shown as subscripts: (1) "an$_4$na$_{1.5}$ see$_6$" → [ˈæ̃ ˈsi]; (2) "bot$_4$tle$_{1.5}$ time$_6$" → [ˈbɑbɑ ˈtaɪm]; (3) "lay$_3$ down$_8$" → [ˈle ˈjaʊn]. In the first example, the syllable with the lowest prominence value is omitted; in the second example, the syllable with the lowest prominence value is weakened via reduplication; in the third example, weakening through neutralization of the consonant in the onset occurs on the syllable with the highest prominence value given that the word "down" shares both nuclear accent (four points) and phrase final position (two points). In total, 704 target syllables were analyzed, of which 15% were omitted, 7% were weakened, and 78% were completed. Overall the mean prominence scale value was 1.48 for omitted syllables, 2.71 for weakened syllables, and 3.96 for complete syllables. Furthermore, the prominence hypothesis accounted for more than 90% of the syllable reductions in the children's speech whereas the trochaic production template hypothesis accounted for approximately 50% of the syllable reductions observed. Snow concluded that the perceptual salience of syllables plays a key role in phonological development and that metrical templates in child speech have their origins in the child's perception of the input.

The **prominence hypothesis** accounted for more than 90% of the syllable reductions in the children's speech.

Taken together, the studies presented here show that it is difficult to determine with certainty when in development weak syllables should be acquired. Whether or not a syllable will be reduced depends on the prominence of the syllable, the complexity of the word in which the syllable occurs, and the prosodic structure of the phrase that contains the word. These factors probably account for the discrepancy between the Porter and Hodson (2001) study in which good syllable marking was observed in 2-year-olds and the Haelsig and Madison (1986) study in which weak syllable deletion was observed as late as age 4;6. Furthermore, Klein (1981), Snow (1998), and Echols (1993) show that the child's knowledge of weak syllables is not categorical; rather, children's use of syllable maintaining strategies indicates that they have partial representations of these syllables. Furthermore, Carter and Gerken (2004) demonstrated that toddlers leave "acoustic traces" of syllables that are perceived by the adult listener to be deleted. Specifically, they observed that the duration of the between-word boundary was longer in sequences such as "pushed (Cas)sandra" than between "pushed Sandy" when the phonetic content of the weak syllable in "Cassandra" was omitted by the child. This finding suggests that the syllable is represented to some extent on the syllable tier and that the phonetic content is delinked at a lower level of the phonological hierarchy. In older children these partial representations manifest themselves in the form of segment deletions. James, van Doorn, McLeod, and Esterman (2008) examined interactions between the skeletal and syllable tiers of the phonological hierarchy by describing segment deletions as a function of word shape and phonotactic variables. Their findings are considered in greater detail after

The child's knowledge of weak syllables is not categorical; rather, children's use of syllable maintaining strategies indicates that they have partial representations of these syllables.

first discussing cluster reduction and the development of complex onsets and codas.

Multilinear phonological analysis illuminates the process by which children acquire underlying knowledge of **complex onsets and codas** and achieve mastery of these forms at the surface level. Furthermore, this type of analysis shows clearly that the process of cluster reduction does not provide a complete account of children's strategies for producing these forms.

Although a large proportion of the world's languages allow consonant clusters in at least some word positions, English presents a particular challenge for phonological development due to the extraordinary variety and complexity of clusters that occur in onsets and codas in word-initial, word-final, and within-word positions (McLeod, Van Doorn, & Reed, 2001b). Multilinear phonological analysis illuminates the process by which children acquire underlying knowledge of complex onsets and codas and achieve mastery of these forms at the surface level. Chin and Dinnsen (1992) used a spontaneous picture naming task to probe the production of word-initial consonant clusters by preschool-age children with speech sound disorders. They observed 17 different types of cluster realizations, listed with examples from their research participants in Table 4–12. This table shows clearly that the process of cluster reduction does not provide a complete account of children's strategies for producing these forms. Cluster realization types 1 through 8 are examples of cluster reduction but types 1 and 2 involve a completely null onset and types 7 and 8 exemplify a complex variant of cluster reduction called coalescence which is related to assimilation, shown in types 13 and 14. Cluster realization types 9 through 12 are examples of cluster simplifications in which one segment in the cluster is simplified or distorted. Cluster realization type 15 evidences epenthesis, meaning the addition of a segment, in this case a vowel in between the two consonants in the onset which necessitates a resyllabification of the word. Not shown in Table 4–12 is metathesis, probably because reversal of segments is more common in codas, for example, "ask" → [æks].

Metathesis describes a reversal of elements within the cluster.

Chin and Dinnsen demonstrated how a multilinear analysis that takes into account interactions at the segmental and prosodic levels of the phonological hierarchy can be employed to explain the multiple types of cluster realizations. Figure 4–12 illustrates some of these cluster realization types with diagrams inspired by but not taken directly from Chin and Dinnsen's paper. The example shown in Figure 4–12A corresponds to cluster realization type 5 and assumes that the child does not represent complex onsets at the underlying level. Acoustic evidence that the child's productions of words such as "grow" and "go" are phonetically identical along with poor perceptual identification of these minimal pairs would lend weight to the hypothesis that this child has no underlying phonological knowledge of complex onsets. In this case, the skeletal tier is diagrammed with a single timing unit in the onset and the surface form of every cluster in the child's sample is reduced. Cluster realization type 4 is illustrated in Figure 4–12B. In this example clusters are not prohibited per se as evidenced by the appearance of a complex onset in the word "brush"; rather, the child does not produce sibilants in complex onsets and thus delinking of these elements occurs below the level of the skeletal tier. It is very likely

Table 4–12. *Various Cluster Realization Types Produced by Preschool-Age Children with Speech Sound Disorders*

#	*Type*	*Example*
1	$sC_1 = \emptyset$	"spoon" → [ʊn]
2	$pC_1 = \emptyset$	"play" → [eɪ]
3	$sC_1 = s$	"sleep" → [sip]
4	$sC_1 = C_1$	"spoon" → [pʊn]
5	$pC_1 = p$	"play" → [peɪ]
6	$pC_1 = C_1$	"pray" → [ɹeɪ]
7	$sC_1 = C_2$	"swim" → [fɪm]
8	$pC_1 = C_2$	"pew" → [ɸu]
9	$sC_1 = sC_2$	"sky" → [staɪ]
10	$pC_1 = pC_2$	"pray" → [pweɪ]
11	$sC_1 = C_2C_1$	"star" → [θta]
12	$pC_1 = C_2C_1$	"growing" → [dɹoin]
13	$sC_1 = C_2C_3$	"sleep" → [fwip]
14	$pC_1 = C_2C_3$	"treehouse" → [fwihaʊs]
15	$pC_1 = pVC_1$	"queen" → [gəwin]
16	$sC_1 = sC_1$	"stove" → [stov]
17	$pC_1 = pC_1$	"pray" → [pɹeɪ]

Note: Target clusters are shown to the left of the "=" and child surface forms are represented to the right. In the cluster realization type column [s] represents any fricative, [p] represents any stop, C_1 represents the target form of the second element of the cluster, and C_2 and C_3 represent nontarget forms of this element.

Source: From Chin and Dinnsen (1992). Consonant clusters in disordered speech: constraints and correspondence patterns. *Journal of Child Language* by Cambridge University Press, 19, Table I, p. 263. Reproduced with permission of Cambridge University Press.

in a case such as this that acoustic analysis would show evidence of a covert contrast between words such "sleep" and "weep"; for example, imperceptible temporal features might reveal traces of a timing slot for the missing sibilants confirming partial knowledge of the complex onset in the underlying representation (see McLeod et al., 2001b for a brief review of acosutic studies of cluster reduction). Null onsets as shown in cluster realization 1 and diagramed in Figure 4–12C can result from multiple constraints. In this example, singleton but not complex onsets are represented underlyingly;

A. No Clusters in the UR

- [pei] "play"
- [pei] "pray"
- [gou] "grow"
- [pun] "spoon"

PW
F
σ
O R
N
C V V
g o u

B. Delinking of Elements

- [tʌn] "sun"
- [bwʌs] "brush"
- [wip] "sleep"
- [pun] "spoon"

PW
F
σ
O R
N Co
C C V C
p u n

C. Null Onsets

- [ei] "pray"
- [bʌt] "brush"
- [gou] "grow"
- [un] "spoon"

PW
F
σ
O R
N Co
C V C
t u n

D. Spreading of Features

- [fwip] "sweep"
- [fwɪm] "swim"
- [fwip] "sleep"
- [bwʌm] "drum"

σ
O R
N Co
C C
[+con] [+son] [+con]
[+vc] [+nas]
Labial Labial
b w ʌ m

E. Coalescence

- [fun] "spoon"
- [fip] "sleep"
- [fip] "sweep"
- [feɪo] "smell"

σ
O R
N Co
C C
[+con] [+son] [+con]
[+cont]
Labial Labial
f i p

F. Epenthesis

- [bəlu] "blue"
- [bəwʌs] "brush"
- [səwip] "sleep"
- [səpun] "spoon"

PW
F
σ_w σ_s
O R O R
N N
C V C V
b ə l u

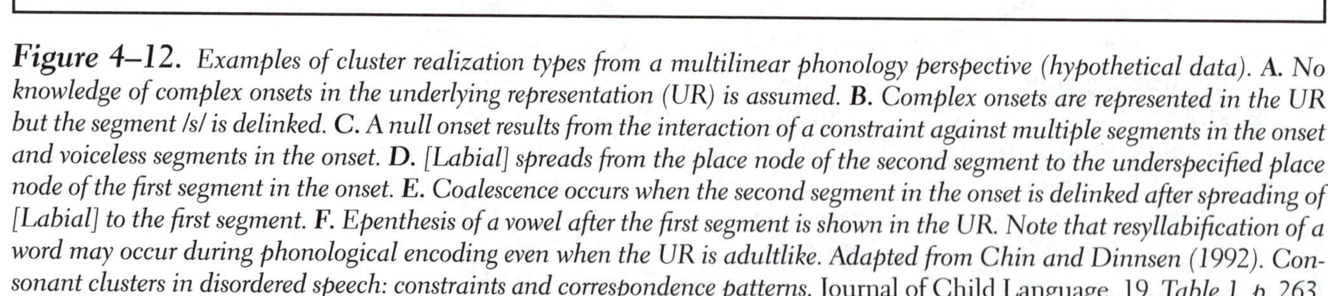

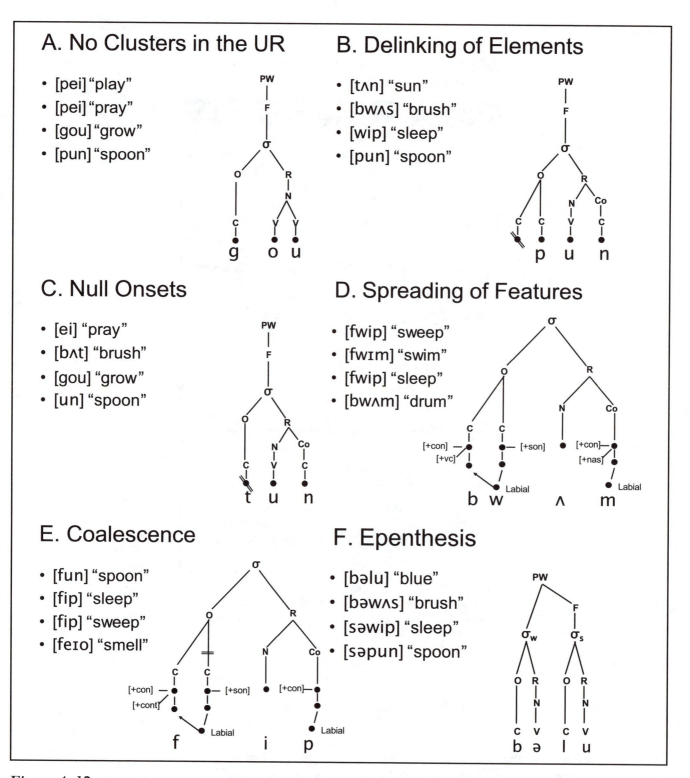

Figure 4–12. *Examples of cluster realization types from a multilinear phonology perspective (hypothetical data).* **A.** *No knowledge of complex onsets in the underlying representation (UR) is assumed.* **B.** *Complex onsets are represented in the UR but the segment /s/ is delinked.* **C.** *A null onset results from the interaction of a constraint against multiple segments in the onset and voiceless segments in the onset.* **D.** *[Labial] spreads from the place node of the second segment to the underspecified place node of the first segment in the onset.* **E.** *Coalescence occurs when the second segment in the onset is delinked after spreading of [Labial] to the first segment.* **F.** *Epenthesis of a vowel after the first segment is shown in the UR. Note that resyllabification of a word may occur during phonological encoding even when the UR is adultlike. Adapted from Chin and Dinnsen (1992). Consonant clusters in disordered speech: constraints and correspondence patterns.* Journal of Child Language, 19, *Table 1, p.* 263.

a single segment, hypothesized to be /t/ in place of the /s/ in the adult target, is represented in the onset but it is delinked at the root node because voiceless phones are not permitted in this position, yielding a null onset in the surface form. Although highly atypical in English, a pattern of consistent onset deletion can occur but in this case both complex and simple onsets are vulnerable to delinking from the skeletal tier. More commonly in English, delinking of codas leads to null codas in both singleton and cluster contexts. Figure 4–12D shows spreading of features within the onset of the child's realization of the word "drum," with the child's productions in this example corresponding to cluster realization types 13 and 14. The child's underlying representation for the cluster in the word "drum" is /dw/ as indicated by the feature tree which shows a consonant unspecified for place and a sonorant specified as a labial. Spreading of [Labial] from the place node of the second element in the cluster to the place node of the first element yields [bwʌm] in the output. Coalescence corresponds to cluster realization types 7 and 8 and is illustrated in Figure 4–12E. Coalescence also involves spreading of features from one element within the cluster to another but one element is subsequently delinked yielding a segment in the output that is a mix of the features from the segments that are present in the underlying representation. In this example, the word "sweep" is realized as [fip] after spreading of [Labial] to the /s/ and delinking of the /w/. In the final example, Figure 4–12F illustrates Epenthesis, corresponding to cluster realization type 15. In this case the child is aware of the two segments /b/ and /l/ at the beginning of the word "blue" but they are represented in separate syllables as a strategy that avoids a structure not yet possible in the child's underlying system. The diagram shows two syllables in the underlying representation but it is possible that the underlying representation in the lexicon is adultlike, that is, a single syllable with a complex onset; in this case, the resyllabification occurs during phonological encoding (see Plate 5 and associated discussion).

Coalescence involves spreading of features from one element within the cluster to another but one element is subsequently delinked yielding a segment in the output that is a mix of the features from the segments that are present in the underlying representation.

Epenthesis involves the addition of a vowel between the consonants in the cluster.

McLeod et al. (2001b) reviewed the literature on the acquisition of clusters from the acoustic, phonetic and phonologic perspectives, yielding the following summary of findings (p. 107):

A summary of findings on cluster development reveals a gradual and roughly predictable developmental sequence despite regressions and reversals within individual children and variability between individual children.

1. Two-year-old children can produce consonant clusters, but these clusters may not be of the same form as the ambient language.
2. Word-final consonant clusters generally appear in inventories earlier than word-initial clusters. Children's production of word-final consonant clusters is increased by the emergence of grammatical morphemes (e.g., plurals and past tense) and consequently the creation of morphophonological consonant clusters (e.g., [-ts] as in *cats*).
3. Two-element consonant clusters are generally produced and mastered earlier than three-element clusters. There is inconclusive evidence regarding whether phonemes are mastered in singleton contexts before they can be accurately produced in clustered contexts.

4. Consonant clusters containing stops (e.g., /pl/, /kw/) are acquired generally before consonant clusters containing fricatives (e.g., /st/, /θr/).
5. Young children typically delete one element of a consonant cluster (cluster reduction), and this deletion may be explained by principles of markedness and sonority.
6. Homonymy occurs in young children's attempts to produce consonant clusters. Homonymy frequently occurs as a result of cluster reduction; however, homonyms can also occur as a result of cluster creation.
7. There are a number of other non-adult realizations of consonant clusters; the most common is cluster simplification, with others including epenthesis and coalescence. Metathesis is rare.
8. The acquisition of consonant clusters is gradual, and there is a typical developmental sequence. It is not an all-or-nothing process. For word-initial clusters, children may initially delete a member of a consonant cluster (one-element realization), then preserve the members while producing one in a non-adult manner (two-element realization), and finally they will produce the consonant cluster correctly (correct realization). Other developmental sequences are possible, particularly for word-final consonant clusters.
9. There is an interrelationship between cluster reduction, cluster simplification, and correct productions of consonant clusters. Initially, most children reduce consonant clusters. Over time, the occurrence of cluster reduction diminishes, whereas the occurrence of cluster simplification increases. Simultaneously, the occurrence of correct productions increases, until eventually production is mastered.
10. Despite there being a typical developmental sequence, the acquisition of consonant clusters is marked by reversals and revisions with considerable individual variation.

McLeod, van Doorn, and Reed (2001a) described cluster development longitudinally in 16 toddlers learning Australian English. Figure 4–13 shows individual data for one of the participants in this study. The variability and reversals in this child's production of the words "clock" and "clocks" over time was typical of the participants in this study and illustrates that the acquisition of complex onsets is not a straightforward process.

Now we return to the topic of interactions between the syllable and skeletal tiers. James et al. (2008) described patterns of consonant deletion in children as a function of word shape. In their study, all consonant deletions were taken into account including deletions of segments from singleton and cluster onsets and codas and deletions of segments from consonants sequences that cross syllable boundaries. They administered the Assessment of Children's Articulation and Phonology to 283 children aged 3 to 7 years.

2;3	2;4	2;5	2;6	2;7	2;8
tɒk	k^{ǂ}lɒk	lɒk	dɒk	t^{ǂ}lɒk	flɒk
tɒk	lɒk	lɒk	dɒk	lɒk^{h}	θlɒk
	k^{ǂ}lɒk	lɒk^{h}	k^{ǂ}lɒkθ	θlɒkθ	θlɒk
	θlɒk	flɒkθ			
		flɒkθ			
		klɒkθ			

Figure 4–13. *Productions of the words "clock" and "clocks" by Participant 5 in the longitudinal study of cluster development. From McLeod et al. (2001a). Consonant cluster development in two-year-olds: General trends and individual difference.* Journal of Speech, Language, and Hearing Research, 44, *Table 4 (corrected), p. 1158. Used with permission of the American Speech-Hearing-Language Association.*

This picture naming test targets a large proportion of multisyllabic words including difficult words such as "ambulance," "computer," and "vegetables." They found that consonant deletions were rare in monosyllabic words at all age levels, but significantly more frequent in disyllabic and polysyllabic words. Even though consonant deletions significantly declined with age, 72% of 7-year-olds deleted consonants in some disyllabic and polysyllabic words. The authors concluded that multiple segmental and prosodic factors interacted to reduce the prominence of specific syllables making them particularly vulnerable to consonant deletions, specifically: a nonfinal weak syllable in a polysyllabic context, sonorant sounds within a consonant sequence, or a within word consonant sequence requiring an anterior-to-posterior articulatory gesture. Some examples of deletions produced by 7-year-old children in this study are shown in Figure 4–14.

Multiple segmental and prosodic factors interact to reduce the prominence of specific syllables in difficult words, accounting for the fact that 72% of 7-year-olds delete consonants in some disyllabic and polysyllabic words.

Clinical Application of Normative Data with Older Children

Detailed information about assessment and speech analysis procedures for diagnostic and treatment planning purposes is provided in Chapters 5 and 6. We provide a brief discussion of a child's speech sample here in order to highlight the complexities of using normative

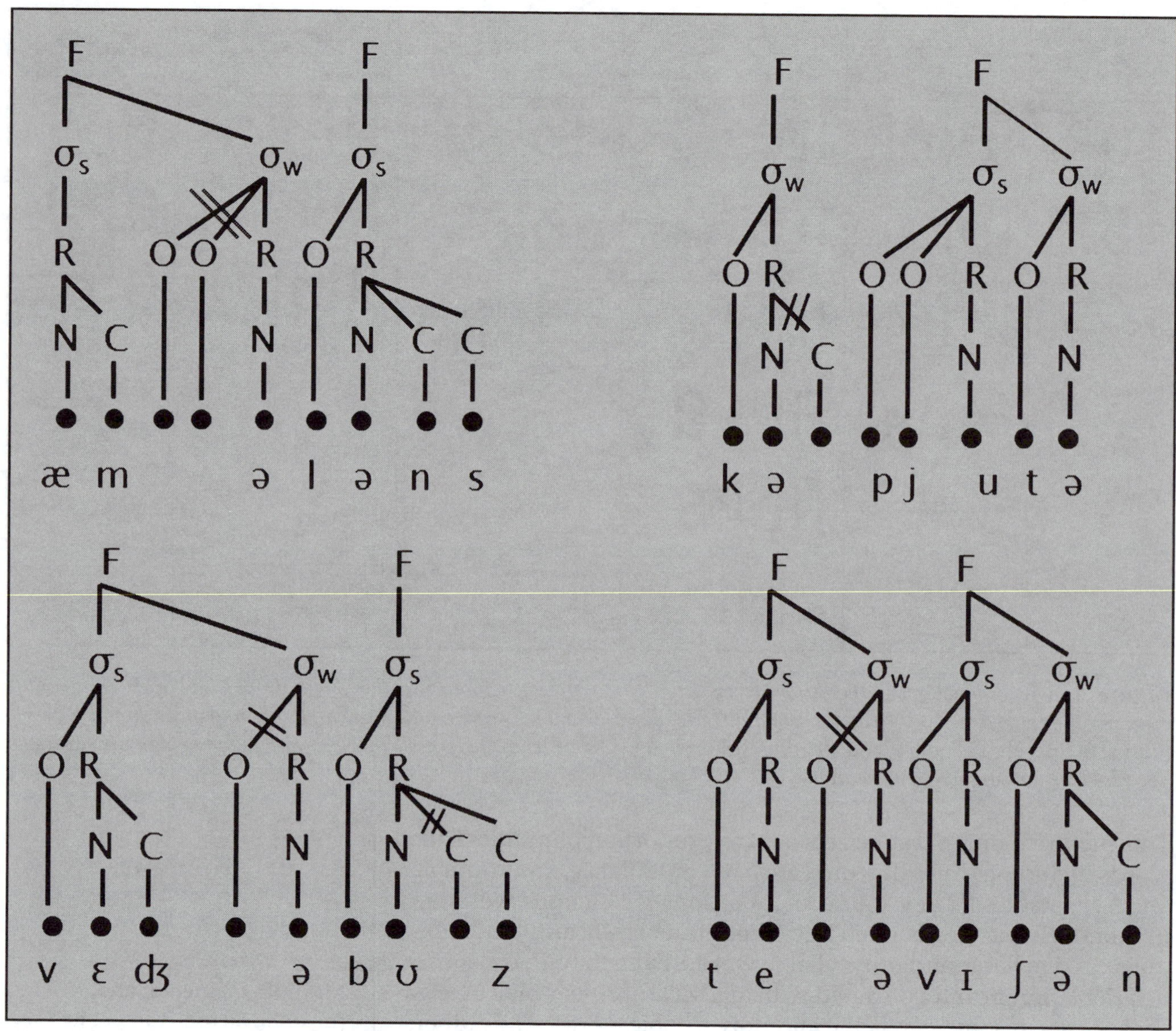

Figure 4–14. *Examples of segment deletion errors produced by 7-year-old children while producing polysyllabic words (ambulance, computer, vegetables, television). Figures created from data reported in James, D. G. H. (2006).* Hippopotamus is hard to say: Children's acquisition of polysyllabic words. *Unpublished doctoral dissertation. The University of Sydney, Sydney, Australia.*

data to determine if a child's speech development is progressing along the expected trajectory. Table 4–13 contains a phonetic transcription of a language sample recorded from a male child aged 4;11 while he was describing the events taking place in a wordless storybook called *Good Dog, Carl* (Day, 1998). Table 4–14 contains picture naming responses from the same child, obtained from administration of the Goldman-Fristoe Test of Articulation-2 (GTFA-2; Goldman & Fristoe, 2000). This child was developing normally except for concerns about his speech and language abilities. His hearing and receptive language abilities were assessed and found to be within normal limits.

Table 4–13. Language Sample Recorded from a Male Child Aged 4;11 (PA232)

	Sentence	Transcription
1	A little baby.	æ lɪdl bebi
2	A little baby has	æ lɪdl bebi hæ
3	There's nothing on there.	ðɛɪz nʊθtɪŋ ɑn dɛʊ
4	A little baby wakes up and get out of bed.	æ lɪdl bebi wekθ ʌp ænd dɛt aʊt ʌ bɛd
5	And the doggie looking out the window and the doggie leave him alone.	ænd ðə dɑgi lʊkɪŋ aʊt ðə wɪndo ænd ðə dɑgi liv hɪm alon
6	And the dog give him a ride.	ænd ðə dɑd dɪv hɪm a wɑɪd
7	And the dog put him on his mommy's bed.	ænd ðə dɑd pʊt hɪm ɑn tɪz mʌmiz bɛd
8	And a little baby look nice.	ænd æ lɪdl bebi lʊk nɑɪs
9	And the dog look nice.	ænd ə dɑg lʊk nɑɪs
10	And them going down the slide.	ænd dɛm doɪŋ daʊn də slɑɪd
11	And a little dog and the baby is scared.	æn æ lɪdl dɑg ænd ə bebi ɪz stɛʊd
12	Save him.	sev hɪm
13	And he put him back on the ride.	ænd hi pʊk hɪm bæk ɑn ə wɑɪd
14	And him fall in the water with the fish.	ænd hɪm fɑl ɪn ə wadɚ wɪf ə fɪʃ
15	And he make a big big mess.	ænd hi mek æ bɪg bɪg mɛs
16	And he standing up look like people.	ænd hi tænɪŋ ʌp lʊk lɑɪk pipl
17	Standing he want to watch something.	tændɪŋ hi wɑnt tu wɑtʃ sʌmtɪŋ
18	And he want to eat and he turn around and he mommy's there.	ænd hi wɑnt it ænd hi tɝn æwaʊnd ænd hi mʌmiz dɛʊ
19	And he and the little baby let him eat some sausage.	ænd hi ænd ðə lɪdl bebi lɛt hɪm it sʌm dadɪd
20	And the little baby eating grapes and the dog gave him some milk.	ænd ə lɪdl bebi idɪŋ gwepz ænd də dɑg gev hɪm sʌm mɪlk
21	And he giving him some soup.	ænd hi gɪvɪŋ hɪm sʌm sup
22	And them made a big mess and eat.	ænd dɛm med æ bɪg mɛs ænd it
23	And them go back up the stairs.	ænd dɛm do bæk ʌpstɛɪs
24	And him poured some XX on him.	ænd hɪm pod sʌm XX ɑn hɪm
25	Yep.	jɛp
26	And he put him and he want him go in the water.	ænd hi pʊt hɪm ænd hi wɑnt hɪm do ɪn də wadə
26	And he make him sink.	æn hi mek hɪm sɪŋk
28	And him put something there.	ænd hɪm pʊt sʌmtɪŋ dɛɪ
29	And he had some bubbles in his mouth.	ænd hi hæd sʌm bʌblz ɪn hɪz maʊf
30	How many?	haʊ mɛni

continues

Table 4–13. continued

	Sentence	Transcription
31	One two three four.	wʌn tu wi foɹ
32	And he's making something and put him back in bed.	ænd hiz mekɪŋ sʌmtɪŋ ænd pʊt hɪm bæk in bɛd
33	And and he go sleep.	ænd ænd hi do tslip
34	And he cleaning up.	ænd hi tinɪ ʌp
35	And he all done.	ænd hi ɑl dʌn
36	And he put that back in there.	ænd hi pʊt dæt bæk ɪn dɛɹ
37	Three more left.	twi moɹ lɛft
38	And he looked out the window and he put some powder on him.	ænd hi lʊkd aʊt də wɪndo ænd hi pʊt sʌm paʊdɚ ɑn hɪm
39	And he put some things on that in his mommy XX.	ænd hi pʊt sʌm θɪŋz ɑn dæt ɪn hɪz mʌmi XX
40	And his mommy bought a new dog.	ænd hɪz mʌmi bɑt æ nu dɑg
41	And he looking out the window.	ænd hi lʊkɪŋ aʊ ə wɪndo
42	And the baby going a sleep and he lying down.	ænd ə bebi doɪŋ æ tip ænd hi laɪɪŋ daʊn
43	And he is lying down again.	ænd hi laɪɪŋ daʊn ægɪn
44	And he's sitting down and mommy pet him.	ænd hiz sɪdɪŋ daʊn ænd mʌmi pɛt hɪm
45	The end!	ðə ɛnd

Table 4–14. Single Word Sample Recorded from Male Child Aged 4;11 (PA232)

house	haʊs	tree	ti	window	wɪndo	telephone	tɛfon
cup	tʌp	knife	naɪf	spoon	spun	girl	gɛu
ball	bɑl	wagon	wægən	shovel	sʌvo	monkey	mʌŋki
banana	bənænʌ	zipper	ʃipo	scissors	sɪzoz	duck	dʌk
quack	kwæk	yellow	jɛdo	vacuum	fætjum	watch	wɑtʃ
plane	pen	swimming	tɪmɪŋ	watches	wɑtʃiz	lamp	læmp
car	kɑɝ	blue	blu	rabbit	wæbɪt	carrot	tæwɪt
orange	ɔwɪndʒ	fishing	fɪʃɪŋ	chair	tɛɝ	feather	fɛdo
pencils	pɛnsəlz	this	ðɪs	bathtub	bæθtʌb	bath	bæθ
ring	wɪŋ	finger	fɪŋgo	thumb	fʌm	jumping	dʌmpɪŋ
pajamas	pədæməz	flowers	faʊwɚz	brush	bɹʌʃ	drum	dlʌm
frog	fɔg	green	blin	clown	kaʊn	balloons	bəlunz
crying	prɑɪ.ɪŋ	glasses	dæsɪz	slide	s̬laid	star	stɑɝz
five	faɪv						

The sample in Table 4–13 can be used to determine that the Percent Consonants Correct is approximately 87%; given that the sample contains 98 unique word types, which is close to the 100 required for this analysis, his PCC can be compared to the reference data presented in Table 4–7, revealing that this level of articulation accuracy is within the normal limits for his age. There are only two unintelligible words (marked as "XX" in the transcript) which is also a positive indicator. However, in order to determine if he has mastered all of the consonants that are expected given his age it is necessary to examine the single word data presented in Table 4–14. The connected speech sample provides both too little and too much information for this purpose. On the one hand, not all of the consonants are represented in all word positions in the language sample. For example, there are no opportunities to produce the /v/ or /ʃ/ phoneme in the word-initial position. The distribution of phonemes across word positions is uneven so that there is one opportunity to produce singleton /k/ in the word-initial position but 4 in word-final, an unfortunate imbalance because velars seem to be most problematic for this child in the word-initial position. These kinds of imbalances can create ambiguities when comparing clinical data, which often involves a moderately large but sometimes unstructured data set from a single child, to normative data, which is based on small structured sets of data aggregated across large numbers of children. The situation is improved somewhat by including the words from the picture naming sample showed in Table 4–14 which at least ensures sampling of most phonemes in three-word positions.

The GFTA results shown in Table 4–14 attest to errors on the phonemes /k ɹ l tʃ ʃ z dʒ v θ ð/ in singleton contexts. According to the Sander (1972) normative chart, displayed in Figure 4–3, we should be concerned about /k/ whereas the other errors are probably developmental. The Iowa-Nebraska norms (Smit et al., 1990), shown in Table 4–8, also suggest that the acquisition ages for all of these phonemes except the /k/ are later than age 5 and thus not of concern. The Sander chart shows the median and 90th percentile ages for the achievement of customary production. Customary production implies greater than 50% accuracy for a given sound although this concept was specifically operationalized by Sander as mastery in two out of three word positions because this yielded a percent correct score of approximately 66% correct in the normative studies that provided the data for the chart, given sampling of two responses in each of 3 word positions. Setting aside the clusters, the single word productions targeting /k/ in Table 4–14 reveal 1/3 correct productions in word-initial position, 1/1 correct productions in word-medial position, and 2/2 correct productions in word-final position. Therefore, /k/ does not achieve either mastery or customary production in word-initial position. The elicitation conditions do not quite replicate the procedures used by the researchers who provided the normative data, as they collected two productions in each word position. Overall, however, the rate of correct production is 66% which suggests customary production. If the data from the language sample are included, the rate of correct production rises to 83% with 1/3, 3/3, and 6/6 correct productions in the initial, medial, and final positions of words. With these additional data we can confirm that this phoneme is mastered in at least two word positions and thus not of concern according to Sander's criteria. Interestingly, all singleton /g/ targets are articulated correctly in all word positions on the picture naming task but [d] is substituted for /g/ 4/6 times in word-initial position during the language sample. Nonetheless, this phoneme too meets the criteria for customary production with 75% correct production across the two sampling conditions and mastery in medial and final word positions.

Smit (1993b) further suggests examining the types of errors. We have already established that most of the phonemes that are misarticulated by this child are developmental because he is younger than the recommended age of acquisition given 90th percentile cutoff ages. However, we might be concerned about these errors if the errors types were atypical. Most of the child's errors are typical substitution errors however as can be seen by comparing these errors to Table 4–9: t/k, d/g, w/ɹ, t/tʃ, s/ʃ, d/dʒ, f/v, and f/θ. Some of the errors produced while picture naming do appear to be unusual, however: d/l and ʃ/z occur in singleton contexts, whereas pɹ/kɹ and s̪l/sl occur in clusters. The language sample reveals some additional unusual substitutions, t/h and k/t as well as an addition error, θt/θ, and an affrication error tsl/sl. Some of these errors may be assimilations but the number of atypical substitutions could be concerning although the lack of consistently atypical patterns in the child's sample is encouraging.

Several highly typical patterns occur that can be considered in relation to the phonological process norms. A detailed phonological process analysis is not undertaken here (phonological analysis is covered in greater detail in Chapter 6). However, some of the more obvious patterns will be examined to determine whether they occur with greater than 20% frequency. We have already noted the substitution of t/k and d/g, examples of fronting. Considering /k g ŋ ʃ tʃ dʒ/ in all word positions in singleton and cluster contexts there are 70 opportunities for fronting to occur and 17 unambiguous instances of fronting when aggregating across the picture naming and narrative language samples. The overall frequency of occurrence at approximately 24% is greater than observed in other children his age as reported by Haelsig and Madison, (1986), Lowe et al. (1985), and Porter and Hodson (2001). Fronting at a frequency higher than 20% allows us to unambiguously credit him with the fronting process which suggests that his speech development is delayed relative to norms which indicate that fronting should be suppressed by the age of 3;0. Liquid gliding is an interesting case, as this process does not apply to both liquids calling into question the status of the error pattern as a "phonological process." Considering both sampling conditions and prevocalic singleton liquids only, gliding does not apply to any /l/ targets although 2 misarticulations of this phoneme occur in word-medial position. In contrast, all 6 singleton /ɹ/ targets are produced as the glide /w/. The overall frequency of gliding is 30% for singleton targets in syllable onsets, falling to 23% when complex onsets (clusters) are included. Although mastery of /ɹ/ is not expected until age 8 years, gliding of liquids should be suppressed by age 4;6 according to the data provided by Haelsig and Madison (1986). The frequency and consistency of gliding of this phoneme in word-initial and word-medial positions does appear to be reason for concern but at the same time the emerging use of /ɹ/ in clusters and the appearance of /ɝ ɚ/ word finally suggest that further gains may occur spontaneously in this sound class.

Finally, we describe this child's realization of consonant clusters in word-initial and word-final position. This task is complicated by the obvious problems with morphosyntax that are so pervasive that we elected to count an obligatory context for a word-final cluster only for monomorphemic words or bimorphemic words where it was clear that the child intended to include the bound morpheme (e.g., third person singular, plural morpheme, or past tense morpheme). We observed that he produced the cluster correctly in 46% of obligatory contexts; misarticulations of the clusters included 55% cluster reduction with the remaining errors split between simplifications and assimilations. Spreading of features is quite common within complex onsets. Take, for example, the unusual realization of the /kɹ/ cluster in "crying": in this word the frequent pattern of velar fronting allows us to hypothesize that the underlying representation for the target /k/ segment is unspecified for place; the feature [+round] spreads from the second segment in the cluster to the first yielding [pɹ] in the output. The realization of /gɹ/ as [bl] is a little more difficult to explain but it seems possible that this is a partial regressive idiom (compare to progressive idioms discussed earlier in this chapter): in other words, the substitution of b/g has persisted in this word after resolution of an earlier pattern of substituting the rounded glide [w] for /l/. On the other hand, as in the longitudinal example shown in Figure 4–13, there may be no spreading-based explanation for this error in which case the child's underlying representation for the word is very unusual reflecting an inability to work out the appropriate feature specifications for the segments in the word.

It is not uncommon for speech-language pathologists to make diagnostic decisions by "eye-balling" speech sample data and interpreting it in relation to their knowledge of the developmental norms. As shown in this case however this procedure rarely provides an unambiguous answer as to the question of whether the child's speech performance falls below normal limits. It is impossible to replicate the exact conditions under which the normative data were collected, and, as mentioned earlier, even small differences in the nature of the words, elicitation procedures or scoring protocol can have a significant difference on the outcome (Edwards & Beckman, 2008). It is essential to combine this analysis with objective standardized test results as discussed further in the next chapter. In fact, this child scored within the average range on the GFTA and thus (if we disregard the issues with morphosyntax) he would not be eligible for treatment solely for the purpose of correcting his speech errors. Monitoring of his speech development might be warranted due to concerns about the high frequency of phonological processes in a child much older than the age 3;6 as well as the presence of some unusual substitution errors. Indeed, this child was enrolled in a longitudinal follow-up study and 2 years later his score on the GFTA fell below normal limits due to the persistence of fronting of palatals and the f/θ substitution.

Theoretical Issues in Phonological Development

4.3.1. Describe the similarities and differences among the three formal linguistic theories: natural phonology, generative phonology, and optimality theory.

4.3.2. Identify 3 weaknesses of formal linguistic theories as theories of phonological development.

4.3.3. Describe the mechanisms that are thought to underly the emergence of phonological knowledge from the cognitive-linguistic perspective.

In the first section of this chapter, children's speech development was described by presenting data from cross-sectional studies covering a variety of units of analysis at the segmental and prosodic tiers of the phonological hierarchy. Certain generalizations can be made. During the toddler period the number of phones and the complexity of syllable shapes increases. Words gradually come to approximate the adult targets more closely and speech becomes more intelligible. Children typically are fully intelligible by the age of 4 years. Stops, nasals, and glides are mastered at relatively young ages whereas affricates and liquids are mastered at relatively late ages and most phonemes are mastered by age 6. Variability in the age of acquisition for late developing phonemes can be very high as is exemplified by the 5-year spread between the 50th and 90th percentile ages for the achievement of customary production of /s/. Despite this variability, certain patterns are predictable as shown by the age-dependent distribution of phonological processes, distortions, and correct productions for certain natural classes of phonemes. For example, stopping of fricatives is relatively common among toddlers but should not be observed with noticeable frequency in children older than 2 years; distortions of sibilants may be observed with greater than 20% frequency in some children as old as 8 years, however. Children's misarticulations typically serve to simplify the child's form relative to the adult target; in a related point, the child's system is usually a restricted version of the adult system with (for example) non-English phones and structures not typically appearing in the system of an English-learning child. Throughout childhood the number of correctly produced consonants and vowels increases, reaching adult levels by approximately age 9 years.

This large body of descriptive data does little to illuminate the processes that underly the acquisition of an adultlike phonological system. Consider, for example, Ferguson and Farwell's (1975) description of the infant's apparently word-based phonology in the earliest days of phonological development. In what way is this early phonological system related to the complex underlying phonological structure that permits the feature spreading that leads to coalescence errors as described by Chin and Dinnsen (1992) for 4-year-olds? What are the processes that explain both continuity and change between these two periods in phonological development? Two broad classes of explanation are available: formal linguistic theories that propose a sharp delineation between competence and performance can be contrasted with cognitive linguistic models in which phonological structure emerges from the "cognitive organization of one's experience with language" (Bybee, 2006, p. 711).

A **phonological theory** must account for *continuity* and *change* in phonological development between infancy and late childhood.

Formal linguistic theories propose a sharp delineation between *competence* and *performance.*

Formal Linguistic Theories

All formal linguistic theories assume an innate component, usually called the universal grammar, which specifies what is possible in the language system as well as what is minimally required. Language development itself is also credited to an innate component, typically viewed as being encapsulated in a domain specific module. This "language acquisition device (LAD)" has responsibility for moving the child from the minimally required system, which contains only unmarked elements, toward the adult model which contains both unmarked and marked elements, without passing through any impossible systems during the developmental process. We do not survey the many different varieties of linguistic theory here, nor do we attempt to detail the formal components of any theory; we refer the reader to other sources such as Ball, Müller, and Rutter (2010) and Bernhardt and Stemberger (1998) for more specific information. However, we provide a broad outline of three theories that are influential in speech-language pathology.

The **universal grammar** is an innate linguistic module that specifies what is possible in the language system as well as what is minimally required.

The **language acquisition device (LAD)** is viewed as a domain specific module that moves the child from the minimally required system toward the adult model.

Barlow and Gierut (1999) state that the purpose of a phonological theory is to explain how the grammar gets from a mental or underlying representation (UR), which reflects the speaker's competence, to the surface representation (SR). The UR of a word is presumed to contain only unpredictable and contrastive information. For example, the UR for the word "pumpkin," shown here for

The **underlying representation (UR)** contains only unpredictable and contrastive information and reflects the speaker's competence.

convenience as a sequence of segments—/pʌmpkɪn/—is actually represented in terms of hierarchically organized unpredictable and nondefault features; default features such as the [-voice] feature of the stops or the [coronal] place of the nasal remain unspecified along with redundant features such as the voicing of the vowels and nasals (see Chapter 1 for further discussion of default specification). The SR of the word contains all details necessary to construct a complete motor plan for articulation of the word and is different from the UR in many ways: [p^{h}ʌ̃ŋkn̩]. Subsequent to the transformation of the UR into the SR performance factors come into play during phonological encoding and motor execution that account for the actual pronunciation of the word.

The **surface representation (SR)** of the word contains all the details necessary to construct a complete motor plan for articulation of the word.

Natural phonology accounts for the discrepancy between the UR and the SF of the word "pumpkin" by positing phonological processes that transform the UR and account for the discrepancy between underlying knowledge of the word form and the way that it is actually pronounced (Ball et al., 2010). Theoretically, there is a distinction between phonological rules that account for changes that are idiosyncratic to the language being spoken and phonological processes that are said to be "natural" in that they occur universally in child and adult speech across many languages and reflect the limitations of the articulatory system. There may also be distinctions drawn between phonological rules and lower level phonetic rules that apply after the transformation of the UR into the SR. In practice, these distinctions are difficult even for researchers to draw and speech-language pathologists rarely make the effort. Despite these complexities, in the "pumpkin" example, reduction of the cluster /mp/ to yield [p^{h}ʌ̃ŋkn̩] could reasonably be attributed to a natural phonological process from the natural phonology perspective. Developmentally, the theory assumes that the child's URs are adultlike from the earliest stages of language development. Phonological processes are provided to the child as innate mental strategies for coping with an immature articulatory mechanism by ensuring that URs are simplified in the SR. As the child gets older, phonological processes are successively suppressed allowing for the appearance of increasingly complex forms in the SR. Common natural phonological processes such as reduplication, cluster reduction and final consonant deletion could explain the productions listed in the categories "stop structure" and "nasal structure" in Figure 4–3 as produced by an 18-month-old boy. Notice, however, that this child's productions show evidence of other patterns that are not so "natural" such as "backing" and "initial consonant deletion." Both of these patterns are supposed to be unusual developmentally and cross-linguistically; in fact they are unusual in the speech of older normally developing children learning English but cross-linguistic child language studies show that "backing" of /ç/ is typical in Japanese (Li, Edwards, & Beckman, 2009) and initial consonant deletion is not uncommon in French (Vihman, 2006). Furthermore, reduplication is generally considered to be problematic

Phonological processes are provided to the child as innate mental strategies for coping with an immature articulatory mechanism by ensuring that URs are simplified in the SR.

as an example of a "natural process" despite its common occurrence in child speech because this process is not observed in adult speech. Ball et al. (2010) have questioned the validity of the theory on the grounds that there is no agreed upon list of "natural processes." Bernhardt and Stemberger (1998) criticized this theoretical perspective because processes have the explicit goal of altering the intended output of the system from an accurate pronunciation of a word to a production that is simplified to the point of bearing little relationship to the adult target or UR. They state that this is as absurd as positing a process for "falling down" that must be suppressed in order for infants to achieve bipedal locomotion. Intuitively, it makes sense to align phonological theory with other domains of development in which the child is seen as moving from simple to complex behaviors through a positive additive process rather than a negative "progression" of process suppression (Bernhardt & Stoel-Gammon, 1994).

Generative phonological theories also account for the discrepancy between the UR and the SR by positing rules that apply to segments sharing specified features appearing in a given context such as the rule that obligates context-specific nasalization of the /ʌ/ preceding /m/ in our example (Ball et al., 2010). From the perspective of generative phonology, however, the developing child might have URs that are much different from those of the adult talker of the language. The way in which the child's underlying system is different from the adult's is constrained by linguistic universals called "principles" (Pinker, 1984) that are embedded in the universal grammar and ensure that the child's underlying grammar conforms to the universal properties of language; at the same time an open set of parameters that are sensitive to language input allow for variation within finite limits (Eisenbeiβ, 2009). The word "pumpkin" is characterized by a trochaic foot structure and underlyingly oral vowels, reflecting the default settings for the corresponding parameters; a child learning French would receive evidence from the language input that specifically sets these parameters to allow for iambic feet and contrastive use of oral versus nasal vowels. The complex coda /mp/ in the word "pumpkin" is a nondefault structure that will not be represented underlyingly until input from the environment sets the corresponding parameter to the nondefault position, thus allowing for both singleton and complex codas in the UR. The child's underlying phonology may prohibit complex onsets generally or the child may be unaware of the /mp/ sequence in the word "pumpkin" specifically; in either case the omission of the /p/ would be consistent with the child's UR rather than the result of a phonological rule altering the UR to a discrepant output. As we described in Chapter 1, from the perspective of a generative analysis, one can distinguish between allophonic rules, in which case a given contrast is not represented underlyingly, and neutralization rules, in which case the contrast is represented underlyingly but a rule prevents it from surfacing in particular contexts. Eisenbeiβ

Generative phonology allows for child URs that are different from the adult URs but the differences are constrained by linguistic universals called *"principles."*

An open set of **parameters** that are sensitive to language input allow for variation within finite limits.

According to **optimality theory** all possible outputs for a given input are evaluated in relation to a set of universal constraints, yielding the selection of the highest ranked output for production.

Faithfulness constraints stipulate that the output be similar to the input by (for example) proscribing deletions and insertions of elements.

Markedness constraints require that only the unmarked properties of the language surface in the output.

explicitly links this "principles and parameters" model of language acquisition to aspects of visual development in which environmental input serves to activate cells that are responsive to certain stimuli (e.g., horizontal bars) but the absence of appropriate input leads to inactivation of this feature detection ability. Recall that the same feature detector model was initially thought to explain early speech perception development (see Chapter 2) but this model has since proven to be a simplistic and inaccurate view of the means by which children gain sensitivity to language-specific phonetic contrasts.

The most current phonological theory, optimality theory, relies exclusively on the notion of constraints in place of rules (Barlow & Gierut, 1999; Bernhardt & Stemberger, 1998). By this account, the relationship between URs, known as inputs, and SRs, known as outputs, is mediated by a generator and an evaluator. When an input form is fed to the generator, it sends a list of possible pronunciations of the word to the evaluator. The output is selected from this list of possibilities after evaluating them in relation to a set of universal constraints. Faithfulness constraints stipulate that the output be similar to the input by (for example) proscribing deletions and insertions of elements. Markedness constraints require that only the unmarked properties of the language surface in the output. Although these two sets of antagonistic constraints are universal,[2] their ranking is unique to each individual and changes with language experience. All candidate versions of an output that are generated for a given input will violate at least one constraint. The evaluation process will select the candidate that violates the least number of highly ranked constraints. If the output does not match the input, constraints will be reranked and over time, gradual changes in the ranking of the constraints will allow more complex forms to surface in the output. Differences between individuals in the pronunciation of a word reflect differences in the ranking of the constraints. Improvements by an individual in the pronunciation of a word reflect demotion of highly ranked markedness constraints relative to faithfulness constraints. Barlow and Gierut (1999) provide an elegant demonstration of how cluster reduction can result from high ranking of a markedness constraint against complex onsets in relation to three faithfulness constraints that specifically proscribe deletion of segments, insertion of segments, and coalescence of segments in the output. They further show how epenthesis and coalescence can be explained by different rankings of the same set of four constraints. One particularly interesting feature of

[2]Several theorists have described nonnativist versions of optimality theory (Bernhardt & Stemberger, 1998; Fikkert & de Hoop, 2009) in which the set of constraints are not universal; in these theories the constraints are functional and thus grounded in phonetic, communicative, or information processing factors. A critique of these forms of optimality theory is beyond the scope of this book. Classical optimality theory is explicitly nativist.

their analysis is that multiple patterns of cluster realization by the same child (as observed in the child who produced the sample given in Table 4–13) can also be explained with the same set of constraints by assuming tied rankings of certain constraints. This theory has excited much attention from developmental phonologists because it accounts for continuity by proposing a universal set of constraints while allowing for much inter- and intraindividual variability via the person-specific ranking and re-ranking of violable constraints.

In many respects, optimality theory suffers from some of the same difficulties as natural phonology as a theory of phonological development. Just as natural phonology theory assumes adultlike URs, optimality theory assumes perfect perception of adult surface forms, thus ensuring adultlike inputs to the generator (Boersma & Hayes, 2001; Fikkert & de Hoop, 2009). According to Barlow and Gierut (1999), an adultlike input is provided to the generator which provides an infinite list of candidate outputs. The candidates are evaluated with respect to the constraints and if the markedness constraints are ranked too highly in relation to the faithfulness constraints, the ultimate output will not match the input. As learning is error driven according to the theory, mismatched outputs will persist until the child begins to notice the difference between the input and output, which motivates a reranking of the constraints (Ball et al., 2010). However, if the child does not have the ability to notice mismatches between the input and output, it is not clear where an adultlike input to feed to the generator might come from! Some learning algorithms from the constraint-based perspective assume that mismatches are noticed each time they occur; change is gradual because many small changes in the positioning of many different constraints are required before the matching output will surface (e.g., Boersma & Hayes, 2001). However, we have shown in Chapter 2 and argue further in this chapter that children's perception of the input is imperfect and early organization of phonological knowledge appears to be far from adultlike.

Historically, natural phonology as a theory was weakened by the weight of "invented processes" that were proposed to deal with phenomena that arose in both typical and atypical child development data. Similarly, child data present challenges for optimality theory that have led to the questionable invention of constraints. Ball, Müller, and Rutter (2010) discuss the issue of consonant harmony, a process that is common in the speech produced by children but not adults, leading some theorists to suggest that some constraints may "come and go" during language acquisition, a proposition that seems unsustainable. The fact that the constraint ranking appears to vary with lexical properties such as word frequency and neighborhood density has led to the invention of constraints (Gierut, 2001) to solve problems that should lead one to question the viability of the underlying assumptions of the theory itself. One

One of the fundamental assumptions of optimality theory is that innate **markedness relationships** are built into the grammar but research has revealed no agreed upon universal hierarchy of markedness relationships.

of the fundamental assumptions is that innate markedness relationships are built into the grammar. However, cross-linguistics studies have not revealed a universal hierarchy of markedness relationships (Menn, Schmidt, & Nicholas, 2009).

Another similarity with natural phonology is the essentially negative conception of development whereby phonological acquisition occurs via the demotion of a potentially infinite number of prohibitive constraints rather than the positive acquisition of new skills or knowledge (Berg, 2000). The notion of faithfulness constraints in tension with markedness constraints is appealing but, ultimately, the theory does not propose that development is a matter of achieving outputs that are faithful to the input. Rather, the goal of phonological development is a progressive reranking of the constraints until the ranking approximates that of the adult language user. From the psycholinguistic perspective, the theory seems no less problematic than its predecessors in that the processing load associated with generating an infinite number of candidate productions for each word, evaluating them in relation to the ranked constraints and then selecting the optimum candidate seems no less onerous than the rule-based procedures of earlier theories (for a discussion of the "100 step problem," see Chapter 1, Bernhardt & Stemberger, 1998).

Formal linguistic theories view language as fundamentally unlearnable and thus do not motivate effective strategies for teaching language to children who are not acquiring language at the normal rate.

Perhaps the most unsatisfying feature of formal linguistic theories is that they are essential adevelopmental. Language competence is viewed as a complex and abstract system of context-free rules and constraints that is unlearnable in the absence of negative evidence that is not provided by the language input. Linguistic theories have helped speech-language pathologists discover the underlying order in children's phonological knowledge and identify efficient targets for intervention. Theories that claim language is fundamentally unlearnable do not provide a coherent explanation for atypical phonological development or motivate valid strategies for helping children learn to use language effectively (Evans, 2001).

Cognitive Linguistic Models

Usage-based theories propose that language is a complex, dynamic system that emerges from the child's experience with the use of language across multiple levels of representation in many contexts.

In stark contrast to the notion that language is unlearnable, usage-based accounts propose that language is a complex, dynamic system that emerges from the child's experience with the use of language across multiple levels of representation in many contexts (Bybee, 2001, 2006; Bybee & McClelland, 2005). Regularity and systematicity emerge, not as rules, but as patterns of statistical probabilities within and among networks of particular forms in multiple domains. With linguistic theories, rules operate at an abstract symbolic level and are independent of the particular words that are impacted by the rule. According to emergentist accounts such as usage-based phonology, linguistic generalizations can never be independent of the specific forms from which they emerge. Therefore, from this perspective exemplar representations of words are required at an initial level of representation and the linkage of word forms across multiple levels of representation is a key developmental process; abstract phonological representations emerge from the act of storing and organizing these representations in the lexicon. Here we return to Plate 1 in which we introduced the multiple levels of representation and the linkages between them.

According to **emergentist accounts** such as usage-based phonology, abstract phonological representations emerge from the act of storing and organizing exemplar representations of words in the lexicon.

The most important influence on a child's language development is the language input that is provided by adults in the environment (Hart & Risley, 1992; Hoff & Naigles, 2002; Huttenlocher, 1998). We illustrate language input as starting at birth in part A of the schematic in Plate 1 but in fact language input begins to impact on the infant's knowledge of the sound system even before birth as we outlined in Chapter 2. It is estimated that the infant will hear 600 to 2600 words per hour (with variance correlated with the family's social class). These words are stored as exemplars that preserve increasing amounts of acoustic detail with repeated exposure. In this example, some of those stored exemplars will be the child's name, pronounced as [su] by the mother, the father and an older sibling (B). Other words containing the vowel [u] will also be heard by the infant. The statistical learning mechanism discussed in Chapter 2 will allow the infant to derive phonetic categories from these detailed exemplars of words (Lacerda, 2003; Pierrehumbert, 2003). The acoustic-phonetic representation for the vowel will be a region of the vowel space (C) that reflects the frequency with which vowels containing a closely spaced F1-F2 are heard and the distribution of vowels in this part of the vowel space relative to other vowels in the input language. Notice that the category is exemplified by the distribution of the feature "graveness" as abstracted from the whole word acoustic-phonetic representations (for further discussion of feature abstraction in relation to episodic models of perception, see Poeppel, Idsardi, & van Wassenhove, 2008). This learning model does not imply that the infant's brain is a blank slate or an "unconstrained learning device" (Spencer et al., 2009). It is clear that infants are especially attracted to speech in general and to [u] vowels in particular; however, this attraction to the vowel [u] is quickly modified by the input so that (for example) French-learning infants lose their preference for [u] over [y] whereas this preference is enhanced in English-learning infants. The acoustic-phonetic details of the categories are unique to the language that the infant is learning and language-specific perceptual representations emerge as gradient categories during the first year of life (McMurray & Aslin, 2005), with vowel categories emerging as early as 6 months of age.

The most important influence on a child's language development is the language input that is provided by adults in the environment.

We propose that the input is stored as **exemplars** that preserve increasing amounts of acoustic detail with repeated exposure.

Acoustic-phonetic representations are language-specific gradient categories that emerge from the distribution of acoustic cues in the stored exemplars.

The infant also begins to babble during the first year of life, usually at 7 months of age. As discussed in Chapter 3, early speech development is also constrained by biological phonetic factors related to differences in oral structure and limitations on speech motor control. Nonetheless, the infant is capable of producing rhythmically organized syllables in both repetitive and variegated strings composed of labial and coronal stops and nasals combined with a variety of vowels. Vihman and Velleman (2000) suggest that the infant implicitly matches frequently used babbling patterns to roughly similar word forms in the input lexicon, accounting for selection effects in early word use and continuity in the phonetic characteristics of the child's babble and meaningful speech. They further claim that a frequently occurring babbling pattern will act as an "articulatory filter" that makes similar patterns in the input stand out as unusually salient. Vihman (2002) has gone so far as to claim that the infant's production patterns directly impact perception of speech but this seems unlikely given that language specific changes in speech perception precede the emergence of babbling and first words. However, it seems very plausible that the proposed "articulatory filter" enhances the likelihood of developing linkages between a given acoustic-phonetic representation in the input (B/C), a gestural score (E) for the production of the word and the semantic representation in the lexicon (F).

A frequently occurring babbling pattern may act as an **articulatory filter** that makes similar patterns in the input stand out as unusually salient, enhancing linkages between gestural scores and acoustic-phonetic representations for syllables and words.

A **gestural score** specifies a spatiotemporal pattern of articulator specific gestures that is abstract but context specific.

Dynamic systems theory and connectionist modelers highlight associative learning as a core developmental mechanism; indeed, from these perspectives, learning is essentially the process of making and strengthening linkages between sensorimotor domains and levels of representation (Hockema & Smith, 2009; Vihman, DePaolis, & Keren-Portnoy, 2009; Westermann & Reck Miranda, 2004). Connectionist models and behavioral studies with children and adults further demonstrate how the process of linking surface regularities across multiple domains leads to the emergence of higher order regularities. Complex structure emerges from the gradual accrual of information from the environment over time in a dynamic nonlinear process that is highly sensitive to small details such as the order in which words are learned. We consider a hypothetical example of the emergence of early phonological structure, as illustrated in Figure 4–15.

Dynamic systems theory explains how phonological structure in the form of **abstract phonological representations** can emerge from the accrual and linkage of information across multiple sensorimotor domains and levels of representation.

In the example in Figure 4–15 we revisit the 4 levels of representation shown in Plate 1 (semantic, acoustic-phonetic, phonological, and articulatory-phonetic). To save space in the diagram our imagined representations for the hypothetical child's lexicon at three time points take the form of traditional orthography for semantic representation and phonetic symbols for the acoustic-phonetic and articulatory-phonetic representational levels. Furthermore, the direct links from semantic to articulatory-phonetic representations are not shown but are implied. The phonological level of representation emerges from the linkages between items within the lexicon itself. As explained in Chapter 2, infants have good perceptual abilities at the phonetic level, so much so that they can recognize subtle mispronunciations of familiar words (see Figure 2–6; Swingley, 2008). Phonemic perception abilities are another matter however; toddlers are not sure which alternative productions of a word form can be appropriately linked to a known semantic representation;

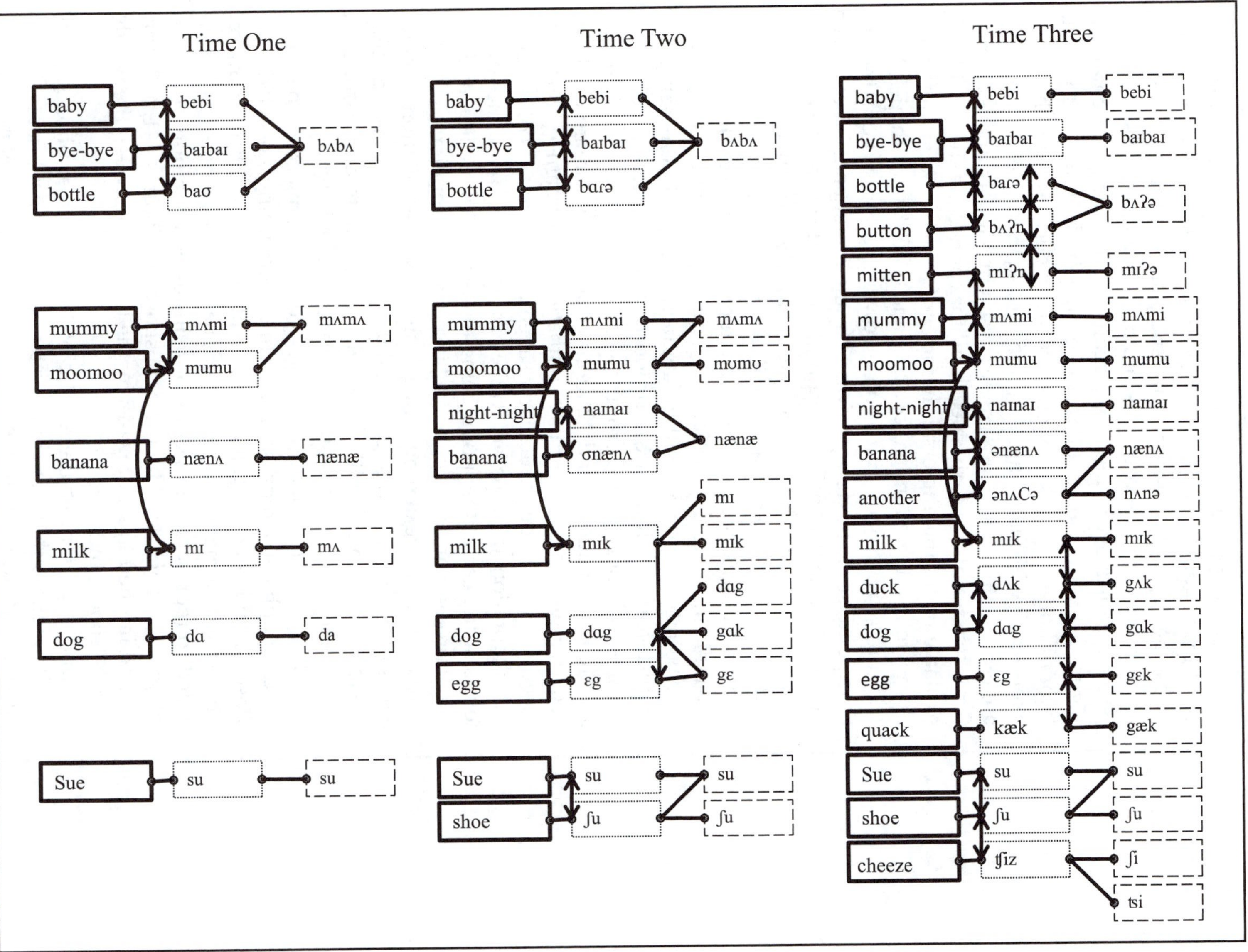

Figure 4–15. *Hypothetical example of emerging phonological structure in the lexicon. Semantic representations shown as traditional orthographic spelling enclosed in solid boxes. Acoustic-phonetic representations shown as phonetic transcriptions enclosed in dotted boxes. Articulatory-phonetic representations shown as phonetic representations enclosed in dashed boxes. Linkages between levels of representation have rounded connectors (links from semantic to articulatory-phonetic representations are hypothesized but not shown due to space restrictions). Linkages between word forms in the lexicon have arrow-headed connectors. See text for discussion. Printed with permission from Susan Rvachew.*

when learning new words and connecting them to semantic referents the child might not store sufficient phonetic detail to support accurate production of all segments and syllables, at least not until many repetitions of the word form have been experienced. These perceptual constraints are suggested in Figure 4–15 by the appearance of final consonants and the specification of segments in weak syllables over time in the acoustic-phonetic representations. Figure 4–15 also shows changes over time in the linkages to articulatory-phonetic representations which are derived from the child's experience with babbling. A number of developmental processes are represented here that were discussed previously in this chapter. First, constraints on early speech motor control are the most likely explanation for the universal character of the early sound inventory as shown in the predominance of CV and CVCV word shapes, labial and coronal obstruents, and central vowels. Furthermore, at the first time point, some tendency toward "frame dominance" is observed in the consonant-vowel correspondence patterns as described in Chapter 3. Although fricatives are relatively infrequent in babble and early words on average, we find that all infants produce them in babble at least some of the time in our laboratory. There is considerable individual variation in the production of fricatives however both between and within language groups. In one sample of English-learning infants the proportion of fricatives among consonants in babble varied from fewer than 10% to more than 50% among infants aged 8 and 12 months (Rvachew, Creighton, Feldman, & Sauve, 2005). For this hypothetical infant named "Sue," the fricative /s/ may be particularly salient. The processes of selection and adaptation are apparent in the example with avoidance of VC forms at the early time point being evidence of selection, and the initial production of "egg" as [gɛ] indicating adaptation to the preferred CV structure at time 2. Regressive velar assimilation emerges not as a rule but as a kind of accident reflecting the high-frequency of stored exemplars with final-velar consonants and associated strong connections to a gestural score for the [gʊk] word shape. The overall organization of the child's lexicon and connections between words graphically represent the child's emerging knowledge of prosodic and segmental structure. Although difficult to show on a two-dimensional drawing, additional linkages could have been added to represent knowledge of features. Recognition of feature categories is suggested by the data shown in Figures 4–1, 4–2, and 4–3 and implied in Figure 4–15 by the linkages between the words "Sue," "shoe," and "cheeze."

One important characteristic of this model of phonological development is that the child system can be considerably different from the adult system even though continuity is maintained throughout development from infancy through adulthood. Representations do not begin as "whole word templates" only to suddenly restructure themselves as segmentalized phonemic representations at some later time. Rather, as proposed by Ferguson and Farwell (1975) and confirmed by recent research on spoken word processing, the listener stores detailed word-based acoustic-phonetic representations throughout the life span; although the details are elaborated with experience, it is the "phonic core" of these stored representations that forms the foundation of phonological knowledge. Phonological structure emerges, not by restructuring the acoustic-phonetic representation itself, but by gradually reorganizing these representations within the lexicon. This reorganization reflects the child's accumulating knowledge of the phonetic characteristics of the individual word forms, the similarities and differences among word forms in the lexicon and the overall structure of the lexicon itself. Research that investigates the impact of the child's phonetic experience and lexical knowledge on phonological development is reviewed in the final section of this chapter.

Phonological structure emerges by gradually reorganizing phonetic representations within the lexicon. This reorganization reflects the child's accumulating knowledge of the phonetic characteristics of the individual word forms, the similarities and differences among word forms in the lexicon, and the overall structure of the lexicon itself.

Environmental Influences and Physiological Constraints on Phonological Development

4.4.1. Define "implicational hierarchy."

4.4.2. Describe 3 factors that account for the order of acquisition of phones across language groups.

4.4.3. Describe laboratory evidence that shows that children do not always have adultlike perceptual representations for words that they mispronounce. Explain why anecdotal reports of accurate perception for misarticulated phonemic contrasts in normal phonological development can be misleading.

4.4.4. Describe the relationship between segment accuracy and movement variability in the production of weak and strong syllables in varying prosodic contexts.

4.4.5. Define word frequency, phonotactic probability, and neighborhood density. Describe the impact of these variables on speech production accuracy and phonological awareness.

A common strategy for studying the interplay of environmental influences and physiological constraints on phonological development is to examine the similarities and differences among children learning different languages. This section begins with a brief discussion of research on feature development in English, Spanish, Cantonese, Arabic, and Dutch. Subsequently, studies that investigated the impact of the child's phonetic experience and lexical knowledge on phonological development are reviewed.

Cross-Linguistic Studies of Feature Development

An **implicational feature hierarchy** lists feature distinctions according to implicational relationships so that the presence of any given feature in an individual's phonology requires that all lower level feature distinctions must also be present in the talker's system.

Dinnsen (1992), following ideas previously put forward by Jacobson, proposed that universality in phonological development could be revealed by describing acquisition in terms of a small and finite set of phonetic features whereby the child increases the size and complexity of the phonetic inventory by adding marked features according to the given order. An implicational relationship between the ordered features was proposed such that the presence of any feature distinction required that all lower level feature distinctions also be present in the hierarchy. He proposed the hierarchy shown in the leftmost column of Table 4–15. The presence of the feature distinctions is determined by examining the child's phonetic inventory, obtained as described in Chapter 1, and noting the presence of at least one member of each contrasting pair for a given feature distinction at each level. Notice that this analysis is concerned with phonetic rather than phonemic features; in other words, the child does not have to demonstrate contrastive use of phones for contrasting feature pairs; rather, the phones simply have to be present in the phonetic inventory. At level A, [consonantal] denotes the presence of a glide and a true consonant (e.g., [w] and [b] or [j] and [n]), [sonorant] indicates the presence of an obstruent and a sonorant which is predictably a nasal at this level (e.g., [b] and [m]), and

Table 4–15. Proposed Implicational Feature Hierarchies for English, Spanish, and Cantonese (see text for details)

Level	English	Spanish	Cantonese
A	[consonantal] [sonorant] [coronal]	[coronal] [sonorant] [nasal]	[consonantal [syllabic] [sonorant]
B	[voice]	[voice] [anterior]	[labial] [coronal] [delayed release]
C	[continuant] and/or [delayed release]	[continuant] and/or [delayed release]	[continuant] [spread glottis]
D	[nasal]	[strident] and/or [lateral]	
E	[strident] and/or [lateral]	[tense]	

[coronal] is credited if coronal and noncoronal place is represented (e.g., [d] and [b]). Level B inventories are characterized by the addition of a [voice] distinction. Level C is attained when the child adds [continuant] in the form of a fricative or [delayed release] with the appearance of an affricate or both a fricative and an affricate. Level D inventories add the feature distinction [nasal] by including a liquid, usually [l], which creates a division within the sonorant class between nasals and liquids. The most complex inventories, placed at Level E, contain strident and nonstrident consonants (e.g., [θ] and [s]) and/or the lateral versus nonlateral liquid (e.g., [l] and [ɹ]). Note that variable inventories are consistent with every level of the hierarchy. Multiple paths from one level to the next are possible because the order of feature acquisition is constrained but the order of segment acquisition is not. Thus, [p b t d m n f s w j ʔ h] is a Level C inventory but this larger inventory is also ranked at Level C because it lacks liquids and nonstrident fricatives: [p b t d k g m n ŋ f v s z ʃ tʃ dʒ w j ʔ h]. Dinnsen (1992) conducted a retrospective review of diary studies of children learning different languages and reported that the data were consistent with this hierarchy. Dinnsen, Chin, Elbert, and Powell (1990) reported that the phonetic inventories derived from the speech of 39 of 40 children with speech delay could be assigned to one of these levels.

Subsequently, the universality of the hierarchy has been tested in studies of children learning other languages. Catano, Barlow, and Moyo (2009) described the phonetic repertoires of 16 Spanish-speaking children, aged 0;11 to 5;1. They found that the feature hierarchy had to be adjusted to account for the different inventory of Spanish and the early emergence of /l/ in Spanish-speaking children. The proposed hierarchy of phonetic feature contrasts is shown in the second column of Table 4–15. The simplest Level A inventory in their sample was [b t m n β l]. They explain that the spirant [β] functions like an approximant in Spanish and thus its presence along with [b] distinguishes sonorants from consonants and the [t n] in contrast to [b m] represents coronal. In English the division within the sonorant class between nasals and liquids would be delayed until Level D but in Spanish children the [nasal] feature distinction emerged early. In fact, every inventory included [l] but some excluded glides or spirants. The addition of [anterior] at Level B differentiates [l] from [j]. The nonlateral liquid added at Level D is a tap [ɾ]. At Level E the new [tense] feature allows for the emergence of the trill [r].

As shown in Table 4–15, Stokes and To (2002) also found that the hierarchy required considerable modification to account for data collected from 122 Cantonese-speaking children, with the addition of the features [labial] and [spread glottis] and relatively early emergence of affricates and late emergence of the Cantonese aspiration contrast (e.g., [p] versus [pʰ]) in comparison to the English voice contrast. On the other hand, Amayreh and Dyson (2000) reported that Dinnsen's (1992) typology worked well for Arabic, despite earlier emergence of /l/ relative to English. However, they recommended the addition of a Level F to account for the emergence of emphatic consonants.

Cross-linguistic studies do not confirm a universal feature hierarchy for phonetic feature development.

Overall, this cross-linguistic review of feature acquisition reinforces a sense of order despite variability within language groups but does not confirm a universal feature hierarchy for phonetic feature development. Children across these four language groups appeared to expand their phonetic repertoires by adding feature contrasts in a gradual fashion and the implicational hierarchy between levels within a language group was upheld. However, the features that were important and the ordering of those features was unique to each language group. Therefore, even the least complex repertoires across languages could not be reliably attributed to a "universal grammar" that defines the unmarked and marked properties of the language. Nor could the developmental order of feature or segment emergence be explained by a simple appeal to phonetic tendencies based on universal physiological constraints.

One factor that may explain the order of segment acquisition is **input frequency**, the frequency with which a given phone occurs in the language being learned by the child.

Functional load indexes the importance of a given phoneme in a language in terms of the information that would be lost if the phoneme merged with all similar phonemes.

Stokes and Surendran (2005) hypothesized that the order of segment acquisition within language groups might be explained by interactions among three factors: input frequency, functional load, and articulatory complexity. In their study, they examined the frequency of word initial consonants specifically, arguing that word onsets are particularly salient perceptually and that the child's preference for CV syllable shapes means that these consonants may receive the most articulatory practice. Functional load indexes the importance of a given phoneme in a language in terms of the information that would be lost if the phoneme merged with all similar phonemes. For example, in English, merging of the contrast /ð/-/d/ would have very little impact despite the high frequency of /ð/ because there are very few minimal pairs that are distinguished by these segments. This is true for all consonants with which /ð/ might merge and therefore, the phoneme /ð/ has low functional load in English. Mathematically, functional load of a given phoneme is calculated to be the sum of functional load of the binary oppositions between the phoneme and the other phonemes with which it is likely to merge, weighted by the frequency of the other phonemes. Stokes and Surendran again chose to focus specifically on word onsets in their calculation of functional load. Finally, they ranked phonemes in terms of relative articulatory complexity, using a scale proposed by Kent (1992). According to this schema, for the three languages studied by Stokes and Surendran, [m p w h n] are at the first level of articulatory complexity, voiced stops, /f/ and /k/ are added at the next level, liquids are added at level 3 and the remaining sibilants and affricates are the most complex segments.

Articulatory complexity is another variable that may explain order of segment acquisition but it is difficult to objectively determine complexity independently of acquisition order.

Stokes and Surendran (2005) examined the impact of these three factors on word-initial consonant acquisition by children speaking English, Dutch and Cantonese. The data sets that they used provided information about age of emergence of consonants in toddlers learning English and Cantonese and about accuracy of consonant production for preschoolers learning English and Dutch. The best predictor of age of emergence in Cantonese was frequency of the consonant in the language input. They explained that Cantonese has a small inventory of consonants with relatively low articulatory complexity. Furthermore, the vowels and tones in Cantonese have greater functional load than the consonants. Therefore, it made sense that input frequency would be the most important predictor of the age that consonants emerge in this language. Turning to the English data, functional load was found to be the best predictor of age of emergence of word-initial consonants in the youngest children. However, articulatory complexity explained accuracy of production in older children. Therefore, when a language has a large and relatively complex consonant inventory, functional load is likely to explain the emergence of the child's early phonological knowledge and then articulatory complexity will play a role in the time required for mastery of production accuracy thereafter. Finally, for Dutch, a language that has a smaller inventory of word-initial consonants than English, the best predictor of accuracy of production was frequency of the consonant in the input.

When a language has a large and relatively complex consonant inventory, functional load is likely to explain the emergence of the child's early phonological knowledge and then articulatory complexity will play a role in the time required for mastery of production accuracy thereafter.

Input variables such as frequency or functional load appear to explain much of the variance in acquisition patterns between language groups. In other words, these kinds of variables can help to explain why a child learning Spanish might begin to produce /l/ at an earlier age than a child learning English. However, it is not clear that input variables alone can explain individual differences within language groups. Why might one child learning English begin to produce /l/ at age 2, whereas another persists in gliding target /l/ until age 7 years? Why does the age of customary production for /s/ vary from age 3 to 8 years among English-speaking children? To answer these questions it is necessary to consider factors that are specific to individual children. We begin with differences in speech perception abilities in the next section.

Speech Perception Skills and Phonological Development

Theorists in child phonology typically begin with the assumption that children perceive speech perfectly, thus assuring adult-like underlying representations (Altvater-Mackensen & Fikkert, 2010). For example, from the perspective of generative phonology, Eisenbeiβ (2009) claimed that categorical perception in infancy supports the "parameter and principles" model of phonological development:

> Studies on phonological development have not only shown the usefulness of the parameter concept, but also provided support for an innate selective LAD: Immediately after birth, infants can discriminate sounds along all the dimensions used by human languages . . . children do not develop capacities to make phonological distinction in adaptation to their environment, but are

> equipped with the capacity for categorical perception, which provides them with distinctions from which they can choose —and which become unavailable if they are not useful for processing the input. (p. 293)

This perspective is directly tied to the initial view of speech perception development as a process of maintenance and loss of innate feature detectors, a hypothesis that we showed to be unsupported by the research in Chapter 2. In fact, every underlying assumption in the paragraph quoted above was shown to be untenable in Chapter 2. Infants are not able to perceive every contrast, some infants have difficulty perceiving many contrasts, and all infants require extraordinary manipulations of laboratory conditions to ensure that memory, attentional, and other cognitive and sensory limitations do not prevent their success on perceptual tasks. Neither infants nor adults actually lose the ability to perceive acoustic-phonetic features, whether present or absent in the input language; however, a statistical learning mechanism allows the infant to develop a language-specific strategy for organizing the input. In other words, category prototypes and boundaries are an emergent property of the distribution of acoustic-phonetic information in the speech input to the child and as such are built up gradually through experience with that input. Thus, it is clear that individual differences in phonological development might arise from differences in the nature of the input or differences in the child's access to that input. Access to the input may be impacted by variables that are internal to the infant such as hearing acuity or maturity of auditory processing, phonological processing, or attentional mechanisms. Access to the input may also be impaired by environmental variables such as excessive background noise.

Individual differences in phonological development might arise from differences in the nature of the language input or differences in the child's access to that input due to environmental or child-related variables such as problems with auditory or phonological processing or attentional mechanisms.

Theorists who do not necessarily adopt a nativist approach to phonological development, such as Bernhardt and Stemberger (1998), have also assumed that "mispronunciations are largely due to production factors rather than perceptual factors" (p. 13). This conclusion is based on anecdotal reports of children's responses to adult live-voice productions of minimal pair words (such as [sip] and [ʃip]) or adult simulations of children's production errors (such as [fɪs] in place of "fish"). Children's discrimination responses to such stimuli do not provide an accurate picture of their phonemic perception abilities, however, and it is phonemic perception that is critical to the accuracy of the child's productive output. The ability to discriminate the acoustic differences between well-produced versions of [sip] and [ʃip] is not sufficient perceptual knowledge to ensure mastery of these phonemes is production. The child may be making this perceptual judgment by attending to transitional rather than spectral cues; the child may have an overly broad or misplaced boundary between the /s/ and /ʃ/ categories; the child may not be aware that [tʃip] and [θip] are not acceptable variants of /ʃip/. Studies that have employed word identification tasks that directly correspond to children typical substitution errors show a clear link between children's perceptual and productive knowledge of phonemes. Many of these studies involve comparisons of children with normal and delayed phonological development and will therefore be reviewed in Chapter 7. Two studies of children whose speech is developing normally are described here.

Studies that have employed word identification tasks that directly correspond to children typical substitution errors show a clear link between children's perceptual and productive knowledge of phonemes.

Eilers and Oller (1976) observed the speech perception abilities of children aged 22 to 26 months by asking the children to find the candy hidden in one of two opaque boxes topped with a real or nonsense object, after being told (for example), "It's under the fish" or "It's under the thish." The child was credited with accurate perception of the contrast if 7 of 8 trials were completed correctly (with random order of trials and stimulus placement). The word pairs "[k^{h}aʊ]-[paʊ]," "[k^{h}aɹ]-[kaɹ]," and "[p^{h}ɪg]-[t^{h}ɪg]" were the easiest for all the children to perceive. The pairs "[plɔk]-[lɔk]," "[plɔk]-[pɔk]," and "[ɹæbɪt]-[wæbɪt]" were moderately difficult with some children not reaching criterion (note that the phone transcribed by the authors as phonetically [p] is phonemically /b/). None of the children were able to reach criterion for the pairs "[mʌnki]-[mʌki]," and "[fɪʃ]-[θɪʃ]." Production ability was also assessed, not only in terms of the ability to produce the target phoneme in the real word but also as the ability the label both the real and the nonsense objects so as to differentiate the contrast between the minimal pair words. Five word pairs were chosen to target commonly occurring misarticulation patterns (k/k^h, p/pl, w/ɹ, k/mk, and θ/f). For these words, the most common pattern was simultaneous absence of perceptual and productive knowledge; however, good perceptual knowledge in the absence of productive knowledge was also very common. Three word pairs were chosen to represent unlikely production errors (t^h/p^h, l/pl and p/k^h). Accurate perception and production was nearly always observed for these pairs but some instances of accurate production with poor perceptual performance was also observed especially for the [p^{h}ɪg]-[t^{h}ɪg] pair. It is possible that these mismatches between perception and production for words that are apparently well known reflect differences in the strength of the connections between real and nonsense words and the corresponding acoustic-phonetic and articulatory-phonetic representations. Lexical effects on perception performance are well known (Polka, Jusczyk, & Rvachew, 1995) and lexical effects on production will be discussed later in this chapter. In any case, despite the small number of anomalies, the authors concluded that "perceptual confusions probably play a substantial part in childhood speech errors but that not all errors are related to perceptual difficulties" (p. 328).

Ohberg (2006) described the acoustic characteristics of /s/ and /θ/ productions recorded from normally developing 5-year-old children and quantified the distance between each child's /s/ and /θ/ categories on the basis of spectral and temporal cues. Restricting the analysis to those children who were stimulable for /s/, 4 clusters of children were revealed: 11 children who achieved 89%

correct production of /s/ by differentiating the categories on the basis of both centroid and duration; 13 children who achieved 88% correct by differentiating the categories on the basis of centroid but not duration; 11 children who achieved 68% correct by differentiating the categories on the basis of duration but not centroid; and 6 children who achieved 47% correct productions but who did not differentiate the categories on the basis of centroid or duration. The children's perception of /s/ was also assessed with the "Sue" module of the Speech Assessment and Interactive Learning System (SAILS), a mispronunciation detection task. This module has three levels: mispronunciations at Level 1 are stop and affricate substitutions; mispronunciations at Level 2 are fricative substitutions; mispronunciations at Level 3 are distortions of the /s/ target. The results are shown in Figure 4–16. Although all of the children were

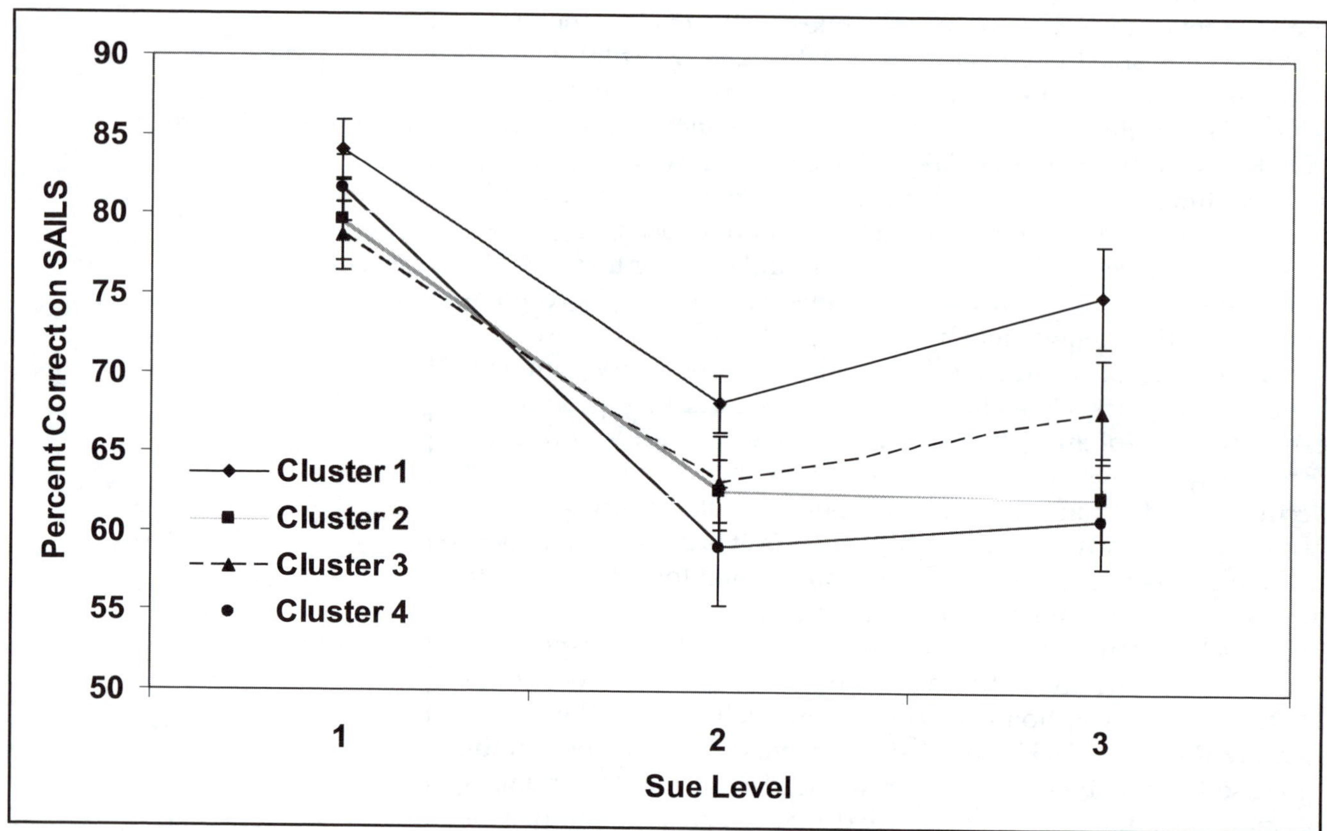

Figure 4–16. *Mean percent correct mispronunciation detection performance on the Speech Assessment and Interactive Learning System (SAILS) at Level 1 (stop and affricate substitutions), Level 2 (fricative substitutions), and Level 3 (distortions). Clusters of children were identified by their performance on a probe of /s/ production accuracy as described using acoustic analysis: Cluster 1 achieved 89% correct by differentiating the categories on the basis of both centroid and duration; Cluster 2 achieved 88% correct by differentiating the categories on the basis of centroid but not duration; Cluster 3 achieved 68% correct by differentiating the categories on the basis of duration but not centroid; and Cluster 4 achieved 47% correct productions but did not reliably differentiate the categories on the basis of centroid or duration. From Ohberg (2006). Articulatory, perceptual, and phonological determinants of accurate production of /s/. Figure 8, p. 54. Used with permission.*

able to identify mispronunciations that involved stop substitutions with reasonable accuracy, it is clear that only the children that differentiated their productions on the basis of both spectral and temporal cues were able to achieve above chance level performance on all three levels of the perceptual test (i.e., Cluster 1). Interestingly, Cluster 3 children who differentiated their /s/ and /θ/ on the basis of duration only achieved better perception task performance at Level 3 than Cluster 2 children who differentiated their productions on the basis of centroid only. Attending to duration can be reasonably effective for perception because /θ/ is reliably shorter than /s/ but this strategy does not help to achieve a high level of accuracy in production because it does not relate to the stridency feature (which requires a grooved tongue shape) or place of articulation difference between the two phonemes. A failure to determine the acoustic (and other) cues that children are using in perception and production has led many observers, on the basis of anecdotal evidence, to conclude incorrectly that some children have perceptual knowledge that they do not, and that other children have production knowledge that leads or exceeds their perceptual knowledge. However, as shown in Chapter 2, perceptual knowledge is acquired gradually and does not achieve adultlike levels until late childhood. Detailed knowledge of the acoustic-phonetic characteristics of a phoneme category is a prerequisite for mastery of production accuracy. The clinical implications of this fact are explored fully in Chapter 9 and factors that account for individual differences in perceptual abilities are discussed in Chapter 7.

Detailed knowledge of the acoustic-phonetic characteristics of a phoneme category is a prerequisite for mastery of production accuracy.

Motoric Factors and Phonological Development

Continuity between the phonetic content of babble and first words (Vihman, Macken, Miller, Simmons, & Miller, 1985) is often taken as evidence of the impact of motoric factors on early speech development. Vihman (Vihman, 2002; Vihman, de Boysson-Bardies, Durand, & Sundberg, 1994) has proposed that babbled utterances act as an articulatory filter, enhancing the salience of matching input and leading to the selection of words with similar phonetic content. Davis and MacNeilage (Davis & MacNeilage, 1995; MacNeilage & Davis, 2000; MacNeilage, Davis, Kinney, & Matyear, 2000) have argued that the phonetic content of both babble and early words is constrained by the limitations on speech motor control that prevent independence of the tongue from the jaw in speech gestures throughout the infant and toddler periods. These studies are characterized by a common weakness: assumptions are made about the child's knowledge at multiple representational levels using a single metric, specifically phonetic transcription of the child's speech output. In the previous section we showed how this practice can yield an inaccurate picture of children's perceptual knowledge at the acoustic-phonetic representational level. It is similarly unsafe to

Continuity between the phonetic content of babble and first words is often taken as evidence of the impact of motoric factors on early speech development.

make assumptions about the role of articulatory factors on phonological development without direct measures of the child's performance at multiple levels of representation.

Goffman, Gerken, and Lucchesi (2007) studied the impact of syllable prominence and underlying hierarchical prosodic structure on the segmental and motoric aspects of speech production in nonword sequences designed to induce output of SWSW, WSWS, and SWWS nonsense words within longer utterances. Earlier, we reviewed two hypotheses about children's tendency to omit or weaken weak syllables in the context of iambic sequences. The prominence hypothesis is that syllables with lower acoustic prominence will be most vulnerable to weakening (Snow, 1998), an effect attributed to the interaction of perceptual and input factors (Echols, 1993). Referencing the model sketched in Plate 1 and Figure 4–15, we would suggest that young children's acoustic-phonetic representations for these syllables are insufficiently detailed, as shown in the examples "banana" and "another." The prosodic account (the trochaic template hypothesis) is that syllables that are "unfooted" in the underlying representational hierarchy are most vulnerable to omission (Gerken, 1996). Again referencing the model sketched in Plate 1 and Figure 4–15, we would suggest that children's knowledge of the prosodic tiers of the phonological hierarchy emerges within the lexicon as a function of the accumulation of perceptual and productive knowledge of these forms, the frequency of these lexical forms within the lexicon (which would be influenced by their frequency in the input), and by the child's organization of those forms within the lexicon. Goffman et al. (2007) examined three outcome measures for weak syllables that were included in the imitated utterances: segment accuracy, segment variability, and a modification of the spatiotemporal index (see Chapters 1 and 3) called the convergence index. The convergence index quantified stability of movement patterns for a given syllable regardless of whether it was produced with accurate segmental content. Normally developing 4-year-old children demonstrated more segmental errors and greater motoric variability when producing weak syllables in comparison with strong syllables, a result that was consistent with the prominence account. When examining weak syllables specifically, segment accuracy and variability was degraded in WSWS and SWWS contexts compared to SWSW contexts; motoric variability was not influenced by these different prosodic contexts however. These results strongly suggest that both phonological (i.e., prosodic structure) and phonetic (i.e., acoustic-phonetic prominence) factors played a role in segmental accuracy and variability, confirming the importance of attending to multiple levels of representation when describing children's phonological development.

Kinematic and phonetic descriptions of weak syllable production by children suggest that both phonological (i.e., prosodic structure) and phonetic (i.e., acoustic-phonetic prominence) factors play a role in segmental accuracy and variability.

An equally important finding in this study was the lack of correspondence between segmental variability and motoric variability in the production of weak syllables in prosodically vulnerable contexts. Normally developing 4-year-olds demonstrated significantly lower segment accuracy for the unfooted first syllable in the WSWS nonsense word compared to any other context. Segment variability was also high in vulnerable syllables, specifically the second weak syllables of WSWS and SWWS nonsense words, in comparison to the second weak syllable of SWSW nonsense words. However, there were no significant differences in movement variability across these contexts or across weak syllables within these nonsense words. The authors caution that "interactions across phonological and motor levels are complex and that inferences need to be made carefully about one domain based on direct observation of the other; increased variability in one domain does not imply increased variability in another" (p. 456). They go on to discuss the implications of these findings for assumptions about subtypes of developmental disorders as discussed further in Chapter 7. Clearly, subtypes that are characterized by variable segment productions cannot be assumed to be based on an underlying substrate of increased motor variability and the source of variability in child speech cannot be determined from phonetic transcription alone.

Kinematic studies reveal a lack of correspondence between segment variability and motor variability in some contexts indicating that interactions across phonological and motor levels are complex.

We would further argue that it is perilous to assume that immature speech motor control explains nonadultlike phonological systems in young children. It may just as well be that the child's efforts to achieve an adultlike phonological system motivate practice of increasingly complex forms, ultimately driving the child toward mature speech motor control. In other words, we might just as well hypothesize that it is language development that causes speech motor development rather than assume that it is speech motor development that limits language output.

Lexical Effects on Phonological Development

In the final section of this chapter we examine the effect of the growing lexicon on phonological development, considering this relationship in the context of productive phonology and phonological awareness. We begin by defining three specific constructs that emerge from the lexicon as a whole: word frequency, phonotactic probability, and neighborhood density. Studies of the impact of these variables on word learning and spoken word processing provide empirical evidence that lexical and phonological development are strongly interdependent (Storkel & Morrisette, 2002).

Lexical and phonological development are strongly interdependent.

Every word that we hear has phonetic properties that are inherent to the word itself as well as phonological and lexical properties that are entirely dependent upon the relationship between the word and all the other words that are stored in the lexicon. One lexical variable that can make a difference is word frequency: for example, databases of child speech indicate that the word "baby" is about 15 times more frequently occurring than the word "bottle" (Storkel & Hoover, 2010), which is why we can reasonably imagine that our hypothetical infant has an incomplete acoustic-phonetic representation

Word frequency is the frequency with which a given word occurs in the input language, usually expressed as log frequency.

Phonotactic probability relates to the frequency of occurrence of specific sound sequences.

Neighborhood density is defined as the number of words that differ from the target word by all but one phoneme addition, substitution, or deletion.

Word frequency is a very powerful variable having a facilitatory effect on speed of access to a word in the lexicon and thus increasing accuracy and speed of word comprehension.

Commonly occurring phonotactic sequences are much easier to remember and to repeat than rare phonotactic sequences.

for the final syllable in "bottle" at Time 1 (see Figure 4–15). Phonotactic probability relates to the frequency of occurrence of specific sound sequences. Typically, these are calculated for sequences of two contiguous phones. For example, the word "duck" contains two biphone sequences, [dʌ] and [ʌk]; in relation to the number of words in the input that have biphones in the same positions, the first sequence is somewhat more likely to occur in English than the second; furthermore, the sequence [dʌ] occurs more than twice as often at the beginning of words in child speech than the sequence [gʌ]. The third construct, neighborhood density, is defined as the number of words that differ from the target word by all but one phoneme addition, substitution or deletion. In our hypothetical lexicon, the words "Sue" and "shoe" are neighbors because they differ by a single phoneme. As this child's lexicon grows, she will add new words to this particular neighborhood such as "see," "two," and "soup." According to databases of child speech, the word "Sue" has 25 neighbors and the word "shoe" has 19 neighbors (Storkel & Hoover, 2010); therefore, "Sue" has a slightly more dense neighborhood than "shoe"; in comparison, the word "milk" resides in a very sparse neighborhood containing only three other words that differ by a single phone.

Storkel and Morisette (2002) summarize the impact of these variables on spoken word processing and on speech production learning. In brief, word frequency is a very powerful variable having a facilitatory effect on speed of access to a word in the lexicon and thus increasing accuracy and speed of word comprehension. Children also learn to produce new sounds and generalize this learning more readily when the new sounds are taught in frequently occurring words. As we reported in Chapter 2, even very young infants are sensitive to the phonotactic characteristics of speech input. Commonly occurring phonotactic sequences are much easier to remember and to repeat than rare phonotactic sequences. Neighborhood density effects are more complicated to describe because they vary with the specific task and interact with other word characteristics. In general, a word from a dense neighborhood can be more difficult to access during receptive tasks as a consequence of competition from similar sounding neighbors. Therefore, the listener will be slower to comprehend the word or might confuse the word with a neighbor especially in difficult listening conditions. In some circumstances, words from sparse neighborhoods are easier to learn to produce and words from dense neighborhoods are more difficult to learn to produce. We describe a few studies in detail that have investigated lexical variables on nonword repetition and phonological awareness performance. The clinical implications of this research are discussed in Chapter 11.

Edwards, Beckman, and Munson (2004) described children's ability to repeat nonwords containing high probability phonotactic sequences versus low probability phonotactic sequences. For example, given the pair /ˈmoipəd/ and /ˈmæbɛp/, the sequence /mæ/ occurs with higher frequency than /moi/; similarly, given the pair /ˈauftəˌgɑ/ and /ˈauntəˌko /, the sequence /aun/ occurs with higher frequency than /auf/. Normally developing children, aged 3 to 8 years, and adult participants, repeated 2 and 3 syllable nonwords presented in semirandom order. Repetition accuracy was scored by awarding points for correct production of the features of each phoneme in the target sequence. The results, as shown in Figure 4–17, revealed that production accuracy was greatest for high-frequency sequences but children were more sensitive to sequence frequency than adults. Additional analyses revealed that expressive vocabulary size predicted both repetition accuracy and the size of the difference in accuracy between low- and high-frequency sequences;

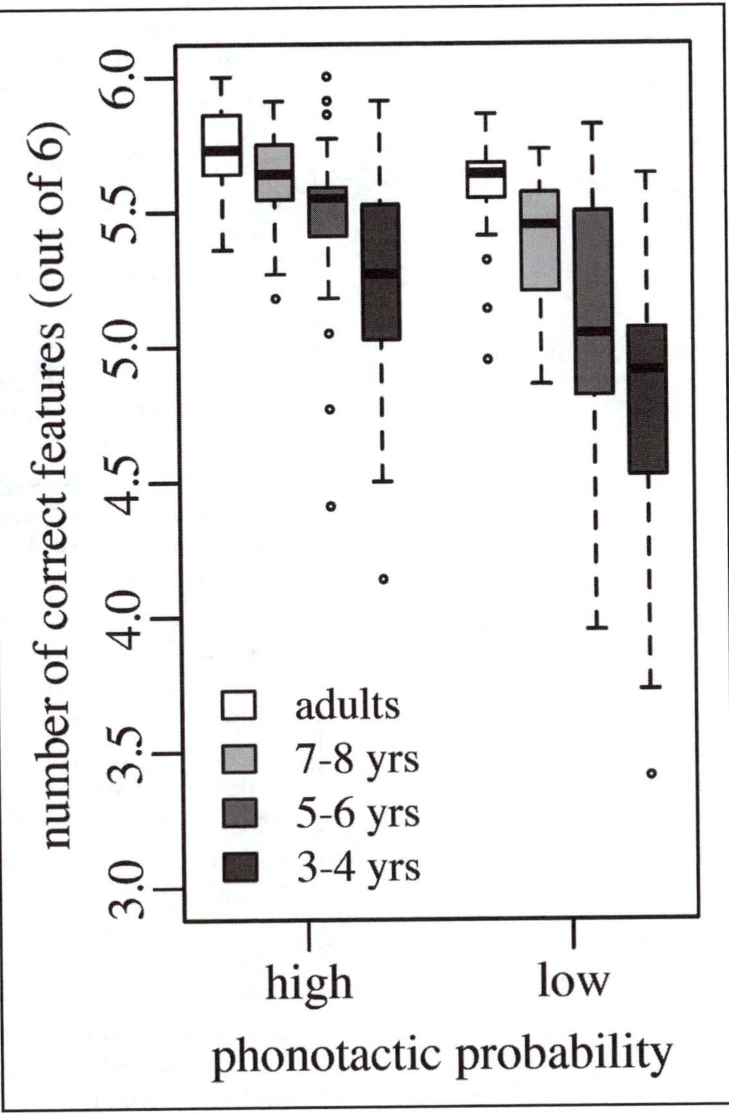

Figure 4–17. *Box plots showing medians and distributions of biphone accuracy scores obtained during a nonword repetition task. Accuracy was measured in terms of number of correctly reproduced features for the consonant and vowel in each biphone sequence (see text for details). Results are shown separately by age group for sequences with high versus low phonotactic probability summarizing data reported in Edwards, Beckman, and Munson (2004). Copyright © 2011 Edwards, Beckman, and Munson. All rights reserved. Used with permission.*

In studies of nonword repetition accuracy, the child's vocabulary size explained repetition accuracy and differences in accuracy between words containing phone sequences with low versus high phonotactic probability.

in fact, these analyses showed that it was vocabulary size rather than age that explained the ability to repeat nonwords, especially those with low phonotactic probability. The authors explain that there are two possible reasons for this finding: children with large vocabularies may have more experience listening to and producing words that contain rare biphone sequences; alternatively, children with large vocabularies may have abstracted more robust and generalized phonological knowledge at the phoneme level from their experience with specific words and syllables, allowing them to flexibly combine those phoneme-sized units into novel patterns. In order to test these alternative hypotheses, they compared repetition accuracy for rare sequences versus sequences that never occur in English. The results supported the second hypothesis in that children with smaller vocabulary sizes had considerably more difficulty with sequences that they had never encountered before in comparison to rare sequences; children with larger vocabulary sizes were more accurate overall indicating that they had robust phonological representations at the level of individual phonemes.

Richtsmeier, Goffman, and Hogan (2009) point out that the effect of phonotactic probability on nonword repetition accuracy may reflect production practice or perceptual learning on the part of the child, prior to the child's participation in the laboratory nonword repetition experiment. They designed an experiment to examine these variables independently by manipulating phonotactic probability of the nonwords (i.e., past exposure prior to the experiment) and input frequency during the experiment. Normally developing 4-year-olds were presented with drawings of nonsense animals and recordings of corresponding nonsense names for those animals such as [fospəm], [mæfpəm], [fæmpɪm], and [bopkəm]. Note that [sp] and [mp] are high probability sequences whereas [fp] and [pk] are low probability sequences. The picture-word pairs were presented to the children in random order with frequency varied so that half of the high probability and half of the low probability sequences occurred 10 times, whereas the remaining words were presented only once; in this example [fospəm] and [bopkəm] would be presented 10 times but [mæfpəm] and [fæmpɪm] would be presented once each. In the first experiment, all spoken words were presented in the same voice. After the children listened to the words as they were paired with the corresponding animal pictures, the animal pictures were represented and they were asked to imitate the corresponding animal "name." In the single voice experiment, improved production accuracy was observed for high frequency sequences (i.e., greater phonotactic probability) regardless of amount of in-laboratory exposure. In other words, greater accuracy would be obtained for [fospəm] and [fæmpɪm] than for [mæfpəm] and [bopkəm] in our example. Then the experiment was repeated with a new sample of 4-year-old children. This time the procedure was the same except that the spoken words were recorded from multiple talkers; for example, if the child heard [fospəm] ten times, the word was spoken by a different talker each time. The results were very different in this experiment: a greater amount of in-laboratory exposure to a word led to improved production, regardless of phonotactic probability; in other words, given the example words above, greatest accuracy would be observed for both [fospəm] and [bopkəm]. This study confirmed that perceptual learning plays an important role in production accuracy. Furthermore, it demonstrated that exposure to multitalker speech input facilitated production learning for unfamiliar sound sequences in new words. The clinical implications of this finding are clear and are explored further in Chapter 9.

Improved speech production accuracy is just one manifestation of phonological development. Another indicator is the acquisition of phonological awareness, as discussed in Chapter 2. Indeed, more refined phonological representations are required for reading and spelling than are required for accurate production of speech (Lewis, O'Donnell, Freebairn, & Taylor, 1998). Recall that phonological awareness is the child's implicit or explicit knowledge of the sublexical components of words: syllables, onset and rimes, and phonemes. Metsala and Walley (1998) proposed the Lexical Restructuring Hypothesis as an explanation for the emergence of children's phonological awareness abilities. Specifically, they proposed that changes in the developing lexicon, both global (increased size) and local (increased density within specific neighborhoods), drove the child toward increasingly segmentalized phonological knowledge of words; consequently, children would be able to succeed at tasks that required more explicit manipulations of smaller and smaller units within words as their vocabulary size grew. Their hypothesis also led to predictions based on the specific properties of words such as word frequency, age of acquisition, lexical status, and neighborhood density. Furthermore, these lexical characteristics were expected to impact performance on other spoken word processing tasks such as recognition of gated words and nonword repetition. Their predictions have been supported in a large number of studies conducted with children and adults. One of these studies is reviewed here.

Lexical Restructuring Hypothesis: changes in the developing lexicon, both global (increased size) and local (increased density within specific neighborhoods), drive the child toward increasingly segmentalized phonological knowledge of words.

Metsala (1999) studied phonological awareness in 4- and 5-year-old children using two tasks: a task in which the children blended an onset and a rime into a whole word or nonsense syllable and a task in which the children identified and pronounced the first sound in a real or nonsense word. The children's performance was examined in relation to lexical status (real word or nonword) and age of acquisition (early acquired versus late acquired words). Two potential predictors of the children's performance were also examined: vocabulary size and nonword repetition performance. The results showed that older children had higher accuracy on the tasks than younger children but that all children achieved greater accuracy with real words than nonwords and early acquired words than later acquired words. Furthermore, the children's performance on these tasks was predicted by vocabulary size. Although this result

Children's phonological awareness performance is better for real words than nonwords and for early acquired words than later acquired words.

is consistent with the lexical restructuring hypothesis, it might also support an alternative view that both phonological awareness and vocabulary are facilitated by strong phonological short-term memory skills. Nonword repetition is believed to be a measure of phonological short-term memory (Gathercole & Baddeley, 1993) even though it is often found to be more closely associated with speech production accuracy (for discussion, see Rvachew & Grawburg, 2008). Metsala (1999) was able to demonstrate, however, that nonword repetition did not explain the children's phonological awareness performance after vocabulary size was taken into account. Rather, a growing vocabulary size facilitates both phonological awareness and nonword repetition skills by allowing the child to abstract robust representations for phonemes through lexical restructuring, a finding fully compatible with the conclusions cited above from Edwards et al. (2004).

A growing vocabulary size facilitates both phonological awareness and nonword repetition skills by allowing the child to abstract robust representations for phonemes through lexical restructuring.

Summary

Phonological knowledge is not only crucial to accurate speech production but a key component of oral and written language development. We have traced its origins to the infant's earliest experiences with the phonetic characteristics of words. We have proposed that phonological representations emerge from the linkages between acoustic-phonetic, articulatory-phonetic, and semantic representations. Phonological representations become increasingly fine grained with a rapidly growing vocabulary as the child organizes and restructures the lexicon to facilitate efficient lexical access, flexible construction of novel word forms, and the acquisition of metaphonological knowledge to support literacy development. The clinical implications of this approach to phonological development are explored in depth as we move from the "foundations" to the "clinical" parts of this book. A detailed description of a multiple representations approach to assessment and diagnosis of developmental disorders is covered in Part II.

References

Altvater-Mackensen, N., & Fikkert, P. (2010). The acquisition of the stop-fricative contrast in perception and production. *Lingua, 120*, 1898–1909.

Amayreh, M. M., & Dyson, A. T. (2000). Phonetic inventories of young Arabic-speaking children. *Clinical Linguistics & Phonetics, 14*(3), 193–215.

Austin, D., & Shriberg, L. D. (1997). *Lifespan reference data for ten measures of articulation competence using the speech disorders classification system (SDSC)*: Waisman Center on Mental Retardation and Human Development, University of Wisconsin-Madison.

Ball, M. J., Müller, N., & Rutter, B. (2010). *Phonology for communication disorders*. New York, NY: Psychology Press.

Barlow, J. A., & Gierut, J. A. (1999). Optimality theory in phonological acquisition. *Journal of Speech, Language, and Hearing Research, 42*(6), 1482–1498.

Berg, T. (2000). A local connectionist account of consonant harmony in child language. *Cognitive Science, 24*, 123–149.

Bernhardt, B., & Stemberger, J. P. (1998). *Handbook of phonological development from the perspective of constraint-based phonology.* San Diego, CA: Academic Press.

Bernhardt, B., & Stoel-Gammon, C. (1994). Nonlinear phonology: Introduction and clinical application. *Journal of Speech and Hearing Research, 37*, 123–143.

Boersma, P., & Hayes, B. (2001). Empirical tests of the gradual learning algorithm. *Linguistic Inquiry, 32*, 45–86.

Bunta, F., Davidovich, I., & Ingram, D. (2006). The relationship between the phonological complexity of a bilingual child's words and those of the target languages. *International Journal of Bilingualism, 10*, 71–88.

Bunta, F., Fabiano-Smith, L., Goldstein, B., & Ingram, D. (2009). Phonological whole-word measures in 3-year-old bilingual children and their age-matched monolingual peers. *Clinical Linguistics & Phonetics, 23*, 156–175.

Burrows, L., & Goldstein, B. A. (2010). Whole word measures in bilingual children with speech sound disorders. *Clinical Linguistics & Phonetics, 24*, 357–368.

Bybee, J. (2001). *Phonology and language use.* Cambridge, UK: Cambridge University Press.

Bybee, J. (2006). From usage to grammar: The mind's response to repetition. *Language, 82*, 711–733.

Bybee, J., & McClelland, J. L. (2005). Alternatives to the combinatorial paradigm of linguistic theory based on domain general principles of human cognition. *Linguistic Review, 22*, 381–410.

Cahill Haelsig, P., & Madison, C. L. (1986). A study of phonological processes exhibited by 3- 4- and 5-year-old children. *Language, Speech, and Hearing Services in Schools, 17*, 107–114.

Carter, A., & Gerken, L. (2004). Do children's omissions leave traces? *Journal of Child Language, 31*, 561–586.

Catano, L., Barlow, J. A., & Moyo, M. (2009). A retrospective study of phonetic inventory complexity in acquisition of Spanish: Implications for phonological universals. *Clinical Linguistics & Phonetics, 23*, 446–472.

Chin, S. B., & Dinnsen, D. A. (1992). Consonant clusters in disordered speech: constraints and correspondence patterns. *Journal of Child Language, 19*, 259–285.

Coplan, J., & Gleason, J. R. (1988). Unclear speech: Recognition and significance of unintelligible speech in preschool children. *Pediatrics, 82*, 447–452.

Davis, B. L., & MacNeilage, P. F. (1995). The articulatory basis of babbling. *Journal of Speech and Hearing Research, 38*, 1199–1211.

Day, A. (1998). *Good dog, Carl.* New York, NY: Farrar Straus Giroux.

Dinnsen, D. A. (1992). Variation in developing and fully developed phonetic inventories. In C. A. Ferguson, L. Menn, & C. Stoel-Gammon (Eds.), *Phonological development: Models, research and implications* (pp. 191–210). Timonium, MD: York Press.

Dinnsen, D. A., Chin, S. B., Elbert, M., & Powell, T. W. (1990). Some constraints on functionally disordered phonologies: Phonetic inventories and phonotactics. *Journal of Speech and Hearing Research, 33*(1), 28–37.

Dodd, B., Holm, A., Hua, Z., & Crosbie, S. (2003). Phonological development: A normative study of British English-speaking children. *Clinical Linguistics & Phonetics, 17*(8), 617–643.

Echols, C. H. (1993). A perceptually-based model of children's earliest productions. *Cognition, 46*, 245–296.

Edwards, J., & Beckman, M. E. (2008). Methodological questions in studying consonant acquisition. *Clinical Linguistics & Phonetics, 22*, 937–956.

Edwards, J., Beckman, M. E., & Munson, B. (2004). The interaction between vocabulary size and phonotactic probability effects on children's production accuracy and fluency in nonword repetition. *Journal of Speech, Language, and Hearing Research, 47*, 421–436.

Eilers, R. E., & Oller, D. K. (1976). The role of speech discrimination in developmental sound substitutions. *Journal of Child Language, 3*, 319–329.

Eisenbeiβ, S. (2009). Generative approaches to language learning. *Linguistics, 47*, 273–310.

Evans, J. L. (2001). An emergent account of language impairments in children with SLI: Implications for assessment and intervention. *Journal of Communication Disorders, 34*, 39–54.

Ferguson, C., & Farwell, C. B. (1975). Words and sounds in early acquisition. *Language, 51*(2), 419–439.

Fikkert, P., & de Hoop, H. (2009). Language acquisition in optimality theory. *Linguistics, 47*, 311–357.

Gathercole, S. E., & Baddeley, A. D. (1993). *Working memory and language*. Hove, UK: Lawrence Erlbaum.

Gerken, L. (1996). Prosodic structure in young children's language production. *Language, 72*, 683–712.

Gierut, J. (2001). A model of lexical diffusion in phonological acquisition. *Clinical Linguistics & Phonetics, 15*, 19–22.

Goffman, L., Gerken, L., & Lucchesi, J. (2007). Relations between segmental and motor variability in prosodically complex nonword sequences. *Journal of Speech, Language, and Hearing Research, 50*, 444–458.

Goldman, R., & Fristoe, M. (2000). *Goldman-Fristoe Test of Articulation* (2nd ed.). Circle Pines, MN: American Guidance Service.

Haelsig, P. C., & Madison, C. L. (1986). A study of phonological processes exhibited by 3-, 4-, and 5-year-old children. *Language, Speech, and Hearing Services in Schools, 17*, 107–114.

Hart, B., & Risley, T. (1992). American parenting of language-learning children: Persisting differences in family-child interactions observed in natural home environments. *Developmental Psychology, 28*, 1096–1105.

Hockema, S. A., & Smith, L. B. (2009). Learning your language, outside-in and inside-out. *Linguistics, 47*, 453–479.

Hodson, B. W. (2004). *Hodson Assessment of Phonological Patterns* (3rd ed.). Austin, TX: Pro-Ed.

Hoff, E., & Naigles, L. (2002). How children use input to acquire a lexicon. *Child Development, 73*(2), 418–433.

Hoffman, P. R., Schuckers, G. H., & Daniloff, R. G. (1980). Developmental trends in correct /r/ articulation as a function of allophone type. *Journal of Speech and Hearing Research, 23*, 746–756.

Huttenlocher, J. (1998). Language input and language growth. *Preventive Medicine, 27*, 195–199.

Ingram, D. (1975). Surface contrast in phonology: Evidence from children's speech. *Journal of Child Language, 2*, 287–292.

Ingram, D. (2002). The measurement of whole-word productions. *Journal of Child Language, 29*, 713–733.

Ingram, D., & Ingram, K. D. (2001). A whole-word approach to phonological analysis and intervention. *Language, Speech, and Hearing Services in Schools, 32*, 271–283.

James, D. G. H. (2006). *Hippopotamus is hard to say: Children's acquisition of polysyllabic words.* Unpublished doctoral dissertation. University of Sydney, Sydney, Australia.

James, D. G. H., van Doorn, J., McLeod, S., & Esterman, A. (2008). Patterns of consonant deletion in typical developing children aged 3 to 7 years. *International Journal of Speech-Language Pathology, 10*, 179–192.

Kay-Raining Bird, E., & Chapman, R. S. (1998). Partial representations and phonological selectivity in the comprehension of 13- to 16-month-olds. *First Language, 18*, 105–127.

Kent, R. D., & Bauer, H. R. (1985). Vocalizations of one-year-olds. *Journal of Child Language, 12*, 491–526.

Klein, H. B. (1981). Productive strategies for the pronunciation of early polysyllabic lexical items. *Journal of Speech and Hearing Research, 24*, 389–405.

Lacerda, F. (2003). Phonology: An emergent consequence of memory contraints and sensory input. *Reading and Writing: An Interdisciplinary Journal, 16*, 41–59.

Lewis, B. A., O'Donnell, B., Freebairn, L., & Taylor, H. G. (1998). Spoken language and written expression—interplay of delays. *American Journal of Speech-Language Pathology, 7*, 77–84.

Li, F., Edwards, J., & Beckman, M. E. (2009). Contrast and covert contrast: The phonetic development of voiceless sibilant fricatives in English and Japanese toddlers. *Journal of Phonetics, 37*(1), 111–124.

Lowe, R. J., Knutson, P. J., & Monson, M. A. (1985). Incidence of fronting in preschool children. *Language, Speech, and Hearing Services in Schools, 16*, 119–123.

MacLeod, A. N., Laukys, K., & Rvachew, S. (2011). Impact of bilingual language learning on whole-word complexity and segmental accuracy among preschoolers. *International Journal of Speech-Language Pathology, 13(6)*, 490–499.

MacNeilage, P. F., & Davis, B. L. (2000). On the origin of internal structure structure of word forms. *Science, 288*, 527–531.

MacNeilage, P. F., Davis, B. L., Kinney, A., & Matyear, C. L. (2000). The motor core of speech: A comparison of serial organization patterns in infants and languages. *Child Development, 71*(1), 153–163.

McIntosh, B., & Dodd, B. J. (2008). Two-year-old's phonological acquisition: Normative data. *International Journal of Speech-Language Pathology, 10*, 460–469.

McLeod, S., Van Doorn, J., & Reed, V. A. (2001a). Consonant cluster development in two-year-olds: General trends and individual difference. *Journal of Speech, Language, and Hearing Research, 44*, 1144–1171.

McLeod, S., Van Doorn, J., & Reed, V. A. (2001b). Normal acquisition of consonant clusters. *American Journal of Speech-Language Pathology, 10*, 99–110.

McMurray, B., & Aslin, R. N. (2005). Infants are sensitive to within-category variation in speech perception. *Cognition, 95*, B15–B26.

Menn, L., Schmidt, E., & Nicholas, B. (2009). Conspiracy and sabotage in the acquisition of phonology: Dense data undermine existing theories, provide scaffolding for a new one. *Language Sciences, 31*(2–3), 285–304.

Metsala, J. L. (1999). Young children's phonological awareness and non-word repetition as a function of vocabulary development. *Journal of Educational Psychology, 91*(1), 3–19.

Metsala, J. L., & Walley, A. C. (1998). Spoken vocabulary growth and the segmental restructuring of lexical representations: Precursors to phonemic awareness and early reading ability. In J. L. Metsala & L. C. Ehri (Eds.), *Word recognition in beginning reading* (pp. 89–120). Mahwah, NJ: Lawrence Erlbaum.

Ohberg, A. (2006). *Articulatory, perceptual, and phonological determinants of accurate production of /s/.* Unpublished masters thesis, McGill University, Montreal, Quebec.

Pierrehumbert, J. (2003). Phonetic diversity, statistical learning, and acquisition of phonology. *Language and Speech, 46*, 115–154.

Pinker, S. (1984). *Language Learnability and Language Development*. Cambridge, MA: Harvard University Press.

Poeppel, D., Idsardi, W. J., & van Wassenhove, V. (2008). Speech perception at the interface of neurobiology and linguistics. *Philosophical Transactions of the Royal Society, 363*, 1071–1086.

Polka, L., Jusczyk, P. W., & Rvachew, S. (1995). Methods for studying speech perception in infants and children. In W. Strange (Ed.), *Speech perception and linguistic experience: Issues in cross-language research* (pp. 49–89). Timomium, MD: York.

Pollock, K. E., & Berni, M. C. (2003). Incidence of non-rhotic vowel errors in children: data from the Memphis Vowel Project. *Clinical Linguistics & Phonetics, 17*, 393–401.

Porter, J. H., & Hodson, B. W. (2001). Clinical forum. Collaborating to obtain phonological acquisition data for local schools. *Language, Speech, and Hearing Services in Schools, 32*(3), 165.

Prather, E. M., Hedrick, D. L., & Kern, C. A. (1975). Articulation development in children aged two to four years. *Journal of Speech and Hearing Disorders, 40*, 179–191.

Preisser, D. A., Hodson, B. W., & Paden, E. P. (1988). Developmental phonology: 18–29 months. *Journal of Speech and Hearing Disorders, 53*, 125–130.

Richtsmeier, P. T., Gerken, L., Goffman, L., & Hogan, T. (2009). Statistical frequency in perception affects children's lexical production. *Cognition, 111*, 372–377.

Rvachew, S., Creighton, D., Feldman, N., & Sauve, R. (2005). Vocal development of infants with very low birth weight. *Clinical Linguistics & Phonetics, 19*(4), 275–294.

Rvachew, S., & Grawburg, M. (2008). Reflections on phonological working memory, letter knowledge and phonological awareness: A reply to Hartmann (2008). *Journal of Speech, Language, and Hearing Research, 51*, 1219–1226.

Saaristo-Helin, K., & Savinainen-Makkonen, T. (2006). The phonological mean length of utterance: methodological challenges from a cross-linguistic perspective. *Journal of Child Language, 33*, 179–190.

Sander, E. (1972). Do we know when speech sounds are learned? *Journal of Speech and Hearing Disorders, 37*, 55–63.

Schmitt, L. S., Howard, B. H., & Schmitt, J. F. (1983). Conversational speech sampling in the assessment of articulation proficiency. *Language, Speech, and Hearing Services in Schools, 14*, 210–214.

Schwartz, R., & Leonard, L. (1982). Do children pick and choose? An examination of selection and avoidance in early lexical acquisition. *Journal of Child Language, 9*, 319–336.

Schwartz, R., Leonard, L., Loeb, D., & Swanson, L. (1987). Attempted sounds are sometimes not: An expanded view of phonological selection and avoidance. *Journal of Child Language, 14*, 411–418.

Selby, J. C., Robb, M. P., & Gilbert, H. R. (2000). Normal vowel articulations between 15 and 36 months of age. *Clinical Linguistics & Phonetics, 14*(4), 255–265.

Shriberg, L. D., Austin, D., Lewis, B. A., McSweeny, J. L., & Wilson, D. L. (1997). The Speech Disorders Classification System (SDCS): Extensions and lifespan reference data. *Journal of Speech, Language, and Hearing Research, 40*(4), 723–740.

Shriberg, L. D., & Kwiatkowski, J. (1982). Phonological Disorders III: A procedure for assessing severity of involvement. *Journal of Speech and Hearing Disorders, 47*, 256–270.

Smit, A. B. (1993a). Phonological error distributions in the Iowa-Nebraska Articulation Norms Project: Consonant singletons. *Journal of Speech and Hearing Research, 36*, 533–547.

Smit, A. B. (1993b). Phonological error distributions in the Iowa-Nebraska articulation norms project: Word-initial consonant clusters. *Journal of Speech and Hearing Research, 36*, 931–947.

Smit, A. B., Hand, L., Freilinger, J. J., Bernthal, J. E., & Bird, A. (1990). The Iowa articulation norms project and its Nebraska replication. *Journal of Speech and Hearing Disorders, 55*, 779–798.

Snow, D. (1998). A prominence account of syllable reduction in early speech development: the child's prosodic phonology of tiger and giraffe. *Journal of Speech, Language, and Hearing Research, 41*, 1171–1184.

Spencer, J. P., Blumberg, M. S., McMurray, B., Robinson, S. R., Samuelson, L. K., & Tomblin, J. B. (2009). Short arms and talking eggs: Why we should no longer abide the nativist-empiricist debate. *Child Development Perspectives, 3*(2), 79–87.

Stoel-Gammon, C. (1985). Phonetic inventories, 15–24 months: A longitudinal study. *Journal of Speech and Hearing Research, 28*, 50–512.

Stoel-Gammon, C. (1987). Phonological skills of 2-year-olds. *Language, Speech, and Hearing Services in Schools, 18*, 323–329.

Stoel-Gammon, C. (2001). Transcribing the speech of young children. *Topics in Language Disorders, 21*, 12–21.

Stokes, S. F., & Suredran, D. (2005). Articulatory complexity, ambient frequency, and functional load as predictors of consonant development in children. *Journal of Speech, Language, and Hearing Research, 48*, 577–591.

Stokes, S. F., & To, C. K. S. (2002). Feature development in Cantonese. *Clinical Linguistics & Phonetics, 16*, 443–459.

Storkel, H. L., & Hoover, J. R. (2010). An online calculator to compute phonotactic probability and neighborhood density on the basis of child corpora of spoken American English. *Behavior Research Methods, 42*, 497–506.

Storkel, H. L., & Morrisette, M. L. (2002). The lexicon and phonology: Interactions in language acquisition. *Language, Speech, and Hearing Services in Schools, 33*, 24–37.

Swingley, D. (2008). The roots of the early vocabulary in infants' learning from speech. *Current Directions in Psychological Science, 17*, 308–312.

Taelman, H., Durieux, G., & Gillis, S. (2005). Notes on Ingram's whole-word measures for phonological development. *Journal of Child Language, 32*, 391–405.

Vihman, M. M. (2002). The role of mirror neurons in the ontogeny of speech. In M. Stamenov & V. Gallese (Eds.), *Mirror neurons and the evolution of brain and language* (pp. 305–314). Amsterdam, Netherlands: John Benjamin.

Vihman, M. M. (2006, June 29 to July 1, 2006). *Phonological templates in early words: A cross-linguistic study*. Paper presented at the 10th Conference on Laboratory Phonology, Paris, France.

Vihman, M. M., & Croft, W. (2007). Phonological development: Toward a "radical" templatic phonology. *Linguistics: An Interdisciplinary Journal of the Language Sciences*, FindArticles.com. 02 Nov 2008. http://findarticles.com/p/articles/mi_hb2195/is_2004_2045/ai_n29373777

Vihman, M. M., de Boysson-Bardies, B., Durand, C., & Sundberg, U. (1994). External sources of individual differences? A cross-linguistic analysis of the phonetics of mothers' speech to 1-year-old children. *Developmental Psychology, 30*(5), 651–662.

Vihman, M. M., DePaolis, R. A., & Keren-Portnoy, T. (2009). Babbling and words: A Dynamic Systems perspective on phonological development. In E. L. Bavin (Ed.), *The Cambridge handbook of child language*. Cambridge, UK: Cambridge University Press.

Vihman, M. M., Macken, M. A., Miller, R., Simmons, H., & Miller, J. (1985). From babbling to speech: A re-assessment of the continuity issue. *Language, 61*(2), 397–445.

Vihman, M. M., & Velleman, S. L. (2000). The construction of a first phonology. *Phonetica, 57*, 255–266.

Waterson, N. (1971). Child phonology: A prosodic view. *Journal of Linguistics, 7*, 179–211.

Weiner, F. F. (1979). *Phonological process analysis*. Baltimore, MD: University Park Press.

Westermann, G., & Reck Miranda, E. (2004). A new model of sensorimotor coupling in the development of speech. *Brain and Language, 89*(2), 393–400.

Part II

A Holistic Approach to Diagnosis and Treatment Planning

The course of normal phonological development, as described in Part I, involves the integration of increasingly complex knowledge at multiple levels of representation, resulting in observable markers of the child's progress toward the achievement of adultlike competency. The average child will produce speechlike babble at approximately 7 months of age, recognizable words around the time of the first birthday, fully intelligible speech by the age of 4 years, and adultlike accuracy in the production of spoken language before the age of 9 years. These achievements make an important contribution to social-emotional and cognitive development, allowing the child to form social relationships with others, accomplish instrumental goals, learn new skills, achieve independence, and participate fully in socially appropriate family and community contexts. When someone in the child's environment perceives that these events have not occurred within expected timeframes the speech-language pathologist (SLP) may be asked to intervene.

Parents often bring their child to the SLP when there has been a change in the environmental context that challenges their child's capacity to function or participate in their home or community. Transition from home to daycare may provide opportunities to note differences in the child's speech relative to peers. A new child in the family may serve as a contrast to the first child's slower rate of speech development. Upcoming school entry may heighten latent anxieties about the child's tendency to shy away from social interactions with peers. The child may express frustration during communication breakdowns with new playmates after a move to a new neighborhood. Regardless of the trigger for the parents' visit they will arrive in the SLP's office with a description of their concerns

The World Health Organization's **International Classification of Functioning, Disability and Health (ICF)** was endorsed by the World Health Assembly on May 22, 2001 as the international standard for measuring health and disability at both individual and population levels.

that has components that align with the World Health Organization's framework for the Classification of Functioning, Disability and Health (McCormack, McLeod, Harrison, & McAllister, 2010; McCormack, McLeod, McAllister, & Harrison, 2010; Thomas-Stonell, Oddson, Robertson, & Rosenbaum, 2009). Parents will identify a problem with the clarity or accuracy of the child's speech. This description will necessarily have a comparative or normative aspect: the child is not speaking as clearly as the parent expects, perhaps in relation to other children of the same age. Parents may also express concern about the potential for future problems such as the likelihood of social or academic problems once the child starts school. In some cases, the parent may not be concerned but the expectations of another family member or the child's teachers for greater speech clarity on the part of the child are the impetus for the referral. Some parents may propose an explanation for the child's speech problem such as ear infections, "tongue tie," or a family history of speech difficulties. The parent will also describe the problem in terms of the limitations on the child's ability to communicate effectively and the restrictions that this limitation may place on the child's participation in socially expected roles such as playing with siblings, attending birthday parties, or making the transition to preschool. Personal factors such as the child's frustration during communication breakdowns or, alternatively, the child's apparent lack of awareness of the problem as perceived by the parent, will also form part of the picture. Finally, the parent may be aware that the nature of the problem changes depending on the environment. When the parent arrives in the SLP's office with this multifaceted description of their concerns about their child's speech, the SLP's response should be based on a similar holistic framework but in fact diagnostic assessment protocols tend to focus on the issue of whether the child presents with impaired speech. These assessment practices flow directly from a medical model of disability that situates the problem within the child. In our introduction to Part II we introduce a biopsychosocial model of disability in an effort to counter this tendency and align your approach to assessment, diagnosis, and treatment planning with the parents' view of their child's speech problem as situated within a complex dynamic of the child in interaction with the family and community.

Assessment protocols in SLP often flow from a **medical model** that focuses on diagnosis of impairment within the child.

A **biopsychosocial model** of disability situates the child's speech problem within a complex dynamic of the child in interaction with the family and community.

ICF-CY

The medical perspective classifies speech problems according to a clinical diagnosis (Bishop & Rosenbloom, 1987). For example, an infant may be diagnosed with cleft lip and/or palate which are craniofacial anomalies causing speech and resonance problems. The medical approach aims to define the medical condition underlying the speech problem with the expectation that the diagnosis itself will identify the appropriate medical intervention (e.g., surgical correction of the cleft) as well as information regarding prognosis (Stackhouse, 1993). However, there are disadvantages to the medical approach. First, it is not always possible to make a clinical diagnosis, as in most cases of developmental phonological disorder (Baker, Croot, McLeod, & Paul, 2001). Second, a medical diagnosis does not specify the speech and language difficulties and the degree of severity that a child is likely to have (Stackhouse, 1993). For instance, two children with a cleft palate may exhibit markedly different profiles of speech accuracy and as many as 46% of children with cleft lip and/or palate also have language and learning disabilities (Broder, Richman, & Matheson, 1998). Furthermore, the diagnosis does not in fact provide clear direction for the selection of type or intensity of service; neither does it predict the child's likelihood of social, academic and vocational success in the future. Continuing with the example of cleft lip and/or palate, approximately half of this population will achieve normal speech and language functioning following the initial surgical correction of the craniofacial anomaly alone whereas the remainder will require additional surgical, orthodontic and therapeutic interventions of varying intensity to achieve a good outcome (Blakeley & Brockman, 1995).

Disadvantages of the medical approach include the difficulty of making a clinical diagnosis and the lack of clear links between diagnosis and intervention strategies.

In contrast to the medical model, the International Classification of Functioning, Disability and Health (ICF; World Health Organization, 2001) provides an interdisciplinary and international framework to describe health issues that challenges how we view disability. The World Health Organization (WHO) defines *health* as "a state of complete physical, mental, and social well-being and not merely the absence of disease or infirmity" (World Health Organization, 2006). The ICF is intended for the collection of statistical data, research, clinical and social policy use. In other words, the ICF is not an assessment measure or a formal model, but rather a classification system based on a holistic and person-centered approach (Threats, 2008). The International Classification of Functioning, Disability and Health for Children and Youth (ICF-CY; World Health Organization, 2007) was later developed specifically for individuals from birth to 17 years, and contains the same structure as the ICF.

The World Health Organization (WHO) defines **health** as "a state of complete physical, mental, and social well-being and not merely the absence of disease or infirmity."

The **International Classification of Functioning, Disability and Health for Children and Youth (ICF-CY)** is a holistic and person-specific framework developed specifically for individuals aged birth to 17 years.

According to the ICF, disability is not viewed as arising solely from impairments in biological structures or functions attributed to the individual. Rather, the disability arises from complex interactions between biological and psychological factors within the individual and the physical and social context within which the individual lives. The framework permits a description of the individual's functioning as an interaction between health conditions and contextual factors that can be used to identify interventions to maximize the individual's functioning and evaluate the outcome of those interventions. The description of the individual's functioning and disability begins with the identification of impairments in body structures and body functions that are relevant to the health condition (i.e., disease or disorder) of interest. There are literally

The ICF-CY framework permits a description of the individual's functioning as an interaction between health conditions and contextual factors that can be used to identify interventions to maximize the individual's functioning and evaluate the outcome of those interventions.

Impairments in **body structures** and **body functions** are rated on a 5-point severity scale (no impairment, mild, moderate, severe, complete).

Difficulties with the execution of **activities** and restrictions on **participation** in life situations are rated in relation to capacity and performance.

hundreds of codes to choose from and a broad variety relate to speech, language, and communication disorders (McCormack & Worrall, 2008). Impairment is rated on a 5-point severity scale (no impairment, mild, moderate, severe, complete). The description of the individual's functioning and disability further requires that the impact on activity limitations and participation restrictions be assessed. Difficulties with the execution of activities and restrictions on involvement in life situations are rated in relation to capacity and performance. The distinction between capacity and performance is important, with capacity requiring standardized test conditions to determine the person's highest probable level of functioning and the performance evaluation revealing typical performance in the child's every day environments, with or without assistance or assistive devices. Notice that there can be disparities between capacity and performance in either direction. The child's performance on standardized tests in a quiet test environment with a single evaluator may overestimate the child's performance in a noisy classroom with multiple conversation partners. On the other hand, a gregarious and creative child who is unintelligible to strangers may communicate effectively in a supportive preschool environment that is well adapted to the child's needs. This leads into the importance of considering the contextual factors as contributors to the health problem itself and as potential targets of the intervention strategies that may be planned to maximize the child's functioning. These contextual factors include aspects of the physical environment, the social network that the child is connected to, the attitudes of the people in that network, as well as systems and policies that impact on the child's functioning and access to services (McCormack, McLeod, Harrison, et al., 2010). These factors are rated as barriers or facilitators of the child's performance. Finally, personal factors such as the child's awareness of the problem, gender, race, age, temperament, coping styles, and other health conditions must be taken into account, again as barriers or facilitators of the child's functioning.

It is important to consider **contextual factors** as contributors to the health problem itself and as potential targets of the intervention strategies that may be planned to maximize the child's functioning.

Developmental Phonological Disorders as the Diagnostic Term

As we discuss the application of the ICF framework in the context of DPD, we must be begin by unpacking the term "developmental phonological disorder" and justifying this choice of terminology to describe this health condition. Since the dawn of our profession, many terms have been used to describe children who have unintelligible or inaccurate speech, with all of the terms reflecting the tongue-in-cheek perspective of Compton (1970) who compared the diagnostic role of the SLP to that of a "TV repairman"! The diagnostic term that is applied specifies the "part" that is presumed to need fixing, either "articulation," "phonology," or "speech," with these terms all in current use although, historically, earlier usages focused on articulation problems and current preference in North America is to refer to "speech" as a cover term that is presumed to include both the articulatory and phonological aspects of the child's difficulty. We feel, however, that "speech" is too broad a term because it is often used as a cover term for difficulties with articulation, stuttering and voice in epidemiological studies, as seen in Chapter 7. Furthermore, in the developmental context there is no possibility of separating articulation from other aspects of phonological knowledge. Children who appear to have a motor speech problem called childhood apraxia of speech have significant difficulties with various aspects of phonological processing (see Chapter 7 for further discussion of this point). Returning to the topic of cleft lip and/or palate, this structural disorder that might appear at first glance to cause a purely articulatory problem, actually results in speech patterns that are best described and treated with phonological approaches (Howard, 1993; Pamplona, Ysunza, & Espinoza, 1999). Therefore, it is our preference to identify the central issue as being in the child's developing phonological system, stressing as we do throughout this book, that phonology comprises interlocking components at multiple levels of representation.

In using the term **developmental phonological disorder** we identify the central issue as being in the child's developing phonological system, stressing that phonology comprises interlocking components at multiple levels of representation.

The diagnostic term also requires one or more modifiers that indicate a specific type of phonological problem. We use the term "developmental" to simply denote that we are referring to children whose phonological systems are still developing. Furthermore, as shown in Chapter 7, the most likely causal factors in the majority of cases are interacting genetic and environmental variables that impact primary neurodevelopmental processes. The modifier "functional" was used for many decades, sometimes replaced with the phrase "of unknown origin," to differentiate problems that had a known biological cause from those that did not and were therefore presumed to reflect an unexplained failure to learn the required articulatory gestures or an unexplained delay in the suppression of phonological processes. We reject these terms on the grounds that distinguishing between biological causes that are currently known and those yet to be discovered is nonsensical and that, furthermore, we cannot force a pure demarcation between biological and environmental causes. For example, so-called functional speech problems are indeed associated with sociodemographic disadvantages (for discussion, see Shriberg, Tomblin, & McSweeny, 1999) but these sociodemographic conditions are themselves associated with biological causal-correlates such as increased risk of otitis media, fetal and child exposure to parental smoking, and low birth weight. Furthermore, environmental variables and biological maturation are reciprocally related as discussed in Part I: maturation of brain function in areas associated with language and reading development is driven in part by exposure to high quality language input. In another example, Noble, Wolmetz, Ochs, Farah, and McCandliss

The term **developmental** constrains the population of interest to children younger than age 9 years whose phonological systems are still developing.

(2006) demonstrated that socioeconomic status significantly moderates the relationship between brain function and phonological processing even when phonological abilities are controlled across advantaged and disadvantaged groups. The nature of the relationship is such that high quality inputs for children in advantaged homes buffers them from the ill effects of poor phonological processing abilities, allowing them to achieve higher reading levels and higher activations in areas of the brain important to reading than would be predicted on the basis of their phonological processing abilities alone. Disadvantaged children show a correspondence between brain activation and reading ability that is linearly predicted by their phonological processing skills, however. These kinds of studies support a dynamic systems approach to phonological disorders and highlight the joint causal influences of intrinsic and extrinsic factors on children's linguistic functioning (issues that are revisited in Chapter 7 when we discuss approaches to the subtyping of phonological disorders). For these reasons we prefer the modifier "developmental" rather than "functional" or any other term that strictly demarcates biological and nonbiological causes of phonological difficulties.

Recognizing the joint causal influences of intrinsic and extrinsic factors on development, the use of terms such as **functional** that demarcate biological and nonbiological causes of phonological difficulties are avoided.

Some classification systems explicitly differentiate between **speech delay versus speech disorder** but this distinction exists more on a continuum of severity than a sharply delineated dichotomy.

Some children's speech delay is severe enough that it places them at risk for current or future activity limitations and participation restrictions in which case the problem deserves the appellation "disorder."

Finally, there continues to be some controversy about whether the problem should be referred to as a "disorder" or a "delay." In fact, as we discuss further in Chapter 7, some classification systems explicitly differentiate between children whose speech appears to be delayed by virtue of having characteristics similar to younger normally developing children and those whose speech has characteristics deemed to be atypical. We argue as we move through Part II that the diagnostic and prognostic implications of this distinction are uncertain and that the delay-disorder classification exists more on a continuum of severity than a sharply delineated categorical distinction. We take the position that some children's speech delay is severe enough that it places them at risk for current or future activity limitations and participation restrictions in which case the problem deserves the appellation "disorder." This is essentially the position of the ICF-CY (McLeod & Threats, 2008).

Developmental phonological disorder (DPD) can be contrasted with **normal speech acquisition**, differentiating those children whose speech development is progressing as expected from those children who, at ages younger than 9 years, are producing more speech errors than would be expected for their age.

Nondevelopmental phonological disorder denotes those cases where the speech difficulty has its onset after 9 years of age.

Speech differences arise from cultural and linguistic diversity and are not considered to be a speech impairment.

Ultimately, this brings us to the diagnostic term developmental phonological disorder (DPD), which corresponds to one of the superordinate categories in the Speech Disorders Classification System as originally formulated (Shriberg, Austin, Lewis, McSweeny, & Wilson, 1997). DPD can be contrasted with normal (or normalized) speech acquisition, differentiating those children whose speech development is progressing as expected from those children who, at ages younger than 9 years, are producing more speech errors than would be expected for their age. Nondevelopmental phonological disorders denotes those cases where the speech difficulty has its onset after 9 years of age. Speech differences arise from cultural and linguistic diversity and are not considered to be a speech impairment (although a speech difference may overlap with a coexisting health problem and may have functional consequences for an individual's participation in some environments). The outcome of the initial assessment of a child who is referred due to concerns regarding speech accuracy or intelligibility should be a diagnosis with respect to one of these 4 major categories. Subsequent to an initial diagnosis of DPD the SLP may also diagnose a specific subtype of DPD, as discussed in Chapter 7.

We point out here that throughout Parts II and III we remain focused on those cases where the child's primary difficulty is with speech (and/or language and/or reading). We do not specifically cover secondary phonological disorders in which the child's speech delay is directly associated with impairments of sensory systems, cognitive deficits, craniofacial anomalies or other developmental disorders. The assessment and treatment procedures to be described are applicable to children with secondary speech delay with modifications to take these specific developmental conditions into account however.

Application of the ICF-CY to Diagnosis and Treatment Planning in the Context of DPD

In Part II we discuss assessment as the gathering of information with respect to the three levels of human functioning as classified by the ICF-CY: the body or body part revealing information about impairment; the whole child revealing the presence of activity limitations; and the child in his or her social context thus describing participation and participation restrictions in those contexts. At all three levels the information can be interpreted for diagnostic or treatment planning purposes. Diagnostic questions include the following: Does the child have a DPD? If so, what type of DPD? Are there other concomitant impairments? Treatment planning questions include the following: Is it advisable to provide an intervention? If so, what are the goals of the intervention? What approach to therapy is best suited to the child's needs? What service delivery model is best suited to the child's needs? A number of different kinds of assessment procedures that can be employed to address these questions are shown in Table II–1.

Assessment data gathered about impairment, activity limitations, or participation restrictions can be interpreted for diagnostic or treatment planning purposes.

In speech-language pathology, there are many standardized tests for the assessment of the child's speech accuracy during the production of single words relative to other children of the same age, such as the Goldman-Fristoe Test of Articulation (GFTA-2; Goldman & Fristoe, 2000). Sometimes, tests such as these are criticized because they do not provide a sample that is deep enough for the purpose of treatment planning (which is true) and thus the SLP may be inclined to omit such tests in favor of phonological measures such as the Hodson Assessment of Phonological Patterns (HAPP-3; Hodson, 2004). This practice represents a confusion of aims, however. A standardized assessment tool is essential for determining whether the child presents with DPD and assigning a severity rank-

A standardized assessment tool is essential for determining whether the child presents with a speech impairment.

Table II–1. *General Types of Assessment Tools Organized by the Three Levels of Human Functioning as Classified by the ICF-CY and by Diagnostic or Treatment Planning Purposes*

	Diagnosis Does the child have a DPD? If so what type and severity of DPD? Are there concomitant impairments in other domains?	*Treatment Planning* Need treatment? Treatment goals? Treatment approach? Service delivery model?
Body or Body Part (Impairment)	Standardized measures of treatment accuracy Measures of functioning in other speech domains (voice, resonance, fluency) Standardized measures of function in other language domains Standardized measures of functioning in other areas of development (cognitive, motor, social, etc.) Measures of hearing acuity and possibly central auditory function Standardized measures of oral motor structure and function	Measures of knowledge of linguistic units at multiple levels of the phonological hierarchy at three levels of phonological representation (requires analysis of single word and connected speech samples) Stimulability testing Measures of phonological processing that tap multiple levels of phonological knowledge and varying linguistic units (e.g., phonemic perception, phonological awareness of onsets, rimes, phonemes, nonword repetition)
Whole Child (Activity Limitations)	Measures of speech accuracy in connected speech (e.g., PCC) Standardized measures of speech intelligibility Ratings of speech intelligibility in everyday environments	Measures of speech accuracy in connected speech (e.g., PCC) Standardized measures of speech intelligibility Ratings of speech intelligibility in everyday environments
Child in Social Context (Participation Restrictions)	Structured measures of participation (e.g., FOCUS) Parent, teacher, and child interviews Case history form	Structured measures of participation (e.g., FOCUS) Observation of child in multiple contexts Diagnostic therapy

ing to the child's degree of delay relative to an appropriate normative group of age peers; therefore, a standardized test such as the GFTA-2 is an essential component of the assessment, especially the initial diagnostic assessment (this argument is developed further with case examples in Chapter 8). Subsequent to determining that the child's delay is severe enough to warrant a DPD diagnosis and the implementation of an intervention, more in-depth sampling, and analysis of the child's phonological knowledge is required to determine treatment goals and for this purpose the use of a standard protocol for sampling phonological units at multiple levels of the phonological hierarchy is essential.

In-depth sampling and analysis of the child's phonological knowledge is required to determine treatment goals.

Additional standardized assessments will determine if there are impairments in other structures or functions that contribute to the DPD, aiding in the diagnosis of a primary or secondary disorder. It is also necessary to determine if there are concomitant developmental delays in linguistic, cognitive, motor, or other domains of functioning. As indicated in Chapter 4, children who are initially referred due to late talking or unintelligible speech often prove to present with other difficulties and the SLP must be alert to the need to refer the child for assessment by other professionals when necessary. In addition to contributing to the diagnosis, in-depth assessment of the child's functioning across multiple domains will help to determine the approach to intervention that is best suited to the underlying nature of the child's DPD.

Activity limitations may be revealed by assessing speech intelligibility in natural connected speech contexts in the home and school environment.

Moving to the assessment of activity limitations, it is necessary to gather information about the child's speech accuracy and speech intelligibility in more naturalistic connected speech contexts such as conversation or narrative production. Collection of such speech samples with controlled materials in the clinic provide information about capacity whereas observations of the child's speech accuracy and intelligibility in his or her home and school environments provide information about typical levels of functioning. Discrepancies between the child's capacity as revealed by standardized tests at the single word level and performance in conversation as well as discrepancies in performance across varied environments can be of diagnostic significance. Such discrepancies may also impact on the choice of treatment goals, treatment approach, and service delivery model.

Discrepancies in performance across varied speaking contexts and environments may be explained by the extent to which contextual variables serve as barriers to or facilitators of the child's performance.

Discrepancies in performance across varied speaking contexts and environments may be explained by the extent to which contextual variables serve as barriers to or facilitators of the child's performance. These may be revealed by standard protocols such as the FOCUS (Thomas-Stonell, Oddson, Robertson, & Rosenbaum, 2009) or by interviewing the child, family and school personnel or by direct observation of the child in varying environments. Thorough examination of the child's birth, health, developmental, and academic history is also essential.

Further detail on the administration of these assessment tools and information about the interpretation of assessment results for diagnostic purposes are covered in Chapter 5. Procedures for in-depth analysis of speech samples to aid treatment planning are presented in Chapter 6. Chapter 7 provides a review of the scientific literature on possible subtypes of DPD, providing background for the interpretation of assessment data for the purpose of determining the underlying nature of the child's DPD for diagnostic and treatment planning purposes. The final chapter in Part II, Chapter 8, covers treatment planning in detail by presenting a framework for deciding which children to treat, evaluating the efficacy of selected service delivery practices and outlining evidence-based approaches to the selection of treatment goals.

References

Baker, E., Croot, K., McLeod, S., & Paul, R. (2001). Psycholinguistic models of speech development and their application to clinical practice. *Journal of Speech, Language, and Hearing Research, 44*, 685–702.

Bishop, D., & Rosenbloom, L. (1987). Classification of childhood language disorders. In W. Yule & M. Rutter (Eds.), *Language development and disorders* (pp. 16–41). London, UK: Mac Keith Press.

Blakeley, R. W., & Brockman, J. H. (1995). Normal speech and hearing by age 5 as a goal for children with cleft palate: A demonstration project. *American Journal of Speech-Language Pathology, 4*(1), 25–32.

Broder, H. L., Richman, L. C., & Matheson, P. B. (1998). Learning disability, school achievement, and grade retention among children with cleft: A two-center study. *Cleft Palate-Craniofacial Journal, 35*(2), 127–131.

Compton, A. J. (1970). Generative studies of children's phonological disorders. *Journal of Speech and Hearing Disorders, 35*(4), 315–339.

Goldman, R., & Fristoe, M. (2000). *Goldman-Fristoe Test of Articulation* (2nd ed.). Circle Pines, MN: American Guidance Service.

Hodson, B. W. (2004). *Hodson Assessment of Phonological Patterns—Third Edition*. Austin, TX: Pro-Ed.

Howard, S. J. (1993). Articulatory constraints on a phonological system: A case study of cleft palate speech. *Clinical Linguistics and Phonetics, 7*, 299–317.

McCormack, J., McLeod, S., Harrison, L. J., & McAllister, L. (2010). The impact of speech impairment in early childhood: Investigating parents' and speech-language pathologists' perspectives using the ICF-CY. *Journal of Communication Disorders, 43*, 378–396.

McCormack, J., McLeod, S., McAllister, L., & Harrison, L. J. (2010). My speech problem, your listening problem, and my frustration: The experience of living with childhood speech impairment. *Language, Speech, and Hearing Services in Schools, 41*, 379–392.

McCormack, J., & Worrall, L. E. (2008). The ICF Body Functions and Structures related to speech-language pathology. *International Journal of Speech-Language Pathology, 10*, 9–17.

McLeod, S., & Threats, T. T. (2008). The ICF-CY and children with communication disabilities. *International Journal of Speech-Language Pathology, 10*, 92–109.

Noble, K. G., Wolmetz, M. E., Ochs, L. G., Farah, M. J., & McCandliss, B. (2006). Brain-behavior relationships in reading acquisition are modulated by socioeconomic factors. *Developmental Science, 9*, 642–654.

Pamplona, M. C., Ysunza, A., & Espinoza, J. (1999). A comparative trial of two modalities of speech intervention for compensatory articulation in cleft palate children: Phonological approach versus articulatory approach. *International Journal of Pediatric Otorhinolaryngology, 49*, 21–26.

Shriberg, L. D., Austin, D., Lewis, B. A., McSweeny, J. L., & Wilson, D. L. (1997). The Speech Disorders Classification System (SDCS): Extensions and lifespan reference data. *Journal of Speech, Language, and Hearing Research, 40*(4), 723–740.

Shriberg, L. D., Tomblin, J. B., & McSweeny, J. L. (1999). Prevalence of speech delay in 6-year-old children and comorbidity with language impairment. *Journal of Speech, Language, and Hearing Research, 42*(6), 1461–1481.

Stackhouse, J. (1993). Psycholinguistic assessment of developmental speech disorders. *European Journal of Disorders of Communication, 28*(4), 331.

Thomas-Stonell, N., Oddson, B., Robertson, B., & Rosenbaum, P. (2009). Predicted and observed outcomes in preschool children following speech and language treatment: Parent and clinician perspectives. *Journal of Communication Disorders, 42*(1), 29–42.

Thomas-Stonell, N. L., Oddson, B., Robertson, B., & Rosenbaum, P. L. (2009). Development of the FOCUS (Focus on the Outcomes of Communication Under Six), a communication outcome measure for preschool children. *Developmental Medicine and Child Neurology, 52*(1), 47–53.

Threats, T. T. (2008). Use of the ICF for clinical practice in speech-language pathology. *International Journal of Speech-Language Pathology, 10*(1–2), 50–60.

World Health Organization. (2001). *International Classification of Functioning, Disability and Health (ICF)*. Geneva, Switzerland: Author.

World Health Organization. (2006). *World Health Organization Constitution*. Geneva, Switzerland: Author.

World Health Organization. (2007). *International Classification of Functioning, Disability and Health for Children and Youth (ICF-CY)*. Geneva, Switzerland: Author.

Chapter 5

Assessment of Children with Developmental Phonological Disorders

A critical aspect of the assessment process is the balance of thoroughness versus time constraints. Several factors have been suggested that could prevent clinicians from completing a thorough assessment. These include caseload size and required paperwork in the clinical setting, the limited amount of time a child can realistically cooperate during the assessment session, and limited finances of parents (Tyler et al., 2002). However, a comprehensive evaluation represents the foundation on which the clinician will design intervention strategies. "Our treatment programs follow directly from the assessment and diagnosis of the disorder and therefore, can only be as effective as the assessment is thorough and the diagnosis is accurate" (Gierut, 1986, p. 1). Although the main goal of the initial speech assessment is to identify whether the child's performance is below expectations for his age, additional goals of the evaluation include determining the severity level if difficulties are present, identifying possible etiological factors, evaluating prognosis for change, and determining a direction for intervention (Prezas & Hodson, 2007). In other words, at the end of the assessment session, parents should have an understanding of whether their child's performance is within normal limits, and if not, what possibly caused the speech difficulties, the potential for improvement, and recommendations for intervention (Tyler & Tolbert, 2002).

A **comprehensive evaluation** represents the foundation on which the clinician will design intervention strategies.

The **main goal** of the initial speech assessment is to identify whether the child is performing below age expectations.

Additional goals of the assessment include: determining the severity level, identifying etiological factors, evaluating the prognosis, and determining a direction for intervention.

In order to meet these goals, an in-depth and multifaceted assessment of the child is necessary. Sufficient information at multiple levels of representation needs to be collected in order to reach an appropriate diagnosis; on the other hand, collecting information that is not valuable in the diagnosis or treatment planning processes represent a waste of time for you, the child, and the parents. Skahan,

Information at multiple levels of representation needs to be collected to reach an appropriate diagnosis; the balance of thoroughness versus time constraint is a critical aspect of the assessment process.

Watson, and Loft (2007) recently investigated the assessment procedures used by SLPs for children suspected of having a DPD. Their questionnaire of 1,000 SLPs working with children revealed that more than 50% of them completed the direct assessment in less than 51 minutes. Most SLPs assessed speech production skills, intelligibility, and integrity of the oral-motor mechanism during the initial assessment session. However, the most important outcome goals for children and their parents are the achievement of better participation in daily life activities. The holistic nature of the ICF inherently associates the impact of the communication impairment on life activities, which allows the SLPs to align their goals with those of the client (Threats, 2010).

Although it is clear that you cannot answer all of the diagnostic and treatment planning questions shown in Table II–1 in less than an hour, we recognize that assessment is an ongoing process. Typically, the main goal of the initial assessment session is to determine if the child presents with an impairment that warrants ongoing assessment or follow-up by the SLP and/or other professionals. Remaining components that were not assessed during the initial visit can be evaluated at a later time, during the first therapy sessions, or a second assessment session. In addition, the child's performance during intervention can be compared to the baseline measures obtained during the initial assessment, as response to intervention can also help in differential diagnosis. An exciting part of the speech-language assessment is that a cookbook approach cannot be used; each child is individual and although we recommend essential assessment components, several tasks will be optional depending on each child. Taking into account the mandated requirements for an assessment and the time constraints in typical clinical practice we recommend an assessment plan as illustrated in Figure 5–1. The first section of the chapter illustrates how to evaluate Environmental and Personal Barriers and Facilitators. The second section covers the components of the assessment related to Body Functions and Structures, including standardized measures of speech accuracy; stimulability testing; measures of phonological processing such as speech perception, phonological awareness, and nonword repetition; measures of functioning in other speech and language domains; cognitive development; measures of hearing acuity and auditory processing; and standardized measures of oral motor function. The third part describes Activity Limitations, such as standardized measures and rating scales of speech intelligibility, as well as structured measures of Participation Restrictions. The fourth section addresses considerations for dialect speakers, children speaking English as a second language, and multilingual children. Finally, a case study of a preschool child with suspected DPD is presented. Measures of speech accuracy in connected speech and techniques to analyze the speech sample in depth to support treatment planning are presented in Chapter 6.

The assessment plan we recommend is illustrated in **Figure 5–1**; several tasks will be optional depending on each individual child.

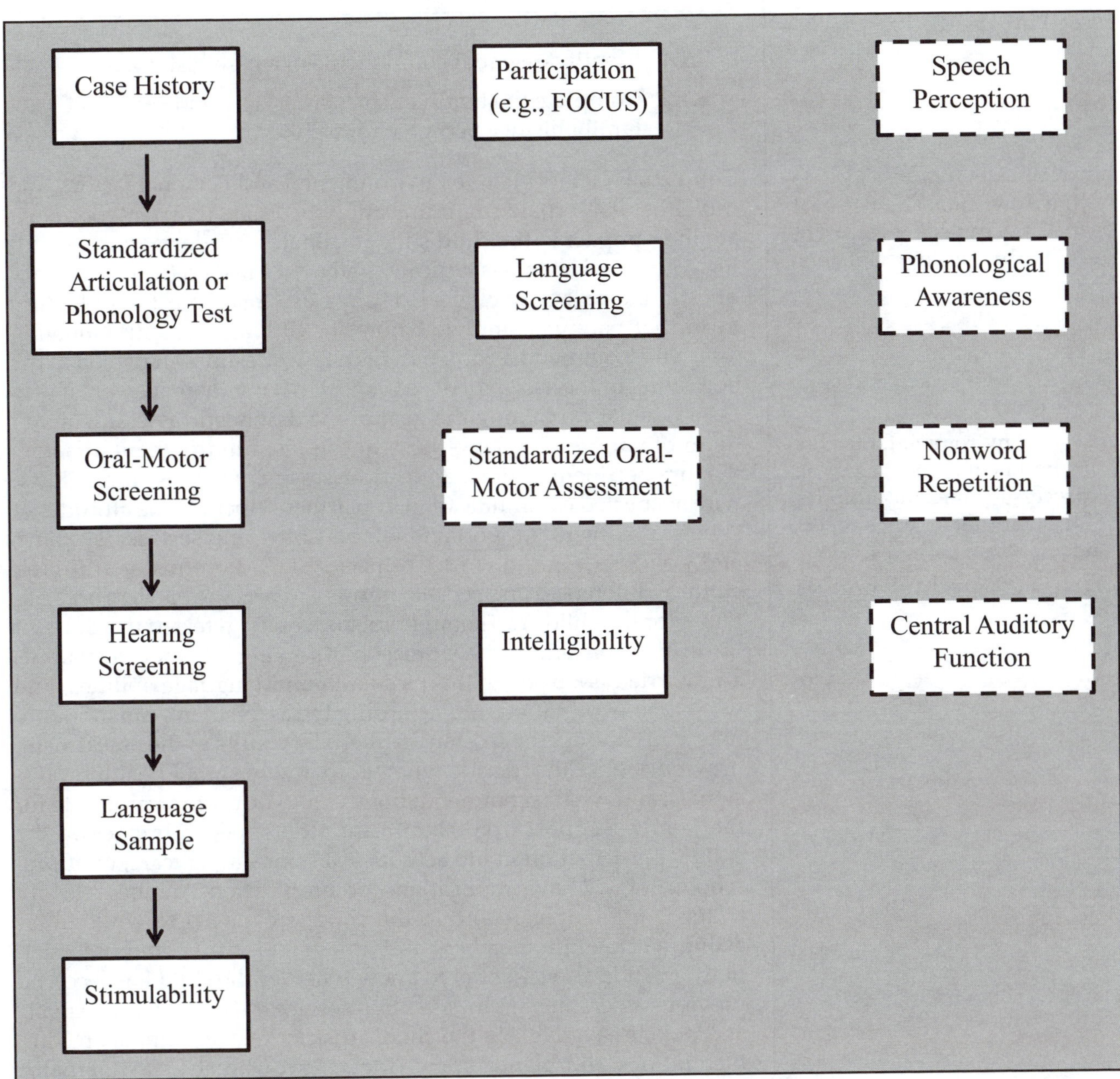

Figure 5–1. *Recommended assessment plan. Solid boxes indicate necessary components; boxes with a dashed line indicate components that are optional depending on the individual profile of the child. Left column represents the recommended sequence of tasks to be administered during the initial assessment session (75–90 minutes). Tasks in the middle column could be administered during the initial assessment session if time permits and if the child is collaborating, or during a second assessment session. Tasks in boxes with dashed lines may be useful to decide whether referrals to other health professionals such as family physicians, ENTs, psychologists, or occupational therapists are warranted for the child. Tasks in the right column could be administered during the initial therapy session to help in treatment planning.*

Contextual Barriers and Facilitators

5.1.1. Identify essential components of a case history.

5.1.2. Complete the family history interview and construct a family history pedigree for a child.

Contextual factors include Environmental and Personal factors, and can either consist of barriers or facilitators.

Environmental factors pertinent in the diagnostic process include: the attitudes of significant others; support and relationships; and services, systems, and policies.

Gathering of information from the child's case history, as well as observations made during the initial assessment and results of informal and formal testing, allow for the formulation of hypotheses, particularly regarding the etiology of the DPD and its prognosis.

Contextual factors include Environmental and Personal factors, and can either exacerbate communication disorders (barriers) or alleviate their impact in the child's life (facilitators). Information regarding contextual factors is typically gathered through the case history questionnaire. Many clinical settings use a standard case history form that parents complete before the SLP assessment. Nonetheless, we recommend asking parents a few questions in person at the beginning of the assessment session, clarifying their answers if necessary, while explaining the goal of the diagnostic assessment and the motivation for asking these questions. Environmental factors that are pertinent in the diagnostic assessment process for children with suspected communication impairments include the attitudes of significant others; support and relationships; and services, systems, and policies (McLeod & McCormack, 2007). In terms of attitudes, cultural differences and societal norms can become barriers or facilitators for the child. You should first know who referred the child for the evaluation, and for what reason. Knowing whether the parents are worried about their child's speech and language abilities, and what their expectations are regarding the assessment, can influence how you conduct the session; explain the results of the assessment; provide counseling; decide whether to involve other health professionals; and what recommendations would be more appropriate for the family. Support from significant others has an impact on the child's participation in life activities at home, at daycare, or at preschool and will have implications for intervention. Another relevant factor is the language(s) that the child is exposed to while interacting with family members and other significant communication partners. It is also essential to know whether the child has received previous assessment or intervention services. The services, systems, and policies available in the child's district will also impact recommendations and management (McLeod & Threats, 2008). Finally, personal factors such as the child's age, gender, disposition, and coping styles should also be taken into account.

Gathering of information from the child's case history, as well as observations made during the initial assessment and results of informal and formal testing, allow for the formulation of hypotheses, particularly regarding the etiology of the DPD and its prognosis (Tyler & Tolbert, 2002). The case history usually covers the following general categories: birth and medical history; developmental history; family history; education history; and social development (Bleile, 2002). Specific questions for each of these categories, in relation to the Contextual factors of the ICF, are presented in Table 5–1.

Table 5–1. *Case History: Contextual Factors and Sample Questions*

Contextual Factors	*Sample Questions*
Environmental Factors	
Attitudes and Support	Are you concerned about your child's speech and language development? Do you think your child has difficulties communicating with significant others, peers, and/or other adults?
Social Situation	Who is your child living with? Who are the main people your child interacts with?
Languages	What language(s) is your child exposed to?
Family History	Did other family members present with a speech or language impairment? Do other family members present with developmental delays? Are there other family members receiving intervention services?
Education History	Is your child currently attending, or has he previously attended daycare or preschool? Is your child currently receiving special services?
Personal Factors	
Birth History	Were there complications during pregnancy or at birth? Was your child born at term? How long was your child hospitalized after birth?
Medical History	How would you describe your child's health? Has your child been diagnosed with a medical condition? Is your child taking medication? Has your child been hospitalized, or has he had surgeries? Has your child had ear infections? If so, how many, and when? Has your child's hearing been assessed?
Developmental History	Do you have concerns about your child's development? When did your child start walking? At what age did your child start babbling? Produce his first few words? His first word combinations on a consistent basis? Produce his first short sentences?
Social Development	Do you have concerns about your child's social development? Does your child have friends? Do you have concerns about how you child interacts with friends, school mates, or family members?

Regarding the birth and medical history, special attention should be paid to hospitalizations; medications; allergies; surgeries; and diagnoses the child may have received. Parents should be asked about whether their child has had otitis media, and if so, further information about age of onset, frequency, and treatment history should be gathered. Procedures to follow if the child's hearing has not yet been assessed are discussed in the second section of this chapter. In terms of the developmental history, information about the age at which general motor and language milestones were attained, as well as whether there have been recent improvements or less progress recently, may indicate the need to obtain more information regarding other aspects of development (Hodson, Scherz, & Strattman, 2002). For instance, between 40 and 60% of children receiving treatment for DPD also present with language difficulties; receptive and expressive language may therefore also need to be assessed (Tyler & Tolbert, 2002). As seen in Chapter 7 a significant proportion of children with DPD have a positive family history of speech, language, reading, spelling, and/or learning disability. A family history for three generations should be collected (the child, siblings, and cousins being generation one; parents, uncles, and aunts being generation two; and grandparents being generation three). Lewis and Freebairn (1993) developed a tool to systematically assess family history for speech, language, and learning disorders. Their family history interview can be administered in approximately 15 minutes and collects extensive information on the nuclear family of the child, as well as on the paternal and maternal sides of the family, which is then used to draw a pedigree. The percentage of family members presenting with a speech, language and/or learning disorder can then be calculated, with a percentage higher than 10% indicating a familial basis to the DPD. Appendix 5–1 presents an adaptation of the family history interview developed by Lewis and Freebairn and instructions on how to administer the questionnaire. In brief, presence of speech-language difficulties, stuttering, reading, spelling, and learning disabilities is indicated for each biological family member of three generations.

A significant proportion of children with DPD have a positive family history of speech, language, reading, spelling, and/or learning disability. A **family history for three generations** should be collected; **Appendix 5–1** presents and adaptation of the family history interview developed by Lewis and Freebairn to do so.

During the education history, parents should be asked whether their child is attending school or daycare, and has received or is receiving special services. In addition, questions about social development allow determination of whether the child has opportunities to interact and communicate with different partners. The child could be exposed to other languages at home or with other family members outside of the home, at daycare or school, or with peers in the neighborhood. By asking parents which languages the child is exposed to, at which frequency and in which contexts, exposure or proficiency in another language, as well as dialectal differences, can be taken into account.

Parents should be asked which language(s) their child is exposed to, at which frequency and in which contexts in order to take these differences into account in the assessment process.

Family Pedigree

Demonstration 5–1 describes how to draw the pedigree for a francophone child age 4;3 who was assessed in our laboratory. Parents

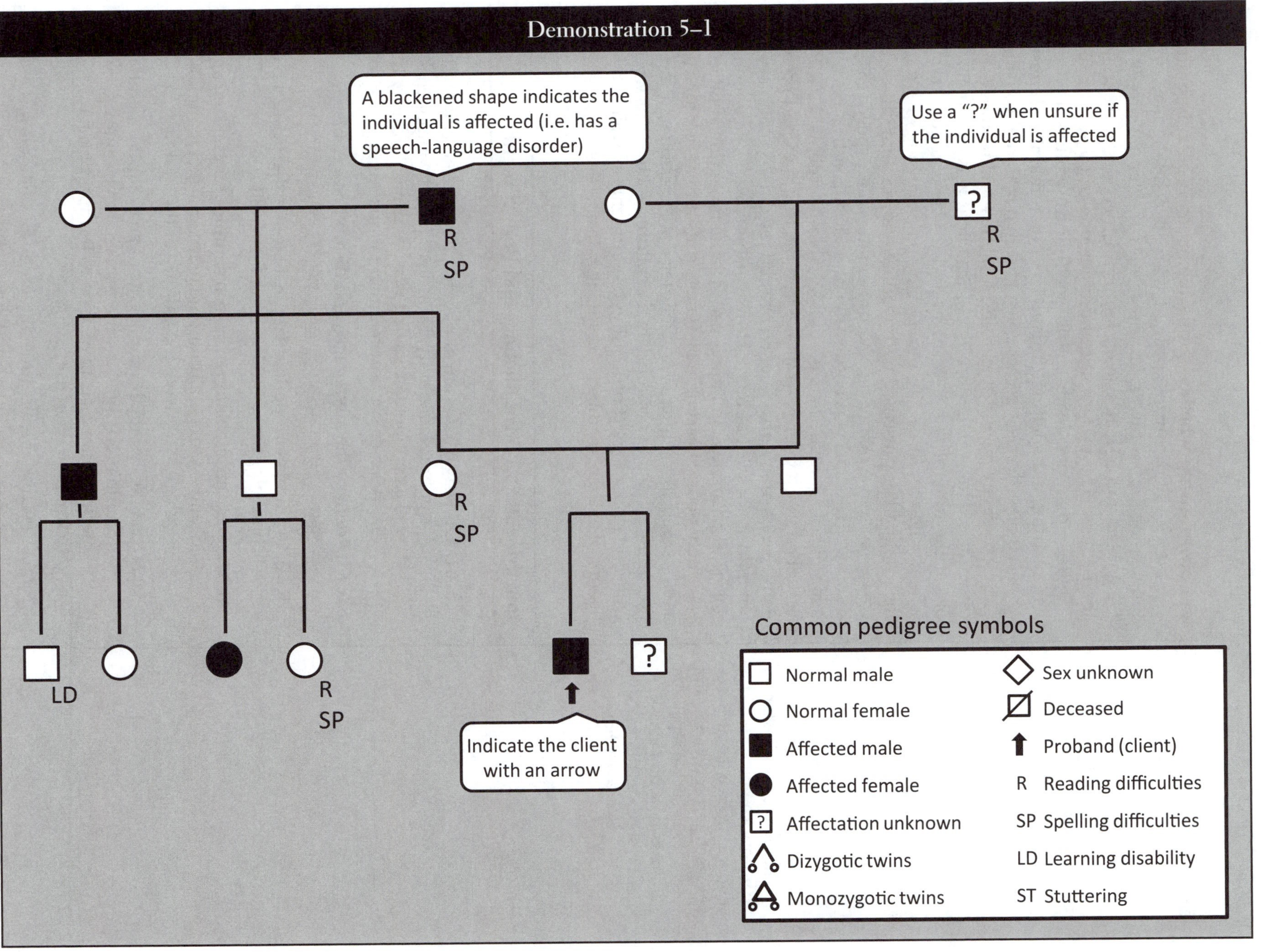
Demonstration 5–1
A blackened shape indicates the individual is affected (i.e. has a speech-language disorder)
Use a "?" when unsure if the individual is affected
?
R
SP
R
SP
R
SP
LD
R
SP
?
Indicate the client with an arrow
Common pedigree symbols
Normal male
Normal female
Affected male
Affected female
?
Affectation unknown
Dizygotic twins
Monozygotic twins
Sex unknown
Deceased
Proband (client)
R Reading difficulties
SP Spelling difficulties
LD Learning disability
ST Stuttering

are often unsure whether family members, especially grandparents, uncles and cousins, present with speech-language or communication impairments. In the case of the family presented in Demonstration 5–1, however, family history was well known to the parents. The maternal grandfather presented with a speech-language disorder, reading and spelling difficulties; the mother had reading and spelling difficulties, a maternal uncle presented a speech disorder as a preschooler, and two maternal cousins presented respectively with a learning disability and reading/spelling difficulties. The younger brother of the client was less than 2 years old at the time of the assessment and it was therefore unknown whether he would be affected. On the paternal side of the family, the grandfather presented with reading and spelling difficulties; it was unknown whether he also presented with a speech-language disorder. The child was enrolled in a randomized trial of different interventions to remediate phonological impairments (ECRIP trial) described in Chapter 9. At intake into the trial the child presented with average nonverbal intelligence and receptive vocabulary skills but mild speech impairment. However, his speech perception, phonological awareness and nonsense syllable repetition abilities were extremely poor. This profile of deficits puts him at risk for dyslexia as discussed in Chapter 7. In Chapter 9 we describe an intervention approach that is appropriate for children such as this who have DPD and phonological processing impairments as well as a family history of speech, reading, and spelling disabilities.

The child's positive family history, combined with his poor performance on measures of speech perception, PA, and nonsense syllable repetition tasks puts him at risk for **dyslexia** as discussed in Chapter 7.

Impairments in Body Functions and Body Structure

5.2.1. Design an assessment plan for a 4-year-old child referred for poor intelligibility. Include required components as well as optional tasks that may be useful to clarify the diagnosis or support treatment planning.

5.2.2. Identify the advantages and disadvantages of standardized single-word tests.

5.2.3. Administer a standardized single-word articulation or phonology test and interpret the results.

5.2.4. Plan the elicitation of speech samples for children aged 3, 5, and 7 years including the preparation of materials and strategies to ensure the validity of the sample.

5.2.5. List the essential components of an oral-peripheral examination. Interpret the results of maximum performance tests in relation to the appropriate normative reference.

5.2.6. Describe at least three different types of tools for assessing a child's phonological processing skills.

Depending on your specific clinical setting, you may have the opportunity to complete the assessment of the child's speech and language abilities over a few sessions. In Figure 5–1 we have recommended tasks that should be completed during the initial assessment visit(s), as well as tasks that can be administered during the first therapy sessions. Nonetheless, the beginning of the assessment process starts before the child comes to your office; for example when you receive the case history questionnaire from the parents, ask the referring teacher about any concerns regarding the child's speech, or meet the family and the child in the waiting room. Information gathered at that time will influence how to conduct the assessment, and in particular may have an impact on the specific order of the tasks during the assessment session(s). For instance, in Figure 5–1 we recommend administering a standardized single-word citation form test after completing the case history. However, if the parents or teacher have mentioned that the child is shy and the child has not yet talked, you could start with the receptive language test instead of moving on to the articulation or phonology test, so that the child has more time to warm up before being required to talk. At times, it may be useful to then complete the language sample, using strategies described later in this chapter for children who are reluctant to produce spontaneous speech "on demand," thus allowing the child to interact with you for a longer period of time before being required to complete the standardized articulation or phonology test. On the other hand, you could start with all the formal testing tasks right away if the child seems very active and the parent mentions the child has a very short attention span. Typically in this case we explain to the child he will first complete the articulation test, oral-motor screening, and hearing screening (if necessary) which should take about 30 minutes, and then he will play with the clinician. In general, however, we recommend conducting the case history at the beginning of the session which allows you not only to clarify the expectations of the parents regarding your assessment and their concerns about their child's speech and language abilities, but also to observe the child while playing and interacting with his parents. This initial observation will help you decide in what particular order you plan to administer the assessment tasks; behavior of the child and his performance during each task may also lead you to make changes later on in the session.

The beginning of the assessment starts before the child comes to your office: information gathered before the assessment visit and when meeting the child in the waiting room will influence how you conduct the assessment, and particularly the specific order of the tasks.

Standardized Single-Word Citation-Form Tests

The administration of a norm-referenced, single-word standardized articulation/phonology test is an essential part of the assessment process. The purpose of a standardized articulation test is to compare the performance of the child to a normative sample of same age peers to determine if a DPD is present, with a percentile rank less than 16 indicating the presence of speech impairment. Percen-

Administering a norm-referenced, single-word standardized articulation test is essential and allows one to compare the performance of the child to a normative sample of age peers to determine if a DPD is present.

tile ranks derived from the test also allow the clinician to assign a severity ranking of the child's speech difficulties and are very convenient for showing parents how their child is performing in comparison to peers. Finally, percentile ranks are sometimes required to qualify for services or third-party payments (Tyler & Tolbert, 2002).

An additional advantage of **single-word tests** is that the target words are known, allowing one to collect data from children whose speech is largely unintelligible and thus not easily analyzable with other speech sampling methods.

Standardized single-word tests typically elicit spontaneous production of single words by having the child name pictures or photographs to sample consonants, consonant clusters, and at times vowels and diphthongs. Single-word articulation tests provide a comparison of the child's performance with that of the normative group in a time-efficient and standardized manner. An additional advantage of single-word tests is that the target words are known, which facilitates transcription and comparison of the child's production to the adult form (Bernhardt & Holdgrapher, 2001; Hodson et al., 2002). Most, and often all, English consonants are targeted in the initial and final positions; several tests also target consonants in the medial position. As mentioned previously, vowels are rarely targeted, as most children master production of vowels by the age of 3 (see Chapter 4; Dodd, Holm, Hua, & Crosbie, 2003; Donegan, 2002; Pollock & Berni, 2003). However, as discussed in Chapter 4, some children with DPD do produce vowel errors and these errors have diagnostic significance, especially for the identification of motor speech disorders. As vowels are rarely targeted in single-word articulation tests, and most of them record the production of one instance of each consonant in each word position, Klein (1984) recommended transcribing all the sounds in each test item. Although not all sounds transcribed will contribute toward the score obtained on the test, the whole-word transcriptions are informative and can help determine intervention goals in combination with other sampling procedures such as the connected speech sample. This is discussed later in this chapter and in detail in Chapter 6. Information regarding the most common standardized single-word articulation and phonology tests is presented in Table 5–2.

Transcribe all the sounds in each test item of single-word articulation tests. Not all sounds transcribed will contribute toward the score on the test, but the **whole-word transcriptions** can help determine intervention goals in combination with other sampling methods.

Several criticisms of single-word tests have been reported. For instance, most of the test items are nouns, as they are easier to represent by drawings or pictures (Bernhardt & Holdgrapher, 2001). Similarly, single words cannot assess the effects of coarticulation, and the child's ability to produce certain sounds in single words may not be representative of the child's ability to produce the same sounds in different contexts. Moreover, most articulation tests do not distinguish between substitutions, omissions, distortions, and additions (SODA). This system of scoring is also commonly referred to as five-way scoring, with correct responses representing one category and the different types of errors representing the other four categories (as shown in Figure 1–22). In most single-word articulation tests, two-way scoring is used (correct or incorrect); the score corresponds to the total number of speech sound errors produced by the child even if the various types of errors impact intelligibility differently. For example, omissions of consonants will have quite

Most articulation tests do not distinguish between **SODA** (substitutions, omissions, distortions, and additions). Usually, **two-way scoring** is used instead: correct or incorrect.

Table 5–2. *Standardized Single-Word Tests of Articulation and Phonology Published Since 1990*

Name of Test	*Authors & Year*	*Publisher*	*Age Range (norms)*	*Number of words*	*Consonant Positions*
Arizona Articulation Proficiency Scale, 3rd ed. (AAPS-3)	Fudala, 2000	Western Psychological Services	1;6–18;0	42	IF
Bankson-Bernthal Test of Phonology (BBTOP)	Bankson & Bernthal, 1990	Special Press	3;0–9;0	80	IF
Clinical Assessment of Articulation and Phonology (CAAP)	Secord & Donahue, 2002	Super Duper® Publications	2;6–8;11	44	IF
Diagnostic Evaluation of Articulation and Phonology (DEAP)	Dodd, Hua, Crosbie, Holm, & Ozanne, 2003	Psychological Corporation®	3;0–6;11	30	IF
Goldman-Fristoe Test of Articulation, 2nd ed. (GFTA-2)	Goldman & Fristoe, 2000	Pearson	2;0–21;11	53	IMF
Hodson Assessment of Phonological Patterns (HAPP-3)	Hodson, 2004	Pro-Ed	3;0–8;0	50	n/a
Khan-Lewis Phonological Analysis, 2nd ed. (KLPA-2)	Khan & Lewis, 2002	American Guidance Service	2;0–21;11	53	n/a
LinguiSystems Articulation Test (LAT)	Bowers & Huisingh, 2010	LinguiSystems	3;0–21;11	52	IMF
Photo-Articulation Test, 3rd ed. (PAT-3)	Lippke, Dickey, Selmar, & Soder, 1997	Pro-Ed	3;0–8;11	77	IMF
Smit-Hand Articulation and Phonology Evaluation (SHAPE)	Smit & Hand, 1997	Western Psychological Services®	3;0–9;0	81	IF
Structured Photographic Articulation Test, 2nd ed. (SPAT–II)	Dawson & Tattersall, 2001	Janelle Publications	3;0–9;0	45	IMF

Note: The AAPS-3, DEAP, and HAPP-3 also measure the accuracy of vowels.

a detrimental effect on intelligibility whereas distortions such as interdental lisps may not significantly diminish intelligibility (Prezas & Hodson, 2007). As there are no distinctions between SODA on single-word articulation tests, it is also difficult to notice progress after intervention if the child no longer omits consonants but rather substitutes or distorts them.

Another criticism of single-word articulation and/or phonology tests is that the child's performance on each specific test item may be related to factors other than the child's true capacity. As the goal of the test is to determine whether the child's performance is within normal limits, the particular target words selected on the test may not be appropriate by themselves to determine sounds missing from the child's phonetic inventory. For example, word-initial consonants are more likely to be mispronounced in unstressed than stressed syllables and word-initial fricatives are more likely to be produced accurately in monosyllabic than longer words (Ingram, Christensen, Veach, & Webster, 1980). Recently, Eisenberg and Hitchcock (2010) compared all occurrences of word-initial and word-final singleton consonants and vowels on 11 standardized single-word tests of articulation and phonology. They found that none of the tests targeted all consonants and/or vowels in at least two "phonetically controlled words." For singleton consonants, they defined a phonetically controlled word as having the following characteristics: (1) monosyllabic or bisyllabic word; (2) target consonant different from the consonants in the other positions; (3) target consonant in the stressed syllable if bisyllabic word; and (4) target consonant not part of a separate morpheme for word-final consonants. The authors therefore did not recommend using only the whole-word transcriptions from a single-word articulation test to complete the phonetic inventory and select intervention goals.

Standardized articulation/phonology tests do not target all consonants and/or vowels in phonetically controlled contexts. Whole-word transcriptions of items on these tests should not be used by themselves to derive a phonetic inventory and select intervention goals.

Although we agree with all of the criticisms as reviewed above, the goal of the single-word test is to compare the performance of the child to a normative sample to identify whether DPD is present. McCauley and Swisher (1984) discussed the misuse of normative tests and noted that they should not be used to select intervention goals or make conclusions about the efficacy of the intervention. Single-word tests provide a comparison of the child's performance with the performance of the normative group in a time-efficient manner. They also allow obtaining data from children with a wide range of severity of DPD, including children whose speech is largely unintelligible and thus not easily analyzable with other speech sampling methods. Although there are disadvantages with regards to the phonetic contexts sampled and limited representativeness of connected speech, transcriptions of whole words are a valuable sampling procedure that can be used in combination with the speech sample.

Normative tests should not be used to select intervention goals or make conclusions about the efficacy of the intervention.

Scoring of a Standardized Articulation Test

Demonstration 5–2 shows the scored Sound-In-Words subtest of the Goldman-Fristoe Test of Articulation-2 (Goldman & Fristoe, 2000) for PA 218. As can be seen in the demonstration, we did not calculate the age equivalent for the child, as it should not be used for making diagnostic or intervention decisions due to inherent psychometric problems with this measure (Bracken, 1988). Percentile ranks are the preferred score to use to make clinical decisions as error scores from articulation and phonology tests are not normally distributed.

The **age-equivalent measure** cannot be used for making diagnostic or intervention decisions due to psychometric problems.

Demonstration 5–2

Online age calculators and applications are available to ensure accurate calculation of the age of the child. Alternatively, confirm the age of the child in years and months with the parent.

Age Calculation

	Year	Month	Day
Test Date	2002	05	28
Birth Date	1997	06	22
Chronological Age	4	11	6

Verify whether the age of the child is to be rounded up if the number of days exceeds 15.

Scoring of the stimulus words

Plate			
1.	/haʊs/ → [haʊt]	/tri/ → [tʃiv]	/wɪndo/ → [wɪndo]
2.	/tɛləfon/ → [won]		
3.	/kʌp/ → [kʌp]	/naɪf/ → [naɪt]	/spun/ → [bun]
4.	/gɝl / → [gɝəl]	/bɔl/ → [bəl]	
5.	/wægən/ → [wægən]	/ʃʌvəl/ → [jəʃəl]	
6.	/mʌŋki/ → [mʌŋki]	/bənænə/ → [minænæ]	
7.	/zɪpɚ/ → [jɪpoɚ]		
8.	/sɪzɚz/ → [jɪdɚd]		
9.	/dʌk/ → [dʌk]	/kwæk/ → [kæk]	/jɛlo/ → [lɛlo]
10.	/vækjum/ → [wækjum]		
11.	/watʃ/ → [wat]		
12.	/plen/ → [pen]		
13.	/swɪmɪŋ/ → [wɪmɪŋ]		
14.	/watʃɪz/ → [wat]		

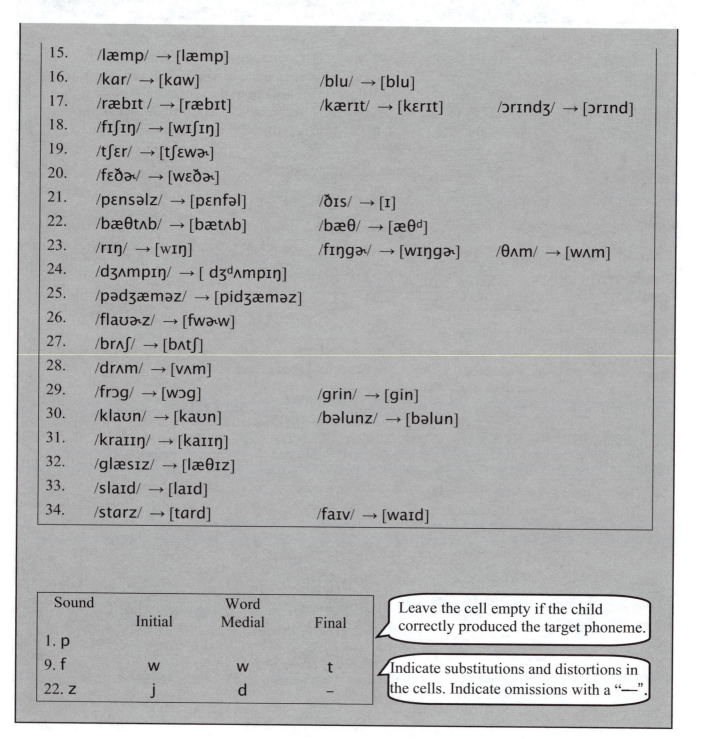

15.	/læmp/ → [læmp]		
16.	/kɑr/ → [kɑw]	/blu/ → [blu]	
17.	/ræbɪt / → [ræbɪt]	/kærɪt/ → [kɛrɪt]	/ɔrɪndʒ/ → [ɔrɪnd]
18.	/fɪʃɪŋ/ → [wɪʃɪŋ]		
19.	/tʃɛr/ → [tʃɛwɚ]		
20.	/fɛðɚ/ → [wɛðɚ]		
21.	/pɛnsəlz/ → [pɛnfəl]	/ðɪs/ → [ɪ]	
22.	/bæθtʌb/ → [bætʌb]	/bæθ/ → [æθ^{d}]	
23.	/rɪŋ/ → [wɪŋ]	/fɪŋgɚ/ → [wɪŋgɚ]	/θʌm/ → [wʌm]
24.	/dʒʌmpɪŋ/ → [dʒ^{d}ʌmpɪŋ]		
25.	/pədʒæməz/ → [pidʒæməz]		
26.	/flaʊɚz/ → [fwɚw]		
27.	/brʌʃ/ → [bʌtʃ]		
28.	/drʌm/ → [vʌm]		
29.	/frɔg/ → [wɔg]	/grin/ → [gin]	
30.	/klaʊn/ → [kaʊn]	/bəlunz/ → [bəlun]	
31.	/kraɪɪŋ/ → [kaɪɪŋ]		
32.	/glæsɪz/ → [læθɪz]		
33.	/slaɪd/ → [laɪd]		
34.	/stɑrz/ → [tɑrd]	/faɪv/ → [waɪd]	

Sound	Initial	Word Medial	Final
1. p			
9. f	w	w	t
22. z	j	d	–

Leave the cell empty if the child correctly produced the target phoneme.

Indicate substitutions and distortions in the cells. Indicate omissions with a "—".

This peculiarity of articulation tests occurs because the total scores are error scores (rather than number of correct responses) and because the words have not been selected to become more difficult as the test participants become older (as is the case with a vocabulary test for example). However, some service providers require that a child fall below a certain standard score, such as 84 or 77, in order to qualify for services. If a standard score is required, you must use the table provided in the test manual; do not transform it manually from the percentile rank. As the distribution of the raw scores is not normally distributed, a percentile rank of 16 will not necessarily correspond to a standard score of 84 and a *z*-score of −1 as would be the case for normed tests where the total scores correspond to a normal distribution. In the case of PA218, age 4;11, a percentile rank of 4 on the GFTA-2 corresponds to a standard score of 65 in the test manual, whereas it would indicate a standard score of 74 or 75 on the normal curve.

You cannot manually transform the standard score from the percentile rank for articulation/ phonology tests because the distribution of raw scores is not normally distributed.

Connected Speech Sample

The speech sample is a crucial part of the assessment process and should always be collected. However, only about one-third of clinicians consistently elicit a connected speech sample when assessing children suspected of presenting DPD (Skahan et al., 2007) probably because of perceived time constraints and lack of transcription skills. Although obtaining a speech sample from a child who is conscious of his speech difficulties and does not want to talk much can sometimes be a challenge, it is feasible to obtain an adequate speech sample in 10 to 15 minutes. Connected speech samples present several advantages over single-word samples. First, they are more ecologically valid and allow analysis of the accuracy of speech sound production in conversation, which represents the long-term intervention goal for children with DPD. Furthermore, they allow assessment of intelligibility in conversation, informal assessment of prosody, voice, resonance, fluency as well as pragmatics and expressive language skills, as discussed later in this chapter (Bernhardt & Holdgrafer, 2001; Miccio, 2002; Tyler & Tolbert, 2002). In fact, obtaining a speech sample allows an appraisal of several skills in a short period of time.

The **speech sample** has several advantages: it is more ecologically valid and allows for the appraisal of speech production accuracy, voice, resonance, fluency, pragmatics, and expressive language skills in conversation.

Obtaining a good speech sample requires carefully planning the elicitation strategy to maximize the information obtained in the time available. Shriberg and Kwiatkowski (1985) identified four potential threats to the validity of the speech sample: (1) productivity: the child may not speak much; (2) intelligibility: unintelligible speech makes it very difficult to gloss the sample and transcribe what the child is saying; (3) representativeness: the utterances produced by the child will not necessarily contain a representative sample of English phonemes and word shapes; and (4) reactivity: children may react to the stimuli used during the speech sample and use unusual speaking registers that will affect the analyses. Finally, in the context of conversation, the probability of the child deleting, substituting or assimilating phonemes is increased relative to the single-word context (Morisson & Shriberg, 1992). It is therefore recommended that both types of sample be elicited as their respective advantages complement each other and there might be discrepancies between the two types of samples, which are informative for diagnosis

There are several potential **threats to the validity** of the speech sample: productivity, intelligibility, representativeness, and reactivity.

and treatment planning purposes. We first review recommendations regarding the size and characteristics of the speech sample, followed by descriptions of different manners of eliciting the speech sample to minimize the potential threats to their validity, and, last, how best to record the speech sample.

Size of the Speech Sample

Speech sample size has been frequently discussed in the literature (e.g., Andrews & Fey, 1986; Bernhardt & Holdgrafer, 2001; Dinnsen & Elbert, 1984; Morrison & Shriberg, 1992). There is no clear consensus as to what minimum sample length provides a maximum of information; however, according to Grunwell, "a comprehensive analysis requires a minimum of 100 different words" (1985, p.7). Typically developing 3- to 5-year-old children produce an average of 148 syllables per minute (range 109 to 183 syllables/min) in conversation (Pindzola, Jenkins, & Lokken, 1989), which corresponds to 60 to 100 words per minute depending on their length. Taking into account the fact that the clinician will interact with the child during the sample collection and that the child may at times remain silent, eliciting a speech sample of 100 to 200 words with children should not take more than 10 to 15 minutes.

We recommend eliciting a speech sample of 100 to 200 words. Specific strategies to elicit the conversational speech sample within 10 to 15 minutes are presented in **Table 5–3**.

In Chapter 6 we demonstrate how to conduct a nonlinear phonology analysis on the speech sample. In order to conduct such an in-depth analysis, the speech sample should meet specific criteria. As the key remains the balance of time-constraints versus effectiveness, collecting a longer speech sample than the typical 100 to 200 words may not be efficient to select treatment goals for children with a few error patterns or consistent error patterns. For children with inconstant productions or complex error patterns, it may be necessary to supplement the speech sample with a list of words targeting specific features or word shapes in order to select the optimal intervention goals for them (Bernhardt & Holdgrafer, 2001b). In brief, the sample should provide information for all levels of the phonological hierarchy and using both the single-word articulation or phonology test and words obtained in the connected speech sample is preferable. For instance, the standard phrasal-stress patterns are stressed-unstressed (strong-weak; S-w); unstressed-stressed (w-S) and stressed-unstresssed-unstressed-stressed (S-w-w-S). Words or syllables may be deleted by the child when they fall in an unstressed position (Bernhardt & Stemberger, 1998) and words can be contrasted according to their stress patterns. In terms of word shapes, mono- and bisyllabic words are the most frequently occurring word lengths in English. Single-word citation-form tests rarely probe multisyllabic words, and some children avoid producing longer words in their spontaneous speech sample; for them it may be necessary to elicit three and four-syllable words. It is also useful to compare two-syllable and longer words that are monomorphemic (such as *dinosaur*) and words that have more than one morpheme (such as *eating*

The speech sample should provide information for all levels of the phonological hierarchy. An example of when and how you can **supplement the speech sample** for an in-depth phonological analysis is presented in **Chapter 6**.

or *bathtub*). The word shapes CVC, CCVC, CVCC, and CVC.CVC should be included, targeting liquids, nasals, stops, and fricatives in singleton and complex onsets and codas. You can verify whether various word shapes, all consonant manners and places, sequences of place, voicing contrast, and various vowels (high and low, front and back, diphthongs) are present in the language sample once it has been collected. Specific tools are available to supplement the sample if needed. For example, McLeod and Hand (1991) developed a comprehensive single word test of consonant clusters. The test contains 72 words; each word-initial and word-final cluster commonly used in Australian English is elicited twice. This test may be useful if the child you are assessing produced very few clusters during the language sample. The test was designed to assess whether consonant clusters are produced differently by the child depending on their word position, number of elements in the consonant cluster, and features of the consonants in the cluster. Instructions on how to administer the test, scoring form, and target pictures are available free of cost at http://athene.riv.csu.edu.au/~smcleod/Consonantclustertest.pdf. Readers are referred to the two companion articles by Bernhardt and Holdgrafer (2001; 2001b) for further details of the sampling needs for an in-depth nonlinear phonological analysis. In the next chapter an example of when and how it would be appropriate to supplement the original speech sample with a list of words is provided.

Specific tools are available to supplement the sample if required, such as the **single word test of consonant clusters** developed by McLeod and Hand (1991).

Eliciting the Continuous Sample

The preferred method in the field of speech-language pathology for obtaining a continuous speech sample consists of spontaneous conversation, and there is some debate as to whether imitative responses should be used (Goldstein, Fabiano, & Iglesias, 2004). Several studies have investigated whether speech sound accuracy is different in imitative responses from spontaneous responses in normally developing preschoolers (e.g., Paynter & Bumpas, 1977; Siegel, Winitz, & Conkey, 1963; Templin, 1947). Overall, the results obtained from imitative procedures in these studies were not appreciably different from spontaneous responses. As mentioned previously, however, the particular stimuli used to elicit the sample, such as stress, word shape, and neighboring phonemes can have an impact on speech sound accuracy. Therefore, Kenney, Prather, Mooney, and Jeruzal (1984) controlled the phonetic context and semantic difficulty of three sampling procedures, namely delayed imitation in a picture naming task, direct imitation in a nonsense word naming task, and conversation in a story retell task. A total of 30 typically developing children age 4;4 to 4;8 participated in the task. The outcome measure was the accuracy of production of the phonemes /ɹ,s,l,tʃ,ʃ,k,f,t/ in each of the sampling tasks. Results showed no significant differences in the number or types of errors across the sampling tasks although there was a trend toward more

The preferred method to elicit the continuous speech sample consists of **spontaneous conversation**.

errors with the direct imitation of nonsense words. In short, use of an imitative sampling procedure when the phonetic complexity of the stimuli was controlled did not improve the performance of the children. Fewer studies, however, have investigated whether the use of imitative or spontaneous sampling procedures affects the accuracy of the speech sound productions of preschool children with DPD. Goldstein, Fabiano, and Iglesias (2004) asked 12 Spanish-speaking children age 3;1 to 4;9 and with mild-moderate DPD (as determined by percentage of consonants correct, or PCC, values of 65 to 85%) to name a picture spontaneously; if there was a speech sound error in the spontaneous production a second response was obtained using delayed imitation. The children's productions were identical under both sampling tasks 62% of the time. Words produced spontaneously were more accurate than in delayed imitation in 12% of cases, and imitative productions were more accurate than spontaneous productions in 25% of the words. There were differences between children, indicating that child-specific factors play a role in whether imitative productions are more accurate than spontaneous productions. Although overall the result indicates that using imitative responses is appropriate, we must keep in mind that older children and children who have previously received speech therapy may very well perform better in imitation than in spontaneous productions. Therefore, we recommend, as is the consensus in the field, to use spontaneous conversation to elicit the speech sample. If the child is not sufficiently talkative and you have used the strategies described at the end of this section without obtaining an adequate length of speech sample in about 10 minutes, do not hesitate to use sentence imitation if necessary.

Although we recommend eliciting the speech sample in conversation, do not hesitate to use **sentence imitation** if the child is not sufficiently talkative.

The usual elicitation procedure to obtain the continuous sample consists of engaging the child in spontaneous conversation. Various methods can be used to do so, and Shriberg and Kwiatkowski (1985) noted that questions used by the examiner and the materials presented to the child could have an impact on the productivity, intelligibility, representativeness, and reactivity of the child during the collection of the speech sample. They compared five sampling conditions in 12 children age 2;10 to 4;6 with DPD (PCC values ranging from 62 to 77%). The sampling conditions were (1) free: child-selected toys, few instructions or prompts provided by the examiner; (2) story: child made picture with "Muppet" reusable stickers and background board, examiner used nondirective comments related to the materials such as, "Tell me about your picture," "I don't know anything about this one. Can you tell me something about him?"; (3) routines: house setup, examiner asked questions and commented on the materials such as "I am putting the girl in the bed. Now your turn to tell me what you need and where you will put it" and "What is this boy doing in the kitchen?"; (4) interview: no materials, examiner asked open-ended questions about the child, his favorite activities and interests; and (5) scripted: picture

The specific questions and materials you use while collecting the speech sample can impact the child's productivity, intelligibility, representativeness, and reactivity.

book selected by the examiner who used a script to prompt specific words and phrases. There were no significant differences in terms of productivity, as measured by the total number of words and number of different words used by the child. The percentage of intelligible words also did not significantly differ between the sampling conditions. In addition, there were no significant differences regarding representativeness, as measured in terms of the parts of speech used by the child, types of intended consonants and types of intended syllable and word shapes. Differences were found regarding reactivity: children were more likely to use a reduced register (whispering or mumbling), playful register (different voices for the play characters), or sound effects (for example, animal and vehicle noises) during the free play, story, and routine conditions. However, these differences in reactivity did not impact the phonetic accuracy of the children's utterances and therefore the differences between these five sampling conditions were clinically nonsignificant. In other words, any of these five sampling conditions can be used with the child being assessed.

There were **no clinically significant differences between sampling conditions**. Free play, routines, telling a story, asking the child open-ended questions, or following a script could be used to obtain the speech sample.

We have found in our laboratory that wordless books such as *Good Dog Carl*, by Alexandra Day, are very useful in eliciting a narrative language sample with preschool children with DPD, a strategy also recommended by Tyler and Tolbert (2002). Using a playhouse and accessories to obtain the language sample is also usually successful; Miccio (2002) recommends asking the child to talk about familiar activities, using sabotage strategies during tabletop activities, such as forgetting to give the child all the necessary materials or mixing up materials from another game, as children who do not engage in pretend play may be engaged by daily living activities such as making cookies.

Shriberg and Kwiatkowski (1985) recommend being flexible and ready to modify the sampling procedure as necessary during the session to ensure that the child will keep talking. Monitor representativeness of the sample as you proceed and use questions or prompts or introduce materials as necessary to ensure coverage of the distribution of the English phonemes. Most importantly, to collect an adequate speech sample with children, the amount of talking from the examiner should be kept to a minimum; for very shy children the proportion of examiner to child talking time might be closer to 50%, but you should not be talking more than the child. Although it can feel awkward, remaining silent for several seconds or more is a strategy we have found to be successful with many children who did not seem talkative at the beginning of the speech sample collection. On very rare occasions, once we felt we had tried all these strategies, we have left the child and the parent alone in the assessment room with a wordless book and toys, recorded their conversation, and stood by the door, transcribing what the child said. A summary of recommendations to obtain an adequate speech sample in 10 to 15 minutes is presented in Table 5–3.

While collecting the language sample, the amount of talking from the examiner should be kept at a minimum and **not exceed 50%**.

Table 5–3. Useful Strategies to Obtain a Speech Sample

Strategies
Ask open-ended questions about a familiar topic of conversation (the child's pets, favorite movie, television show, or activity).
Ask the child to describe how to make cookies, build a snowman, etc.
Ask a choice question by providing two answers, one of which is clearly the correct answer.
Use fill-in-the-blank completion prompts.
Avoid yes-no questions.
Remain silent for several seconds or more if necessary while waiting for the child to respond.
Follow the child's lead when replying to the child's response.
Do not comment on or correct the accuracy of the child's speech.

Recording the Speech Sample

Transcribe on-line as much as possible and **recast** the utterances understood by the adults when collecting the language sample in order to decrease the amount of time required to complete the transcription at a later time.

The quality of the recording of the speech sample can **only be as good as the weakest step in the recording process** (microphone, cabling, preamplifier, and recording device).

You should transcribe online as much as possible to decrease the amount of time necessary to complete the transcription at a later time. For unintelligible children, it is also very useful to recast in a natural way the utterances understood by the adults in the room: the flow of conversation will not be broken, and the recasts will prove helpful to transcribe what the child said when listening to the recording. Vogel and Morgan (2009) recently discussed the methodological factors related to the selection of hardware and recording software, microphone, recording environment, and sampling rate. In certain cases it may be useful to record speech for acoustic analyses, which will require very good quality sound recordings. As explained by Vogel and Morgan, "the quality of the recording is only as good as the weakest link" (2009, p. 432). In other words, if the microphone, cabling, preamplifier, or recording device is not optimal the sound quality will be limited by that particular step in the recording process regardless of the quality of the other components. Although the best configuration consists of recording in a sound room with a stand-alone hard disk recorder, high-caliber microphone, independent mixer to lessen the input, and insulated wiring, other configurations that take into account limited budget, need for portability and use with children can be perfectly adequate for recording and transcribing speech samples and conducting some acoustic measures. In terms of hardware, it is best if the recording level can be adjusted. If using the computer to record, the software typically allows controlling the sampling rate (approximately 22 kHz is recommended to capture all the frequencies of speech), mono or stereo input, and file format (.wav, .avi, or .aif are recommended as they do not compress the signal and reduce the quality of the recording). The microphone is a crucial component of the recording process: its sensitivity and frequency response, as well as the distance to the talker and angle of recording, can all have a significant effect on signal quality. The frequency response of the microphone, which ideally would remain constant across all speech frequencies, can particularly modify the acoustic signal (Parsa, Jamieson, & Pretty, 2001). Clinically, we have found that when collecting speech samples from children it is best to use a unidirectional microphone and position it so that the children will not touch it with their hands or mouth, or breathe directly into it. The recording environment is often problematic, as assessment rooms with lots of reverberation are often the norm (e.g. due to little furniture and/or no carpet), siblings are sometimes present in the room during the recording and other children can be playing loudly in the hallway. By using a unidirectional microphone, positioning it properly and ensuring that extraneous noise is limited as much as possible (for instance by asking the parent to step out of the room with the younger sibling and trying to plan the language sample collection for a time at which there are no other children playing in the hallway), it is possible to record high-quality speech samples.

In terms of the hardware, adjustable recording levels, a sampling rate of 22 kHz and .wav, .avi, or .aif file formats are recommended.

Stimulability Testing

Stimulability is the child's ability to correctly imitate a phoneme following the model of the clinician (Miccio, 2002; Rvachew, 2005). In most cases, the child is asked to watch the clinician's face and listen to what she says (Lof, 1996). If the child is not readily stimulable given audiovisual input, the SLP may supplement with verbal placement instructions and tactile cues in order to determine the level of support that the child needs in order to produce the sound correctly (Glaspey & Stoel-Gammon, 2007). The results of the stimulability assessment provide valuable information regarding prognosis. It is more likely the child will make more rapid progress mastering a phoneme when it is stimulable (e.g., Miccio, Elbert, & Forrest, 1999; Tyler, 1996). There is, however, controversy as to how the results of the stimulability assessment should be taken into account for selecting treatment targets, and more specifically, over whether stimulable or nonstimulable sounds should be treated first (Tyler & MacRae, 2010). This issue is discussed in Chapter 8.

Stimulability is the child's ability to correctly imitate a phoneme when provided with an audiovisual model; additionally, verbal placement instructions and tactile cues can be used.

Stimulability is usually assessed in different linguistic environments. Tyler and Tolbert (2002) use a short stimulability task that varies with the child's articulation competence for each phoneme: (1) if the sound is absent from the inventory, assess stimulability in isolation and if correct, then in CV and VC syllables; (2) if the sound is incorrectly produced in a particular word position, assess stimulability in that position in syllables and words; and (3) if the sound is inconsistently produced accurately in words, assess stimulability of the sound at the word and sentence level. The Glaspey Dynamic Assessment of Phonology (GDAP), formerly the Scaffolding Scale of Stimulability described in Glaspey and Stoel-Gammon (2007), elicits all phonemes in initial and final word positions and /ɹ/, /s/, /l/ clusters. If the child accurately produces the target, the linguistic environment is systematically made more complex; conversely if the child mispronounces the target, cues are gradually added in a cumulative and additive fashion, meaning that if a cue is used it can be used again, but not removed. Four different cue levels and six linguistic environments are included, as shown in Figure 5–2. The administration of the GDAP starts at the word level, without cues. If the child incorrectly produces the target in this context, the SLP moves to the right of the chart to add cues. If the child continues to incorrectly produce the target the SLP moves down to the isolation context. If the child correctly produces the target in a word when asked "What's this?" the SLP moves up the chart to sentences. We recommend using this protocol for potential or actual treatment targets only, as it is most useful as a systematic means of collecting information to aid in decisions such as selecting treatment targets, deciding when to terminate treatment for a given sound, or when to introduce treatment for a new sound. The tool is also very useful to document progress on treated sounds and generalization of treatment effects to untreated sounds.

The **Glaspey Dynamic Assessment of Phonology** (GDAP) systematically varies cue levels and linguistic environments to assess stimulability, and is shown in **Figure 5–2**. We recommend using this protocol for potential or actual treatment targets.

Standardized Measures of Oral-Motor Function

The oral peripheral examination is an important part of the differential diagnostic process and may be particularly useful in the identification of etiological factors or underlying speech processes. The role of the SLP is not to diagnose a specific condition but rather to examine the structure and function of the articulators to determine if they are adequate for the production of speech. It is important to remember that "because the speech mechanism is highly flexible and adaptable, only gross abnormalities interfere with speech production" (Bleile, 2002, p. 248). On the other hand, even small structural or functional abnormalities can sometimes form part of a larger syndrome that may have broader developmental and health implications for the child. In fact, three-fourths of all congenital birth defects in humans involve craniofacial malformations (Chai & Maxson, 2006). If any suspected abnormalities are found, the child should be referred to other professionals such as the referring physician, family physician, pediatrician, dentist, or otorhinolaryngologist (ENT) according to the specific guidelines of the clinical setting.

The **oral peripheral examination** is particularly useful in the identification of etiological factors or underlying speech processes.

Although only gross abnormalities in the oral peripheral mechanism interfere with speech production, **small structural or functional abnormalities can form part of a larger syndrome** and have broader developmental and health implications for the child.

Environments	Cues			
	Level 0	**Level 1**	**Level 2**	**Level 3**
	No cues	Instruction & verbal model	Instruction, verbal model, prolongation, segmentation	Instruction, verbal model, prolongation, segmentation visual-tactile representations
Connected Speech	1			
2-Target Sentence	2	3		
4-Word Sentence	4	5		
3-Word Sentence	6	7	8	9
Word	10	11	12	13
Isolation				14
Not Adaptable				15

Environments:
Isolation: the target is elicited by itself or in a CV or VC context.
Word: the SLP shows a picture of a CVC word (CCVC or CVCC for clusters) to the child and asks "What's this?"
3-Word Sentence: the same picture is used, and the child is asked "Tell me about that." The child should produce the target at the end of a three word sentence.
4-Word Sentence: the same picture is used, and the SLP asks the child "Tell me about that." The child should produce the target in the middle of a 4-word sentence.
2-Target Sentence: a second picture is added and the child is asked "Tell me about these." The child is expected to produce at least one of the two targets in the middle of a 4- to 5-word sentence.
Connected Speech: the child is presented a picture scene containing many objects with the target consonant or cluster, and asked "Tell me about the picture." To successfully achieve this level, the child should correctly produce the target twice.

Cue Levels:
Level 0: no cues are used.
Level 1: the SLP provides instructions about the articulatory placement of the target and a verbal model.
Level 2: the SLP can produce the target consonant or cluster separately from the rest of the word (segmentation), and/or prolong the target consonant (prolongation).
Level 3: the SLP can give visual-tactile representations.

Figure 5–2. *Glaspey Dynamic Assessment of Phonology. Printed with permission from Dr. Amy Glaspey.*

The **oral peripheral examination** consists of observation of: (1) facial characteristics; (2) dentition; (3) the tongue; (4) palatal and pharyngeal areas; and (5) maximum performance tasks. An example screening form is presented in **Appendix 5–2**.

The oral peripheral examination routinely consists of observation of: (1) facial characteristics; (2) dentition; (3) the tongue; (4) palatal and pharyngeal areas; and (5) maximum performance tasks. Each will be discussed in turn, first with regard to structure (size, shape, symmetry) and then to function (speed and precision of movement, range of motion, and coordination of the movements of the articulators); an example screening form is presented in Appendix 5–2. A more detailed assessment was described by Robbins and Klee (1987) and is shown with the associated norms for children age 2;6 to 6;11 in Appendix 5–3. The Oral Speech Mechanism Screening Evaluation (St. Louis & Ruscello, 2000) is a commercially available tool that provides normative data for the age range 5 through 78 years. Either one of these two normative tasks, or other commercially available standardized measure of oral-motor function, should be administered to the child if the screening reveals concerns suggesting the need for further testing regarding the child's oral-motor structure or function. It is often difficult for students, as well as junior clinicians, to have an internal standard against which to judge the appropriateness of aspects of the oral-motor mechanism such as size, symmetry and carriage. Clinicians need to look at many oral cavities to gain an appreciation of what is normal and what is not. When in doubt, do not hesitate to ask a more senior colleague to take a look at the child you are assessing to decide whether a more in-depth assessment or referrals are warranted.

Facial Characteristics

Facial characteristics are observed at rest to appraise the child's overall expression and appearance, size, shape and symmetry of the head and facial structures.

Facial characteristics are observed at rest to appraise the child's overall expression and appearance, size, shape and symmetry of the head and facial structures. Guidelines, or canons, of the ideal facial proportions were developed by painters and sculptors many centuries ago, including Polycleitus's Canon, 5th century BC; Marcus Vitruvius Pollio, 1st century BC; and Leonardo da Vinci's Male Head in Profile with Proportions, circa 1490 (Naini, Moss, & Gill, 2006). According to these guidelines, the face should be "five eyes wide": the two eyes, one between the inside corners of the two eyes, and the last two between the outside corners of the eyes to their closest ear. The face should be divided into thirds horizontally, from the top of the head to the eyebrows, the eyebrows to the middle of the nose, and the middle of the nose to the bottom of the chin. Vertically, the tip of the nose, lips, and chin should fall along the same line. Of course these are overall guidelines and may not reflect the specific ratios of the child. However, significant deviations from these may indicate the presence of a syndrome. For instance, short palpebral fissures (the area between the eye lids), thin upper lip, high arched eyebrows, and microcephaly are characteristics of fetal alcohol syndrome (Hoyme et al., 2005). At rest, the lips should be closed with the left and right edges even. Lips that remain partly open or drooping lips can be indicative of decreased muscle tone, and neuromuscular dysfunction could be present should there be fasciculations ("muscle twitch").

In terms of function, the child is generally asked to complete a few movements that probe lip rounding, such as "blowing a kiss," biting the lower lip, and saying [u], as well as movements that probe lip spreading, such as smiling and saying [i]. These movements are elicited by providing a verbal instruction (using language that is appropriate for the age of the child), supplemented with an imitative model when necessary to help the child understand the instruction. Asymmetry in the retraction of the lips during production of [i] is indicative of unilateral nervous system or muscular dysfunction (Miccio, 2002).

In terms of **function**, the child is asked to complete movements that probe lip rounding and lip spreading.

Dentition

Dental deviations may not have an impact on articulation as children can compensate surprisingly well for missing teeth or a malocclusion. Nonetheless, structural deviations, supernumerary teeth or dental appliances could interfere with accurate speech production and their presence should be noted. Provide a model to the child by opening your mouth and keeping the teeth in the closed position and say, "Show me your teeth like this." Note tooth decay, gaps, missing teeth, and misalignment of the back teeth in order to assess dental occlusion. Normal molar occlusion is defined by the bite, which is the relationship between upper and lower molars. The lower first molars should be slightly ahead of the upper first molars. The maxillary central incisors should extend by about one-fourth of an inch over the mandibular central incisors (Newman & Creaghead, 1989). Figure 5–3A presents the normal occlusion.

Normal molar occlusion is defined by the bite, which is the relationship between upper and lower molars. The normal occlusion is shown in Figure 5–3A.

Malocclusions are often hereditary (Litton, Ackermann, Isaacson, & Shapiro, 1970; Stoddard, 1947) but can also be acquired from finger or thumb sucking, tongue thrusting, early loss of teeth, or jaw fractures following an accident. Class I malocclusion, the most common, occurs when the molar relationship is normal but the upper teeth are slightly overlapping with the lower teeth. Class II malocclusion, also called retrognathism, occurs when the upper jaw or teeth project ahead of the lower jaw or teeth (Figure 5–3B). Class III malocclusion, called prognathism, consists of the protrusion of the lower jaw and teeth in front of the upper jaw and teeth (Figure 5–3C). Figure 5–3D presents the measurement of the overbite, the vertical overlap of the upper central incisors over the lower central incisors and the measurement of the overjet, the horizontal distance between the upper anterior teeth and the lower anterior teeth.

Class I malocclusion occurs when the upper teeth are slightly overlapping with the lower teeth. **Class II malocclusion** (retrognathism) occurs when the upper jaw or teeth project ahead of the lower jaw or teeth. **Class III malocclusion** (prognathism) refers to the protrusion of the lower jaw and teeth in front of the upper jaw or teeth.

Open bite, also called apertognathia, occurs when there is normal occlusion of the posterior teeth with no occlusion of the front teeth. A cross-bite consists of one or more teeth being in a more buccal or lingual position than its corresponding tooth in the upper or lower jaw; for example, the lower left canine being closer to the cheek than the upper left canine represents a cross-bite.

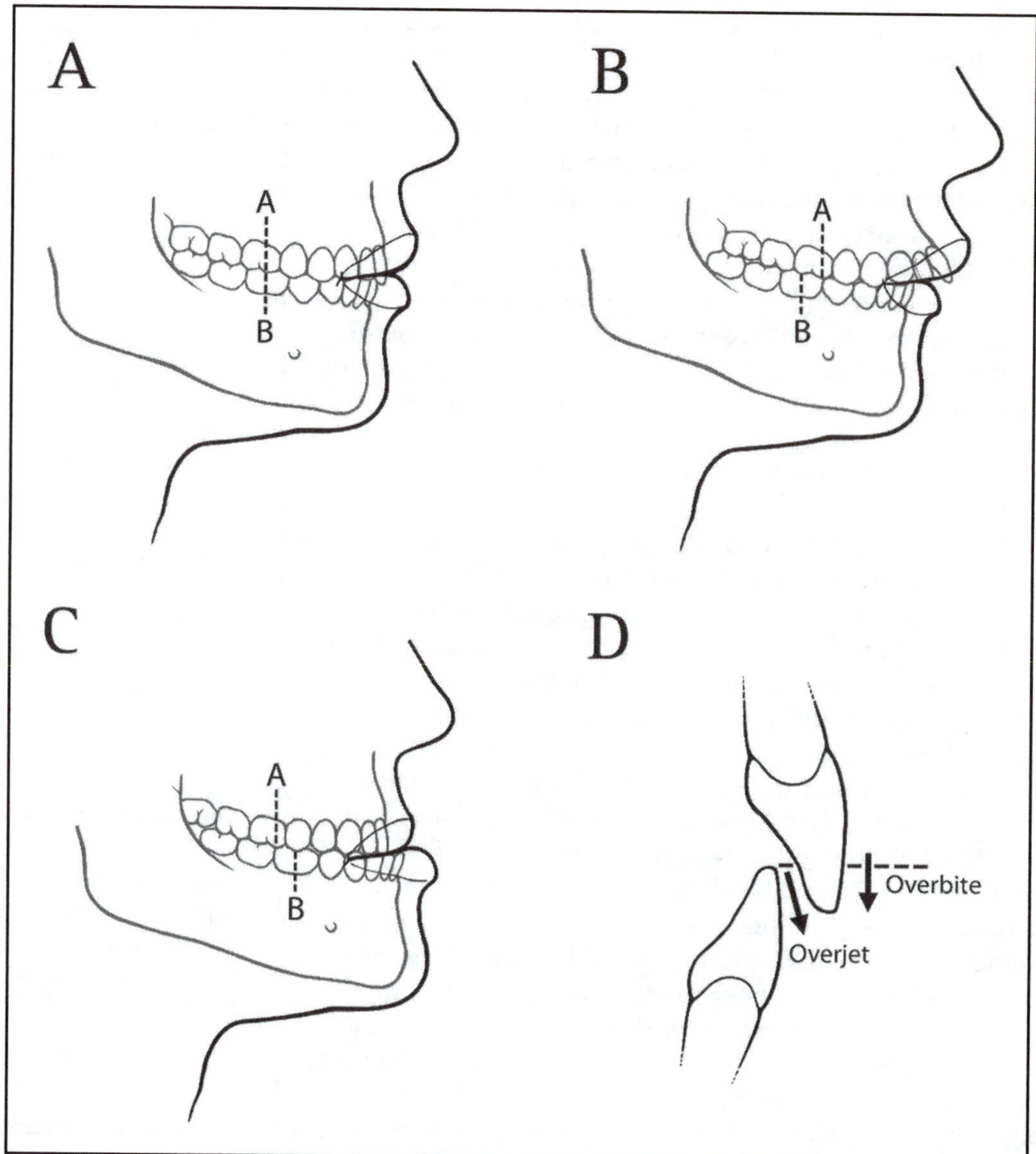

Figure 5–3. *Dental occlusions. Normal molar occlusion is represented in panel A. Class II malocclusion (retrognathism) is depicted in panel B. Class III malocclusion (prognathism) is depicted in panel C. Overbite and overjet are represented in panel D. From* Sleep Medicine, *by K. L. Yaremchuk and P. A. Wardrop, San Diego, CA: Plural, p. 43. Copyright © 2011 Plural Publishing, Inc. All rights reserved. Reprinted with permission.*

The Tongue

Essentially all speech sounds require **tongue** movement. In terms of **structure**, it is inspected for the presence of lesions or growth, general size, symmetry and absence of fasciculations.

Essentially all speech sounds require tongue movement. In terms of structure, the tongue should be first inspected for the presence of lesions or growths and general size and appearance. Its position at rest in the mouth can be quickly observed to assess symmetry and absence of fasciculations. In terms of function, the speed and range of motion of lateral and horizontal movements are typically assessed by prompting the child to protrude the tongue out of the mouth, then upward and downward, then moving it side to side and finally touching the tongue tip to the alveolar ridge. The initial prompt is provided by using a tongue blade as a target for tongue tip motion, positioning the tongue blade centrally and outside the mouth, and then touching the upper and lower lip, and then the left and right corners of the mouth. Imitative models of the desired tongue movements may be added if necessary.

In terms of **function,** the speed and range of motion of lateral and horizontal movements of the tongue are assessed.

The lingual frenum (also called frenulum) is the narrow fold of mucous membrane connecting the base of the tongue to the floor of the mouth. Ankyloglossia, or tongue-tie, occurs when the lingual frenum is short, or when it is attached near the tip of the tongue. Individuals with tongue-tie are usually unable to protrude the tongue tip beyond the edges of the lower incisors or to the maxillary alveolar ridge, behind the upper incisors. When a child with tongue-tie attempts to protrude the tongue it forms a heart-shaped edge or a 'W' shape. Ankyloglossia is usually noted at birth. It is quite common, with recent studies reporting a prevalence of 4 to 5% in newborns (Messner, Lalakea, Aby, Macmahon, & Bair, 2000; Ricke, 2005). Lingual frenotomy (clipping the frenum without anesthesia or under local anesthesia) is often performed immediately, as approximately 25% of newborns experience difficulties with breastfeeding, although there are no clear guidelines as to the indications for the surgery. The functional effects of ankyloglossia tend to diminish as the child gets older; the oral cavity's shape changes and increases in size, and the frenum draws back.

Children with **ankyloglossia** (tongue-tie) are usually unable to protrude the tongue tip beyond the edges of the lower incisors or behind the upper incisors. When they protrude their tongue it forms a heart-shape or "W" shape.

Tongue-tie surgery for toddlers and children is called lingual frenectomy and occurs under general anesthesia. Many health professionals think there is a causal link between ankyloglossia and articulation difficulties; 60% of ENTs, 50% of SLPs, and 23% of pediatricians surveyed by Messner and colleagues (2000) believed there is such a link despite the lack of scientific evidence in the literature. In fact, children with ankyloglossia often do not have speech difficulties since most speech sounds can be produced with minimal movement of the tongue. Focusing on production of /l/ and other lingual-alveolar sounds, as well as the dental fricatives /θ/ and /ð/, is particularly useful to help determine if ankyloglossia has an effect on speech: if the child is unable to correctly produce these sounds while correctly articulating other consonants, ankyloglossia could be having an impact on speech. However, "most experienced speech-language pathologists would conclude that is rarely indicated for speech reasons unless it is very severe or there are concomitant oral-motor problems" (Kummer, 2005, p. 30). Should parents or the child himself opt for the surgery, they may require preoperative exercises, and most will require postoperative exercises to develop new tongue movements and increase awareness of the range of movements of the tongue (Bowen, 2000).

Tongue-tie surgery for toddlers and children is called lingual **frenectomy** and occurs under general anesthesia. It is rarely indicated for speech reasons.

Children with ankyloglossia often do not have speech difficulties. To determine whether ankyloglossia has an effect on speech, **focusing on production of /l/** and other lingual-alveolar sounds as well as **/θ/ and /ð/** is particularly useful.

Coordination of oral movements. The child should also be asked to complete sequences of two movements because children

Children who can complete simple movements but who have difficulty combining them into sequences may have a specific motor speech disorder called **Childhood Apraxia of Speech** as discussed in greater depth in Chapter 7.

who can complete simple movements but who have difficulty combining them into sequences may have a specific motor speech disorder called Childhood Apraxia of Speech, as discussed in greater depth in Chapter 7. A recent study investigated the language, speech, and oro-motor differences of 3 groups of 10 children aged 4 to 6 years: children with suspected Childhood Apraxia of Speech (CAS), children with phonological disorder, and children with typical speech and language development (Aziz, Shodi, Osman, & Habib, 2010). Children were asked to blow a kiss, smile, protrude the tongue, and pucker the cheeks, as well as four combinations of two of these movements (kiss and protrude the tongue; smile and pucker the cheeks, protrude the tongue and smile; pucker the cheeks and protrude the tongue). Children with CAS were differentiated from children with speech delay by their performance on tasks requiring two sequential oral movements but not on the single movements. Nonspeech oral movement performance of the three groups is presented in Table 5–4.

Palatal and Pharyngeal Areas

Abnormalities in the **hard palate** are not always obvious. Particular attention should be paid to its coloration, with a red palate pointing to inflammation and a blue tint being indicative of the absence of tissue such as a **submucous cleft**.

Examination of these two areas should be performed to ensure the structures involved in velopharyngeal closure function properly. Abnormalities in the hard palate are not always obvious and could be indicated by changes in coloration. For example, a red palate points to inflammation and a blue tint close to the midline of the palate is indicative of the absence of tissue such as in the case of a submucous cleft. Fistulae or tiny holes in the palate can be caused by inappropriate postsurgical healing (Miccio, 2002; Newman &

Table 5–4. *Nonspeech Oral Movement Performance of Children With Speech Delay (SD), Motor Speech Disorder—Apraxia of Speech (MSD-AOS), and Normal Speech Development (Normal)*[a]

		SD	MSD-AOS	Normal
Single movement	Mean score/examination/child	39.5	38.5±	40
	Standard deviation	1.52	2.67	0
Two sequential movements	Mean score/examination/child	39*	12.33±	40
	Standard deviation	2.03	7.15	0

[a]See Figure 7-3 for a framework for describing subtypes of DPD.

Note: The child's response was rated on a 3-point scale; 10 points were awarded for a correct response, 5 points for an emerging response with groping and 0 point for an incorrect response for each movement. The 3 trials of each group were averaged to give the final score (out of 40) of the 4 single and the 4 sequential movements of each group.

* Means a significant difference between MPD and CAS groups, p value < 0.01.

± Means a significant difference between CAS and normal groups, p value < 0.01.

Source: Reprinted from A. A. Aziz, S. Shohdi, D. M. Osman, and E. I. Habib, 2010, "Childhood Apraxia of Speech and Multiple Phonological Disorders in Cairo-Egyptian Arabic Speaking Children: Language, Speech, and Oro-Motor Differences," *International Journal of Pediatric Otorhinolaryngology*, 74(6), Table 3, p. 581. Reproduced with permission of Elsevier Ltd.

Creaghead, 1989). The soft palate, or velum, acts as a valve which allows the buildup of intraoral pressure required for production of many consonants, and controls nasal resonance. Its overall size, shape, and symmetry should be examined. General length and symmetry of the velum can be observed while the child produces the sound /a/ in a prolonged manner and then in successive and sudden bursts; the velum should raise symmetrically in a posterior direction. The overall size, shape, and appearance of the uvula, faucial pillars, and palatine tonsils should also be inspected. Among others, the presence of obstructions of the air passage such as overly enlarged tonsils or a bifid (divided) uvula may be noted (Newman & Creaghead, 1989).

The general length and symmetry of the **velum** can be observed while the child prolongs the sound /a/ and then produce it in successive and sudden bursts. The overall size, shape, and appearance of the uvula, faucial pillars, and palatine tonsils should also be inspected.

Maximum Performance Tasks (MPTs)

MPTs are particularly useful in helping determine whether there is a motor component to the speech disorder. MPTs consist of two broad categories of tasks: maximum phonation duration (MPD; how long a sound can be sustained) and maximum repetition rate (MRR; how fast and accurately syllables can be repeated). MPD for the vowel /a/ is typically assessed; production of fricatives such as /f/, /s/ and /z/ is also commonly assessed. MRR is further divided in two types of stimuli: diadochokinetic (DDK) rate for repetitions of monosyllables and alternate motion rate (AMR) for repetitions of syllable sequences. Kent, Kent, and Rosenbeck (1987) found that the most common DDK were /pə/, /tə/, and /kə/ or their voiced counterparts, and the most common syllable sequence was /pətəkə/. It is preferable to use nonmeaningful stimuli as the purpose of MRR is to measure speech motor abilities and the use of meaningful words or phrases such as "patticake" or "pat-a-cake" may tap into linguistic competences (Williams & Stackhouse, 2000).

Maximum performance tasks (MPTs) consist of two broad categories of tasks: **maximum phonation duration (MPD**; how long a sound can be sustained) and **maximum repetition rate (MRR**; how fast and accurately syllables can be repeated).

MRR is further divided in two types of stimuli: **diadochokinetic (DDK)** rate for repetitions of monosyllables and **alternate motion rate (AMR)** for repetitions of syllable sequences.

MPTs are commonly used for older children and adults. Thoonen, Maassen, Wit, Gabreëls, and Schreuder (1996) showed how MPD and MRR could be used with children 6 to 10 years old to differentiate them into groups of children with typically developing speech, spastic dysarthria, or CAS. Although MPTs are very useful for differential diagnosis as discussed in Chapter 8, they are not routinely used with preschool-age children, possibly because normative data regarding performance on MPTs by normally developing children age 8 and younger has only recently been available, because young children may not be motivated to complete the tasks, and/or because they may have difficulties understanding the tasks or demonstrate great variability in performance from one trial to another (Rvachew, Hodge, & Ohberg, 2005). Nonetheless, several normative data sets of children's MPT abilities are now available to SLPs (e.g., Kent et al., 1987; Robbins & Klee, 1987; Rvachew, Ohberg, & Savage, 2006; Thoonen, Maassen, Gabreëls, & Schreuder, 1999; Thoonen et al., 1996; Williams & Stackhouse, 2000). Robbins and Klee's data set (1987) is particularly important, as it provides normative data for

Several normative data sets of children's MPT abilities are available to SLPs. **Appendix 5–3** presents the protocol and normative data from Robbins & Klee (1987), which can be used for children as young as 2;6.

oral structure and function for children age 2;6 to 6;11. A total of 90 typically developing children participated in the study; five boys and five girls were included at each 6-month age interval. Although the inclusion of very young children is a significant strength of this study, clear administration instructions are lacking for certain items. The resulting Oral and Speech Motor Control Protocol and accompanying normative data for oral structure, oral function and maximum performance tasks are presented in Appendix 5–3. In terms of MPTs, maximum phonation of the vowel /a/ (in seconds) was calculated for MPD; diadochokinetic rates for /pʌ/, /tʌ/, and /kʌ/ and alternate motion rates for /pərəkək/ and "patticake" were calculated for MRR. The children were instructed to repeat each of the items as quickly as possible over a 3-second interval.

When measuring repetition rates **standardized instructions and procedures** will minimize variability in performance from one trial to another and variability across young children. Recording MPT responses and using acoustic waveform measurements is also recommended to decrease measurement error.

Kent and colleagues (1987) recommended using standardized instructions and procedures to minimize variability in performance from one trial to another and variability across young children. Moreover, they recommended recording MPT responses and using acoustic waveform measurements to decrease measurement error. Rvachew, Hodge, and Ohberg (2005) described a standard protocol for obtaining MPTs for children based on the protocol developed by Thoonen and colleagues, using software to increase the cooperation of children and to facilitate recording and measurement of their responses. The TOCS+ ™MPT Recorder© version1 (Hodge & Daniels, 2004; http://www.tocs.plus.ualberta.ca/software_TOCS_MPT.html) was developed to aid the SLP administering the MPTs by displaying the instructions at the beginning of each task, providing the correct number of practice and test trials. A short tone and small icon on the screen indicate to the child when it is time to start each task, ensuring that the responses are recorded while minimizing chances of the SLP talking at the same time as the child. The child's responses on each trial are saved as a .wav file. A total of nine tasks are administered: MPD (prolongation of [a] and [mama]); maximum fricative duration (MFD; prolongation of [f], [s], [z]); DDK (repetition of the syllables [pa], [ta], [ka]); AMR (repetition of the syllable sequence [pataka]). In addition, two outcome measures are derived from the performance of the child on the AMR task: a score indicating whether the child successfully achieved a correct [pataka] sequence and the number of attempts beyond the first three trials necessary for the child to achieve the correct trisyllable sequence. The instructions for administering the testing protocol and combining the results to obtain the six outcome measures are presented in Appendix 5–4. Rvachew, Ohberg, and Savage (2006) reported performance of 20 children age 4 to 6 with typical speech on the standard protocol described in Appendix 5–4 using the TOCS+ ™MPT Recorder© version1 software (Hodge & Daniels, 2004). The 20 children completed all tasks, indicating that the protocol can be used with preschool-age children, although the authors reported that maximum prolongation tasks were less reliable and infor-

Appendix 5–4 presents the instructions to administer a standard MPT protocol to preschool-age children.

mative with preschool-age children. Therefore, Thoonen et al.'s scoring protocol for differentiating speech delay from CAS was modified to focus on repetition rates for single and multiple syllable sequences.

Accurate production of the syllable /ka/ is required to score the measure according to Thoonen et al.'s protocol, which young children with DPD may not be able to do. In this case you can use the normative data provided by Williams and Stackhouse (2000), who investigated the performance of 30 typically developing children age 3 to 5 on DDK and AMR tasks. Williams and Stackhouse measured accuracy, rate, and consistency independently for the syllable sequence /pataka/ and found that accuracy and consistency of the children's performance were more sensitive measures than rate of production. For young children, consistent production of the syllable /ka/ → [ta] in the trisyllable sequence (e.g., producing it as [patata]) at a rate of at least 3 repetitions per second would not be of concern.

Accurate production of /ka/ is required to score the protocol presented in Appendix 5-4. When children with DPD cannot accurately produce /ka/, you can use the normative data provided by **Williams and Stackhouse (2000).**

Fletcher (1972) obtained time-by-count norms from 384 children 6 to 13 years old (24 boys and 24 girls each at one-year interval). These were obtained and scored differently: the child was told to say some sounds, such as /pʌ/, as fast as possible. The clinician provided a model, then produced the sequence [pʌ, pʌ, pʌ, . . . pʌ] with the child, and then asked the child to do it once more and start and stop when told to do so. The mean scores in seconds and standard deviations are provided for the time required for 20 repetitions of the single syllables (/pʌ/, /tʌ/, /kʌ/, /fʌ/, /lʌ/), 15 repetitions of the bisyllables (/pʌtə/, /pʌkə/, /tʌkə/) and 10 repetitions of the trisyllable /pʌtʌkʌ/. These norms are presented in Appendix 5–5.

Appendix 5–5 presents the time-by-count norms obtained by Fletcher (1972) for children 6 to 13 years old.

In a recent review of standardized nonverbal and speech motor performance tests commercially available, McCauley and Strand (2008) found six instruments for children. Among them, only the Verbal Motor Production Assessment for Children (VMPAC; Hayden & Square, 1999) provided adequate descriptive information regarding its normative sample. Oral structure was described by only two tests, namely, the VMPAC and the Oral Speech Mechanism Screening Examination, Third Edition (OSMSE-3; Louis & Ruscello, 2000). Five of the six tests reviewed included both nonverbal oral motor and speech motor tasks. None of the tests reported sufficient information regarding the psychometric properties of the test, although McCauley and Strand state that the relevant information was probably available to the authors of each test and may be reported in future versions.

Measurement of MRRmono and MRRtri in a Sound File Editor

Demonstration 5–3 presents two examples of the measurement of MRRmono and MRRtri in a sound file editor, according to the protocol put forth in Appendix 5–4.

Demonstration 5–3

This demonstration shows the measurement of MRRmono and MRRtri for two children who participated in the ECRIP trial; the first child passed both measures; the second child passed the MRRmono but failed the MRRtri. The sound wave is loaded into a separate waveform editor such as Praat, Audacity, or WavePad to visually inspect the waveform, listen to the recording, and measure the duration, and, when appropriate, the number of syllable repetitions.

The procedure for measuring MRRmono consists of loading the sound wave into the waveform display window and identifying 10 syllables produced on a single expiration, excluding the first syllable following an inspiration or the last syllable before an inspiration.

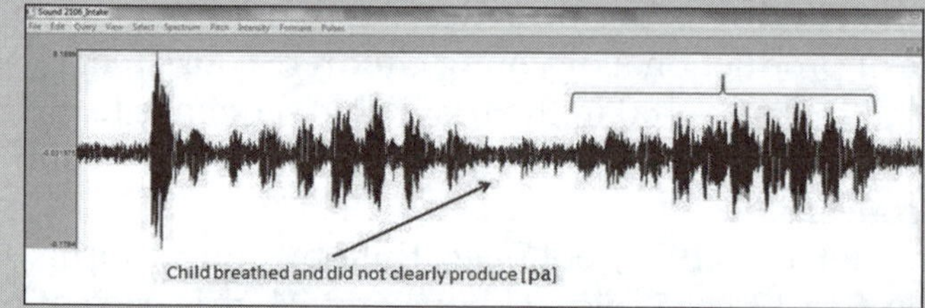

The first example is child 2106, who was 4;1 at the intake and was among the youngest participants in the trial. Child 2106 produced 19 repetitions of the syllable [pa]; the first one was excluded and usually the next 10 would be selected. In this case, however, the child breathed in the middle of the sequence and did not clearly produce [pa] on repetitions 8 and 9; therefore the last 10 clear repetitions of [pa] were selected, as shown in the figure.

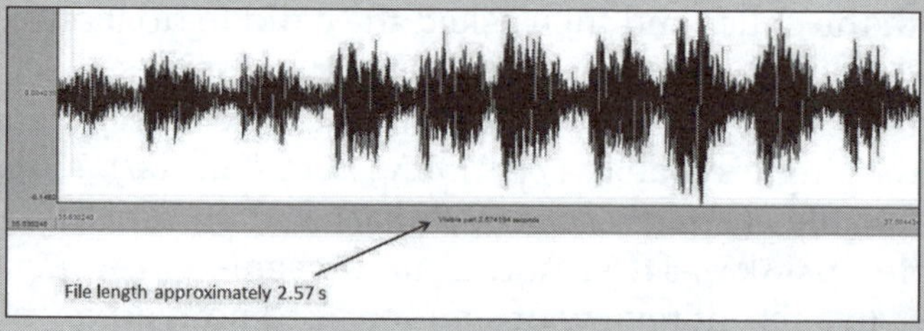

The portion of the waveform representing the 10 syllables chosen is selected; depending on the waveform editor you are using duration will be displayed in seconds or milliseconds. According to the protocol developed by Thoonen et al. the number of syllables produced by second needs to be calculated, which is achieved by dividing the 10 repetitions by the total time in seconds. In the example provided, duration for the 10 repetitions of [pa] was 2.57 seconds, as indicated by the arrow; therefore MRRmono for [pa] on this trial was $10/2.57 = 3.89$ repetitions per second.

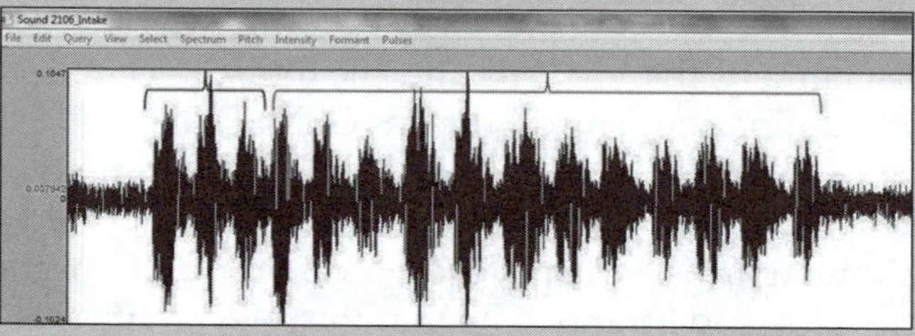

To determine MRRtri, the same procedure as MRRmono is employed, except that 4 consecutive repetitions of [pataka] need to be selected. In the figure the first [pataka] sequence is indicated by the small bracket and was omitted, and the next 4 sequences were selected.

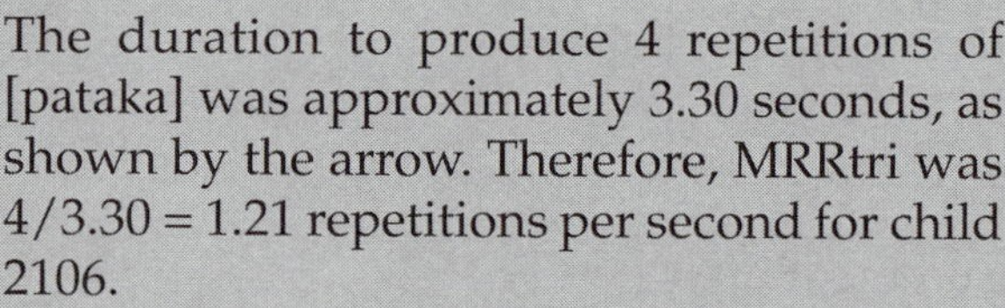

The duration to produce 4 repetitions of [pataka] was approximately 3.30 seconds, as shown by the arrow. Therefore, MRRtri was $4/3.30 = 1.21$ repetitions per second for child 2106.

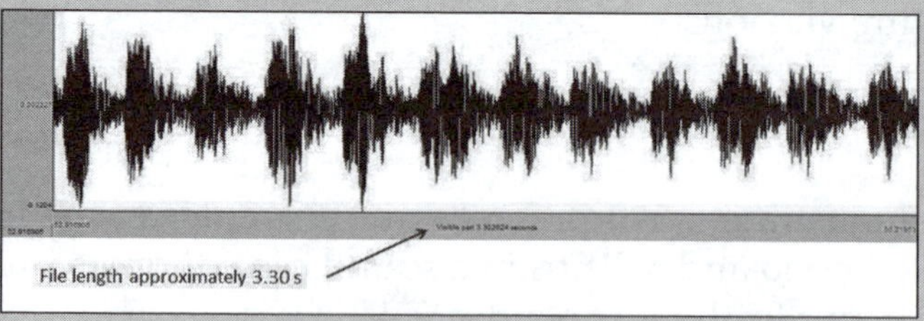

In the second example, child 2108 was 5;3 at the age of the intake assessment. He produced 17 repetitions of [ka] and 10 of these were selected.

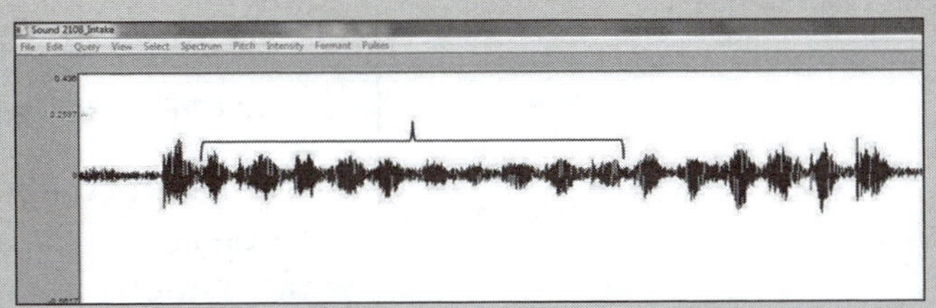

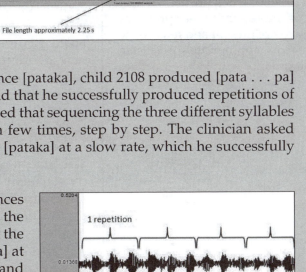

The total duration for the 10 repetitions of [ka] was approximately 2.25 seconds. The MRRmono for [ka] is therefore 4.44 repetitions per second.

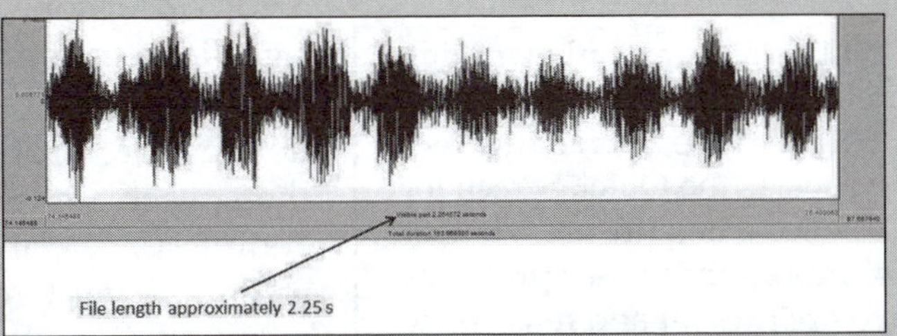

When first attempting the repetitions of the sequence [pataka], child 2108 produced [pata . . . pa] and said "This is hard." The SLP reminded the child that he successfully produced repetitions of each of these syllables in turn. The SLP acknowledged that sequencing the three different syllables is hard, and told the child they would try again a few times, step by step. The clinician asked child 2108 once again to produce one repetition of [pataka] at a slow rate, which he successfully achieved.

She then asked the child to produce two sequences at a slow rate, and the child was able to produce the sequence [patakapataka]. With another model from the SLP, the child produced three sequences of [pataka] at a rate of approximately 1 repetition per second, and then produced four repetitions at about the same rate, as shown in the figure.

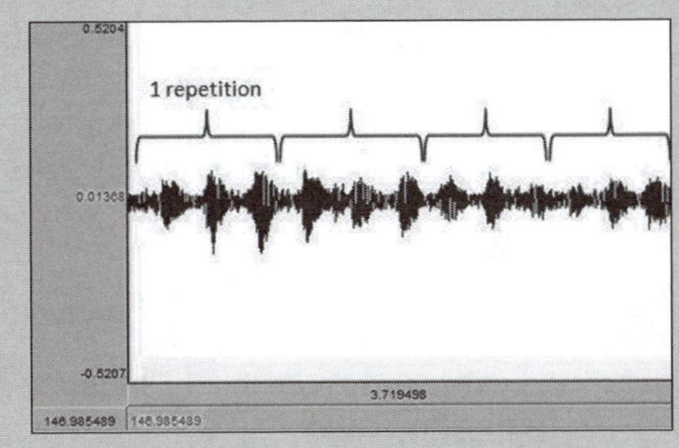

The SLP then modeled five repetitions of the sequence as fast as possible, but child 2108 produced repetitions of [paka] or [pata] when attempting to do the same. The SLP gave two additional trials to the child, then repeated the steps and allowed three additional attempts to produce correct sequences of [pataka] as fast as possible. The child always produced the repetitions as [paka] or [pata], and failed the MRRtri.

Other Speech and Language Domains

Voice and Resonance

SLPs not commonly working in the area of **voice** may find it useful to use a **screening tool** such as the Quick Screen for Voice when unsure whether more subtle voice problems are present and refer to the appropriate specialist in accordance with local guidelines and procedures.

As mentioned above, parameters of voice, resonance, and fluency can be assessed informally, whereas collecting the speech sample; information obtained during the oral-motor screening, such as maximum phonation time, is also useful in identifying the presence of a voice or resonance disorder. Although children who present with significantly abnormal voice quality will be readily identified, SLPs not commonly working in the area of voice may find it difficult to detect more subtle voice problems by listening to the child during the speech sample. The Quick Screen for Voice described in Lee, Temple, Glaze, and Kelchner (2004) assesses respiration, phonation, resonance, and vocal flexibility in 5 to 10 minutes; the screening is failed if a difficulty is found in any of these four areas. Briefly, in terms of respiration, inhalatory stridor, expiratory wheezing, limited breath support for speech, and reduced loudness should be absent. Unusual voice qualities include hoarseness, breathiness, and the presence of glottal fry or aphonia, as well as limited pitch or loudness variability. Hyponasality signals a blockage in the entrance to the nasal cavity or in the nasopharynx; if the child has a cold and is congested during the assessment, hyponasality will be present during production of nasal consonants. On the other hand, hypernasality is more noticeable during production of vowels and liquids, and reflects a velopharyngeal dysfunction that allows air to enter the nasal cavity. The child should be referred to the appropriate specialists for a complete SLP and medical assessment in accordance with local guidelines and procedures for any concerns about voice and/or resonance skills.

Fluency

Fluency disorders refer to **stuttering** and cluttering. **Cluttering** is less common and is characterized by a rapid rate of dysrhythmic and disorganized speech.

Children aged 2 to 4 sometimes repeat sounds, syllables, or words. Children who stutter display an **abnormally high frequency of disfluencies and often repeat only parts of words,** especially the first phoneme or first syllable. There are usually three or more repetitions per syllable that last up to a full second. Sound prolongations may also be present.

Fluency disorders refer to two conditions, stuttering and cluttering. Cluttering is less common and is characterized by a rapid rate of dysrhythmic and disorganized speech, often causing the child to be unintelligible, and may be present in children who stutter (Baker & Blackwell, 2004). Stuttering is a neurodevelopmental disorder that affects the timing and sequencing of the speech articulators, which results in disfluencies such as sound repetitions, sound prolongations, and/or blocks of speech (Guitar, 2006). Children 2 to 4 years old sometimes repeat sounds, syllables, or words and these episodes are considered normal disfluencies (Yairi & Ambrose, 1999); often, these are present with the child is excited, tired, or trying to produce complex sentences. Children who stutter, on the other hand, display an abnormally high frequency of disfluencies. In these children often only parts of the word will be repeated, especially the first phoneme or syllable (e.g., "m-m-m-mommy" or "mo-mo-mo-mommy"), and there are usually three or more repetitions per syllable; repetitions tend to last from half a second to one second. Sound prolongations (e.g., "sssssee") may be present, and occasionally speech blocks and secondary behaviors such as facial grimaces, facial tension, eye blinks, and body stiffening may be noted (Baker & Blackwell, 2004; Donaher, Deery, & Vogel, 2011). If disfluencies in the child's speech are noted during the assessment session, note their number and type. Normally disfluent children tend to repeat whole words or parts of the sentence once or twice as opposed to parts of the word three times or more. An adjunct observation of the child's fluency in the conversational speech sample is the Preschool Stuttering Screen for Healthcare Professionals (Donaher et al., 2011), a nonstandardized checklist with 10 yes/no questions that assesses the risk of persistent stuttering.

Language Skills

SLI and other language impairments are frequently comorbid with DPD in preschool-age children, especially in clinical samples (e.g. Baker & Cantwell, 1982; Shriberg, Tomblin, & McSweeny, 1999; see Chapter 7), therefore, at the very least a language screening measure such as the Kindergarten Language Screening Test-2 (Gauthier & Madison, 1998) should be administered. Preferably, a comprehensive language assessment should be completed, especially if the child fails the language screen. A comprehensive assessment will include standardized measures of the child's receptive and expressive abilities in the domains of vocabulary and syntax and, for school-age children, narrative skills (Tomblin, Records, & Zhang, 1996).

SLI and other language impairments are frequently comorbid with DPD in preschool children. A comprehensive language assessment or at the very least a language screening measure should be administered.

The speech-language sample obtained previously during the session can once again be used for further expressive language analysis. Tyler and Tolbert (2002), for instance, calculate mean length of utterance (MLU) based on 50 representative utterances to compare the child's performance to normative data from Miller and Chapman (1981). In addition, the child's production of pronouns and finite morphemes such as third person singular, auxiliaries, and regular past tense "-ed" provides information about morphosyntactic skills. For very unintelligible children or those who did not produce many sentences during the language sample, a formal expressive language screening instrument or assessment test such as the Expressive Language subtest of the Test of Early Language Development-3 (TELD-3; Hresko, Reid, & Hammill, 1991) might be more appropriate. The Sentence Imitation Test (SIT-61) has recently been developed to assess the expressive morphosyntactic skills of children with speech difficulties and is described in Seeff-Gabriel, Chiat, and Dodd (2010). The stimuli consist of 61 sentences in which the phonotactic structures, phonemes, and word length are developmentally simple; the effects of word frequency and vocabulary familiarity were also taken into account. A supplementary scoring system is also provided for children who are unintelligible in order to credit them with production of morphemes if they are misarticulated. The SIT-61 was administered to 4 groups of children aged 4 to 6 years: 33 typically developing children, 13 children with SLI, and 2 groups of 14 children with inconsistent and consistent

The speech-language sample can be used for further expressive language analysis such as the **mean length of utterance (MLU)**.

The **Sentence Imitation Test (SIT-61)** has recently been developed to assess the expressive morphosyntaxic skills of children with speech difficulties and contain sentences in which the phonotactic structures, phonemes, and word length are developmentally simple.

phonological disorder (this classification system for DPD is discussed in Chapter 7). Differences in performance on this test were found between the typically developing children and the three groups of children with speech or language impairments. The Early Repetition Battery, a shorter version of the SIT-61 has been standardized in the UK (Seeff-Gabriel, Chiat, & Roy, 2008).

Cognitive Development

SLPs do not have the qualifications to formally assess **cognitive skills**; however, in certain cases you may need to refer the child for a cognitive assessment.

SLPs do not have the qualifications to assess cognitive skills formally. However, in certain cases you may need to refer the child for a cognitive assessment to help in differential diagnosis or treatment planning, or because it is a requirement to access certain speech-language services at a rehabilitation center or at school. Most IQ tests are designed for children who do not have speech, language, or motor impairments. For instance, verbal responses are usually required and therefore children with DPD who are not always intelligible are at a disadvantage. In addition, many children with DPD also have language difficulties; performance of children with language impairments on verbal IQ tests may be biased due to their communication difficulties (Swisher, Plante, & Lowell, 1994). Although IQ tests that include both a verbal and a nonverbal scale are preferable and may provide a better estimate of the child's cognitive skills, they are not completely language free. Performance of children with language impairments vary, depending on the particular nonverbal test selected (Francis, Fletcher, Shaywitz, Shaywitz, & Rourke, 1996). These may involve fine motor tasks, such as manipulating puzzle pieces and replicating or matching block patterns and thus would be even more difficult to interpret for children with fine motor difficulties. Finally, standardized IQ tests were not historically sensitive to children from culturally and linguistically diverse backgrounds. Although more recent tests have standardization samples that are representative of the US population, the percentages for many cultures are very small and performance of children on IQ tests is still influenced by culture and language background (Swisher et al., 1994). Interpreting cognitive results for children with speech and language impairments, and for children from culturally and linguistically diverse backgrounds, is problematic and caution should be exercised for these populations.

Interpreting cognitive results for children with speech and language impairments, and children from culturally and linguistically diverse backgrounds is **problematic** and caution should be exercised for these populations.

Hearing and Auditory Processing

Hearing Acuity

If hearing has not been tested, a **hearing screening** as per the Guidelines for Audiologic Screening (ASHA, 1996) should be completed.

If hearing has not yet been assessed and the child is not scheduled to have an audiology assessment very shortly after the speech assessment, a hearing screening as per the Guidelines for Audiologic Screening (ASHA, 1996) should be completed. For preschool children, screening procedures involve visual inspection of the ear, tympanometry, and identification audiometry. Depending on procedures specific to your clinical setting, children should be referred to the family doctor, referring physician, ENT, or the audiologist in the following situations or circumstances: (1) if ear drainage or ear canal abnormalities such as impacted cerumen, secretions, or perforation are observed; (2) if the tympanometric equivalent ear canal volume is greater than 1.0 cm^3 in the presence of a flat tympanogram unless pressure equalization tubes (also known as tympanostomy tubes) are in place; and (3) with earphones, if the child cannot reliably be conditioned to complete play audiometry or if the child does not provide reliable responses at least 2 out of 3 times at 1000, 2000, and 4000 Hz tones at 20 dB HL in each ear.

Depending on procedures specific to your clinical setting, children should be referred to the family doctor, referring physician, ENT, or audiologist if visual inspection of the ear, tympanometry, or identification audiometry reveal concerns.

Auditory Processing

In the past decade there has been a significant increase in awareness regarding auditory processing disorders. However speech-language pathologists and audiologists are often confused as to how what Auditory Processing Disorder is (APD, also referred to as Central Auditory Processing Disorder), how it is identified, and how it is treated (Nelson, 2000). Auditory processing refers to "the perceptual processing of auditory information in the central nervous system and neurobiologic activity that underlies that processing and gives rise to electrophysiologic auditory potentials" (ASHA, 2005, p. 2). APD is present when the central nervous system does not adequately use auditory information; manifestations of APD include difficulties with sound localization and lateralization, temporal integration, auditory discrimination, listening and understanding verbal instructions in challenging environments, processing rapid acoustic stimuli or degraded stimuli (ASHA, 1996; Hind, 2006). The high distractibility and poor attention associated with APD in turn impact on the child's communication, language, and academic skills. APD is often comorbid with other disorders that also impact on the child's ability to attend, listen, comprehend language, and learn. These may include speech and language disorders, attention deficit disorder, learning disabilities, and hearing loss (Bellis, 2003; Jerger & Musiek, 2000). APD results from auditory deficits and not from other higher-order cognitive, language or attention processes; therefore, weak phonological awareness abilities, comprehension of auditory information, and attention to auditory stimuli, for example, would not be part of the APD but rather caused by higher-order processes that also rely on intact function of the central nervous system (ASHA, 2005). In other words, children with poor attention, high distractibility, learning difficulties, and difficulties understanding oral instructions should only receive a diagnosis of APD if it is demonstrated that the neural processing of auditory input is deficient.

Auditory Processing Disorder (APD) is present when the central nervous system does not adequately use auditory information. Manifestations include difficulties with sound localization and lateralization, temporal integration, auditory discrimination, listening, and understanding verbal instructions in challenging environments, and processing rapid acoustic stimuli or degraded stimuli.

APD results from **auditory deficits** and not from other higher-order cognitive, language, or attention processes. Therefore, weak phonological awareness abilities, comprehension of auditory information, and attention to auditory stimuli, for example, would not be part of the APD but rather caused by higher-order processes that also rely on intact function of the central nervous system.

Differential diagnosis is confounded not only by higher-order cognitive processes and comorbidity with developmental disorders, but also by the fact that there currently is not a gold standard for assessment of APD (Jerger & Musiek, 2000). In fact, approximately 35 different APD assessment measures are listed in the ASHA technical report on APD (ASHA, 2005) but audiology clinics across the US and in the UK do not have clear indications as to when a measure should be used and with which population (Emanuel, Ficca, & Korczak, 2011). Fergusson and colleagues (2011) investigated whether measures of cognitive and language abilities and parent report of their child's communication, listening, and behavioral skills would differentiate children who were previously diagnosed with SLI from children who were diagnosed with APD. A total of 88 children aged 6 to 13 years with normal hearing and normal middle ear function were included in the analyses; 22 children recruited through a community health speech and language clinic who had been identified as presenting with SLI; 19 children recruited through the local audiology or ENT clinic and who were prospectively identified as presenting with APD based on parent report of symptoms; and a random sample of 47 children attending local elementary schools. There were no significant differences between the performance of the children diagnosed with SLI and with APD on measures of verbal and nonverbal IQ, digit span, nonsense word repetition, spoonerisms, reading, grammar, and intelligibility, or between questionnaires on their behavior and communication and listening skills that had been completed by their parents. Both groups obtained significantly lower scores on each measure compared to the children attending mainstream elementary schools. The authors concluded that the children received either a diagnosis of SLI or APD based on whether they had been referred to a speech and language clinic or an audiology or ENT clinic. In other words, it had not been established that children diagnosed with APD presented with impaired neural processing of auditory input. Some parents will ask the SLP conducting the initial speech-language evaluation whether it is possible that the communication difficulties experienced by their child is caused by APD; other parents will have heard about APD from their family doctor, pediatrician, or the media. Although there is currently no universally accepted screening tool for APD, several screening test protocols, checklists, and questionnaires have been proposed and can help you decide for which children it would be appropriate to complete a referral for APD testing. According to the ASHA technical report on APD (ASHA, 2005), audiologists, SLPs, psychologists, and other professionals can perform a screening for APD, but the audiologist is the only professional who should diagnose APD. As per the ASHA Scope of Practice in Speech-Language Pathology, the SLP may be involved in the assessment process by "collaborating in the assessment of (central) auditory processing disorders and providing intervention where there is evidence of

SLPs, along with audiologists, psychologists, and other professionals can perform a **screening** for APD but only audiologists should diagnose the condition.

speech, language, and/or other cognitive-communication disorders" (ASHA, 2001, p. 5).

Screening instruments for APD typically probe auditory behaviors involved in listening skills, communication, and academic achievement. Emmanuel, Ficca, and Korczak (2011) conducted a survey of audiologists' protocols for diagnosing and managing APD; 195 ASHA audiology members who listed APD as an area of expertise and members of the Educational Audiology Association completed the survey. In terms of screening, 69% of the respondents used the SCAN-A: Test for Auditory Processing Disorders in Adolescents and Adults (Keith, 1994) or SCAN-C: Test for Auditory Processing Disorders in Children—Revised (Keith, 1999). Newer versions of these screening instruments are now available, the SCAN-3A and SCAN-3C (Keith, 2009a).

Phonological Processing

As covered in Chapter 4, the accurate production of speech requires detailed acoustic-phonetic representations for words; as seen in Chapter 7, many children with DPD have significant phonological processing difficulties. Recall that it was previously suggested that the child develops increasingly detailed, fine-grained phonological representations and stores them in long-term memory as the number of words in the lexicon expands. This lexical restructuring allows the child to retrieve words more efficiently and achieve more complex phonological processing, such as phonological awareness, which requires accessing sublexical units (Claessen, Heath, Fletcher, Hogben, & Leitao, 2009). Several tasks tap into the child's phonological processing skills; the assessment of speech perception, phonological awareness, and nonword repetition are discussed below.

Many children have phonological processing difficulties, as seen in Chapter 7. Several tasks tap **phonological processing skills**, including speech perception, phonological awareness, and nonword repetition.

Speech Perception Skills

As a group, children with DPD have difficulties with speech perception relative to their typically developing peers (Broen, Strange, Doyle, & Heller, 1983; Hoffman, Daniloff, Bengoa, & schuckers, 1985; Rvachew & Jamieson, 1989); Chapter 7 further describes studies that have investigated the speech perception skills of children with DPD and Chapter 9 elaborates on which children with DPD would particularly benefit from incorporating speech perception intervention in therapy. In brief, as many children with DPD have speech perception difficulties, the inclusion of a measure of speech perception skills in the assessment is important. Skahan el al. (2007) found that few SLPs routinely assess speech perception skills; there are few well-designed speech perception assessment tools available to clinicians, which could in part explain why speech perception skills are seldom considered in the diagnostic assessment process.

The goal of the speech perception assessment is to determine whether the child's **underlying acoustic-phonetic representation is accurate** by requiring the child to access his acoustic-phonetic representation and compare it to a spoken stimulus.

The assessment measure should examine the **child's perception of the target in relation to the misarticulated sound**.

The assessment measure should consist of an **identification** task.

The assessment measure should contain **multiple trials and control items**.

The goal of the speech perception assessment is to determine whether the child's underlying acoustic-phonetic representation is accurate by requiring the child to access his acoustic-phonetic representation and compare it to a spoken stimulus (Claessen et al., 2009). In order to reach this goal, the assessment measure has to meet several conditions (Locke, 1980a). First, the child's perception of the target sound should be examined in relation to the misarticulated sound. For instance, if the child substitutes [w] for /ɹ/ as in "rake" → [wek], then it would be appropriate to contrast these two words to assess the child's perception of the phoneme /ɹ/. However, Locke found that perception tests typically contrasted "rake" and "lake" even though this contrast does not correspond to most children's error pattern for these liquids. Second, the assessment measure should consist of an identification task rather than a discrimination task, so that the test is tapping the quality of the child's internal representation for the target word as discussed in Chapters 1 and 2. Third, there should be multiple trials. If a child produces the error /f/ → [p] but answers correctly on the only trial contrasting /p/ and /f/ on the speech perception test, no conclusions can be made as to whether his perception of /f/ is appropriate or whether the child obtained the correct response by chance, in which case perception of /f/ should actually be treated. In addition, control items, which are perceptually similar to the adult target but different from the child's mispronunciations, should be included in the assessment measure. Available speech perception tests examined by Locke either did not include control items, or included control items that were entirely different from the relevant phoneme contrast. In the first case, when no control items are included at all, it is impossible to determine whether the child understands the task and is attentive but does not perceive the difference in the two sounds presented, or is inattentive or does not understand the task. In the second case, when control items which are perceptually unrelated to the target contrast are included (such as /t/ - /k/ for the child who produces /f/ → [p]), it can only be determined whether the child understands the instructions and is at least somewhat attentive. The problem of determining whether the child can discriminate /f/ from other sounds he does not replace it with, but which are perceptually similar, such as /v/ or /b/, remains.

Finally, the assessment measure needs to be appropriate for children with regard to the vocabulary it uses, and in particular, the task paradigm and type of responses required (Locke, 1980a; Vance, Rosen, & Coleman, 2009). Some assessment measures use a same/different task, in which children hear two words and have to say whether these words are the same or different. However, the concept of same-different is not easily understood by children, who may perceive differences between pairs of words but make mistakes on the test. Moreover, if the test contains pairs of words that are perceptually similar, as recommended, it is difficult for children and adults alike to decide how similar the two items have to be to be considered as "same." Locke (1980b) specifically recommended using either a mispronunciation detection task or an ABX task. Two studies have compared performance levels on these two types of task leading to the conclusion that the mispronunciation task is easier for preschool-age children to perform (Bountress, Sever, & Williams, 1989; Vance et al., 2009).

Finally, it is very important to ensure that the speech stimuli used in the test match the language and dialect spoken by the child. As indicated in Chapter 2, there are several mispronunciation detection tasks now available for different dialects of English, specifically British English (McNeil & Hesketh, 2010; Vance et al., 2009), Australian English (Claessen et al., 2009), and midwestern North American English (Speech Assessment and Interactive Learning System). SAILS is a computer-based tool that was developed for treating speech perception deficits (e.g., Rvachew, 1994). Recently, it was used as an assessment tool in a longitudinal follow-up study of children with speech delay that also included a control group of 35 children recruited from daycares and preschools. SAILS scores as obtained from these children at the end of the school year during the three successive years of the study are shown in Table 5–5.

If no test is available for the dialect that your clients speak, such a test can be developed locally by recording words from children whose speech is delayed or developing normally so as to represent the typical range of correct and incorrect productions that occur. One strategy for stimulus presentation is to insert edited recordings of each word into PowerPoint slides along with a picture of the intended word and ask children to listen to the audio stimulus and

A **mispronunciation detection task** or an **ABX task** is most appropriate for assessing children's speech perception skills; the mispronunciation task is easier for preschool-age children.

The speech stimuli used in the speech perception test should match the language and dialect spoken by the child.

Table 5–5. *Expected Performance on the SAILS Modules* lake, cat, rat, *and* Sue

	Prekindergarten (mean age: 59 months)		*Kindergarten (mean age: 71 months)*		*First Grade (mean age: 89 months)*	
Module	*Mean*	*S.D.*	*Mean*	*S.D.*	*Mean*	*S.D.*
/l/: lake	87.00	8.06	91.92	10.96	92.29	10.31
/k/: cat	78.60	7.17	77.31	10.79	81.43	12.87
/ɹ/: rat	79.46	10.92	82.31	8.51	85.70	12.61
/s/: Sue	71.52	8.64	80.26	8.38	81.24	7.59
All four	77.70	6.60	82.09	6.10	84.12	6.68

Note: Normative data were collected from 35 middle-class Canadian children who were normally developing and spoke English as their first language according to their parents and teachers. Thirteen of the children attended French immersion schools. Goldman-Fristoe Test of Articulation percentiles were within normal limits (M = 45.03; SD = 18.53). Peabody Picture Vocabulary Test standard scores were average or above average (M = 112.43; SD = 11.02). The mean score reflects the child's percent correct score, averaged across all of the test blocks for the module as shown (after omitting the score for practice blocks). The scores are expressed as percent correct responses per module. This assessment and treatment tool can be obtained by contacting the authors (see http://www.medicine.mcgill.ca/srvachew for more information).

judge whether it represents the pictured word or not. A small set of words targeting commonly misarticulated phonemes in the onset or coda position of words that match the typical prosodic structure of the language will suffice. The words should be chosen so that it is likely that only the target phoneme will be misarticulated by the children who produce the word for your recordings. Commonly available recording and waveform editing software can be used for this task (e.g., Audacity).

If no speech perception test exists for your client's dialect, such a test can be developed or you can use the **Speech Perception Production Task**.

Another alternative is the *Speech Production Perception Task*, a live-voice procedure developed by Locke (1980b) so that assessment could be customized to each child's pattern of speech production errors. The clinician first needs to identify the child's speech sound errors; the adult target is the stimulus phoneme (SP), the child's error is the response phoneme (RP) and the control phoneme (CP) consists of a perceptually similar target. For each error phoneme, 18 items are constructed: 6 repetitions of the SP (e.g., /ɹ/), 6 of the RP (e.g., /w/), and 6 of the CP (e.g., /m/), presented in random order. The clinician administers the task live-voice by presenting a picture of the stimulus to the child (e.g., a picture of a rake), and then asking on each trial: *Is this ____ (e.g., "rake," "wake," or "make")?* and circling the child's response. Administration of each 18-item test takes approximately 5 minutes. An example of a test protocol is presented as part of Case Study 5–1 at the end of this chapter.

Phonological Awareness Skills and Emergent Literacy

As a group, individuals with DPD have deficits in PA; however, there is **no significant correlation between the severity of the DPD and PA abilities**.

As seen in Table 7–9, several studies have demonstrated that, as a group, children and adults with DPD have deficits in phonological awareness (PA), a crucial factor in early literacy development (e.g., Bird, Bishop, & Freeman, 1995; Larivee & Catts, 1999; Lewis, Freebairn, & Taylor, 2002; Nathan, Stackhouse, Goulandris, & Snowling, 2004; Rvachew, 2007; Rvachew, Ohberg, Grawburg, & Heyding, 2003). However, there is no significant correlation between the severity of the speech sound production difficulties and PA abilities. In other words, some children have poor articulation accuracy and average PA skills, and some children have mild articulation accuracy difficulties yet perform well below normal limits on measures of PA (Hesketh, 2004; Holm, Farrier, & Dodd, 2008; Rvachew, Chiang, & Evans, 2007; Sutherland & Gillon, 2005). Children with resolved speech difficulties may also have poor PA skills and be at risk for dyslexia (Raitano, Pennington, Tunik, Boada, & Shriberg, 2004). Therefore, if assessing a child who presents with mild articulation errors, or resolved speech production difficulties, it is nonetheless important to assess PA skills. Furthermore, children with poor reading skills in first grade are very likely to have reading difficulties throughout school. For instance, Juel (1988) followed 54 children from first grade to fourth grade. Eighty-eight percent of the poor readers in first grade remained poor readers in fourth grade and at the end of the study had not achieved the level of

PA skills should also be assessed for children with mild or resolved speech production difficulties.

decoding skills that the good readers possessed at the beginning of second grade. Another longitudinal study demonstrated that the reading achievement gap between good readers and poor readers is quite stable from first grade through high school (Francis, Stuebing, Shaywitz, & Fletcher, 1996). Measures of early literacy, such as letter knowledge, letter-sound correspondence knowledge, and invented spelling at the ages of 3 to 6 years also predict the later literacy skills of school-age children. Catts, Fey, Zhang, and Tomblin (2001) administered measures of language, early literacy, and nonverbal cognition to 604 children in kindergarten. They also administered measures of reading in second grade. Logistic regression analyses showed that five kindergarten variables uniquely predicted later reading outcome with 93% accuracy, namely, letter identification, sentence imitation, PA, rapid naming, and mother's education. The inclusion of a PA and emergent literacy measure in the assessment of children with DPD and/or language difficulties is therefore necessary to identify children who are at risk of later reading difficulties. This assessment could take place during the initial diagnostic assessment session or later, during the first intervention sessions. Assessing PA skills of young children referred for speech and/or language difficulties allows the SLP to establish a baseline and track progress in this essential skill prior to the onset of formal reading instruction. Furthermore, significant delays may be rectified with appropriate early interventions if necessary. Interventions for PA and emergent literacy skills are covered in Chapter 11.

There is a wide diversity of tasks to assess PA skills, and the usefulness of each of them is dependent on the age and level of PA skills of the child. Adams (1990) described five levels of development of PA skills: (1) sensitivity to rhyme; (2) rhyme detection and comparison; (3) syllable blending and segmentation; (4) phoneme counting; and (5) phoneme manipulation tasks (e.g., phoneme addition, deletion, or displacement). Schatschneider, Francis, Foorman, Fletcher, and Mehta (1999) administered seven different PA tasks to a total of 945 children attending kindergarten, first grade, or second grade, and found that comparing initial sounds was the easiest task and most appropriate for young children along with blending syllables; blending onsets and rimes was relatively easy and appropriate for children in the first half of kindergarten; phoneme blending was recommended to discriminate abilities of children in the second half of kindergarten and beginning of first grade. Phoneme segmentation and deleting phonemes were the most difficult tasks.

There is a wide diversity of tasks to assess PA skills, and the usefulness of each of them is dependent on the age and level of PA skills of the child.

There are several standardized PA assessments currently available, although the standardization samples may not all be relevant to the particular child you are assessing. For instance, the Comprehensive Test of Phonological Processing (CTOPP; Wagner, Torgensen, & Rashotte, 1999) was normed on a US sample and consists of two versions: children aged 5 and 6 years and individuals aged 7 to 24 years. The Preschool and Primary Inventory of Phonological Awareness (PIPA: Dodd, Crosbie, McIntosh, Teizel, & Ozanne,

There are several standardized PA assessments currently available, although the standardization samples may not all be relevant to the particular child you are assessing.

2000), on the other hand, consists of six subtests and measures syllable segmentation, rhyme awareness, alliteration awareness, phoneme isolation, phoneme segmentation, and letter knowledge. It has a UK and Australian standardization sample of children age 3;0 to 6;11 and may not be appropriate for American or Canadian children, as the ages of school entry and literacy instruction practices are different in these countries.

PA tasks that require a nonverbal or a yes/no response should be used for children with DPD who may be unintelligible.

Various standardized and informal PA assessment measures are available for preschool children and for young school-age children. However, specific considerations other than the standardization sample also need to be taken into account for children with DPD. As these children have difficulties accurately producing target words and can be unintelligible, tasks that require a nonverbal or a yes/no response should be used to avoid difficulty in interpreting their verbal responses. Furthermore, visual stimuli and the use of one or two syllable target words are also recommended, as they help diminish the load on phonological short-term memory. The Phonological Awareness Test was developed by Bird, Bishop, and Freeman (1995) for research purposes and uses nonverbal responses. It consists of three subtests: rime matching, onset matching, and onset segmentation and matching. In the rime matching subtest, the child is shown a puppet, told its name, and told that the puppet "likes things that sound like his name." The child is then asked which of four pictures he would like. The clinician names each of the pictures while pointing them and the child is then required to point to the correct picture. In the onset matching subtest, the child is shown a puppet and told that the puppet likes "everything he owns to start with the same sound." The clinician produces the phoneme, and the child is asked to select the correct picture among four items. Finally, in the onset and segmentation subtest the child is presented with a puppet, told its name, and told that the puppet "likes things that start with the same sound as her name," without specifying the target sound. There are five practice items at the beginning of each subtest during which feedback is provided to the child; the rime matching subtest has 14 test items and the remaining two subtests each have ten test items. The test items are not well controlled for global similarity as would be the case with more recently developed tests (see Chapter 2 for discussion). Nonetheless, the test has several advantages including a long history of usage with the DPD population because of the nonverbal response mode and the many practice items that ensure that young children understand the task. Many studies have shown that the responses of preschool-age children with DPD on this test are associated with later literacy outcomes as described in Bird et al. (1995) in the UK and by Rvachew and colleagues (e.g., Rvachew, 2006; Rvachew & Grawburg, 2006) in Canada and by Pennington and colleagues (e.g., Peterson, Pennington, Shriberg, & Boada, 2009; Raitano et al., 2004) in the US. A recent study of the PA skills in preschool children with DPD also adapted the test developed by Bird and colleagues but presented the pic-

The **Phonological Awareness Test** (Bird, Bishop, and Freeman, 1995) is often used with children with DPD because of its nonverbal response mode and because many practice items ensure that young children understand the task.

tures on a computer with previously recorded audio stimuli (Preston & Edwards, 2010). We have used this test extensively in our own research, using a live-voice presentation format, and present the test items and normative data from this research in Appendix 5–6.

Claessen, Leitao, and Barrett (2010) recently developed the Silent Deletion of Phonemes Task (SDPT) which assesses children's ability to silently delete or manipulate sounds in their own stored phonological representation. This task also minimizes the impact of articulation difficulties and is appropriate for school-age children with DPD. The SDPT is computer-administered and contains two training items and 35 test items; test items consist of five of each of the following types of stimuli: part of a compound word is deleted (e.g., "starfish" → "star"); initial phoneme is deleted (e.g., "tie" → "eye"); final phoneme is deleted (e.g., "beak" → "bee"); initial phoneme of a word initial cluster is deleted (e.g., "block" → "lock"); final phoneme of a word initial cluster is deleted (e.g., "snail" → "nail"); initial phoneme of a word final cluster is deleted (e.g., "nest" → "net"); and final phoneme of a word final cluster is deleted (e.g., "lamp" → "lamb"). Throughout the task the name of the item is not said in the prerecorded instructions, or by the child. During administration of the task the child is shown a picture on the computer and verbally instructed to look at the picture and think of the name of the picture without saying it aloud. The child is then asked to delete a phoneme or syllable from the word and choose the correct response from four pictures by clicking on it with the computer mouse. The child then sees four pictures: the target (e.g., "bee"), a semantic foil (e.g., "bird"), and two phonological foils (e.g., "E" and "key"). The task is useful for children in the first grades of school; performance of normally developing children from the ages of 7;2 to 8;1 is normally distributed and was not at the basal or ceiling levels, and was correlated with measures of PA. In combination with a traditional measure of PA requiring verbal responses, it provides a more detailed representation of the child's phonological representations. For instance, a child who performs well on the SDPT but not on a standard measure of PA would be considered to have detailed phonological representations but difficulties at the output level, whereas a child who does not perform well on either task could indicate poorly defined phonological representations. Claessen and colleagues are currently investigating the integrity of phonological representations using the SDPT in children with SLI, age-matched, and language-matched peers.

The **Silent Deletion of Phonemes Task (SDPT)** assesses children's ability to silently delete or manipulate sounds in their own stored phonological representation. It minimizes the impact of articulation difficulties and is appropriate for school-age children with DPD.

As mentioned earlier, emergent literacy skills should be assessed. Justice, Invernizzi, and Meier (2002) recommended assessing written language awareness, letter name knowledge, grapheme-phoneme correspondence, literacy motivation, and home literacy environment. They also provided guidelines and strategies for developing an emerging literacy and PA screening instrument. The example screening tool from Justice et al. (2002) for children aged 4 to 5 years is presented in Table 5–6.

In terms of **emergent literacy**, written language awareness, letter name knowledge, grapheme-phoneme correspondence, literacy motivation, and home literacy environment can be assessed.

Table 5–6. *Example of a Preschool Early Literacy Screening Protocol*

Target	*Task*
Written language awareness	Preschool Word and Print Awareness task (Justice & Ezell, 2001) Name Writing task of the Phonological Awareness Literacy Screening–PreK (Invernizzi, Sullivan, & Meier, 2001)
Phonological awareness	Rhyming Production, Sentence Segmentation, and Initial Sound Isolation tasks of the Phonological Awareness Test (Robertson & Salter, 1997)
Letter name knowledge	Upper-Case Alphabet Knowledge of the PALS–PreK (Invernizzi et al., 2001)
Grapheme–phoneme correspondence[a]	
Literacy motivation	Classroom observation (2 activities) with Likert-type rating (Kaderavek & Sulzby, 1998)
Home literacy	Parent questionnaire

[a]Grapheme–phoneme correspondence tasks typically are not administered to preschool children.

Source: From L. M. Justice, M. A. Invernizzi, & J. D. Meier, 2002, "Designing and Implementing an Early Literacy Screening Protocol: Suggestions for the Speech-Language Pathologist," *Language, Speech, and Hearing Services in Schools*, 33, Table 3, p. 95. Reprinted with permission of the American Speech-Language-Hearing Association.

Implicit and explicit awareness of the properties of written language consist of a wide range of knowledge about the function of print, properties of print (such as the fact that the direction of print is from left to right in English), and how to interact with books (for example, holding the book the correct way). The Written Language Awareness Checklist developed by Justice and Ezell (2001) is presented in Table 5–7. To assess letter knowledge, the child is typically presented with upper and/or lowercase letters and asked to point to the letter named by the clinician (receptive knowledge) or asked to name the letters (expressive knowledge). Younger children or children having difficulties identifying letters could be asked to recite the alphabet. Although preschool children's exposure to formal literacy instruction varies considerably from one school district to another, parent interview data of 8,549 preschool children obtained by the National Center for Education Statistics (1999) indicate that 28% of children age 4 and 36% of children age 5 are able to recognize all letters of the alphabet. Knowledge of grapheme-phoneme correspondences requires letter name knowledge as well as skills related to written language and phonological awareness, and is therefore not typically assessed in children who have not acquired these prerequisite skills or received some formal reading instruction. Preschool-age children may nonetheless know the grapheme-phoneme correspondence for some letters that are highly significant to them, such as the first letter of their name, and be able to produce

Table 5–7. *The Written Language Awareness Checklist (Justice & Ezell, 2001)*

Child's Name: ______________________ Date: ______________

Child's Age: ____________ Birth Date: __________ Examiner: ______________

Directions: Observe the child in an array of early literacy activities (for example, one-on-one shared storybook reading, and whole class writing and reading activities). Check each of the following that applies.

_______	Child recognizes that print runs from left to right.
_______	Child distinguishes scribbles ("writing") from pictures in drawings.
_______	Child knows that words are comprised of letters.
_______	Child uses a print vocabulary, such as read, word, write, and letter.
_______	Child responds to signs in the classroom.
_______	Child recognizes common logos, such as store names or a sports team.
_______	Child shows interest in what items say in the classroom.
_______	Child differentiates between pictures and print on posters and signs.
_______	Child asks for help to "read" signs and words in environment.
_______	Child understands that print has a different role than pictures on signs.
_______	Child is interested in reading and sharing books.
_______	Child identifies the front and back of a book.
_______	Child holds books the correct way (right side up, front side forward).
_______	Child can tell title of favorite books.
_______	Child turns pages of a book from front to back.
_______	Child knows that print tells the story.

Source: From L. M. Justice, M. A. Invernizzi, & J. D. Meier, 2002, "Designing and Implementing an Early Literacy Screening Protocol: Suggestions for the Speech-Language Pathologist," *Language, Speech, and Hearing Services in Schools,* 33, Appendix, p. 101. Reprinted with permission of the American Speech-Language-Hearing Association.

the sound that goes with that particular letter, or name the corresponding letter when the adult produces that specific sound. Children's interest or motivation toward print-related tasks has been shown to impact their performance on early literacy tasks (Frijters, Barron, & Brunello, 2000), and is rarely assessed in commercially available emergent literacy screening and assessment tools. Justice and colleagues (2002) recommend rating the child's engagement on a scale from 0 (no engagement) to 4 (total engagement) during one classroom and one individual literacy activity. To assess the home literacy environment, parents may be asked to complete a questionnaire such as the one used by Dickinson and DeTemple (1998) to determine if the child has access to, and participates in, literacy activities at home, presented in Table 5–8.

Table 5–8. Questionnaire to Assess the Home Literacy Environment in Preschoolers

Child's Name: ____________________		Date: ____________________	
Child's Birth Date: ____________________		Child's Age: ____________________	
Home Support for Emergent Literacy (circle correct answer)			
Do you read to your child?	YES		NO
Daily?	YES		NO
Does anyone else read to your child?	YES		NO
If so, how often?	1–2 times/week		3+ times/week
How many children's books do you own?	1–10	11–25	25+
Do you get books from the library?	YES		NO
Do you get books from a bookstore?	YES		NO
Do you read anything else with your child?	YES		NO
Cartoons?	YES		NO
Catalogues	YES		NO
Children's magazines	YES		NO
Newspapers	YES		NO
Child's Emergent Literacy Skills (circle correct answer)			
Reading			
Can your child recognize and name letters?	YES		NO
Does your child pretend to read alone?	YES		NO
Does your child pretend to read to others?	YES		NO
Has your child memorized any books?	YES		NO
Does your child have a favorite book?	YES		NO
Does your child recognize any sign?	YES		NO
Writing			
Does your child pretend to write?	YES		NO
Does your child pretend to write texts?	YES		NO
Does your child pretend to write other names or words?	YES		NO
Can your child write some letters?	YES		NO
Can your child write all letters?	YES		NO
Can your child write his or her own name?	YES		NO

Source: Adapted from D. K. Dickinson and J. DeTemple, 1998, "Putting Parents in the Picture: Maternal Reports of Preschoolers' Literacy as a Predictor of Early Reading," *Early Childhood Research Quarterly*, *13*(2), Tables 1 and 2, p. 248. Reproduced with permission of Pergamon.

Nonword Repetition

In the past few years nonword repetition has often been used as a measure of phonological memory. However, there is growing consensus that nonword repetition taps into many processes, including speech perception, encoding of the phonological representation, phonological memory, motor planning, and articulation (Coady & Evans, 2008; Rvachew & Grawburg, 2008). The Nonword Repetition Task (NRT; Dollagan & Campbell, 1998) was developed to minimize the impact on performance of language knowledge and potential articulation difficulties. The task contains 4 items each of 1-, 2-, 3-, and 4-syllables; none of the syllables represent an English word and do not include consonant clusters or any of the "8 late-developing" consonants. The stimuli are presented in Table 5–9. The child is instructed, "Now I will say some made-up words. Say them after me exactly the way that I say them," The child hears each previously recorded stimulus only once, under earphones. Scoring is based on the percentage of consonants correct (PCC) system and calculated for each nonword length and for the entire test.

Nonword repetition taps into many processes, including speech perception, encoding of the phonological representation, phonological memory, motor planning, and articulation.

The **Nonword Repetition Task (NRT)** was developed to minimize the impact on performance of language knowledge and potential articulation difficulties.

Although the NRT does not contain any of the later developing consonants, it includes nine vowels and 11 different consonants. For young children or children with DPD it is likely that they will misarticulate some of the target phonemes, which further complicates the interpretation of their performance on the nonword repetition task. Therefore, Shriberg and colleagues (2009) recently developed the Syllable Repetition Task (SRT). It contains only one vowel (/ɑ/) and 4 consonants (/b/, /d/, /m/, /n/). These particular phonemes were selected because 100% of children with moderate to severe DPD (PCC scores lower than 65%) who had participated in other studies at the Phonology Project and Clinic, Waisman Center, University of Wisconsin-Madison had spontaneously and accurately produced the phonemes /ɑ, b, m, n/ in a language sample, and 99.3% of the children had at least one instance of /d/ in a conversational language sample. The SRT contains eight 2-syllable items (CVCV, such as *dama*), six 3-syllable items (CVCVCV, such as *bamana*) and four

The **Syllable Repetition Task (SRT)** contains only one vowel and four consonants that are accurately produced by young children with DPD.

Table 5–9. *Stimuli of the Nonword Repetition Task*

One syllable	*Two syllables*	*Three syllables*	*Four syllables*
nɑɪb	tervɑk	tʃinɔɪtɑʊb	veitɑtʃɑɪdɔɪp
voʊp	tʃoʊvæg	nɑɪtʃoʊveɪb	dævoʊnɔɪtʃig
toʊdʒ	vætʃɑɪp	dɔɪtɑʊvæb	nɑɪtʃɔɪtɑʊvub
dɔɪf	nɔɪtɑʊf	tervɔɪtʃɑɪg	tævɑtʃinɑɪg

Source: From C. A. Dollaghan and T. F. Campbell, 1998, "Nonword Repetition and Child Language Impairment," *Journal of Speech, Language, and Hearing Research, 41*, Table 2, p. 1138. Reprinted with permission of the American Speech-Language-Hearing Association.

Table 5–10. *Stimuli of the Syllable Repetition Task (SRT)*

Two syllables	*Three syllables*	*Four syllables*
bada	bamana	bamadana
dama	dabama	danabama
bama	madaba	manabada
mada	nabada	nadamaba
naba	banada	
daba	manaba	
nada		
maba		

Source: The scoring form and scoring instructions are available in the Technical Report No. 14 by Shriberg and Lohmeier (2008) at http://www.waisman.wisc.edu/phonology

4-syllable items (CVCVCVCV, such as *manabada*). The 18 items of the SRT are presented in Table 5–10. The vowel is not scored. Consonants are scored as correct if both the manner feature (stop or nasal) and place feature (labial or alveolar) are identical to the target; cognate substitutions, such as /b/ → [p], are scored as correct, as are distortions. Omissions or substitutions of another consonant with a different place or manner feature are scored as incorrect. Technical report 14 (Shriberg & Lohmeier, 2008) includes detailed scoring instructions for the SRT, a PowerPoint presentation to present the audio stimuli, the scoring form and psychometric data on the SRT. Technical report 17 (Lohmeier & Shriberg, 2011) presents reference data for children aged 3 to 17 years with typical speech and typical language skills; children aged 3 to 8 years with speech delay and typical language skills; children aged 4 to 5 years with typical speech and language impairment; and children aged 3 to 7 years with speech delay and language impairment. These technical reports are available free of cost from the Phonology Project website (http://www.waisman.wisc.edu/phonology). From the main page of the Phonology Project and Clinic, click on: Phonology Project, then Publications & Presentations, and finally Technical Reports.

Activity Limitations and Participation Restrictions

5.3.1. Define intelligibility and describe at least one valid procedure for measuring speech intelligibility.

5.3.2. Distinguish measures of participation from measures of impairment, that is, in relation to the ICF-CY framework.

Historically, when assessing children with communication disorders, SLPs focused on Body Functions and Body Structures; few assessment tools were available for Activities and Participation, Environmental Factors and Personal Factors (McLeod & McCormack, 2007). The publication of the ICF-CY in 2007 assisted in changing the focus of assessment toward the inclusion of measures of the impact of the child's communication impairments on activity limitations and participation restrictions to identify barriers and facilitators, which in turn allows implementation of strategies that will maximize the child's functioning in real-life situations. During the case history, the parents may have mentioned activity limitations and participation restrictions they have noticed their child experience, or are worried their child will experience with environment changes, such as attending kindergarten. Impairments in body functions and body structures, contextual factors, and personal factors interact in an intricate manner and impact how the child can participate in daily life activities (McLeod & Threats, 2008; Threats, 2008). The components of the assessment described in the previous section of this book were clearly related to impairments in body functions and body structures. Some measures, such as intelligibility, belong less clearly in a specific category; for instance, intelligibility has been classified both under Activities (McLeod, 2004) and under Body Functions (Ma, Worrall, & Threats, 2007). A child who is not very intelligible to unfamiliar adults but whose parents and siblings generally understand may not experience many activity limitations and participation restrictions at home, but may have significant difficulties interacting with peers at daycare. In this section we describe measures of intelligibility and outcome measures for preschool children with communication impairments that capture participation in life activities.

The publication of the ICF-CY in 2007 assisted in changing the focus of assessment toward the inclusion of measures of the impact of the child's communication impairments on **activity limitations** and **participation restrictions**. This allows implementation of strategies that will maximize the child's functioning in real-life situations.

Measures of Intelligibility

Intelligibility represents the degree to which a person is understood. For children with DPD, being intelligible is generally their long-term goal. Intelligibility is often confused with accuracy, which is a related but different concept. As discussed in Chapter 4, mothers of normally developing 4-year-old children report that their children are completely intelligible to a stranger (Coplan & Gleason, 1988), but they do not necessarily produce all speech sounds accurately (Smit, Hand, Frellinger, Bernthal, & Bird, 1990). Conversely, a speaker could accurately produce all speech sounds but not be very intelligible due to inappropriate prosody, syntactic and grammatical mistakes, and difficulties staying on topic. In clinical practice, SLPs do not usually measure intelligibility directly but rather make an informal estimate from responses on an articulation or phonology test and/or from the conversational sample they obtained during

Intelligibility represents the degree to which a person is understood. It is often confused with **accuracy**, a related but different concept.

The use of **rating scales** for measuring intelligibility is problematic as listeners do not divide the intervals of the scale equally and because there is variability across listeners, particularly in the middle part of the scale.

the assessment session. Simple rating scales may be used to quantify the estimate, such as the conversational rating scale proposed by Bleile (1995). However, problems with the use of rating scales for measuring intelligibility were identified by Schiavetti (1992). First, listeners do not divide the intervals of the scale equally and therefore scales cannot reliably be used to compare children with different intelligibility levels, or to monitor the progress of one child as it is difficult to quantify how much change in intelligibility is required to move from one level of the scale to another. Second, there is considerable variability across listeners, in particular in the middle part of the scale, making it very difficult to interpret values such as "somewhat intelligible in conversation" across individuals. Estimating intelligibility from the conversational sample is problematic as it lacks reliability and precision, relying heavily on memory, and varying considerably from one clinician to another, as unfamiliar listeners are not equally capable of understanding what a marginally intelligible child is saying. Finally, rating scales do not identify possible sources of breakdown causing the intelligibility deficit.

The articulation score obtained on the GFTA-2 accounted for only 25% of the variance in the intelligibility scores.

Ertmer (2010) recently investigated whether intelligibility could accurately be derived from performance on the GFTA-2 (Goldman & Fristoe, 2000) Sounds in Words subtest. The articulation test was administered to 44 children age 2;10 to 15;5 with mild to profound bilateral hearing loss; all children used hearing aids or cochlear implants. A sentence repetition task was also used to obtain a connected speech sample. Three adults listened to the audio recordings of the sentences obtained from each child, wrote down the words they understood, and indicated every unintelligible word with an "X." The percentage of words correctly identified for each child was calculated. Results showed that the articulation score obtained on the GFTA-2 accounted for only 25% of the variance in the intelligibility scores, demonstrating the importance of measuring speech intelligibility directly. There are two specific scenarios where precise measurement of the child's intelligibility may be required. First, some children will present with poor intelligibility despite scoring within the average range on tests of articulation accuracy. In these rare cases, it is necessary to document carefully the degree of unintelligibility and identify the sources of the child's difficulties with the achievement of intelligible speech, in order to justify intervention and plan the therapy program. Second, when children present with severe speech delay, direct measurement of intelligibility may be necessary to document functional changes as a result of intervention, because a long period of speech therapy may be required before measurable change will be detected with tests of speech accuracy.

Precise measurement of the child's intelligibility may be required for: (1) children who score within normal limits on articulation tests but have poor intelligibility; and (2) children with severe speech delay for which a long period of speech therapy may be required before measurable changes will be detected on tests of speech accuracy.

Word identification tasks or write-down procedures can be used at different linguistic levels (single words, phrases, sentences, conversation) to generate intelligibility percentages and do not present the same disadvantages as rating scales (Gordon-Brannan, 1994; Schiavetti, 1992). The listener identifies the words spoken by the child, either by transcribing orthographically or phonetically what was said (an open-set word identification task), or by selecting what was said from a selection of responses (a closed-set word identification task). Several tools are available to assess intelligibility formally at the word level, including the *Children's Speech Intelligibility Measure* (CSIM; Wilcox & Morris, 1999). The CSIM was developed for use with children age 3 to 10, and takes approximately 20 minutes to administer and score. Each stimulus word has 11 phonetically similar words; the examiner randomly selects 50 stimulus words and the child's imitation of these is audio-recorded. One or preferably two unfamiliar listeners then either write down the 50 words produced by the child (open-set word identification) or select the multiple choice option from the stimulus word and the 11 phonetically similar foils (closed-set word identification). Intelligibility is calculated by dividing the number of correctly identified words by 50 and multiplying by 100. The *Beginner's Intelligibility Test* (BIT; Osberger, Robbins, Todd, & Riley, 1994) is one of the tools available to assess intelligibility at the sentence level. It was developed for use with young children with cochlear implants but can be used with other populations, including young children with DPD who are very unintelligible. It consists of lists of 10 short sentences containing simple, one or two syllable words; the child imitates or reads the sentences that are audio-recorded. Ideally, three unfamiliar listeners write down the child's productions, and the percentage of target words correctly identified, averaged across the listeners, is calculated. Hodge implemented a similar procedure on a computer platform for easy administration and scoring (the TOCS+ Plus version 5.3; Hodge & Daniels, 2007; http://www.tocs.plus.ualberta.ca/software_Intelligibility.html).

Word-identification tasks or **write-own procedures** do not present the same disadvantages as rating scales. Several tools are available to assess intelligibility formally at the word level, including the Children's Speech Intelligibility Measure (CSIM).

The Beginner's Intelligibility Test (BIT) is one of the tools available to assess intelligibility at the sentence level.

Despite the fact that write-down procedures have several advantages over rating scales, clinicians do not commonly use them to assess intelligibility in conversation. Yet "conversational speech is the most socially valid context for evaluating speech intelligibility" (Flipsen, 2006, p. 303). Unlike the write-down procedures at the word or sentence levels described above, the number of words produced in conversation is unknown for children who are unintelligible and for whom word boundaries are difficult to perceive. This problem represents a significant obstacle for clinicians, and along with time constraints, is probably the reason why intelligibility in conversation is rarely assessed for children with DPD. Test administration procedures for measures such as the CSIM and the BIT described above specify that unfamiliar listeners should be used as judges. To assess intelligibility, including in conversation using a measure of Intelligibility Index, it is always best to use an unfamiliar listener. In clinical practice the SLP could ask a colleague who is not familiar with his client to act as a judge, and do the same for her clients. Scoring of intelligibility measures is an appropriate role for communication disorders assistants or other paraprofessionals and student speech-language pathologists. During the assessment

It is always best to use **unfamiliar listeners** to judge intelligibility. An SLP colleague, communication disorders assistants, other paraprofessionals, or student SLPs could score the intelligibility measure.

session you will have become more familiar with the child's speech difficulties and may therefore be able to understand words that would be unintelligible to an unfamiliar listener. Similarly, it is not recommended to ask the client's parents or siblings to judge intelligibility, as they can likely understand your client much better than unfamiliar listeners (Flipsen, 1995).

Structured Measures of Participation

Appropriate outcomes measures of functional communication are needed to assess the impact of the intervention on the child's participation in daily life.

The Focus on the Outcomes of Communication Under Six (FOCUS) measure was specifically developed to provide a measure of functional communication skills for preschool children based on the ICF-FY framework.

The shift from the medical model, which assesses impairment, to a more holistic paradigm such as the ICF, which focuses on the whole child, has motivated health professionals to develop interventions that enhance the child's functional communication skills. In order to assess the impact of the intervention on the child's participation in daily life, appropriate outcome measures of functional communication are needed. Very few speech-language pathology outcome measures are available for preschool children. The American Speech-Language-Hearing Association National Outcome Measure System (Pre-K NOMS; ASHA, 1996) is commonly used in the US; however, there are no studies on the reliability and validity of the Pre-K NOMS measure, and a recent study found that it underestimated functional changes following speech-language intervention (Thomas-Stonell, McConney-Ellis, Oddson, Robertson, & Rosenbaum, 2007). The Therapy Outcome Measures (TOM; Enderby, 1997) were developed in England based on an earlier model of the WHO framework and later adapted for Australia (Australian Therapy Outcomes Measures; AusTOMS). The Focus on the Outcomes of Communication Under Six (FOCUS) measure was specifically developed to provide a measure of functional communication skills for preschool children based on the ICF-FY framework. In other words, the FOCUS was designed to capture the performance of the child in life activities and the level of assistance required to successfully participate in the activity rather than only measuring the communication impairment. Internal consistency, test-restest reliability, content, and construct validity have been established and sensitivity to change over short intervals of intervention has been demonstrated with large samples of preschool-age children receiving speech and language interventions (Thomas-Stonell, Oddson, Robertson, & Rosenbaum, 2010). Both a clinician and parent version of the FOCUS are currently available; they contain the same items but the clinician version includes an area for specifying if the information was obtained directly or through parental report. Completion time is 10 minutes, or longer if clinicians use parent interview to complete the questionnaire. The FOCUS is sensitive to changes that occur following one block of intervention lasting on average 6 to 8 weeks; a validation study to assess the usefulness of the tool for documenting long-term change is ongoing. The FOCUS includes many items related to the ICF-CY domains of activities and participation, such as "My child is included in play activities by other children," "My child makes friends easily," "My child participates in group activities," and "My child will sit and listen to stories." Clinicians currently using the FOCUS have reported collecting more information about the child's participation abilities in the community and selecting more treatment goals related to increasing participation levels and decreasing participation restrictions (Thomas-Stonell et al., 2010). Further information about the FOCUS can be found at http://www.hollandbloorview.ca/research/focusmeasurement.

Considerations for Dialect Speakers, Children Speaking English as a Second Language, and Multilingual Children

5.4.1. Describe five steps to assess second language learners of English and bilingual children.

An exciting part of the diagnostic process in phonological assessment is that a cookbook approach cannot be used; although core general components of the assessment will be similar as described earlier in this chapter, each child we assess is unique. Individual differences need to be identified and considered to differentiate whether the child presents with a DPD or whether the segmental and prosodic patterns we observe are typical of the child's linguistic community (ASHA, 2004). Although General American English (GAE) is the dialect promoted in the education system in the United States and the one typically present in the media, several English dialects are spoken in the US, including Eastern American English, Southern American English, Appalachian English, Ozark English, and African American English (AAE). Furthermore, one in five school-age children is not a native speaker of English (US Bureau of the Census, 2000). These students have a wide variety of native languages, including Spanish (79%) and Asian languages such as Vietnamese (2%), Hmong (1,6%), Cantonese (1%), and Korean (1%). Other languages account for less than 1% of nonnative English speaking students in the US but may be the first language in importance spoken after English in certain states, such as Yup'ik in Alaska, French in Maine, Blackfoot in Montana, and Croatian in Vermont (Office of English Language Acquisition, 2002). Only 6 states accounted for roughly three-quarters of immigrants in 2000 (California, Texas, New York, Florida, Illinois, and New Jersey) but the number of immigrants in other states has increased considerably since 1990 (Ruiz-de-Velasco & Fix, 2000). In Canada, the 2006 Census revealed that approximately 20% of the population was born in a foreign country; 70% of them declared their maternal language to be different than English or French, the two official Canadian languages, in the following proportions: Chinese (19%), Italian (7%), Pendjabi (6%), Spanish (6%), German (5%), Tagalog (5%), and Arabic (5%).

Individual differences need to be identified and considered to differentiate whether the child presents with a DPD or whether the segmental and prosodic patterns we observe are typical of the child's linguistic community.

SLPs across North America, as elsewhere in the world, therefore, are very likely to have children who are not proficient in English and/or speak more than one language in their caseload. As the mobility level of society increases, it is also possible to encounter a child who speaks a dialect unusually present in the geographical area of your clinical setting. It is important to be aware of characteristics of the local dialect(s). We briefly review the most common dialects of English in the United States in this chapter. Two sources of information may be particularly useful for SLPs practicing around the globe: (1) the International guide to speech acquisition (McLeod, 2007) provides information about 12 dialects of English and 24 languages other than English, including assessment and intervention tools commonly used for each of these languages and dialects; and (2) Multilingual aspects of speech sound disorders in children (McLeod & Goldstein, 2012) addresses multilingual speech acquisition and translates research into clinical practice for specified regional or linguistic contexts.

Speakers of Dialects of English

The term **dialect** refers to varied forms of a language shared by speakers of a geographical region, ethnic group or social class. We all speak a dialect of English and vary our **register** depending on the interlocutor, topic of conversation, and social setting.

The term *dialect* refers to varied forms of a language shared by speakers of a geographical region, ethnic group or social class. No dialect is superior to another, although the "standard" dialect of a language, GAE in the US, is promoted in the educational system and considered more prestigious than other dialects of the language (Adler, 1984). We all speak a dialect of English and use different registers of the dialect depending on our interlocutor, topic of conversation and social setting. For instance, speakers of GAE tend to use a formal register in writing and during formal speaking situations but an informal register when talking to family and friends. Regional variability in pronunciation and vocabulary will be accepted as part of the continuum of the standard dialects of a language, whereas dialects that contain grammatical structures that are socially stigmatized will be considered outside the informal range of the standard dialect. These are called *vernacular dialects* and sometimes social or ethnic dialects as they are usually related to ethnicity and/or socioeconomic status. Examples of nonstandard English grammatical structures include omission of the copula (e.g., "Who you?"), double negation (e.g., "I don't know nothing") and lack of subject-verb agreement (e.g., "They was sleeping"). The recently published Atlas of North American English (Labov, Ash, & Boberg, 2006) describes the pronunciation and vowel systems of English dialects in the US and Canada and maps their ongoing sound changes. Data was obtained by conducting phone interviews with 762 speakers of small and big cities across North America, with special attention given to adults between the ages of 20 and 40. IPA transcriptions of vowels elicited in minimal pairs were completed, and additionally acoustic analyses were performed on 439 of the speech samples.

Four major regions of distinctive varieties of English pronunciation were identified in the US: North, South, West, and Midland. We now turn to a brief description of these four regional dialects; their common dialectal variations are summarized in Table 5–11. A more in-depth description of African American English, the most common vernacular dialect in the US, follows.

North

The northern dialect, also called *Eastern American English,* runs from Vermont to New Jersey, including parts of Iowa and Minnesota to the West (Wolfram & Schilling-Estes, 2006). Labov, Yaeger, and Steiner (1973) first described the Northern Cities Vowel Shift, a vowel rotation pattern in which each of a chain of vowels receives a new place of articulation in terms of tongue advancement and height. More specifically, the long vowels move forward and upward, whereas the short vowels move downward and backward (Wolfram & Schilling-Estes, 2006). In other words, /ɔ/ is raised, tensed, and lengthened

Table 5–11. *Common Dialectal Variations of Standard American English Dialects Other Than the North and South Vowel Shifts*

Phonological Pattern	*Example*		*Dialect(s)*
/ɹ/ and /l/ reduction or loss after a vowel	/ɹ/ → [ə] or [ː] /l/ → [ʊ]	"sister" → [sɪstə] "car" → [kaː] "still" → [stɪʊ]	North, South
Loss of postconsonantal /ɹ/	/ɹ/ → [Ø]	"throw → [θoʊ]	Appalachian, Ozark
Loss of intervocalic /ɹ/	/ɹ/ → [Ø]	"carrot" → [kæət]	Appalachian, Ozark
Rhotacization of /ə/, often if the following word starts with a vowel	/ə/ → [ɚ]	"Linda" → [lɪndɚ]	North
Loss of /l/ before labials	/l/ → [Ø]	"help" → [hɛp]	Appalachian, Ozark
Initial [w] reduction	/w/ → [Ø]	"wall" → [ɒl]	Appalachian, Ozark
Deletion of initial unstressed syllable	IUS → [Ø]	"aloud" → [laʊd]	Appalachian, Ozark
Epenthesis in clusters	/CCC#/ → [CCəC#]	"tests" → [tɛstəs]	Appalachian, Ozark
Stopping of /θ/ and /ð/ word initially	/θ/ → [t]; /ð/ → [d]	"thing" → [tɪŋ] "this" → [dɪs]	North, Appalachian, Ozark
Intrusive /t/	/s/# → [st] /f/# → [ft]	 "cliff" → [klɪft]	Appalachian
Epenthesis of /i/ before /u/	/u/ → /iu/	"new" → /niu/	South

Source: Data summarized from Small (2012), Wolfram and Schilling-Estes (2006), and Christian, Wolfram, & Dube (1988).

and moves forward in the direction of /ɑ/; /ɑ/ in turns moves toward /ae/; and /ae/ moves toward the vowel /ɛ/. The merger of the low back vowel /ɔ/ and low back/central vowel /ɑ/ results in words such as "caught" and "cot" being pronounced the same way and is a main characteristic of regions in Eastern New England and Western Pennsylvania. Major cities throughout the country, such as New York and Philadelphia in the North, have developed their own regional dialects. Common differences in the production of consonants in the North are presented in Table 5–11.

South

The Southern American English dialect runs approximately from Maryland to the north, Florida to the south, and Texas to the west (Wolfram & Schilling-Estes, 2006). The Southern Vowel Shift is also a rotation pattern, but in this case the short front vowels shift upward and often become diphthongized (e.g. /ɪ/ → [i]; /ɛ/ → [e] or [eɪ]). At the same time, the long front vowels move backward and downward (e.g., /e/ → [ɛ]; /i/ → [ɪ]) and the back vowels move forward (e.g., /u/ → [ʊ]; /o/ → [ʌ]). This vowel shift is not present in all regions of the South, and in particular is absent in Charleston, South Carolina and Savannah, Georgia. Differences in the production of consonants in the Southern dialect include /ŋ/ → [n] and voicing assimilations (Small, 2004; Wolfram & Schilling-Estes, 2006). Two common regional dialects are present in the South: Appalachian English (parts of Kentucky, Tennessee, West Virginia, Virginia, and North Carolina) and Ozark English (southern Missouri, northern Arkansas, and northwestern Oklahoma (Christian, Wolfram, & Dube, 1988). The major phonological patterns associated with Southern American English, Appalachian English, and Ozark English are also presented in Table 5–11.

Midland

A common feature in the Midland region is the lack of participation in the North and South vowel shifts. Fronting of /uʊ/, /oʊ/, and /aʊ/ is very frequent; however, each of the main cities has developed its own regional patterns, such that Philadelphia, Pittsburg, Cincinnati, Columbus, Indianapolis, St. Louis, and Kansas City have their own urban dialects (Labov et al, 2006).

West

As we move to the West there is a diffusion of the characteristics of the North, South, and Midland that results in little dialectal diversity (Labov et al, 2006). The merger of the low back vowel /ɔ/ and low back/central vowel /ɑ/ is the most prominent feature of the West, although it is also present in the North. However the merger of these two vowels, in combination with the fronting of /u/, is more frequent in the West than elsewhere in the US.

African American English (AAE)

Many African Americans, but not all, speak AAE, and speakers of AAE vary in the degree to which they use characteristic features of AAE. Other groups in the US who are geographically close to speakers of AAE will exhibit features of AAE in their speech. For example, Wolfram (1974) found that Puerto Rican children speaking English in Harlem, New York, were using more features of AAE in their speech if they had close contact with African Americans. Most African American children entering kindergarten speak AAE and will acquire GAE in school. Phonological features of AAE often persist longer than morphological, syntactic, and semantic characteristics (Craig, Thompson, Washington, & Potter, 2003), and as many as 50% of children who spoke AAE in kindergarten still use some phonological features of AAE in fifth grade (Craig & Washington, 2004). Recent studies on AAE phonological milestones and phonological skills of AAE-speaking children with DPD provide crucial information which helps the SLP distinguish phonological differences from signs of DPD in speakers of this dialect. Pearson, Velleman, Bryant, and Charko (2009) provided phonological milestones for AAE-speaking children who were learning GAE as a second dialect. A total of 854 normally developing children aged 4 to 12 years participated in the study: 537 were acquiring AAE as a first dialect and 317 were acquiring GAE. The participants completed the Dialect Sensitive Language Test (DSLT; Seymour, Roeper, & de Villiers, 2000), which is an unpublished pilot edition of the Diagnostic Evaluation of Language Variation (DELV; Seymour, Roeper, & de Villiers, 2003, 2005). Pearson and colleagues calculated the age of mastery (90% production accuracy) of singletons and clusters in initial and final position. Both groups of participants mastered production of the following phonemes in initial position at age 4: /b/, /t/, /d/, /k/, /g/, /m/, /n/, /h/, /j/, /w/, /f/, /dʒ/, /tʃ/, /ʃ/, and /l/ (initial /p/ was omitted by mistake from the study). Initial /v/ and /z/ were mastered at age 5 and /θ/ at age 6 in both groups. Children acquiring AAE mastered initial /ɹ/ and /s/ at age 4, 2 years earlier than GAE-speaking children. In the final position, the phonemes /m/, /n/, /p/, /ŋ/, /f/, /ʃ/, /tʃ/, and /ɹ/ were mastered at age 4 by both groups. Children speaking AAE mastered final /s/ and /z/ at the age of 4 compared to the age of 6 for speakers of GAE. However, children speaking GAE mastered several final consonants at age 4 which were mastered by AAE speaking-children at age 5 (/b/, /dʒ/, /l/), age 6 (/k/, /g/, /v/), and age 8 (/t/, /d/). AAE-speaking children mastered several initial clusters earlier: /kl/ and /pl/ at age 4 compared to 5 for speakers of GAE; /kɹ/ at 4 compared to 6; /pɹ/, /gɹ/, /sp/, and /st/ at age 5 compared to age 6; and /skɹ/ at age 7 compared to age 8. Children speaking GAE mastered initial /tɹ/, /stɹ/, /ʃɹ/, and /θɹ/ at a younger age. Final consonant clusters were generally mastered by speakers of GAE earlier than by speakers of AAE. The disparity between groups was greatest for the phoneme /ð/ as it was mastered at age 12 by speakers of AAE, 4 years later

Many African Americans, but not all, speak **AAE**, and speakers of AAE vary in the degree to which they use characteristic features of AAE.

Phonological features of AAE often persist longer than morphological, syntactic, and semantic characteristics. Up to 50% of children using AAE in kindergarten will still use some phonological features of the dialect in fifth grade.

Pearson, Velleman, Bryant, and Charko (2009) provided phonological **milestones for AAE-speaking children** who were learning GAE as a second dialect that help SLPs distinguish phonological differences from a DPD.

than speakers of GAE in the initial position and 2 years later in the final position.

Differences between the phonological systems of GAE and AAE are present mostly at the **prosodic level**.

Further inspection of the differences between the phonological systems of GAE and AAE reveal that they are present mostly at the phonotactic (prosodic) level. The syllable and word structures influence in what context and how often segments are used, as seen in Table 5–12. The authors noted that according to Velleman, Pear-

Table 5–12. *Phonetic (Segmental) and Phonotactic (Prosodic) Differences Between AAE and GAE*

Difference	*Example*
Phonetic differences	
Final obstruents (stops, fricatives, and affricates): Devoiced	"cage" → [ketʃ]
Final /d/: Glottalized	"mad" → [mæʔ]
/l/: Vowelized or absent, especially in final position and before labials	"help" → [hɛp]
/r/: Vowelized or absent	
intersyllabically	"story" → [stoʊi]
in syllabic contexts	"butter" → [bʌɾə]
postvocalically	"hard" → [hɑd]
in clusters, specifically after /θ/ and in unstressed syllables	"throw" → [θo]
Hyperarticulated postvocalically	"chair" → [tʃɛrə]
Interdental fricatives (/θ/, /ð/): replaced by	
alveolar stops in initial position	"these" → [diz]
labial fricatives or alveolar stops in medial and final contexts	"bath" → [bæf]
Specific initial clusters substituted	
/str-/ realized as [skr-]	"street" → [skrit]
/kj-/ realized as [kr-]	"cute" → [krut]
Phonotactic differences	
Final consonants absent, especially	
obstruents, especially voiced, coronal, and/or stop	
vowel lengthening preserved if voiced	"mad" → [mæː]
nasals; vowel nasalization preserved	"can" → [kæ̃ː]
Final clusters reduced	"fast" → [fæs]
Initial weak syllables absent from iambic words	"about" → [baʊʔ]
Medial weak syllables absent, particularly in reduplicated contexts	"Mississippi" → "Missippi"
Initial weak syllables stressed (trochaicization)	"poLICE" → "POlice"
[final] /s/ + stop metathesized—lexically specified?	"asks" → [æks]

Source: From S. L. Velleman and B. Z. Pearson, 2010, "Differentiating Speech Sound Disorders From Phonological Dialect Differences: Implications for Assessment and Intervention," *Topics in Language Disorders*, 30(3), Table 1, p. 177. Reproduced with permission of Lippincott, Williams & Wilkins.

son, Bryant, and Charko (submitted) there is a different tradeoff between the segmental and the prosodic level in speakers of these two dialects. Children acquiring AAE are more likely to simplify the phonotactic word structure, for instance, by reducing consonant clusters or inserting a vowel between the two consonants. These simplifications allow them to achieve greater accuracy of later-developing consonants. Children acquiring GAE, on the other hand, do not tend to simplify complex word structures and are less accurate in producing segments.

There seems to be a **different tradeoff between the segmental and the prosodic level** in speakers of GAE and AAE, with AAE children achieving greater accuracy of later-developing consonants while being more likely to simplify the phonotactic word structure.

Velleman and Pearson (2010) investigated whether the differences seen between normally developing children acquiring GAE and AAE would also be seen in children who present with a speech sound delay or disorder. The participants were 72 children acquiring GAE and 76 children acquiring AAE, age 4 to 12, who were identified by the school SLP as presenting with speech delay/disorder and who scored more than 1 SD below the mean on the phonology subtest of the DELV-Norm Referenced (Seymour et al., 2005). Children with speech delays/disorders were delayed in their mastery of many initial consonants compared to normally developing children, but some dialectal differences remained. For example, AAE children with speech sound disorder/delay mastered /f/, /j/, and /s/ at age 6 compared to age 8 and /v/, /tʃ/, and /dʒ/ at age 8 compared to age 10 for children speaking GAE with DPD. Both groups of children with DPD mastered initial consonant clusters at a much later age than typically developing children. Dialectal differences were also observed for clusters; AAE-speakers with DPD mastered several clusters at earlier ages than GAE-children with DPD. For instance, AAE-DPD speakers mastered /bɹ/, /dɹ/, /tɹ/, /gl/, and /θɹ/ clusters at age 10 compared to age 12 or later for GAE speaking children with DPD. The results of this study confirm the value in using a dialect-neutral phonology test such as the DELV-NR to differentiate dialectal differences from DPD in children speaking dialects of English.

Children with DPD speaking either GAE or AAE were delayed in their mastery of initial consonants and consonant clusters compared to normally developing children. However, some **dialectal differences remained**, with AAE speaking children with DPD mastering some initial consonants and consonant clusters earlier than children speaking GAE with DPD.

Children Speaking English as a Second Language, Bilingual and Multilingual Children

Taking dialectal variations into account when analyzing the phonological system of children from culturally and linguistically diverse backgrounds ensures correctly identifying children who present with a DPD and require intervention, although not erroneously diagnosing normally developing children as presenting with a DPD. Ideally the SLP would be proficient in each of the child's languages, but that is not often the case. If you are a monolingual SLP, or are not proficient in the language(s) spoken by the child, you could consider using interpreters/translators (I/Ts), hiring bilingual consultants, or working in collaboration with bilingual communication disorders assistants (Langdon & Cheng, 2002). When using interpreters,

For accurate diagnosis, it is important to take dialectal variations into consideration when assessing children from culturally and linguistically diverse backgrounds.

Working in collaboration with **interpreters/translators, bilingual consultants, or bilingual communication disorders assistants** is recommended if you are not proficient in the child's languages. It is best to avoid using parents or other family members as interpreters/translators.

it is recommended to verify whether they are trained and/or have experience helping SLPs conduct speech and language assessments, are proficient in the same dialects as the family, can relate to their cultural group, and understand their role and professional responsibilities (Langdon & Cheng, 2002). As opposed to most other situations interpreters encounter, during the SLP assessment they have to be very careful not to use repetitions, body language, synonyms, or semantic clues that may affect the performance of the child. Before the assessment it is useful to meet with the I/Ts, and clarify what they will do if the parents seek advice during or after the SLP assessment; if they disagree with what the SLP says or how the questions are formulated; and what are things you can do to help them. It is preferable not to use parents, siblings, or other family members as I/Ts, as they are not trained, may leave out information, and may be uncomfortable in this role (Lynch, 2004). If you do not speak the language(s) of a child with very limited or no proficiency in English, and there are no bilingual professionals available, you may conduct the hearing screening, oral-peripheral examination, and nonverbal assessment measures (ASHA, 1985).

If there are no bilingual professionals available and you are not proficient in the language(s) of a child with very limited or no English proficiency, you may conduct the hearing screening, oral-peripheral examination, and nonverbal assessment measures.

Although SLPs are aware of the importance of considering dialectal variations, exactly how to do so during the assessment process is often unclear. Children learning English as a second language and multilingual children are exposed to English in different proportions and have different degrees of English proficiency. The phonological development of bilingual children is similar to that of monolingual children in each of their languages, but not quite identical (Goldstein, 2004; Goldstein et al., 2005). In other words, bilingual children are not "two monolingual children in one." Like monolingual children, as they get older and with continued exposure to their languages, bilingual children will develop more precise perceptual, articulatory, phonological, and suprasegmental knowledge, eventually achieving adultlike pronunciation in each of their languages. However, it may be challenging for the SLP to determine whether a young bilingual child presents with speech sound errors that are due to a DPD, due to cross-linguistic effects, or due to normal development (Yavas & Goldstein, 1998). Similarly, in school age children it may be difficult to determine whether a bilingual or multilingual child simply presents with an accent, or whether the child actually presents with residual errors due to a DPD that will require intervention.

The phonological development of bilingual children is similar to that of monolingual children in each of their languages, but **not quite identical**. It may be challenging for an SLP to determine whether a young bilingual child presents with speech sound errors that are due to a DPD, cross-linguistic effects, or normal development.

Clinicians now have access to a growing body of knowledge concerning the phonological systems and normal phonological development for a variety of languages. Table 5–13 lists sources of information for the most common languages other than English in the US, namely, Spanish, Vietnamese, Hmong, Cantonese, and Korean. The identification of DPD in children from linguistically diverse backgrounds often starts by looking at the phonemic inventories of the child's language(s), and comparing them to English.

Table 5–13. *Useful Sources of Information Regarding Normal and Disordered Phonological Development, As Well As the Adult Phonological Systems of the Most Common Languages Other Than English in the US*

Language	*Phonological Development*	*Children with DPD*	*Adult Phonological System*
Spanish			
Hispanic	Goldstein (1995, 2000, 2007a)	Goldstein & Pollock (2000); Goldstein (2007b)	Goldstein (1995); Hammond (2001)
Cuban American			Hidalgo (1987)
Puerto Rican		Goldstein (2007b)	Zentella (2000)
Nicaraguan			Lipski (2000)
Vietnamese		Tang & Barlow (2006)	Hwa-Froelich, Hodson, & Edwards (2002)
Cantonese	So & Dodd (1995)	So & Dodd (1994)	Bauer & Benedict (1997)
Hmong			Mortensen (2004); Ratliff (1992)
Korean	Ha, Johnson, & Kuehn (2009)		Ladefoged & Maddieson (1996); Lee (1999)

However, we caution that this will not be sufficient to determine which English sounds may be difficult for the child to learn. Multiple acoustic cues may signal each phonological contrast, but some cues are more relevant than others and influence perception to a greater degree. For example, when distinguishing English /b/ from /d/, formant transitions are more important than the spectral characteristics of the burst, whereas when discriminating English /s/ from /ʃ/ in English, the spectral characteristics of the frication has a greater influence than the formant transitions (Nittrouer, 2002). The cues also differ by language, such that different cues may be important for the same phoneme across languages. Nonetheless identifying DPD in children from linguistically diverse backgrounds relies on determining which speech errors are possibly due to influence from the child's other language(s) (Yavas & Goldstein, 1998). There are several ways in which the phonology of one of the child's language will influence another language (Goldstein, 2007). Some phonemes will only be present in the phonemic inventory of English, and the child may then substitute another phoneme from the native language that has similar acoustic or articulatory characteristics to the sound in English. For example, /ɹ/ and /l/ are not present in Japanese, and are assimilated to the flap /ɾ/, which is present in the Japanese phonemic inventory. Differences also exist in terms of the place of articulation of a consonant across languages; for example native speakers of Spanish may produce English /d/ with a dental rather than alveolar place of articulation, as Spanish /d/ is produced dentally (Perez, 1994). The contexts in which phonemes

Although looking at the phonemic inventories of the child's language(s) and comparing them to English is a good start, it is **not sufficient** to determine which English sounds may be difficult for the child to learn.

are allowed also vary across languages, such that some sounds are not allowed in certain word positions. For instance, in Japanese only nasal codas are allowed, and Japanese-speaking children learning English will often omit or weaken English codas (e.g., Dickerson, 1975).

The challenges for the SLP include deciding in which language(s) to conduct the assessment, and which assessment measures to use. A detailed phonological assessment consists of a combination of formal and informal measures. Unfortunately, few tools are available to formally assess articulation or phonology skills in languages other than English and Spanish. In this case the parents, and often the interpreter as well, can help determining to what extent is the child intelligible and whether the child produces vowels and consonants in the same way as other children speaking the same language. Goldstein and Fabiano (2007) described five steps to assessing second language learners of English and bilingual children. The first step is to gather specific information during the case history regarding past and current number of hours per week the child hears each of his languages, and past and current number of hours the child uses each language. Step two consists of obtaining single-word and connected speech samples in each of the languages of bilingual children and second language learners who have some or good proficiency in English. For second language learners of English who have no or little proficiency of English, the language sample should be collected in their native language(s). Step three is the independent analysis, as described in Chapter 4 (e.g., organizing the phonetic inventory of each language by place and manner of articulation). Step four consists of performing a relational analysis to determine: how accurate the child is in producing vowels and consonants that are common to both languages, and vowels and consonants that are unique to each language. The relational analysis also includes looking at phonological patterns, keeping in mind the type and frequency of patterns normally occurring in each language. The final step, step five, is the substitution error analysis. Accounting for dialectal differences at this step involves giving credit to the child if an error can be due to dialectal differences or cross-linguistic factors. For example, if a Japanese second language learner of English produces English /ɹ, l/ → /ɾ/, these would be scored as a dialectally appropriate.

Goldstein and Fabiano (2007) described **five steps** to assessing second language learners of English and bilingual children.

Preston and Seki (2011) recently described a method to correctly identify residual errors in a bilingual child by presenting the case study of KT, an 11-year-old Japanese-English bilingual boy. The authors recommend first conducting a relational speech analysis in each of the child's languages to identify differences in production that may be due to transfer of the native language to the second language. In the case of KT a single-word test of articulation was administered in each language, the GFTA-2 in English

Preston and Seki (2011) recently described a method to correctly identify residual errors in bilingual children. This method combines a **relational speech analysis** with measures of **speech motor control** and **phonological awareness**.

and the Japanese Articulation Test-Revised (Japanese Speech-Language-Hearing Association, 1994). A conversational speech sample and sentence imitation were also elicited in each language. In English, the relational analysis involved looking at the sounds and syllable shapes present in English but not in Japanese, and giving him credit if the errors could be due to cross-linguistic transfer. The PCC and PCC-R based on the production of the single words of the GFTA-2, scoring possible transfer errors as correct, was outside the normal range for 11-year-olds. The authors then looked at whether KT's errors were context-specific and predictable, and could be due to phonological rules developed by KT. However, several errors did not seem consistent or highly systematic. In Japanese, errors typically seen in children younger than age 6 were present in picture-naming, sentence repetition and conversational speech. Similarities between error patterns in English and in Japanese were then examined. Preston and Seki supplemented the results of the relational speech analysis with measures of speech motor control and phonological awareness. Although PA was a relative strength for KT in both languages, difficulties were present with repeated productions of English and Japanese multisyllabic/multimoraic words, as well as in the repetition of the syllable sequence /pʌtʌkʌ/. Based on these results they concluded that KT presents with residual errors that appeared to reflect difficulties with speech motor control.

Putting It All Together

In this chapter we have discussed assessment tools that can be used over a series of assessment sessions to gather information for diagnostic purposes at the level of impairment, activity limitations, and participation limitations. In Case Study 5–1, we present the results of an initial assessment that lasted 90 minutes and describe the interpretation of this information. The child to be featured in this case study, PA 218, was referred to a major children's hospital for assessment by his family doctor. He was then recruited into a longitudinal follow-up study of children with speech delay; PA 218 was 4;11 at the time of the assessment. The results of the assessment measures administered are presented below. A brief interpretation of the assessment results follow; in Chapter 8 we provide a detailed discussion of how to integrate assessment test scores with other information in order to make decisions about when to provide intervention to children with DPD.

Case Study 5–1

Case History

Parents are concerned about their son's intelligibility compared to other children his age. His impending enrollment in kindergarten heightened their level of concern.

Birth: unremarkable (no complications during pregnancy or at birth).

Medical: uneventful (no hospitalizations, medication, allergies or surgeries).

Developmental: delayed language milestones (first words around 18 months; word combinations with verbs around age 3;0).

Family history: father (speech difficulties as preschooler); maternal uncle (language difficulties). Both parents completed high school and are currently working.

Summary of Scores Obtained at Initial Assessment (CA = 4;11)

PPVT-III	61st percentile
MLU	2.53
GFTA-2	4th percentile
PCC	71.77%, $z = -1.07$
SAILS	60.42%, $z = -2.62$
PAT	Raw score = 10, $z = -2.49$
Letters	Raw score = 8
Literacy Knowledge	Raw score = 1

Notes: PPVT-III = Peabody Picture Vocabulary Test-III (Dunn & Dunn, 1997); MLU = Mean Length of Utterance (in morphemes); GFTA-2 = Goldman-Fristoe Test of Articulation—2 (Goldman & Fristoe, 2000); PCC = Percent Consonants Correct, assessed in conversation (see Chapters 4 and 5); SAILS = Speech Assessment and Interactive Learning System (measure of speech perception skills; see http://www.medicine.mcgill.ca/srvachew); PAT = Phonological Awareness Test (Bird, Bishop, & Freeman, 1995); Letters = number of letters named; Literacy Knowledge = adaptation of an early literacy assessment protocol used by Jerry L. Johns at Northern Illinois University.

Speech Sample

A dog.
æ dɑg.

No.
no.

A baby.
æ bebi.

A lady.
æ ledi.

Shop/ing.
jɑpɪŋ.

A dog.
æ dɑg.

He pull/ing the dog (EW: dog/Z) ear.
hi pʌlɪŋ ʌ dɑg iə.

A baby come/d (EW: came) out.
æ bebi kʌmd aut.

In here.
ɪn hiə.

Turn/ing on a light.
tərɪŋ ɑn ɑ lait.

Him (EW: he's) put/ing the baby in a truck.
hɪm pʊtɪŋ ʌ bebi ɑ ɪn æ trʌ.

Him (EW: he's) push/ing him.
hɪm pʊtʃɪŋ hɪm.

I *don't know.
æ no.

Him (EW: he's) bite/ing him there.
hɪm baiɪŋ hɪm de.

Yeah.
jɛ.

In a library.
ɪn ɑ laibəwi.

Read/ing *a book.
wiɪŋ bʊ.

No.
no.

I *don't know.
æ no.

Put/ing on *a hat.
pʊtɪŋ an hæt.

I *don't know.
æ no.

I *don't know.
æ no.

A TV store.
æ ti wi do.

A baby.
æ bebi.

A dog.
æ dɑg.

(A a) a mitten.
æ æ æ mɪdɛn.

Glove.
gʌb.

Cry/ing.
kɑaiɪn.

Him (EW: he's) go/ing in a (e) elevator.
him goɪŋ ɪn æ ɛ ɛwɑgedər.

And sleep/ing.
æn lipɪŋ

I *don't know.
æ no.

Eat.
ɪt.

Cheese.
tʃid.

Eat/ing.
itɪŋ.

Him (EW: he's) look/ing at the pet
hɪm lʊkɪŋ æt dʌ pɛt.

Parrot.
pewɑt.

Dog.
dɑg.

Cat.
kæ.

Dog.
dɑg.

Dog.
dɑg.

Bunny.
bʌni.

They *are let/ing them out.
de lɛtɪŋ dɛm aʊt.

I *don't know.
æ no.

A chicken.
æ tʃɪkən.

I *don't know.
æ no.

Hu/ging him.
hʌgɪŋ ɪm.

(On him) on the box.
ɑn hɪm ɑn ʌ bɑt.

Him (EW: he's) walk/ing.
hɪm wɑkɪŋ.

(R r) run/ing.
w w wʌnɪŋ.

Walk/ing.
wɑkɪŋ.

A (EW: an) elevator.
æ æwɪgedər.

And him (EW: he) run/ed (EW: ran).
æn hɪm wʌnd.

Note: The speech sample was obtained with the wordless book *Carl Goes Shopping,* by Alexandra Day. The sample was also analyzed using the Systematic Analysis of Language Transcripts (SALT; Miller & Chapman, 1996); the coding scheme for SALT is presented in the orthographic gloss of the sample; the summary of the results of the word and morphemes analysis is presented below.

Word and Morphemes Summary for the Speech Sample Analyzed Using SALT

MLU in Words	2.19
MLU in Morphemes	2.53
Brown's Stage	III
Expected Age Range (mos.)	24–41
Type Token Ratio	0.50
No. Diff. Word Roots	52
No. Main Body Words	103
No. Bound Morphemes	16
No. Maze Words	3
No. Omitted Words	12
No. Omitted Bound Morphemes	4

Speech Perception Assessment

Four modules of SAILS were administered to PA 218. Demonstration 5–4 shows how to transform the child's raw scores on these modules into z-scores to compare his performance to the normative sample.

The SAILS computer program does not allow for assessment of all of the phonemes that this child misarticulated. For example, the error /v/ → [w] in onsets can be seen on the GFTA-2 protocol for PA 218, but SAILS does not contain modules for any voiced phonemes. An example scoring sheet, individualized to the error patterns observed in PA 218's speech, is presented in Table 5–14 with appropriate stimulus, response and control phonemes for testing perception of /v/ and /z/.

Interpretation of the Results

In terms of language skills, receptive vocabulary as measured by the PPVT-III, was well within normal limits, with a standard score of 104 and a percentile rank of 61. The mean length of utterance for the spontaneous language sample of 64 utterances was 2.53, significantly lower than the expected value of 5.32 to 5.63 for children between the ages of 4;9 and 5;0 (Miller & Chapman, 1981). Difficulties with morphosyntax included: omission of the auxiliary (obligatory); omission of articles and pronouns (frequent); difficulties with pronoun use (such as using *him* for *he* and *she*); difficulties with irregular past tense (example: *a baby comed out*), production

Demonstration 5–4
Calculation of the *z*-Scores Obtained by Child PA 218 on Certain SAILS Modules During the Prekindergarten Assessment

	Norms			
Module	**Mean**	**SD**	**Mean score[a]**	***z*-score[b]**
Cat	87.00	8.06	70.00	−2.11
Lake	78.60	7.17	60.00	−2.59
Rat	79.46	10.92	55.00	−2.24
Sue	71.52	8.64	56.67	−1.72

[a]Mean score is the child's percent correct score averaged across the test blocks for the module

[b]To calculate the z-score: (child's mean score – mean) / SD
Example: for "cat" module, z-score = (70 – 87) / 8.06 = −2.11

Table 5–14. Sample Speech Perception Production Task Filled in for Child PA 218

Child's Name: PA 218 ____ Sex: M Birthdate: ____ Age: 4 yrs. 11 mos.

Date ____		Date ____		Date ____	
Production Task		Production Task		Production Task	
Stimulus	Response*	Stimulus	Response*	Stimulus	Response*
/v a n/ →	[w a n]	/z ɪ p/ →	[j ɪ p]	/ / →	[ ]
SP /v/ RP /w/	CP /b/	SP /z/ RP /j/	CP /s/	SP RP	CP
Stimulus-Class	*Response*	*Stimulus-Class*	*Response*	*Stimulus-Class*	*Response*
1 /b/ - CP	yes NO	1 /z/ - SP	YES no		
2 /w/ - RP	yes NO	2 /s/ - CP	yes NO		
3 /v/ - SP	YES no	3 /j/ - RP	yes NO		
4 /v/ - SP	YES no	4 /s/ - CP	yes NO		
5 /w/ - RP	yes NO	5 /z/ - SP	YES no		
6 /b/ - CP	yes NO	6 /z/ - SP	YES no		
7 /b/ - CP	yes NO	7 /j/ - RP	yes NO		
8 /v/ - SP	YES no	8 /s/ - CP	yes NO		
9 /w/ - RP	yes NO	9 /s/ - CP	yes NO		
10 /v/ - SP	YES no	10 /z/ - SP	YES no		
11 /w/ - RP	yes NO	11 /j/ - RP	yes NO		
12 /b/ - CP	yes NO	12 /j/ - RP	yes NO		
13 /b/ - CP	yes NO	13 /z/ - SP	YES no		
14 /w/ - RP	yes NO	14 /j/ - RP	yes NO		
15 /v/ - SP	YES no	15 /s/ - CP	yes NO		
16 /b/ - CP	yes NO	16 /j/ - RP	yes NO		
17 /v/ - SP	YES no	17 /z/ - SP	YES no		
18 /w/ - RP	yes NO	18 /s/ - CP	yes NO		
RP ____ CP ____	SP ____	RP ____ CP ____	SP ____	RP ____ CP ____	SP ____

*The correct response is in uppercase letters.

Source: From J. L. Locke, 1980, "The Inference of Speech Perception in the Phonologically Disordered Child. Part II: Some Clinically Novel Procedures, Their Use, Some Findings," *Journal of Speech and Hearing Disorders*, 45(4), Figure 1, p. 447. Adapted with permission of the American Speech-Language and Hearing Association.

of very few sentences of the form *Subject* + *Verb* + *Object* and no production of more complex sentences. Parameters of voice, resonance, fluency and pragmatics were within normal limits as subjectively assessed during the speech sample. He passed the hearing screening and no significant issues were raised during the oral-peripheral examination.

As seen in Demonstration 5–2, PA 218 obtained a percentile rank of 4 on the GFTA-2, which according to the standardized test corresponds to a severity ranking of moderate.

The PCC for the speech sample was 71.77%, which corresponds to a severity level of "mild-moderate" as recommended by Shriberg and Kwiatkowski (1982). However, "moderate" or even "moderate-severe" is clearly a more appropriate ranking when one considers the child's error patterns. Closer examination of his error patterns on the GFTA-2 and in connected speech reveal the presence of atypical errors, especially pervasive gliding of many fricatives in onsets and occasional affrication of /tʃ/ in ambisyllabic and coda contexts. Frequent stopping of fricatives, a phonological process that should be resolved before the age of 3 years is also a significant concern. Although it is not uncommon for production of consonant clusters to not be mastered yet in a child aged 4;11, the fact that he produced only one cluster (/fɹ/ →[fw]) is worrisome.

His performance on the four modules of SAILS was well below normal limits for his age, with *z*-scores ranging from −1.72 to −2.59 standard deviations from the means (see Demonstration 5–4). The child obtained a raw score of 10/34 on the Phonological Awareness Test (Bird, Bishop, & Freeman, 1995), a score that is more than one standard deviation below the mean compared to other children his age (refer to Appendix 5–6). The Early Literacy Assessment used in this research project, an adaptation of a protocol by Jerry L. Johns at Northern Illinois University, indicated that PA 218 identified 8/12 letters and did not identify any words such as "a," "to," "in." The child obtained a score of 1/10 on Literacy Knowledge: among others he did not show the front of the book, the title, a letter, or a word.

We can interpret these assessment results with reference to the framework shown in Table II–1. In the first column we asked questions relating to diagnosis, specifically, does the child have DPD? For PA218, we can be certain of this diagnosis from his performance on the GFTA, with converging evidence from his PCC, showing standardized scores below normal limits for speech accuracy. The presence of nondevelopmental phoneme errors (e.g., /f/) and phonological processes (e.g., stopping of fricatives), as well as atypical phonological patterns (e.g., gliding and affrication of fricatives) further confirms the diagnosis of DPD. The question about type of DPD requires integration of this information with further research evidence about subtypes of DPD to be presented in Chapter 7. However, in this case the assessment results reveal significant problems with phonological processing (below average performance on measures of speech perception and phonological awareness) as well as poor emergent literacy skills and a family history of speech and language problems. These are important clues as to the underlying nature of his speech impairment. On the other hand, there are no indications of motor speech disorder or hearing difficulties. As to the issue of concomitant problems in other domains, he has significant difficulties with expressive language but no issues with social, cognitive, or motor skills were raised during the assessment. Overall, no reasons to refer to other specialists arose during the assessment, although further standardized assessment of his receptive language abilities would be advisable. Additional assessment is also necessary to systematically explore activity limitations and participation restrictions, thus providing a baseline against which to measure future progress. Informally, it is clear that the atypical error patterns impact his speech intelligibility and that his parents' primary and justified concern is the likelihood that he will suffer participation restrictions when he enters kindergarten. In addition to the barriers that may arise as a consequence of his poor speech intelligibility and delayed language skills, he demonstrates poor readiness for the academic demands of the kindergarten classroom by virtue of his poor emergent literacy skills. Finally, further sampling of his speech followed by an in-depth phonological analysis is required for treatment planning purposes. An analysis of the speech sample, as seen in Chapter 6, would help describe his phonological system in more detail to select specific intervention goals for him.

References

American Speech-Language-Hearing Association. (1996). *Guidelines for audiologic screening*. Rockville Pike, MD: Author.

American Speech-Language Hearing Association. (2011). *National Outcome Measurement System (NOMS) for Pre-Kindergarten*. Rockville Pike, MD: Author.

Adams, M. J. (1990). *Beginning to read: Thinking and learning about print*. Cambridge, MA: MIT Press.

Adler, S. (1984). *Cultural language differences: Their educational and professional implications*. Springfield, IL: Charles C Thomas.

Andrews, N., & Fey, M. (1986). Analysis of the speech of phonologically impaired children in two sampling conditions. *Language, Speech, and Hearing Services in Schools, 17*, 187–198.

Aziz, A. A., Shohdi, S., Osman, D. M., & Habib, E. I. (2010). Childhood apraxia of speech and multiple phonological disorders in Cairo-Egyptian Arabic speaking children: Language, speech, and oro-motor differences. *International Journal of Pediatric Otorhinolaryngology, 74*(6), 578–585.

Baker, B. M., & Blackwell, P. B. (2004). Identification and remediation of pediatric fluency and voice disorders. *Journal of Pediatric Health Care, 18*(2), 87–94.

Baker, L., & Cantwell, D. P. (1982). Developmental, social and behavioral characteristics of speech and language disordered children. *Child Psychiatry and Human Development, 12*, 195–206.

Bankson, N., & Bernthal, J. (1990). *Bankson-Bernthal Test of Phonology.* Austin, TX: Pro-Ed.

Bauer, R. S., & Benedict, P. K. (1997). *Modern Cantonese phonology (Trends in Linguistics. Studies and Monographs; 102).* Berlin, Germany: Mouton/de Gruyer.

Bellis, T. J. (2003). *Assessment and management of central auditory processing disorders in the educational setting: From science to practice* (2nd ed.). Clifton Park, NY: Delmar Learning.

Bernhardt, B. H., & Holdgrafer, G. (2001a). Beyond the basics I: The need for strategic sampling for in-depth phonological analysis. *Language, Speech, and Hearing Services in Schools, 32*(1), 18–27.

Bernhardt, B. H., & Holdgrafer, G. (2001b). Beyond the basics II: Supplemental sampling for in-depth phonological analysis. *Language, Speech, and Hearing Services in Schools, 32*(1), 28–37.

Bernhardt, B. H., & Stemberger, J. P. (1998). *Handbook of phonological development from the perspective of constraint-based nonlinear phonology.* San Diego, CA: Academic Press.

Bird, J. Bishop, D. V. M., & Freeman, N. H. (1995). Phonological awareness and literacy development in children with expressive phonological impairments. *Journal of Speech and Hearing Research, 38*(2), 446–462.

Bleile, K. (1995). *Manual of articulation and phonological disorders.* San Diego, CA: Singular.

Bleile, K. (2002). Evaluating articulation and phonological disorders when the clock is running. *American Journal of Speech-Language Pathology, 11*(3), 243–249.

Bountress, N. G., Sever, J. C., & Williams, J. (1989). Relationship between two nontraditional procedures for assessing speech-sound discrimination. *Perceptual and Motor Skills, 69*, 499–503.

Bowen, C. (2000). Tongue-tie, ankyloglossia or short fraenum. Retrieved December 22, 2010, from http://www.speech-language-therapy.com/tonguetie.html

Bowers, L., & Huisingh, R. (2010). *LinguiSystems Articulation Test (LAT).* East Moline, IL: LinguiSystems.

Bracken, B. A. (1988). Ten psychometric reasons why similar tests produce dissimilar results. *Journal of Psychology, 26*, 155–166.

Broen, P. A., Strange, W., Doyle, S. S., & Heller, J. H. (1983). Perception and production of approximant consonants by normal and articulation-delayed preschool children. *Journal of Speech and Hearing Research, 26*(4), 601–608.

Catts, H. W., Fey, M. E., Zhang, X., & Tomblin, J. B. (2001). Estimating the risk of future reading difficulties in kindergarten children: A research-based model and its clinical implementation. *Language, Speech, and Hearing Services in Schools, 32*(1), 38–50.

Chai, Y., & Maxson, R. E. (2006). Recent advances in craniofacial morphogenesis. *Developmental Dynamics, 235*(9), 2353–2375.

Christian, D., Wolfram, W., & Dube, N. (1988). *Variation and change in geographically isolated communities: Appalachian English and Ozark English.* Tuscaloosa: University of Alabama Press.

Claessen, M., Heath, S., Fletcher, J. M., Hogben, J., & Leitao, S. (2009). Quality of phonological representations: a window into the lexicon? *International Journal of Language & Communication Disorders, 44*(2), 121–144.

Claessen, M., Leitao, S., & Barrett, N. (2010). Investigating children's ability to reflect on stored phonological representations: the Silent Deletion of Phonemes Task. *International Journal of Language & Communication Disorders, 45*(4), 411–423.

Coady, J. A., & Evans, J. L. (2008). Uses and interpretations of nonword repetition tasks in children with and without specific language impairments (SLI). *International Journal of Language & Communication Disorders, 43*(1), 1–40.

Coplan, J., & Gleason, J. R. (1988). Unclear speech: Recognition and significance of unintelligible speech in preschool children. *Pediatrics, 82*(3), 447–452.

Craig, H. K., Thompson, C. A., Washington, J. A., & Potter, S. L. (2003). Phonological features of child African American English. *Journal of Speech, Language, and Hearing Research, 46*, 623–635.

Craig, H. K., & Washington, J. A. (2004). Grade-related changes in the production of African American English. *Journal of Speech, Language, and Hearing Research, 47*, 450–463.

Dawson, J. I., & Tattersall, P. J. (2001). *Structured Photographic Articulation Test* (2nd ed.). DeKalb, IL: Janelle.

Dickerson, L. J. (1975). The learner's interlanguage as a system of variable rules, *TESOL Quarterfly, 9*. 401–408.

Dickinson, D. K., & DeTemple, J. (1998). Putting parents in the picture: Maternal reports of preschoolers' literacy as a predictor of early reading. *Early Childhood Research Quarterly, 13*(2), 241–261.

Dinnsen, D., & Elbert, M. (1984). On the relationship between phonology and learning. In M. Elbert, D. Dinnsen, & G. Weismer (Eds.), *Phonological theory and the misarticulating child.* (ASHA Monographs, Number 22, pp. 59–68). Rockville, MD: American Speech-Language-Hearing Association.

Dodd, B., Crosbie, S., McIntosh, B., Teitzel, T., & Ozanne, A. (2000). *Preschool and Primary Inventory of Phonological Awareness*. London, UK: Pearson PsychCorp.

Dodd, B., Holm, A., Hua, Z., & Crosbie, S. (2003). Phonological development: A normative study of British English-speaking children. *Clinical Linguistics & Phonetics, 17*(8), 617–643.

Dodd, B., Hua, Z., Crosbie, S., Holm, A., & Ozanne, A. (2003). *Diagnostic evaluation of articulation and phonology*. London, UK: Psychological Corporation.

Dollaghan, C. A., & Campbell, T. F. (1998). Nonword repetition and child language impairment. *Journal of Speech, Language, and Hearing Research, 41*, 1136–1146.

Donaher, J., Deery, C., & Vogel, S. (2011). The Preschool Stuttering Screen for health care professionals. *Perspectives on Fluency and Fluency Disorders, 21*, 59–62.

Donegan, P. (2002). Normal vowel development. In M. J. Ball & F. Gibbons (Eds.), *Vowel disorders* (pp. 1–35). Woburn, MA: Butterworth-Heinemann.

Dunn, L. M., & Dunn, L. M. (1997). *Peabody Picture Vocabulary Test* (3rd ed.). Circle Pines, MN: American Guidance Service.

Eisenberg, S. L., & Hitchcock, E. R. (2010). Using standardized tests to inventory consonant and vowel production: A comparison of 11 tests of articulation and phonology. *Language, Speech, and Hearing Services in Schools, 41*(4), 488–503.

Emanuel, D. C., Ficca, K. N., & Korczak, P. (2011). Survey of the diagnosis and management of auditory processing disorder. *American Journal of Audiology, 20*, 48–60.

Enderby, P. (1997). *Therapy outcome measures: Speech-language pathology user's manual*. London, UK: Singular.

Ertmer, D. J. (2010). Relationships between speech intelligibility and word articulation scores in children with hearing loss. *Journal of Speech, Language, and Hearing Research, 53*(5), 1075–1086.

Ferguson, M. A., Hall, R. L., Riley, A., & Moore, D. R. (2011). Communication, listening, cognitive and speech perception skills in children with auditory processing disorder (APD) or specific language impairment (SLI). *Journal of Speech, Language, and Hearing Research, 54*, 211–227.

Fletcher, S. G. (1972). Time-by-count measurement of diadochokinetic syllable rate. *Journal of Speech and Hearing Research, 15*, 763–770.

Flipsen, P. J. (1995). Speaker-listener familiarity: Parents as judges of delayed speech intelligibility. *Journal of Communication Disorders, 28*(1), 3–19.

Flipsen, P. J. (2006). Measuring the intelligibility of conversational speech in children. *Clinical Linguistics & Phonetics, 20*(4), 303–312.

Francis, D. J., Fletcher, J. M., Shaywitz, B. A., Shaywitz, S. E., & Rourke, B. P. (1996). Defining learning and language disabilities: Conceptual and psychometric issues with the use of IQ tests. *Language, Speech, and Hearing Services in Schools, 27*, 132–143.

Francis, D. J., Stuebing, K. K., Shaywitz, S. E., Shaywitz, B. A., & Fletcher, J. M. (1996). Developmental lag versus deficit models of reading disability: A longitudinal, individual growth curves analysis. *Journal of Educational Psychology, 88*(1), 3–17.

Frijters, J. C., Barron, R. W., & Brunello, M. (2000). Direct and mediated influences of home literacy and literacy interest on prereaders' oral vocabulary and early written language skill. *Journal of Educational Psychology, 92*, 466–477.

Fudala, J. B. (2000). *Arizona Articulation Proficiency Scale—Third Edition*. Los Angeles, CA: Western Psychological Services.

Gauthier, S. V., & Madison, C. L. (1998). *Kindergarten Language Screening Test—Second Edition*. Austin, TX: Pro-Ed.

Gierut, J. A. (1986). On the assessment of productive phonological knowledge. *Journal of the National Student Speech-Language-Hearing Association, 14*, 83–100.

Glaspey, A., & Stoel-Gammon, C. (2007). A dynamic approach to phonological assessment. *Advances in Speech Language Pathology, 9*(4), 286–296.

Goldman, R., & Fristoe, M. (2000). *Goldman Fristoe Test of Articulation—Second Edition*. Minneapolis, MN: Pearson Assessments.

Goldstein, B. (1995). Spanish phonological development. In H. Kayser (Ed.), *Bilingual speech-language pathology: An Hispanic focus* (pp.17–38). San Diego, CA: Singular.

Goldstein, B. (2000). *Cultural and linguistic diversity resource guide for speech-language pathology*. San Diego, CA: Singular.

Goldstein, B. A. (2004). *Bilingual language development and disorders in Spanish-English speakers*. Baltimore, MD: Brookes.

Goldstein, B. (2007a). Spanish speech acquisition. In S. McLeod (Ed.), *The International Guide to Speech Acquisition* (pp. 539–553). Clifton Park, NY: Thomson Delmar Learning.

Goldstein, B. (2007b). Phonological skills in Puerto Rican- and Mexican-Spanish speaking children with phonological disorders. *Clinical Linguistics & Phonetics, 21*, 93–109.

Goldstein, B., Fabiano, L., & Iglesias, A. (2004). Spontaneous and imitated productions in Spanish-speaking children with phonological disorders. *Language, Speech, and Hearing Services in Schools, 35*(1), 5–15.

Goldstein, B. A., & Fabiano, L. (2007, February). Assessment and intervention for bilingual children with phonological disorders. *ASHA Leader.*

Goldstein, B., & Pollock, K. (2000). Vowel errors in Spanish-speaking children with phonological disorders: A retrospective, comparative study. *Clinical Linguistics & Phonetics, 14,* 217–234.

Gordon-Brannan, M. (1994). Assessing intelligibility: Children's expressive phonologies. *Topics in Language Disorders, 14*(2), 17–25.

Grunwell, P. (1985). *Phonological assessment of child speech.* San Diego, CA: College-Hill Press.

Guitar, B. (2006). *Stuttering: An integrated approach to its nature and treatment* (3rd ed.). Baltimore, MD: Lippincott, Williams & Wilkins.

Ha, S., Johnson, C. J., & Kuehn, D. P. (2009). Characteristics of Korean phonology: Review, tutorial, and case studies of Korean children speaking English. *Journal of Communication Disorders,* 42, 163–179.

Hammond, R. (2001). *The sounds of Spanish: Analysis and application (with special reference to American English).* Sommerville, MA: Cascadilla Press.

Hayden, D., & Square, P. (1999). *Verbal Motor Production Assessment for Children.* San Antonio, TX: Psychological Corporation.

Hesketh, A. (2004). Early literacy achievement of children with a history of speech problems. *International Journal of Language & Communication Disorders, 39*(4), 453–468.

Hidalgo, M. (1987). On the question of "standard" versus "dialect": Implications for teaching Hispanic college students. *Hispanic Journal of Behavioral Sciences, 9,* 375–395.

Hind, S. (2006). Survey of care pathway for auditory processing disorder. *Audiological Medicine, 4,* 12–24.

Hodge, M., & Daniels, J. D. (2007). *Test of Children's Speech Plus (TOCS+ Plus) ver. 5.3* [Computer program]. Edmonton: University of Alberta.

Hodge, M. M., & Daniels, J. D. (2004). *TOCS + MPT Recorder ver. I.* [Computer software]: Edmonton: University of Alberta.

Hodson, B. (2004). *Hodson Assessment of Phonological Patterns* (3rd ed.). Austin, TX: Pro-Ed.

Hodson, B. W., Scherz, J. A., & Strattman, K. H. (2002). Evaluating communicative abilities of a highly unintelligible preschooler. *American Journal of Speech-Language Pathology, 11*(3), 236–242.

Hoffman, P. R., Daniloff, R. G., Bengoa, D., & Schuckers, G. H. (1985). Misarticulating and normally articulating children's identification and discrimination of synthetic [r] and [w]. *Journal of Speech and Hearing Disorders, 50*(1), 46–53.

Holm, A., Farrier, F., & Dodd, B. (2008). Phonological awareness, reading accuracy and spelling ability of children with inconsistent phonological disorder. *International Journal of Language & Communication Disorders, 43*(3), 300–322.

Hoyme, H. E., May, P. A., Kalberg, W. O., Kodituwakku, P., Gossage, J. P., Trujillo, P. M., . . . Robinson, L. K. (2005). A practical clinical approach to diagnosis of fetal alcohol spectrum disorders: Clarification of the 1996 institute of medicine criteria. *Pediatrics, 115*(1), 39–47.

Hresko, W. P., Reid, D. K., & Hammill, D. D. (1991). *Test of Early Language Development, Third Edition.* Austin, TX: Pro-Ed.

Hwa-Froelich, D., Hodson, B., & Edwards, H. (2002). Characteristics of Vietnamese phonology. *American Journal of Speech-Language Pathology, 11,* 264–273.

Ladefoged, P., & Maddieson, I. (1996). *The sounds of the world's languages.* Oxford, UK: Blackwell.

Ingram, D., Christensen, L., Veach, S., & Webster, B. (1980). The acquisition of word-initial fricatives and affricates in English between 2 and 6 years. In G. H. Yen-Komshian, J. F. Cavanaugh, & C. A. Ferguson (Eds.), *Child phonology: Volume 1 Production* (pp. 169–192). New York, NY: Academic Press.

Invernizzi, M., Sullivan, A., & Meier, J. D. (2001). *Phonological Awareness Literacy Screening: Pre-kindergarten.* Charlottesville: University of Virginia.

Jerger, J., & Musiek, F. (2000). Report of the consensus conference on the diagnosis of auditory processing disorders in school-aged children. *Journal of the American Academy of Audiology, 11*, 467–474.

Juel, C. (1988). Learning to read and write: A longitudinal study of 54 children from first through fourth grades. *Journal of Educational Psychology, 80*(4), 437–447.

Justice, L. M., & Ezell, H. K. (2001). Written language awareness in preschool children from low-income households: A descriptive analysis. *Communication Disorders Quarterly, 22*, 123–134.

Justice, L. M., Invernizzi, M. A., & Meier, J. D. (2002). Designing and implementing an early literacy screening protocol: Suggestions for the speech-language pathologist. *Language, Speech, and Hearing Services in Schools, 33*(2), 84–101.

Kaderavek, J. N., & Sulzby, E. (1998, November). *Low versus high orientation towards literacy in children.* Paper presented at the annual convention of the American Speech-Language-Hearing Association, San Antonio, TX.

Keith, R. W. (1994). *SCAN–A: Test for auditory processing disorders in adolescents and adults.* San Antonio, TX: Psychological Corporation.

Keith, R. W. (1999). *SCAN–C: Test for auditory processing disorders in children–Revised.* San Antonio, TX: Pearson Education.

Keith, R. W. (2009). *SCAN–3 for adolescents and adults: Tests for auditory processing disorders.* San Antonio, TX: Pearson Education.

Kenney, K. W., Prather, E. M., Mooney, M. A., & Jeruzal, N. C. (1984). Comparisons among three articulation sampling procedures with preschool children. *Journal of Speech and Hearing Research, 27*(2), 226–231.

Kent, R. D., Kent, J. F., & Rosenbeck, I. C. (1987). Maximum performance tests of speech production. *Journal of Speech and Hearing Disorders, 52*, 367–387.

Khan, L. M., & Lewis, N. P. (2002). *Khan-Lewis Phonological Analysis* (2nd ed.). Circle Pines, MN: American Guidance Services.

Klein, H. B. (1984). Procedures for maximizing phonological information from single-word responses. *Language, Speech, and Hearing Services in Schools, 15*(4), 267–274.

Kummer, A. W. (2005, December 27). Ankyloglossia: to clip or not to clip? That's the question. *ASHA Leader.*

Labov, W., Ash, S., & Boberg, C. (2006). *The atlas of North American English: Phonetics, phonology and sound change.* Berlin, Germany: Mouton/de Gruyter.

Labov, W., Yaeger, M., & Steiner, R. (1973). *The quantitative study of sound change in progress.* Philadelphia, PA: U.S. Regional Survey.

Langdon, H. W., & Cheng, L. L. (2002). *Collaborating with interpreters and translators. A guide for communication disorders professionals.* Eau Claire, WI: Thinking Publications.

Larrivee, L. S., & Catts, H. W. (1999). Early reading achievement in children with expressive phonological disorders. *American Journal of Speech-Language Pathology, 8*, 118–128.

Lee, H. B. (1999). Korean. In *Handbook of the International Phonetic Association* (pp.120–122). Cambridge: Cambridge University Press.

Lee, L., Stemple, J. C., Glaze, L., & Kelchner, L. N. (2004). Quick Screen for Voice and supplementary documents for identifying pediatric voice disorders. *Language. Speech, and Hearing Services in Schools, 35*, 308–319.

Lewis, B. A., & Freebairn, L. A. (1993). A clinical tool for evaluating the familial basis of speech and language disorders. *American Journal of Speech-Language Pathology, 2*, 38–43.

Lewis, B. A., Freebairn, L. A., & Taylor, H. G. (2002). Correlates of spelling abilities in children with early speech sound disorders. *Reading and Writing, 15*, 389–407.

Lippke, B. A., Dickey, S. E., Selmar, J. W., & Soder, A. L. (1997). *Photo-Articulation Test* (3rd ed.). Austin, TX: Pro-Ed.

Lipski, J. (2000). The linguistic situation of Central Americans. In S. McKay & S. Wong (Eds.), *New immigrants in the United States* (pp. 189–215). Cambridge, UK: Cambridge University Press.

Litton, S. F., Ackermann, L. V., Isaacson, R. J., & Shapiro, B. L. (1970). A genetic study of class III malocclusion. *American Journal of Orthodontics, 58*(6), 565–577. doi: 10.1016/0002-9416(70)90145-4

Locke, J. L. (1980a). The inference of speech perception in the phonologically disordered child. Part 1: A rationale, some criteria, the conventional tests. *Journal of Speech and Hearing Disorders, 45*, 431–444.

Locke, J. L. (1980b). The inference of speech perception in the phonologically disordered child. Part II: Some clinically novel procedures, their use, some findings. *Journal of Speech and Hearing Disorders, 45*, 445–468.

Lof, G. L. (1996). Factors associated with speech-sound stimulability. *Journal of Communication Disorders, 29*(4), 255–278.

Lohmeier, H. L., & Shriberg, L. D. (2011). *Reference data for the Syllable Repetition Task (SRT)* [Technical Report No. 17]. Madison, WI: Waisman Center.

Ma, E. P. M., Worrall, L., & Threats, T. T. (2007). Introduction: The International Classification of Functioning, Disability and Health (ICF) in clinical practice. *Seminars in Speech and Language, 28*(4), 241–243.

McCauley, R. J., & Strand, E. A. (2008). A review of standardized tests of nonverbal oral and speech motor performance in children. *American Journal of Speech-Language Pathology, 17*(1), 81–91.

McCauley, R. J., & Swisher, L. (1984). Use and misuse of norm-referenced test in clinical assessment: A hypothetical case. *Journal of Speech and Hearing Disorders, 49*, 338–348.

McLeod, S. (2004). Speech pathologists' application of the ICF to children with speech impairment. *Advances in Speech Language Pathology, 6*, 75–81.

McLeod, S. (Ed.). (2007). *The international guide to speech acquisition*. Clifton Park, NY: Thomson Delmar Learning.

McLeod, S., & Goldstein, B. A. (Eds.). (2012). *Multilingual aspects of speech sound disorders in children*. Clevedon, UK: Multilingual Matters.

McLeod, S., & Hand, L. (1991). *Single word test of consonant clusters*. Retrieved June 2011 from http://athene.riv.csu.edu.au/~smcleod/Consonantclustertest.pdf

McLeod, S., & McCormack, J. (2007). Application of the ICF and ICF-children and youth in children with speech impairment. *Seminars in Speech and Language, 28*(4), 254–264.

McLeod, S., & Threats, T. (2008). The ICF-CY and children with communication disabilities. *International Journal of Speech-Language Pathology, 10*(1–2), 92–109.

Messner, A. H., Lalakea, L., Aby, J., Macmahon, J., & Bair, E. (2000). Ankyloglossia: Incidence and associated feeding difficulties. *Archives of Otolaryngology-Head and Neck Surgery, 126*(1), 36–39.

Miccio, A. W. (2002). Clinical problem solving: Assessment of phonological disorders. *American Journal of Speech-Language Pathology, 11*(3), 221–229.

Miccio, A. W., Elbert, M., & Forrest, K. (1999). The relationship between stimulability and phonological acquisition in children with normally developing and disordered phonologies. *American Journal of Speech-Language Pathology, 8*(4), 347–363.

Miller, J., & Chapman, R. (1981). Research note: The relation between age and mean length of utterance in morphemes. *Journal of Speech and Hearing Research, 24*, 154–161.

Miller, J., & Chapman, R. (1996). *SALT: Systematic Analysis of Language Transcripts*. Madison: University of Wisconsin.

Morrison, J. A., & Shriberg, L. D. (1992). Articulation testing versus conversational speech sampling. *Journal of Speech and Hearing Research, 35*(2), 259–273.

Mortensen, D. (2004). *Preliminaries to Mong Leng (Hmong Nijua) phonology*. Retrieved August 2011 from http://www.pitt.edu/~drm31/mong_leng_phonology.pdf

Naini, F. B., Moss, J. P., & Gill, D. S. (2006). The enigma of facial beauty: Esthetics, proportions, deformity, and controversy. *American Journal of Orthodontics and Dentofacial Orthopedics, 130*(3), 277–282.

Nathan, L., Stackhouse, J., Goulandris, N., & Snowling, M. J. (2004). The development of early literacy skills among children with speech difficulties: A test of the "critical age hypothesis." *Journal of Speech, Language, and Hearing Research, 47*(2), 377–391.

Nelson, N. W. (2000). Basing eligibility on discrepancy criteria: A bad idea whose time has passed. *Special Interest Division 1 Language Learning and Education, 7*, 8–12.

Newman, P. W., & Creaghead, N. A. (1989). Assessment of artiulatory and phonological disorders. In N. A. Creaghead, P. W. Newman, & W. A. Secord (Eds.), *Assessment and remediation of articulatory and phonological disorders: Second edition* (pp. 69–121). New York, NY: Macmillan.

Nittrouer, S. (2002). Learning to perceive speech: How fricative perception changes, and how it stays the same. *Journal of the Acoustical Society of America, 112*, 711–719.

Osberger, M. J., Robbins, A. M., Todd, S. L., & Riley, A. I. (1994). Speech intelligibility of children with cochlear implants. *Volta Review, 96*(5), 169–180.

Parsa, V., Jamieson, D. G., & Pretty, B. R. (2001). Effects of microphone type on acoustic measures of voice. *Journal of Voice, 15*, 331–343.

Paynter, E. T., & Bumpas, T. C. (1977). Imitative and spontaneous articulatory assessment of 3-year-old children. *Journal of Speech and Hearing Disorders, 42*, 113–118.

Pearson, B. Z., Velleman, S. L., Bryant, T. J., & Charko, T. (2009). Phonological milestones for African American English-speaking children learning mainstream American English as a second dialect. *Language, Speech, and Hearing Services in Schools, 40*, 229–244.

Perez, E. (Ed.). (1994). *Phonological differences among speakers of Spanish-influenced English.* New York, NY: Thieme.

Peterson, R. L., Pennington, B. F., Shriberg, L. D., & Boada, R. (2009). What influences literacy outcome in children with speech sound disorder? *Journal of Speech, Language, and Hearing Research, 52*(5), 1175–1188.

Pindzola, R. H., Jenkins, M. M., & Lokken, K. J. (1989). Speaking rates of young children. *Language, Speech, and Hearing Services in Schools, 20*, 133–138.

Pollock, K. E., & Berni, M. C. (2003). Incidence of non-rhotic vowel errors in children: Data from the Memphis vowel project. *Clinical Linguistics & Phonetics, 17*(4–5), 393–401.

Preston, J., & Edwards, M. L. (2010). Phonological awareness and types of sound errors in preschoolers with speech sound disorders. *Journal of Speech, Language, and Hearing Research, 53*(1), 44–60.

Preston, J. L., & Seki, A. (2011). Identifying residual speech sound disorders in bilingual children: A Japanese-English case study. *American Journal of Speech-Language Pathology, 20*, 73–85.

Prezas, R. F., & Hodson, B. (2007). Diagnostic evaluation of children with speech sound disorders. *Encyclopedia of Language and Literacy Development* (pp. 1–8). London, Ontario, Canada: Canadian Language and Literacy Research Network. Retrieved December 20, 2010, from http://www.literacyencyclopedia.ca/pdfs/topic.php?topld=21.

Raitano, N. A., Pennington, B. F., Tunick, R. A., Boada, R., & Shriberg, L. D. (2004). Pre-literacy skills of subgroups of children with speech sound disorders. *Journal of Child Psychology and Psychiatry, 45*(4), 821–835.

Ratliff, M. (1992). *Meaningful tone: A study of tonal morphology in compounds, form classes, and expressive phrases in White Hmong* (Monograph No. 27, Southeast Asia). De Kalb, IL: Northern Illinois University Center for Southeast Asian Studies.

Ricke, L. A., Baker, N. J., Madlon-Kay, D. J., & DeFor, T. A. (2005). Newborn tongue-tie: Prevalence and effect on breast-feeding. *Journal of the American Board of Family Practice, 18*(1), 1–7.

Robbins, I., & Klee, T. (1987). Clinical assessment of oropharyngeal motor development in young children. *Journal of Speech and Hearing Disorders, 52*, 271–277.

Robertson, C., & Salter, W. (1997). *The Phonological Awareness Test.* East Moline, IL: LinguiSystems.

Ruiz-de-Velasco, J., & Fix, M. (2000). *Overlooked and underserved: Immigrant students in U.S. secondary schools.* Washington, DC: Urban Institute.

Rvachew, S. (2005). Stimulability and treatment success. *Topics in Language Disorders, 25*(3), 207–219.

Rvachew, S. (2006). Longitudinal predictors of implicit phonological awareness skills. *American Journal of Speech-Language Pathology, 15*(2), 165–176.

Rvachew, S. (2007). Phonological processing and reading in children with speech sound disorders. *American Journal of Speech-Language Pathology, 16*(3), 260–270.

Rvachew, S., Chiang, P. Y., & Evans, N. (2007). Characteristics of speech errors produced by children with and without delayed phonological awareness skills. *Language, Speech, and Hearing Services in Schools, 38*(1), 60–71.

Rvachew, S., & Grawburg, M. (2006). Correlates of phonological awareness in preschoolers with speech sound disorders. *Journal of Speech, Language, and Hearing Research, 49*(1), 74–87.

Rvachew, S., & Grawburg, M. (2008). Reflections on phonological working memory, letter knowledge and phonological awareness: A reply to Hartmann. *Journal of Speech, Language, and Hearing Research, 51*, 1219–1226.

Rvachew, S., Hodge, M., & Ohberg, A. (2005). Obtaining and interpreting maximum performance tasks from children: A tutorial. *Journal of Speech-Language Pathology and Audiology, 29*(4), 146–157.

Rvachew, S., & Jamieson, D. G. (1989). Perception of voiceless fricatives by children with a functional articulation disorder. *Journal of Speech and Hearing Disorders, 54*(2), 193–208.

Rvachew, S., Ohberg, A., Grawburg, M., & Heyding, J. (2003). Phonological awareness and phonemic perception in 4-year-old children with delayed expressive phonology skills. *American Journal of Speech-Language Pathology, 12*(4), 463–471.

Rvachew, S., Ohberg, A., & Savage, R. (2006). Young children's responses to maximum performance tasks: Preliminary data and recommendations. *Journal of Speech-Language Pathology and Audiology, 30*(1), 6–13.

Schatschneider, C., Francis, D. J., Foorman, B. R., Fletcher, J. M., & Mehta, P. (1999). The dimensionality of phonological awareness: An application of item response theory. *Journal of Educational Psychology, 91*(3), 439–449.

Schiavetti, N. (1992). Scaling procedures for the measurement of speech intelligibility. In R. D. Kent (Ed.), *Intelligibility in speech disorders* (pp. 11–34). Philadelphia, PA: John Benjamin.

Secord, W., & Donahue, J. (2002). *Clinical Assessment of Articulation and Phonology*. Greenville, SC: Super Duper.

Seeff-Gabriel, B., Chiat, S., & Dodd, B. (2010). Sentence imitation as a tool in identifying expressive morphosyntactic difficulties in children with severe speech difficulties *International Journal of Language & Communication Disorders, 45*, 691–702.

Seeff-Gabriel, B., Chiat, S., & Roy, P. (2008). *Early Repetition Battery*. London, UK: Pearson.

Seymour, H., Roeper, T., & de Villiers, J. (2003). *Diagnostic Evaluation of Language Variation Screening Test*. San Antonio, TX: Psychological Corporation.

Seymour, H., Roeper, T., & de Villiers, J. (2005). *Diagnostic Evaluation of Language Variation Norm-Referenced Test*. San Antonio, TX: Psychological Corporation.

Seymour, H., Roeper, T., & de Villiers, J. G. (2000). *Dialect Sensitive Language Test*. [Unpublished manuscript]. San Antonio, TX: Psychological Corporation.

Shriberg, L. D., & Kwiatkowski, J. (1985). Continuous speech sampling for phonologic analyses of speech-delayed children. *Journal of Speech and Hearing Disorders, 50*(4), 323–334.

Shriberg, L. D., & Lohmeier, H. L. (2008). *The Syllable Repetition Task (SRT)* [Technical Report No. 14]. Madison, WI: Waisman Center.

Shriberg, L. D., Lohmeier, H. L., Campbell, T. F., Dollaghan, C. A., Green, J. R., & Moore, C. A. (2009). A nonword repetition task for speakers with misarticulations: The Syllable Repetition Task (SRT). *Journal of Speech, Language, and Hearing Research, 52*(5), 1189–1212.

Shriberg, L. D., Tomblin, J. B., & McSweeny, J. L. (1999). Prevalence of speech delay in 6-year-old children and comorbidity with language impairment. *Journal of Speech, Language, and Hearing Research, 42*(6), 1461–1481.

Siegel, R., Winitz, H., & Conkey, H. (1963). The influence of testing instruments on articulatory responses of children. *Journal of Speech and Hearing Disorders, 28*, 67–76.

Skahan, S. M., Watson, M., & Lof, G. L. (2007). Speech-language pathologists' assessment practices for children with suspected speech sound disorders: Results of a national survey. *American Journal of Speech-Language Pathology, 16*(3), 246–259.

Small, L. H. (2012). *Fundamentals of phonetics: A practical guide for students* (3rd ed.). Upper Saddle River, NJ: Pearson.

Smit, A. B., & Hand., L. (1997). *Smit-Hand Articulation and Phonology Evaluation*. Los Angeles: Western Psychological Services.

Smit, A. B., Hand, L., Freilinger, J. J., Bernthal, J. E., & Bird, A. (1990). The Iowa articulation norms project and its Nebrasks replication. *Journal of Speech and Hearing Disorders, 55*, 779–798.

So, L., & Dodd, B. (1994). Phonologically disordered Cantonese-speaking children. *Clinical Linguistics & Phonetics, 8*, 235–255.

So, L., & Dodd, B. (1995). The acquisition of phonology by Cantonese-speaking children. *Journal of Child Language, 22*, 473–495.

St. Louis, K. O., & Ruscello, D. (2000). *Oral Speech Mechanism Screening Examination, Third Edition*. Austin, TX: Pro-Ed.

Stoddard, E. S. (1947). Inheritance of malocclusion. *Journal of Heredity, 38*(4), 117–120.

Sutherland, D., & Gillon, G. T. (2005). Assessment of phonological representations in children with speech impairment. *Language, Speech, and Hearing Services in Schools, 36*(4), 294–307.

Swisher, L., Plante, E., & Lowell, S. (1994). Nonlinguistic deficits of children with language disorders complicate the interpretation of their nonverbal IQ scores. *Language, Speech, and Hearing Services in Schools, 25*, 235–240.

Tang, G., & Barlow, J. (2006). Characteristics of the sound systems of monolingual Vietnamese-speaking children with phonological impairment. *Clinical Linguistics & Phonetics, 20*, 423–445.

Templin, M. C. (1947). Spontaneous vs. imitated verbalizations in testing articulation in preschool children. *Journal of Speech and Hearing Disorders, 12*, 293–300.

Thomas-Stonell, N., McConney-Ellis, S., Oddson, B., Robertson, B., & Rosenbaum, P. (2007). An evaluation of the responsiveness of the pre-kindergarden ASHA NOMS. *Canadian Journal of Speech-Language Pathology and Audiology, 31*(2), 74–82.

Thomas-Stonell, N. L., Oddson, B., Robertson, B., & Rosenbaum, P. L. (2010). Development of the FOCUS (Focus on the Outcomes of Communication Under Six), a communication outcome measure for preschool children. *Developmental Medicine and Child Neurology, 52*(1), 47–53.

Thoonen, G., Maassen, B., Gabreëls, F., & Schreuder, R. (1999). Validity of maximum performance tasks to diagnose motor speech disorders in children. *Clinical Linguistics & Phonetics, 13*(1), 1–23.

Thoonen, G., Maassen, B., Wit, J., Gabreels, F., & Schreuder, R. (1996). The integrated use of maximum performance tasks in differential diagnostic evaluations among children with motor speech disorders. *Clinical Linguistics & Phonetics, 10*, 311–336.

Threats, T. T. (2008). Use of the ICF for clinical practice in speech-language pathology. *International Journal of Speech-Language Pathology, 10*(1–2), 50–60.

Threats, T. T. (2010). The ICF and speech-language pathology: Aspiring to a fuller realization of ethical and moral issues. *International Journal of Speech-Language Pathology, 12*(2), 87–93.

Tomblin, J. B., Records, N. L., & Zhang, J. (1996). A system for the diagnosis of Specific Language Impairment in kindergarten children. *Journal of Speech and Hearing Research, 39*, 1284–1294.

Tyler, A. A. (1996). Assessing stimulability in toddlers. *Journal of Communication Disorders, 29*(4), 279–297.

Tyler, A. A., & MacRae, T. (2010). Stimulability: Relationships to other characteristics of children's phonological systems. *Clinical Linguistics & Phonetics, 24*(4–5), 300–310.

Tyler, A. A., & Tolbert, L. C. (2002). Speech-language assessment in the clinical setting. *American Journal of Speech-Language Pathology, 11*(3), 215–220.

Tyler, A. A., Tolbert, L. C., Miccio, A. W., Hoffman, P. R., Norris, J. A., Hodson, B., . . . Bleile, K. (2002). Five views of the elephant: Perspectives on the assessment of articulation and phonology in preschoolers. *American Journal of Speech-Language Pathology, 11*(3), 213–214.

United States Department of Education. (1999). *National household education survey*. Washington, DC.

Vance, M., Rosen, S., & Coleman, M. (2009). Assessing speech perception in young children and relationships with language skills. *International Journal of Audiology, 48*(10), 708–717.

Velleman, S. L., & Pearson, B. Z. (2010). Differentiating speech sound disorders from phonological dialect differences: Implications for assessment and intervention. *Topics in Language Disorders, 30*(3), 176–188.

Velleman, S. L., Pearson, B. Z., Bryant, T. J., & Charko, T. (submitted). Phonotactic versus phonetic development in African American English.

Vogel, A. P., & Morgan, A. T. (2009). Factors affecting the quality of sound recording for speech and voice analysis. *International Journal of Speech-Language Pathology, 11*(6), 431–437.

Wagner, R., Torgensen, J., & Rashotte, C. (1999). *Comprehensive Test of Phonological Processing*. Austin, TX: Pro-Ed.

Wilcox, K., & Morris, S. (1999). *Children's Speech Intelligibility Measure*. San Antonio, TX: Psychological Corporation.

Williams, P., & Stackhouse, J. (2000). Rate, accuracy and consistency: Diadochokinetic performance of young, normally developing children. *Clinical Linguistics & Phonetics, 14*(4), 267–293.

Wolfram, W., & Schilling-Estes, N. (2006). *American English: Dialects and variation*. Cambridge/Oxford, UK: Basil Blackwell.

Yairi, E., & Ambrose, N. (1999). Early childhood stuttering I: Persistency and recovery rates. *Journal of Speech, Language, and Hearing Research, 42*, 1097–1112.

Yavas, M., & Goldstein, B. A. (1998). Phonological assessment and treatment of bilingual speakers. *American Journal of Speech-Language Pathology, 7*, 49–60.

Zentella, A. (2000). Puerto Ricans in the United States: Confronting the linguistic repercussions of colonialism. In S. McKay & S. Wong (Eds.), *New immigrants to the United States* (pp. 137–164). Cambridge, UK: Cambridge University Press.

Appendix 5–1

Family History Questionnaire Adapted from the Family History Interview

Indicate name, age, gender, handedness, and presence of speech, language, stuttering, reading, spelling, or learning disability for each **biological** family member.

Nuclear Family

Individual	Name	Age	Gender	Hand	S	L	ST	R	SP	LD
Client										
Mother										
Father										
Sibling: 1										
2										
3										
4										

Paternal Family. This is all in relation to the client's **father**.

Individual	Name	Age	Gender	Hand	S	L	ST	R	SP	LD
Father										
Mother										
Sibling 1										
Nephew/niece: 1										
2										
3										
4										
Sibling 2										
Nephew/niece: 1										
2										
3										
4										
Sibling 3										
Nephew/niece: 1										
2										
3										
4										

Maternal Family. This is all in relation to the client's **mother**.											
Individual	Name	Age	Gender	Hand	S	L	ST	R	SP	LD
Father										
Mother										
Sibling 1										
Nephew/niece: 1										
2										
3										
4										
Sibling 2										
Nephew/niece: 1										
2										
3										
4										
Sibling 3										
Nephew/niece: 1										
2										
3										
4										

S (speech) and L (language): check if the individual received SLP intervention, was not understood by unfamiliar adults until the age of 5 years or older, or demonstrates below age-appropriate speech-language skills on standardized measures.

ST (stuttering): check if the individual received SLP intervention for stuttering, if there is reported stuttering past the age of 5, or if the individual is currently considered to stutter.

R (reading): check if the individual received a diagnosis of dyslexia or received tutoring for reading.

SP (spelling): check if the individual received a diagnosis of dysorthographia or received tutoring for spelling.

LD (learning disability): check if the individual was enrolled in special education classes in school.

If information is unknown, typically for very young or older family members, indicate a question mark in the box.

Source: Adapted from B. A. Lewis and L. A. Freebairn, 1993, "A Clinical Tool for Evaluating the Familial Basis of Speech and Language Disorders," *American Journal of Speech-Language Pathology*, Appendix A, p.42. Reproduced with permission of the American Speech-Language-Hearing Association.

Appendix 5–2
Sample Oral-Motor Screening Form

Face	Pass	**Describe Deviation from Normal**
Head size and shape		
Symmetry of the face		
Face: absence of drooping		
Appearance of the nose		
Lips		
Contact of the lips at rest		
Smile on demand		
Protrude lips on demand		
Teeth		
Absence of gaps or missing teeth		
Occlusion (indicate type if malocclusion)		
Tongue		
Appearance		
Size in relation to oral cavity		
Protruding the tongue on demand		
Move tongue upward on demand		
Move tongue downward on demand		
Move tongue left to right on demand		
Coordinated Nonspeech Movements		
Alternate lip rounding and retraction		
Alternate lip spreading and tongue protrusion		
Palatal and Pharyngeal Areas		
Appearance of the palate		
Absence of nasal emission		
Appearance of uvula		
Adequate velar movement during production of /a/		
Maximum Performance Tasks		
DKR: production of [papapa]		
AMR: production of [pataka]		

Appendix 5–3

Oral and Speech Motor Control Protocol and Normative Data

Age	*Total Structural Score*					*Total Functional Score*				
	n	*M*	*SD*	*SE*	*Min–Max*	*n*	*M*	*SD*	*SE*	*Min–Max*
2;6–2;11	10	22.5	0.8	0.3	22-24	8	97.0	9.2	3.3	78-106
3;0–3;5	10	23.5	0.8	0.3	22–24	10	99.3	8.5	2.7	86–109
3;6–3;11	10	23.0	1.2	0.4	20–24	8	107.1	3.8	1.3	99–111
4;0–4;5	10	23.4	0.8	0.3	22–24	9	108.1	2.1	0.7	104–111
4;6–4;11	10	22.4	1.7	0.5	20–24	9	109.3	2.1	0.7	106–112
5;0–5;5	10	23.3	0.7	0.2	22–24	8	109.8	2.6	0.9	106–112
5;6–5;11	10	23.0	1.2	0.4	21–24	10	109.8	2.6	0.8	103–112
6;0–6;5	10	22.0	2.0	0.6	18–24	9	110.6	1.3	0.4	108–112
6;6–6;11	10	22.4	1.1	0.3	20–24	10	111.1	1.2	0.4	108–112
TOTAL	90	22.8	1.3	0.1	18–24	81	107.0	6.5	0.7	78–112

Age	*Number of Repetitions per Second*										*Max. Phonation Time*	
	/pʌ/		/tʌ/		/kʌ/		/pətəkək/		Patticake			
	M	*SD*	*M*	*SD*	*M*	*SD*	*M*	*SD*	*M*	*SD*	*M*	*SD*
2;6–2;11	3.70	0.86	3.70	0.76	3.65	0.49	1.0	0.27	1.26	0.11	5.55	1.87
3;0–3;5	4.66	0.80	4.56	1.02	3.82	1.45	1.06	0.29	1.36	0.32	5.51	1.49
3;6–3;11	4.81	1.20	4.78	1.13	4.83	0.57	1.76	0.90	1.75	0.83	7.79	2.37
4;0–4;5	4.89	1.12	4.77	1.05	4.58	1.08	1.37	0.28	1.56	0.25	8.01	2.11
4;6–4;11	4.64	0.82	4.46	0.62	4.29	0.57	1.34	0.27	1.33	0.10	9.22	2.19
5;0–5;5	4.76	0.84	4.82	0.85	4.56	0.94	1.40	0.43	1.58	0.28	8.06	1.97
5;6–5;11	5.09	0.44	5.22	0.45	4.91	0.25	1.58	0.19	1.65	0.21	9.42	1.65
6;0–6;5	5.36	0.64	5.32	0.48	4.94	0.28	1.45	0.25	1.61	0.23	10.99	3.06
6;6–6;11	5.51	0.43	5.37	0.72	4.85	0.71	1.72	0.19	1.64	0.26	11.47	3.02
TOTAL	4.85	0.92	4.80	0.91	0.91	0.88	1.43	0.44	1.54	0.38	8.51	2.91

continues

Robbins & Klee Test Items	S	F
LIPS (CN VII)		
1. Symmetry		
2. Relationship (open vs. closed)		
3. Rounding		
4. Protrusion (blowing)		
5. Retraction		
6. Alternate pucker/smile		
7. Bite lower lip		
8. Lip seal		
9. Puff cheeks		
10. Open–close lips		
11. Rounding /oʊː/		
12. Protrusion /uː/		
13. Retraction /iː/		
14. Alternate /u/, /i/		
15. Bite lower lip /f/		
16. Open–close lips /mʌ/		
MANDIBLE (CN V)		
17. Symmetry		
18. Occlusion		
19. Size (re: facial features)		
20. Excursion (click teeth 5 times)		
MAXILLA		
21. Symmetry		
22. Size		
TEETH		
23. Decay		
24. Alignment		
25. Gaps		
26. Missing		
27. Occlusion (re: maxillary teeth)		

Robbins & Klee Test Items	S	F	R
VELOPHARYNX (CN X)			
42. Symmetry			
43. Uvula			
44. Tonsils			
45. Vault height			
46. Palatal juncture (palpate)			
47. Blow on cold mirror			
48. Suck through straw			
49. /aː/			
50. /ha.ha.ha/			
LARYNX–RESPIRATION (CN X)			
51. Posture during quiet breathing			
52. Cough, laugh, or cry			
81. Maximum phonation time (in sec): /aː/			
53. Pitch variation			
54. Loudness variation			
55. /ha.ha.ha/			
COORDINATED SPEECH MOVEMENTS			
56. (82)[a] /pʌ/ accuracy and repetitions			
57. (83)[a] /tʌ/ accuracy and repetitions			
58. (84)[a] /kʌ/ accuracy and repetitions			
59. (85)[a] /pəɾəkək/ accuracy and repetitions			
60. (86)[a] Pattycake accuracy and repetitions			
61. you			
62. top			
63. beef			
64. fume			
65. cowboy			
66. Band–Aid			
67. halftime			
68. banana			

Robbins & Klee Test Items	S	F	*Robbins & Klee Test Items*	S	F	R
TONGUE (CN XII)			69. kitty cat			
28. Symmetry			70. puppy dog			
29. Carriage			71. communicate			
30. Fasciculations			72. 1950			
31. Furrowing			73. potato head			
32. Atrophy			74. Winnie the Pooh			
33. Hypertrophy			SPEECH SAMPLE (Prosody and voice)			
34. Protrusion			75. Rate			
35. Elevation to alveolar ridge			76. Intonation			
36. Anterior–posterior sweep			77. Pitch			
37. Interdental			78. Loudness			
38. Elevation to alveolar ridge: /n/, /t/, or /l/			79. Voice quality			
39. Lateral edges of tongue to teeth: /s/ or /ʃ/			80. Nasal resonance			
40. Interdental /θ/			**TOTALS**			
41. Posterior tongue to palate: /k/ or /g/						

[a]Items 56 to 60 are scored for articulatory accuracy, and items 82 to 86 for mean number of repetitions per second over 3 seconds.

Notes on Administration: S = oral structure; F = oral function. Structural test items are scored as normal (score = 1) or abnormal (score = 0). Functional test items are scored as adultlike (score = 2), emerging skill (i.e., approximation of the target but lacking adultlike precision; score = 1) or absent function (score = 0). For items 56 to 60, instruct the child to repeat each item as quickly as possible during a 3-second interval and count the mean number of repetitions per second. Items 65 to 74 are scored for articulatory accuracy using the same 3-point scale as for functional test items. Items 75 to 80 are scored from a spontaneous speech sample using the same 3-point scale.

Source: From I. Robbins and T. Klee, 1987, "Clinical Assessment of Oropharyngeal Motor Development in Young Children," *Journal of Speech and Hearing Disorders,* 52, Table 1 and 2, p. 273, Table 3, p. 274, Appendix p. 277. Adapted with permission of the American Speech–Language and Hearing Association.

Appendix 5–4

Instructions for Administration of the Maximum Performance Tasks

Including Maximum Phonation Duration (MPD), Maximum Fricative Duration (MFD), Maximum Repetition Rate for Single Syllables (MRRmono), and Maximum Repetition Rate for Trisyllabic Sequences (MRRtri)

Task	*Instructions*
Maximum Phonation Duration (MPD)	
[a]	1. Produce a prolonged [a] for approximately 2 seconds on one breath in a monotonic manner with normal pitch. Ask the child to imitate your model. Repeat if necessary until the child is successful in imitating your model. 2. As above except model a prolongation of [a] for 4 to 5 seconds and then ask the child to imitate your model. 3. Ask the child to say [a] for as long as possible on one breath (with no model provided in this case). Repeat the instruction two more times, providing the child with a total of three opportunities to prolong [a] for as long as possible.
[mama]	Repeat steps 1, 2, and 3 above except that in this case, model a repetition of the syllables [mama . . .]. Again at step 3, give the child three opportunities to produce [mama . . .] for as long as possible on a single breath.
MPD	MPD is the mean of the longest prolongation of [a] and the longest prolongation of [mama . . .].
Maximum Fricative Duration (MFD)	
[f]	Repeat steps 1, 2, and 3 as described for MPD, in this case modeling a prolonged production of [f]. Again at step 3, give the child three opportunities to prolong [f] for as long as possible on a single breath.
[s]	Repeat steps 1, 2, and 3 as described above, in this case modeling a prolonged production of [s]. Again at step 3, give the child three opportunities to prolong [s] for as long as possible on a single breath.
[z]	Repeat steps 1, 2, and 3 as described above, in this case modeling a prolonged production of [z]. Again at step 3, give the child three opportunities to prolong [z] for as long as possible on a single breath.
MFD	MFD is the mean of the longest prolongation of [f], the longest prolongation of [s] and the longest prolongation of [z].
Maximum Repetition Rate—Monosyllabic (MRRmono)	
[pa]	1. Ask the child to say [pa], and then [papapa], and then [papapapapa]. 2. Model the repetition of approximately 12 [pa] syllables on a single breath at a rate of about four syllables per second and ask the child to imitate your model. 3. Ask the child to repeat step 2 but this time as fast as possible. Stop recording when the child has produced 12 or more syllables. Provide the child with two additional opportunities to maximize the repetition rate.
[ta]	Repeat steps 1, 2, and 3 as described above, in this case modeling repetition of the syllable [ta]. Again at step 3, give the child three opportunities to produce [ta] as fast as possible on a single breath.
[ka]	Repeat steps 1, 2, and 3 as described above, in this case modeling repetition of the syllable [ka]. Again at step 3, give the child three opportunities to produce [ka] as fast as possible on a single breath.
MRRmono	For each trial the repetition rate is calculated as the number of syllables produced per second. MRRmono is the mean repetition rate for the fastest repetition of [pa], the fastest repetition of [ta] and the fastest repetition of [ka].

Task	*Instructions*
Maximum Repetition Rate—Trisyllabic (MRRtri)	
[pataka]	1. Ask the child to say [pataka] at a slow rate. Practice this syllable sequence, breaking it down into its component parts if necessary, until the child can produce a single correct sequence. 2. Produce the sequence twice [patakapataka] fluently and at a slow rate and ask the child to imitate. 3. Produce the sequence three times at a normal speaking rate and ask the child to imitate. 4. Produce the sequence four times at a rate of about four syllables per second and ask the child to imitate. 5. Model a repetition of the sequence, five times and as fast as possible. Ask the child to produce the sequence as fast as possible for as long as possible on a single breath. Give the child two additional trials to perform this task. If the child cannot produce the sequence accurately, repeat the steps and allow three additional attempts to produce a correct sequence as fast as possible and as long as possible on a single breath.
MRRtri	MRRtri is the number of syllables per second produced during the child's fastest attempt at repeating this sequence. The sequence must be produced correctly over 5 repetitions on a trial for it to be used to calculate the MMRtri.
Sequence	Score 1 if the child produces a correct repetition of the sequence. Score 0 if the child does not succeed in producing a correct sequence.
Attempts	This score is the number of additional attempts (beyond the first three) that are required for the child to achieve a correct repetition of the sequence.

Diagnostic Criteria for School-Age Children: Dysarthria Score	
0 = Not dysarthric	MRRmono > 3.5
1 = Undefined	3.0 < MRRmono > 3.5 AND MPD > 7.5
2 = Dysarthric	MRRmono < 3.0 OR 3.0 < MRRmono > 3.5 AND MPD ≤ 7.5
Diagnostic Criteria for School-Age Children: Dyspraxia Score	
0 = Not dyspraxic	MRRtri > 4.4
1 = Undefined	3.4 < MRRtri > 4.4 AND MFD > 11s OR Attempts < 3
2 = Dyspraxic	MRRtri ≤ 3.4 OR Sequence = 0 OR Criteria for 0 or 1 not met
Diagnostic Criteria for Preschool-Age Children: Dysarthria Score	
0 = Not dysarthric	MRRmono > 3.4
1 = Undefined	3.0 < MRRmono > 3.4
2 = Dysarthric	MRRmono < 3.0
Diagnostic Criteria for Preschool-Age Children: Dyspraxia Score	
0 = Not dyspraxic	MRRtri > 3.4
1 = Undefined	3.0 < MRRtri > 3.4
2 = Dyspraxic	MRRtri < 3.0

Note: Instructions and diagnostic criteria for school-age children are summarized from Thoonen, Maassen, Witt, Gabreels, and Schreuder (1996) and Thoonen, Maassen, Gabreels, and Schreuder (1999). The diagnostic criteria were validated from data recorded from school-aged children with normally developing speech, nonspecific speech disorder, apraxia, and dysarthria as presented in Chapter 7 (see Table 7–5). Criteria for preschool-age children are suggested on the basis of data recorded from normally developing children aged 4 to 6 years, as described in Rvachew, Ohberg, and Savage (2006).

Source: From S. Rvachew, M. Hodge, and A. Ohberg, 2005, "Obtaining and Interpreting Maximum Performance Tasks from Children: A Tutorial," *Journal of Speech-Language Pathology and Audiology,* 29(4), Table 1, pp.149–150.

Appendix 5–5

Norms, in Seconds, of the Time Required for 20 Productions of Single Syllables, 15 Productions of Bisyllables, and 10 Productions of the Trisyllable /pataka/

Age		pʌ	tʌ	kʌ	fʌ	lʌ	pʌ tə	pʌ kə	tʌ kə	pʌ tʌ kə
6	Mean	4.8	4.9	5.5	5.5	5.2	7.3	7.9	7.8	10.3
	SD	0.8	1.0	0.9	1.0	0.9	2.0	2.1	1.8	3.1
7	Mean	4.8	4.9	5.3	5.4	5.3	7.6	8.0	8.0	10.0
	SD	1.0	0.9	1.0	1.0	0.8	2.6	1.9	1.8	2.6
8	Mean	4.2	4.4	4.8	4.9	4.6	6.2	7.1	7.2	8.3
	SD	0.7	0.7	0.7	1.0	0.6	1.8	1.5	1.4	2.1
9	Mean	4.0	4.1	4.6	4.6	4.5	5.9	6.6	6.6	7.7
	SD	0.6	0.6	0.7	0.7	0.5	1.6	1.5	1.7	1.9
10	Mean	3.7	3.8	4.3	4.2	4.2	5.5	6.4	6.4	7.1
	SD	0.4	0.4	0.5	0.5	0.5	1.5	1.4	1.2	1.5
11	Mean	3.6	3.6	4.0	4.0	3.8	4.8	5.8	5.8	6.5
	SD	0.6	0.7	0.6	0.6	0.6	1.1	1.2	1.3	1.4
12	Mean	3.4	3.5	3.9	3.7	3.7	4.7	5.7	5.5	6.4
	SD	0.4	0.5	0.6	0.4	0.5	1.2	1.5	1.1	1.6
13	Mean	3.3	3.3	3.7	3.6	3.5	4.2	5.1	5.1	5.7
	SD	0.6	0.5	0.6	0.5	0.5	0.8	1.5	1.3	1.4

Source: From S. G. Fletcher, 1972, "Time-By-Count Measurement of Diadochokinetic Syllable Rate," *Journal of Speech and Hearing Research, 15*, Table 1, p. 765. Reprinted with permission of the American Speech-Language-Hearing Association.

Appendix 5–6

Test Items of the Phonological Awareness Test

Administration Instructions: Show different puppet for each animal name and set of four pictures for each item. Read instruction and then point to and name each picture. Repeat instruction for every item. Assist child during training items but offer no additional support during test items. Include only responses to test items when calculating raw score.

Subtest 1. Rime matching. Raw Score (sum items 6 through 19):				
Paul Training Items: "This animal's name is Paul. Paul likes things that sound like his name. Listen, which one of these things does Paul like?"				
1.	key	ken	map	*ball*
2.	fork	*doll*	comb	boot
Ken Training Items: "This animal's name is Ken. Ken likes things that sound like his name. Listen, which one of these things does Ken like?"				
3.	bird	fish	mop	*hen*
4.	carrot	*men*	bell	tap
5.	worm	fork	*pen*	top
Dan Testing Items: "This animal's name is Dan. Dan likes things that sound like his name. Listen, which one of these things does Dan like?"				
6.	spoon	cup	*pan*	fork
7.	kite	plane	*fan*	bike
8.	vase	*can*	tap	mug
9.	house	boat	car	*van*
Wug Testing Items: "This animal's name is Wug. Wug likes things that sound like her name. Listen, which one of these things does Wug like?"				
10.	chair	bed	table	*rug*
11.	*mug*	plate	knife	cake
12.	pot	cup	*jug*	fork
Pat Testing Items: "This animal's name is Pat. Pat likes things that sound like his name. Listen, which one of these things does Pat like?"				
13.	ham	*hat*	shoe	fish
14.	*cat*	cap	sock	pan
15	*mat*	scarf	book	map
16.	bag	purse	*bat*	comb
Zap Testing Items: "This animal's name is Zap. Zap likes things that sound like her name. Listen, which one of these things does Zap like?"				
17.	top	ball	cat	*cap*
18.	saw	mat	*map*	door
19.	pen	tag	*tap*	book

continues

Appendix 5–6 continued

Subtest 2. Onset matching raw score (sum items 6 through 15)				
/f/ Training Items: "This animal likes everything he owns to begin with the same sound. The sound he likes is /f/. Which one of these will he want?"				
1.	cat	saw	*fork*	ball
2.	mop	*fan*	bee	gun
3.	*fish*	sock	worm	bell
4.	car	dog	ship	*fence*
5.	cake	pen	*feet*	duck
/p/ Testing Items: "This animal likes everything he owns to begin with the same sound. The sound he likes is /p/. Which one of these will he want?"				
6.	*pipe*	fan	kite	house
7.	fork	*pan*	cup	vase
8.	key	hen	watch	*pig*
9.	jug	hand	*purse*	ring
10.	car	*pen*	saw	duck
/tʃ/ Testing Items: "This animal likes everything he owns to begin with the same sound. The sound he likes is /tʃ/. Which one of these will he want?"				
11.	bike	peg	*chair*	map
12.	bell	*chain*	key	net
13.	*chips*	fan	fish	cat
14.	carrot	pig	tap	*chicken*
15.	worm	tree	dog	*cherry*
Subtest 3. Onset segmentation and matching raw score (sum items 6 through 15):				
Marg Training Items: "This animal's name is Marg. Marg likes things that start with the same sound as her name. Which one of these things will Marg want?"				
1.	spoon	*mat*	vase	bed
2.	*map*	chicken	purse	kite
3.	tag	boat	*mug*	door
4.	house	key	bee	*mop*
5.	hen	sock	*meat*	boot
Tom Testing Items: "This animal's name is Tom. Tom likes things that start with the same sound as his name. Which one of these things will Tom want?"				
6.	sock	*tie*	pipe	hat
7.	bird	*teddy*	book	doll
8.	*table*	cake	shoe	fence
9.	gun	ship	van	*tap*
10.	*tea*	box	mug	lamp

Sam Testing Items: "This animal's name is Sam. Sam likes things that start with the same sound as his name. Which one of these things will Sam want?"				
11.	*sun*	car	fan	ball
12.	bee	tie	*saw*	hat
13.	boot	pen	mop	*sock*
14.	cup	*soup*	knife	fork
15.	table	bed	*soap*[a]	mat

[a]"settee" was replaced with "soap" for testing in North America as in Rvachew, 2006; Rvachew & Grawburg, 2006.

Performance on the Bird, Bishop, and Freeman (1995) Phonological Awareness Test Obtained from 35 Normally Developing Children in Early Spring of 3 Successive Years

	Prekindergarten (mean age: 59 months)		*Kindergarten (mean age: 71 months)*		*First Grade (mean age: 89 months)*	
Subtest	*Mean*	*S.D.*	*Mean*	*S.D.*	*Mean*	*S.D.*
1	9.29	2.28	11.69	2.20	12.77	1.09
2	7.03	1.85	9.23	0.95	9.74	0.51
3	5.53	1.73	7.90	2.84	9.80	0.58
Total	21.54	4.63	28.85	3.97	32.31	1.60

Note: The scores are expressed as number of correct responses per subtest. Normative data was collected from the same sample of children who provided the SAILS normative data in Table 5–5. These children were part of a longitudinal follow-up study reported in Rvachew and Grawburg (2006) and Rvachew (2007).

Source: From J. Bird, D. V. M. Bishop, and N. H. Freeman, 1995, "Phonological Awareness and Literacy Development in Children with Expressive Phonological Impairments," *Journal of Speech and Hearing Research*, 38, Appendix, p. 462. Adapted with permission of the American Speech-Language-Hearing Association.

Chapter 6

Speech Sample Analysis

Analysis of the speech sample at multiple levels of representation will allow for the identification of mismatches in the child's phonological knowledge in relation to the adult system for all levels of the phonological hierarchy. In other words, the analysis focuses on what the child can do, and what is absent from the child's system (Bernhardt & Stemberger, 2000). The results of this in-depth phonological analysis are particularly useful to: (1) select treatment targets; (2) track treatment progress; and (3) help predict which error patterns may change without treatment. Each of these is discussed in turn, with case studies providing examples and demonstrations of how to complete the speech sample analysis.

In-depth analysis of the speech sample will identify mismatches in the child's phonological knowledge in relation to the adult system for all levels of the phonological hierarchy.

Analyses to Select Treatment Goals

6.1.1. Collect a speech sample, evaluate its adequacy for a multilinear analysis, and plan strategies to supplement the sample if necessary.

6.1.2. Given a transcribed sample of child speech, complete the quick version of the multilinear analysis to yield an overview of the child's strengths and needs at multiple levels of the phonological hierarchy.

6.1.3. Given a transcribed sample of child speech, complete an in-depth multilinear analysis to provide a systematic description of the child's strengths and needs at multiple levels of the phonological hierarchy.

6.1.4. Describe the goals of the phonetic and phonotactic assessment for young children.

Clinicians often complete a phonological process analysis to describe the child's error patterns, an approach which became very popular in the late 1970s and 1980s (e.g., Shriberg & Kwiatkowski, 1980). This analysis is based on Natural Phonology theory (Stampe, 1973), which assumes that natural phonetic constraints, which simplify articulation, are typical of the speech of young children. According to the theory, adults have learned to suppress these phonological processes and achieve a more complex phonological system. Ultimately, this theory failed to explain production errors, but SLPs commonly use phonological processes to describe children's phonological errors (Fey, 1992; Kamhi, 1992). Lof (2002) argued that phonological process analysis should be modified, in part because more contemporary theories of phonology have since been developed, and also because phonological processes result in labels that are not descriptive enough. For example, "cluster reduction" is a single label often used by SLPs to describe various types of errors, including producing both consonants of the cluster but simplifying liquids (e.g., "green" → [gwin]; "slide" → [swaɪd]), consistently omitting the second consonant (e.g., "green" → [gin]; "slide" → [saɪd]), omitting the first consonant only if it belongs to a certain class of sounds (e.g., "green" → [ɡɹin]; "slide" → [laɪd]), and merging consonants as in the case of coalescence (e.g., "swim" → [fɪm]). In other words, a phonological process is the symptom of the underlying DPD but does not explain why the errors occur.

Phonological processes is not the best option to describe children's phonological errors, in part because Natural Phonology theory failed to explain productive errors and phonological processes labels are insufficiently descriptive.

Phonological Patterns

The *Hodson Assessment of Phonological Patterns, Third Edition* (HAPP-3; Hodson, 2004) is the revision of the *Assessment of Phonological Processes* (APP; Hodson, 1980) and *Assessment of Phonological Processes-Revised* (APP-R; Hodson, 1986). The major improvement of the latest version of the test is the inclusion of normative scores. The test also includes a preschool phonological screening and a multisyllabic word screening form. A total of 50 target words are elicited and transcribed, and can be entered in the Hodson Computerized Analysis of Phonological Patterns (HCAPP) or scored manually. Major phonological deviations are analyzed in terms of word/syllable structures (omission of syllables; of consonants in sequences/clusters, with or without stridents; of consonant singletons in the prevocalic, intervocalic, and postvocalic positions) and in terms of consonant category deficiencies (substitutions and omissions of sonorants, stridents, velars, and others). A total of 28 different substitutions, distortions, additions and position changes in a word, such as stopping, fronting, labial assimilation, and reduplication, are recorded on the Substitutions and Other Strategies Analysis Form. Although the HAPP-3 provides several labels that are more descriptive than phonological processes, and incorporates some analyses of syllable and word structures, a multilinear analysis has advan-

The HAPP-3 is an analysis of phonological patterns that provides several labels that are more descriptive than phonological processes and incorporates some analyses of syllable and word structures.

tages over a phonological patterns analysis. Nonetheless, for some children with fairly consistent deviation patterns, such as the real child presented in Case Study 6–1, the HAPP-3 allows for a quick and complete analysis of phonological patterns in order to identify intervention targets. The case study identifies issues with word structure (consonant sequences, intervocalic consonants) and with major consonant class deficiencies (liquids, stridents, velars) that warrant immediate attention. When the word productions shown in Case Study 6–1 were submitted to The Hodson Computerized Analysis of Phonological Patterns (HCAPP), his speech deficit was rated as "high severe" due to a total occurrence of 142 major phonological deviations. With regard to issues with word/syllable structures, major findings included omissions of consonant sequences/clusters (100%), and omission of intervocalic and postvocalic singleton consonants, and of syllables. A summary of the findings using the terminology of the Major Phonological Deviations Analysis and Substitutions and Other Strategies Analysis forms of the HAPP-3 is shown in the left side of Table 6–1. The right side of Table 6–1 represents the data from Case Study 6–1 in terms of a multilinear analysis as described in the sections to follow. We return to Table 6–1 later in the chapter.

For children with fairly consistent deviation patterns, the HAPP-3 allows for a quick and complete analysis of phonological patterns in order to identify intervention targets.

Multilinear Analysis

A multilinear (or nonlinear) analysis has the advantage of examining the relationships among the units of the phonological hierarchy, which provides a more systematic description of the child's underlying representations (Bernhardt & Stoel-Gammon, 1994). Although phonological process analysis or the assessment of phonological patterns includes both substitution and syllable structure processes, nonlinear analysis provides a more systematic description of underlying representations at the syllable, word, and phrase structure levels and the hierarchical relationships among these levels in the child's phonological system. As seen in Chapter 5, the mismatches of children with DPD who are speakers of African American English (AAE) occur frequently at the prosodic level. A recent study described the consonant inventory of typically developing Quebec French-speaking children 20 to 53 months (McLeod et al., 2011). Results indicated earlier acquisition of phonemes than English, a similar pattern to that observed between children speaking English and children speaking AAE. We have found that DPD manifests itself differently in French than in English: whereas incomplete inventories are characteristic of preschool English-speaking children with DPD (e.g., Dinnsen et al., 1990; Schwartz et al., 1980), French-speaking children with DPD have difficulties at the prosodic level, as illustrated by their wide variety of errors that alter the syllable structure of the word (Brosseau-Lapré, Rvachew, & Laukys, 2010). The difference in the manifestation of DPD in French compared to English could be due to differences at the prosodic level.

A **multilinear analysis** has the advantage of examining the relationships among the units of the phonological hierarchy (syllable, word, phrase structure levels). This provides a more systematic description of the child's underlying representations at each of these levels.

Case Study 6–1

Case History: Boy aged 5;1 was referred for severe speech sound production difficulties. Birth, developmental, medical, and family history unremarkable.

Pretreatment transcriptions of the stimulus words of the HAPP-3.

Target word	Child's production	Target word	Child's production
1. basket	bæɪʔ	26. shoe	du
2. boats	boʔs	27. slide	laɪd
3. candle	kæ	28. smoke	moʔ
4. chair	tɛɚ	29. snake	nɛʔ
5. clouds	kaʊ	30. sofa	doʔ
6. cowboy hat	kæbɔɪhæ	31. spoon	bun
7. feather	fɛ	32. square	wɛɚ
8. fish	fɪʃ	33. star	dɑɚ
9. flower	faʊwɛ	34. string	wɪŋ
10. fork	fɔɚ	35. swimming	wɪmɪŋ
11. glasses	dæɪz	36. television	tɛvɪn
12. glove	gʌ	37. toothbrush	tubʌʃ
13. gum	gʌm	38. truck	fwʌʔ
14. hanger	hæɚ	39. vase	bɔs
15. horse	hɔɚs	40. watch	wɑʃ
16. ice cubes	aɪtu	41. yo-yo	ojo
17. jumping	dʌʔɪŋ	42. zip	lɪʔ
18. leaf	liʔ	43. crayon	fwenz
19. mark	mæs	44. black	bæʔ
20. music box	muɪʔbɑ	45. green	fwin
21. page	pez	46. yellow	tɛlo
22. (air) plane	pen	47. three	fwi
23. queen	twin	48. thumb	fʌn
24. rock	wɑʔ	49. nose	noz
25. screwdriver	wuwaɪɚ	50. mouth	maʊs

Major Potential Target Patterns for Goal Statement according to the Hodson Computerized Analysis of Phonological Patterns (HCAPP):

Facilitate emergence of the following phonological patterns:

- Consonant sequences/clusters
- Intervocalic singletons
- Prevocalic liquids
- Stridents
- Velars

Table 6–1. *Summary of Frequently Occurring Patterns Identified by the HAPP-3 and a Multilinear Analysis for Case Study 6–1*

HAPP-3	*Multilinear Analysis*
Weak syllable deletion	Delinking of weak syllables (in trochees and iambs)
Deletion of intervocalic singletons	Delinking or weakening of simple and complex onsets in ambisyllabic contexts
Deletion or glottal stop replacement of final consonants	In the coda, [−continuant] and [−nasal] obstruents are either delinked at the root node (leading to an omission), or the supralaryngeal place node is delinked (leading to a glottal stop replacement)
Consonant sequences/ cluster reduction	Delinking of elements within complex onsets and codas
Fronting of velars	Dorsal is sometimes delinked yielding the default Coronal
Stopping of fricatives	Delinking of [+continuant] from obstruents in the onset position
Gliding of liquids	Deletion of [+consonantal] from /ɹ/, leading to production of /w/
Deaffrication	Delinking of [+continuant] in the onset position; delinking of the [−continuant] branch in coda position

French, like Spanish, is a syllable-timed language, meaning that every syllable has roughly the same duration and equal stress. English, however, is a stress-timed language: on average, the amount of time between consecutive stressed syllables is constant. Multilinear analysis therefore is more appropriate for selecting the optimal treatment targets for children speaking a variety of dialects and languages; as seen later with Case Study 6–2 it also offers advantages for the description of the phonological systems of English-speaking children.

Multilinear analysis is more appropriate for selecting the optimal treatment targets for children speaking a variety of dialects and languages; it also offers advantages for the description of the phonological systems of English-speaking children.

Bernhardt and colleagues have been using a multilinear approach to assessment and intervention of children with DPD since the 1990s (e.g., Bernhardt, 1990, 1992; Bernhardt & Gilbert, 1992; Bernhardt & Stemberger, 1998). As discussed in Chapter 5, we are aware of the balance of thoroughness versus time constraints during the assessment process. Many SLPs whom we have worked with in the past decade have told us they do not feel capable of performing a multilinear speech sample analysis in a short period of time and therefore prefer to use a phonological process analysis as they can complete it rapidly. The first author has been teaching multilinear phonology analysis to graduate SLP students for many years, including to the second author more than a decade ago. As explained by Bernhardt and Stemberger (2000), completing a multilinear analysis for phonological intervention may take a couple of hours the first time; with practice it can be completed in as little as

Although completing a multilinear analysis may be time consuming at first, it can be completed efficiently in a short period of time once you are more familiar with the approach.

The concepts of **prosodic hierarchy, phonological features, feature geometry, and basic rules (delinking and spreading)** are fundamental to a multilinear analysis. We recommend reviewing the section Multilinear Phonology of Chapter 1 if necessary.

A key feature of multilinear phonology, the **prosodic hierarchy**, is the hierarchical organization of words, syllables, segments, and features.

Ambisyllabic consonants, such as the /p/ of the word "happy," link to the coda of the first syllable and the onset of the second syllable.

20 minutes, depending on the complexity and length of the speech sample. It has been our experience, as well as that of students and colleagues who have worked with us, that multilinear analysis can be completed efficiently in a short period of time once you are more familiar with the approach.

Short Tutorial on Multilinear Phonology

This chapter demonstrates how an analysis at all levels of the phonological hierarchy can be completed efficiently for daily use in clinical practice. Application of the analysis requires comprehension of a few important concepts that were presented in Chapter 1 and thus they are reviewed very briefly in this section: prosodic hierarchy, phonological features and feature geometry, and basic rules (delinking and spreading). We strongly recommend revising the section Multilinear Phonology of Chapter 1 if needed.

Prosodic Hierarchy. A key feature of multilinear phonology is the hierarchical organization of words, syllables, segments and features. The word, which is part of a phrase or a sentence, is composed of progressively smaller units, each represented on their own level or "tier." From the bottom up, segments are first grouped together into syllables. A syllable consists of a peak of sonority, also called the syllabic nucleus, which is usually the vowel. The nucleus is the only obligatory component of the syllable. The longest permissible sequence of consonants to the left of the nucleus makes up the onset (e.g., /stɹ/ and /spl/ are permissible onsets in English; /pk/ is not). Remaining consonants at the right of the nucleus make up the coda. The rime consists of the nucleus and the coda (O'Grady & Dobrovolsky, 1997; see Figure 6–1). Some of you may be aware that the /s/ in consonant clusters in the onset and coda positions is considered by some phonologists to be an appendix and not truly part of the onset or coda. We have decided to ignore this and assume, as did O'Grady and Dobrovolsky, that in words such as "stops," the initial /st/ and the final /ps/ are both consonant clusters.

In English, words with two syllables such as "giraffe" are fairly easy to syllabify, with /dʒə/ consisting of the onset and the nucleus of the first syllable, and /ɹæf/ being the onset, nucleus and coda of the second syllable. For some words such as "happy," however, most speakers of English are unsure whether the phoneme /p/ belongs to the onset of the second syllable, or whether it belongs to the first syllable. In this case the intervocalic consonant is called *ambisyllabic*, meaning that it belongs to both syllables (Figure 6–2).

Consonant clusters can also be ambisyllabic, as long as they are permissible both in the onset and coda position. For example, "system" contains an ambisyllabic cluster, as the sequence /st/ is legal in the onset position (e.g., "steam") and in the coda position (e.g., "cyst"). Ingram (1981) described four rules to define the

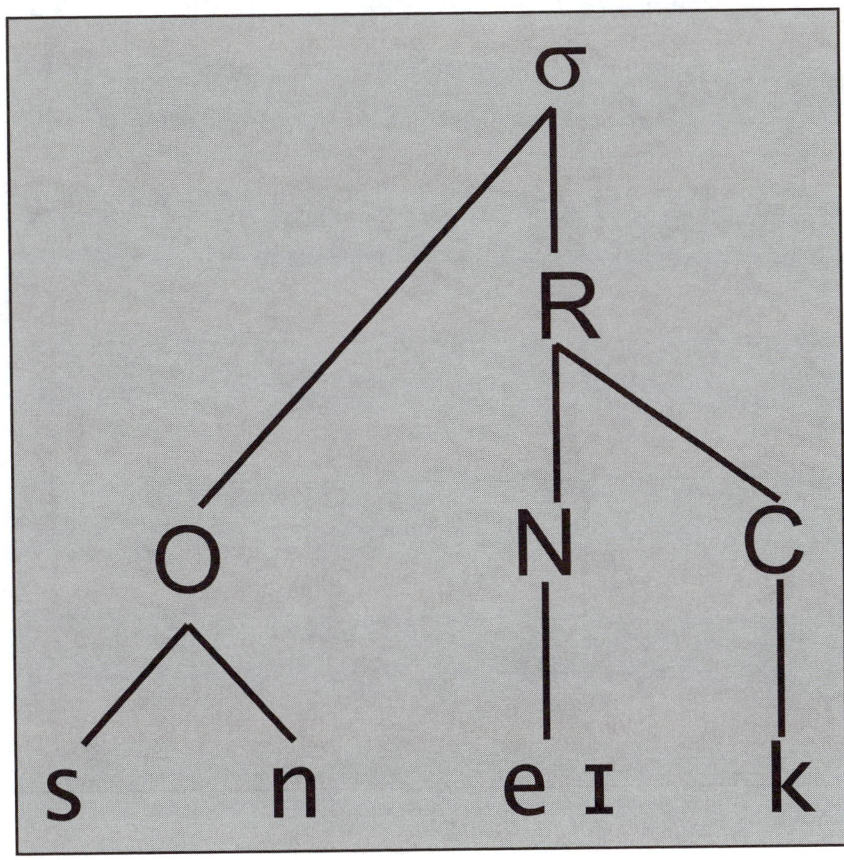

Figure 6–1. *Syllabification of the word "snake."*

syllable positions of consonants. Rule 1 is to place a syllable boundary after an unstressed syllable if it precedes a stressed syllable, such as in "ba/nana" (/bə.nænə/) and "tele/phone" (/tɛlə.fon/). Rule 2 is to place a syllable boundary between syllables of compound words, as they both carry stress (e.g., "school/bag": /skul.bæg/; "bath/tub": /bæθ.tʌb/). Rule 3 is to place a syllable boundary between consonants in the medial position if they are not legal final clusters in English. For instance, a boundary is placed in the word "nap/kin" as English words cannot end in the consonant sequence /pk/. The cluster /sk/, on the other hand, is permissible as a word-final consonant sequence in English and therefore in a word such as "basket" a syllable boundary is not required, resulting in an ambisyllabic /sk/ cluster. Rule 4 is to consider all remaining consonants between vowels to be ambisyllabic. Regarding word-medial consonant clusters, O'Grady and Dobrovolsky (1997) put a syllable boundary between the two consonants if they are not a permissible cluster in both the onset and coda position (Figure 6–3). In other words, whereas "candle" would be syllabified as /kændəl/ by Ingram because [nd] is a permissible coda in English, it would be syllabified as /kæn.dəl/ by O;Grady and Dobrovolsky as [nd] is not a permissible onset in English.

Ingram (1981) described four rules to define the syllable positions of consonants.

Word medial consonant clusters are classified as **ambisyllabic** if they are permissible word finally according to Ingram. O'Grady, and Dobrovolsky (1997) only allow ambisyllabic consonant clusters if they are permissible both in the onset and coda position.

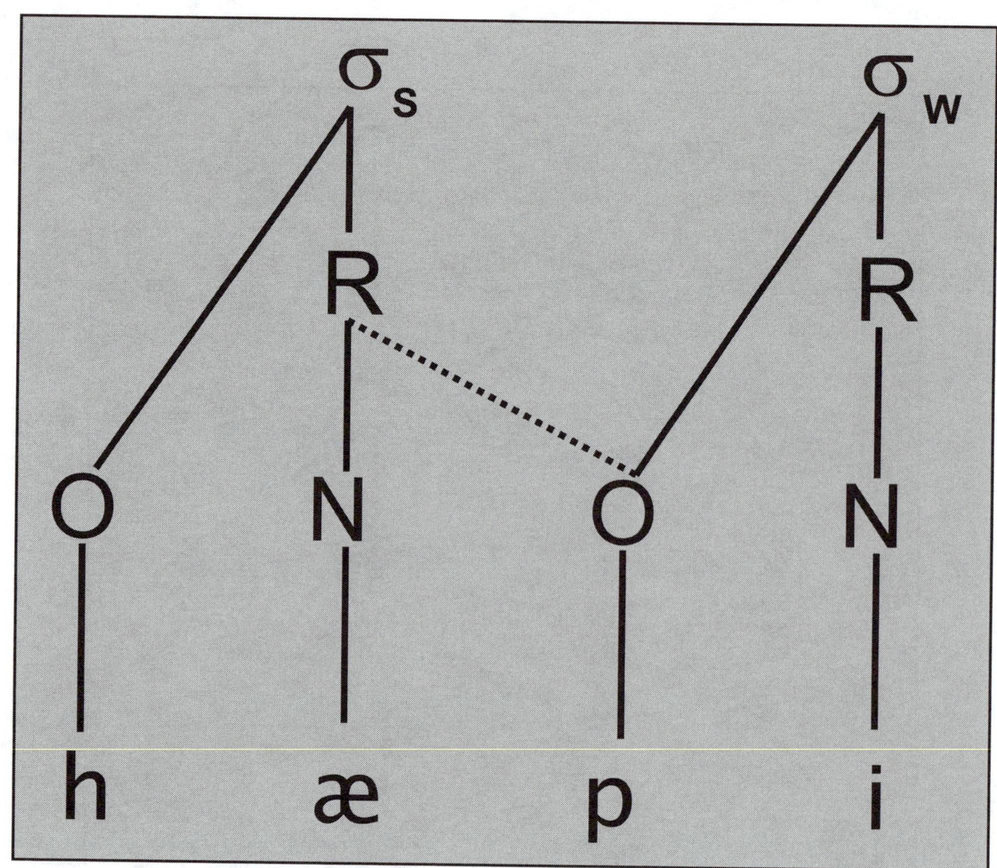

Figure 6–2. Syllabification of the word "happy."

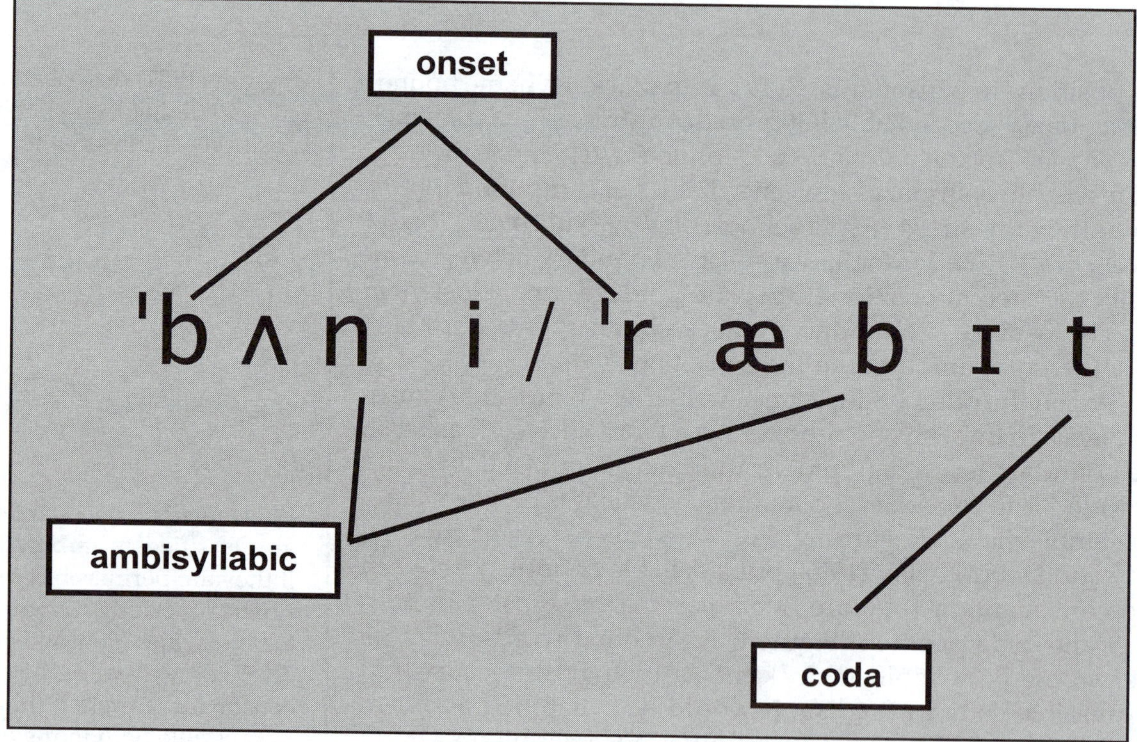

Figure 6–3. The positions of the consonants in the word "bunny rabbit."

Stressed syllables are more prominent than others and are usually called "strong" (S) whereas unstressed syllables are called "weak" (W). Syllables are grouped in units called *feet*, with each foot containing only one stressed syllable. In English most 2-syllable words are strong-weak, or "Sw." Feet are in turn grouped to form the prosodic word (Figure 6–4).

Syllables are grouped in units called **feet**, which in turn are grouped to form the prosodic word.

Timing units are additional elements that indicate that a segment is present. English adult consonants and short vowels contain one timing unit; the long vowels [iː] and [uː], and probably the vowels [æː], [ɑː], and [ɔː] each have two timing units, as do diphthongs (/eɪ/, /oʊ/, /ɑɪ/, /ɑʊ/, and /ɔɪ/). Children sometimes produce one long consonant with two timing units in place of a consonant cluster. Figure 6–5 shows the timing units for the words "bit," "beat," "no," and "snow," demonstrating these various possibilities. Children often have constraints and repairs related to timing

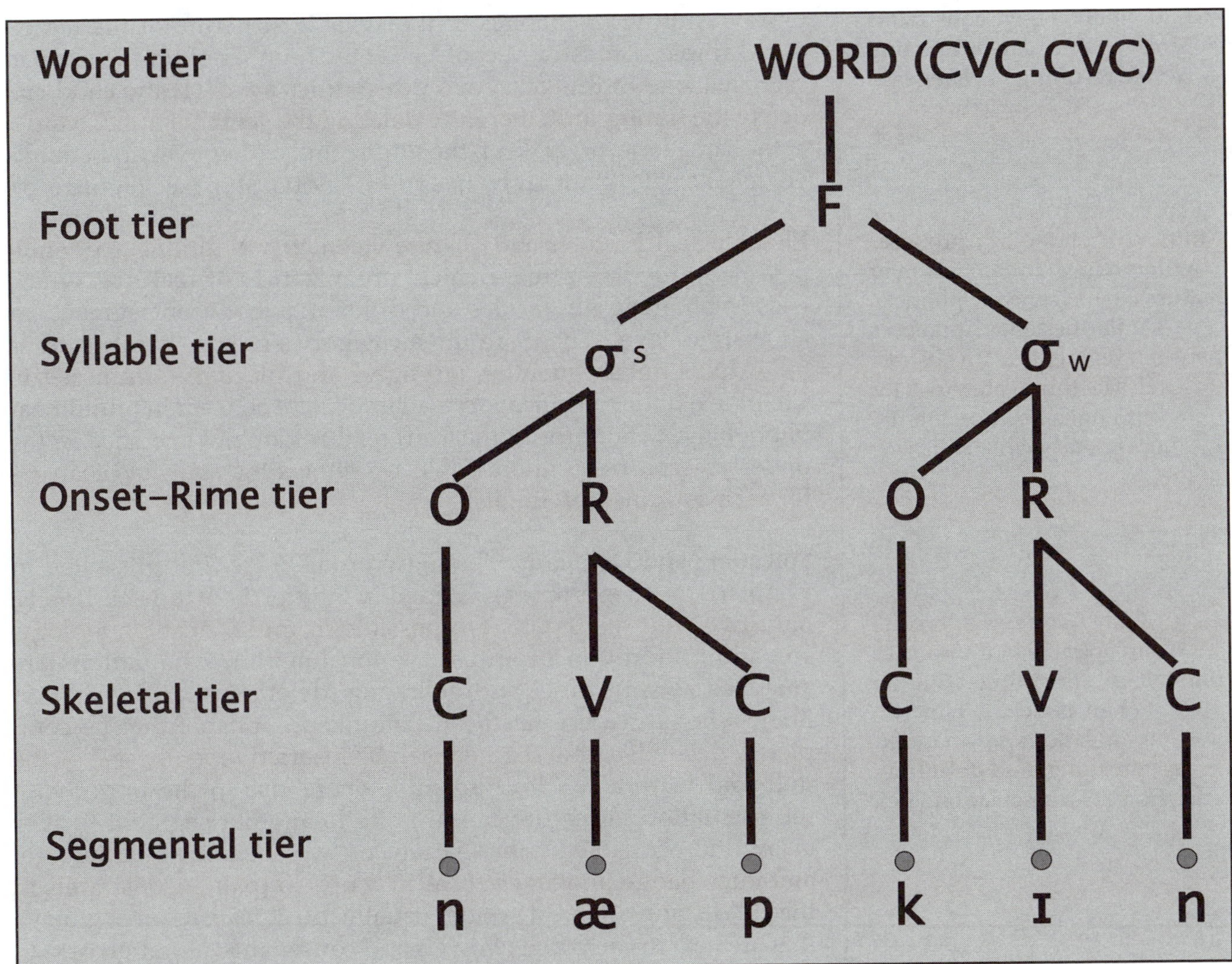

Figure 6–4. *Hierarchical representation of the prosodic word "napkin."*

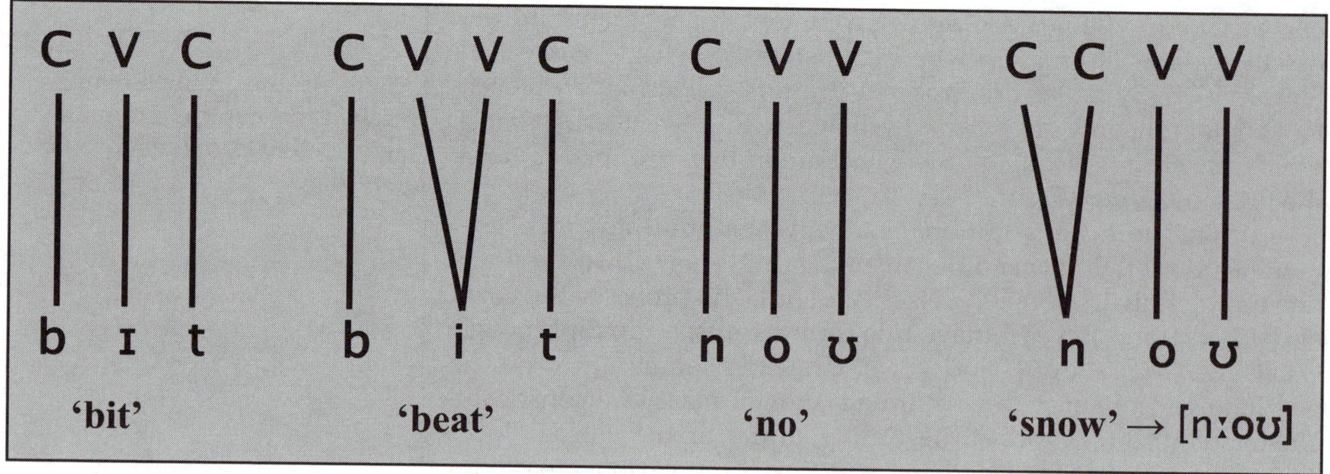

Figure 6–5. *Timing units for the words "bit," "beat," "no," and "snow."*

Children often have constraints and repairs related to **timing units**, resulting in changes in the syllable structure of the target.

units, resulting in changes in the syllable structure of the target. For example, a constraint could limit the number of timing units in each syllable. In this case, two possibilities arise: (1) the child can delete the timing unit, therefore deleting the segment attached to it at the same time, or; (2) keep the timing unit, either by lengthening a vowel or a consonant, or by inserting a glottal stop (see Figure 6–5).

Multilinear phonology proposes a **hierarchical organization of features**, which encode phonetic similarities and differences between segments at an abstract level. The three categories for adult English consonants are *manner*, *laryngeal*, and *place*.

Phonological Features and Feature Geometry. Multilinear phonology also proposes a hierarchical organization of features, which encode phonetic similarities and differences between segments at an abstract level. There are three categories of consonant features for Adult English: manner, laryngeal and place. As discussed in Chapter 1, underspecification is an important concept in multilinear phonology: default (or unmarked) features are not specified in the underlying representation. Table 1–2 shows the specified features for each consonant in English.

Only two rules or repairs are possible in multilinear phonology: **spreading** (addition of an association line; all assimilations are analyzed as spreading) and **delinking** (deletion of an association line).

Spreading and Delinking. These two rules were first presented in Chapter 1, with examples provided in Figures 1–29 to 1–31. Briefly, only two rules or repairs are possible in multilinear phonology: spreading (addition of an association line; all assimilations are analyzed as spreading) and delinking (deletion of an association line). When a feature has been "unlinked," it can either be completely deleted; a new segment can be inserted (epenthesis); or the unlinked feature can link up somewhere else in the underlying representation. A feature can migrate to another segment further away, and occasionally the features of two segments will migrate and interchange (metathesize, as in "cup" → [pʌk]). Constraints in the child's phonological system usually affect features or segments that are next to each other. Vowels and consonants, although next to one another in the CV strings, are assumed to be on different planes of the representation. The analogy of a parking lot presented by Bernhardt and Stemberger has also helped many students understand that although the hierarchies are presented visually in two-dimensions, in multilinear phonology features and segments are not organized in a linear fashion and are not necessarily "next to" one another. In a parking lot, some cars are parked in adjacent spots and there is no space to park another car between them: these cars are clearly "next to" one another. Other cars have an empty space between them but could be considered to be "next to" one another for some purposes. Figure 6–6 presents possible examples of delinking for a child who has a constraint that prevents the sequence of the places of articulation Dorsal – Labial in consonants. Figure 6–7 presents examples of spreading to the default consonant [t] which is highly susceptible to assimilation, in which nondefault features such as Labial and [+voice] replace the unspecified Coronal, [−voice] defaults.

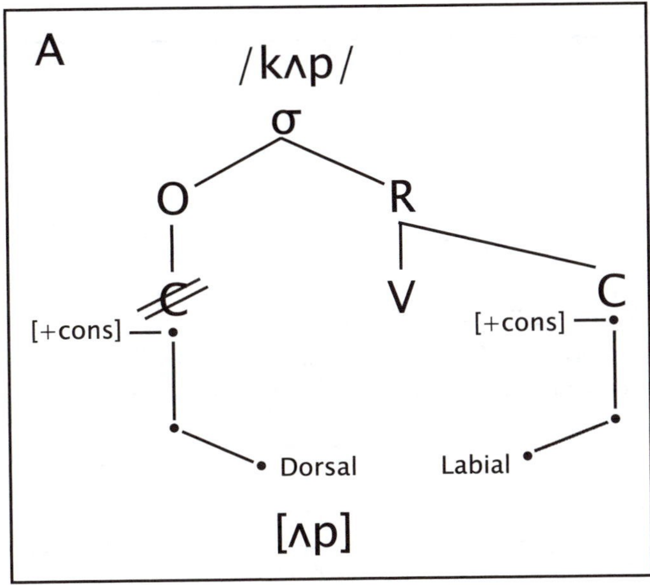

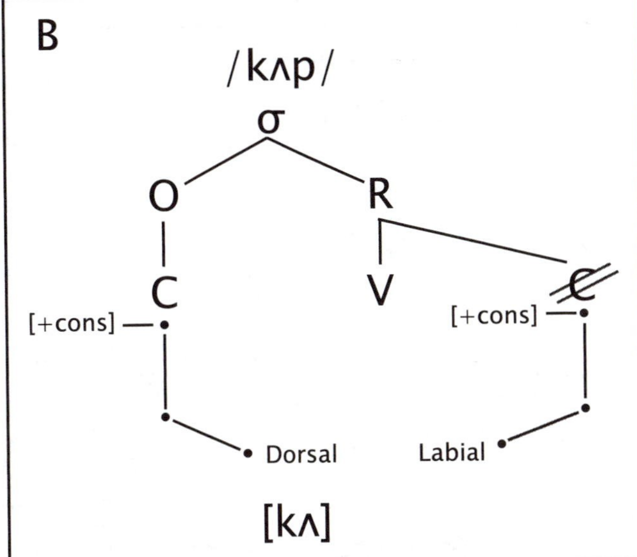

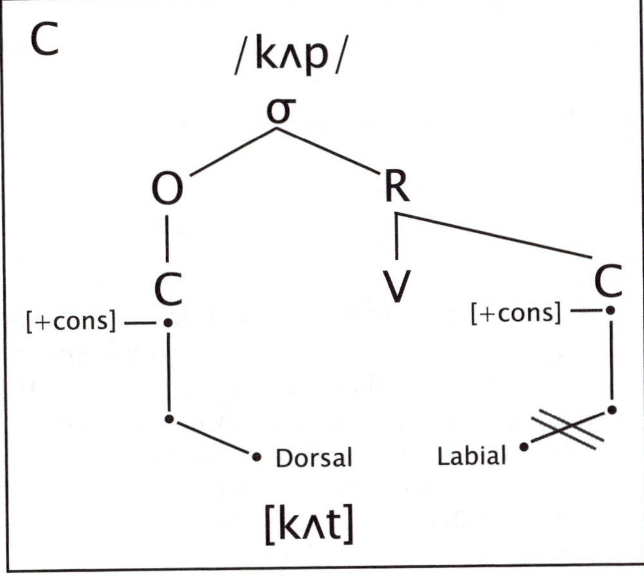

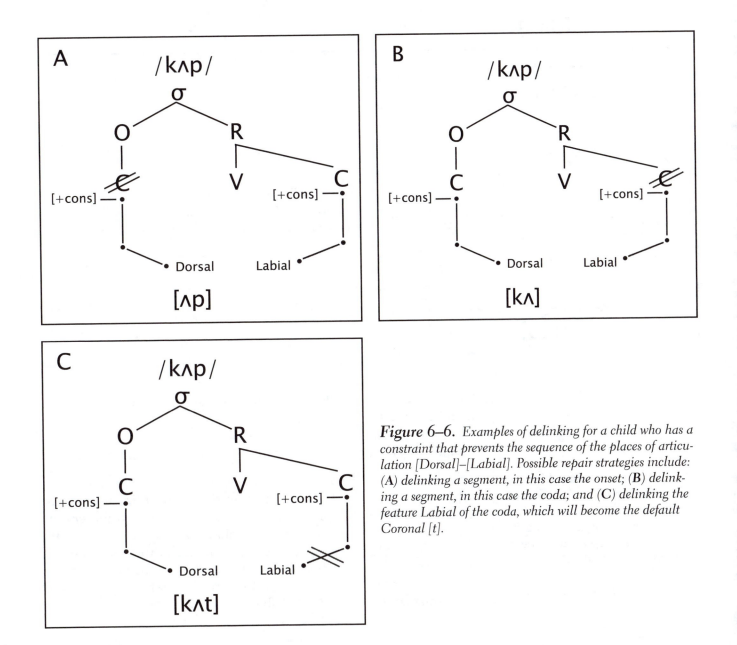

Figure 6–6. *Examples of delinking for a child who has a constraint that prevents the sequence of the places of articulation [Dorsal]–[Labial]. Possible repair strategies include: (**A**) delinking a segment, in this case the onset; (**B**) delinking a segment, in this case the coda; and (**C**) delinking the feature Labial of the coda, which will become the default Coronal [t].*

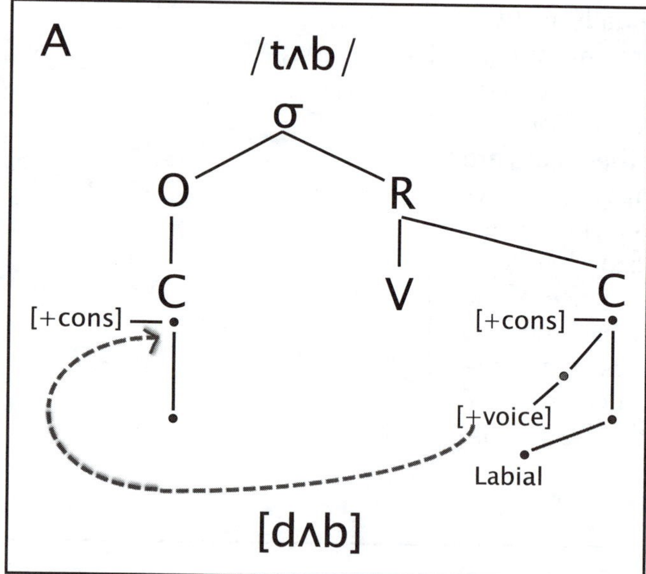

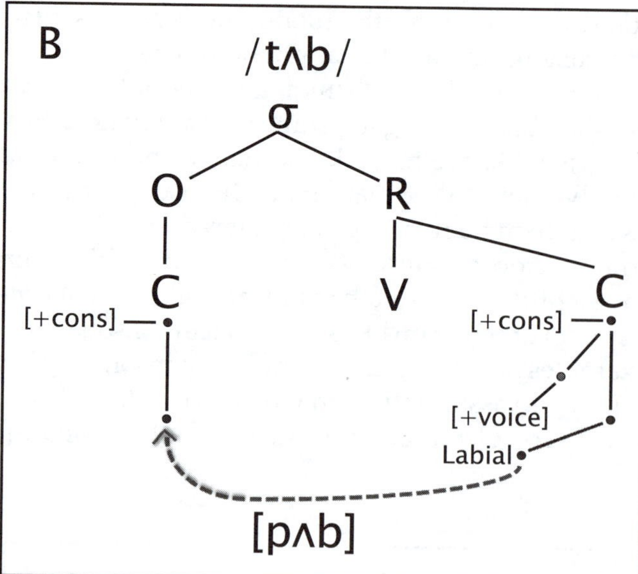

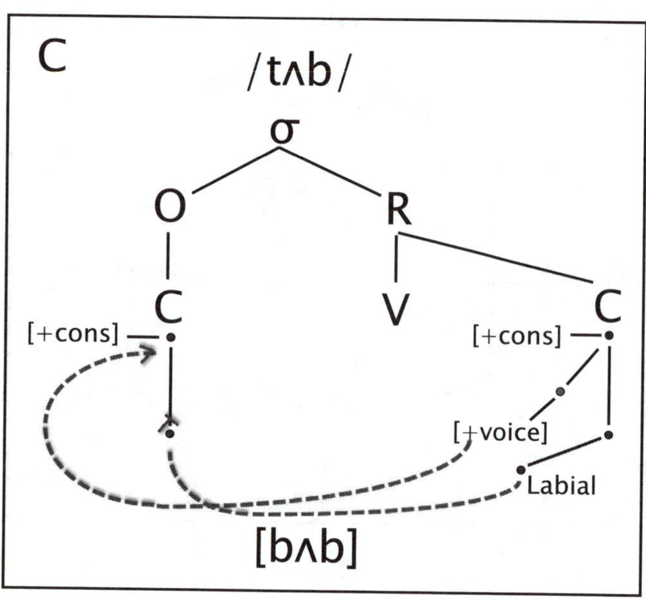

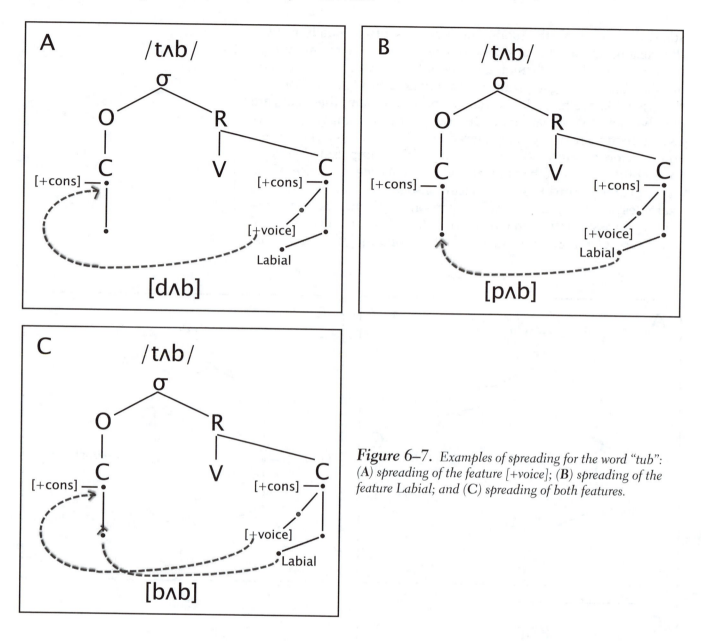

Figure 6–7. *Examples of spreading for the word "tub": (**A**) spreading of the feature [+voice]; (**B**) spreading of the feature Labial; and (**C**) spreading of both features.*

Further examples of delinking and spreading are demonstrated with Case Study 6–2 (Amber).

Adequacy of the Speech Sample for a Multilinear Analysis

The speech sample should meet specific criteria that **ensure sufficient coverage of phones and syllable shapes** in order to conduct an in-depth multilinear analysis to describe the child's phonological system and select intervention goals.

As discussed in Chapter 5, the speech sample should meet specific criteria in order to conduct an in-depth multilinear analysis to describe the child's phonological system and select intervention goals. The checklist presented by Bernhardt and Holdgrafer (2001) was completed for the speech sample of Case Study 6–2, and is presented in Table 6–2. Bernhardt and Holdgrafer also recommend answering a few questions related to word shape structures and the segmental content of the word shapes, as presented in Table 6–3.

Case Study 6–2

Pretreatment speech sample of a girl age 4;8 with severely disordered phonological skills.

#	Orthographic Gloss	Adult Form	Child's Production	#	Orthographic Gloss	Adult Form	Child's Production
1	banana	bə.nænʌ	bʌnɑijʌ	30	nailpolish	nɛl.pɑlɪʃ	nepɑjɪs
2	basket	bæskɪt	bæsɪt	31	newspaper	nus.pepɚ	nuspese
3	black	blæk	bæt	32	pages	pedʒəz	pesəs
4	blue	blu	bu	33	pajamas	pə.dʒæməz	paijʌs
5	brush	bɹʌʃ	bʌs	34	pencils	pɛnsəlz	pætes
6	bunny rabbit	bʌni.ɹæbɪt	bʌjiwæjɪt	35	raining	ɹenɪŋ	weije
7	candle	kændəl	tɑije	36	rocket	ɹɑkɪt	wɑtɛt
8	car	kɑɝ	tɑn	37	Santa Claus	sæntə.klɔz	tʌjeitas
9	carrots	kɛɝɹʌts	tejʌts	38	scissors	sɪzɚz	dɪsəs
10	chair	tʃɛɝ	tei	39	screwdriver	skɹu.dɹɑɪvɚ	tudɑiwe
11	chicken	tʃɪkən	tɪtən	40	shovel	ʃʌvəl	pʌjei
12	coffee cup	kɑfi.kʌp	pɑsitʌp	41	sleeping	slipɪŋ	pitɪn
13	drum	dɹʌm	dʌmə	42	smoke	smok	pot
14	duck	dʌk	dʌt	43	snake	snek	tet
15	feather	fɛðɚ	pɑije	44	soap	sop	top
16	finger	fɪŋ.gɚ	peje	45	sock	sɑk	tɑt
17	fish	fɪʃ	pɪs	46	squirrel	skwɝɹəl	tʌwe
18	glasses	glæsəz	dæsəs	47	stove	stov	pos
19	glove	glʌv	dʌv	48	table	tebəl	tewe
20	gun	gʌn	dʌnə	49	toothbrush	tuθ.bɹʌʃ	tufbʌs
21	gum	gʌm	dʌm	50	up	ʌp	ʌp
22	half	hæf	hæf	51	vacuum cleaner	vækjum. klinɚ	bætum tijes
23	jump rope	dʒʌmp.ɹop	dʌpwop	52	vase	ves	bes
24	keep	kip	pit	53	wagon	wægən	wɑjən
25	knife	nɑɪf	nʌf	54	window	wɪndo	wɪje
26	ladder	lædɚ	nʌje	55	yawning	jɑnɪŋ	nɑji
27	looking	lʊkɪŋ	nʊtɪn	56	yellow	jɛlo	nʌje
28	matches	mætʃəz	nʌtɛs	57	zipper	zɪpɚ	pɪte
29	mouth	mɑʊθ	mʌf				

Table 6–2. *Completed Checklist for Segments (phonemes) and Context for the Speech Sample of Case Study 6–2*

Segment	Word-Initial	First Vowel	Cross-V Place Sequence	Word-Medial			Word-Final	Word Shape
				SI	IV	SF		
p	✓✓✓	e, ɛ, ə	Lab-Cor-Cor Lab-Cor-Lab-Cor	✓✓	✓✓✓	✓	✓✓✓✓ ✓	CVCV.CVC, CVC, CVCC.CVC, CVCVC CVC.CVCVC, VC, CVC.CVCV, CVCV CV,CVCVC, CVCCVCC, CCVCVC
b	✓✓✓✓✓✓	ə, æ, ʌ, u	Lab-Cor-Cor; Lab-Cor Lab-Cor-Cor-Lab-Cor	✓	✓✓			CV.CVCV, CVCCVC, CCVC, CCV CVCV.CVCVC, CVC.CCVC
t	✓✓	e, u	Cor-Lab-Cor Cor-Cor-Cor		✓✓	✓	✓✓✓	CVCCVC, CVCVC, CVCV.CVCVC CVVCVCC, CCVC, CVCC.CCVC CVC.CCVC
d	✓✓	ʌ, aɪ	Cor-Lab; Cor-Dor Cor-Lab	✓	✓✓✓			CVCCVC, CVC, CCVC, CVCV, CCCV.CCVVCV, CVCCV
k	✓✓✓✓✓	æ, ɑ, ɛ, i	Dor-Cor-Cor Dor-Lab-Dor-Lab; Dor-Lab	✓✓✓✓ ✓	✓✓✓✓ ✓		✓✓✓✓ ✓	CVCCVC, CCVC, CVV, CVVCVCC CVCVC, CVCV.CVC, CVC, CCCVCVC CVCCV.CCVC, CCCV.CCVVCV CVCCVC.CCVCV
g	✓✓✓✓	æ, ʌ	Dor-Cor-Cor; Dor-Lab; Dor-Cor	✓	✓			CVC.CV, CCVCVC, CCVC, CVC, CVCVC
m	✓✓	æ, aʊ	Lab-Cor-Cor; Lab-Cor	✓	✓✓	✓	✓✓	CCVC, CVC, CVVC, CVCVC, CV.CVCVC CVCC.CVC, CVCCVC.CCVC
n	✓✓✓	ɑɪ, ɛ, u	Cor-Lab; Cor-Cor-Lab-Lab Cor-Cor-Lab-Cor-Cor	✓✓	✓✓✓✓ ✓✓✓✓ ✓		✓✓✓	CV.CVCV, CVC, CVCV.CVCVC CVCCVC, CVVC, CVCVC, CVCCVCC CVC.CVCVC, CVC.CVCV, CVCVC CVCCV.CCVC, CCVC, CVCCV CVCCVC.CCVCV
ŋ						✓	✓✓✓✓	CVC.CV, CVCVC, CCVCVC
f	✓✓✓	ɛ, ɪ	Lab-Cor; Lab-Dor		✓		✓✓	CVCV, CVC.CV, CVC, CVVC

Segment	Word-Initial	First Vowel	Cross-V Place Sequence	Word-Medial SI	Word-Medial IV	Word-Medial SF	Word-Final	Word Shape
v	✓✓	æ, e	Lab-Dor-Lab-Dor-Cor Lab-Cor		✓		✓✓	CVC, CCVC, CVCVC CVCCVC.CCVCV, CCCV.CCVVCV
θ						✓	✓	CVVC, CVC.CCVC
ð					✓			CVCV
s	✓✓✓✓✓ ✓✓✓✓✓	æ, ɪ, u, i, o, e, ɑ, ɝ	Cor-Cor-Dor-Cor; Cor-Cor-Cor; Cor-Lab-Dor; Cor-Lab; Cor-Cor-Lab; Cor-Dor		✓✓✓	✓	✓✓	CVCCVC, CVVCVCC, CCVCVC CVC.CVCV, CVCCVCC, CVCVC CCCV.CCVVCV, CCVC, CVC CCCVCVC
z	✓	ɪ	Cor-Lab		✓		✓✓✓✓ ✓✓✓	CVCV, CCVCVC, CVCVC, CV.CVCVC CVCCVCC, CVCCV.CCVC
ʃ	✓	ʌ	Cor-Lab-Cor				✓✓✓✓	CVC.CVCVC, CVC, CVC.CCVC, CCVC, CVCVC
ʒ								
tʃ	✓✓	ɛ, ɪ	Cor-Dor-Cor		✓			CVV, CVCVC
dʒ	✓	ʌ	Cor-Lab-Cor-Lab	✓	✓			CCVC.CVC, CVCVC, CV.CVCVC
w	✓✓	æ, ɪ	Lab-Dor-Cor; Lab-Cor	✓				CVCVC, CVCCV, CCCVCVC
j	✓✓	ɑ, ɛ	Cor-Cor-Dor; Cor-Cor		✓			CVCVC, CVCV, CVCCVC.CCVCV
l	✓✓	æ, ʊ	Cor-Cor; Cor-Dor-Dor	✓✓✓✓ ✓✓✓	✓✓	✓✓	✓✓✓✓	CCVC, CCV, CVCCVC, CCVCVC CCVC, CVCV, CVCVC, CVC.CVCVC CVCCVCC, CVCCV.CCVC, CCCVCVC CVCCVC.CCVCV
r	✓✓	e, ɑ	Cor-Cor-Dor; Cor-Dor-Cor	✓✓✓✓ ✓✓✓	✓✓			CCVC, CVCV.CVCVC, CVVCVCC CVCC.CVC, CVCVC, CCCV.CCVVCV CCCVCVC, CVC.CCVC
h	✓	æ	Cor-Lab					CVC

Source: From Bernhardt and Holdgrapher (2001). Beyond the basics II: Supplemental sampling for in-depth phonological analysis. *Language, Speech and Hearing Services in Schools*, 32, Figure 1, p. 29. Adapted with permission of the American Speech-Language-Hearing Association.

Table 6–3. Questions Recommended by Bernhardt and Holdgrapher (2001) to Evaluate the Adequacy of Syllable Shapes in the Speech Sample to Conduct an In-Depth Multilinear Analysis

Word Shape Structures
Are there enough words to establish a pretreatment baseline performance for the various word shapes?
Are there complexity effects related to the number of consonants in the word?
Differences between vowel-initial and consonant-initial variants of words?
Differences between vowel-final and consonant-final variants of words, such as CCV versus CCVC?
Do diphthongs affect the production of a particular word shape, such as CVC versus CVVC?
Segmental Content of Word Shapes
Is a variety of segments represented in the multiple tokens of the same word shape?
Is the accurate production of words facilitated by segment similarity, such as C_1VC_1 versus C_1VC_2?
Do morphological endings facilitate production of a word shape, such as CVC word more likely to be produced accurately when the final consonant is a plural /s/?

Source: Adapted from Bernhardt and Holdgrapher (2001). Beyond the basics II: Supplemental sampling for in-depth phonological analysis. *Language, Speech and Hearing Services in Schools, 32,* p. 31.

The speech sample should contain a minimum of 10 tokens each of CVC, CCV(C), CVCV, and CVCVC word shapes, as well as at least 5 tokens each of (C)V(V), (C)VCC, CVCCV(C), and (C)VCVCC, with a minimum of 5 vowel-initial words.

The speech sample should contain a minimum of ten tokens each of CVC, CCV(C), CVCV, and CVCVC word shapes, as well as at least five tokens each of (C)V(V), (C)VCC, CVCCV(C) and (C)VCVCC, with a minimum of five vowel-initial words. As described in Chapter 5 the recommended speech sample length for multilinear analysis is 100 to 150 words. For demonstration purposes, however, we present an abbreviated sample of only 57 words here while retaining representativeness for the speech typically produced by Amber (Case Study 6–2) when she was 4 years old. When we examine the adult targets of the words that Amber attempted, we notice that most consonant-initial word shapes are represented in sufficient number in the short Amber sample; therefore, complexity effects related to the number of consonants can be examined, for example by comparing Amber's production of CCV and CCVC words. There are also several words with diphthongs; however, there is only one vowel-initial word resulting in one vowel-initial and consonant-initial variant of the same word in the entire sample (i.e., "up" versus "cup"). In terms of the segmental content of word shapes, a variety of segments is represented in various instances of the same word shape. Nonetheless, as seen in Table 6–2, some phonemes are not well represented in the sample (specifically, /θ, ð, ʒ, h/). There are several instances of the plural "–s" and present progressive "–ing" endings, which allows us to examine whether morphological endings facilitate production of certain word shapes. These questions about word shape and syllable structures probe the child's production of a variety of word shapes without considering the particular features and segments present in these various word shapes.

Questions about word shape and syllable structures probe the child's production of a variety of word shapes without considering the particular features and segments present in these various word shapes.

In conversation, each sound is produced in a variety of phonetic contexts; adjacent phonemes, word length, and word shape complexity affect the accuracy of the production of the word. The sample should therefore contain various manner, place, and voicing features and segments to determine whether they affect the production of various word shapes. As seen in Table 6–2, there are gaps in the Amber sample. One option is to administer a *deep test* such as the Deep Test of Articulation (McDonald, 1964), which systematically varies the consonant and/or vowel preceding or following the target sound, allowing the assessment of each individual phoneme in approximately 50 contexts. Each test item consists of two monosyllable words, one of which contains the target phoneme, such as "duck-sun." The Deep Test of Articulation could be administered for phonemes that are not well represented in the speech sample, especially if they are correctly produced in some words and not others, with no clear pattern of contexts that facilitate production of the target.

When there are gaps in the speech sample regarding the variety of phonetic contexts, you can administer a **deep test of articulation** which systematically varies the consonant and/or vowel preceding or following the target sound.

Another option to supplement the Amber sample would be to follow some of the suggestions made by Bernhardt and Holdgrafer (2001), summarized in Table 6–4. In Amber's case, supplemental probing of VC or VCC words, increasing segmental variety in the onset and coda positions (such as probing CVC, CVCV, and CCV(C) words containing fricatives and liquids) and probing words with final clusters from a variety of categories would be most appropriate. As Amber's sample contains several CVC words with a variety of final consonants, and as she produced a final consonant for the vast majority of these words, supplemental probing of CVC and CVVC words would not give us more information to select treatment targets. In terms of /ɹ/ clusters in the onset position, the sample contains only two instances each of /bɹ/ and /dɹ/ clusters; it could be interesting to probe whether target clusters with voicing similarity (e.g, /gɹ/) or manner similarity (e.g., /fɹ/) increase the probability of producing a complex onset.

Another option to supplement the speech sample is to follow the suggestions summarized in Table 6–4.

Quick Version of the Multilinear Analysis (Figure 6–8)

The quick version of the multilinear analysis involves no or limited counting, and can be performed by scanning the speech sample. The goal of the multilinear analysis is to quickly identify major weaknesses in the child's phonology as potential intervention goals for the child; the quick version of the analysis might be enough to derive a complete intervention plan for children who present with straightforward phonological patterns but it is preferable to complete the full multilinear analysis for children with complex patterns of mismatches to the adult targets. We first demonstrate how to complete the quick version of the analysis, considering both Case Studies 6–1 and 6–2, before proceeding to the full version of the multilinear analysis for Case Study 6–2 (Amber).

The goal of the **multilinear analysis** is to quickly identify major weaknesses in the child's phonology as potential intervention goals for the child.

The **quick version of the multilinear analysis** can be completed efficiently for daily use in clinical practice; however, it is always preferable to complete the full analysis for children with complex patterns of mismatches to the adult targets.

Although a detailed discussion of goal selection occurs in Chapter 8, a very brief description of the general principles of goal

Table 6–4. Supplemental Sampling Strategies

(C)V(V)C and longer words with final consonants	
Probe additional VC or VVC words	"in," "on," "out," "up," "all," etc.
Probe additional CVC or CVVC words	"sit," "bike," "ball," "nose," "foot," etc.
Probe near-minimal pairs V(V)C and CV(V)C	"up" and "pup;" "ice" and "dice," "eat" and "meat," etc.
Probe whether diphthongs affect the production of the final consonant	"eat" and "ate;" "done" and "down;" "cut" and "kite," etc.
Increase segmental variety in onset and coda; liquids and fricatives in the coda position are often underrepresented	"ball," "bear," "knife," "mouse," "bus," etc.
Probe whether consonant similarity facilitates production of final consonants	"dad" and "dog;" "pop" and "pot;" "cake" and "cage;" "sauce" and "sock;" etc.
Probe differences in production of final consonants that are part of the word and final grammatical morphemes	"bees" and "buzz;" "towed" and "toad," etc.
CCV(C) words	
Probe words with clusters from a variety of categories	s-clusters: /sm/, /sn/, /sl/, /st/, /sp/, /sk/, sw/ stop-glide clusters: /kw/, /tw/, /fj/, /pj/, /mj/, /hj/, /bj/ r-clusters: /pɹ/, /bɹ/, /tɹ/, /dɹ/, /kɹ/, /gɹ/, /fɹ/, /θɹ/ l-clusters: /pl/, /bl/, /kl/, /gl/, /fl/
Probe whether longer words or words with final consonants decrease the probability of accurate initial-cluster production	"spy," "spoon," "spider;" "play," "plate," "playing,", etc.
Probe whether similarity of features in the cluster facilitates or inhibits production of the cluster	voicing similarity: /gɹ/, /sp/, /bl/ manner similarity: /fɹ/, /fl/, /sw/, / θɹ/ place similarity: /st/, /sn/, /sl/
Probe whether vowel features impact consonant cluster production	Do round vowels increase substitution of /r/ by /w/ in words such as "troll" vs. "truck;" "grow" vs. "green?"

Source: Adapted from Bernhardt and Holdgrafer (2001). Beyond the basics II: Supplemental sampling for in-depth phonological analysis. *Language, Speech and Hearing Services in Schools*, 32.

Default structures are the *least marked* forms at each level of the phonological hierarchy.

selection in multilinear phonology will help in understanding the purpose of the analysis. Briefly, the strengths and weaknesses at all levels of the phonological hierarchy (phrase, word, syllable structure, segment, feature, and associations between tiers) are examined in the multilinear phonology analysis of the child's speech. Both prosodic and segmental goals are targeted in multilinear phonology, with the child's strengths supporting the needs such that new syllable structures are targeted with segments that the child produces well whereas new segments or features are targeted in established syllable or word structures. The multilinear phonology analysis also identifies the child's default structures, which may not always correspond to the adult default structures.

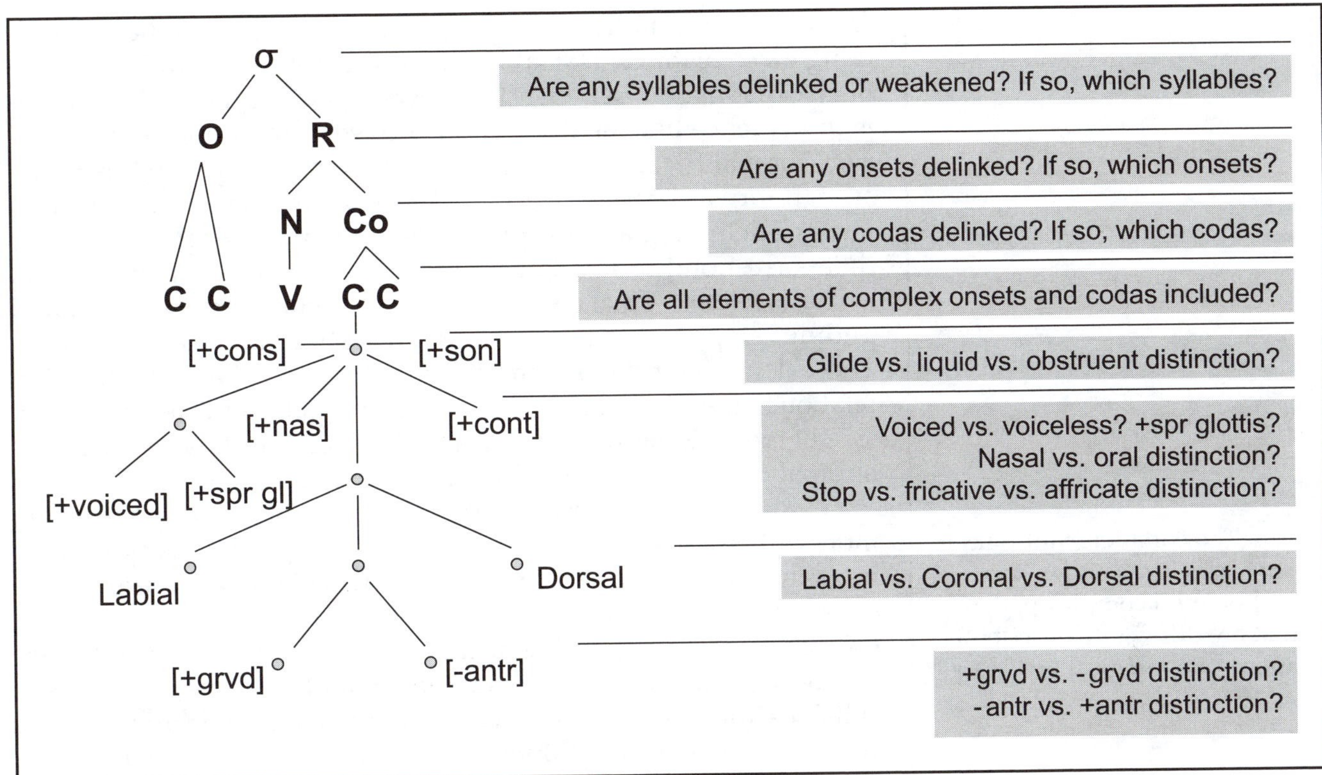
σ
O
R
N
Co
C C
V
C C
[+cons]
[+son]
[+nas]
[+cont]
[+voiced]
[+spr gl]
Labial
Dorsal
[+grvd]
[-antr]
Are any syllables delinked or weakened? If so, which syllables?
Are any onsets delinked? If so, which onsets?
Are any codas delinked? If so, which codas?
Are all elements of complex onsets and codas included?
Glide vs. liquid vs. obstruent distinction?
Voiced vs. voiceless? +spr glottis?
Nasal vs. oral distinction?
Stop vs. fricative vs. affricate distinction?
Labial vs. Coronal vs. Dorsal distinction?
+grvd vs. - grvd distinction?
- antr vs. +antr distinction?

Figure 6–8. *Quick version of a multilinear analysis.*

The quick version of the multilinear phonology analysis first examines the syllable tier to identify whether any of them are delinked or weakened. Considering Case Study 6–1, this child occasional delinks the weak syllable in trochees and iambs which is somewhat unusual (e.g., "basket" → [bæɪʔ]). Moving to onsets, these are often delinked in the ambisyllabic position, although it is possible that the absent ambisyllabic segments are treated as codas by the child (e.g, target /z/ in "music box"→ [muɪʔbɑ]). Codas are sometimes delinked (e.g., "glove" → [gʌ]) or weakened by delinking of the supralaryngeal place node leaving a glottal stop in both word final and word internal coda contexts (e.g., "leaf" → [liʔ]). Elements within complex onsets and codas are usually delinked although some /ɹ/ clusters were produced with 2 elements (e.g., "three" → [fwi]). Moving on to the feature aspects of this child's phonology, it can be seen that all major sound classes are represented and there is only one unexpected cross-class confusion ("zip" → [lɪʔ]) although liquids are sometimes produced as glides. The voicing contrast is established and [+spread glottis] is present. The nasal-oral distinction is also preserved. Delinking of [+continuant] from obstruents in the onset position occurs frequently but is usually retained in the coda (e.g., compare "shoe" to "fish"). Deaffrication is consistent but the pattern is position dependent with [branching continuant] delinked in the onset (e.g., "chair" → [tɛɚ]) but the [+continuant]

The quick version of the multilinear phonology analysis consists of a systematic scan of the speech sample to identify missing elements or obvious weaknesses at multiple levels of the phonological hierarchy.

feature retained in the coda (e.g., "watch" → [wɑʃ]). When considering place features, Dorsal is sometimes delinked. No knowledge of the distinction between [−grooved] and [+grooved] fricatives is in evidence but the distinction between [+anterior] and [−anterior] coronal fricatives is well established in the coda. In this rather straightforward case, a very quick scan of the sample reveals patterns of delinking at multiple levels of the phonological hierarchy that correspond to familiar phonological processes, that is, weak syllable deletion, final consonant deletion, cluster reduction, liquid gliding, stopping of fricatives, deaffrication, and velar fronting. These delinking rules, summarized on the right side of Table 6–1 in relation to the corresponding phonological patterns listed on the left side of the table, show that this child is a clear candidate for a cycles approach to intervention as described in Chapter 11.

The complete multilinear analysis is recommended for children with complex patterns that are difficult to describe as natural phonological processes.

Some children present with more complex patterns that are more difficult to describe as natural phonological processes. Turning now to Case Study 6–2, we see that syllable shapes are a relative strength for Amber, as only "pajamas" (CV.CVCVC) is reduced to a CVVCVC (/pɑijʌs/). At the next tier, we consider onsets and rimes and notice that Amber does not delink singleton onsets in stressed syllables. Many instances of weakening can be seen in ambisyllabic contexts, however (e.g., /ɹenɪŋ/ → [weije]; /wægən/ → [wɑjən]). Within the rime, however, codas sometimes present a problem as singleton /l/ codas are consistently delinked and most /ŋ/ codas are also delinked. Moving to the skeletal tier, complex onsets never occur; Amber also delinks one of the segments from complex codas, with one exception: /kɛɝɹʌts/ → [tejʌts]. We can now examine the use of segments and features beginning with the major sound class features attached to the root node of the feature hierarchy. Although [+consonantal] and [+sonorant] features appear, there are many instances in which glides are substituted for obstruents—an unusual pattern in English that signals the need for a more in-depth analysis. She did not produce any /l/ or /ɹ/ segments indicating the absence of the feature combination [+consonantal] [+sonorant] from her underlying representations. In terms of the laryngeal node, many mismatches involving these features are apparent in the sample although both [+voice] and [−voice] phones are present; the feature [+spread glottis] is emerging with a single instance of /h/. The distinction between the oral and nasal places of articulation is also present but substitutions of glides for nasals indicate some delinking of [+nasal] that requires further investigation. Stops and fricatives are present, but not affricates. The contrast between [+continuant] and [−continuant] obstruents is clearly conditioned by position of the consonant within the syllable, however. Shifting focus to the place nodes, it is clear that Amber produces both Labial and Coronal places of articulation but not always as expected (e.g., "stove" → [pos], "zipper" → [pɪtə]) and thus her use of these place features requires deeper analysis. There is an inventory constraint against Dorsal consonants. Finally, at the bottom of

Inventory constraints refer to phonemes or sound classes that are completely absent from the repertoire.

the hierarchy, Amber also did not produce any [+distributed] or [−anterior] obstruents.

A very close look at the Amber sample reveals the vestiges of a constraint against closed syllables that manifests itself as the addition of a vowel, resyllabifying CVC → CVCV (e.g., "gun" → [gʌnə]). These kinds of syllable structure constraints are not uncommon. Some children might have a constraint against open syllables for example, which leads to the addition of a default consonant in the onset position for VC syllables and coda position for CV syllables. Another possibility is the use of a default or filler syllable used in place of all syllables of a given type, usually weak syllables. An example of a child using this latter strategy is presented in Demonstration 11–2. Finally, when scanning the sample for feature contrasts it is useful to look for position dependent patterns of which there are several in Amber's sample. Although a quick scan of her sample revealed much information it is clear that in her case a more in-depth analysis will be required for treatment planning purposes.

Syllable structure constraints refer to restrictions on the kinds of syllable shapes that can occur in the child's inventory.

Complete Multilinear Analysis

The goal of the complete multilinear analysis is to provide a systematic description of the child's underlying representations at all levels of the phonological hierarchy, as well as the relationship between these levels. In other words, mismatches in the child's phonological knowledge in relation to the adult system are identified for all levels of the phonological hierarchy (phrase, word, syllable, segment, feature, and associations between tiers). A deep and detailed description of the child's system will lead to a more successful and time-efficient intervention. The results of the multilinear analysis are used to select both prosodic and segmental treatment goals in which the child's strengths are used to target the weaknesses. Different steps in the process provide crucial information on the child's phonological system, specifically the syllable/word shape inventory, and then the segmental and feature analyses which include a phonetic inventory by syllable position and feature match ratios, also by syllable position. The multilinear analysis itself consists of the interpretation of this information to yield a picture of the structures that are present in the child's underlying system along with delinking and spreading rules that explain the child's productive output.

A deep and detailed description of the child's system will lead to a more successful and time-efficient intervention.

The multilinear analysis consists of the **interpretation** of the information gathered during the three main steps of the process: (1) syllable/word shape inventory, (2) segmental analysis, and (3) feature analysis.

Identification of the *syllable* and *word shape inventory* is an important first step because these can be used as vehicles for targeting weaknesses with the production of segments or features. Absent word and syllable structures will usually have the most striking negative impact on the child's intelligibility and will themselves be important early targets for intervention. Note that if the adult target words of the speech sample are not diversified in terms of syllable shapes, supplemental sampling as discussed above may be necessary. The syllable and word shapes produced by the child, regardless of the adult target, are listed in a table. Consonants are identified by

The **syllable and word shape inventory** is an important first step because these can be used as vehicles for targeting weaknesses with the production of segments or features.

"C", vowels by "V," and diphthongs by "VV." Although the stress pattern for the adult target is known, it is sometimes difficult to decide whether the child produced a similar pattern as the target. For instance, the word structure for "pajamas" is CV.'CVCVC; as Amber produced [paijʌs] we need to note whether the syllable shape she produced is 'CVVCVC or CVV.'CVC or 'CVV.'CVC before we can attempt to match up the consonants that she produced with the segments in the target. The rest of the sample generally gives clues as to the likely substitution pattern; as we will see later in the complete multilinear analysis, Amber weakens ambisyllabic voiced consonants and produces the glide [j] in their place. Therefore, with this clue and information from the intonation contour heard in the original recording we can propose that she produced the word shape 'CVVCVC with the ambisyllabic "C" → [j] corresponding to the ambisyllabic "m" in the word "pajamas." The inventory of syllable/word shapes for Amber is presented in Table 6–5.

The goals of the **segmental and feature analyses** are to identify individual features and combinations of features that are established, emerging, or absent in the child's phonological system.

The goals of the *segmental and feature analyses* are to identify individual features and combinations of features that are established, emerging, or absent in the child's phonological system. Information gathered during these analyses also provides cues as to what the child's defaults might be; whereas the adult default features are those of [t], these may or may not be the default features of the child. Finally, information obtained from the segmental and feature analyses also provide insight into what rules (delinking, spreading) explain the child's production of target words. The steps in the segmental and feature analyses are as follows: (1) identify substitution patterns; (2) complete a phonetic inventory by syllable position; (3) calculate feature-match ratios for individual features and some combinations of features by syllable position; and (4) describe interactions between the feature/segmental and prosodic tiers of the phonological hierarchy. Each of these is discussed in turn, and demonstrated with the sample from Case Study 6–2 (Amber).

Table 6–5. *Syllable/Word Shapes Inventory for Case Study 6–2*

Syllable/word shapes	
(VC)	CV.CVVCV
(CV), (CVV)	(CV.CVCVC)
CVC	CVC.CVC
(CV.CV), CVCV, CVVCV, (CVCVV)	(CVC.CVCV)
CVCVC	(CVCV.CVC), (CVCVV.CVC)
(CVCVCC)	(CVCV.CVCVC)
(CVV.CVC)	(CVCVC.CVCVC)

Note: Syllable/word structures that occur only once are identified in brackets.

Demonstration 6–1: Substitution Analysis for Case Study 6–2

The first step is a *substitution analysis*, with the procedures shown for Amber's speech sample in Demonstration 6–1. The outcome of the procedure is a summary of Amber's productions for each consonant and consonant cluster by syllable position (onset, ambisyllabic, and coda): this summary is then used to quickly and more easily complete the remaining steps of the analysis.

Demonstration 6–1 describes how to fill out the Substitution Analysis Form which contains cells for each consonant and syllable position. As shown in the demonstration, omission, distortion and substitution errors along with correct productions are logged for each consonant in every word of the sample. The substitution analysis procedure is somewhat iterative because decisions about how to syllabify Amber's productions relative to the adult targets depend on her overall phonological patterns and cannot always be made on the basis of a single word in isolation from the rest of the sample. The first example in the demonstration, "banana" → [bʌnɑijʌ] is quite straightforward in terms of matching up the consonants produced by Amber with their intended targets. Previously, we mentioned the difficulty with the word "pajamas" → [pɑijʌs]; we

The first step in the segmental and feature analyses is the **substitution analysis**: the summary of the child's production of consonants and consonant clusters by syllable position. This summary is then used to quickly and more easily complete the remaining steps of the analysis.

Demonstration 6–1
Completing the Substitution Analysis Form

The substitution analysis form lists all singleton consonants and /l/, /ɹ/, /s/, and /n, m/ consonant clusters in the syllable onset, ambisyllabic, and syllable coda positions. Correct productions of the phoneme are marked with a checkmark; omissions with a dash; distortions with the IPA diacritic or a capital "D"; and substitutions indicated by writing in the substituted phoneme. For example, for item 1 Amber produced /bə.nænʌ/ → [bʌnɑijʌ] and therefore the following would be indicated in the substitution form:

Substitution of [j] for ambisyllabic /n/. For all error types the number of the item in the speech sample is written in superscripted brackets.

	Syllable Onset	% √	Ambisyllabic	% √	Syllable Coda	% √
n	✓		j[(1)]			
b	✓					

Clusters are coded separately, at the bottom of the form. In Amber's case we have coded the words "candle," "pencils," "Santa," and "window" as if they contain an ambisyllabic consonant cluster and therefore the substitution form would contain the following entries for ambisyllabic clusters:

Notice that the /ns/ cluster (item 34) is coded both under /m,n/ and /s/ clusters.

	Syllable Onset	% √	Ambisyllabic	% √	Syllable Coda	% √
m, n			j-/nd(7,54) j-/ŋg(16) -t/ns(34) j-/nt(37)			
s			s-/sk(2) -t/ns(34)			

When the consonants of all the words of the speech sample have been coded, divide the number of checkmarks inside a cell by the total number of marks in this cells. The result obtained is the percent correct for each phoneme in each word position. The abbreviation "n/a" is used to denote cells for which there are no possible entries in English; "nd" is written when no data were available from the speech sample. For example, in Amber's case the substitution analysis chart for the phonemes /ʃ/ and /j/ would indicate:

The speech sample did not contain any words with /ʃ/ in the ambisyllabic position, such as "cushion" or "fisherman."

	Syllable Onset	% √	Ambisyllabic	% √	Syllable Coda	% √
ʃ	p(40)	0		nd	s(5,17,30,49)	0
j	n(55,56)	0		n/a		n/a

/j/ is not permissible in the ambisyllabic and coda positions in English.

When all words have been coded the cells in the columns headed "% √" can be filled in. In most cases, these cells are calculated to represent the percentage of correct productions for that consonant in that syllable position. Alternative indicators are "nd" for "no data" and "n/a" when the consonant does not occur in English in a given syllable position.

proposed on the basis of global syllable shape patterns in Amber's speech that this production probably corresponds to the trochaic target /dʒæməz/ leading us to conclude that the [p] was substituted for the /dʒ/ in this word. Determining the correct syllabification of target words containing consonant sequences also requires special attention. It is important to make sure that only sequences that are truly consonant clusters are recorded in the "cluster" cells of the form. In other words, all members of the sequence need to be part of the same onset or coda to form a true cluster. For example, the word "napkin" does not contain a /pk/ cluster, as the /p/ is in the coda of the first syllable and the /k/ is in the onset of the second syllable. On the other hand, the word "basket" clearly has an ambisyllabic cluster because /sk/ is a legal onset and a legal coda in English, following O'Grady and Dobrovolsky (1997).

To complete the substitution analysis, the child's productions need to be syllabified relative to the adult targets. Special attention is required when determining the correct syllabification of target words containing consonant sequences to make sure that all members of the sequence belong to the same onset or coda.

When the child did not produce all elements of the cluster, the clinician needs to decide which sound(s) were delinked. In the case of the 3-element cluster "string" → [wɪŋ], we would decide that [w] was substituted for /ɹ/ rather than /s/ or /t/ because of the relative closeness of the substituted sound to the presumed target on the sonorancy hierarchy described in Chapter 1. The nasal clusters are ambiguous in English because they constitute a legal coda but not a legal onset allowing them to be ambisyllabic clusters according to Ingram's rule (1981) but not according to Dobrovolsy and O'Grady's rule as mentioned above. In cases like this where the solution is not clear from the published literature, the child's pattern is the best guide. In Amber's case, she produced 1/1 ambisyllabic singleton /m/ → [j] and 5/5 ambisyllabic /n/ → [j]. She also produced the ambisyllabic nasal clusters as glides, /kændəl/ → [tɑije] and /wɪndo/ → [wɪje]. We have two possible explanations for Amber's treatment of words with a nasal sequence between vowels in a trochee: we can assume she delinked the second consonant and substituted [j] for the ambisyllabic nasal phoneme; alternatively, complex onsets and codas are not permitted in her underlying representations and thus these words are represented as containing an underlying ambisyllabic singleton consonant that is expressed in the output as a glide. In either case, we code the [j] substitutions in cells of the form corresponding to ambisyllabic target clusters (rather than assuming that the sequence is split between two syllables). We caution, however, that some children might treat nasal sequences in this context as if the two elements of the sequence should be split between the two syllables and thus the analysis must be individualized to each child.

In cases where it is not clear how to syllabify the child's production of clusters from the literature (for example, when phonemes are omitted in nasal clusters), the child's pattern is the best guide.

When all the target words have been coded, the completed substitution analysis form is a very convenient tool that can be used to rapidly and more easily complete the phonetic inventory by syllable position and calculate feature-match ratios. Table 6–6 presents the completed form for Amber; the data obtained could also be used to classify speech errors as typical or atypical and developmental or nondevelopmental as described in Chapter 4.

Table 6–6. Completed Substitution Analysis Form for Case Study 6–2

	Syllable Onset	% √	Ambisyllabic	% √	Syllable Coda	% √
m	✓ n[28]	50	j[33]	0	✓✓ mə[13]	67
n	✓✓✓✓	100	j[1,6,35,51,55]	0	✓✓ nə[20]	67
ŋ		n/a		n/a	n[27,41] _[35, 55]	0
p	✓✓✓✓ _[33]	80	s[31] t[41,57]	0	✓✓✓✓ t[24]	80
b	✓✓✓	100	j[6] w[48]	0		nd
t	✓✓	100		nd	✓✓✓	100
d	✓	100	j[26]	0		nd
k	t[7,8,9,12] p[12,24]	0	t[11,27,36,51]	0	t[3,14,42,43,45]	0
g	d[20,21]	0	j[53]	0		nd
f	p[15,16,17]	0	s[12]	0	✓✓	100
v	b[51, 52]	0	w[39] j[40]	0	✓ s[47]	50
θ		nd		nd	f[29, 49]	0
ð		nd	j[15]	0		nd
s	t[37,44,45] d[38]	0	✓	100	✓✓	100
z	p[57]	0	s[38]	0	s[18,28,32,33,37,38]	0
ʃ	p[40]	0		nd	s[5,17,30,49]	0
ʒ		nd		nd		nd
tʃ	t[10,11]	0	t[28]	0		nd
dʒ	d[23] p[33]	0	s[32]	0		nd
h	✓	100		n/a		n/a
w	✓✓	100		n/a		n/a
j	n[55,56]	0		n/a		n/a
l	n[26,27]	0	j[30,56]	0	e[7] _[30,40,46,48]	0
ɹ	w[6,23,35,36]	0	j[9] w[46]	0	n[8] i[10]	0
l	b-/bl[3,4] d-/gl[18,19] t-/kl[37,51] p-/sl[41]	0		nd	-s/lz[34]	0
ɹ	b-/bɹ[5,49] d-/dɹ[13,39] -t-/skɹ[39]	0		nd		nd
m, n	p-/sm[42] t-/sn[43]	0	j-/nd[7,54] j-/ŋg[16] -t/ns[34] j-/nt[37]	0	-p/mp[23]	0
s	-t-/skɹ[39] p-/sl[41] p-/sm[42] t-/sn[43] -t-/skw[46] p-/st[47]	0	s-/sk[2]	0	✓/ts	100

Demonstration 6–2: Phonetic Inventory by Syllable Position for Case Study 6–2

The completed Substitution Analysis Form makes it easy to construct the *phonetic inventory by syllable position*, as shown in Demonstration 6–2. The result allows us to identify features and phonemes that are completely absent from the child's repertoire, indicating inventory constraints (what is probably absent from the underlying representation). It will also identify interactions between the prosodic and segmental tiers: for example interactions between the syllable position and feature use, such as when a specific feature is present in certain positions but absent in others, pointing to the presence of delinking rules. The phonetic inventory consists of the phones produced by the child, correctly or incorrectly, phonemic in the child's language or not. The consonants are organized by place and manner of articulation as shown in Demonstration 6–2.

The second step in the segmental and feature analyses is to complete a **phonetic inventory by syllable position**. The result allows us to identify features and phonemes that are completely absent from the child's repertoire, as well as interactions between the prosodic and segmental tiers.

From the phonetic inventory by syllable position we can list features that are completely absent and features that are emerging in the child's phonological system. In Amber's case, we note that the phonemes /ŋ, k, g/ are never produced, meaning that the feature Dorsal is probably absent from her underlying representation. Similarly, Amber never produced the phonemes /l, ɹ/ in any word position signaling a constraint against the combination of [+consonantal] [+sonorant]. Delinking of [+continuant] in the onset position is revealed by the absence of fricatives in syllable onsets despite their appearance in the ambisyllabic and coda positions. We also note that Amber did not produce any nasal consonant or voiced obstruent consonants in the ambisyllabic position; interpretation of the complete multilinear analysis will identify the delinking rule which explains this pattern.

From the phonetic inventory by syllable position we can list features that are never produced, and probably absent from the child's UR.

The calculation of feature-match ratios sheds light on what otherwise would look like variable patterns in the child's speech. For instance, simply by looking at the substitution form, Amber's production of /v/ seems inconsistent across positions (/v/ → [b] in onset position, /v/ → [w, j] in ambisyllabic position, and /v/ → [v, s] in the coda position). Although some patterns of delinking were noted in Amber's case by completing the phonetic inventory by syllable position, the quantitative analysis resulting from calculating the correct proportion of use of every feature by syllable position further allows us to compare the relative degree of correct use of various features and feature combinations in comparison to one another.

The third step in the segmental and feature analyses is to calculate **feature-match ratios**, allowing a comparison of the relative degree of correct use of various features and feature combinations in comparison to one another as a function of syllable position.

Feature-match ratios are calculated by comparing the features associated with every target phoneme to the features associated with the phonemes produced by the child. An illustration of a feature-match ratio tally is shown in Figure 6–9. In this case Amber produced /bʌni.ɹæbɪt/ → [bʌjiwæjɪt]. The figure shows the feature specification for each target consonant, taken from the Default Underspecification Matrix in Table 1–2. The features associated with the /b/ from "bunny" are [+consonantal], [+voice], [+labial];

Feature-match ratios are calculated by comparing the features associated with every target phoneme to the features associated with the phonemes produced by the child.

Demonstration 6–2
Phonetic Repertoire by Syllable Position

Indicate the phonemes that were produced by the child in each of the three positions. Phonemes that were produced only once in a position are indicated with brackets. As explained in Chapters 1 and 4, the phones do not have be produced correctly or produced in the appropriate target positions because this is an independent rather than relational analysis.

Although Amber only produced one correct instance of [d] in the onset position she produced this phoneme a few times in place of /g/ and /dʒ/ and therefore there are no brackets for [d] in onset position in the inventory.

Syllable onset position:

	Bilabial	**Labio-dental**	**Dental**	**Alveolar**	**Post-alveolar**	**Palatal**	**Velar**	**Glottal**
Plosive	p b			t d				
Nasal	(m)			n				
Fricative								(h)
Affricate								
Glide	w							
Liquid								

Ambisyllabic position:

	Bilabial	**Labio-dental**	**Dental**	**Alveolar**	**Post-alveolar**	**Palatal**	**Velar**	**Glottal**
Plosive				t				
Nasal								
Fricative				s				
Affricate								
Glide						j		
Liquid								

Coda position:

	Bilabial	Labio-dental	Dental	Alveolar	Post-alveolar	Palatal	Velar	Glottal
Plosive	p			t				
Nasal	(m)			n				
Fricative		f (v)		s				
Affricate								
Glide								
Liquid								

There were no opportunities to produce /b/ and /d/ in the coda position in the sample (i.e., there were no target words ending in these consonants). As they were produced accurately in the initial position and [p] and [t] are present in the syllable coda inventory, they might have been in the syllable coda inventory given a longer and more diverse speech sample.

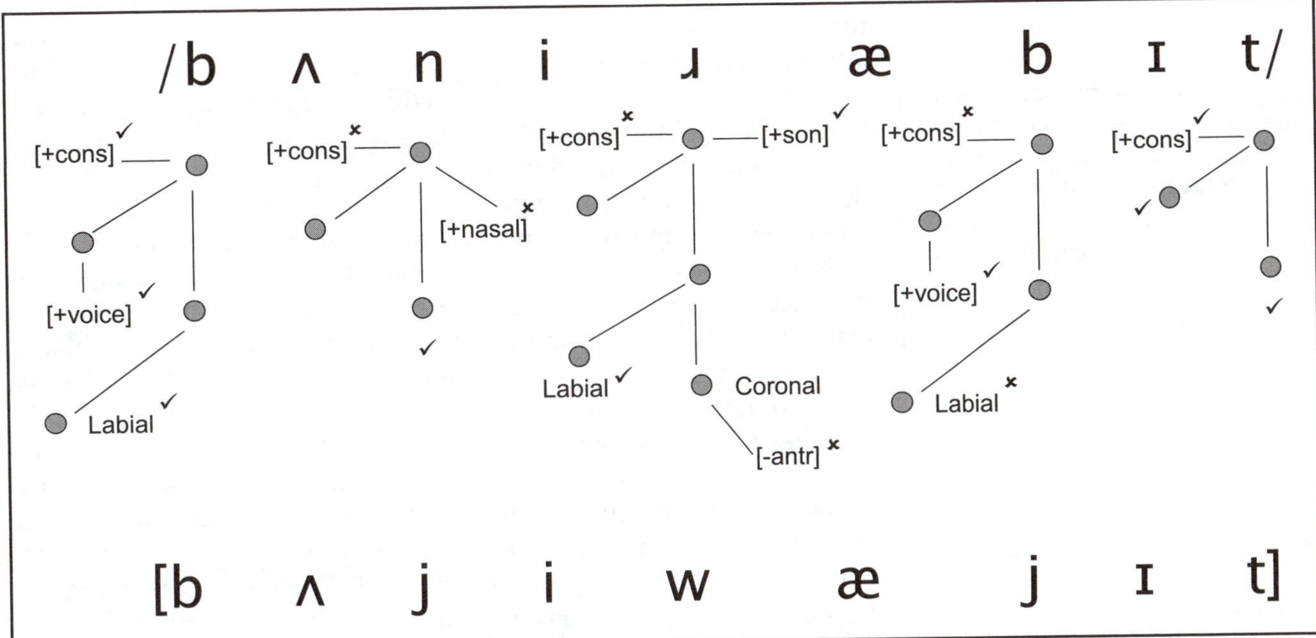

Figure 6–9. *Visual representation of the feature match calculation for the word "bunny rabbit" produced by Amber. The features associated with each of the target consonants are presented in the hierarchy; for each feature a match is indicated with a checkmark whereas a mismatch is indicated with an "x."*

as Amber accurately produced this phoneme, she receives a match for each of these features (indicated by the checkmarks). She receives a match only for Coronal for her production of /n/ → [j] as /j/ is not [+consonantal] or [+nasal]. Ultimately, match data will be aggregated across segments by feature. For example, in the word "bunny rabbit" Amber matches [+consonantal] in 2 segments but fails to match this feature in 3 segments. Continuing with this process for every consonant in every word would allow us to calculate the proportion of matches to the total number of matches and mismatches per feature, yielding the feature-match ratio for each feature and place node. This analysis can be calculated separately for each syllable position and for singleton versus cluster consonants or it can be aggregated across all consonants in the sample.

Feature-match ratios are calculated by comparing the features associated with every target phoneme to the features associated with the phonemes produced by the child.

A complete feature-match ratio calculation can be accomplished by hand for each word contained in the sample, or as will be shown shortly, by using a more automated process such as an Excel workbook. In either case, the calculation process remains the same. Furthermore, efficiency is increased by working from the data in the Substitution Analysis Form rather than counting the feature matches word-by-word. Regardless of the method used for calculating the match ratios (i.e., hand tally or worksheet), you must decide which features to focus on for this analysis. You might restrict yourself to only those represented by radical underspecification principles or consider all the features in the fully specified feature matrix. We have created a spreadsheet that calculates the match ratios that correspond roughly to the Default Underspecified Feature Matrix presented in Table 1–2 for each of the consonants with a few divergences. We have allowed some additions to the default underspecified matrix so that we will notice if the child is failing to match some of the default features, which may be a sign that the child has idiosyncratic defaults. For example, although Coronal is the default place feature for adult English, we have decided to note when the child matches this place as shown by the checkmark indicating that the child matched Coronal when the word final /t/ was produced correctly in Figure 6–9. Not all children conform to the expected defaults; hearing-impaired children often have Labial as the default place and some children with DPD appear to use Dorsal as the default place. We therefore keep track of matches and mismatches for the Coronal place feature, with a very low match ratio for Coronal indicating that the child's place default may be Labial or Dorsal. Alternatively, low match ratios for the default place may indicate frequent appearance of spreading rules. Similarly, [−voiced] is the voicing default in adult English and is not specified in Table 1–2, but it is coded in the spreadsheet. Second, we do not code the phoneme /h/ as its status as a consonant or a glide is debated and not all children treat the phoneme in the same manner. For instance, Amber never produced a [+continuant] consonant in the onset position, but produced /h/ in this context and therefore seems to treat it like a glide. A possibility would be to code for /h/

Frequent mismatches for certain default features could be a sign that the child has **idiosyncratic defaults** or that there is an unusually high occurrence of spreading rules.

and modify its coded features depending on the child. Interpretation of the results of the feature-match ratio sheets must take into account the decisions you have made when coding feature matches. For instance, all sonorants are [+continuant] by default; if the child glides fricatives and produces /v/ → [j], you could decide to code a match for [+continuant] because [j] is [+continuant][+sonorant] or you could decide to not match [+continuant] because the child has failed to match the [+continuant][+consonantal] combination. In either case, the child's constraints regarding combinations of features must be taken into account in the final analysis.

Demonstration 6–3: Calculation of the Feature-Match Ratios for Case Study 6–2

Feature-match ratios for individual features and some combinations of features can be calculated using the completed Substitution Analysis Form and an electronic worksheet as shown in Demonstration 6–3. Our Excel Workbook contains a total of six worksheets: one each for singletons in the onset, ambisyllabic, and coda positions, one each for clusters in the onset and coda positions, and a worksheet in which the totals for each features are calculated. Each worksheet is a table consisting of 23 rows (1 for each consonant to be coded) plus an additional row at the top for the headings and three additional rows at the bottom for calculations. Two columns are provided for each of the features to be coded: consonantal, sonorant, nasal, continuant, voiced, voiceless, labial, round, coronal, grooved, anterior, and dorsal. The first column in each pair is for counting matches whereas the second is for counting mismatches. The three rows for calculations consist of the sum of matches, the sum of mismatches, and the number of matches divided by the total number of matches and mismatches to yield the proportion of matched features. The spreadsheet has been formatted so that only the cells in each row that correspond to the default underspecified features are unlocked; all other cells are locked and not open for the addition of data. In other words, in the row corresponding to the consonant target /t/, it is only possible to add match and mismatch data to the columns representing consonantal, voiceless, and coronal. All consonants except for /h/ are represented, and features for which match ratios are calculated for each consonant are indicated in yellow. A table, whether constructed in paper form or electronically, can be used to calculate match ratios via hand tally from the Substitution Analysis Form. For example, Table 6–6 indicates 6 correct productions of /n/ and therefore 6 should be entered into the match columns in the /n/ row for the cells corresponding to the features consonantal, nasal, and coronal. Demonstration 6–3 presents exact instructions on how to use our Workbook which accomplishes this task using an Excel form (and which is available from the authors); alternatively you can construct your own Workbook using other computer software.

Demonstration 6–3

1. Open the Excel document entitled *Nonlinear Analysis Workbook*. Notice that there are a total of six worksheets: one each for syllable onset singletons [*onset*], ambisyllabic singletons [*ambi*], syllable coda singletons [*coda*], complex onsets [*onsetcl*], and complex codas [*codacl*]. We generally ignore ambisyllabic clusters for this analysis, as it is complicated to decide which clusters the child treats as ambisyllabic clusters.

2. Use the completed Substitution Analysis Form rather than the language sample to fill out the Excel worksheets, which significantly reduces the amount of time required to calculate the feature match ratios.

3. If the **Form** button is not displayed in the Quick Access Toolbar at the top left of your screen, click the arrow next to the Quick Access Toolbar at the top left of your screen, and click on **More Commands**.

   The following pop-up menu will appear: select **All Commands**. In the list box, select the **Form** button, click **Add**, and then **Ok**.

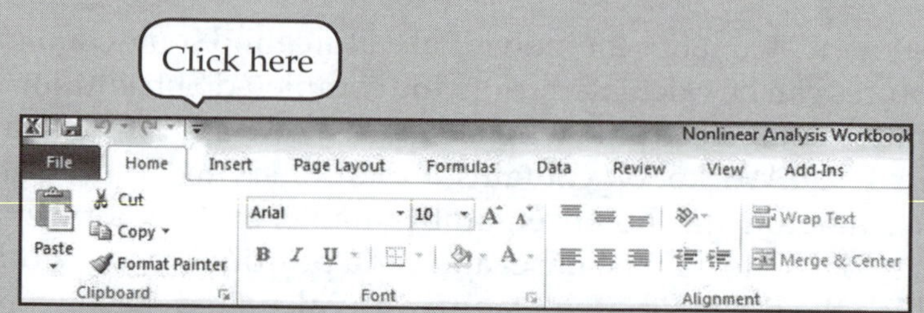

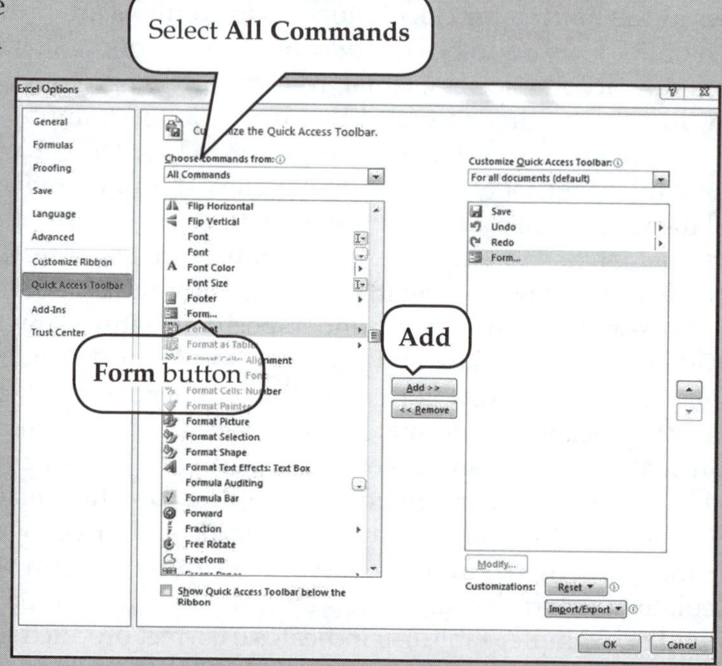

4. Begin with the first cell of the Substitution Analysis Form, that is, /m/ in syllable onset position.

	Syllable Onset	% √
m	✓ n(28)	50

5. Place your cursor in cell B13. Click on the **Form** button in the Quick Access Toolbar at the top left of your screen, then on **Ok**. A data form will pop up, as displayed in the figure. Notice that the form is labeled "m" at the top and that only the cells corresponding to the features defining /m/ are open.

   Notice that there are two cells for each feature, one labeled "m" for match and one labeled "mm" for mismatch.

6. Begin by coding the one correct production of /m/ by indicating "1" in the cells "cons m," "nasal m" and "labial m" as all three features were matched for this correct production.

onset
m
1 of 26
New
Delete
Restore
Find Prev
Find Next
Criteria
Close
cons m:
cons mm:
son m:
son mm:
nasal m:
nasal mm:
cont m:
cont mm:
vd m:
vd mm:
vless m:
vless mm:
labial m:
labial mm:
round m:
round mm:
coronal m:
coronal mm:
grovd m:
grovd mm:
antr m:
antr mm:
dorsal m:
dorsal mm:

7. The [n] substitution represents a match for consonantal and nasal, but a mismatch for labial. Change the value in the cells "cons m" and "nasal m" to "2" and indicate "1" for "labial mm."

8. Continue to code all the cells of the 'Syllable Onset' column of the Substitution Analysis Form. Notice at the top of the pop-up data menu that the sheet for "m" indicates 1 of 26; use the scroll-down menu to change the page until you see the appropriate label at the top of the form. If a cell contains no entries ("n/a" or "n/d,") do not enter values in the data form for this phoneme.

9. Select the worksheet labeled *ambi* and repeat the same steps for all the ambisyllabic consonants.

10. Select the worksheet labeled *coda* and repeat for all the final consonants.

11. Select the worksheet called *onsetcl* and code all of the consonants in this position. For example, Amber's production of syllable initial /l/ clusters is presented in the figure.

    We recommend coding all the consonants one at a time, alternating between the various corresponding pages of the data form. As you work your way down the cells, take care to not code the same cluster twice. For instance, for /l/ clusters the following would be coded in their corresponding data forms: matches for all the features associated with /b/ (twice); /g/ → [d] (twice); /k/ → [l] (twice); /s/ → [p] (once); and mismatches for all features associated with /l/ will be coded a total of seven times as shown in the figure.

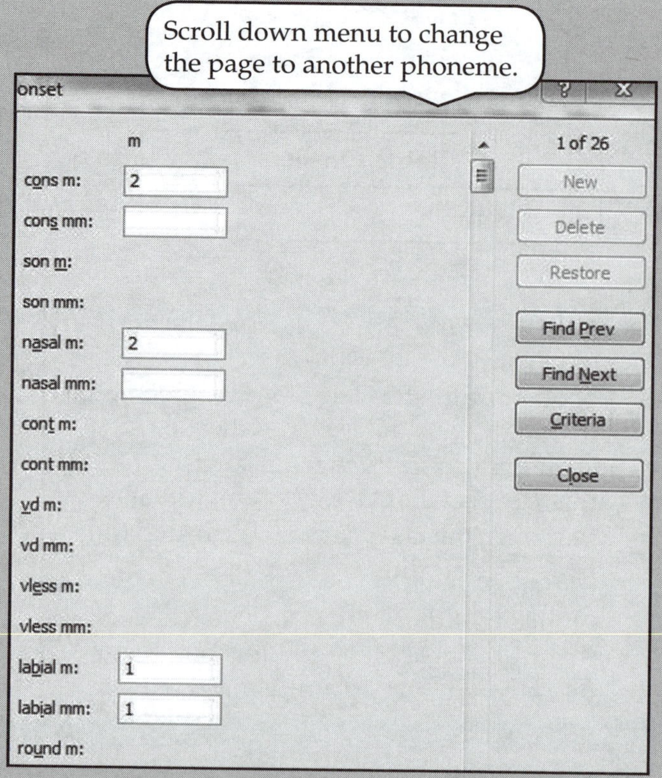

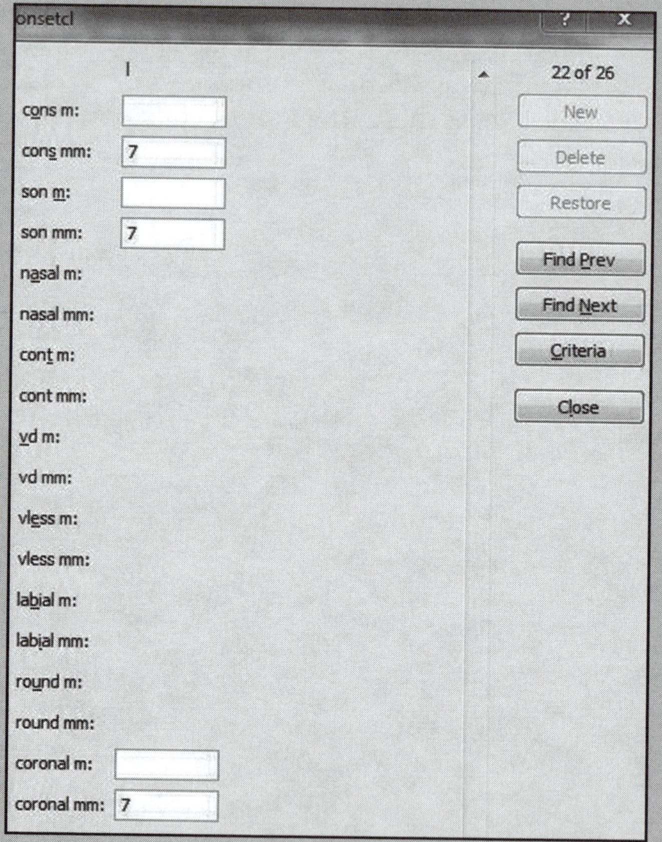

Scroll down menu to change the page to another phoneme.

onset

m

1 of 26

cons m: 2
cons mm:
son m:
son mm:
nasal m: 2
nasal mm:
cont m:
cont mm:
vd m:
vd mm:
vless m:
vless mm:
labial m: 1
labial mm: 1
round m:

New
Delete
Restore
Find Prev
Find Next
Criteria
Close

onsetcl

l

22 of 26

cons m:
cons mm: 7
son m:
son mm: 7
nasal m:
nasal mm:
cont m:
cont mm:
vd m:
vd mm:
vless m:
vless mm:
labial m:
labial mm:
round m:
round mm:
coronal m:
coronal mm: 7

New
Delete
Restore
Find Prev
Find Next
Criteria
Close

Therefore, when reaching the cell for initial /s/ cluster, /sl/ → [p-] would not be coded again because it was coded first when coding the /l/ clusters.

	Syllable Onset	% √
l	b-/bl[3,4] d-/gl[18,19] t-/kl[37,51] p-/sl[41]	0

12. Follow the same steps for all clusters on the form. For initial /s/ clusters, the final tally on the "onsetcl /s/" data form would be as represented in the figure. On two occasions Amber omitted the /s/ and therefore 2 mismatches would be coded for all the features associated with /s/. The four other substitutions she produced were /s/ → [p] (3 times) and /s/ → [t] (once). We thus would add: 4 matches for [+consonantal], 4 additional mismatches for [+continuant], 4 matches for [+voiceless], and 1 match and 3 additional mismatches for Coronal.

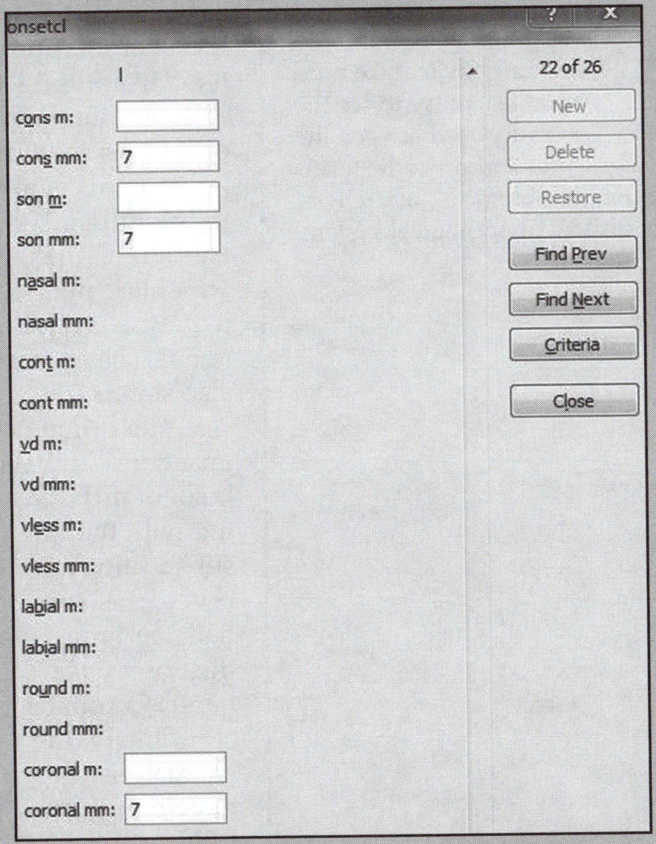

onsetcl

l

cons m:
cons mm: 7
son m:
son mm: 7
nasal m:
nasal mm:
cont m:
cont mm:
vd m:
vd mm:
vless m:
vless mm:
labial m:
labial mm:
round m:
round mm:
coronal m:
coronal mm: 7

22 of 26
New
Delete
Restore
Find Prev
Find Next
Criteria
Close

13. When you have finished coding all of the consonants, the final match ratios by feature will be shown in the sheet labeled *totals*.

14. The final match ratios by feature can be used to draw feature trees for each syllable position, as shown in Demonstration 6–4.

	Syllable Onset	% √
s	-t-/skɹ[39] p-/sl[41] p-/sm[42] t-/sn[43] -t-/skw[46] p-/st[47]	0

When the cells of the feature match worksheets have been filled out it will be possible to calculate the feature ratios, aggregated across all segments by word position (individually for singleton and cluster contexts if you wish). This information can be presented in numerical form or diagrams can be constructed for a visual representation of the child's use of features.

Demonstration 6–4: Feature Trees by Syllable Position

The feature ratios, aggregated across all segments by word position, can be represented visually by feature trees that make it easy to see the interactions between the segmental and prosodic levels of the phonological hierarchy in the child's phonological system.

Demonstration 6–4 illustrates the outcome of the feature-match ratio calculations in visual form; the feature-match trees make it easy to see the interactions between the segmental and prosodic levels of the phonological hierarchy in Amber's phonological system. Examining the singleton consonant contexts, it is immediately obvious that a large part of the system is established in the onset position. The feature [+consonantal] is fully established and [+sonorant] is also developing although it is not established due to the difficulty with the [+consonantal][+sonorant] combination. Nasal is also established as is the voiced/voiceless distinction. The only place node that is established is Labial with Dorsal being completely absent and mismatches for Coronal being unusually frequent. The absence of the [+consonantal][+continuant] combination also stands out in the onset position.

The difference between the feature trees when comparing the onset and ambisyllabic positions is striking. In ambisyllabic it is [+sonorant] that is established whereas [+consonantal] is developing with the low match ratio reflecting the high frequency of glide substitutions in this context. Nasal is completely absent. Although [−voice] is consistently matched, [+voice] is only matched about half the time. In stark contrast to the absence of [+continuant] in the onset position, this feature is developing in ambisyllabic consonants. Coronal is established but Labial is only emerging.

Finally, the feature tree for the coda position reveals unique characteristics again, with Nasal, [+voice], Labial and Coronal only developing but [+consonantal], [−voice], and [+continuant] are fully established.

A quick scan of Amber's cluster productions reveals that a feature-match analysis would not yield any new information. Most mismatches involve delinking of a complete segment from the skeletal tier. Some mismatches reflect absent features that have already been noted in the analysis of the singleton consonants, that is, complete absence of Dorsal, delinking of [+continuant] from obstruents in the onset position and the constraint against the [+consonantal][+sonorant] combination. Therefore, the feature-match analysis for complex onsets and codas was not strictly necessary although it is provided in Demonstration 6–4 for completeness.

Demonstration 6–4

When the final match ratios have been calculated in the excel workbook, they can be used to draw feature trees for each syllable position. Features or nodes that are never matched should not appear on the tree, indicating features that are *absent* from the child's productive output and probably from the underlying representations as well. If the match ratio is between 2 and 20 percent, include the node/feature with a dotted line, highlighting *emerging* features that are the most likely treatment targets. Use a dashed line for nodes/features that are matched between 21 and 80 percent of the time to indicate features that are *developing*. Use a solid line to include nodes/features that are matched with greater than 80% frequency to identify *established* features that would normally be excluded as possible treatment targets. (These cutoff points are somewhat arbitrary and could be adjusted in some cases.)

In Amber's case, the percentages for matching the features in the onset position were:

cons	son	nasal	cont	voiced	vless	labial	round	coronal	grvd	antr	dorsal
93%	50%	100%	0	82%	91%	89%	100%	78%	n/d	0	0

In the Onset position, the feature tree therefore would be:

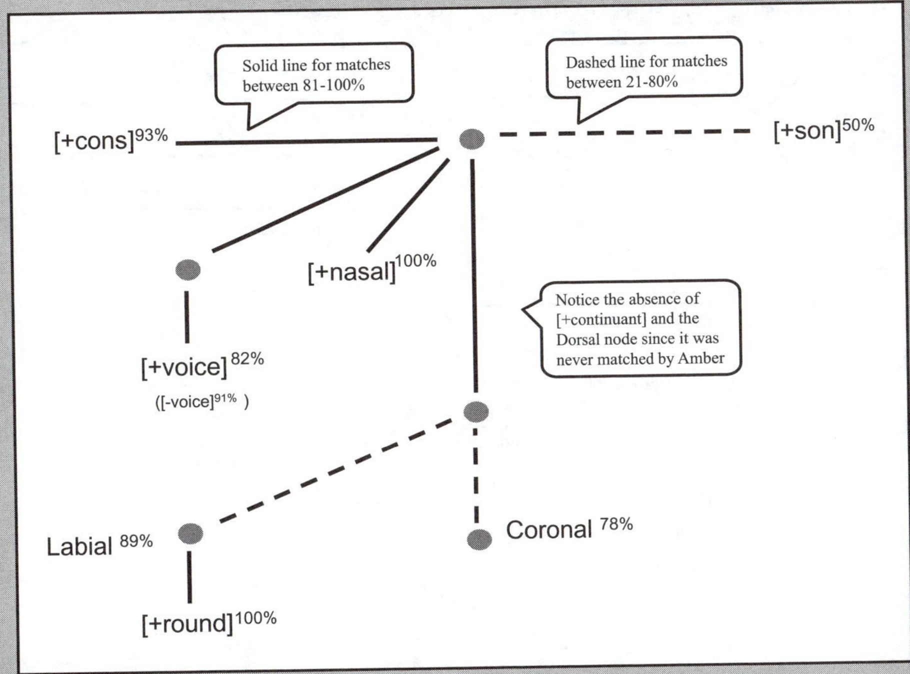

For ambisyllabic singletons, the match ratios and the feature tree for Amber are:

cons	son	nasal	cont	voiced	vless	labial	round	coronal	grvd	antr	dorsal
44%	100%	0	88%	67%	100%	22%	50%	93%	0	0	0

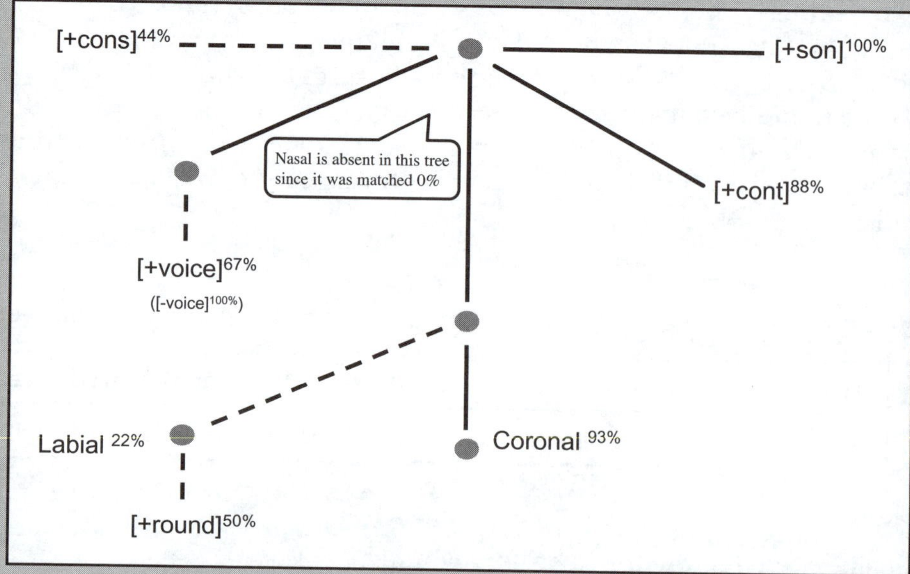

For singletons in the coda position, the match ratios and the feature tree for Amber are:

cons	son	nasal	cont	voiced	vless	labial	round	coronal	grvd	antr	dorsal
81%	0	80%	100%	50%	100%	71%	0	62%	0	0	0

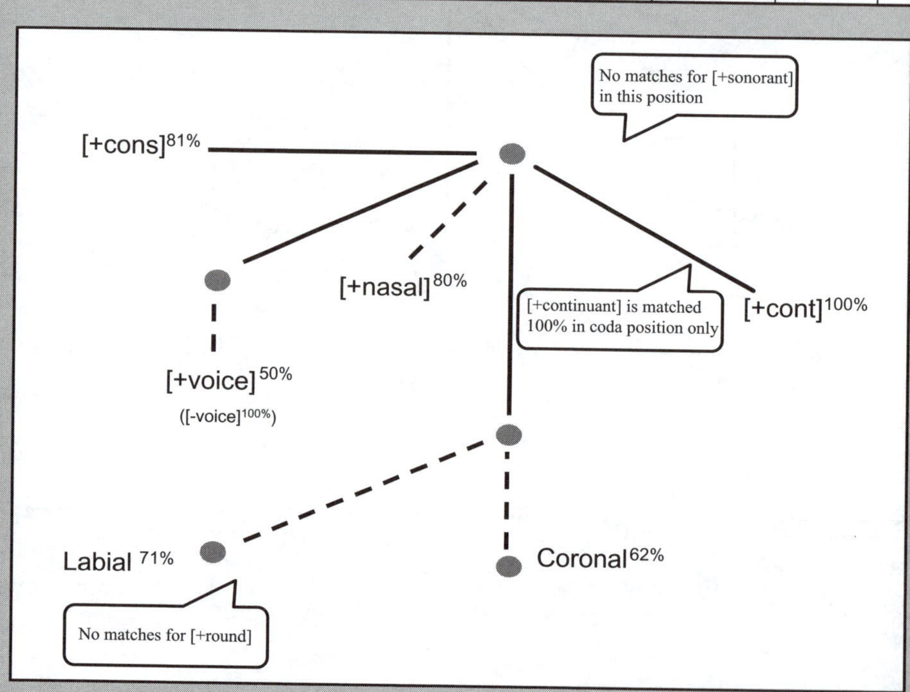

For complex onsets, the match ratios and the feature tree for Amber are:

cons	son	nasal	cont	voiced	vless	labial	round	coronal	grvd	antr	dorsal
41%	0	0	0	100%	73%	0%	0	14%	n/d	0	0

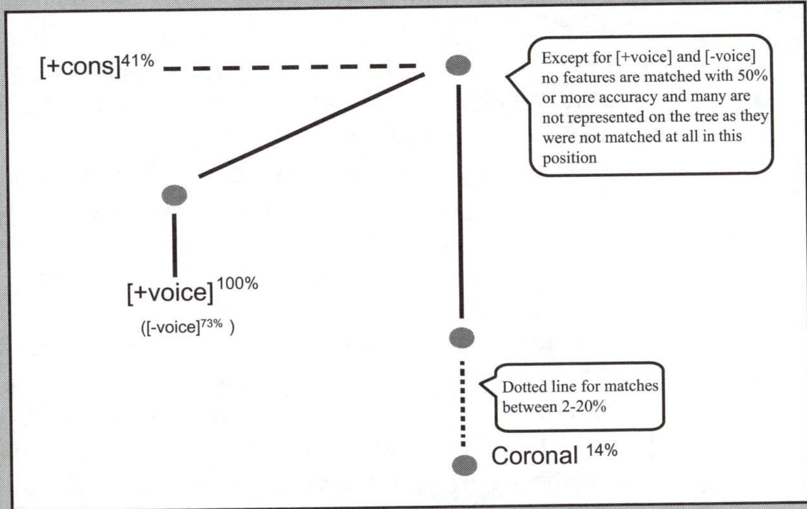

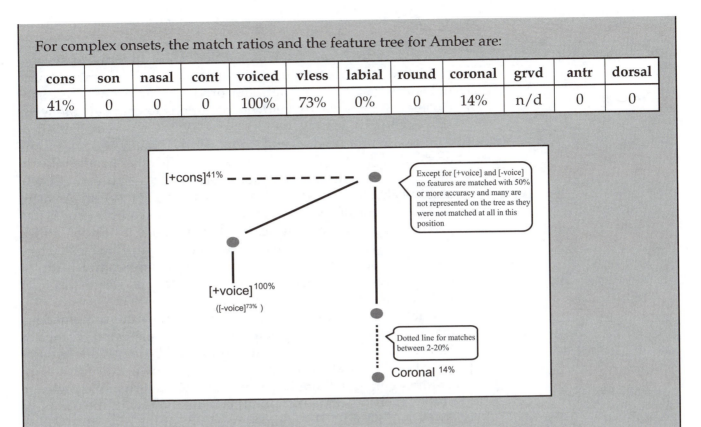

For complex codas, the match ratios and the feature tree for Amber are:

cons	son	nasal	cont	voiced	vless	labial	round	coronal	grvd	antr	dorsal
67%	0	0	100%	0	100%	50%	n/d	75%	n/d	n/d	n/d

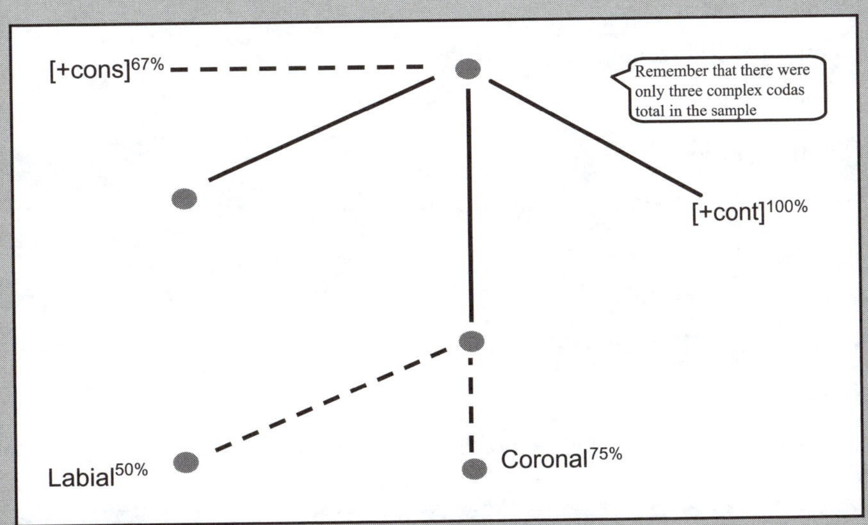

Multilinear Interpretation and Analysis for Case Study 6–2

Amber is a girl, aged 4;8, with a severe DPD. In terms of syllable and word shapes, strengths have been identified in Amber's phonological system. Although she produced only one consonant cluster, which is clearly below expectations for her age, the word shapes CV(V), CVC, CV(V)CV(V), and CVCVC are well established. Amber also produced several longer word structures on at least one occasion each. Her phonetic inventory, on the other hand, is clearly restricted in all singleton positions: onset ([p, b, t, d, (m), n, (h), w]); ambisyllabic ([t, s, j, w]), and coda ([p, t, (m), n, f, (v), s]). As mentioned previously, Amber produced only one complex coda, [ts], and no complex onsets. The feature trees by syllable position drawn from the final feature-match ratios are a very compelling visual representation of Amber's system. The findings of the complete multilinear analysis (syllable/word shape inventory and segmental and feature analyses) are presented in Table 6–7.

Table 6–7 begins with the features and feature combinations that are absent from her system. Dorsal never appeared in stops or nasals and although perception testing would confirm our hypothesis, it is likely that she has no underlying knowledge of this place feature. Similarly, there is no evidence of underlying knowledge of the [+consonantal][+sonorant] combination, with the complete absence of liquids. The complete absence of interdental fricatives

Table 6–7. *Summary of Multilinear Analysis for Case Study 6–2*

Structures Absent from the Underlying Representation
Dorsal
[+consonantal] [+sonorant]
[−grooved]
Delinking Rules
[+continuant] from obstruents in the onset position
[+voice] in [+continuant] codas
[+consonantal] in ambisyllabic voiced nasal and obstruent consonants
Second consonant in complex onsets, complex codas, and ambisyllabic clusters
Spreading Rule
Inconsistent spreading of Labial to syllable initial consonants that are unspecified for place
Resyllabification
Inconsistent resyllabification of /m/ → [mə] and /n/ → [nə] in the coda position

indicates that there is no distinction between [–grooved] and [+grooved] fricatives.

Moving to delinking rules, it is clear from an examination of the feature trees that [+continuant] is delinked in the onset (from obstruent targets) because it is matched consistently in the coda. Delinking of [+voice] from obstruents in the coda position is also fairly straightforward, for example, "glasses" → [dæsəs]. The more complex pattern to discern is the delinking of [+consonantal] from ambisyllabic voiced consonants, yielding a glide substitution; this rule also applies to nasals that are voiced by default. This pattern revealed itself by the high frequency of glide substitutions apparent on the substitution form; the high match ratio for [+sonorant] combined with the low match ratios for [+nasal] and [+voice] on the ambisyllabic feature tree confirmed the pattern.

The decision to code the cluster reduction errors as delinking of a segment from within the complex coda or complex onset (as opposed to a constraint against these structures in the underlying representation) stems from two observations. First, there is a single example of a complex coda in the sample. Second, and more compelling, coalescence errors occur within complex onsets (e.g., "smoke" → [pot]) providing clear evidence that Amber represented the features of both segments within the onset.

Coalescence, as described in Chapter 1, involves spreading of features between segments. Spreading occurs quite frequently in Amber's sample and accounts for many of the more unusual production patterns. These instances of spreading serve to preserve Amber's preference for Labial in word onsets and Coronal in later word positions. For example, in the word "zipper," Labial is spread from the /p/ in the ambisyllabic position to the unspecified place node of the consonant in the onset, yielding [pɪte] after delinking of [+continuant] and [Labial] from the ambisyllabic segment.

Coalescence, as described in Chapter 1, involves spreading of features between segments.

Amber's production of the sampled words can at times be explained by one of the absent structures or delinking and spreading rules summarized in Table 6–7. However, more often than not a combination of these rules explains her production of target words. For instance, the combined absence of [+consonantal] [+sonorant] and Dorsal from the underlying representation explain "looking" → [nʊtɪn]; in this particular case Amber's underlying representation and her productive output are identical (Figure 6–10). As shown in Figure 6–11, a total of four operations explain "candle" → [taije]: (1) Dorsal is absent from the UR and therefore the consonant in the onset position is both represented as /t/ and produced as [t]; (2) delinking of the second consonant in nasal clusters explains the omission of [d]; (3) the remaining first consonant of the cluster is treated as an ambisyllabic nasal consonant and [+consonantal] is delinked, resulting in /n/ → [j]; and (4) the combination of [+consonantal] [+sonorant] is absent from the representation and therefore the syllabic /l/ is represented as a vowel. Similarly, a total of four

Inaccurate production of words by children with DPD at times can be explained by one of their absent structures or delinking and spreading rules. However, frequently a combination of these rules explains their productions.

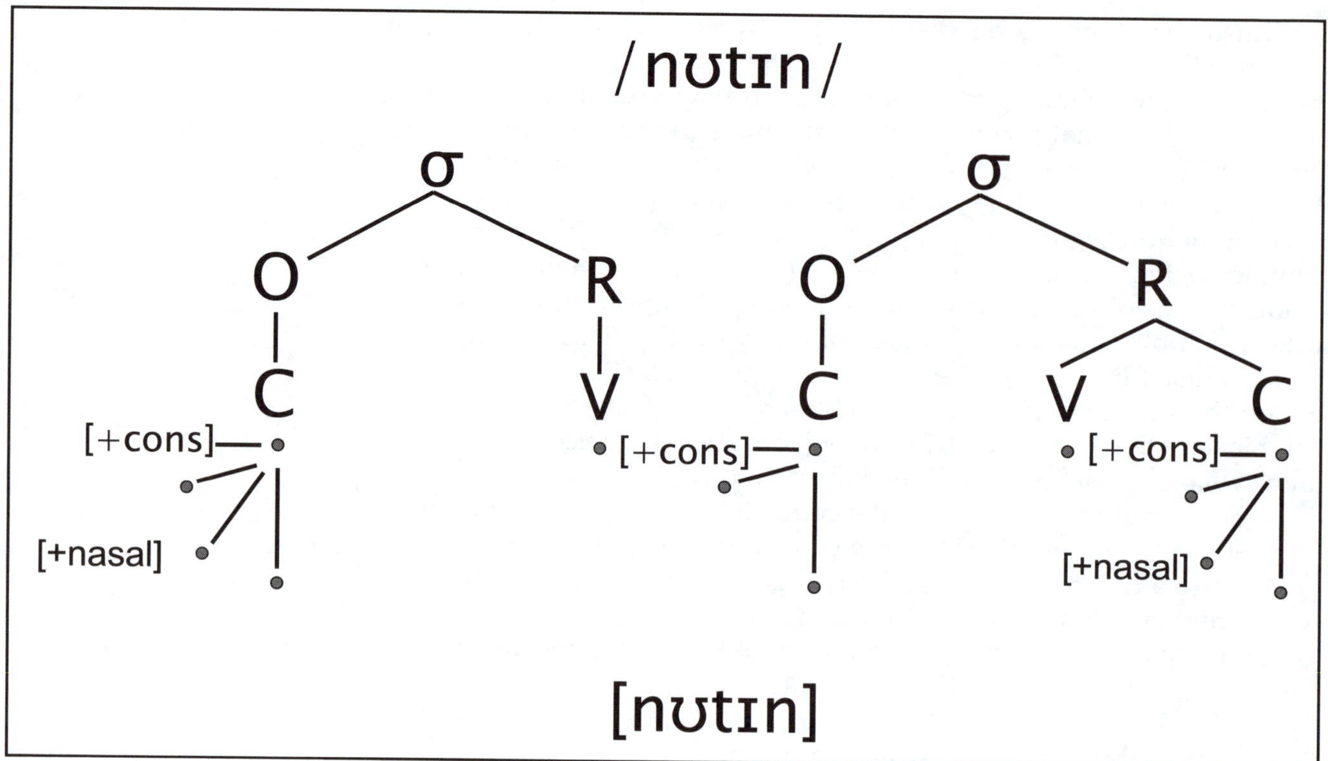

Figure 6–10. *Feature tree for Amber's production of "looking." The combination of [+consonantal] [+sonorant] and Dorsal being absent from her underlying representation explain her production of this word.*

rules explain "stove" → [pos] as shown in Figure 6–12: (1) the second consonant of the complex onset is delinked; (2) [+continuant] is delinked from the remaining singleton /s/ in the onset position; (3) Labial spreads from the /v/ to the onset which was not specified for place and (4) [+voice] is delinked from the coda. Other complex productions in Amber's sample can be explained with combinations of delinking and spreading rules in this fashion. We invite the reader to explain her production of the word "pajama," for example.

Phonetic and Phonotactic Assessment

Young children with immature phonological systems often demonstrate difficulties with both **phonetic and phonotactic components of speech**.

The multilinear analysis provides an in-depth description of underlying representations at the various units of the phonological hierarchy of the child's phonological system. However, a language sample of approximately 100 to 150 words is recommended to complete a multilinear assessment. For very young children or children with developmental delays and disorders who are almost nonverbal or have a small expressive vocabulary, completing a multilinear analysis is not yet possible. The main advantage of multilinear phonology is that the strengths and weaknesses of the child's at the phrase, word, syllable structure, segment, feature, and associations between tiers are examined. Children with phonological delays or disorders,

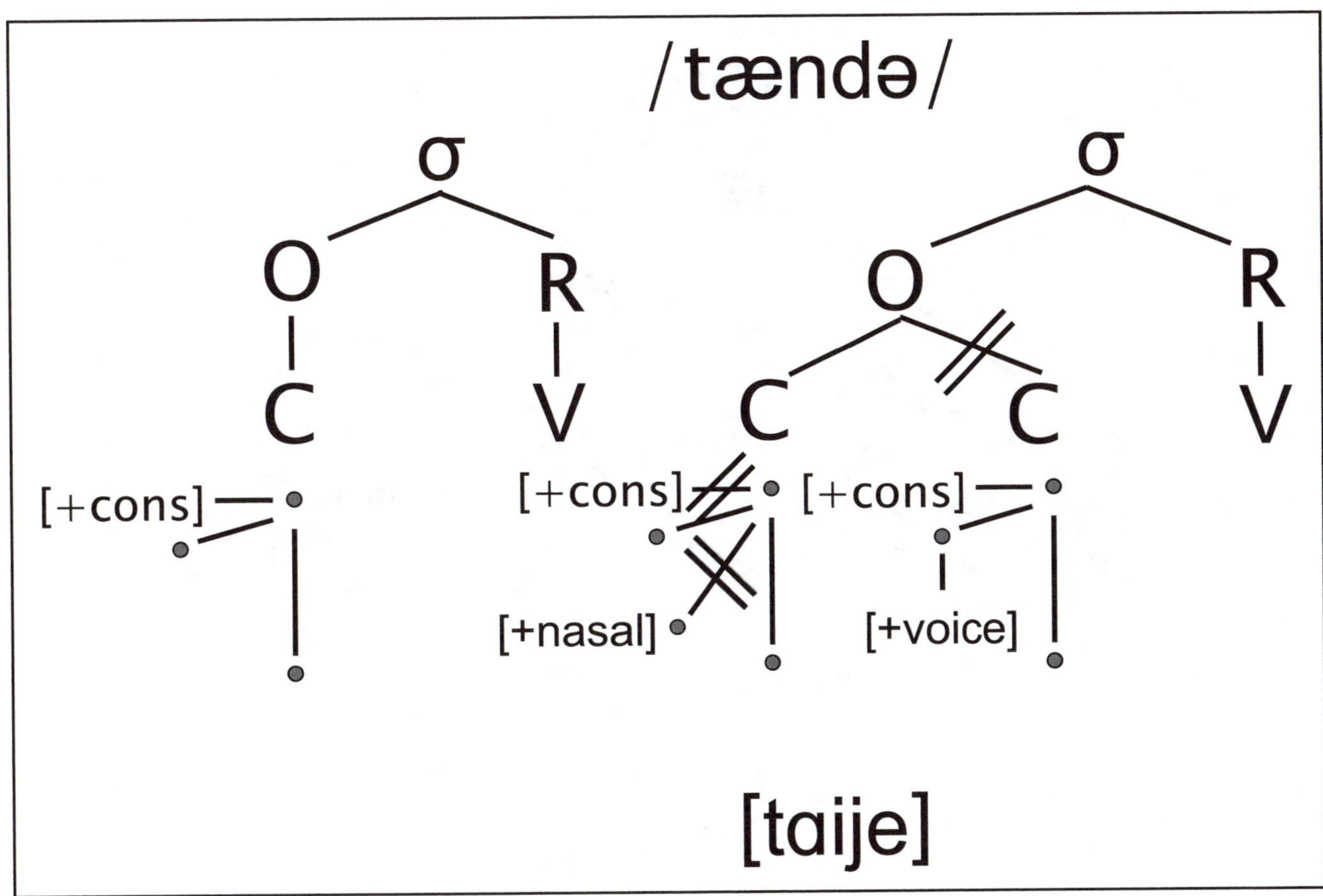

Figure 6–11. *Feature tree for Amber's production of "candle," explained by a total of four operations: (1) the consonant in the onset position is both represented as /t/ and produced as [t] since Dorsal is absent from the UR; (2) [d] is omitted due to delinking of the second consonant in nasal clusters; (3) the remaining first consonant of the cluster is treated as an ambisyllabic nasal consonant and [+consonantal] is delinked, resulting in /n/ → [j]; and (4) the syllabic /l/ is represented as a vowel as the combination of [+consonantal] [+sonorant] is absent from the UR.*

including young children with immature phonological systems, often demonstrate difficulties with both phonetic and phonotactic components of speech, the latter referring to the frame of the words, or in other words the syllable/word shape and the sequencing of the speech sounds within the word (Velleman, 2002). For children with limited speech output, information should be obtained at both the phonetic and phonotactic levels. A phonetic inventory and a phonotactic assessment including syllable/word shape inventory, phonotactic constraints, and, when possible, syllable stress inventory and constraints can be completed: children cannot be too young or not have enough phonological development yet for these analyses. In turn, the results of these analyses can be used to select their initial treatment goals. Carefully choosing the treatment goals and specific stimuli for these children can make a significant difference in the amount and rate of progress they will make. As reviewed in Chapter 4, young children often expand their expressive vocabulary by

Phonotactic components of speech refer to the frame of the words, or in other words the syllable/word shape and the sequencing of the speech sounds within the word.

Children cannot be too young nor have enough phonological development to complete a phonetic inventory and a **phonotactic assessment** including syllable/word shape inventory, phonotactic constraints, and, when possible syllable, stress inventory and constraints.

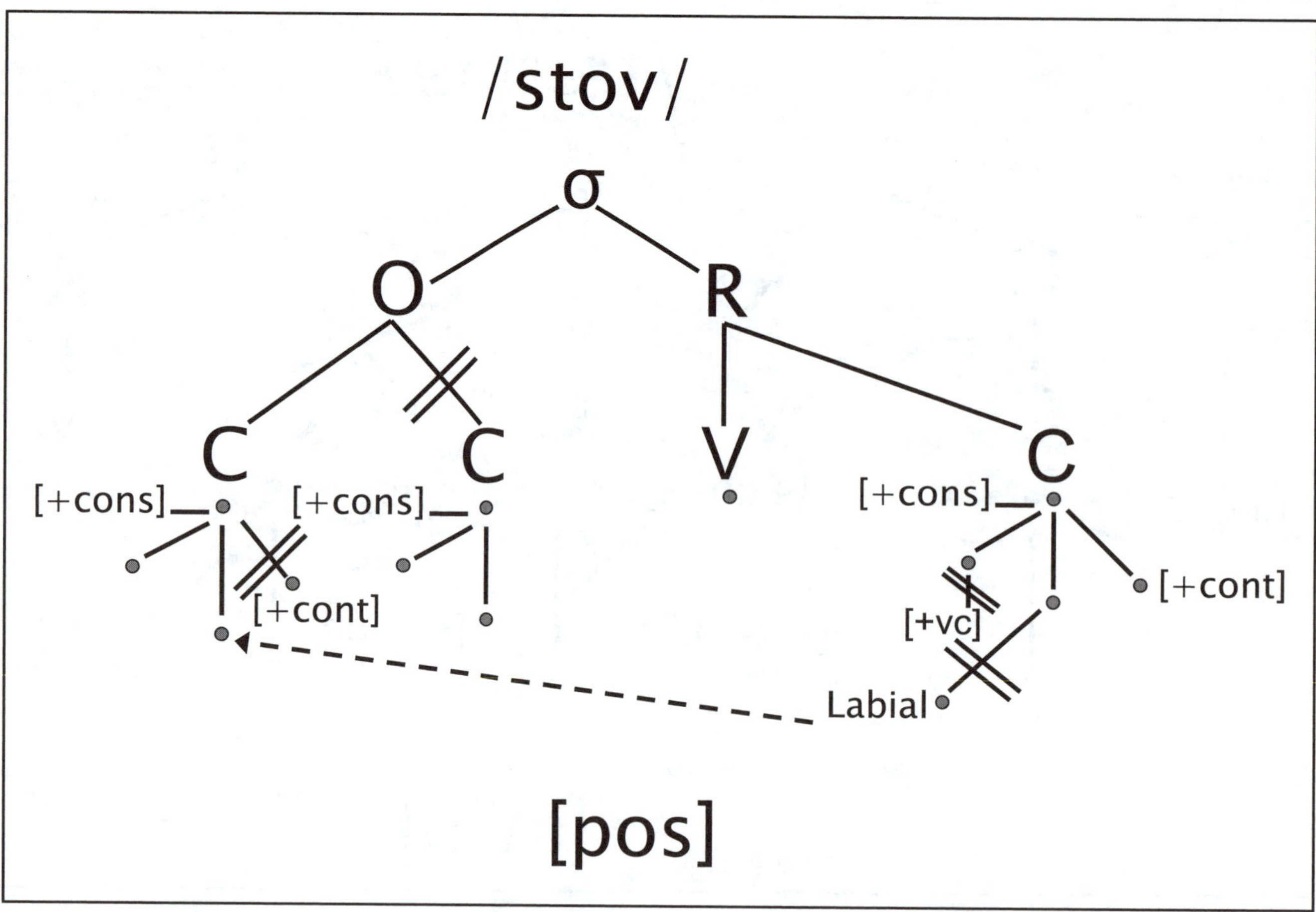

Figure 6–12. *Feature tree for Amber's production of "stove," explained by a total of four rules: (1) the second consonant of the complex onset is delinked; (2) [+continuant] is delinked from the remaining singleton /s/ in the onset position; (3) Labial spreads from the /v/ to the onset which was not specified for place; and (4) [+voice] is delinked from the coda.*

adding new items within preferred templates and the SLP can take advantage of this principle when selecting early treatment goals; eventually, the child can be encouraged to expand the repertoire of phonetic and phonotactic structures providing new opportunities for productive output as described further in Part III. We demonstrate how to complete the phonetic and phonotactic assessment with Case Study 6–3, which presents the entire expressive vocabulary of a 22-month-old girl.

The phonetic inventory identifies phones that are absent from and those that are present in the child's repertoire. Subsequently, this information can be used to carefully select target words such that strengths will be used to support weaknesses.

The phonetic inventory identifies phones that are absent from and those that are present in the child's repertoire (Table 6–8). Subsequently, this information can be used to carefully select target words such that strengths will be used to support weaknesses. Although the focus here is on how to analyze the speech sample to select treatment targets, the assessment should also lead to a hypothesis regarding the underlying nature of the DPD. There are

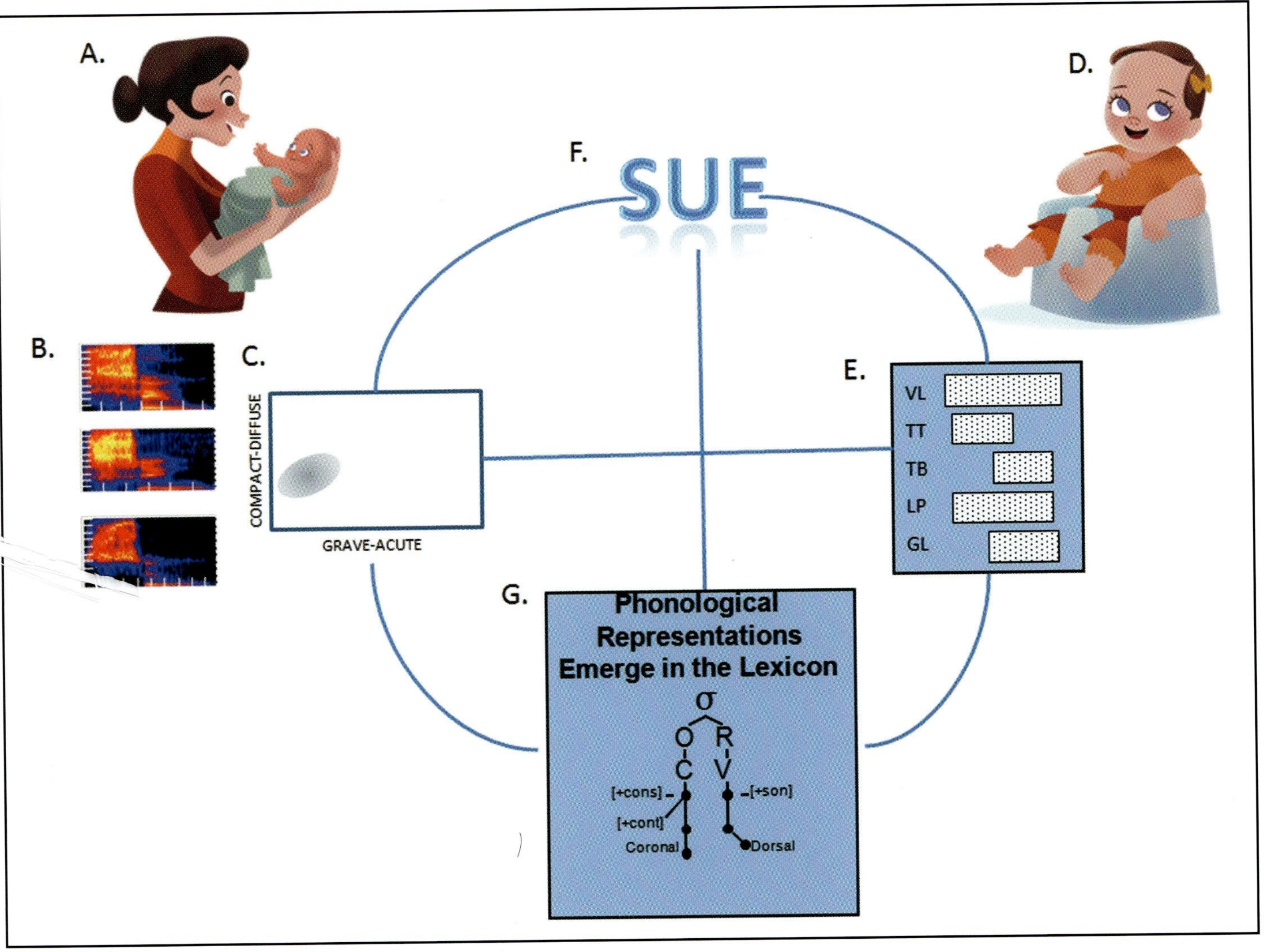

Plate 1. *Schematic of the emergence of phonological representations from the child's experience with language at multiple levels of representation:* (**A**) *language input;* (**B**) *stored acoustic exemplars, in this hypothetical example, the child's name as produced by the mother, the father and an older sibling;* (**C**) *acoustic-phonetic representations of linguistic units, in this example the vowel* [u] *derived from the distribution of F1-F2 values in the grave corner of the vowel space;* (**D**) *the child's experience with speech in the form of babbled syllables,* (**E**) *a gestural score for a CV syllable comprised of a coronal sibilant combined with a rounded grave vowel;* (**F**) *the semantic representation for "Sue" stored in the lexicon; and* (**G**) *an emergent phonological representation for the word that reflects the child's experience with the phonetic characteristics of the word, the linkages between the representations of the word in multiple domains and the similarities and differences between this word and others in the lexicon at multiple levels of the phonological hierarchy. The concepts and processes are elaborated throughout the first four chapters of this book* (Part I).

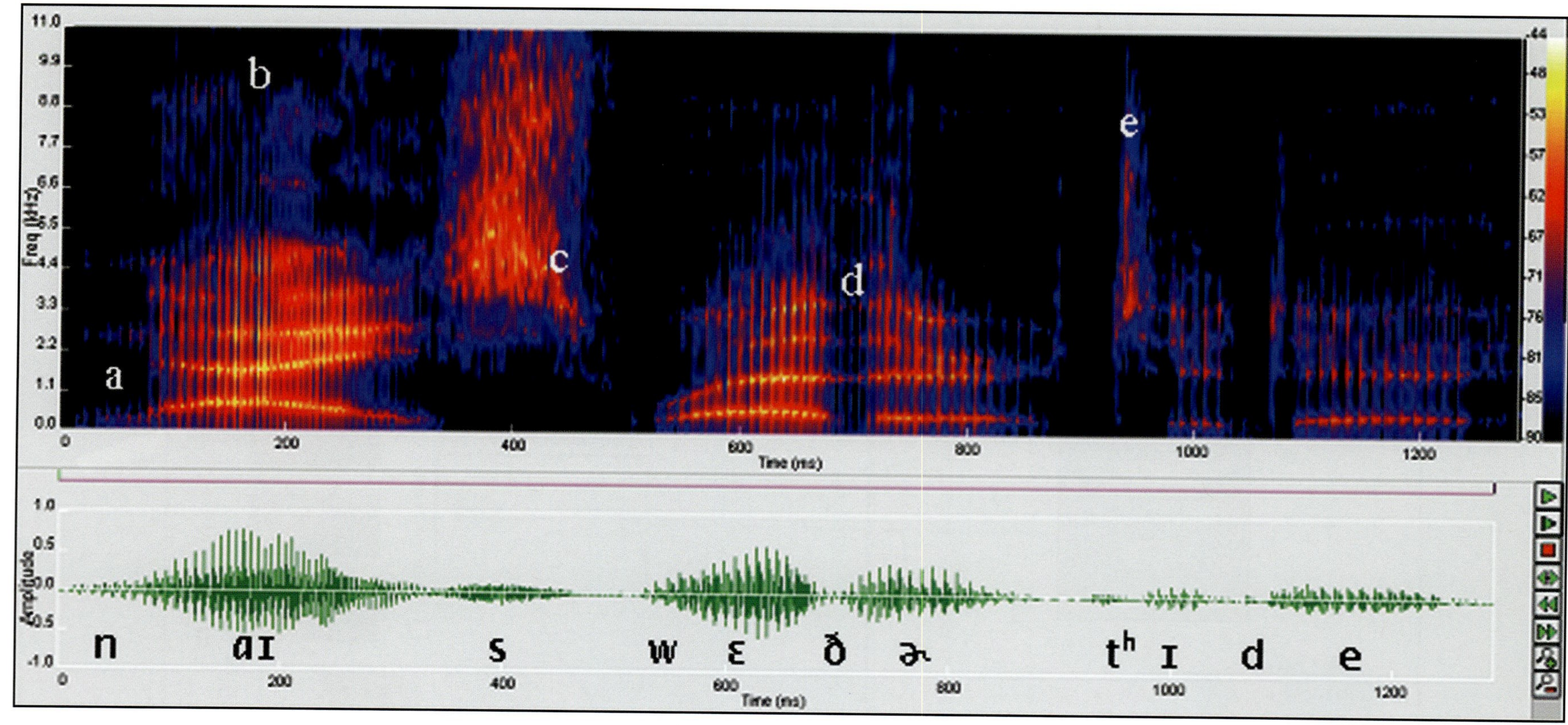

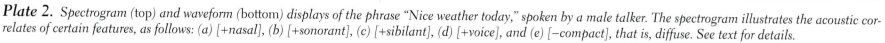

Plate 2. *Spectrogram* (top) *and waveform* (bottom) *displays of the phrase "Nice weather today," spoken by a male talker. The spectrogram illustrates the acoustic correlates of certain features, as follows: (a) [+nasal], (b) [+sonorant], (c) [+sibilant], (d) [+voice], and (e) [−compact], that is, diffuse. See text for details.*

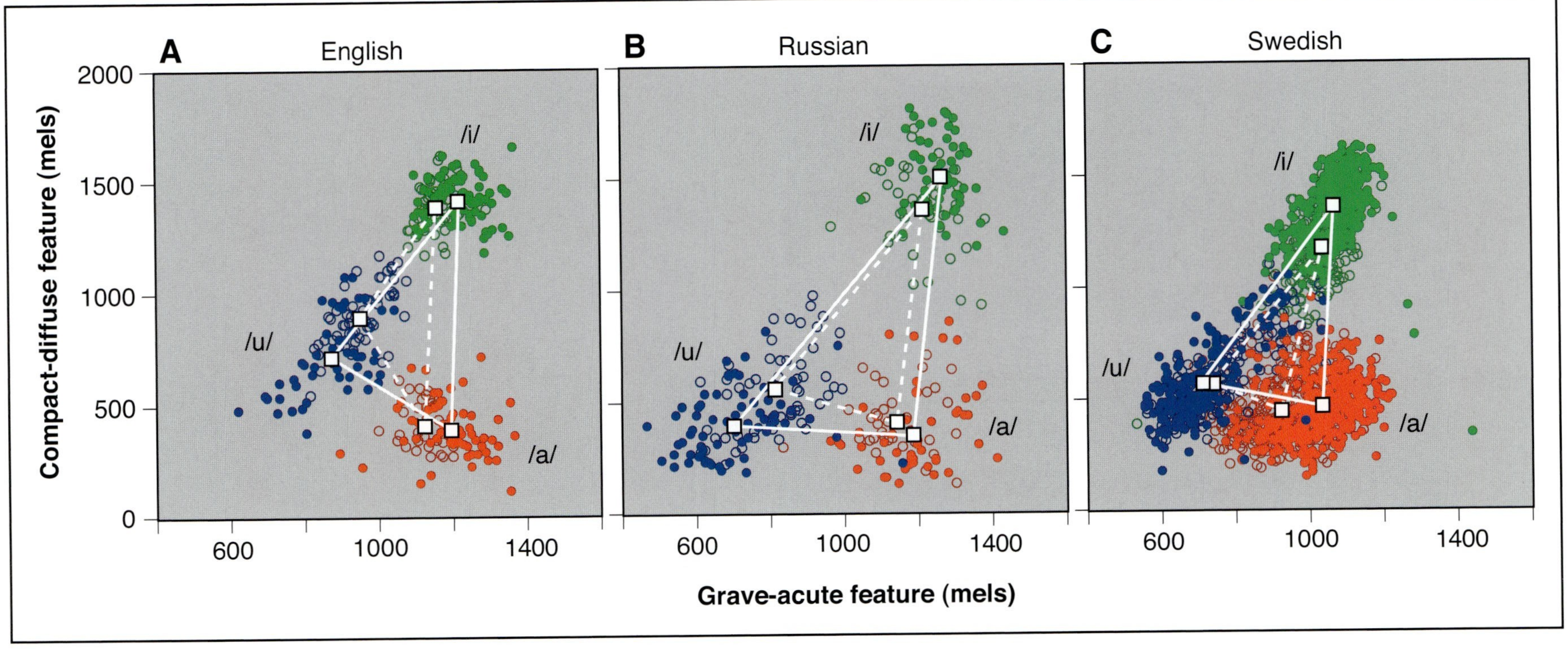

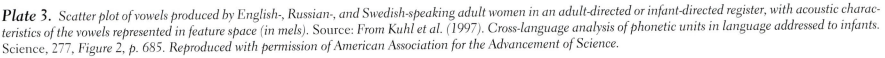

Plate 3. *Scatter plot of vowels produced by English-, Russian-, and Swedish-speaking adult women in an adult-directed or infant-directed register, with acoustic characteristics of the vowels represented in feature space (in mels).* Source: *From Kuhl et al. (1997). Cross-language analysis of phonetic units in language addressed to infants.* Science, 277, *Figure 2, p. 685. Reproduced with permission of American Association for the Advancement of Science.*

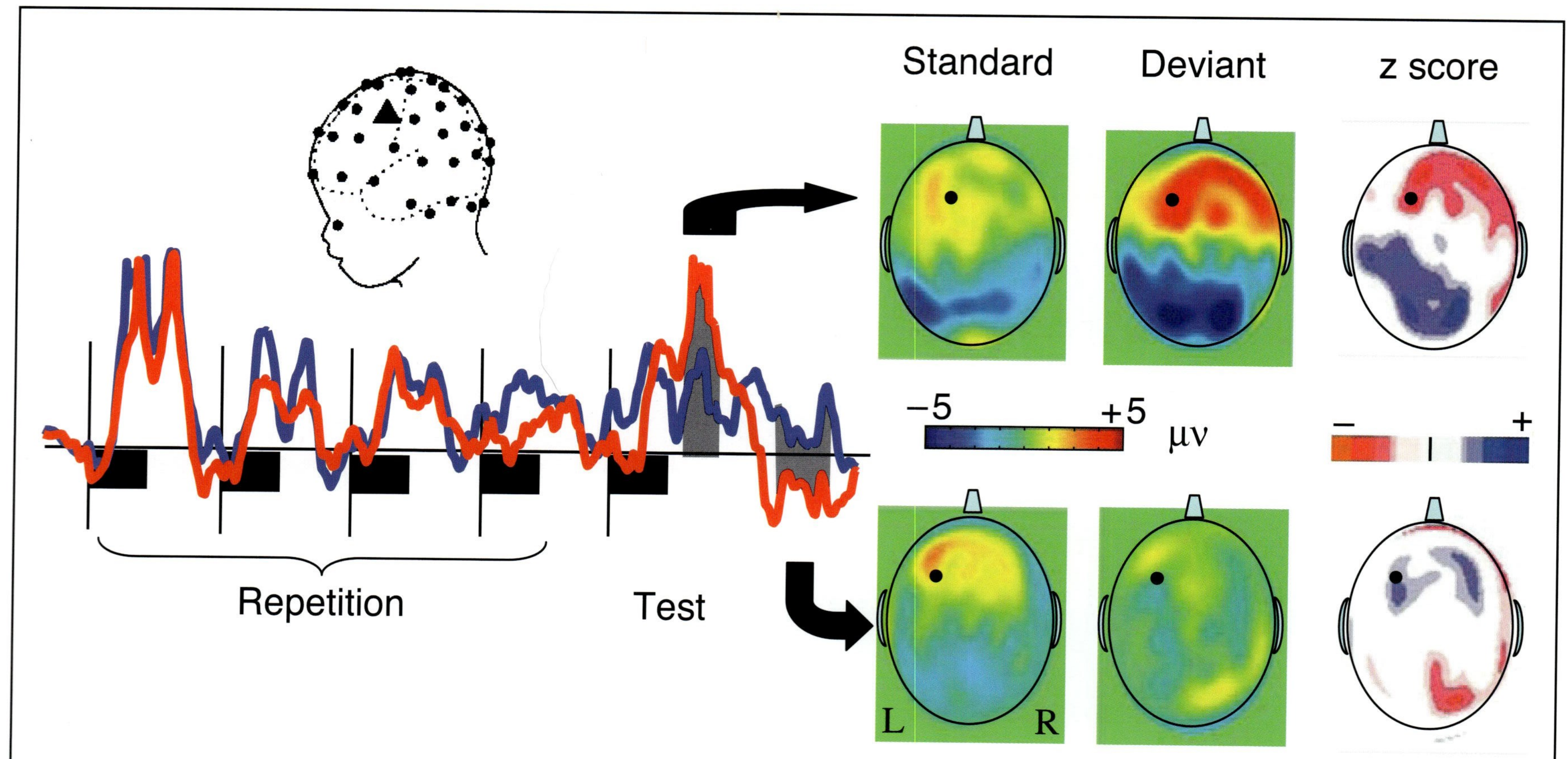

Plate 4. *Grand average recorded from a left frontal electrode in 16 3-month-old infants during an entire trial for the standard* (blue line) *and deviant condition* (red line). *Mismatch responses are marked with gray bars at approximately 400 ms (originating from the temporal lobes) and 600 ms (originating over the frontal areas) after the test stimulus.* Source: *From Dehaene-Lambertz and Gliga (Copyright 2004). Common neural basis for phoneme processing in infants and adults.* Journal of Cognitive Neuroscience *by Cognitive Neuroscience Institute (Norwich, Vt.), 16(8), Figure 2, p. 1379. Reproduced with permission of MIT Press—Journals.*

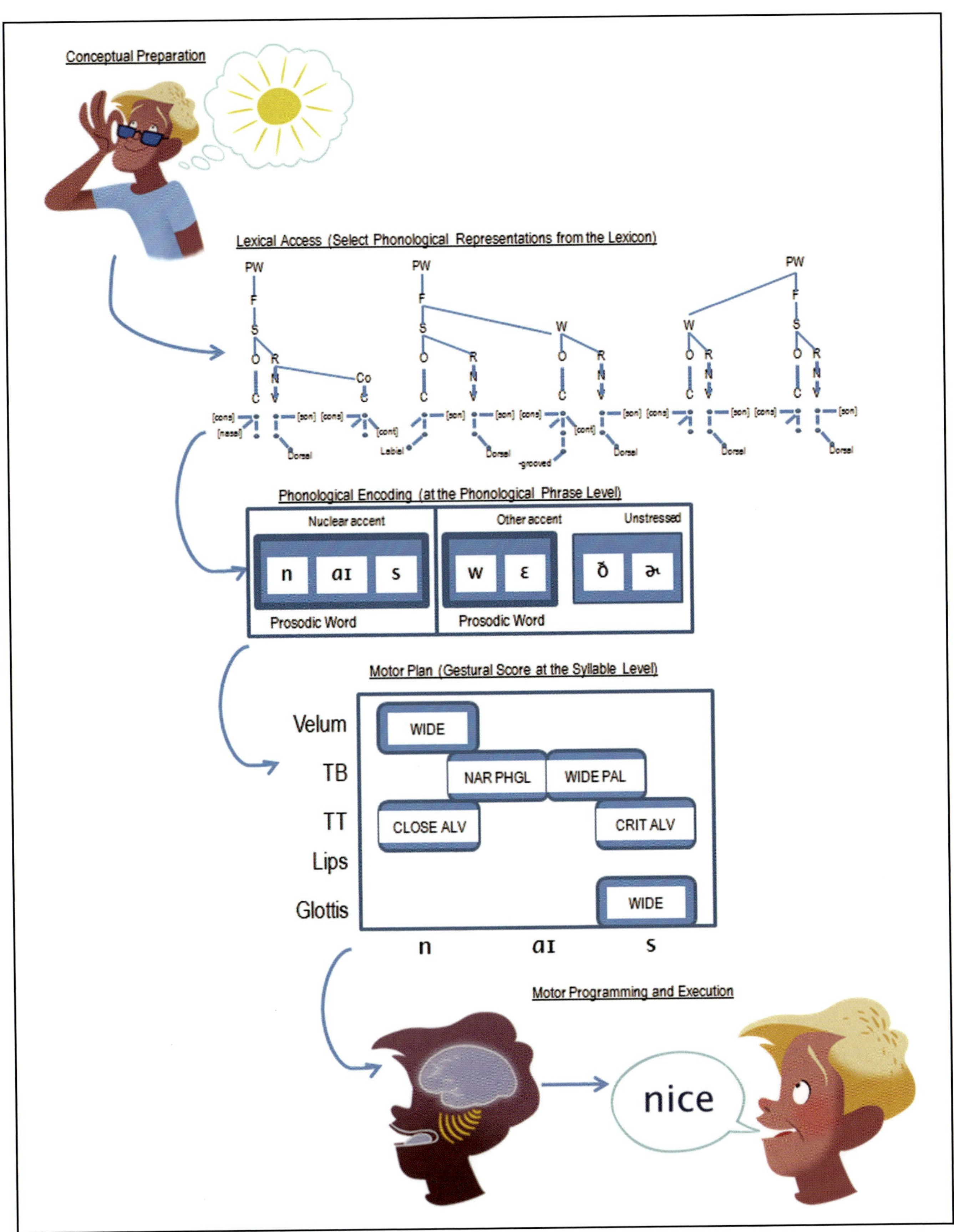

Plate 5. *Graphical representation of a highly simplified psycholinguistic model of the speech production process (see text for details).*

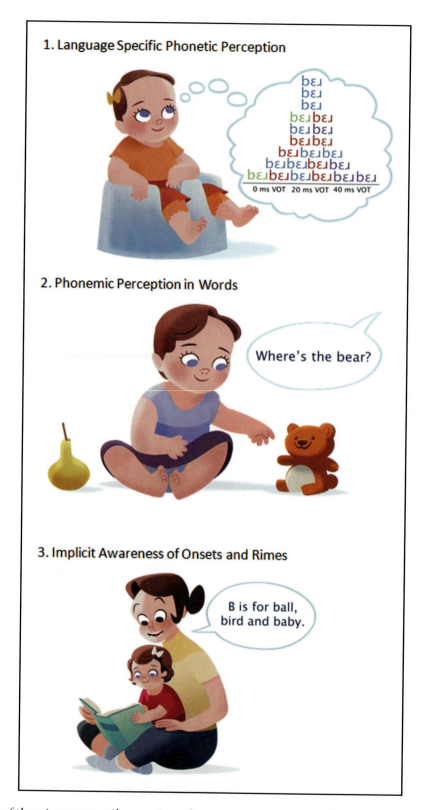

Plate 6. *Illustration of three important milestones in early speech perception and phonological processing skills (see Chapter 2 for details). 1. During the first year of life, the infant shifts from language general to language-specific processing of phonetic categories that are abstracted from exemplars in the input using statistical learning mechanisms. 2. During the second year of life the toddler learns to use phonetic categories to acquire and differentiate meaningful words leading to the emergence of perceptual knowledge of phonemic contrasts. 3. During the third year the child demonstrates implicit phonological awareness in the form of a beginning awareness of similarities among words based on shared onsets or rimes.*

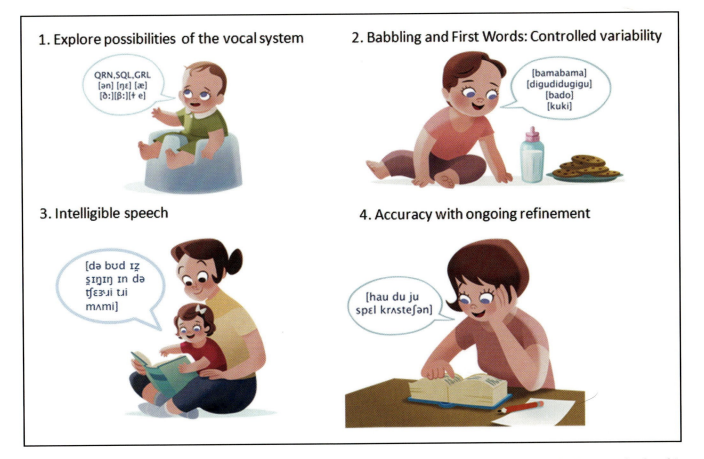

Plate 7. *Illustration of important milestones in the achievement of speech motor control (see text and Chapter 3 for details). 1. Expansion stage—explore possibilities of the vocal system including variations in pitch, loudness, resonance, and different places of vocal tract closure; production of fully resonant vowels and marginal babble. 2. Integrative stage—integration of lip, tongue, velar, and laryngeal movements into an increasingly stable jaw trajectory for the production of syllable sequences that include a range of place and manner classes in babbling, jargon, and early words. 3. Intelligible speech—differentiation of early speech templates to accurately produce the full range of segments in the target language. 4. Refinements in accuracy and precision—achievement of adultlike minima in variability for phonetic accuracy, fundamental frequency, vowel formants, and other speech parameters.*

1. Word-based phonology, followed by emerging phonological structure

2. Successive reorganizations of phonological structure in the lexicon contribute to speech accuracy and increasingly complex language use

3. Metaphonological ability permits acquisition of literacy skills

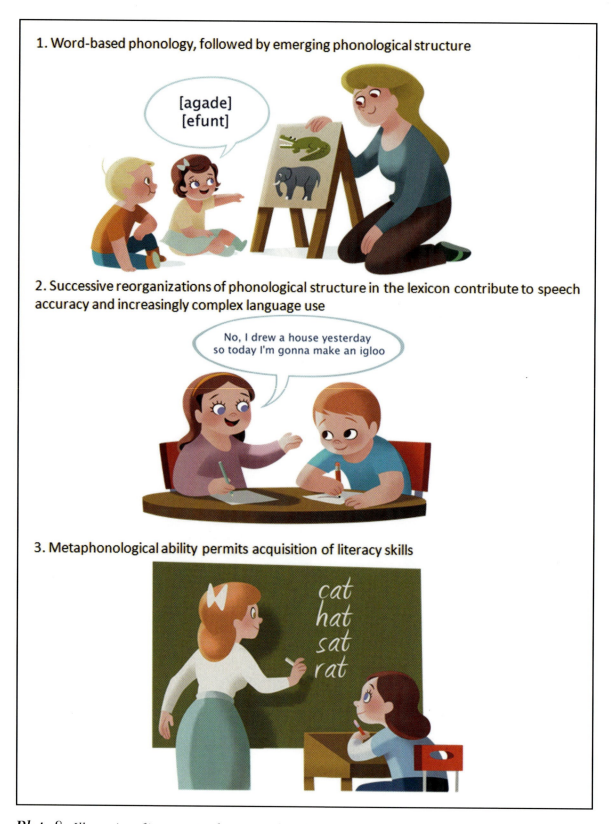

Plate 8. *Illustration of important milestones in the achievement of phonological knowledge. (1) A word based phonology is gradually superseded by emerging phonological structure leading to increasingly predictable patterns in the child's speech. (2) Successive reorganizations of phonological structure in the lexicon lead to the achievement of phonological and morphological proficiency. (3) Metaphonological ability (explicit access to phonological structure) permits acquisition of decoding and spelling abilities.*

Case Study 6–3

Case History: Birth and family history unremarkable. In terms of medical history, the child had recurrent otitis media and was diagnosed with developmental coordination disorder.

Speech sample at 22 months of age (entire expressive vocabulary).

Orthographic Gloss	Adult Form	Child's Production	Orthographic Gloss	Adult Form	Child's Production
1. bath	bæθ	bæ	7. egg	ɛg	gəgə
2. banana	bə.nænə	nænʌ	8. grandpa	grændpɑ	bæpʌ
3. bear	bɛɹ	bɛ	9. meow	miaw	au
4. bottle	bɑɾəl	bɑpo	10. pablum	pæbləm	pæbu
5. cracker	kɹækɚ	kækə	11. puppy	pʌpi	bʌpu
6. daddy	dædi	dædi	12. up	ʌp	bʌ

Table 6–8. *Consonant and Vowel Phonetic Repertoires for Case Study 6–3*

	Bilabial	*Labio-dental*	*Dental*	*Alveolar*	*Post-alveolar*	*Palatal*	*Velar*	*Glottal*	*Labiovelar*
Plosive	p b			d			k g		
Nasal				n					
Fricative									
Affricate									
Glide									
Liquid									

	Front	*Central*	*Back*
Close	i y		u
Close-mid		ə	o
Open-mid	ɛ æ		ʌ
Open	a		ɑ

only 12 words in this toddler's expressive vocabulary and therefore we completed a consonant and vowel phonetic inventory aggregated across syllable positions. The first observation is that a variety of front and back vowels are present even though her consonant inventory is limited. The varied vowel repertoire is one of several clues that can help to differentiate between the various subtypes of DPD, as discussed in Chapter 7.

The **phonotactic inventory** identifies strengths and weaknesses with regard to the sequencing of the speech sounds within a word.

The phonotactic inventory identifies strengths and weaknesses with regard to the sequencing of the speech sounds within a word. The completed syllable/word shape inventory and phonotactic repertoire are similar to some components of the multilinear analysis. Case Study 6–3 has a very restricted inventory of syllable/word shapes: (VV), CV, CVCV, and (CVCVV). Stoel-Gammon (1987) described the phonological skills of 33 English monolingual children aged 24 months by collecting two 30-minute conversational speech samples for each child. On the basis of her data as presented in Table 4–2, we would expect Case Study 6–3, who was 22 months old when she was assessed, to have a well-established CVC shape and possibly produce CVCVC and CCV words.

The main **phonotactic patterns** that should be assessed are similar to the first few tiers of the quick version of the multilinear analysis: omission of syllables and omission of consonants in the onset position of syllables; omission of consonants in the coda position of syllables; omission of segments of complex onsets and codas.

The main phonotactic patterns that should be assessed are similar to the first few tiers of the quick version of the multilinear analysis: omission of syllables, and if so, which ones; omission of consonants in the onset position of syllables; omission of consonants in the coda position of syllables; omission of segments of complex onsets and codas. Finally attention should also be paid to harmony and reduplication, and to word stress patterns.

Reduplication occurs when the same syllable is repeated in the word.

Harmony refers to the same consonant or the same vowel being repeated.

Reduplication occurs when the same syllable is repeated in the word; Case Study 6–3 only has one instance of reduplication, "egg" → [gəgə]. Harmony refers to the same consonant or the same vowel being repeated; there are no instances of vowel harmony in the very small speech sample produced by Case Study 6–3 but consonant harmony is pervasive with three examples of complete harmony: [nænʌ], [kækə] , and [dædi]. The remaining words show partial harmony involving [p] and [b], keeping constant the manner and place of articulation. It is very difficult to assess stress patterns in such a small sample that does not contain three-syllable words. However, we note that Case Study 6–3 seems to produce only strong-weak two syllable words.

Case Study 6–3 produced monosyllabic open syllables, disyllabic reduplicated open syllables, and disyllabic open syllables with consonant harmony (Table 6–9). Treatment goals and specific stimuli words that would be appropriate for Case Study 6–3 are presented in Chapter 9; briefly, syllable shapes that she prefers and phonemes already in her inventory will be used to increase her expressive vocabulary; phonemes that are not yet in her inventory are introduced using syllable shapes that she prefers, and new syllable shapes (particularly final consonants) will be introduced using phonemes that she already produces.

Table 6–9. Hierarchy of Phonotactic Difficulty

Syllable shape	Description	Examples
CV, CVV	Monosyllabic open syllables	"go," "me," "zoo," "boy"
$C_1V_1C_1V_1$	Disyllabic, reduplicated open syllables	"mama," "yo-yo," "bye-bye," "tutu"
$C_1V_1C_1V_2$ $C_1V_1C_2V_1$	Disyllabic, nonreduplicated open syllables with harmonization of vowels or consonants	"daddy," "cookie," "paper" "macaw," "lava," "polo," "tiny"
$C_1V_1C_2V_2$	Disyllabic open syllables without reduplication or harmonization	"sofa," "movie," "pillow"
C_1VC_1	Harmonized closed syllables	"dad," "mom," "cake," "pop"
C_1VC_2	Closed syllables without harmonization	"ball," "nose," "sun," "duck"
CVCVC CVCCVC	Disyllabic closed syllables with or without reduplication and/or harmonization	$C_1V_1C_2V_1C_1$: "kayak" $C_1V_1C_1V_2C_2$: "baboon" $C_1V_1C_2V_1C_3$: "robot" C_1V_1 $C_2C_1V_2C_2$: "hip-hop" C_1V_1 $C_2C_1V_2C_3$: "mailman"
CC	Words with initial, ambisyllabic, and/or final consonant clusters	CCV: "play"; CCVC: "spoon" CCVCVC: "crayon" CVCC: "boats" CVCCVC: "basket" CVCVCC: "mittens"

Source: Adapted from Velleman (2002). Phonotactic therapy. *Seminars in Speech and Language*, 23(1).

Analyses to Track Treatment Progress

6.2.1. List the characteristics that measures to track treatment progress should possess, and explain why standardized single-word articulation tests are not adequate to measure progress following intervention.

6.2.2. Perform the Syllable Stucture Level analysis for a speech sample obtained from a toddler.

6.2.3. Calculate the pMLU for a speech sample obtained from a child at the early stages of phonological development.

6.2.4. Identify the advantages of the Weighted Speech Sound Accuracy Measure.

Measures used to track treatment progress should be sensitive enough to detect change following phonological intervention over typical intervention block durations. Additionally, they should

Measures used to **track treatment progress** should be sensitive enough to detect change following phonological intervention over typical intervention block durations. Additionally, they should show little change when used twice in a short time interval during which the child is not receiving intervention (test-retest reliability) and yield similar results if completed by different clinicians (interrater reliability).

Standardized single-word articulation tests should not be used to measure progress following intervention.

Intelligibility and other functional measures could be used to document progress due to intervention as children with severe DPD may need a long period of therapy before gains are detected on measures of speech accuracy.

show little change when used twice in a short time interval during which the child is not receiving intervention (test-retest reliability) and yield similar results if completed by different clinicians (inter-rater reliability). In Chapter 5 we explained that standardized single-word articulation tests were designed to compare the performance of the child to a normative sample and should not be used to measure progress following intervention (McCauley & Swisher, 1984). One option available to clinicians to measure treatment progress is the Focus on the Outcomes of Communication Under Six (FOCUS) described in Chapter 5, as it is sensitive to change over short intervals of intervention (Thomas-Stonell, Oddson, Robertson, & Rosenbaum, 2010); assessment of the usefulness of the measure to document long-term change is ongoing. The FOCUS also has good internal consistency, test-restest reliability, content, and construct validity. Intelligibility measures such as the *Children's Speech Intelligibility Measure* (CSIM; Wilcox & Morris, 1999) developed to assess intelligibility at the word level with children age 3 to 10 and the *Beginner's Intelligibility Test* (BIT; Osberger, Robbins, Todd, & Riley, 1994) to assess intelligibility at the sentence level were also described in Chapter 5. They could be used by clinicians to document progress due to intervention as children with severe DPD may need a long period of therapy before gains are detected on measures of speech accuracy. There also are measures derived from the language sample that can be used to track treatment progress during or following intervention. These include independent measures such as the phonetic inventory and relational measures such as the Phonological Mean Length of Utterance (pMLU) and the Weighted Speech Sound Accuracy (WSSA) measure which are discussed below.

Independent Measures

Recently, Morris (2009) investigated the temporal stability of independent measures such as phonetic inventory and word shape analyses to determine whether they are reliable tools to measure treatment progress by looking at their test-retest reliability. In other words, if the results of independent analyses conducted on two language samples collected from the same child within a few days of each other are markedly different, then progress seen on independent measures following a period of intervention might not indicate treatment progress but rather might be due to the unstable nature of the measure. The language samples of 10 monolingual children 18 to 22 months old with typical language skills were recorded while they played with their mothers during 20 minutes on two occasions within 2 to 7 days. Only the first two variable productions of the same word and only intelligible words were included in the language samples. The test-retest reliability of four different independent analyses was measured: the phonetic inventory (number of consonants in word-initial and word-final positions), the number of different syllable/word shapes, the Syllable Structure Level (SSL; Paul & Jennings, 1992) and the Index of Phonetic Complexity (IPC; Jakielski, Maytasse, & Doyle, 2006). The SSL obtained a high significant test-retest correlation. The IPC had a nonsignificant high correlation, the number of consonants in word-final position and number of syllable/word shapes achieved nonsignificant moderately high correlations and the number of initial consonants obtained a low test-retest correlation. Therefore, although the phonetic inventory and word shape analyses are very useful to select treatment goals, their temporal stability is limited and should not be used to measure treatment progress.

Although the phonetic inventory and word shape analyses are very useful to select treatment goals, their temporal stability is limited and therefore they should not be used to measure treatment progress.

Syllable Structure Level (Table 6–10)

The Syllable Structure Level (SSL) combines information from the phonetic inventory and the syllable shape analysis into one score (Demonstration 6–5). The Mean Babbling Level (MBL) was initially described by Stoel-Gammon (1987) to assess the phonetic diversity of children who produce mostly babbling and very few meaningful words. Paul and Jennings (1992) adapted the MBL's levels to word-like utterances and meaningful words and changed the name to SSL for use with toddlers. One of three levels of syllable structure development is assigned to each word produced by the child based on its shape and the sounds contained in the word.

The **Syllable Structure Level (SSL)** combines information from the phonetic inventory and the syllable shape analysis into one score.

Table 6–10. *Syllable Structure Levels*

Level	*Description*
1	Words including only a vowel (e.g., [aʊ], [ɛ]), a syllabic consonant (e.g., [m̩]), or a consonant vowel (CV) or vowel consonant (VC) word in which the only consonant type is a glottal (e.g., [ʔu] or [hi]) or glide (e.g., [wi] or [ju]).
2	Words containing at least one CV or VC sequence in which the consonant is a true consonant (not a glide or glottal) (e.g., [be], [ve]). The place and manner feature of multiple true consonants within the word cannot change (e.g., [mɑm], [dædi]), but the voicing feature may change (e.g., [bɑpɑ]).
3	Words containing two or more true consonants (e.g., [degi], [kup], [fɪn]) that differ in place or manner of articulation.

Source: Adapted from Morris (2010). Clinical application of the mean babbling level and syllable structure level. *Language, Speech and Hearing Services in Schools, 41*, Appendix B, p. 230. Originally adapted from Stoel-Gammon's (1989) procedure.

Demonstration 6–5

The complete expressive vocabulary of Case Study 6–3 at the time of the initial assessment contained only 12 words, and her consonantal phonetic inventory was quite limited. The Syllable Structure Level is a good option to track treatment progress during intervention for this child. Eventually when her phonetic inventory and vocabulary are more developed and almost all the utterances she produces are at Level 3 of the SSL, the relational measures to be described later in this chapter could be used instead to measure treatment progress.

Child's Production	SSL Level	
au	1	Word including only a vowel.
bæ	2	CV word with one true consonant.
bɛ	2	
bʌ	2	
nænʌ	2	CVCV with true consonants; place and manner features of the consonants are the same.
bɑpo	2	
kækə	2	
dædi	2	
gəgə	2	
bæpʌ	2	
pæbu	2	
bʌpu	2	
	Total SSL = 1.92	

The total SSL is calculated by dividing the sum of all word values by the total number of words.

Phonological Mean Length of Utterance

The whole-word measures (Ingram, 2002; Ingram & Ingram, 2001) described in Chapter 4 were designed to track changes in the complexity and consistency of the word productions attempted by the child, and their increasing proximity to the adult target. In particular, the Phonological Mean Length of Utterance (pMLU) describes the length of the child's production (number of consonants and vowels regardless of accuracy), plus the number of correct consonants, divided by the total number of words. Similar to the SSL, the pMLU is designed for young children or children in early stages of phonological development. The analysis requires the selection of 25 to 50 words from the broadly transcribed language sample (Sample Size rule), which may consist of all the words produced by the child during the language sample collection. The words selected should be representative of the entire language sample, such that if the child produced 75 words during the language sample, two out of every three words could be selected. Only common nouns, verbs, adjectives, prepositions and adverbs used in adult conversation are included in the analysis; child words such as "daddy" and "mama" are excluded (Lexical Class rule). The Compound Word rule states that compound words spelled as one word count as one-word tokens (e.g., "cowboy"), whereas compounds spelled as two words count as two word tokens (e.g., "teddy bear"). Only a single production of a lexical item is included (Variability rule). If the child produced more than one production for the same word, the most frequent one only is included in the sample to be analyzed. If no production of the same word is more frequent than others, the last production only is counted.

The **Phonological Mean Length of Utterance (pMLU)** describes the length of the child's production (number of consonants and vowels regardless of accuracy), plus the number of correct consonants, divided by the total number of words.

The **Sample Size rule** refers to the fact that the pMLU analysis requires the selection of 25 to 50 words from the broadly transcribed language sample.

The **Lexical Class rule** states that only common nouns, verbs, adjectives, prepositions, and adverbs used in adult conversation are included in the analysis.

According to the **Compound Word rule** compound words spelled as one word count as one word token whereas compounds spelled as two words count as two word tokens.

The **Variability rule** specifies that only a single production of a lexical item is included. The most frequent production of the same word is included; if no production is more frequent than others, the last one is counted.

Calculating the exact pMLU value for each word token involves the application of two rules. The Production rule states that one point is counted for each consonant and vowel occurring in the child's production. Syllabic consonants receive one point: when /l/, /ɹ/, and /n/ are transcribed with a schwa following the consonant, the combination of the two should only count as one consonantal segment. For instance, the word "bottle" could be transcribed as either [bɑdl] or [bɑdəl]: in both cases the total for the production rule would be 4 (one point each for [b, ɑ, d, l]). Segments produced by the child that are in addition to the total number of segments counted in the adult target are not awarded points. For example, if the child produced /kʌp/ → [twʌp] he would only get credit for two consonants produced, not three. One additional point is assigned for each correct consonant (Consonant Correct rule). Vowel accuracy is not included in the pMLU calculation because interrater reliability on vowel transcription is typically lower than for consonants.

The **Production rule** states that one point is counted for each consonant and vowel occurring in the child's production.

Following the **Consonant Correct rule,** one additional point is assigned for each correct consonant.

Although Ingram's rules are quite detailed, there remains some ambiguity regarding the specific ordering of the consonants. Taelman, Durieux, and Gillis (2005) suggested awarding points according to the Consonants Correct rule only for consonants produced in the correct word position and order (e.g., /kʌp/ → [pʌk] would be scored as 3 points for the Production rule and 0 points for the Consonant Correct rule). They also did not award points for a correct consonant produced next to an added consonant (e.g., /fɪʃ/ → [fpɪs] would yield a score of 3 for the Production rule because points are not awarded for segments produced by the child that are in addition to the total number of points in the adult form, and a score of 0 for the Consonants Correct rule since the final [s] is incorrect and the [f] is also considered incorrect, being produced adjacent to the added [p].

The final pMLU value is the average of the pMLU values for each word token included in the sample to be analyzed. The pMLU is sensitive to the word shapes attempted by the child, with longer and more complex words getting more points in the Production rule than shorter words and/or words with less complex syllable shapes. However, the Consonant Correct rule moderates the effect of the exact syllable shapes attempted by the child, such that the pMLU for a CVC word structure produced accurately yields a score of 5 whereas the pMLU for a CVCVCV word with only one consonant correct would result in a score of 4.

Demonstration 6–6 presents the pMLU calculation for the speech samples obtained from a young boy at the initial assessment, and at a follow-up visit 4 months later. The child was referred for a speech-language assessment at a young age since he had been followed regularly by a team of nurses, physicians and other health care professionals through a neonatal clinic. The boy had been born prematurely by caesarean section at 31 weeks gestation due to placenta previa.

The pMLU obtained in the initial assessment sample presented in the demonstration was 2.32. Although there are no English monolingual mean pMLU values for children age 25 months in Table 4–4, we see that typically developing English monolingual children age 19 months have an average pMLU of 3.29, a value superior to that obtained by the child from the demonstration who is in fact six months older than this comparison sample. Although the pMLU value obtained four months later at the follow-up visit remains below what would be expected for his age, a nice progression on this measure can be seen, with the child now obtaining a pMLU value of 3.18 at 29 months.

Demonstration 6–6

Calculation of the pMLU for the language sample (initial assessment, age 25 months):

Orthographic gloss	Adult form	Child's production	Production rule	Consonants Correct rule	pMLU for the word
again	[əgɛn]	[ədɛ]	3	0	3
apple	[æpəl]	[æə]	2	0	2
baby	[bebi]	[bei]	3	1	4
ball	[bɔl]	[bɔ]	2	1	3
boat	[bot]	[bo]	2	1	3
bye	[baj]	[ba]	2	1	3
car	[kɑɹ]	[tɑ]	2	0	2
cat	[kæt]	[tæ]	2	0	2
cookie	[kʊki]	[ʊi]	2	0	2
dog	[dag]	[da]	2	1	3
down	[daʊn]	[da]	2	1	3
fall	[fɑl]	[pɑ]	2	0	2
go	[go]	[do]	2	0	2
hat	[hæt]	[æ]	1	0	1
hello	[həlo]	[əo]	2	0	2
me	[mi]	[mi]	—	—	—
me	[mi]	[mi]	2	1	3
meow	[miau]	[iau]	—	—	—
milk	[mɪlk]	[ɪ]	1	0	1
mommy	[mɑmi]	[ɑi]	—	—	—

Only the last production of "me" is included (Variability rule).

"Meow" and "mommy" are excluded from the sample (Lexical Class rule).

Orthographic gloss	Adult form	Child's production	Production rule	Consonants Correct rule	pMLU for the word
more	[mɔɹ]	[mɔ]	2	1	3
no	[no]	[no]	2	1	3
no	[no]	[no]	—	—	—
no	[no]	[o]	—	—	—
open	[opən]	[oə]	2	0	2
phone	[fon]	[po]	2	0	2
plane	[plen]	[e]	1	0	1
puzzle	[pʌzəl]	[ʌə]	2	0	2
shoes	[ʃuz]	[tu]	2	0	2
sit	[sɪt]	[tɪ]	2	0	2
this	[ðɪs]	[ɪ]	1	0	1
train	[tɹen]	[en]	2	1	3
up	[ʌp]	[ʌp]	2	1	3

Only one instance of the most frequent production of "no" is kept in the sample (Variability rule).

Average pMLU for the initial assessment sample:

Sum of pMLU scores	Number of words in the analyzed sample	Average pMLU
65	28	65/28 = 2.32

The average pMLU is obtained by dividing the total of the individual pMLU values by the number of words in the analyzed sample.

Calculation of the pMLU for the language sample (follow-up visit, age 29 months):

Orthographic gloss	Adult form	Child's production	Production rule	Consonants Correct rule	pMLU for the word
again	[əgɛn]	[ədɛ]	3	0	3
baby	[bebi]	[bei]	3	1	4
ball	[bɔl]	[bɔʊ]	3	1	4
balloons	[bəlunz]	[bəu]	3	1	4
big	[bɪg]	[bɪ]	2	1	3
bird	[bəɹd]	[bə]	2	1	3
blue	[blu]	[bu]	2	1	3
bunny	[bʌni]	[bʌni]	4	2	6
bye	[baj]	[ba]	2	1	3
car	[kɑɹ]	[tɑ]	2	0	2
cat	[kæt]	[tæt]	3	1	4
chicken	[tʃɪkən]	[tɪə]	3	0	3
cow	[kaʊ]	[taʊ]	3	1	4
cup	[kʌp]	[tʌ]	2	0	2
dog	[dag]	[da]	2	1	3
duck	[dʌk]	[dʌ]	2	1	3
frog	[fɹɑg]	[pɑp]	3	0	3
go	[go]	[do]	2	0	2
hello	[həlo]	[əwo]	3	0	3
horse	[hɔɹs]	[hɔ]	2	1	3

Orthographic gloss	Adult form	Child's production	Production rule	Consonants Correct rule	pMLU for the word
house	[haʊs]	[ha]	2	1	3
me	[mi]	[mi]	2	1	3
mine	[majn]	[ma]	2	1	3
more	[mɔɹ]	[mɔ]	2	1	3
mouse	[maʊs]	[maʊ]	3	2	5
no	[no]	[no]	2	1	3
open	[opən]	[oə]	2	0	2
pig	[pɪg]	[pɪ]	2	1	3
play	[plei]	[pei]	2	1	3
puzzle	[pʌzəl]	[pʌə]	3	1	4
this	[ðɪs]	[ɪ]	1	0	1
truck	[tɹʌk]	[tʌt]	3	1	4
up	[ʌp]	[ʌp]	2	1	3

Average pMLU for the follow-up visit sample:

Sum of pMLU scores	Number of words in the analyzed sample	Average pMLU
105	33	105 / 33 = 3.18

Weighted Speech Sound Accuracy Measure

Most standardized articulation tests and other measures of productive phonology use two-way scoring (correct or incorrect). However, various types of speech sound errors affect intelligibility differently. For instance, distortions such as interdental lisps may not significantly reduce intelligibility, whereas atypical errors such as glottal replacement will have much greater impact (Prezas & Hodson, 2007). Changes to the syllable structure considerably diminish intelligibility, with deletion of final consonants having more of a detrimental effect on intelligibility than substitutions affecting the manner or place of articulation such as stopping of fricatives and velar fronting (Klein & Flint, 2006). Segment additions change syllable structure and therefore may also affect intelligibility considerably (Dodd & Iacano, 1989). Improvements in the child's speech following intervention may therefore not be captured by measures of phonetic accuracy that assign the same weights to substitutions, omissions, distortions, and additions, as the child could have fewer omissions and additions in his speech but nonetheless obtain an incorrect score due the presence of substitutions and distortions. Furthermore, most tools for the assessment of speech sound production accuracy do not take into account vowels; as mentioned in Chapter 4 some children with DPD do produce vowel errors, and these errors also have diagnostic significance.

Measures of phonetic accuracy that assign the same weights to substitutions, omissions, distortions, and additions may not capture improvements in the child's speech following intervention.

The Weighted Speech Sound Accuracy (WSSA) was recently developed to address the limitations of currently available measures of phonetic accuracy (Preston et al., 2011). It assigns different numerical values to different types of speech errors and takes into account both consonant and vowel production. The WSSA is intended to distinguish children with SSD from normally developing children at various ages, be sensitive to developmental growth and changes following intervention, show little change if the same child is tested within a short time interval or if a smaller language sample from the same child is analyzed, and have strong correlations between transcribers.

The **Weighted Speech Sound Accuracy (WSSA)** was recently developed to provide a valid and reliable measure of speech accuracy. It assigns different numerical values to different types of speech errors and takes into account both consonant and vowel production.

Oller and Ramsdell (2006) developed a weighted reliability measure for phonetic transcription and introduced three different concepts: the global structural agreement score, the featural agreement score and the multiplication of these two which results in the overall transcription agreement score. The WSSA calculates three similar scores as described below, although adaptations were made to Oller and Ramsdell's scoring system. In both cases the agreement scores were calculated through the Logical International Phonetics Program (LIPP; Oller & Delgado, 1999) which is available commercially at Intelligent Hearing Systems. The first step to calculate the WSSA is to align the transcription of the target with the transcription of the child's production in different slots, as shown in Table 6–11. The adult target production can be modified to be the same as the child's production in cases of dialectally acceptable variations

***Table 6–11.** Alignment of the Target and Child's Productions of "Play With my Alligator"*

Target	[p l e ɪ	w ɪ θ	m a ɪ	ʔ æ l ə g e ɪ ɾ ɚ]
Child's production	/ p e ɪ	w ɪ t	m ə	ʔ ɛ d ə ɾ ə /
GSA score	2.5/3.5 = 0.71	1.0	2/2.5 = 0.80	5.5/8 = 0.69

In the word "alligator," the child's production of [d] is matched with /g/, as the two phonemes are closer phonetically than /l/ → [d], resulting in an empty slot for /l/. Weak consonants and vowels are worth 0.5 points for the global structural agreement score, such as the glottal stop in "alligator" and the weak vowel in the diphthongs of "play," "my," and "alligator."

such that a mismatch between the two transcriptions will not be computed. There are four alignment principles to standardize the alignment process: (1) *strict order* does not allow for reordering the order of segments in the target or child's productions; (2) *nucleus alignment* first dictates ordering of vowels before consonants; (3) the *matched segments* principle ensures simple alignment of consonants and vowels when the target and the child's production contain the same number of consonants and vowels produced in the same order; and 4) when obvious matching is impossible, the *minimal discrepancy* principle mandates alignment of segments that are phonetically similar.

The child's production of the target needs to be aligned with the transcription of the target to calculate the WSSA. There are four **alignment principles**: (1) *strict order*; (2) *nucleus alignment first*; (3) *matched segments*; and (4) *minimal discrepancy*.

The global structural alignment score is the proportion of slots that are filled both in the target and child's production. Each slot containing a strong consonant or vowel is awarded a score of 1.0; each slot containing a weak segment, defined as such as glottals, glides and weak vowels, is awarded a score of 0.5 points. Slots that are filled on both lines receive full points, 1.0 or 0.5 depending on the target sound. The penalty for deletions or additions of strong segments is 1.0; the penalty for deletions or additions of weak segments is 0.5 points.

The **global structural alignment score** is the proportion of slots that are filled both in the target and child's production.

The featural agreement is then calculated for the slots that contain both an adult target and a phoneme produced by the child. Each slot is allotted a score of 1.0, and deductions are applied for vowel and consonant substitutions. Smaller deductions are applied to errors that are closer to the target than substitutions that are farther from the target. The featural agreement would be 1.0 if the child produced all non-omitted segments accurately. The WSSA, which is the multiplication of the global structural agreement score by the featural agreement score, would in this case account for the fact that the child omitted phonemes. Substitutions of consonants are coded in terms of place, manner, and voicing; each of these is worth a total of 0.33 points. Penalties are deducted for teeny, small, big, or huge errors as shown in Table 6–12. The direction of change has an impact on the deduction applied, with atypical errors such as backing receiving a steeper deduction than errors seen in normal phonological development such as fronting.

The **featural agreement score** refers to the application of deductions for vowel and consonant substitutions from a score of 1.0 allowed to each slot in the alignment of the child's and target transcriptions.

The **WSSA** is the multiplication of the global structural agreement score by the featural agreement score.

Table 6–12. Consonant Features and Penalties for Errors

Consonant feature (weight)		Penalty			Example
Manner (0.333)	Huge manner	−0.3333	Plosive	→	Fric. or affric./#____
	Uncommon errors, damaging to intelligibility		Glide	→	Liquid
			Nasal	→	Nonnasal
			Semivowel	→	Nasal
	Big manner		Sonorant	↔	Obstruent
	Less common in phonological development	−0.25	Plosive	→	Fric. or affric./C or V____
			Fric. or affric.	→	Lateral fric. or affric.
	Small manner				
	Common errors in phonological development	−0.1666	Fric. or affric.	→	Plosive
			Fric.	↔	Affric.
	Teeny manner		Liquid	→	Glide or tap
	Minor phonetic errors	−0.0833	Nonspecific distortion		
Place (0.333)	Huge place	−0.3333	Dorsal	↔	Labial
	Uncommon, very damaging to intelligibility		Glottal	↔	Nonglottal
	Big place	−0.25	Coronal	↔	Labial
	Less common in phonological development		Coronal	→	Dorsal
			Alveolar	→	Palatal
			Palatal	→	Dental
			Retroflex	↔	Not retroflex
	Small place	−0.1666	Linguadental	↔	Labiodental
	Typical error in phonological development		Dental	↔	Alveolar
			Palatal	→	Alveolar
			Dorsal	→	Coronal
	Teeny place	−0.0833	Bilabial	↔	Labiodental
	Phonetic errors in English, based on small changes in tongue placement		Lips not spread	↔	Lips spread
			Lips not round	↔	Lips round
			Labialization		
			Blading		
			Tongue advance/ retract		
Voicing (0.333)	Huge voicing	−0.3333	Word-initial or medial devoicing		
	Uncommon		Word-final voicing		
	Small voicing	−0.2222	Word-final devoicing		
	Common		Word-initial voicing		
	Teeny voicing	−0.1111	Aspiration of nonaspirated C (e.g., ste → st^he)		
	Phonetic changes				

Note: Fric. = fricative; Affric. = affricate; C = consonant, V = vowel.

Source: From Preston et al. (2011). Developing a weighted measure of speech sound accuracy. *Journal of Speech, Language, and Hearing Research*, *54*, Table 1, p. 6. Reprinted with permission of the American Speech-Language-Hearing Association.

Accurately produced vowels receive a featural agreement score of 1.0: vowel features are coded along four dimensions: tongue height (0.4 credit), tongue advancement (0.4 credit), rounding (0.1 credit), and nasalization (0.1 credit). Common error weights for vowel substitutions are presented in Table 6–13.

Finally, vowels can be substituted for consonants, and consonants substituted for vowels. Obstruent-vowel alternations receive a deduction of 1.0; vowel-syllabic unvoiced obstruent alternations, as well as alternations between high or low vowels and mid-semivowels, receive a 0.75 point deduction. The penalty for substituting any nonglide vowel for a liquid or vice versa is 0.5; alternations between vowels and syllabic liquids is 0.25.

Preston et al. (2011) calculated the WSSA for transcribed speech samples recorded from normally developing toddlers and preschoolers and young adolescents with and without SSD. Psychometric data obtained to date indicate that the WSSA correlated with SLPs' judgments of the severity of the speech disorder, with other measures of speech sound accuracy such as the Percentage of Consonants Correct (PCC) and raw scores obtained on the GFTA-2; at the same time, the WSSA was more sensitive to atypical speech errors than these other measures demonstrating the advantage of the weighted scoring over the traditional SODA approach to documenting speech accuracy. WSSA scores distinguished children developing normally from children with SSD and increased with age, indicating that it captured growth in toddlers' phonetic accuracy.

The child featured in Case Study 6–4, PA 224, was referred for a speech-language assessment by his family doctor to a children's hospital. He was then recruited into a longitudinal follow-up study of children with speech delay. PA 224 was 4;9 at the time of the initial assessment; results of the measures and the language sample collected are presented below. PA 224 received intervention to remediate his sound production difficulties, with the number of sessions, frequency, and duration determined by his treating SLP at the hospital.

Table 6–13. *Vowel Feature Weights and Penalties for Errors*

Vowel feature	*Weight*		*Penalties*		*Example*
Height	(0.40)	Huge height	−0.40	4-step height change	/i/ ↔ [ɑ]
		Big height	−0.30	3-step height change	/ɪ/ ↔ [ɑ]
		Small height	−0.20	2-step height change	/i/ ↔ [e]
		Teeny height	−0.10	1-step height change	/ɑ/ ↔ [ɛ]
Advancement	(0.40)	Big front	−0.40	Front ↔ Back	/o/ ↔ [e]
		Small front	−0.20	Front ↔ Central or Back ↔ Central	/i/ ↔ [ə]
Nasalization	(0.1)	Small nasal	−0.10	Not nasal → Nasal	/ɑ/ ↔ [ɑ̃]
Rounding	(0.1)	Small rounding	−0.10	Round ↔ Not round	/ʌ/ ↔ [ɔ]

Source: From Preston et al. (2011). Developing a weighted measure of speech sound accuracy. *Journal of Speech, Language, and Hearing Research*, 54, Table 2, p. 7. Reprinted with permission of the American Speech-Language-Hearing Association.

Case Study 6–4

Case History: Child (PA224) was born at 36 weeks following an uneventful pregnancy and birth. Developmental, medical, and family history are unremarkable.

Summary of Scores Obtained at Initial Assessment (CA = 4;9)

PPVT-III	94th percentile
MLU	7.69
GFTA-2	4th percentile
PCC	73.8%, z = −0.81
SAILS	75.7%, z = −0.30
PAT	Raw score = 19, z = −0.55
Letters	Raw score = 10
Literacy Knowledge	Raw score = 6

Summary of Scores Obtained at Follow-Up Reassessment (CA = 5;10)

PPVT-III	96th percentile
MLU	6.58
GFTA-2	5th percentile
PCC	81.6%, z = −0.67
SAILS	74.3%, z = −1.28
PAT	Raw score = 26, z = −0.72
Letters	Raw score = 12
Literacy Knowledge	Raw score = 7

Notes. PPVT-III = Peabody Picture Vocabulary Test-III (Dunn & Dunn, 1997); MLU = Mean Length of Utterance (in morphemes); GFTA-2 = Goldman-Fristoe Test of Articulation-2 (Goldman & Fristoe, 2000); PCC = Percent Consonants Correct, assessed in conversation (see Chapters 4 and 5); SAILS = Speech Assessment and Interactive Learning System (measure of speech perception skills; see http://www.medicine.mcgill.ca/srvachew); PAT = Phonological Awareness Test (Bird, Bishop, & Freeman, 1995); Letters = number of letters named; Literacy Knowledge = adaptation of an early literacy assessment protocol used by Jerry L. Johns at Northern Illinois University

Speech Sample at Intake Assessment

The dog's laying down.
də dɔgz leɪŋ daʊn.

The baby's getting out.
də beɪbiz dɛtɪŋ aʊt.

And the baby's foot is on the dog.
ænd də beɪbiz fʊt ɪz ɑn də dɑg.

Looking out the window.
lʊkɪŋ aʊt də wɪndo.

The baby falled down on the bed and the dog's standing up.
də beɪbiʃ faʊld daʊn ɑn də bɛd ænd də dɑgz stændɪŋ ʌp.

And the baby is riding the dog like a horse.
ænd də beɪbi ɪz waɪdɪŋ də dɑg laɪk æ hows.

And the baby putting makeup stuff on him.
ænd də beɪbi pʊɾɪŋ mekʌp fʊs ɑn hɪm.

They look in the mirror.
de wʊk ɪn də miwəɹ.

And the dog's jumping down the stairs.
ænd də dɑgz dʌmpɪŋ daʊn də dɛwz.

The baby was looking down the stairs.
də beɪbi wɑz wʊkɪŋ daʊn də dɛwz.

And the dog was right there.
ænd də dɑg wɑz waɪt dɛɹ.

Hey where's his other leg?
he wɛɹz hɪz ʊdəɹ wɛg.

Maybe you just can't see them.
mebi ju dʌs kæn ti dɛm.

The baby finds the dog.
də beɪbi faɪndz də dɑg.

And the baby's riding him like a horse again.
ænd də beɪbiʒ waɪdɪn hɪm waɪk æ hows ædɪn.

And the baby's swimming and the dog's trying to get in I think.
ænd də beɪbiz dɪmɪŋ ænd də dɑgz baɪɪŋ tu dɛt ɪn ɑɪ tɪŋk.

In the fish tank.
ɪn də dɪsdænk.

I think.
ɑɪ tɪŋk.

And he's turning on the radio and he's dancing.
ænd hiz dɛnɪŋ ɑn də wedio ænd hiz dænsɪŋ.

And he's trying to opening the fridge and they're eating.
ænd hiz daɪŋ tu opɛnɪŋ bɪdʒ ænd dɛɹ idɪŋ.

And they're pouring coffee and milk.
ænd dɛɹ powɪŋ dɑsi ænd mɪlk.

Yeah and they are eating some things.
jæ ænd de ɑɹ idɪŋ dʌm tɪŋz.

And they made a big mess.
ænd de med æ bɪg mɛs.

And they're walking back upstairs.
ænd dɛɹ wɑkɪŋ bæk ʌpdɛwz.

And he's dropping him in the tub.
ænd hiz dʌpɪŋ hɪm ɪn də dʌb.

Don't know.
dont no.

Then he's spraying him off with the hose or the dryer.
dɛn hiz speɪŋ hɪm ɑf wɪs də hoz oɹ də baɪəɹ.

Yeah and putting him back in his cage.
jæ ænd butɪn hɪm bæk ɪn hɪz tedz.

And the dog's washing the floor.
ænd də dɑgz waʃɪŋ də boɹ.

And then he looks out the window again.
ænd dɛn hi wukz aʊt də wɪndo ædɪn.

And he's putting all away the things and cleaning up the mess.
ænd hiz pʊrɪŋ æl æwe də dɪŋz ænd tinɪŋ ʌp də mɛs.

And mom comes home with a dog I think.
ænd mɑm dɑm hom wɪs æ dɑg ɑɪ dɪŋk.

Speech Sample at Follow-Up Re-Assessment

Look after the baby Carl.
lʊk æftəɹ də beɪbi kawl.

I'll be back shortly.
aɪl bi bæk ʃoɹtwi.

The mum's leaving.
də mʌmz wivɪŋ.

And the baby's awake.
ænd də beɪbiz ʌweɪk.

Guard him.
gaɹd n.

It would be better if it was a gorilla.
ɪt wʊd bi bɛtow ɪf ɪt wʌz ɑ gowɪwɑ.

The baby climbs.
də beɪbi kwaɪmz.

The baby's standing up and the dog's looking out the window.
də beɪbiz stændɪŋ ʌp ænd də dɑgz wʊkɪŋ aʊt də wɪndo.

Then the baby's coming out.
dɛn də beɪbiz kʌmɪŋ aʊt.

The thing on the dog.
ðə sɪŋ ɑn də dɑg.

And then the dog goes in the mum's room.
ænd dɛn də dɑg goʊz ɪn də mʌmz rum.

And then the baby falls down.
ænd dɛn də beɪbi fɑwz daʊn.

And the baby's using some of the mum's stuff.
ænd də beɪbiz juzɪŋ sʌm ʌv də mʌmz stʌf.

And then he wants to play dress up.
ænd dɛn hi wɑnts tu pweɪ dwɛs ʌp.

And then he wants go in the laundry.
ænd dɛn hi wɑnts goʊ ɪn ðə wɑndwi.

And then the dog's always downstairs.
ænd dɛn də dɑgz ɑwweɪz daʊnstɛwz.

And then the baby's in the basement and the dog's on the stairs.
ænd dɛn də beɪbiz ɪn də beɪsmɪnt ænd də dɑgz ɑn də stɛwz.

And the dog helps get the baby out.
ænd də dɑg hɛlps gɛt də beɪbi aʊt.

And then the dog gets in the fish tank.
ænd dɛn də dɑg gɛts ɪn də fɪʃ tæŋk.

And the baby does too.
ænd də beɪbi dʌz tu.

I think the dog doesn't.
aɪ θɪŋk də dɑg dʌznt.

And then the dog turns on the radio.
ænd dɛn də dɑg tʌwnz ɑn də weɪdio.

And then the dog dances.
ænd ðɛn də dɑg dænsɪz.

And then he gets something to eat.
ænd dɛn hi gɛts sʌmθɪŋ tu it.

He gets a bread thing then eats some bread.
hi gɛts ɑ bwɛd sɪŋ dɛn its sʌm bwɛd.

And then he opens some cookies.
ænd dɛn hi opɛnz sʌm kʊkiz.

He then some grapes, soda, cookies.
hi dɛn sʌm gweɪps soʊdɑ kʊkiz.

And then they go upstairs.
ænd dɛn deɪ goʊ ʌpstɛwz.

Then the dog puts him in the bathtub.
dɛn də dɑg pʌts hɪm ɪn də bæftʌb.

Then washes him.
dɛn wɑʃɪz hɪm.

Out.
aʊt.

Then he dries him off.
dɛn hi draiz hɪm ɑf.

Then he has bubbles coming out of his mouth.
dɛn hi hæz bʌblz kʌmɪŋ aʊt ʌp hɪz maʊf.

And the dog tries to get the bubbles out of his mouth.
ænd də dɑg twaɪz to gɛt də bʌblz kʌmɪŋ aʊt ʌ hɪz maʊf.

Then the dog looks out the window.
dɛn də dɑg wʊks aʊt də wɪndo.

And then he uses some of his mum's stuff.
ænd dɛn hi juzɪz sʌm ʌv hɪz mʌmz stʌf.

And then he sees his mom coming home.
ænd dɛn hi siz hɪz mʌm kʌmɪŋ hoʊm.

And then he's down.
ænd dɛn hiz daʊn.

And then the mum does something to the dog.
ænd dɛn də mʌm dʌz sʌmθɪŋ tu də dɑg.

Note: The speech samples were obtained with the wordless book *Carl Goes Shopping,* by Alexandra Day.

He was reassessed in the context of the research project at the age of 5;10, toward the end of the kindergarten school year. The results obtained and the language sample collected during the follow-up reassessment session are presented above.

PA 224 obtained almost the same percentile rank on the GFTA-2 administered on two occasions one year apart (4th and 5th percentile ranks); as explained in Chapter 5 and briefly mentioned in this chapter, standardized articulation tests compare the child's performance with same age peers and should not be used to make conclusions about intervention efficacy. PA 224's answers on the items of the GFTA-2 were much closer to the targets at the follow-up assessment. For instance, he produced the consonant clusters /bl/, /bɹ/, /fl/, /fɹ/, /gɹ/, /kɹ/, /sp/, and /tɹ/ → [b] and all other clusters tested on the GFTA-2 as either [d] or [p] at the initial assessment. At the follow-up assessment, on the other hand, he produced four clusters accurately (/kw/, /sp/, /st/, /sw/), produced the first consonant of all other clusters accurately, omitted one second consonant /l/, and produced all other second consonant /l, ɹ/ → [w]. Although PA 224's production of the targets on the GFTA-2 at the reassessment contained fewer omissions and atypical errors, the percentile rank remained the same as during the assessment as different types of errors are not weighed differently on the GFTA-2 and as PA 224 was one year older and most children age 5;10 rarely produce speech sound errors.

Demonstration 6–7: Calculation of the WSSA Scores for Case Study 6–4

The PCC derived from the language samples obtained with the wordless book *Carl Goes Shopping* by Alexandra Day increased by almost 8 points from the assessment to the reassessment visit. However, the PCC does not assign different numerical values to different types of speech errors and does not give us information about both the prosodic and segmental progress made by PA 224 between the two assessment points. We therefore calculated the WSSA for PA 224, as shown in Demonstration 6–7. In the demonstration we included one instance of each production of a token and calculated the global structural agreement score, the featural agreement score, and the WSSA (the multiplication of these two scores) by hand. Case Study 6–4 has very few vowel substitutions and consonant-vowel or vowel-consonant substitutions. The LIPP software program is available commercially, and the analysis routine to implement the WSSA is available from Jonathan Preston at Haskins Laboratory. Completing the analysis by hand was moderately time-consuming and therefore using the LIPP software would be more practical for children with many typical and atypical speech errors. The full calculations for the WSSA at the Intake Assessment are demonstrated; a less detailed and therefore less time-consuming manner of calculating the WSSA is shown for the language sample obtained during the follow-up reassessment.

Demonstration 6–7

Calculation of the WSSA for the language sample obtained from Case Study 6–4 at the Initial Assessment (age 4;9). The alignment of the target and child production, as well as the score obtained for the GSA and FA, are provided only for two correctly produced words at the top of the demonstration ("all" and "and"); other words produced accurately in the language sample are listed in a table below.

Target	/	æ	l		æ	n	d		æ	g	ɪ	n	/
Child production	[	æ	l		æ	n	d		æ	d	ɪ	n	]
GSA		1.0			1.0				1.0				
FA		1.0	1.0		1.0	1.0	1.0		1.0	0.83	1.0	1.0	

The addition of [ʃ] is taken into account in the GSA but not the FA as both slots are not filled.

Target	/	k	æ	n	t		b	e	ɪ	b	i		/
Child production	[	k	æ	n			b	e	ɪ	b	i	ʃ	]
GSA		3/4 = 0.75					4.5/5.5 = 0.82						
FA		1.0	1.0	1.0	n/a		1.0	1.0	1.0	1.0	1.0	n/a	

Featural agreement /g/ → [d]: small place deduction of −0.1666; FA = 0.8334

Target	/	k	e	dʒ		b	e	ɪ	b	i	z		/
Child production	[	t	e	dz		b	e	ɪ	b	i	ʒ		]
GSA		1.0				1.0							
FA		0.83	1.0	0.83		1.0	1.0	1.0	1.0	1.0	0.83		

Featural agreement /k/ → [t]: small place deduction of −0.1666; FA = 0.8334

Featural agreement /dʒ/ → [dz]: small place deduction of −0.1666; FA = 0.8334

Featural agreement /z/ → [ʒ]: small place deduction of −0.1666; FA = 0.8334

Target	/	k	l	i	n	ɪ	ŋ		k	ɑ	f	i	/
Child production	[	t		i	n	ɪ	ŋ		d	ɑ	s	i	]
GSA		5/6 = 0.834							1.0				
FA		0.83	n/a	1.0	1.0	1.0	1.0		0.61	1.0	0.75	1.0	

The FA for /k/ → [d] was described above and therefore is not listed again here.

Featural agreement /k/ → [d]: small place deduction of –0.1666; small voicing deduction of –0.2222; FA = 0.6112

Featural agreement /f/ → [s]: big place deduction of –0.25; FA = 0.75

Target	/	k	ɑ	m	z		d	ɹ	ʌ	p	ɪ	ŋ	/
Child production	[	d	ɑ	m			d		ʌ	p	ɪ	ŋ	]
GSA		3/4 = 0.75					5/6 = 0.834						
FA		0.61	1.0	1.0	n/a		1.0	n/a	1.0	1.0	1.0	1.0	

Target	/	s	i		ð	ə		g	ɛ	d	ɪ	ŋ	/
Child production	[	t	i		d	ə		d	ɛ	d	ɪ	ŋ	]
GSA		1.0			1.0			1.0					
FA		0.83	1.0		0.67	1.0		0.83	1.0	1.0	1.0	1.0	

Featural agreement /s/ → [t]: small manner deduction of –0.1666; FA = 0.8334

Featural agreement /ð/ → [d]: small manner deduction of –0.1666; small place deduction of –0.1666; FA = 0.6668

Target	/	f	ɹ	ɪ	dʒ		dʒ	ʌ	m	p	ɪ	ŋ	/
Child production	[	b		ɪ	dʒ		d	ʌ	m	p	ɪ	ŋ	]
GSA		3/4 = 0.75					1.0						
FA		0.67	n/a	1.0	1.0		0.67	1.0	1.0	1.0	1.0	1.0	

Featural agreement /f/ → [b]: small manner deduction of –0.1666; teeny place deduction of –0.0833; FA = 0.6668

Featural agreement /dʒ/ → [d]: small manner deduction of –0.1666; small place deduction of –0.1666; FA = 0.6668

Target	/	f	ɪ	ʃ		g	ɛ	t		l	ɛ	g	/
Child production	[	d	ɪ	s		d	ɛ	t		w	ɛ	g	]
GSA		1.0				1.0				1.0			
FA		0.58	1.0	0.83		0.83	1.0	1.0		0.67	1.0	1.0	

Featural agreement /f/ → [d]: small manner deduction of −0.1666; big place deduction of −0.25; FA = 0.5834

Featural agreement /ʃ/ → [s]: small place deduction of −0.1666; FA = 0.8334

Target	/	f	l	o	ɹ		s	w	ɪ	m	ɪ	ŋ	/
Child production	[	b		o	ɹ		d		ɪ	m	ɪ	ŋ	]
GSA		3/4 = 0.75					5/5.5 = 0.909						
FA		0.75	n/a	1.0	1.0		0.61	n/a	1.0	1.0	1.0	1.0	

Featural agreement /s/ → [d]: small manner deduction of −0.1666; small voicing deduction of −0.2222; FA = 0.6112

Target	/	h	o	ɹ	s		s	p	ɹ	e	ɪ	ŋ	/
Child production	[	h	o	w	s		s	p		e	ɪ	ŋ	]
GSA		1.0					5/6 = 0.84						
FA		1.0	1.0	0.83	1.0		1.0	1.0	n/a	1.0	1.0	1.0	

Featural agreement /ɹ/ → [w]: small manner deduction of −0.1666; FA = 0.8334

Target	/	l	ʊ	k	z		l	ʊ	k	ɪ	ŋ		/
Child production	[	w	ʊ	k	z		w	ʊ	k	ɪ	ŋ		]
GSA		1.0					1.0						
FA		0.75	1.0	1.0	1.0		0.67	1.0	1.0	1.0	1.0		

Featural agreement /l/ → [w]: small manner deduction of −0.1666; teeny place deduction of −0.883; FA = 0.7501

Target	/	dʒ	ʌ	s	t		d	ɹ	a	ɪ	e	ɹ	/
Child production	[	d	ʌ	s			b		a	ɪ	e	ɹ	]
GSA		3/4 = 0.75					4.5/5.5 = 0.818						
FA		0.67	1.0	1.0	n/a		0.75	n/a	1.0	1.0	1.0	1.0	

Featural agreement /d/ → [b]: big place deduction of –0.25; FA = 0.75

Target	/	m	i	ɹ	ə	ɹ		p	o	ɹ	ɪ	ŋ	/
Child production	[	m	i	w	ə	ɹ		p	o	w	ɪ	ŋ	]
GSA		1.0						1.0					
FA		1.0	1.0	0.83	1.0	1.0		1.0	1.0	0.83	1.0	1.0	

Target	/	ɹ	e	d	i	o		p	u	t	ɪ	ŋ	/
Child production	[	w	e	d	i	o		b	u	t	ɪ	n	]
GSA		1.0						1.0					
FA		0.83	1.0	1.0	1.0	1.0		0.78	1.0	1.0	1.0	0.83	

Featural agreement /p/ → [b]: small voicing deduction of –0.2222; FA = 0.7778

Featural agreement /ŋ/ → [n]: small place deduction of –0.1666; FA = 0.8334

Target	/	ʊ	ð	ə	ɹ		ɹ	ɑ	ɪ	d	ɪ	ŋ	/
Child production	[	ʊ	d	ə	ɹ		w	ɑ	ɪ	d	ɪ	ŋ	]
GSA		1.0					1.0						
FA		1.0	0.67	1.0	1.0		0.83	1.0	1.0	1.0	1.0	1.0	

Target	/	ɹ	ɑ	ɪ	d	ɪ	ŋ		ɹ	ɑ	ɪ	t	/
Child production	[	w	ɑ	ɪ	d	ɪ	n		w	ɑ	ɪ	t	]
GSA		1.0							1.0				
FA		0.83	1.0	1.0	1.0	1.0	0.83		0.83	1.0	1.0	1.0	

Target	/	s	ʌ	m		ð	ɛ	m		ð	ɛ	n	/
Child production	[	d	ʌ	m		d	ɛ	m		d	ɛ	n	]
GSA		1.0				1.0				1.0			
FA		0.61	1.0	1.0		0.67	1.0	1.0		0.67	1.0	1.0	

Target	/	s	t	ɛ	ɹ	z		l	ɑ	ɪ	k		/
Child production	[		d	ɛ	w	z		w	ɑ	ɪ	k		]
GSA		4/5 = 0.8						1.0					
FA		n/a	0.78	1.0	0.83	1.0		0.67	1.0	1.0	1.0		

Featural agreement /t/ → [b]: big place deduction of −0.25; small voicing deduction of −0.2222; FA = 0.5278

Target	/	s	t	ʊ	f		t	ɛ	ɹ	n	ɪ	ŋ	/
Child production	[	f		ʊ	s		d	ɛ		n	ɪ	ŋ	]
GSA		3/4= 0.75					5/6 = 0.84						
FA		0.75	n/a	1.0	0.75		0.78	1.0	n/a	1.0	1.0	1.0	

Featural agreement /s/ → [f]: big place deduction of −0.25; FA = 0.75

Target	/	t	æ	n	k		t	ɛ	ɹ	n	ɪ	ŋ	/
Child production	[	d	æ	n	k		d	ɑ			ɪ	ŋ	]
GSA		1.0					4/6 = 0.667						
FA		0.78	1.0	1.0	1.0		0.78	0.70	n/a	n/a	1.0	1.0	

Featural agreement /ɛ/ → [ɑ]: teeny height deduction of 0.1; small front deduction of 0.2; FA = 0.7

Target	/	w	ɪ	θ		ð	ɛ	ɹ		ð	ə	ɹ	/
Child production	[	w	ɪ	s		d	ɛ	ɹ		d	ə	ɹ	]
GSA		1.0				1.0				1.0			
FA		1.0	1.0	0.83		0.67	1.0	1.0		0.67	1.0	1.0	

Featural agreement /θ/ → [s]: small place deduction of −0.1666; FA = 0.8334

Target	/	θ	ɪ	ŋ	z		θ	ɪ	ŋ	z			/
Child production	[	t	ɪ	ŋ	z		d	ɪ	ŋ	z			]
GSA		1.0					1.0						
FA		0.67	1.0	1.0	1.0		0.44	1.0	1.0	1.0			

Featural agreement /θ/ → [t]: small manner deduction of −0.1666; small place deduction of −0.1666; FA = 0.6668

Featural agreement /θ/ → [d]: small manner deduction of −0.1666; small place deduction of −0.1666; small voicing deduction of −0.2222; FA = 0.4446

Target	/	θ	ɪ	ŋ	k		θ	ɪ	ŋ	k			/
Child production	[	t	ɪ	ŋ	k		d	ɪ	ŋ	k			]
GSA		1.0					1.0						
FA		0.67	1.0	1.0	1.0		0.44	1.0	1.0	1.0			

Target	/	θ	ɪ	ŋ	k		t	ɹ	ɑ	ɪ	ɪ	ŋ	/
Child production	[	d	ɪ	ŋ	k		b		ɑ	ɪ	ɪ	ŋ	]
GSA		1.0					4.5/5.5 = 0.818						
FA		0.44	1.0	1.0	1.0		0.53	n/a	1.0	1.0	1.0	1.0	

Featural agreement /t/ → [d]: small voicing deduction of −0.2222; FA = 0.7778

Target	/	ʌ	p	s	t	ɛ	ɹ	z		l	ʊ	k	/
Child production	[	ʌ	p		d	ɛ	w	z		w	ʊ	k	]
GSA		6/7 = 0.857								1.0			
FA		1.0	1.0	n/a	0.78	1.0	0.83	1.0		0.75	1.0	1.0	

List of words produced accurately:

Number of slots filled in both the Target and Child Production lines

Target	GSA	FA
"are" → [ɑɹ]	1.0	2.0
"away" → [æwe]	1.0	3.0
"baby" → [beɪbi]	1.0	5.0
"baby's" → [beɪbiz]	1.0	6.0
"back" → [bæk]	1.0	3.0
"bed'"→ [bɛd]	1.0	3.0
"big" → [bɪg]	1.0	3.0
"dancing" → [dænsɪŋ]	1.0	6.0
"dog" → [dɑg]	1.0	3.0
"dog's" → [dɑgz]	1.0	4.0
"don't" → [dont]	1.0	4.0
"down" → [daʊn]	1.0	4.0
"eating" → [idɪŋ]	1.0	4.0
"falled" → [faʊld]	1.0	5.0
"finds" → [faɪndz]	1.0	6.0
"foot" → [fʊt]	1.0	3.0
"he" → [hi]	1.0	2.0
"he's" → [hiz]	1.0	3.0
"hey" → [he]	1.0	2.0
"him" → [him]	1.0	3.0
"his" → [hiz]	1.0	3.0
"home" → [hom]	1.0	3.0
"hose" → [hoz]	1.0	3.0
"in" → [ɪn]	1.0	2.0
"is" → [ɪz]	1.0	2.0
"know" → [no]	1.0	2.0

Target	GSA	FA
"laying" → [leɪŋ]	1.0	4.0
"like" → [laɪk]	1.0	4.0
"looking" → [lʊkɪŋ]	1.0	5.0
"made" → [med]	1.0	3.0
"makeup" → [mekʌp]	1.0	5.0
"maybe" → [mebi]	1.0	4.0
"mess" → [mɛs]	1.0	3.0
"milk" → [mɪlk]	1.0	4.0
"mom" → [mɑm]	1.0	3.0
"off" → [ɑf]	1.0	2.0
"on" → [ɑn]	1.0	2.0
"opening" → [opɛnɪŋ]	1.0	6.0
"or" → [oɹ]	1.0	2.0
"out" → [aʊt]	1.0	3.0
"putting" → [pʊɾɪŋ]	1.0	5.0
"standing" → [stændɪŋ]	1.0	7.0
"to" → [tu]	1.0	2.0
"up" → [ʌp]	1.0	2.0
"was" → [wɑz]	1.0	3.0
"walking" → [wɑkɪŋ]	1.0	5.0
"washing" → [wɑʃɪŋ]	1.0	5.0
"where's" → [wɛɪz]	1.0	4.0
"window" → [wɪndo]	1.0	5.0
"yeah" → [jæ]	1.0	2.0
"you" → [ju]	1.0	2.0

Total of the GSA scores for each word

Total number of words in the sample

Total Global Structural Agreement score: 102.541 / 106 = 0.9674

Total of the GSA scores for each word

Total number of words in the sample

Total Featural Agreement score: 378.10 / 393 = 0.9621

Total GSA multiplied by Total FA

WSSA: 0.9674 × 0.9621 = 0.9307

WSSA for the language sample obtained from Case Study 6–4 at the Follow-Up Assessment (age 5;10).

Words produced inaccurately:

Item	Target	Child's Production	GSA	FA
"always"	/ɑlweɪz/	[ɑwweɪz]	1.0	1+0.75+1+1+1+1= 5.75
"bath"	/bæθ/	[bæf]	1.0	1+1+0.83= 2.83
"bread"	/bɹɛd/	[bwɛd]	1.0	1+0.83+1+1= 3.83
"Carl"	/kaɹl/	[kawl]	1.0	1+1+0.83+1= 3.83
"climbs"	/klaɪmz/	[kwaɪmz]	1.0	1+0.75+1+1+1+1= 5.75
"downstairs"	/daʊnstɛɪz/	[daʊnstɛwz]	1.0	1+1+1+1+1+1+1+0.75+1= 8.75
"dress"	/dɹɛs/	[dwɛs]	1.0	1+0.83+1+1= 3.83
"falls"	/fɑlz/	[fɑwz]	1.0	1+1+0.75+1= 3.75
"gorilla"	/goɹɪlɑ/	[gowɪwɑ]	1.0	1+1+0.83+1+0.75+1= 5.58
"grapes"	/gɹeɪps/	[gweɪps]	1.0	1+0.83+1+1+1+1= 5.83
"him"	/hɪm/	[n]	1/3 = 0.67	0.75
"I'll"	/aɪl/	[aɪw]	1.0	1+1+0.75= 2.75
"laundry"	/lɑndɹi/	[wɑndwi]	1.0	0.75+1+1+1+0.83+1= 5.58
"leaving"	/livɪŋ/	[wivɪŋ]	1.0	0.75+1+1+1+1= 4.75

Item	Target	Child's Production	GSA	FA
"looks"	/lʊks/	[wʊks]	1.0	0.75+1+1+1= 3.75
"looking"	/lʊkɪŋ/	[wʊkɪŋ]	1.0	0.75+1+1+1+1= 4.75
"mouth"	/maʊθ/	[maʊf]	1.0	1+1+1+0.83= 3.83
"of"	/ʌv/	[ʌ]	1/2= 0.50	1
"play"	/pleɪ/	[pweɪ]	1.0	1+0.75+1+1= 3.75
"radio"	/ɹeɪdio/	[weɪdio]	1.0	0.83+1+1+1+1+1= 5.83
"shortly"	/ʃoɹtli/	[ʃoɹtwi]	1.0	1+1+1+1+0.75+1= 5.75
"stairs"	/stɛɹz/	[stɛwz]	1.0	1+1+1+0.83+1= 4.83
"the"	/ðə/	[də]	1.0	0.67+1= 1.67
"then"	/ðɛn/	[dɛn]	1.0	0.67+1+1= 2.67
"they"	/ðeɪ/	[deɪ]	1.0	0.67+1+1= 2.67
"thing"	/θɪŋ/	[sɪŋ]	1.0	0.83+1+1= 2.83
"tries"	/tɹaɪz/	[twaɪz]	1.0	1+0.83+1+1+1= 4.83
"turns"	/tʌɹnz/	[tʌwnz]	1.0	1+1+0.83+1+1= 4.83
"upstairs"	/ʌpstɛɹz/	[ʌpstɛwz]	1.0	1+1+1+1+1+0.83+1= 6.83

Words produced accurately:

Target	GSA	FA
"after" → [æftəɹ]	1.0	5.0
"and" → [ænd]	1.0	3.0
"awake" → [ʌweɪk]	1.0	5.0
"baby" → [beɪbi]	1.0	5.0
"baby's" → [beɪbiz]	1.0	5.0
"back" → [bæk]	1.0	3.0
"basement" → [beɪsmɪnt]	1.0	8.0
"be" → [bi]	1.0	2.0
"bubbles" → [bʌblz]	1.0	5.0

Target	GSA	FA
"in" → [ɪn]	1.0	5.0
"it" → [ɪt]	1.0	2.0
"look" → [lʊk]	1.0	3.0
"mom" → [mʌm]	1.0	3.0
"mom's" → [mʌmz]	1.0	3.0
"of" → [ʌv]	1.0	4.0
"off" → [ɑf]	1.0	3.0
"on" → [ɑn]	1.0	4.0
"opens" → [opɛnz]	1.0	4.0

Target	GSA	FA
"coming" → [kʌmɪŋ]	1.0	5.0
"cookies" → [kʊkiz]	1.0	5.0
"dances" → [dænsɪz]	1.0	6.0
"does" → [dʌz]	1.0	3.0
"doesn't" → [dʌznt]	1.0	5.0
"dog" → [dɑg]	1.0	3.0
"dog's" → [dɑgz]	1.0	4.0
"down" → [daʊn]	1.0	4.0
"dries" → [draiz]	1.0	5.0
"eat" → [it]	1.0	2.0
"eats" → [its]	1.0	3.0
"fish" → [fiʃ]	1.0	3.0
"get" → [gɛt]	1.0	3.0
"gets" → [gɛts]	1.0	4.0
"go" → [goʊ]	1.0	3.0
"goes" → [goʊz]	1.0	4.0
"guard" → [gɑɹd]	1.0	4.0
"has" → [hæz]	1.0	3.0
"he" → [hi]	1.0	2.0
"helps" → [hɛlps]	1.0	4.0
"him" → [him]	1.0	3.0
"his" → [hiz]	1.0	3.0
"home" → [hom]	1.0	3.0
"if" → [ɪf]	1.0	2.0

Target	GSA	FA
"out" → [aʊt]	1.0	3.0
"puts" → [pʌts]	1.0	2.0
"room" → [rum]	1.0	4.0
"sees" → [siz]	1.0	3.0
"soda" → [soʊdɑ]	1.0	3.0
"some" → [sʌm]	1.0	3.0
"something" → [sʌmθɪŋ]	1.0	2.0
"standing" → [stændɪŋ]	1.0	5.0
"stuff" → [stʌf]	1.0	4.0
"tank" → [tæŋk]	1.0	4.0
"the" → [ðə]	1.0	2.0
"then" → [ðɛn]	1.0	3.0
"think" → [θɪŋk]	1.0	4.0
"to" → [tu]	1.0	2.0
"too" → [tu]	1.0	2.0
"tub" → [tʌb]	1.0	3.0
"up" → [ʌp]	1.0	2.0
"uses" → [juzɪz]	1.0	5.0
"using" → [juzɪŋ]	1.0	5.0
"was" → [wʌz]	1.0	3.0
"wants" → [wɑnts]	1.0	5.0
"washes" → [wɑʃɪz]	1.0	5.0
"window" → [wɪndo]	1.0	5.0
"would" → [wʊd]	1.0	3.0

Total GSA score: 94.17 / 95 = 0.9913

Total FA score: 363.38 / 370 = 0.9821

WSSA: 0.9736

PA 224 obtained a WSSA score of 0.9307 at Intake, and a score of 0.9736 one year later, showing improvement in his speech. In particular, whereas PA 224 omitted segments from complex onsets and codas at intake, he only omitted segments on two occasions at the reassessment. The segments omitted then are well mastered by PA 224, and are in words he had properly produced on a few occasions; therefore, these errors might be due to coarticulation and a fast rate of speech (/hɪm/ → [n]; /ʌv/ → [v]). Closer inspection of the language sample at the follow-up reveals that the only segmental speech errors remaining were /l/ → [w], /ɹ/ → [w], /ð/ → [d], /θ/ → [f], and /θ/ → [s], with no prosodic errors other than the two instances mentioned previously. Of particular interest for PA 224 is the result obtained on SAILS at the time of the re-assessment (74.3%); performance on the /l/, /k/, /ɹ/, and /s/ modules for children in kindergarten should be 82.09%, with a standard deviation of 6.10 (see Table 5–5). PA 224's *z*-score therefore is −1.28 and input-focused intervention methods to be covered in Chapter 9 might be most appropriate for him.

Analyses to Help Predict Error Patterns That May Change Without Intervention

6.3.1. Describe the protocol for predictive assessment of distortions of sibilants proposed by Smit, Hand, Freilinger, Bernthal, and Bird (1990).

6.3.2. Identify two strategies that are helpful in determining whether a covert contrast is present in the child's speech.

A detailed analysis of the speech sample reveals what is present in the child system and what is absent; in addition it helps predict what is absent but may emerge without treatment, and what is emerging but may become mastered without intervention. This information is useful for diagnostic purposes and to decide whether the child should receive intervention and, if so, which treatment targets should be selected. The last section of this chapter is concerned with the predictive value of the speech sample analysis for diagnostic purposes and its general usefulness for selecting treatment goals; in particular the protocol for predictive assessment proposed by Smit, Hand, Freilinger, Bernthal, and Bird (1990) and covert contrast will be discussed below. Decisions as to whether the child should receive an intervention and detailed treatment planning including goal selection goal attack strategies are covered in Chapter 8.

Detailed analysis of the speech sample may also have **predictive value** that is helpful for diagnostic purposes and the selection of treatment goals.

Protocol for Predictive Assessment

Smith et al. (1990) had difficulty determining a clear expected age of acquisition for /s/ and /z/, since their growth curves were unstable between the ages of 6 and 9. Standardized articulation tests typically probe for production of these phonemes on one occasion in the initial, medial, and final positions; a preschool-age child may therefore obtain a percentile rank indicating a phonological delay if all singleton sibilants and consonant clusters containing sibilants were produced with a distortion, even though no other articulation errors are recorded during the test administration. Not all error types are equally worrisome; for instance, dental distortions of sibilants are typical and may resolve spontaneously whereas lateral distortions are atypical and unlikely to resolve without intervention. Nonetheless, on a standardized articulation test a child would obtain the same score whether sibilants were produced with a dental or lateral distortion. Smit and colleagues therefore proposed a predictive assessment to decide whether intervention is warranted. The language sample usually provides many more exemplars of production of sibilants, especially in English as the phonemes /s/ and /z/ are frequent and are prominent in the morphology of the language. Case Study 6–5 (PA 201) presents a child who was referred for a speech-language assessment by his family doctor and was enrolled in a longitudinal follow-up study of children with speech delay. PA 201 was first assessed in the spring of the prekindergarten year (age 4;10) and reassessed a year later (age 5;9).

According to the predictive assessment protocol of Smit et al. (1990), a child should not be treated for distortions of sibilants before the age of 7 unless the error pattern is atypical.

At the initial assessment, several speech errors were noted on the GFTA-2; as listed in Case Study 6–5, these errors included omissions, substitutions, and typical and atypical distortion errors, all involving phonemes not yet expected to be mastered by a 4-year-old child. The percentile rank obtained on the GFTA at that time indicated a mild speech delay for the child's age. The SLP must now decide whether to offer treatment or "wait and see" if these errors will correct spontaneously.

At the age of 7 the child should be reassessed; if the child's upper incisors have not yet erupted, if any correct productions of /s/ and /z/ occur in the speech sample, or if the child is stimulable for correct production of these phonemes, treatment should be delayed.

According to the predictive assessment protocol of Smit and colleagues, a child should not be treated for distortions of sibilants before the age of 7 unless the error pattern is atypical. At the age of 7 the child should be reassessed; if the child's upper incisors have not yet erupted, if any correct productions of /s/ and /z/ occur in the speech sample, or if the child is stimulable for correct production of these phonemes, treatment should be delayed. The child should then be reassessed at 8 years and treatment should be initiated if no changes have occurred in the past year or if participation restrictions are present. In other cases, the child should be reassessed at the age of 9 years and treatment should begin if distortions are still present in the child's speech. It is important to note that the predictive assessment applies specifically to distortion errors;

The child should then be reassessed at 8 years and treatment should be initiated if no changes have occurred in the past year or if participation restrictions are present.

In other cases, the child should be reassessed at the age of 9 years and treatment should begin if distortions are still present in the child's speech.

Case Study 6–5

Case History: Child (PA201) was born at term following an uneventful pregnancy and birth. In terms of developmental history, the child walked independently at 14 months and produced his first words at 15 months; word combinations appeared a few months after the age of 2 years. The medical history is unremarkable. The mother received speech therapy in elementary school for articulation difficulties.

Summary of Scores Obtained at Prekindergarten (CA = 4;10)

PPVT-III	86th percentile
MLU	7.72
GFTA-2	11th percentile
PCC	75.5%, z = −0.59
SAILS	63%, z = −2.23
PAT	Raw score = 18, z = −0.76
Letters	Raw score = 12

Summary of Scores Obtained at Kindergarten Assessment (CA = 5;9)

PPVT-III	95th percentile
MLU	5.71
GFTA-2	14th percentile
PCC	75.17%, z = −1.48
SAILS	87%, z = 0.80
PAT	Raw score = 33, z = 1.04
Letters	Raw score = 12

Speech errors noted on GFTA-2

/s/	[s̪] in initial, medial, final positions
/z/	[z̪] in initial, medial, final positions
/ʃ/	[ɬ] in initial, medial, final positions
/tʃ/	[ts̪] in initial, medial, final positions
/dʒ/	[dz̪] in initial, medial, final positions
/θ/	[f] initial and final; omitted medial
/ð/	[d] initial, [v] in medial position
/l/	[l̪] final position
/ɹ/	[w] initial and medial, omitted final
/Cɹ/	[C–] or [Cw] on 4/6 instances
/sC/	[s̪C] on 2/4 instances

Speech errors noted on GFTA-2

/s/	[s̪] in initial, medial, final positions
/ʃ/	[ɬ] in initial, medial, final positions
/tʃ/	[ts] in initial, medial, final positions
/θ/	[f] in initial, medial, final positions
/ð/	[d] initial, [v] in medial position
/ɹ/	[ə] in medial and final positions
/Cɹ/	[Cw] on 4/6 instances
/sC/	[s̪C] on 2/4 instances

Example sentences from prekindergarten speech sample

And the dog's pushing the baby.
ænd də dɑgz̪ pʊɬɪŋ də bebi.

The baby's like playing with those toys.
də bebis̪ laik pleɪŋ wɪ doz toiz̪.

The dog's like has the gloves on his mouth.
də dɑgz̪ laik hæz̪ dæ glʌvz̪ ɑn hɪz̪ maʊf.

The dog pulling like its pajamas and trying to xx.
də dɑg pʊtɪŋ laik ɪts̪ pædz̪æməz̪ æn pɹaiɪŋ tu xx.

And they took all the creatures out.
ænt de tʊk də kɹitjəz aʊ.

Example sentences from kindergarten speech sample

The baby's pulling the dog's ear.
də bebiz pʊlɪŋ də dɑgz ɪɹ.

They're going to a food shop and now they're eating.
dəɹ goɪŋ to e fʊd ɬɑp ænd naw dəɹ itɪŋ.

Little crackers or cookies and he's eating dog biscuits.
lɪtəl kwækəɹz ɔɹ kʊkiz̪ ænd hiz itɪŋ dɑg bɪs̪kəts̪.

Take them out of the cage and play.
teɪk dəm aʊt əv də keɪdʒ ænd pleɪ.

Sometimes on hockey games you see a lot of TVs.
s̪ɑmtaɪmz ɑn hɑki geɪmz ju si ə lɑt əv tiviz.

Notes. PPVT-III = Peabody Picture Vocabulary Test-III (Dunn & Dunn, 1997); MLU = Mean Length of Utterance (in morphemes); GFTA-2 = Goldman-Fristoe Test of Articulation-2 (Goldman & Fristoe, 2000); PCC = Percent Consonants Correct, assessed in conversation (see Chapters 4 and 5); SAILS = Speech Assessment and Interactive Learning System (measure of speech perception skills; see http://www.medicine.mcgill.ca/srvachew); PAT = Phonological Awareness Test (Bird, Bishop, & Freeman, 1995); Letters = number of letters named. The speech samples were obtained with the wordless book *Carl Goes Shopping,* by Alexandra Day.

if the child completely delinks the [+continuant] feature from target sibilants resulting in a stop substitution, treatment should begin much earlier than 7 years of age. In the case of PA 201, treatment would not be initiated on the basis of the dental distortions of /s/ and /z/ alone because these are typical developmental errors for a child of this age; the fact that two correct productions of /z/ were present during the speech sample at the initial assessment further indicates that accurate production of this phoneme is emerging. The errors observed for the interdental fricatives, affricates, and liquids are also typical developmental errors that could be monitored for spontaneous improvement. However, the lateral distortion of /ʃ/ is of significant concern and thus it is not surprising that this child was scheduled to receive treatment in his prekindergarten year. In accordance with the hospital protocol, intervention was rationed to a 4-month block and then he was transferred to the school jurisdiction where he was placed on the wait list for service.

The predictive assessment applies specifically to distortion errors; if the child completely delinks the [+continuant] feature from target sibilants resulting in a stop substitution, treatment should begin much earlier than 7 years of age.

Unfortunately, PA 201 did not make gains for production of /ʃ/ despite the intervention, confirming that lateral distortions are indeed a very difficult error to treat. Validating the predictive assessment protocol however, he showed improvements for /s, z, tʃ, dʒ, ɹ/ even though these phonemes were not the target of the speech therapy intervention. PA 201 did receive intervention specifically aimed at improving his phonological awareness abilities. The reassessment at the age of 5;9 revealed great improvement on the Phonological Awareness Test (PAT; Bird, Bishop, & Freeman, 1995) and on the Speech Assessment and Interactive Learning System (SAILS; AVAAZ Innovations,1994). The percentile rank obtained on the GFTA-2, although it increased by 3 points, continues to indicate a mild speech delay for his age. The PCC in conversation did not change corresponding to a *z*-score −1.5 standard deviations from the mean during the kindergarten assessment. He continues to be a candidate for intervention due to the persistence of this atypical error in his speech. For contrast, we direct the reader to Case Study 8–3, a child whose typical distortion errors resolved gradually and spontaneously.

In brief, Smith et al. offer a predictive assessment protocol for distortions of late developing sibilants and/or liquids (questionable residual errors, to be defined in Chapter 7). For other error patterns similar factors help the clinician decide whether the child is likely to make progress without intervention: is the error pattern typical and developmental?; is the child stimulable for production of the phoneme or syllable shape?; does the child demonstrate knowledge of the contrast and, if so, at which levels of representation?; are any correct productions present in the single-word and/or conversational speech sample? In certain cases closer examination at the acoustic level is necessary to determine whether the child is neutralizing a contrast or whether a covert contrast is present.

Covert Contrasts

Speech samples are transcribed using the IPA, which is a categorical system, and therefore it cannot capture finergrained speech-sound variations.

Covert contrasts occur when children produce acoustic differences between two sounds, but these are perceived by adults as belonging to the same category and therefore are transcribed with the same phonetic symbol.

Kent (1996) suggested supplementing transcription with acoustic analysis to understand the child's phonological knowledge as it provides detailed information about the child's phonological knowledge at the acoustic level which cannot necessarily be perceived by the human ear.

Acoustic analysis is a potentially useful tool to predict whether the child is likely to need intervention to remediate an error pattern (e.g., in the case that there is no covert contrast and the child does not produce the two target phonemes differently).

Speech samples are transcribed using the IPA, which is a categorical system. One limitation due to the categorical nature of the IPA is that it cannot capture finer grained speech-sound variations (Munson, Edwards, Schellinger, Beckman, & Meyer, 2010). Because children's acquisition of speech contrasts is continuous or gradual, they may first produce two targets in exactly the same manner (such as /s/ and /ʃ/), then produce an intermediate production of /ʃ/, and finally produce audibly different productions of both phonemes. Covert contrasts occur when children produce acoustic differences between two sounds, but these are perceived by adults as belonging to the same category and are therefore transcribed with the same phonetic symbol. Macken and Barton (1980) first described covert contrasts for Voiced Onset Times (VOTs) of voiced and voiceless stops (see Figure 3–11 and associated discussion). Covert contrasts have since been found for various contrasts in the speech of normally developing children and children with DPD, including place of articulation of fricatives (e.g., Baum & McNutt, 1990; Li, Edwards, & Beckman, 2009) and place of articulation for stops (e.g., Forrest, Weismer, Hodge, Dinnsen, & Elbert, 1990). The presence of a covert contrast is important clinically because children who exhibit one have been shown to make progress more rapidly during intervention (Tyler, Figurski, & Langdale, 1993). Covert contrasts therefore are useful to predict whether the child is likely to make progress with production of a specific contrast without intervention.

Kent (1996) suggested supplementing transcription with acoustic analysis to understand the child's phonological knowledge. In the example provided in Figure 1–21, productions of /s/ and /θ/ by the 5-year-old girl were all perceived as [θ]; acoustic analysis of the spectral characteristics revealed that she differentiated them on the basis of the duration of the fricative noise but produced them with the same mean centroid. In order to verify the presence or absence of a covert contrast many tokens for a single type of exemplar is necessary. Acoustic analysis has the advantage of providing detailed information about the child's phonological knowledge at the level of articulatory-phonetic and phonological representations, even when the child's expression of this knowledge is not perceptible to the adult listener. Acoustic analysis is a potentially useful tool to predict whether the child is likely to need intervention to remediate an error pattern (e.g., in the case that there is no covert contrast and the child does not produce the two target phonemes differently). However, it is time consuming and we do not advocate routinely conducting acoustic analyses on the child's speech sample.

The acoustic signal contains a wealth of information and many cues typically differentiate between contrasts, but only a few parameters are measured in acoustic analyses. For instance, whereas VOT itself differentiates stop voicing, several cues also play a role in voicing contrast, including ratio of first to second harmonic amplitudes (Kong, 2009) and fundamental frequency at the beginning of the following vowel (Haggard, Summerfield, & Roberts, 1981). Therefore, Stoel-Gammon (2001) and Edwards and Beckman (2008) proposed that transcribers distinguish between clearly accurate productions of a target, intermediate productions, and clear substitutions, creating a continuum of possible listener responses. More specifically, in the Edwards and Beckman study adults transcribed responses as either correct (e.g., /s/ → [s]); clear substitution (e.g., /s/ → [θ]); intermediate between the two sounds ([s]: [θ] for "in between /s/ and /θ/ but more like /s/" and [θ]: [s] for "in between /s/ and /θ/ but more like /θ/"), and distortion (e.g., /s/ → [ɬ]). Another method to create a continuum of possible responses using the phonetic symbols of the IPA is Visual Analog Scaling as described in Urberg-Carlson, Kaiser, and Munson (2008) and shown in Figure 6–13.

Transcribers can distinguish between clearly accurate productions of a target, intermediate productions, and clear substitutions, creating a continuum of possible listener responses.

Another method to create a continuum of possible responses using the phonetic symbols of the IPA is **Visual Analog Scaling** as shown in Figure 6–13.

The continuum of possible transcription responses represents an option which is less time-consuming and more easily implemented when transcribing the speech sample either during the speech-language assessment or when listening to the recording. The information gathered by using the continuum of possible responses provides further information about the child's underlying knowledge of phonological units and phonemic contrasts.

This chapter has stressed that a thorough analysis of the child's speech data is essential to understand the child's underlying phonological system which, in turn, is necessary for selecting treatment goals and monitoring treatment progress. In Chapter 7 we discuss the scientific literature on DPD, indicating how assessment data can be combined with the outcome of the speech sample analysis to generate hypotheses about the underlying nature of the child's speech impairment. Integrating and interpreting all the assessment data in view of what is known about etiological factors in DPD is an important final step before choosing an approach to intervention that is best suited for an individual child.

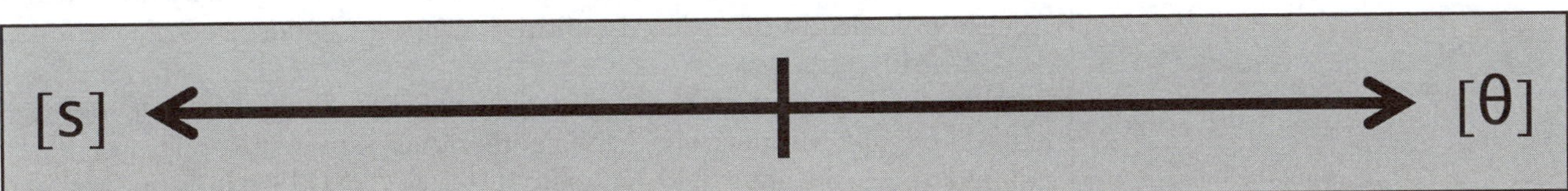

Figure 6–13. *Example of a Visual Analog Scale. A horizontal line is used and the endpoints represent the two contrasting phonemes.*

References

Baum, S. R., & McNutt, J. C. (1990). An acoustic analysis of frontal misarticulation on /s/ in children. *Journal of Phonetics, 18*, 51–63.

Bernhardt, B. (1990). *Application of nonlinear phonological theory to intervention with six phonologically disordered children*. Unpublished PhD dissertation, University of British Columbia, Vancouver.

Bernhardt, B. (1992). The application of nonlinear phonological theory to intervention with one phonologically disordered child. *Clinical Linguistics & Phonetics, 6*(4), 283–316.

Bernhardt, B., & Gilbert, J. (1992). Applying linguistic theory to speech-language pathology: The case for nonlinear phonology. *Clinical Linguistics & Phonetics, 6*(1–2), 123–145.

Bernhardt, B. H., & Holdgrafer, G. (2001b). Beyond the basics II: Supplemental sampling for in-depth phonological analysis. *Language, Speech, and Hearing Services in Schools, 32*(1), 28–37.

Bernhardt, B. H. & Stemberger, J. P. (2000). *Workbook in nonlinear phonology for clinical application*. Austin, TX: Pro-Ed.

Bernhardt, B., & Stoel-Gammon, C. (1994). Nonlinear phonology: Introduction and clinical application. *Journal of Speech and Hearing Research, 37*, 123–143.

Bird, J., Bishop, D. V. M., & Freeman, N. H. (1995). Phonological awareness and literacy development in children with expressive phonological impairments. *Journal of Speech and Hearing Research, 38*(2), 446–462.

Brosseau-Lapré, F., Rvachew, S., & Laukys, K. (2010, November). *Consonant inventory of preschool French-speaking children with speech sound disorders*. Poster session presented at the annual convention of the American Speech-Language-Hearing Association, Philadelphia, PA.

Dinnsen, D. A., Chin, S. B., Elbert, M., & Powell, T. W. (1990). Some constraints on functionally disordered phonologies: Phonetic inventories and phonotactics. *Journal of Speech and Hearing Research, 33*, 28–37.

Dodd, B., & Iacano, T. (1989). Phonological disorders in children: Changes in phonological process use during treatment. *British Journal of Disorders of Communication, 24*, 333–351.

Dunn, L. M., & Dunn, L. M. (1997). *Peabody Picture Vocabulary Test* (3rd ed.). Circle Pines, MN: American Guidance Service.

Edwards, J., & Beckman, M. E. (2008). Methodological questions in studying consonant acquisition. *Clinical Linguistics & Phonetics, 22*, 937–956.

Fey, M. E. (1992). Articulation and phonology: An introduction. *Language, Speech, and Hearing Services in Schools, 23*, 224–232.

Forrest, K., Weismer, G., Hodge, M., Dinnsen, D. A., & Elbert, M. (1990). Statistical analysis of word-initial /k/ and /t/ produced by normal and phonologically disordered children. *Clinical Linguistics & Phonetics, 4*, 327–340.

Goldman, R., & Fristoe, M. (2000). *Goldman Fristoe Test of Articulation—Second Edition*. Minneapolis, MN: Pearson Assessments.

Haggard, M., Summerfield, Q., & Roberts, M. (1981).Psychoacoustical and cultural determinants of phoneme boundaries: evidence from trading f0 cues in the voiced-voiceless distinction. *Journal of Phonetics, 9*, 49–62.

Hodson, B. W. (1980). *The Assessment of Phonological Processes*. Austin, TX: Pro-Ed.

Hodson, B. W. (1986). *The Assessment of Phonological Processes-Revised.* Austin, TX: Pro-Ed.

Hodson, B. (2003). *Hodson Computerized Analysis of Phonological Patterns* (3rd ed.). Wichita, KS: Phonocomp Software.

Hodson, B. W. (2004). *Hodson's Assessment of Phonological Patterns* (3rd ed.). Austin, TX: Pro-Ed.

Ingram, D. (1981). *Procedures for the phonological analysis of children's language*. Baltimore, MD: University Park Press.

Ingram, D. (2002). The measurement of whole-word productions. *Journal of Child Language, 29,* 713–733.

Ingram, D., & Ingram, K. D. (2001). A whole-word approach to phonological analysis and intervention [Clinical forum]. *Language, Speech, and Hearing Services in Schools, 32,* 271–283.

Jakielski, K. J., Maytasse, R., & Doyle, E. (2006, November). *Acquisition of phonetic complexity in children 12 to 36 months of age*. Poster session presented at the annual convention of the American Speech-Language-Hearing Association, Miami, FL.

Kamhi, A. G. (1992). The need for a broad-based model of phonological disorders. *Language, Speech, and Hearing Services in Schools, 23,* 261–268.

Kent, R. (1996). Hearing and believing: some limits to the auditory-perceptual assessment of speech and voice disorders. *American Journal of Speech-Language Pathology, 5,* 7–23.

Klein, E. S., & Flint, C. B. (2006). Measurement of intelligibility in disordered speech. *Language, Speech, and Hearing Services in Schools, 37,* 191–199.

Kong, E. (2009). *The development of phonation-type contrasts in plosives: Cross-linguistic perspectives*. Unpublished PhD dissertation. Department of Linguistics, Ohio State University. Columbus, OH.

Li, F., Edwards, J., & Beckman, M. E. (2009). Contrast and covert contrast: The phonetic development of voiceless sibilant fricatives in English and Japanese toddlers. *Journal of Phonetics, 37,* 111–124.

Lof, G. L. (2002). Special forum on phonology: Two comments on this assessment series. *American Journal of Speech-Language Pathology, 11,* 255–256.

MacLeod, A. A. N., Sutton, A., Trudeau, N., & Thordardottir, E. (2011). The acquisition of consonants in Québécois French: A cross-sectional study of pre-school-aged children. *International Journal of Speech-Language Pathology, 13*(2), 93–109.

Macken, M., & Barton, D. (1980). The acquisition of the voicing contrast in English: A study of voice onset time in word-initial stop consonants. *Journal of Child Language, 7,* 41–74.

McCauley, R. J., & Swisher, L. (1984). Use and misuse of norm-referenced test in clinical assessment: A hypothetical case. *Journal of Speech and Hearing Disorders, 49,* 338–348.

McDonald, E. T. A. (1964). *A Deep Test of Articulation*. Pittsburgh, PA: Stanwix House.

Morris, S. R. (2009). Test–retest reliability of independent measures of phonology in the assessment of toddlers' speech. *Language, Speech, and Hearing Services in Schools, 40,* 46–52.

Morris, S. (2010). Clinical application of the mean babbling level and syllable structure level. *Language, Speech, and Hearing Services in Schools, 41,* 223–230.

Munson, B., Edwards, J., Schellinger, S. K., Beckman, M. E., & Meyer, M. K. (2010). Deconstructing phonetic transcription: covert contrast, perceptual bias, and an extraterrestrial view of Vox Humana. *Clinical Linguistics & Phonetics, 24*, 245–260.

O'Grady, W., & Dobrovolsky, M. (1997). *Contemporary linguistics* (3rd ed.). New York, NY: St. Martin's Press.

Oller, D. K., & Delgado, R. E. (1999). Logical international phonetic programs [Computer program]. Miami, FL: Intelligent Hearing Systems.

Oller, D. K., & Ramsdell, H. L. (2006). A weighted reliability measure for phonetic transcription. *Journal of Speech, Language, and Hearing Research, 49*, 1391–1411.

Osberger, M. J., Robbins, A. M., Todd, S. L., & Riley, A. I. (1994). Speech intelligibility of children with cochlear implants. *Volta Review, 96*(5), 169–180.

Paul, R., & Jennings, P. (1992). Phonological behavior in toddlers with slow expressive language development. *Journal of Speech and Hearing Research, 35*, 99–107.

Preston, J. L., Frost, S. J., Mencl, W. E., Fulbright, R. K., Landi, N., Grigorenko, E., Jacobsen, L. & Pugh, K.R. (2010). Early and late talkers: School-age language, literacy and neurolinguistic differences. *Brain, 133*(8), 2185–2195.

Prezas, R., & Hodson, B. (2007). Diagnostic evaluation of children with speech sound disorders. In S. Rvachew (Ed.), *Encyclopedia of language and literacy development* (Online, pp. 1–7). London, Ontario: Canadian Language and Literacy Research Network (http://www.literacyencyclopedia.ca).

Preston, J. L., Ramsdell, H. L., Oller, D. K., Edwards, M. L., & Tobin, S. J. (2011). Developing a weighted measure of speech sound accuracy. *Journal of Speech, Language, and Hearing Research, 54*, 1–18.

Schwartz, R. G., Leonard, L. B., Folger, M. K., & Wilcox, M. J. (1980). Early phonological behavior in normal-speaking and language disordered children: Evidence for a synergistic view of linguistic disorders. *Journal of Speech and Hearing Disorders, 45*, 357–377.

Shriberg, L. D., & Kwiatkowski, J. (1980). *Natural process analysis: A procedure for phonological analysis of continuous speech samples*. New York, NY: MacMillan.

Smit, A. B. (1993). Phonological error distributions in the Iowa-Nebraska Articulation Norms Project: Consonant singletons. *Journal of Speech and Hearing Research, 36*, 533–547.

Smit, A. B., Hand, L., Freilinger, J. J., Bernthal, J. E., & Bird, A. (1990). The Iowa articulation norms project and its Nebraska replication. *Journal of Speech and Hearing Disorders, 55*, 779–798.

Stampe, D. (1973). *A dissertation on natural phonology*. Unpublished doctoral dissertation, University of Chicago. Also published as: *A dissertation on natural phonology*, New York, NY: Garland Publishing, 1979.

Stoel-Gammon, C. (1987). Phonological skills of 2-year-olds. *Language, Speech, and Hearing Services in Schools, 18*, 323–329.

Stoel-Gammon, C. (1989). Pre-speech and early speech development of two late talkers. *First Language, 9*, 207–223.

Stoel-Gammon, C. (2001). Transcribing the speech of young children. *Topics in Language Disorders, 21*, 12–21.

Taelman, H., Durieux, G., & Gillis, S. (2005). Notes on Ingram's whole-word measures for phonological development. *Journal of Child Language, 32*, 391–405.

Thomas-Stonell, N. L., Oddson, B., Robertson, B., & Rosenbaum, P. L. (2010). Development of the FOCUS (Focus on the Outcomes of Communication Under Six), a communication outcome measure for preschool children. *Developmental Medicine and Child Neurology, 52*(1), 47–53.

Tyler, A. A., Figurski, G. R., & Langdale, T. (1993). Relationships between acoustically determined knowledge of stop place and voicing contrasts and phonological treatment progress. *Journal of Speech and Hearing Research, 36*, 746–759.

Urberg-Carlson, K., Kaiser, E., & Munson, B. (2008, November). *Assessment of children's speech production 2: Testing gradient measures of children's productions*. Poster presented at the annual convention of the American Speech-Language-Hearing Association, Chicago, IL.

Velleman, S. (2002). Phonotactic therapy. *Seminars in Speech and Language, 23*, 43–57.

Wilcox, K., & Morris, S. (1999). *Children's Speech Intelligibility Measure (CSIM)*. San Antonio, TX: Psychological Corporation.

Chapter 7

Nature of Developmental Phonological Disorders

Classification of Developmental Phonological Disorders

In Chapters 5 and 6 of Part II, procedures for assessing the child's phonology at multiple levels of phonological representation were presented. An important outcome of the assessment process is the detailed description of the child's overt speech and underlying phonological system that will emerge from the analysis procedures described in Chapter 6. This is not the end stage of the assessment process, however. It has long been recognized that the population of children with a developmental phonological disorder (DPD) is heterogeneous and it is commonly assumed that subgroups within this population will respond differentially to specific approaches to intervention. Therefore, the assessment should lead to a diagnosis that reflects your best hypothesis about the underlying nature of the child's phonological disorder.

The population of children with a **developmental phonological disorder** is heterogeneous and it is commonly assumed that subgroups within this population will respond differentially to specific approaches to intervention.

Assessment should lead to a **diagnosis** that reflects your best hypothesis about the underlying nature of the child's phonological disorder.

Although it is generally agreed that children with phonological disorders do not form a unitary population, there is no consensus on the criteria by which children might be classified into subtypes. In theory, the different classification schemes that are used by clinicians and researchers are based to a greater or lesser extent on criteria at the linguistic, psycholinguistic, or etiological levels of description. In practice, all of the classification schemes make reference to multiple levels of description because the validation of the scheme typically involves classification of children at one level of description with the assumption that the resulting groups will be distinguished at some other level of description, according to the underlying assumptions of the classification scheme. Three

Different schemes for classifying children with DPD according to subtype are based to a greater or lesser extent on criteria at the **linguistic, psycholinguistic, or etiological levels of description.**

commonly used classification schemes are described in the first section of this chapter, with conclusions about the clinical utility of the criteria used to classify children included in each case. Subsequently, studies that examine the psycholinguistic underpinnings of DPD are described.

The final section of this chapter focuses on epidemiological studies of developmental phonological disorders (DPD). This section includes data regarding prevalence of DPD, a discussion of comorbidity between DPD, specific language impairment (SLI) and reading disability (RD), and information about medium and long-term outcomes for children with DPD.

Linguistic Classification Systems

7.1.1. Evaluate the clinical utility of distinguishing between apparent "phonetic" versus "phonemic" disorder.

7.1.2. Describe the linguistic characteristics associated with the four subtypes of speech delay proposed by Dodd.

Phonetic Versus Phonemic Disorder

A **phonetic disorder** is viewed as a problem derived from "faulty habits of articulation" and may be treated by using sensory-motor procedures to focus on articulatory knowledge of target phonemes.

A **phonemic disorder** is seen as arising from "breakdowns at the cognitive level of linguistic knowledge and organization" and will require an intervention to reorganize the child's phonological knowledge.

The primary marker of a phonetic disorder is presumed to be the presence of **distortion errors** because these do not eliminate meaningful contrasts between words.

The assumption that phonetic errors have an articulatory basis whereas substitution or omission errors have a cognitive-linguistic basis is unsupported by evidence.

Traditionally, children with speech sound errors have been viewed as having a problem that stems from "persistence of faulty habits of articulation" (Morley, 1957, p. 232) or "breakdowns at the cognitive level of linguistic knowledge and organization" (Grunwell, 1981, p. 5). Gierut (1998) referred to the former type as a *phonetic disorder* and the latter type as a *phonemic disorder* while stressing that the two types may not be mutually exclusive. Characterization of the child's disorder as phonetic might lead to the selection of a treatment approach that is specifically designed to improve the child's articulatory knowledge of target phonemes using sensorimotor procedures; in contrast, characterization of the child's disorder as phonemic might lead to the selection of a treatment approach designed to reorganize the child's phonological knowledge (Fey, 1992). The primary marker of a phonetic disorder is presumed to be the presence of distortion errors because these do not eliminate meaningful contrasts between words, as in the example "wake" → [wek], "rake" → [ɹʷek], and "lake" → [lʷek]. Phonemic errors neutralize contrast between words, however, such as in the case of liquid gliding, for example, "wake" → [wek], "rake" → [wek], and "lake" → [wek]. One difficulty with this approach to subtyping is that the difference between a phonetic error and a phonemic error may be more in the ear of the listener than the mind of the talker. Furthermore, the assumption that phonetic errors have an articulatory basis whereas substitution or omission errors have a cognitive-linguistic basis is unsupported by evidence. For example, Shuster found that 7-year-old children just starting therapy for remediation of /ɹ/-distortions, and 12-year-old children, recently discharged due to failure to succeed after 2 years of therapy for remediation of /ɹ/-distortions, were similarly unable to identify correct and incorrect productions of words containing /ɹ/. In other words, both groups of children had inaccurate acoustic-phonetic representations for the target phoneme and thus it is not surprising that they were unable to develop accurate motor plans for the production of /ɹ/. The assumption of the treating clinicians, that the children's /ɹ/-distortions were a phonetic error requiring a treatment approach that focused exclusively on articulatory knowledge of the phoneme, was obviously and tragically wrong! Given that distortion errors frequently coexist with errors that would be described as phonological processes, there is no reason to think that distortion, substitution, and omission errors might not have the same origin in some children.

Rvachew, Chiang, and Evans (2007) described the relationship between types of speech sound errors and the presence of phonological processing difficulties in a sample of 58 children with a developmental phonological disorder who were assessed twice, once before kindergarten entry and again at the end of the kindergarten year. If one assumes that children with phonological awareness difficulties might be particularly likely to have a speech deficit that has a cognitive-linguistic origin, one might expect more phonemic errors and fewer distortion errors among children with phonological awareness deficits. However, distortion errors were relatively rare and the frequency of these errors was the same on average for children who passed a test of phonological awareness compared to children who failed the test. Distortion errors, when present, co-occurred with phonemic errors in the child's speech samples. Most children appeared to "grow out of" their distortion errors in that the frequency of these errors declined along with the frequency of their phonemic errors. A few children showed a slightly different pattern in that the frequency of their phonemic errors declined to negligible levels while the residual distortion errors persisted in their error inventory. Overall, the presence or absence of distortion errors did not appear to have any diagnostic or prognostic significance in this sample (Figure 7–1 presents error type distributions). On the other hand, the presence of atypical errors and syllable structure errors (i.e., omissions that alter word shape such as cluster reduction or final consonant deletion) was significantly associated with a phonological awareness deficit. A more sophisticated linguistic approach to subtyping DPDs that takes type and consistency of the children's errors into account is considered next.

Children with DPD produce relatively few distortion errors compared to substitution and omission errors; however, they do co-occur with phonemic errors and phonological processing difficulties.

Dodd's Linguistic Classification System

Dodd (1995) also recommends subtype classification on the basis of the surface characteristics of the child's speech. However, this scheme takes consistency of the child's word productions over multiple repetitions into account as well as the types of error patterns that are observed in the child's speech. The classification is

Dodd recommends subtype classification on the basis of the surface characteristics of the child's speech while taking consistency and error type into account.

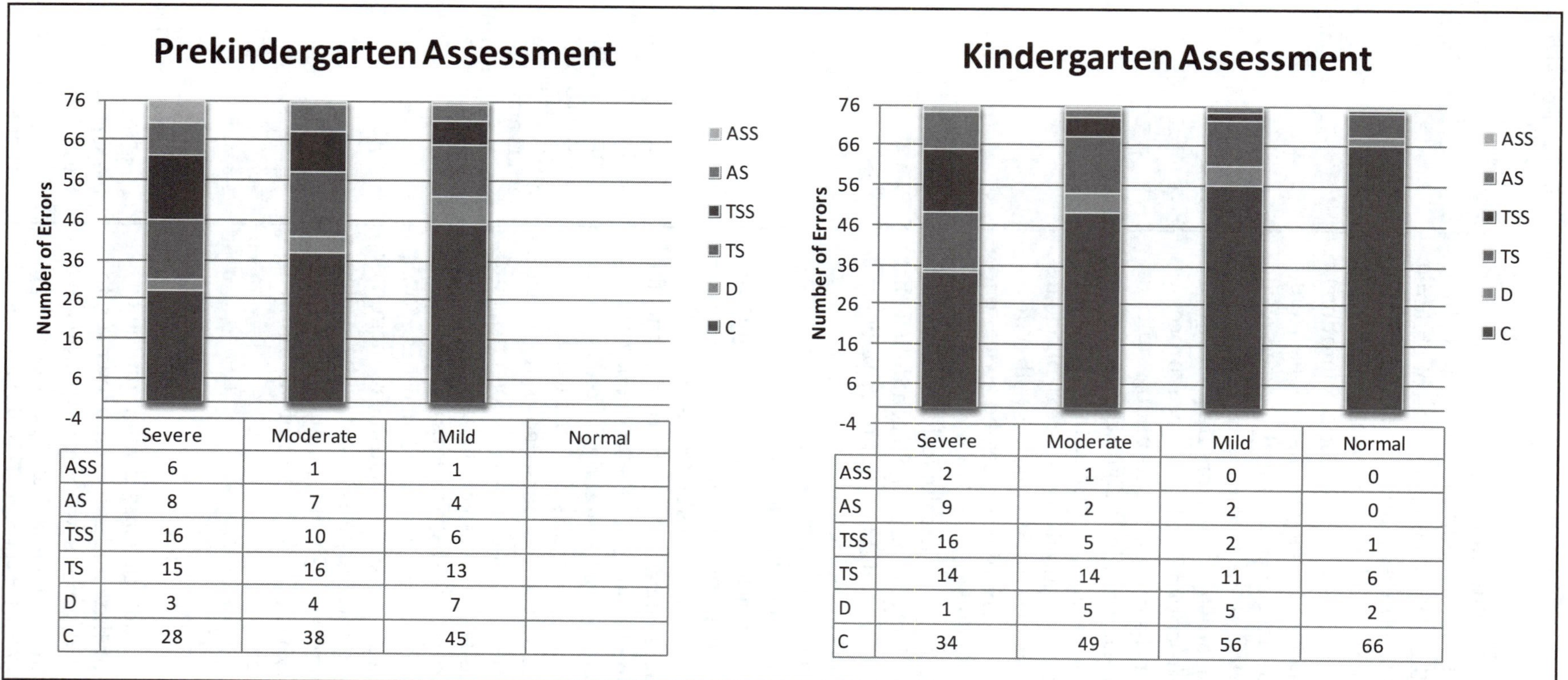

	Severe	Moderate	Mild	Normal
ASS	6	1	1	
AS	8	7	4	
TSS	16	10	6	
TS	15	16	13	
D	3	4	7	
C	28	38	45	

	Severe	Moderate	Mild	Normal
ASS	2	1	0	0
AS	9	2	2	0
TSS	16	5	2	1
TS	14	14	11	6
D	1	5	5	2
C	34	49	56	66

Figure 7–1. *Mean number of consonant errors produced when naming Goldman-Fristoe Test of Articulation-2 stimuli that were coded according to the following categories: Correct (C), Distorted (D), Typical Segment error (TS), Typical Syllable Structure error (TSS), Atypical Segment error (AS), and Atypical Syllable Structure error (ASS). The chart on the left shows data obtained when the children were aged 57 months with mean GFTA-2 percentiles classing 16 children as severe (M = <1), 25 as moderate (M = 4), and 17 as mild (M = 8) with respect to severity of DPD. The chart on the right shows data obtained when the same children were aged 70 months with mean GFTA-2 percentiles classing 6 as severe (M = <1), 21 as moderate (M = 4), 14 as mild (M = 11), and 17 within normal limits (M = 26). Printed with permission from Susan Rvachew.*

expected to ensure exhaustive classification of children with DPD into 4 mutually exclusive categories and to be universally applicable regardless of the child's age or language background. Furthermore, the child's classification should be developmentally stable even as he or she ages and progresses from a more severe to a less severe state of DPD. Although measurement of underlying psycholinguistic abilities is not required for classification because subtyping is determined solely from the linguistic description of the child's speech patterns, certain hypotheses about the underlying cognitive-linguistic basis of each subtype have been proposed. Finally, the children in each subtype are expected to respond differentially to variant treatment strategies. The four subtypes are described in the following paragraphs, summarized from multiple sources (Broomfield & Dodd, 2004; Dodd, Holm, Crosbie, & McCormack, 2005; Fox & Dodd, 2001; Fox, Dodd, & Howard, 2002; So & Dodd, 1994).

An *Articulation Disorder* manifests itself as the inability to articulate a few specific phones. Distortion errors are given as the most common example and thus this category is analogous to the category of phonetic disorder. Descriptions of this type of disorder state specifically that the child must produce the same substitution or distortion for the target phoneme, usually /s/ or /ɹ/, on every attempt. It is our experience that preschool-age children who clearly fall into this category by virtue of the specificity of their error phones can be inconsistent in terms of the error types; for example, dentalized, palatalized, and lateralized variants of coronal sibilants may be produced by the same child but it is not clear how a child with these errors would be classified. The hypothesized level of deficit is stated variously to be learning of the motor movements, phonetic planning, or execution of smooth sequences of gestures.

An **Articulation Disorder** manifests itself as the inability to articulate a few specific phones and may result from a deficit in the learning of motor movements, phonetic planning, or execution of smooth sequences of gestures.

Delayed Phonological Development is characterized by error patterns that would be typical of a normally developing but younger child. Examples of the error patterns are typical phonological processes such as velar fronting or cluster reduction. The child should produce the error patterns consistently across multiple repetitions of the same word. It is also expected that the child's productions will be similar in spontaneous versus imitated naming and in single word versus connected speech contexts. No particular level of breakdown in psycholinguistic processing is hypothesized; rather, the etiology might be slow neurolinguistic maturation or impoverished input.

Delayed Phonological Development is characterized by error patterns that would be typical of a normally developing but younger child, in other words, typical phonological processes that persist due to slow neurolinguistic maturation, or impoverished input.

A child would be classified with *Consistent Deviant Phonological Disorder* if he or she consistently produced atypical phonological error patterns although these will likely co-occur with typical phonological processes. Examples of deviant or atypical error patterns might be consistent deletion of syllable onsets or gliding of fricatives (although we caution that this is specific to English: onset deletion is not deviant in French, for example, so you must use language specific norms for classification of error patterns; see Chapter 4 for further discussion). It is hypothesized that atypical error pat-

A child would be classified with **Consistent Deviant Phonological Disorder** if he or she consistently produced atypical phonological error patterns that likely will co-occur with typical phonological processes.

Dodd proposes that atypical error patterns arise because the child has difficulty abstracting the rules that govern phonology.

terns arise because the child has difficulty abstracting the rules that govern phonology. Consequently, such children have an impaired understanding of their native language phonological system (Dodd, 2011). Dodd et al. (1995) predicted that it would be this subtype that would be associated with a family history of speech difficulties although this prediction was not confirmed; rather, in a subsequent study family history was commonly reported across subtypes (Broomfield & Dodd, 2004).

Dodd et al. (2005) stated that phonological awareness difficulties are specific to the consistent deviant subtype and not observed in children with delayed phonological development or inconsistent deviant phonological disorder (described below). Rvachew, Chiang, and Evans (2007) also found a small trend toward an association between atypical errors and poor phonological awareness test performance among 4- to 6-year-old children with DPD. However, logistic regression analyses showed that phonological error types were not reliable indicators of whether a child would have a phonological processing problem. Furthermore, atypical errors were rare overall with the frequency of typical errors being 3 times greater than atypical errors in both groups.

Inconsistent Deviant Phonological Disorder is manifested by atypical phonological error patterns and inconsistent productions of words over repeated attempts to produce the same word.

Inconsistent Deviant Phonological Disorder is manifested by atypical phonological error patterns and inconsistent productions of words over repeated attempts to produce the same word. A special list of 25 words was developed by Dodd and colleagues to assess consistency of production across multiple productions of the same word. The child is asked to name pictures to elicit the 25-word list 3 times during the same assessment, with other tasks interceding between elicitations of the word set. Children who show variable productions on at least 40% of the words meet the criterion for inconsistency. Furthermore, the inconsistent productions are likely to represent multiple atypical productions of a word rather than alternations between a typical process and the correct production. For example, when attempting the word "vacuum" a child with delayed phonology might alternate between [bækjum] and [vækjum] whereas a child classified in the inconsistent deviant disorder subtype was observed to produce the word as [bækɒf], [bækɪf], and [bækhoʊ] (Dodd et al., 2005, p. 59). Children with inconsistent deviant phonological error patterns have also been shown to achieve higher accuracy in imitated than spontaneous productions of words. It is hypothesized that the level of breakdown is at the phonological planning level (i.e., the level referred to as phonological encoding on Plate 5; notice this is distinct from the motor planning level).

Dodd proposes that inconsistent disorder is caused by a **phonological planning deficit** (i.e., breakdown in phonological encoding).

Studies of English-, German-, Spanish, and Cantonese-speaking children have found that similar proportions of children can be classified into these four categories in each language group, specifically: 10 to 12% articulation disorder; 50 to 60% delayed phonological development; 25 to 30% consistent deviant phonological disorder;

and 10% inconsistent deviant phonological disorder. In terms of the validity of this approach to subtyping, it appears that the system can be used to reliably classify children into the 4 proposed subtypes at a given point in time. No studies have been conducted by Dodd and her colleagues to demonstrate that the categories are stable over time, however. In other domains, it has been shown that classification systems that are based on linguistic symptoms will result in reclassification of children upon retesting. This phenomenon was revealed in a longitudinal study by Conti-Ramsden (1999) who classified children with SLI into six different categories at age 7 years and then assessed the stability of those categories when the children were 2 years older. Although the cluster analysis revealed the same clusters and similar proportions of children in each cluster at the two assessment times, there was considerable movement of children between clusters from the earlier to the later assessment. For example, 20% of the children classified with a lexical-syntactic deficit at time 1 were reclassified as having a phonological-syntactic deficit at time 2. Speech and language disorders are developmental conditions; changes in the surface characteristics of the child's linguistic system reflecting the natural course of the disorder, maturational change, and the impact of parental, educational, and therapeutic interventions are inevitable. Any classification system that does not allow for a developmental perspective is likely to result in unstable categories.

Frequency of occurrence of the subtypes in clinical samples is: 10 to 12% articulation disorder; 50 to 60% delayed phonological development; 25 to 30% consistent deviant phonological disorder; and 10% inconsistent deviant phonological disorder.

In fact, data presented by Dodd and colleagues suggest that the four subtypes reflect the age of the child and the severity of the DPD rather than qualitatively distinct subtypes of phonological disorder. Dodd et al. (2005) report that mean PCC scores vary with subtype as follows: Control, 96; Phonological Delay, 77; Consistent Deviant, 60 and Inconsistent Deviant, 44. Broomfield and Dodd (2004) show a distinct age gradient with subtype as well, with articulation disorder being commonly assigned to children aged 7 years or older and inconsistent deviant disorder almost exclusively assigned to children aged 3 to 5. Children with deviant error patterns were clearly younger on average than children with developmental error patterns. In our own longitudinal study (Rvachew et al., 2007), we observed that error types changed with age and varied with severity: younger and more severely impaired children produced more syllable structure errors and more atypical errors than older and less severely impaired children, as shown in Figure 7–1.

Research suggests that the four subtypes reflect the age of the child and the severity of the DPD rather than qualitatively distinct subtypes of phonological disorder.

In terms of underlying psycholinguistic profile, Dodd et al. (2005) expressed surprise that inconsistent word productions were significantly more frequent among the phonological delay and consistent deviant subtypes in comparison to the typical control group (although as expected, and indeed ensured by definition, variability was greatest for the children in the inconsistent deviant group). Williams and Chiat (1993) compared children with developmental versus deviant error patterns on four tasks tapping output processing, specifically picture naming, word repetition, nonword repetition, and sentence repetition. They concluded that children with consistent deviant error patterns presented with a qualitatively similar profile to children with developmental phonological errors but with a more severe impairment. This conclusion seems consistent with the facts of normal phonological development as laid out in Chapter 4. Rather than being the hallmarks of phonological disorder, inconsistent and unusual matches to adult targets are the primary characteristics of very early phonological development. Certainly, the persistence of these behaviors signals the need for assessment and appropriate follow-up by SLPs but they can be seen to exist on a developmental continuum with later emerging error patterns.

In summary, we conclude that it is possible to reliably classify children's error profiles at a given point in time using this framework. It has not been established that the resulting classifications reflect stable subtypes with respect to underlying psycholinguistic processing deficits. It appears that the classifications may reflect a gradient of severity and developmental level of the child more clearly than qualitative differences in the nature of the child's phonological disorder. We turn now to a classification system that proposes subtypes based on proposed etiologies, a system that includes the developmental course of the disorder as one of the criteria by which diagnostic classifications are assigned.

Shriberg's Framework for Research in Speech Sound Disorders

7.2.1. Describe the three-parameter system for organizing assessment data when classifying children according to the clinical typologies outlined in Shriberg et al.'s framework for research in speech sound disorders.

7.2.2. Diagram the framework for research in speech sound disorders at the levels of Speech Processes and Clinical Typologies.

7.2.3. Distinguish Speech Errors from Speech Delay and Motor Speech Disorders.

7.2.4. For the clinical typologies of SD-Gen and MSD-AOS, describe the proposed etiological factors, underlying speech processes, endophenotype, diagnostic markers, and phenotype.

7.2.5. Predict the likelihood of future psychiatric problems for boys and girls with speech and/or language delay at school entry.

7.2.6. Describe the direct and indirect paths by which chronic OME might result in speech and language delay.

Shriberg (Shriberg, 1994; Shriberg, Austin, Lewis, McSweeny, & Wilson, 1997; Shriberg et al., 2010; Shriberg, Lohmeier, Strand, & Jakielski, submitted; Shriberg et al., 2005) outlines a three-parameter system for gathering and organizing information about a child that permits classification of the child's speech disorder according to a medical model that links observed characteristics of the child's speech to proposed underlying explanatory processes which are in turn linked to putative etiological factors. The first parameter is a description of the child's articulation competence, typically derived from a conversational speech sample (i.e., PCC and PCC-R as described in Chapters 4 and 5). Prosody and voice indexes have also been derived from the speech sample using standardized rating criteria (Shriberg, 1993). Subsequently, additional measures were added to form the Madison Speech Assessment Protocol that samples speech in syllables, words, and longer utterances using imitated and spontaneous evocation methods (Shriberg et al., 2010). Measures of competence, precision, and accuracy are derived.

Shriberg outlines a **three-parameter system** that links observed characteristics of the child's speech to proposed underlying explanatory processes which in turn are linked to putative etiological factors.

The *first parameter* is a description of the child's **articulation competence**, typically derived from a conversational speech sample (i.e., PCC or PCC-R)

The second parameter is a description of the time course of the child's speech delay relative to age norms. Any child's whose speech competence is within normal limits relative to age norms receives the classification of Normal or (in the case of prior speech delay) Normalized Speech Acquisition. Classifications that reflect the developmental trajectory of the child's speech competence are illustrated in Figure 7–2. The growth curve for Normal Speech Acquisition reflects the data shown in Tables 4–7, 4–8, and 4–10 in Chapter 4 whereby consonant accuracy progresses rapidly during the first 3 years, with at least 75% accuracy achieved in conversation along with mastery of some phonemes in all major sound classes except liquids. Gradual refinements occur thereafter with most children achieving adult levels of competence between the ages of 6 and 8 years. Developmental Phonological Disorders[1] is a broad category encompassing both primary and secondary phonological disorders that have their onset before 9 years of age. Therefore, if a child suffered a sudden decline in speech competence secondary to an event such as traumatic brain injury, the classification would be dependent on the child's age at the time of the accident. A Nondevelopmental Speech Disorder would be assigned as the classification if the secondary speech disorder had its onset after the age of 9 years. Within the category of Developmental Phonological Disorders, there are three basic subcategories, Speech Delay (SD), Speech Errors (SE),

The *second parameter* is a description of the **time course** of the child's speech delay relative to age norms.

Within the category of **Developmental Phonological Disorders**, there are three basic subcategories: *Speech Delay (SD)*, *Speech Errors (SE)*, and *Motor Speech Disorder (MSD).*

[1]The Speech Disorders Classification System (SDCS; Shriberg, Austin, et al., 1997) has recently been altered and thus there are some discrepancies among various publications, the description of some elements in this chapter, and Figure 7–3. The original SDCS connected the clinical typologies that we describe here to a superordinate category called Developmental Phonological Disorders which has subsequently been renamed Speech Sound Disorders. We have retained the original superordinate category name (see Introduction to Part II for discussion).

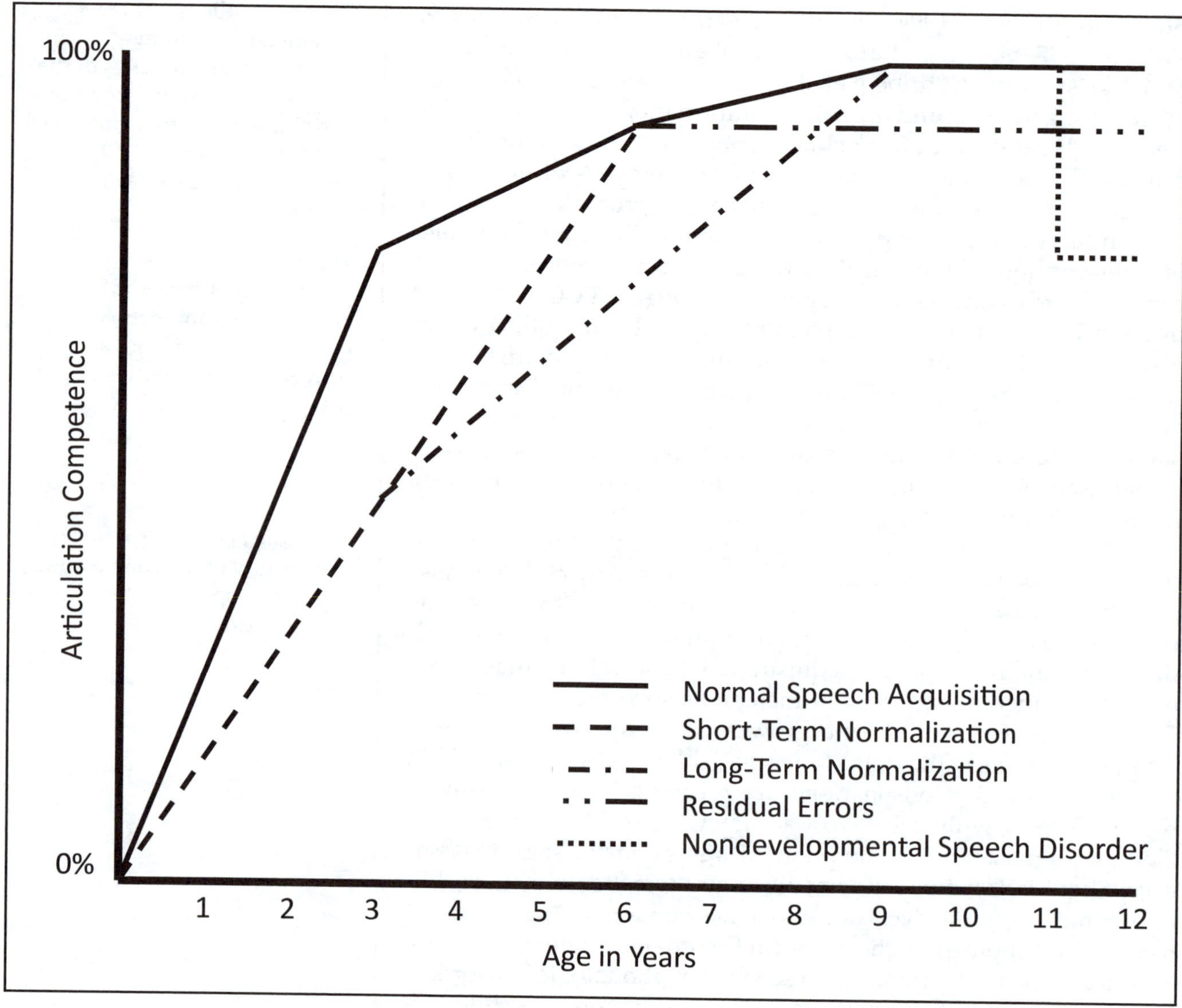

Figure 7–2. *Alternative developmental trajectories for the acquisition of articulation competence that contribute to the diagnosis of clinical typologies within the Speech Disorders Classification System. Adapted from Shriberg (1994).*

and Motor Speech Disorder (MSD).[2] Speech Delay is characterized by persisting substitution and deletion errors and low intelligibility not appropriate for the child's age. These children will begin to show signs of delay at an early age but often evidence a trajectory of

[2]The original SDCS (i.e, Shriberg, 1994; Shriberg et al., 1997) included Speech Delay—Motor Involvement as a subtype of Speech Delay that was roughly synonymous with Childhood Apraxia of Speech. Recently, the SDCS has been reorganized to describe Motor Speech Disorders as a separate category that is distinct from Speech Delay and that includes three subtypes termed apraxia of speech, dysarthria, and motor speech disorder—not otherwise specified (Shriberg et al., 2010). We focus our discussion on apraxia of speech because within the category of primary developmental phonological disorders this variant has received the most research attention.

short-term normalization, achieving age-appropriate speech competence by approximately age 6 years given appropriate intervention (although, as we discuss later in this chapter, other problems in the language and reading domains may persist or emerge after this age). Children with (Residual) Speech Errors produce common distortions of late developing sibilants and/or liquids. This latter group may be composed of children with two distinct developmental trajectories: those whose speech development was essentially normal through age 6 years and those with speech delay but whose substitution and deletion errors resolved before age 6 leaving the distortion errors unresolved thereafter. Although some of these children may show a trajectory of long-term normalization or persistent speech errors into adulthood, there are typically no concomitant academic and vocational concerns provided that the trajectory of speech and language development is otherwise normal. Children with Motor Speech Disorder also demonstrate persisting substitution and deletion errors and low intelligibility not appropriate for the child's age; however, these children will also show evidence of difficulties with speech motor planning or execution and often experience a trajectory of long-term normalization in which progress toward adultlike speech competence is considerably slower than seen in children with SD (Shriberg, Kwiatkowski, & Gruber, 1994); normalization may be delayed until 9 years or later and in some cases the speech disorder may persist into adulthood.

The third parameter is a description of all relevant developmental correlates of the child's speech impairment. This includes a detailed description of the current and historical status of the speech and hearing mechanism, cognitive-linguistic functioning, and psychosocial correlates. This description will emerge from the oral-peripheral mechanism examination, the hearing screening, the case history, and any other medical or developmental assessments that the child has undergone, as described in Chapter 5. These data may reveal the presence of known risk factors for speech or language delay. Campbell et al. (2003) found that speech delay was 7.71 times more likely in a child who had the three risk factors of male sex, mother not graduated from high school, and family history of stuttering, articulation and/or language disorder. This study provides a particularly reliable estimate of risk because it is derived from a large population-based sample with blinded assessment of the 639 participants (meaning that the assessors were unaware of participant/family characteristics when they assessed and judged the child's speech status). Furthermore, the three risk factors revealed by the study have been replicated in other population based studies. As discussed below the heritability of speech disorders is now well established (Bishop & Hayiou-Thomas, 2008; Lewis et al., 2006) and male sex as a risk factor has been replicated in other large sample and population based studies (Shriberg, Tomblin, & McSweeny, 1999; Silva, Justin, McGee, & Williams, 1984; Winitz & Darley, 1980). Low maternal education was interpreted as an index of socioeconomic

The *third parameter* is a description of all relevant **developmental correlates** of speech sound disorder. This includes a detailed description of the current and historical status of the speech and hearing mechanism, cognitive-linguistic functioning, and psychosocial correlates.

Speech delay is 7.71 times more likely in a child who has the three **risk factors** of male sex, mother not graduated from high school, and family history of stuttering, articulation, and/or language disorder.

status, a variable that has been associated with speech delay in other studies conducted in the United States (Winitz & Darley, 1980), although lower social class is more likely to be identified as a correlate if there is concomitant language impairment than in the case of isolated speech disorders (Baker & Cantwell, 1982). In contrast, socioeconomic status was not associated with speech problems in studies conducted in Germany (Fox et al., 2002) and in the United Kingdom (Roulstone, Miller, Wren, & Peters, 2009). It is possible that the correlation between social class and speech delay may be specific to certain countries because the relationship between social class and any outcome that has a social gradient will vary between countries that have differing levels of equality (for explanation, see Wilkinson & Marmot, 2003; Wilkinson & Pickett, 2010). Hoff (2003) has shown that it is quality of the maternal language input to the child that is the specific factor that explains the relationship between family socioeconomic status and language outcomes. The relationship between low maternal education and speech delay may be mediated by any number of biological and environmental variables in a complex fashion. In general, it is important to remember that risk factors are not necessarily causal factors. Possible causes of DPD are discussed in the following sections that describe the classifications proposed in the Speech Disorders Classification System.

Each subtype is described in accordance with the framework illustrated in Figure 7–3, covering each of the 5 levels of description briefly to the extent that data are available. Before proceeding to the description of each subtype it will be helpful to understand this descriptive framework. The framework is clearly based on a medical model, intended to aid research into the genotypic origins of different subtypes of DPD (Shriberg et al., submitted; Shriberg, et al., 2005). At level I, etiological processes are proposed that reflect the interaction of genetic and environmental contributions to the neurobiological underpinnings of speech development. At Level II, a breakdown in a distinct underlying speech process is proposed as the explanation for the child's speech delay, with the caveat that these proposed explanations are fully speculative. Level III, clinical typology, simply refers to the subcategory name. Diagnostic markers are proposed for each category although the validity of these markers is stronger for some categories than others as discussed below.

Etiological processes are proposed that reflect the interaction of genetic and environmental contributions to the neurobiological underpinnings of speech development.

Phenotype refers to observable characteristics that result from the interaction of the genotype and environmental influences.

Phenotype refers to observable characteristics that result from the interaction of the genotype and environmental influences (Gottesman & Gould, 2003). Efforts to identify genetic influences on observed phenotypes are complicated by nonlinear relationships between these levels of analysis: variable phenotypes may arise from a single genotype and similar phenotypes may be traced back to variable genotypes. This is a particularly acute problem in the case of complex neurodevelopmental disorders and thus the concept of the endophenotype has been proposed as an intermediary between the genotype and the observed phenotype. In the case of

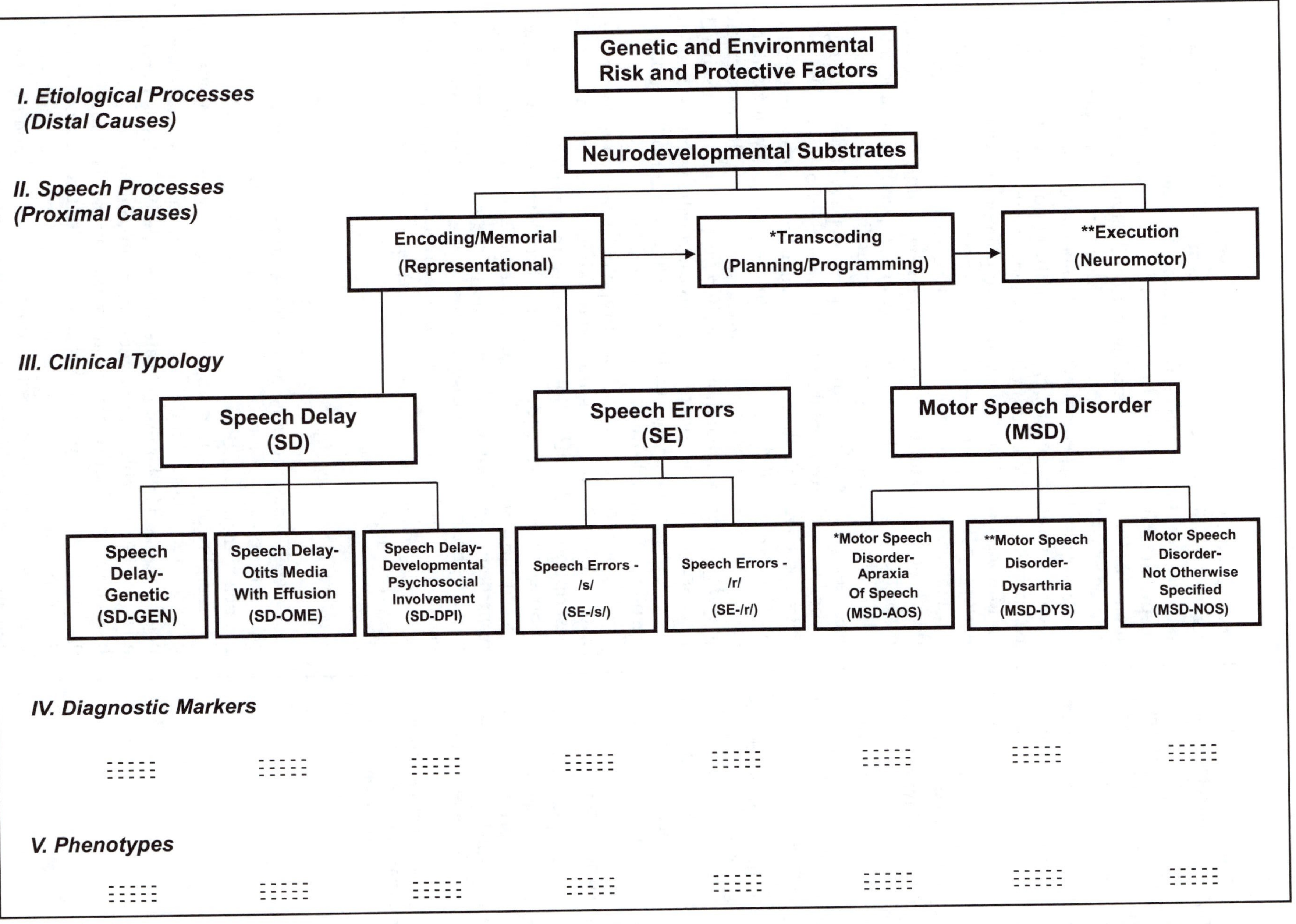

Figure 7–3. *A framework for research in speech sound disorders. Adapted from Shriberg, Lohmeier, Strand, and Jakielski (submitted). Copyright © 2011 L. D. Shriberg. Used with permission.*

The **endophenotype** that is proposed as an intermediary between the genotype and the phenotype should be reliably associated with the condition, heritable, and state-independent.

Differentiating among subtypes may require assessment of endophenotypes or identification of diagnostic markers.

Diagnostic markers are specific speech behaviors that serve to distinguish the subtypes despite considerable overlap in speech characteristics.

Children with **Speech Delay** present with persisting substitution and deletion errors at a higher frequency than is observed in their age peers.

Five subtypes of speech delay are presumed to arise from neurodevelopmental constraints in speech processes that impact phonological representations.

Auditory perceptual encoding refers to the transformation of speech input into acoustic-phonetic or lexical representations.

Speech delay may also involve **memorial processes** (storing and retrieving representations).

monogenic disorders, these relationships can be relatively straightforward (Gottesman & Hanson, 2005) as in the example of phenylketonuria, an autosomal recessive metabolic genetic disorder in which a specific PKU mutation (genotype) interacts with diet (environment) to affect measured intelligence (phenotype) as a consequence of processes related to phenylalanine blood levels (endophenotype). In the case of polygenic neurodevelopmental conditions in which there are multiple genetic influences, the endophenotype may not be specific to the condition in question (in other words, multiple conditions may share the same endophenotype). However, the endophenotype should be reliably associated with the condition, heritable, and state-independent. In the case of DPD, state independence means that the endophenotype will manifest itself regardless of the age of the child or the severity of the speech delay and traces will likely remain present even after normalized speech acquisition has been achieved. In contrast, the phenotype will be changing in response to environmental and maturational influences as the child develops. Given that the phenotype will overlap among the clinical typologies and will change within clinical typologies as the children age, differentiating among subtypes may require: (1) the assessment of endophenotypes that more closely reflect the underlying speech processes, or (2) the identification of diagnostic markers, that are specific speech behaviors which serve to distinguish the subtypes despite considerable overlap in speech characteristics.

We now describe the clinical typologies shown in Figure 7–3 within the context of this framework, beginning with a detailed description of the three subtypes subsumed under the category of Speech Delay and proceeding to a brief discussion of the two Speech Error subtypes. These five subtypes are presumed to arise from neurodevelopmental constraints in speech processes that impact phonological representations, either auditory perceptual encoding (transforming speech input into acoustic-phonetic or lexical representations) or memorial processes (storing and retrieving representations).

Speech Delay—Genetic

The Speech Delay category covers the group of children who present with persisting substitution and deletion errors at a higher frequency than is observed in their age peers along with reduced intelligibility of speech. A trajectory of short-term normalization is expected for children in this category provided appropriate therapeutic inputs. The largest subcategory of Speech Delay is hypothesized to be heritable and of genetic origin (Shriberg et al., 2005). In an effort to identify diagnostic markers for this clinical typology, Shriberg et al. reported that children with two or more family members with a history of speech-language delay were more likely to produce omission errors (in contrast to substitution or distortion errors) and less likely to back /s/ (in contrast to producing a fronted distortion of /s/), relative to children with lower "genetic load." A classification algorithm based on the frequency of these error types proved to have poor sensitivity but reasonable positive predictive value. The authors proposed that the tendency toward omission errors may reflect an absence of phonological knowledge of the omitted phonemes. Earlier accounts attributed this absence of phonological knowledge to a cognitive-linguistic deficit (Shriberg, Austin, et al., 1997) whereas phonological memory and/or auditory-perceptual encoding (Shriberg et al., submitted) have been invoked more recently as explanatory speech processes.

Speech Delay—Genetic is proposed as the largest subcategory of speech delay. A heritable difficulty with phonological memory or auditory-perceptual encoding is suggested as the underlying explanatory process and a tendency toward syllable structure (omission) errors is described as the diagnostic marker.

Family aggregation and twin studies have confirmed that speech delay is heritable. Molecular genetic studies examine the DNA of individuals with speech delay and their family members, looking for specific variants of genes that are associated with the phenotypes or endophenotypes of interest. These studies invariably find that the participants' performance on measures of articulation (e.g., GFTA percentiles, PCC), phonological processing (e.g., phonemic awareness) and phonological memory (e.g., nonword repetition) are highly intercorrelated. Furthermore, a substantial minority of these samples of individuals with speech delay will also have comorbid language impairment and/or reading disability (issues related to comorbidity are discussed later in this chapter). These studies have found that speech delay and reading disability are jointly linked to regions on certain chromosomes, 6p22, 15p21, and 1p36 (Rice, Smith, & Gayán, 2009; Smith, Pennington, Boada, & Shriberg, 2005; Stein et al., 2004). The candidate genes that have been proposed for these chromosome locations are involved in neuronal or axonal migration during early maturation of the central nervous system (for reviews, see Bishop, 2009; Lewis et al., 2006).

Speech delay and reading disability are jointly linked to regions on certain chromosomes (6p22, 15p21, 1p36) involved in neuronal or axonal migration during early maturation of the central nervous system.

Brain imaging studies of children with DPD have just begun to emerge in the research literature. Preston, Felsenfeld, Frost, Fulbright, Mencl, Goen, and Pugh (2012) reported fMRI imaging data for 17 children aged 8;6 to 10;10 who misarticulated sibilants and/or liquids and another subset of children without misarticulations who were matched for age, gender, intelligence, and language performance. The children were required to signal when spoken or printed stimulus words matched a target word presented as a picture. The 80% of stimulus items that did not match the target shared phonological, semantic, or orthographic characteristics with the target. Between-group differences in activation patterns across a number of brain regions were observed including left superior and middle temporal regions and the left insula, suggesting difficulties with the perception of the phonetic properties of speech among children with speech errors. Specifically, the authors concluded that the children with speech errors were relying "more upon several dorsal speech perception regions and less on ventral speech perception regions" (p. 1), referencing the dual-stream model of speech processing (Hickok & Poeppel, 2007) described in Chapter 2.

Neuroimaging studies confirm an underlying deficit in phonological processing for at least some children with a history of speech delay.

Lewis, Chen, Freebairn, Holland, and Tkach (2010) used fMRI to search for the neural correlates of speech production in young adults, 6 of whom had a prior history of delayed phonological development as preschoolers and 7 of whom had normal speech development. Although overt speech production was perceptually normal in both groups and no significant differences were observed on the nonword repetition task that was employed during scanning, less activation in the right inferior frontal gyrus was observed in the participants with a history of DPD relative to those with normal speech development. Relative to controls, hyperactivation was observed in pre- and supplementary motor cortex, inferior parietal, supramarginal gyrus, and cerebellum. The authors concluded that the pattern of hypoactivation reflected a phonological processing deficit whereas the pattern of hyperactivations relative to controls reflected compensatory mechanisms.

These findings are consistent with a large body of literature revealing difficulties with speech perception and phonological processing among children with DPD as discussed in detail in the section on psycholinguistic approaches to subtyping. Furthermore, children with DPD who have difficulties with phonological processing produce more omission errors (i.e., syllable structure errors) and atypical errors than children with DPD who do not have difficulties with phonological processing (Preston & Edwards, 2010; Rvachew et al., 2007). Overall, support for this subtype is very strong at all levels of description in the scientific literature. As discussed in greater detail later in this chapter, a phonological processing deficit is the likely endophenotype given that this deficit contributes to both speech delay and reading difficulties and persists across the life span in this population even when perceptually accurate speech is achieved. Demonstration 5–1 illustrates a candidate for this clinical typology who exemplifies the importance of attending to family history in the assessment of children with DPD as well as being especially alert to the child's therapeutic needs beyond the correction of overt speech errors given the complex nature of the underlying disorder.

Given the common occurrence and complex nature of Speech Delay—Genetic, the SLP must attend to family history in the assessment of children with DPD and be alert to the child's therapeutic needs beyond correction of overt speech errors.

Speech Delay—Otitis Media with Effusion

Otitis media with effusion (OME) is a common correlate of speech delay that may overlap with family history of speech delay.

Shriberg (1994) observed that about a third of children with speech delay have histories of recurrent otitis media with effusion (OME) before the age of 3, a possible correlate of speech delay that may or may not overlap with family history, another risk factor that affects half to two-thirds of the DPD population. Hearing loss during an episode of OME averages only 23 dB (Fria, Cantekin, & Eichler, 1985), however, and many decades of prospective and retrospective studies have failed to establish a direct causal link between ear infections and speech or language disorders (for review, see Roberts et al., 2004). Nonetheless, 5 to 10% of children experience hearing loss as great as 50 dB during an episode of OME and studies employing auditory brain stem response measures have shown abnormal binaural processing subsequent to prolonged OME that is consistent with the predictions of animal models (Popescu & Polley, 2010).

These findings are also consistent with these children's behavioral responses on binaural unmasking release and comodulation release tests, with their responses on these tests signaling long-term difficulties with the perception of speech in noisy environments. Therefore, it is a plausible hypothesis that OME might cause specific central auditory processing deficits that in turn degrade acoustic-phonetic representations for phoneme categories, thus explaining speech delay in children with early-onset and chronic OME. Experimental support for the hypothesis is weak, possibly because few studies of OME impacts provide detailed information about the children's auditory function and speech perception abilities; furthermore, even though some of these studies have had numerically large samples, they have had insufficient power to either support or refute an effect of OME on speech and language development (Roberts, Rosenfeld, & Zeisel, 2004). The absence of differences in outcomes in randomized control trials of the effectiveness of pressure equalization tubes as a treatment for OME has been taken as strong refutation of a link between OME and language development (Paradise et al., 2001). However, in these studies no child received the tubes as early as the infant or toddler periods and yet correlational studies show that the risk of poorer outcomes is linked to chronic OME during the first year of life (Johnson et al., 2000; Teele et al., 1984), as might be expected given what is known about critical periods in auditory system development and the important events in speech perception development that occur during this period (see Chapter 2). The risk for OME is correlated with variables that also place a child at risk for delayed speech and/or language development including low SES, male sex, and bottle feeding/propping (e.g., Paradise et al., 1997); furthermore, children with primary causes of speech and language delay such as cleft palate and Down syndrome are at elevated risk for chronic OME. This confounding of risk factors complicates efforts to isolate the impact of OME-related hearing impairment on developmental outcomes. Therefore, OME as a direct cause of speech delay in a small minority of children with moderate hearing loss secondary to chronic early-onset OME cannot be ruled out.

It is a plausible hypothesis that OME might cause specific central auditory processing deficits that, in turn, degrade acoustic-phonetic representations for phoneme categories, thus explaining speech delay in children with early-onset and chronic OME.

An alternative explanation is that OME interacts with auditory, cognitive, attentional, and linguistic factors to produce mild delays in language skills as well as diffuse effects on speech intelligibility (Shriberg, Friel-Patti, Flipsen, & Brown, 2000). One such model, proposed by Bennett and Haggard (1999), is presented in Figure 7–4. These researchers, in a long-term prospective study, found that ear discharge and hearing problems at age 5 were associated with a small but significantly increased risk of difficulties with speech articulation, vocabulary knowledge, and behavior at ages 5 and 10 years. Polka and colleagues (Polka & Rvachew, 2005; Polka, Rvachew, & Molnar, 2008), in a prospective study of infants, found that early onset OME was associated with poor selective attention to speech in quiet conditions and poorer perception

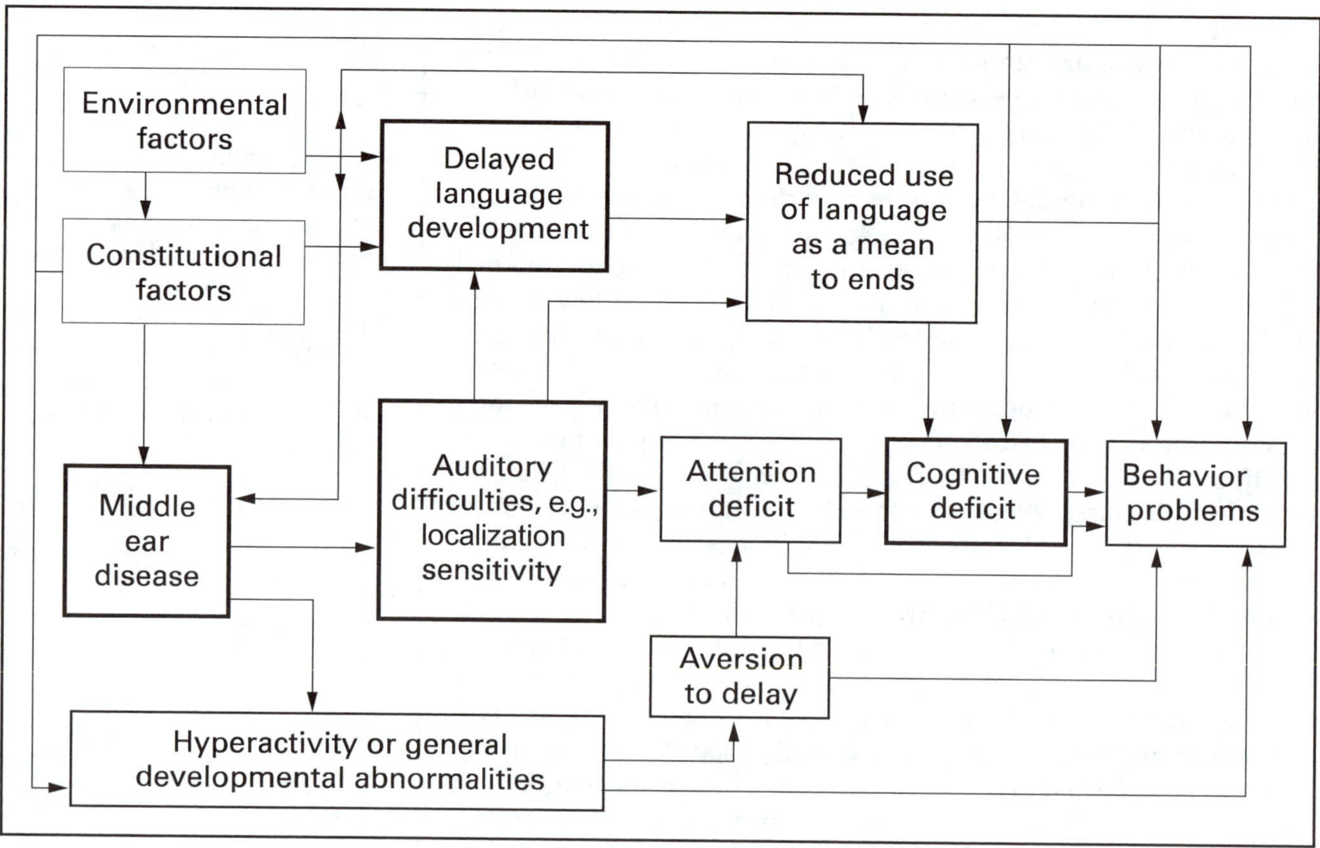

Figure 7–4. Model of the relationship between middle ear disease (OME) and developmental outcomes as mediated by illness, the environment, hearing, and attention factors. From Bennett and Haggard (1999). Behavior and cognitive outcomes from middle ear disease. Archives of Disease in Childhood, 80, *Figure 1, p. 28. Reprinted with permission of BMJ Publishing Group Ltd.*

of CV syllables which may explain small but significant delays in the onset of canonical babbling (Rvachew, Slawinski, Williams, & Green, 1999) and a reduced vowel space in infants with early onset OME (Rvachew, Slawinski, Williams, & Green, 1996; also see Figure 3–18). Vernon-Feagans and colleagues have shown that language outcomes subsequent to recurrent OME are mediated by the quality of communicative interactions between the mother and child (for reviews, see Vernon-Feagans, 1999; Yont, Snow, & Vernon-Feagans, 2003). Altogether, these findings support the hypothesis that OME impacts are mediated by the child's access to the language environment via pathways that are both direct (i.e., child hearing factors) and indirect (child attentional factors and parental input factors). Shriberg, Flipsen, Kwiatkowski, and McSweeny (2003) suggested that one of the diffuse effects that occurs within this matrix of interacting factors is that the child does not learn to adjust speech intelligibility in response to the listener's needs. This effect manifests itself as a gap between overall speech intelligibility and measures of speech accuracy (Shriberg, Flipsen, et al., 2003).

Research findings support the hypothesis that the impacts of OME on speech and language outcomes are mediated by the child's access to the language environment via pathways that are both direct (i.e., child hearing factors) and indirect (child attentional factors and parental input factors).

Such a discrepancy may reflect less precision in the production of vowels and consonants, reminiscent of the restricted vowel space observed in infants with early onset OME.

A gap between speech intelligibility and measures of speech accuracy may be a diagnostic marker for **Speech Delay—OME.**

Tests of this mediated account of the relationship between OME and speech and language outcomes confirm that OME explains significant variation in speech and language outcomes within the normal range (e.g., Klausen, Moller, Holmefjord, Reisaeter, & Asbjornsen, 2007; Paradise et al., 2000). This degree of variation can have significant impacts when combined with biological risk factors. McGrath et al. (2007) examined the interaction between genetic risk for speech disorder, otitis media history, and language outcomes. In this twin study, speech (e.g., articulation accuracy, speech-motor control), language (e.g., picture vocabulary, grammatic understanding), and prereading (e.g., phonological awareness, letter knowledge) phenotypes were linked to risk alleles at chromosome locations 6p22 and 15q21. The result conformed to a diathesis-stress model of a gene-environment interaction whereby the presence of the environmental risk factor increased the risk of language disorder in the presence of genetic risk: specifically, performance on semantic measures was correlated with otitis media history when genetic risk for speech disorder was high; no correlation was observed when there was no genetic risk for speech disorder. In contrast, all the other gene-environment interactions that were investigated in this study conformed to a bioecological model: for example, in homes that provided an enriched literacy environment, phonological awareness performance was highly determined by genetic factors such that children without genetic risk achieved substantially better phonological awareness scores in these homes than children with high genetic risk; in contrast, phonological awareness performance was uniformly low compared to controls, regardless of degree of genetic risk, when the child did not receive optimum environmental input.

The **diathesis-stress model of a gene-environment interaction** predicts that a genetic vulnerability (e.g., genetic predisposition for dyslexia) that is coupled with an environmental stressor (e.g., an OME-related reduction in access to language input) increases probability of a poor outcome (e.g., poor vocabulary skills).

The **bioecological model of a gene-environment interaction** predicts that a genetic vulnerability (e.g., genetic predisposition for dyslexia) is actualized in an optimum environment but masked in a risk environment.

In summary, there is support for the hypothesis that OME is an indirect causal factor in speech delay. However, with the exception of a small minority of cases where severe early-onset OME may directly cause long-term problems with auditory processing, it is likely that this subtype overlaps with the Speech Delay-Genetic subtype. In these cases OME interacts with the underlying genetic substrate and environmental inputs; therefore, the intervening explanatory process is likely to be impaired phonological processing (i.e., auditory-perceptual encoding and associated memorial processes) (Nittrouer, 1996; Nittrouer & Burton, 2005).

Speech Delay—Psychosocial Involvement

The third etiological subtype proposed in the Speech Delay category is associated with psychosocial issues. Hauner, Shriberg, Kwiatkowski, and Allen (2005) acknowledged that many studies linking psychosocial problems to speech delay specifically are older and

Speech Delay—Psychosocial Involvement is hypothesized to arise from genetic factors that explain the co-occurrence of negative affect and speech impairment in some children. This hypothesis has not been verified empirically.

unreliable due to methodological difficulties. They further acknowledge that the nature of this hypothesized link may be complex in any case: speech delay could be a direct cause of psychiatric problems; speech delay could be a symptom of an underlying psychiatric problem; or comorbid psychiatric and speech problems could have a common but unidentified antecedent. That said, they proceeded to suggest that genetic factors that determine temperament explain co-occurring negative affect and speech deficits in some children. On the basis of a retrospective chart review of children who received speech therapy, they estimated that approximately 11% of children with speech delay present with behavioral difficulties associated with either approach-related negative affect (aggressive, angry, manipulative, control-seeking behaviors), or withdrawal-related negative affect (socially withdrawn, shy, fearful, extremely taciturn behaviors). Analysis of conversational speech samples yielded weak evidence of slightly more severe speech deficits for children rated by speech-language pathologists and parents to have negative affect had than children who did not. Unfortunately, no standardized language test scores are presented for these children but all well designed studies on the relationship between communication disorders and psychiatric conditions have identified language delay as a significant factor.

Cantwell and Baker (Baker & Cantwell, 1987a, 1987b; Cantwell & Baker, 1987a, 1987b) described the prevalence of psychiatric problems in a sample of 600 children, aged 2 through 16 years, who were referred to a large community speech and hearing clinic in Los Angeles during the late 1970s, capturing virtually all children who were assessed for speech and language problems at the clinic in a 3-year period. Every child received the same battery of language, cognitive, and psychosocial assessments and the psychiatric and neurological examination was administered by the same psychiatrist who was blind to the speech and language assessment results at the time of testing. The results are represented in Table 7–1. Speech disorder was determined from ratings of conversational speech and the Goldman-Fristoe Test of Articulation and included disorders of articulation, voice, and/or fluency. Language delay was determined from a variety of standardized measures of receptive and expressive language tests covering semantics, morphology, and syntax as well as analysis of a conversational speech sample. Language processing disorder was determined from measures of auditory memory, auditory discrimination, and other skills assessed by the Illinois Test of Psycholinguistic Abilities. Psychiatric diagnoses were based on structured interviews of the parent and child and standardized questionnaires administered to the child's parents and teacher. Psychiatric diagnoses were aggregated into four main types: behavioral disorders, which included attention deficit, conduct, and oppositional disorders; pervasive developmental disorders including autism; emotional disorders including anxiety, adjustment, and

Table 7–1. *Demographic Characteristics, Linguistic Diagnoses, and Psychiatric Diagnoses of 600 Children Aged 2 to 16 Years Referred to a Community Speech and Hearing Clinic*

	Pure Speech Disorder (n = 203)	*Speech and Language Disorder* (n = 352)	*Pure Language Disorder* (n = 45)
Demographic Variables			
Age (*M/SD*)	6.3/2.8	5.0/2.5	8.8/3.8
Sex (% males)	67	70	65
Cognitive measures			
Performance IQ (*M/SD*)	118.7/18.5	95.6/24.6	111.4/24.5
Verbal IQ/PPVT (*M/SD*)	110.7/12.4	86.0/21.4	96.2/18.3
Linguistic Diagnoses (% children affected)			
Any speech disorder	100	100	0
Voice disorder	6	2	0
Articulation disorder	85	96	0
Fluency/rate disorder	12	5	0
Any language disorder	0	100	100
Expressive disorder only	0	32	28
Processing disorder only	0	5	36
Receptive disorder	0	63	36
Psychiatric Diagnoses (% children affected)			
Any psychiatric disorder	31	58	73
Behavioral disorder[c]	14	30	47
Attention deficit	10	23	33
PDD[a]	0	2	2
Emotional Disorders[c]	15	21	31
Affective Disorders	3	3	18
Other Disorders	5	9	9
Psychiatric Diagnoses for Age, Sex, and Performance IQ-Matched Groups (% children affected)			
Any axis I diagnosis[b]	21	79	74
Any behavioral diagnosis	0	37	47
Any emotional diagnosis	11	47	16

[a]Pervasive Developmental Disorder.

[b]In accordance with DSM-III.

[c]See text for definition of behavioral and emotional categories.

Source: Adapted from Cantwell and Baker (1987). Prevalence and type of psychiatric disorder and developmental disorders in three speech and language groups. *Journal of Communication Disorders, 20,* Table 1 (p. 153), Table 2 (p. 155), and Table 4 (p. 157). Used with permission of Elsevier Ltd.

affective disorders; and other disorders, a category that included any disorders not fitting into the previous three such as eating disorders, gender identity disorder, and unspecified mental illness.

Baker and Cantwell described 600 children, aged 2 through 16 years, who were referred to a community speech and hearing clinic; 34% presented with speech disorder alone and 59% presented with concurrent speech and language deficits.

The first observation to draw from Table 7–1 is that few children were observed to have an isolated language disorder so that the majority of children had a speech disorder, specifically 34% with speech disorder alone and 59% with concurrent speech and language deficits. Second, performance IQ was significantly lower among the children with concomitant speech and language delay relative to the other two groups. Verbal intelligence was significantly higher among children with isolated speech deficits relative to the two groups of children with language disorder. When considering the full sample and when examining subgroups matched for age, sex, and performance IQ it is clear that psychiatric problems are significantly more likely among children who had a language disorder than among children who had isolated speech disorder. Behavioral and emotional disorders were frequently observed among children with concomitant speech and language disorders; behavioral disorders were more frequent than emotional disorders among the subgroup with isolated language disorder; in contrast, emotional disorders were the most frequent psychiatric condition observed among children with isolated speech disorders. Other information not shown in Table 7–1 is that socioeconomic status was lowest for the speech and language impaired group and that a quarter of this group was found to have other developmental disorders in addition to speech and language delay.

One difficulty with the data presented in Table 7–1 is that it is not possible to know if the reported rates of psychiatric disorder are higher than might be expected from general population estimates. To answer this question it is necessary to conduct a population based epidemiological study such as that conducted by Beitchman and colleagues in Canada in which children were ascertained at age 5 and then followed until adulthood. Beitchman et al. (1996) found that speech or language disorder at age 5 placed girls at high risk for psychiatric diagnosis at age 12 as shown in Table 7–2. Overall, approximately 45% of children who had a communication disorder at age 5 received a diagnosis of psychiatric disorder at age 12 regardless of whether the diagnosis at age 5 involved the speech-only or speech and language domains. Further follow-up at age 19 years (Beitchman et al., 2001) revealed significantly higher rates of anxiety disorders among those who had a language disorder at age 5 in comparison to the control group. An association between language disorder in boys at age 5 and antisocial personality disorder at age 19 was also revealed in this study.

Epidemiological studies reveal considerably higher rates of **psychiatric problems** among children with speech and/or language delay compared to the rest of the population.

Beitchman and colleagues point out that their studies do not illuminate the causal mechanisms that underly the emergence of psychiatric problems in children with preschool speech and language disorders. Another group of Canadian researchers did attempt to uncover these pathways in a study in which the cognitive, language,

Table 7–2. *Psychiatric Diagnosis (% Children Affected) at Age 12.5 Years as a Function of Speech/Language (S/L) Status at Age 5 Years by Gender*

	Boys		Girls	
	S/L Impaired (n = 61)	S/L Normal (n = 74)	S/L Impaired (n = 30)	S/L Normal (n = 37)
Emotional	13.1	10.8	33.3	2.7
Conduct	8.2	6.8	10.0	5.4
ADHD	19.7	8.1	3.3	2.7

S/L Impaired group includes speech-only (*n* = 29), language-only (*n* = 38), and concomitant speech and language (*n* = 24) diagnoses at age 5 years.

Source: Adapted from Beitchman et al. (1996). Seven-year follow-up of speech/language impaired and control children: Psychiatric outcome. *Journal of Child Psychology and Psychiatry*, 37, Table 5 (p. 965). Used with permission of John Wiley and Sons.

behavioral, and psychiatric characteristics of 399 children, aged 7 to 14 years, were assessed upon referral to a hospital for psychiatric services. Cohen, Davine, Horodezky, Lipsett, and Isaacson (1993) reported that 47% had normally developing language, 28% had a previously identified language disorder, and 34% were identified with a previously unsuspected language impairment with this latter group presenting with the most serious externalizing psychiatric disorders. Psychiatrically disturbed children with language impairments had more difficulties with social cognition than those with normal language skills (Cohen et al., 1998). Subsequently, they used linear structural equation modeling and the data from this sample to test alternative models of the relationships between social cognition, language ability, and externalizing psychopathology (Zadeh, Im Bolter, & Cohen, 2007). In the best fitting model, language ability mediated the relationship between social cognition and externalizing psychopathology. These findings support the hypothesis of a causal role for language in the emergence of psychiatric disorders in children with language impairments. Zadeh et al. (2007) suggested that poor language skills impair the child's ability to successfully resolve social conflicts thus increasing the use of maladaptive verbal or physical social problem solving. Beitchman et al. (1996) suggested that language impairment leads to school failure as well as poor peer relationships thus explaining externalizing psychopathology as secondary effects even after resolution of the language delay. Both studies highlight the importance of identifying and resolving the child's communication deficits prior to school entry in order to prevent these secondary effects and/or to better position the child to benefit from social skills and other psychosocial interventions.

Language delay may play a causal role in the emergence of psychiatric disorders because poor language skills impair the child's ability to successfully resolve **social conflicts** and increase the chance of school failure.

All of these studies lead to the conclusion that a separate category of Speech Delay—Psychosocial Involvement may be unwarranted because, at present, the best evidence suggests that the complex causal pathways involved might increase the risk of psychiatric disorder for any child with a speech and language impairment, regardless of the underlying etiology of the communication deficit (see for example the proposed causal model relating OME to language delay and behavior problems in Figure 7–4). In any case, the SLP needs to be aware of the elevated risk of comorbid psychiatric problems in children who have DPD with concomitant language impairment as well as the elevated risk of these problems in school-age children with a prior history of speech or language delay during the preschool period. The finding that psychiatric difficulties (anxiety disorders in girls and attention deficit in boys in particular) may arise after the communication impairment has been resolved has clinical implications for the appropriate follow-up and management of these children during the school years.

The SLP needs to be aware of the elevated risk of comorbid psychiatric problems in children who have DPD with concomitant language impairment as well as the elevated risk of these problems in school-age children with a prior history of speech or language delay during the preschool period.

Speech Errors

Speech errors refers to the second of three superordinate categories and describes children with persistent distortion errors, usually of /s/ or /ɹ/.

The second of three superordinate categories describes children with persistent distortion errors according to two subtypes depending on whether the child distorts /s/ or /ɹ/. These errors by definition show a course of long-term normalization and may persist into adulthood but the child is not expected to be at risk for developmental delays in other domains. Placement of a child into these subtypes requires differentiation from other subtypes involving the presence of other errors and past history of speech delay. The original SDCS contained 7 different classifications for describing children with residual speech errors that took into account the types of errors and the time course of the child's developmental trajectory toward the achievement of mature speech production abilities (Shriberg, Austin, et al., 1997): among children with residual speech errors, those whose speech development was delayed prior to 6 years of age received the designation of RE-A whereas those who demonstrated a normal developmental course before 6 years of age received the designation of RE-B. Some proportion of both groups of children may present with common distortions of late developing sibilants and liquids after the age of 6 years but environmental antecedents are presumed to play a key role in the case of children with an early normal trajectory whereas the etiology in the case of children with a delayed trajectory from an early age is presumed to be largely genetic. Research into the genetic and environmental origins of DPD and studies of comorbidity between DPD and language, learning, or psychiatric disorders are hampered by the inability to determine whether children with DPD, ascertained at school age, fall into the RE-A or RE-B subcategories. For example, the studies reviewed in the previous section concluded that psychiatric disorders were most likely to co-occur with comorbid speech *and* language delay; at the same time psychiatric disorders at age 12 were predicted by speech *or* language delay at age 5. These kinds of

Children with residual speech errors will include those whose speech development was delayed prior to 6 years of age (**RE-A**) and those who demonstrated a normal developmental course before 6 years of age (**RE-B**).

discrepancies might possibly be explained by the failure to distinguish between children who have distortion errors subsequent to a normal trajectory of speech development as preschoolers from those who have had persistent speech delay from an early age. Shriberg and colleagues have attempted to identify acoustic markers that differentiate the RE-A and RE-B subcategories among children who produce /s/ and /ɹ/ distortions. As these markers are not likely to be used for clinical purposes the details are not provided here. Briefly, Shriberg, Flipsen, Karlsson, and McSweeny (2001) found that children in the RE-A category produced distortions that were less derhotacized than the incorrect /ɝ/ tokens of children in the RE-B category. Karlsson, Shriberg, Flipsen, and McSweeny (2002) reported that the children with an otherwise normal developmental trajectory produced the /s/ phoneme with a narrow range of higher than average centroid values suggesting a fronted or dentalized tongue placement. In contrast, children with a prior history of speech delay produced /s/ in a more acoustically acceptable fashion than children with no prior history of speech delay. The authors speculate that the RE-B distortions arise at a very young age when the child does not have the motoric maturity to produce a more accurate phone; as the distortion is more long-standing and pervasive it is resistant to change in the older children that have had otherwise normal development before the age of 6 years. In contrast, the RE-A group children will have simplified these phones at young ages (substituting glides or stops or deleting them entirely), delaying the attempt to produce these later developing phones until an age when they were able to more closely approximate the target. The difference in treatment history for these children could also be considered in this speculative account: children with a prior history of speech delay may well have received some intervention for remediation of their liquid and sibilant errors, especially in the context of strategies to suppress cluster reduction, at a young age; on the other hand, the children with RE-B distortions may not yet have received any intervention and may be less likely to achieve success in treatment at this late age.

With respect to the etiology of speech errors, environmental antecedents are presumed to play a key role in the RE-B subtype whereas the etiology in the RE-A subtype is presumed to be largely genetic.

The research literature abounds with studies of children with residual distortion errors, many quite contradictory in their findings, but it is rare for the researchers to carefully differentiate these subtypes in their research samples. Validation of the hypothesis that distinct explanatory factors underlie these markedly different developmental trajectories requires longitudinal research that involves direct assessment of psycholinguistic abilities at multiple levels of representation. Some studies verify the linkage shown in Figure 7–3 between residual speech errors and phonological encoding processes, revealing issues with phonemic perception (Shuster, 1998) and phonological awareness (Preston & Edwards, 2007) as previously mentioned. Other studies of older children with distortion errors reveal evidence of a motor speech disorder, however

(Gibbon, 1999; Goozée et al., 2007; McNutt, 1977). We now turn to the third superordinate classification shown in Figure 7–3 to discuss the symptoms of motor speech disorders in detail.

Motor Speech Disorder

A very small minority of children with speech delay, 5% or less, are hypothesized to have a **Motor Speech Disorder (MSD)**.

MSDs encompass a continuum of deficits including linguistic planning, motor programming, and execution of an utterance.

A very small minority of children with speech delay, 5% or less, are hypothesized to have a Motor Speech Disorder (MSD)[3] although the motor involvement may encompass a continuum of deficits that include elements of linguistic planning, motor programming, and execution of an utterance (McNeil, 2003; Ozanne, 1995; Shriberg, 1994; Shriberg, Aram, & Kwiatkowski, 1997). Three subcategories are proposed, Apraxia of Speech (involving difficulties with motor planning), Dysarthria (involving difficulties with motor execution), and MSD—Not otherwise specified (in which case the motor involvement is not specifically apraxia or dysarthria).

Wernicke's aphasia is associated with *phonemic paraphasias*: substitutions and transpositions of phonemes or syllable sized units, that suggest a breakdown at the level of *phonological encoding*.

Substitution errors in **Broca's aphasia** involve miscoordination of the timing among multiple articulatory gestures that suggest breakdown at the level of *motor planning*.

The diagnostic terms, definitions and underlying assumptions are borrowed from the literature on adult neurolinguistic and motor speech disorders. Wernicke's or conduction aphasia caused by left posterior brain damage may be associated with a distinct type of speech error called phonemic paraphasias, characterized by substitutions and transpositions of phonemes or syllable-sized units that suggest a breakdown at the level of phonological encoding (see Plate 5). Broca's aphasia caused by left anterior brain damage may also lead to phoneme substitution errors in addition to difficulties with segment and syllable transitions and abnormal prosody, in this case linked to a breakdown at the level of motor planning (Canter, Trost, & Burns, 1985). In the case of phonemic paraphasias, instrumental analyses reveal that errors involve substitution of one phoneme for another; on the other hand, errors that are perceived as substitutions in the speech of adult apraxic patients involve miscoordination of the timing among multiple articulatory gestures resulting in single feature errors such as oral/nasal and voiced/voiceless confusions. Phonetic transcription and phonological analyses also reveal differences; for example, errors in apraxia are more

[3]In the original SDCS, the category Speech Delay—Speech Motor Involvement was primarily concerned with the disorder referred to as Childhood Apraxia of Speech (CAS) by the American Speech-Language-Hearing Association (American Speech-Language-Hearing Association, 2002) and defined as "a neurological childhood (pediatric) speech sound disorder in which the precision and consistency of movements underlying speech are impaired in the absence of neuromuscular deficits" (pp. 3–4). Currently, the SDCS refers to this subtype as Motor Speech Disorder—Apraxia of Speech (MSD-AOS) but this acronym is used interchangeably with its earlier counterpart CAS in this chapter. Many variants of this diagnostic term are also in use in the scientific literature with Developmental Verbal Dyspraxia being common, especially in the United Kingdom. Much of the research is concerned with distinguishing CAS from other forms of motor speech disorder such as dysarthria and other forms of developmental speech disorder variously termed speech delay of unknown origin, functional articulation disorder, nonspecific speech disorder, phonological delay, or phonological disorder.

likely to occur in word-initial position; errors involving multiple feature differences are comparatively more characteristic of phonemic paraphasias. Overall, it appears that the phonemic paraphasias result from errors in the selection and sequencing of phonological units whereas apraxia results from errors in the selection and phonetic specification of articulatory gestures. Another motor speech disorder, dysarthria, involves more pervasive effects on phonation, resonance, articulation, and prosody secondary to paresis, weakness, or abnormalities of tone in the muscles resulting from damage to the upper or lower motor neurons that innervate those muscles.

Phonemic paraphasias result from errors in the *selection and sequencing of phonological units.*

Apraxia results from errors in the *selection and phonetic specification of articulatory gestures.*

Dysarthria results from a breakdown at the level of *motor execution* and involves more pervasive effects on phonation, resonance, articulation, and prosody secondary to paresis, weakness, or abnormalities of tone in the muscles.

Even among adult patients it is difficult to be sure that these theoretically separate levels of linguistic and motor planning and execution can be discretely implicated (Canter et al., 1985). In the developing child it is even less likely that a discrete locus of deficit, phonological or motoric, could be isolated from a description of the overt characteristics of the child's speech patterns. Although it is possible that developmental disorders might impact the functioning of specific brain regions, modularity of psycholinguistic and perceptuomotor processes emerges with experience (Karmiloff-Smith, 2006). Examination of Figure 3–15 shows that many interacting components are required for the development of speech motor control; the key role of auditory feedback explains why children with sensory-neural hearing losses have a speech deficit that is strikingly similar to apraxia (Osberger & McGarr, 1982; Robb, Hughes, & Frese, 1985). As reviewed in Chapter 3, children with smaller vocabulary sizes have more difficulty repeating novel phoneme sequences than children with larger vocabulary sizes. Therefore, it should not be a surprise to find that lists of diagnostic criteria for the diagnosis of Childhood Apraxia of Speech (CAS) share many characteristics in common with other forms of speech delay or even early normal speech development. Ozanne (2005) investigated the presence or absence of 18 commonly proposed symptoms of a motor speech disorder in 100 children aged 3 to 5 with suspected CAS and conducted a cluster analysis. The clusters are shown in Table 7–3. The first cluster appeared to mirror the subtype referred to by Dodd et al. (2005) as Inconsistent Deviant Disorder and attributed to a deficit at the level of phonological encoding (i.e., assembling the phonological plan). Although there is disagreement about the extent to which CAS might involve problems with phonological encoding (Shriberg et al., 1997), a breakdown at this level typically would not be included in the category of MSD even though inconsistent speech sound errors are often considered to be a primary symptom of apraxia of speech (Betz & Stoel-Gammon, 2005). For example, some data on consistency of word productions are reproduced from Betz and Stoel-Gammon in Table 7–4 from three children, one diagnosed with CAS (GFTA percentile = 1), one diagnosed with phonological disorder, that is, DPD with no motor involvement (GFTA percentile = 8) and one with normally developing speech (GFTA percentile = 81). The child with CAS is clearly much more inconsis-

In the developing child it is unlikely that a discrete locus of deficit, phonological or motoric, can be isolated from a description of the surface characteristics of the child's speech patterns.

Many interacting components are required for the development of speech motor control.

Lists of diagnostic criteria for the diagnosis of **Childhood Apraxia of Speech (CAS)** share many characteristics in common with other forms of speech delay.

Ozanne describes four clusters of children diagnosed with CAS, as shown in Table 7–3.

Table 7–3. *Clusters of Symptoms of Motor Involvement in 100 Children with Speech Delay with Suspected Motor Planning Difficulties*

Cluster	*Symptom*
1. Inconsistent Deviant Disorder	Inconsistent production of the same word
	Increased errors with increased performance load
	Atypical errors not explained by common articulation or phonological process errors
	Poor maintenance of phonotactic structure
	Vowel errors
2. Motor Programming Disorder or Subclinical Dysarthria	Slow diadochokinetic rates
	Poor sequencing ability during diadochokinetic tasks
	Difficulties with nonverbal oral-motor tasks
3. Apraxia	Consonant deletion
	Spontaneous production of phonemes in words that the child is unable to imitate
	Use of phonemes in words that do not contain that phoneme but errors on that phoneme in the appropriate context
	Groping (e.g., trial and error movements while imitating single sounds)
4. Subtype of Apraxia	No history of babbling
	Prosodic differences

Source: Adapted from Ozanne (2005). Childhood apraxia of speech. In B. Dodd (Ed.), *Differential diagnosis and treatment of children with speech disorder* (pp. 71–82). Reprinted with permission of Whurr Publishers.

tent upon repeated productions of the same word overall, although it is interesting to note that the CAS and PD children are equally inconsistent with the word "zebra." It is tempting to assume that the inconsistency observed in Table 7–4 reflects some sort of underlying variability in the production of speech motor movements but recall from Chapter 4 that Goffman, Gerken, and Lucchesi (2007) found that segmental variability and motor variability were not always correlated (see also Preston & Koenig, 2011). They concluded that it is hazardous to infer a motor planning deficit without instrumental measures of speech motor control and that motor output may be "relatively stable and patterned" in children who produce inconsistent speech errors. Therefore, the hypothesis that the level of breakdown is at a higher level of planning in children with inconsistent deviant errors is reasonable although unconfirmed when made on the basis of transcriptional evidence alone.

The *first cluster* of children diagnosed with CAS showed **inconsistent deviant** errors that may arise from a deficit in phonological encoding with little or no motor involvement.

Table 7–4. Examples of Inconsistent Word Productions

Participant	*Target Word*	*Production 1*	*Production 2*	*Production 3*	*Production 4*	*Production 5*	*Production 6*
DAS 1	kite	kætə	gæi	kæt	kætə	kæt	kætə
	spoon	əfunə	fun	fun	fuən	funə	fun
	squirrel	goza	got	gʊdə	kəlʌlə	kəʒ	kuədə
	watch	vwat	wat	wat	waʃə	vwaæ	waʃ
	zebra	tʃibə	ʒibə	dʒibæ	tibæ	dʒizba	dʒibæ
PD 1	kite	kaɪt	kaɪt	kaɪt	kaɪt	kaɪt	kaɪt
	spoon	pun	pun	pun	pun	pun	pun
	squirrel	kwowə	kwowə	kwowə	kwowə	kwowə	kwowə
	watch	watʃ	watʃ	watʃ	watʃ	watʃ	watʃ
	zebra	dibwʃ	givwə	tivwə	dʒibwə	dʒivwə	dzibwa
TD 1	kite	kaɪt	kaɪt	kaɪt	kaɪt	kaɪt	kaɪt
	spoon	spun	spun	spun	spun	spun	spun
	squirrel	skɚl	skɚl	skɚl	skɚl	skwɚl	skɚl
	watch	watʃ	watʃ	watʃ	watʃ	watʃ	watʃ
	zebra	zibrə	zibrə	zibrə	zibrə	zibrə	zibrə

DAS = child diagnosed with developmental (i.e., childhood) apraxia of speech; PD = child diagnosed with phonological disorder (PD); TD = child with typical speech development.

Source: Reprinted with permission from Betz and Stoel-Gammon (2005). Measuring articulatory error consistency in children developmental apraxia of speech. *Clinical Linguistics and Phonetics, 19*, Table III, p. 61.

The second cluster shown in Table 7–3 was described as a Motor Programming Disorder whereby the child selected the correct motor plan but specified the incorrect timing or force parameters (see discussion of generalized motor plans in Chapter 3). It was suggested that in some children this disorder might have elements of a movement execution disorder as well, that is, subclinical dysarthria, with slow diadochokinetic rates being a key indicator of this possibility.

The *second cluster* of children diagnosed with CAS had difficulty with maximum performance tasks suggesting **motor programming** deficits and **subclinical dysarthria**.

The third cluster corresponded to classic definitions of CAS because the symptoms indicate difficulties with voluntary motor control: the problem that is commonly understood to be the core feature of this disorder. The characteristic error pattern that was associated with this cluster, use of phonemes in words that do not contain that phoneme but errors on that phoneme in the appropriate context, was described as a symptom of motor planning difficulty; however, the examples given were suggestive of phonemic paraphasias and thus the difficulty of clearly differentiating these

The *third cluster* corresponded to classic definitions of **CAS** because the symptoms indicate difficulties with **voluntary motor control**.

The *fourth cluster*, marked by **prosodic difficulties**, overlapped the third and was described as a possible subtype of CAS.

processing levels, especially without the aid of instrumental analyses, arises. The fourth cluster, marked by prosodic difficulties, overlapped the third and was described as a possible subtype of apraxia of speech.

Many researchers have attempted to validate the sensitivity and specificity of these kinds of diagnostic markers as a means of differentiating MSD, in particular CAS, from Speech Delay (in this context, often referred to as phonological delay by the researchers for contrast). These efforts are complicated by the lack of consensus on the appropriate diagnostic criteria for selecting a CAS sample for study and the inherent difficulties of studying a low incidence disorder. Furthermore, case studies of children diagnosed with CAS reveal considerable change in the profile of symptoms as the children mature and participate in therapy as well as significant individual differences in symptom clusters between children with the CAS diagnosis (Shriberg, Aram, & Kwiatkowski, 1997; Stackhouse & Snowling, 1992). Nonetheless, we feel that it is absolutely clear from these studies that CAS cannot be differentiated from Speech Delay by describing the child's pattern of speech errors (Shriberg, Aram, et al., 1997; Stackhouse, 1992; Thoonen, Maassen, Gabreels, & Schreuder, 1994). Persistent reports of unusual prosody at the utterance level, in particular equal stressed syllables, appear in the scientific literature (Shriberg, 1997; Yoss & Darley, 1974). However, no perceptual or instrumental measures of lexical stress or prosody have proven to have sufficient specificity or sensitivity to be used as a diagnostic marker for CAS (Shriberg, Campbell, et al., 2003; Shriberg, Green, Campbell, McSweeny, & Scheer, 2003; Velleman & Shriberg, 1999).

In contrast, measures of oral-motor function, whether involving production of single or sequenced oral gestures or the standard diadochokinetic rate and alternate motion rate tasks (see Chapter 5) have revealed differences between CAS and phonological disorder (Lewis, Freebairn, Hansen, Taylor, et al., 2004; Thoonen, Maassen, Gabreels, & Schreuder, 1999; Thoonen, Maassen, Wit, Gabreels, & Schreuder, 1996; Yoss & Darley, 1974). It must be said that there is some circularity in these findings given that poor performance on these tasks corresponds to traditional definitions of CAS and thus would enhance the likelihood of community referral to research clinics for inclusion in these studies. Notwithstanding this issue, it is clear that the population of children with primary speech sound disorders can be differentiated into groups on the basis of oral-motor performance. Two of these studies are discussed in greater detail.

Yoss and Darley (1974) described a sample of 30 children, aged 5 to 9 years, referred to the Mayo Clinic with moderate or severe articulation difficulties of unknown etiology. The children were required to demonstrate average verbal intelligence to be included in the study. Compared to a group of age matched children with error-free speech, these children had poorer speech perception and oral motor skills as a group. The group of children with articulation difficulties was divided into two on the basis of their performance on a test of isolated volitional oral movements (e.g., "Show me how you blow; puff out your cheeks"). Among the children who scored below the group median on this test, 15 of 16 exhibited "soft" neurological signs compared to only 4 of 14 among the children who scored above the group median on this measure. The positive neurological signs that were reported in the neurological examination involved functional fine and gross motor abilities (manipulation of buttons and scissors; riding a bicycle; "clumsiness"). Williams, Ingham, and Rosenthal (1981) reported that they could not replicate this finding. However, despite adopting the Yoss and Darley assessment procedures in their study, their sample selection procedures were different; they recruited children from community clinics and selected more mildly impaired children who scored within the average range on tests of nonverbal (rather than verbal) intelligence. The resulting sample achieved much higher scores on the test of volitional oral movements on average and demonstrated many fewer soft neurological signs than the Yoss and Darley sample overall.

Thoonen and colleagues validated and cross-validated the use of maximum performance tasks (MPTs) as a means of distinguishing between CAS, dysarthria and what they termed "nonspecific" speech sound disorder in two small sample studies (Thoonen et al., 1999; Thoonen et al., 1996). The procedures for administering the MPTs are described in detail in Chapter 5 (see Appendix 5–4). First, the criteria were developed on the basis of data collected from three reference groups composed of children diagnosed with CAS, dysarthria, and normally developing speech; then the criteria were validated with new samples of children diagnosed with CAS, spastic dysarthria, nonspecific speech disorder, and normally developing speech. The children were independently diagnosed by two speech-language pathologists who agreed upon group assignment on the basis of standard diagnostic criteria: high frequency of errors, groping, difficulty with phoneme sequences, and inconsistency were indicators of dyspraxia; slow speech rate, hypernasality, monotonous pitch, and imprecision were indicators of dysarthria. The children in the nonspecific speech disorder group had a primary speech disorder that did not meet the criteria for CAS or dysarthria. This latter group was described as being heterogeneous, potentially including all four of Dodd's subtypes (articulation disorder, phonological delay, consistent deviant, and inconsistent deviant). All children had normal hearing, oral structure, and receptive language skills. Table 7–5 shows the performance of the four groups on the MPTs for the reference samples described in Thoonen et al. (1996) and for the validation samples described in Thoonen et al. (1999). The MPT diagnostic criteria derived from the reference samples are described in detail in Chapter 5. When the criteria for identifying dysarthria were applied to the CAS, dysarthric, and nonspecific speech disorder validation groups, sensitivity was 89%

Table 7–5. *Mean (M) and Standard Deviation (SD) of Group Performance on Maximum Performance Tasks by Children with Childhood Apraxia of Speech (CAS), Spastic Dysarthria (SDys), Nonspecific Speech Disorder (NSD), and Normally Developing Speech (Control)*

Group	N	Age Range (mo)	MRRmono	MPD	MRRtri	MFD
Reference Groups (Thoonen et al., 1996)						
CAS	11	75–99	4.39(0.54)	10.75(2.83)	3.69(0.76)[a]	9.36(3.42)
SDys	9	76–123	3.30(0.65)	3.86(1.95)	2.82(0.55)[a]	3.18(1.47)
Control	11	72–98	4.94(0.51)	13.56(3.37)	4.95(0.72)	14.37(4.30)
Validation Groups (Thoonen et al., 1999)						
CAS	10	53–90	3.80(0.23)	7.10(2.78)	2.44(0.02)[b]	6.76(3.39)
Dys	9	64–197	2.74(0.83)	10.31(5.49)	2.93(0.99)[b]	10.13(5.72)
NSD	11	52–131	4.30(0.57)	10.52(4.54)	3.84(1.20)[b]	10.72(3.84)
Control	11	62–138	5.27(0.57)	14.98 (2.72)	5.33(0.96)	15.01(3.31)

MRRmono = maximum repetition rate, monosyllabic (number of syllables/second); MPD = maximum phonation duration (in seconds); MRRtri = maximum repetition rate, trisyllable sequence (number of syllables/second); MFD = maximum fricative duration (in seconds). See Chapter 5 for details of procedures for obtaining measurements and diagnostic criteria.

[a]These means exclude measures from children who were unable to produce a correct trisyllabic sequence after 6 total trials: 4/11 children in CAS group and 2/9 children with dysarthria.

[b]These means exclude measures from children who were unable to produce a correct trisyllabic sequence after 6 total trials: 8/10 children in CAS group, 1/9 children with dysarthria, and 2/11 children with nonspecific speech disorder.

Source: Adapted from Thoonen et al. (1996). The integrated use of maximum performance tasks in differential diagnostic evaluations among children with motor speech disorders. *Clinical Linguistics and Phonetics, 10,* 311–336 and Thoonen et al. (1999). Validity of maximum performance tasks to diagnose motor speech disorders in children. *Clinical Linguistics and Phonetics, 13,* 1–23. Used with permission of Taylor and Francis Ltd.

Slow **monosyllabic repetition rate** and (in older children) short phonation duration are valid indicators for the diagnosis of *dysarthria*.

Difficulty with the sequencing of speech movements as measured by **multisyllable repetition tasks** is a valid indicator for the diagnosis of *apraxia* of speech.

and specificity was 100%. When the criteria for identifying apraxia of speech were applied to the CAS, nonspecific speech disorder, and control validation groups, sensitivity was 100% and specificity was 91%. The results supported the validity of slow monosyllabic repetition rate and (in older children) short phonation duration as indicators of dysarthria. The results also validated difficulty with the sequencing of speech movements as an indicator of apraxia of speech. Despite the success of the procedure in identifying discrete groups, the performance data shown in Table 7–5 reflect overlap in symptoms among the three groups of children with speech sound disorder, however. Thoonen et al. (1999) reported that the performance of the nonspecific speech disorder group on monosyllabic repetition and maximum phonation duration approached that of the CAS group; at the same time the performance of this group on the trisyllabic repetition and maximum fricative duration tasks approached that of the dysarthric group. The CAS group showed some dysarthric symptoms, especially slow monosyllabic repetition rates in some cases.

Lewis and colleagues also provide evidence that multisyllable repetition is a useful endophenotype for CAS in a longitudinal study of children with CAS, speech delay without language impairment (SD), and speech delay with language impairment (SD+LI). When assessed as preschoolers (Lewis, Freebairn, Hansen, Taylor, et al., 2004), the CAS group had more severe speech delay than the other two groups but their language skills were similar to the SD+LI group. Their speech sound sequencing abilities were significantly poorer than the SD and SD+LI groups. When these groups were reassessed approximately 4 years later (Lewis, Freebairn, Hansen, Iyengar, & Taylor, 2004), all three groups achieved mean speech and language test scores within the average range although the CAS group continued to lag behind the other two groups in this area and several children in this group showed persistent speech deficits. Furthermore, the CAS group demonstrated significant difficulties with the Fletcher time-by-count repetition tasks and poor nonword and multisyllabic word repetition performance, relative to age norms and the other groups.

Longitudinal studies suggest that slow multisyllable repetition rate is a useful endophenotype for CAS because it persists even after speech accuracy has normalized.

The distinctive and severe difficulties that these children evidenced with the repetition of complex syllable sequences, even after resolution of the speech delay in many cases, raises the question of a unique etiology for CAS relative to other forms of speech delay. Lewis, Freebairn, Hansen, Taylor, et al. (2004) investigated the family pedigrees of these three groups of children. Familial aggregation was high in all three groups, although higher in the CAS group than in the other two groups. Nuclear family members were reported and/or tested to be affected by a range of speech and language disorders in all three groups supporting the hypothesis of a general verbal trait deficit with a gradient of genetic loading and severity from the SD through SD+LI and CAS groups. The results also supported a sex-specific threshold model whereby manifestation of the CAS phenotype requires a higher genetic loading in females than in males. The notion of a general verbal trait deficit is consistent with the common disease/common variant model described by Bishop (2009). According to this model, the etiology of speech and language disorders is multifactorial, involving interactions among many genetic and environmental factors that combine to explain the full range of variance in ability levels in these domains. The large number of genes involved, each having small effects, accounts for the phenotypic variation (i.e., heterogeneity) observed within the general population and within diagnostic subgroups.

According to the **common disease/common variant** model, the etiology of speech and language disorders is multifactorial, involving interactions among many genetic and environmental factors that combine to explain the full range of variance in ability levels in these domains.

In contrast to the majority of cases of CAS which may be polygenic in underlying etiology, there is at least one known monogenic cause of developmental apraxia however: these are the rare cases of speech disorder linked to an autosomal dominant mutation of the *FOXP2* gene on chromosome 7q31. The eventual identification of *FOXP2* as the first gene to be linked to speech disorder begins with a series of studies investigating the behavioral, genetic, and neurological characteristics of affected and unaffected members of the KE family (for a summary of these findings, see Vargha-Khadem, Gadian, Copp, & Mishkin, 2005). These studies of three generations of this family reveal 15 of 37 members with a mutation of the *FOXP2*

There is at least one known monogenic cause of developmental apraxia: these are the rare cases of speech disorder linked to an autosomal dominant mutation of the ***FOXP2*** gene on chromosome 7q31.

gene. Although affected family members demonstrated difficulties with every aspect of speech and language, including receptive and expressive deficits in spoken and written language, the most striking characteristics were unintelligible speech and difficulties with expressive morphosyntax (Vargha-Khadem, Watkins, Alcock, Fletcher, & Passingham, 1995). Although verbal intelligence was significantly impaired relative to nonverbal intelligence in affected family members, nonverbal intelligence was significantly lower in affected than unaffected family members, attesting to the pervasive cognitive-linguistic deficits associated with *FOXP2* abnormalities. Considerable overlap in the distribution of scores across affected and unaffected family members was observed for many language and cognitive measures, however. The only two measures that unambiguously differentiated affected and unaffected family members were tests of nonword repetition and orofacial praxis, leading to the conclusion that verbal dyspraxia is the core behavioral phenotype associated with *FOXP2* mutation. It is not clear whether the remaining linguistic and nonverbal cognitive deficits arise from the underlying deficit in orofacial praxis or whether they constitute additional core deficits. Neuroimaging studies revealed bilateral structural abnormalities of motor-related regions including the caudate nucleus, inferior frontal gyrus, precentral gyrus, and cerebellum. Functional neuroimaging studies during covert and overt verb generation tasks and during overt nonword repetition tasks revealed underactivation of the putamen, Broca's area, and its right hemisphere homologue. Subsequently, other *FOXP2* abnormalities have been reported in association with motor speech disorders (MacDermot et al., 2005; Shriberg et al., 2006; Zhao et al., 2010).

Dyspraxia, indexed by deficits in nonword repetition and orofacial praxis, is the core behavioral phenotype associated with *FOXP2* mutation.

In summary, despite overlap of phenotypic characteristics with phonological disorder and heterogeneity within the MSD subtype itself, it is reasonable to posit a distinct diagnostic category for children who have difficulty with maximum performance tasks and/or measures of orofacial praxis. At least in some cases, there will be a unique and distinct monogenic origin but in the majority of cases of MSD the cause is more likely polygenic leading to heterogeneity in phenotype with the underlying explanatory factors involving a continuum of planning deficits at the phonological and motoric levels that may be accompanied by subclinical motor execution difficulties (Ozanne, 2005). In all cases there is a strong likelihood of a pervasive disorder impacting speech production, language expression, phonological memory, and literacy skills (Lewis, Freebairn, Hansen, Taylor, et al., 2004; Lewis, Freebairn, Hansen, Iyengar, et al., 2004; Stackhouse, 1992).

Clinical Value of the Medical Approach to Classifying Speech Sound Disorders

The Speech Disorders Classification System proposes three superordinate classifications that link proposed etiological factors, explanatory speech factors, clinical subtypes, diagnostic markers, phenotypes, and endophenotypes in a coherent fashion. Most children with DPD can be expected to fit into the Speech Delay classification, exhibiting multiple speech substitution and deletion errors arising from impaired phonological representations secondary to inherited neurodevelopmental constraints that are polygenic in nature. This subtype is heterogeneous but may have concomitant difficulties with language and reading. Normalization trajectory is expected to be short term with appropriate intervention. Although three subcategories are suggested there appears to be considerable overlap among them. The second superordinate classification, Speech Errors, describes a profile restricted to persistent distortions of late developing phonemes. Although these distortions may persist into adulthood, concomitant difficulties in other areas of development are not expected. The underlying speech processes and etiological factors in these cases are not clearly illuminated by the literature. Finally, Motor Speech Disorders arise from difficulties with motor planning or execution and are prone to a long-term trajectory of normalization with concomitant difficulties in multiple developmental domains. Etiological factors may be quite heterogeneous with some cases clearly linked to rare monogenic syndromes and others apparently polygenic in origin.

Much of the research conducted within the framework of the Speech Disorders Classification System is intended to support efforts to identify the presumed genetic underpinnings of the proposed clinical subtypes. This work is contributing to exciting developments in neurobiology that implicate specific genes that are involved in fetal brain development, linking speech disorders to dyslexia and illuminating complex neural pathways involved in speech motor control. It is fair to consider the clinical value of the medical model to diagnosis however, especially as clear phenotypic markers for each subtype have not been revealed and medical treatments are not available for the speech component of any of the proposed subtypes (although medical intervention is obviously required for OME and may be required if there are contributing oral structural deficiencies or concomitant psychiatric disorders). The possible benefits and drawbacks of the medical model are discussed here.

The Speech Disorders Classification System was developed to support research. A medical model may also have value for clinical assessment, diagnosis, and intervention in speech-language pathology.

An important consideration is the need of the child's parents for a diagnostic label and an explanation for their child's developmental delay or difference relative to other children. Even when the developmental difficulty is perceived by the health care provider to be relatively trivial, the parent may feel considerable distress and be burdened by concerns about the source of the child's problem. Hallberg, Óskarsdóttir, and Klingberg (2010) describe ambivalence between sorrow and relief as a core theme in parents' responses to receiving a diagnosis of their child's medical condition, especially when uncertainty about the diagnosis has persisted for some time. Poehlmann, Clements, Abbeduto, Farsad, and Ferguson (2005) speculate that long periods of uncertainty before receiving a diagnosis may lead to negative coping strategies as mothers worry that they may have caused their child's developmental delay.

Interviews with parents of children with developmental disabilities reveal *seven perceived benefits of a diagnosis* that include validating the parents' concerns and helping them to access information and services.

Makela, Birch, Friedman, and Marra (2009) identified seven perceived benefits of a diagnosis from interviews with parents of children with a diagnosed or undiagnosed intellectual impairment. The first perceived value was in validation of the parents concern which included confirming that parenting practices were not the cause the child's problems. Second, it is important to realize how much information for parents and other caregivers is organized around diagnostic labels and thus the diagnosis helps the family to learn what to expect from the health care system and what to hope for their child's future. In many jurisdictions the diagnostic label is often the key to accessing medical, educational and therapeutic services. In the case of speech disorders, medical insurance may not cover private therapy except for "medical diagnoses" such as CAS. In schools, it is common to deny services for articulation therapy because of a mistaken impression that articulation errors do not threaten the child's academic outcomes. In these settings a diagnosis may be required regardless of whether it meets the SLP's needs. A full understanding of the medical model and further research from this perspective will help the profession to correct these misguided policies and advocate effectively for the child's needs without engaging in diagnostic practices that are fraudulent or not evidence based. Parents also seek a diagnosis with the hope that their child will receive early intervention. Many parents in these interview studies recall being treated as overanxious or neurotic for seeking a diagnosis when their child was young but given the importance of resolving communication deficits during the preschool period and the frequency with which speech and language delays are associated with other developmental disabilities, parental concerns should never be dismissed lightly. The fifth benefit of a diagnosis is access to support from other people, especially other parents with similar experiences, as with information and intervention services, support groups are often organized around diagnostic labels. Parents reported that their need to know the diagnosis changed over time and they often reached a stage when it was no longer critically important to know the cause of their child's problems but some level of curiosity often persists over the long term. Finally, parents may want more information for family planning purposes. Many times speech problems are early indicators of genetically transmitted developmental problems and parents may wish to be referred for genetic counseling. In any case, they will come across a great deal of formal and informal information about potential genetic etiologies and the SLP must know enough to help parents interpret this information and to refer families for expert advice when appropriate. On the subject of referrals for diagnostic services, however, it is important to remember that it is the parents' right to determine when and if they wish to access these services in pursuit of a medical diagnosis.

Notwithstanding these perceived and tangible benefits of a medical diagnostic label for parents, it is not clear that the diagnostic categories proposed in the Speech Disorders Classification System or any other medical model are helpful to the SLP for the purpose of treatment planning. Even if one were able to assign children with confidence to the proposed subtypes, none of the subtypes suggest a distinct treatment approach. For example, the underlying explanatory process associated with Speech Delay—Genetic is a phonological processing disorder which includes significant difficulties with phonological awareness that elevate the risk of reading disability. This profile is also characteristic of children from disadvantaged social environments and may occur secondary to OME and concurrently with CAS, however. It is not clear whether Speech Errors in the RE-B category are articulatory or perceptual in origin. A treatment approach that targets phonological processing may well be appropriate for at least some of the children assigned to any of these subtypes of speech delay. For these reasons, Stackhouse and Wells (1993) recommend that treatment planning be based on a thorough psycholinguistic investigation of the child's speech processing at multiple levels of representation.

Psycholinguistic Approach to the Description of DPD

7.3.1. Identify three possible causes of speech perception deficits in children with DPD.

7.3.2. List two primary determinants of children's underlying phonological knowledge of the sound system of their language as revealed by tests of phonological awareness or nonword repetition.

7.3.3. Define "undifferentiated lingual gesture."

7.3.4. Describe the three primary patterns of responding to maximum performance tasks observed in children with DPD and interpret these performance patterns in reference to a psycholinguistic model of speech processing and production.

Psycholinguistic models of DPD are hypotheses about the processes that underlie perception, comprehension, and production of speech and the effects that a breakdown in any of these processes may have on speech output. A number of different models have been proposed to guide the assessment of speech processing abilities in children with DPD (Chiat, 2001; Hewlett, Gibbon, & Cohen-McKenzie, 1998; Munson, Edwards, & Beckman, 2005a; Stackhouse & Wells, 1993). The models vary in their details but share components roughly described as input processes, internal representations, and

Psycholinguistic models of DPD are hypotheses about the processes that underly perception, comprehension, and production of speech and the effects that a breakdown in any of these processes may have on speech output.

output processes. Computational and neurolinguistic models have been proposed to test hypotheses about the nature of these specific components and/or the mappings between them and the effects of breakdowns in model components or neural functions (Harm & Seidenberg, 1999; Terband, Maassen, Guenther, & Brumberg, 2009). Research from this perspective is less concerned with discrete etiologies of DPD as it is recognized that multiple etiological factors may lead to breakdown at multiple levels of processing. At the same time, given the interconnectedness of the processing functions across multiple levels of representation, a breakdown at one level of representation is likely to impact processing at all levels of psycholinguistic or neurolinguistic functioning. It is expected that individual children will show idiosyncratic combinations of deficits across multiple areas of psycholinguistic processing and thus case studies are a common research design from this perspective. In the next three sections we review studies that have described children with DPD with a view to determining if the primary level of breakdown is in the realm of input processing, underlying phonological representations, or output processing.

Research from the psycholinguistic perspective is less concerned with discrete etiologies of DPD as it is recognized that multiple etiological factors may lead to breakdown at multiple levels of processing.

Input Processing in Children with DPD

As outlined in Chapter 4, accurate speech production skills are dependent on the development of detailed acoustic-phonetic representations for words. The best measure of the child's abilities in this domain is a word identification task, with the word identification skills that emerge in the second year of life building on language specific speech discrimination skills that develop during the first year (see Chapters 1 and 2 for further discussion of these tasks and early speech perception development). The speech discrimination and word identification skills of children with DPD have been studied repeatedly over the past six decades. Rather than describe this literature in detail we have summarized relevant studies in two tables, with Table 7–6 listing studies using speech discrimination tests and Table 7–7 listing studies using a word identification paradigm. The studies shown on these tables were identified by searching the journal archive of the American Speech, Language, and Hearing Association with the search terms "perception and articulation" or "perception and phonology" and then hand searching the results for studies in which the speech perception abilities of children with a primary developmental phonological disorder were compared to a control group. Subsequently, SCOPUS was used to search for additional papers that cited these papers resulting in one addition to the list. The review is meant to be systematic rather than exhaustive; in other words, it is limited to certain journals but unbiased with respect to study outcome: every study that met these criteria is listed in the tables regardless of the findings.

Table 7–6. Summary of Studies That Compare Speech Discrimination Skills of Children with DPD to a Control Group

Study	*Stimuli*	*Clinical Group*	*Control Group*	*Outcome*
Kronvall & Diehl (1952)	Templin Speech Sound Discrimination Test (recorded natural nonsense syllables).	N = 30; 6–9 yrs; "functional articulation disordered."	N = 30; matched for age, sex, intelligence.	M errors = 28.83 vs. 12.37; $t(29) = 23.56$, $p < .001$; $d = 8.75$.
Carrell & Pendergast (1954)	CV syllables presented live voice.	N = 33;9–13yrs; "delayed speech."	N = 33; matched for age, sex, intelligence and home background.	M errors = 6.94 vs. 5.18; $p < .05$.
Sherman & Geith (1967)	Templin Speech Sound Discrimination Test.	N = 18; kindergarten age; "severe functional articulatory defectives."	N = 18, matched for age, sex, grade and intelligence.	M(SD) errors = 28.83 (4.10) vs. 12.37 (4.10); $t(17) = 23.56$, $p <.001$; $d = 2.09$.
Marquardt & Saxman (1972)	Wepman Auditory Discrimination Test.	N = 30; kindergarten age; "numerous misarticulations."	N = 30; kindergarten age; perfect articulation.	M(SD) errors = 10.00 (4.59) vs. 4.76 (2.96); $t(29) = 17.35$, $p < .001$; $d = 6.44$.
Sommers, Cox, & West (1972)	Wepman Auditory Discrimination Test (live voice presentation of nonsense syllables).	N = 56 in total but speech discrimination results reported for a subset of 22 *r*-misarticulators and 37 *s*-misarticulators; kindergarten and first grade; "defective (multiple errors) or deviant (1 or 2 errors) articulation."	14 kindergarten or first grade children with "superior articulation."	M(SD) errors = 32.34 (3.59) for *r*-misarticulators vs. 34.93 (4.56) for *s*-misarticulators vs. 33.22 (3.07) for controls; no significant differences (statistical analysis not reported).
McReynolds, Kohn, & Williams (1975)	Recordings of naturally produced minimal pair words contrasting distinctive features.	N = 7; aged 3–7 yrs; "functional articulation disorders."	N = 7; aged 5–8 yrs; no phonemes with greater than 80% error on the McDonald Deep Test	M(SD) percent correct = 83.95 (6.11) vs. 94.29 (6.12); $t(6) = 4.51$, $p = .015$; $d = 2.29$.
Hoffman, Daniloff, Bengoa, & Schuckers (1985)	Synthetic "ray"-"way" continuum in which onset frequency of first three formants was manipulated.	N = 22; aged 6 yrs; speech delay and misarticulate [ɹ].	N = 13; aged 6 yrs; normal speech and language development.	M correct percent = 57 vs. 80% (see paper for complex statistical analysis).

continues

Table 7–6. continued

Study	Stimuli	Clinical Group	Control Group	Outcome
Maassen, Groenen, & Crul, (2003)	Synthetic continua: /i/-/ɪ/ and /a/-/ɑ/.	N = 11; age 6;9 to 9;5 yrs; Dutch children with CAS.	N = 12; aged 7;0 to 9;7 yrs; Dutch children with normally developing speech.	CAS group required greater difference between stimuli to discriminate them: /i/-/ɪ/, $t(11.9) = 2.85$, $p = .01$, $d = 1.65$; /a/-/ɑ/, $t(12.2) = 2.82$, $p = .01$, $d = 1.61$).
Nijland (2009)	Nonword discrimination task.	N = 21; aged 5;5 to 7;11 yrs; Dutch children with DPD; 8 with CAS and 9 with mixed CAS and phonological disorder; 4 with DPD alone.	N = 21; normally developing Dutch children matched for age.	CAS group had significantly poorer discrimination performance compared to control group; in contrast the remainder of the clinical group did not have difficulty with speech discrimination but all clinical groups had difficulty with a rhyming task. No raw data provided (see figures and statistical analysis provided in paper).

Table 7–7. Summary of Studies That Compare Word Identification Skills of Children with DPD to a Control Group

Study	Stimuli	Clinical Group	Control Group	Outcome
Raaymakers & Crul (1988)	Continuum constructed from naturally produced speech; digitally altered by inserting a silent interval to create a final /t/-/ts/ contrast in a Dutch CVC word.	N = 7; first graders; speech delay with specific misarticulation of final /ts/.	N = 5; first graders; normally developing speech.	$t(8) = 2.01$, $p < .05$, $d = 1.42$.
Rvachew & Jamieson (1989, Study 1)	Synthetic sheet-seat continuum; manipulation of spectral characteristics of frication noise.	N = 12; age 5 yrs; "functional articulation disorder."	N = 12; age 5 yrs; normal speech development.	Significant difference in A′ scores: $t(22) = 3.16$, $p = .002$, $d = 1.35$.

Table 7–7. continued

Study	*Stimuli*	*Clinical Group*	*Control Group*	*Outcome*
Rvachew & Jamieson (1989, Study 2)	Synthetic sick-thick continuum; manipulation of spectral characteristics of frication noise.	N = 9; age 7 yrs; "functional articulation disorder."	N = 13; age 7 yrs; normally developing speech.	Significant difference in A´ scores: $t(17) = 4.41$, $p = .0006$, $d = 1.93$.
Groenen, Maassen, & Crul (1998)	Synthetic continua manipulating formant transition durations to create place of articulation and voicing contrasts.	Children: N = 10; aged 9 yrs; Adolescents: N = 11; aged 14;11 yrs; both groups have speech delay but normal oral motor function.	Children: N = 10; aged 9 yrs; Adults, N = 10; normal articulation, language and nonverbal IQ.	Significant effect for slope of identification function: $F(3,37) = 5.07$, $p = .005$. Both clinical groups different from both control groups.
Edwards, Fox, & Rogers (2002)	Recordings of naturally produced words digitally altered to gate progressively larger portions of word endings; tap vs. tack; cat vs. cap.	N = 35; aged 56 mos; moderate or severe speech delay but normal receptive vocabulary and nonverbal IQ.	N = 13; matched for age, SES and receptive vocabulary skills.	Significant effect of group: $F(1,68) = 5.52$, $p < .03$.
Maassen, Groenen, & Crul, (2003)	Synthetic continua: /i/-/ɪ/ and /a/-/ɑ/.	N = 11; age 6;9 to 9;5 yrs; Dutch children with CAS.	N = 12; aged 7;0 to 9;7 yrs; Dutch children with normally developing speech.	Multivariate analysis revealed significant difference in identification functions: /i/-/ɪ/, $F(7,15) = 3.12$, $p = .03$; /a/-/ɑ/, $F(7,15) = 4.93$, $p = .004$.
Rvachew, Ohberg, Grawburg, & Heyding (2003)	Natural recordings of correctly and incorrectly produced words (SAILS): lake, cat, rate, Sue.	N = 13; aged 56 mos; moderate or severe speech delay but normal receptive vocabulary skills.	N = 13; matched for age, SES, and receptive vocabulary skills	M(SD) percent correct = 63.08 (9.57) vs. 74.08 (9.57); $t(12) = 2.42$, $p = .01$, $d = 1.40$.
Kenney, Barac-Cikoja, Finnegan, Jeffries, & Ludlow (2006)	Two synthetic say-stay continua; one with manipulation of F1 onset frequency; the other with manipulation of stop gap duration.	N = 9; adults; 12th percentile on GFTA but nonverbal IQ and language test scores in average range.	N = 20; adults with articulation, nonverbal IQ and language scores in average range.	A larger change in F1 onset frequency was required (significant difference in slope of identification functions, $p = .001$, $d = 1.60$). No group differences in response to the temporal manipulation.

Studies consistently find an association between speech perception skills and speech production skills among children with DPD.

The important outcome of the review is that, of the 20 comparisons of speech perception skills across clinical and control groups, only one failed to find an association between speech perception and speech production skills. In the 1950s and 1960s it was generally assumed that speech perception deficits were causally related to misarticulations and the dominant speech therapy approach included "ear training" as a core procedure (see Chapter 9). This was not an unreasonable view given the weight of the evidence but during the seventies opinion changed to the view that speech perception deficits in these children either did not occur or resulted directly from the articulation deficit itself and subsequently SLPs were counseled to avoid intervention approaches that focused on speech perception (Mowrer, 1971; Seymour, Baran, & Peaper, 1981). Some skepticism persists despite continued findings of poor perceptual abilities among children with DPD and thus we discuss these issues in more depth.

Some researchers have discounted even their own findings on the grounds that the differences in perceptual ability between clinical and control groups are so small as to be of no practical significance (McReynolds, Kohn, & Williams, 1975). Indeed, the perceptual difficulties can be so subtle in normal speaking situations that many adults find it difficult to believe that they exist and thus the "fis" anecdote that was discussed in Chapter 4. The notion that the children's perceptual difficulties are not important to their speech and language functioning arises from the mistaken idea that perceptual knowledge of a phoneme contrast is an all-or-nothing affair but we now know that the process of acquiring an efficient and language specific cue-weighting strategy for perceiving a contrast across varied speaking environments requires a long period of refinement even for children with normally developing speech. The small performance differences that are observed in speech discrimination tests involving natural speech stimuli occur because the child is not attending to or weighting appropriately the right set of cues for perceiving the contrast in question, a problem that is magnified during more difficult tasks such as identification of synthetic speech in which the acoustic cues have been carefully controlled. Figure 7–5 shows the individual word identification functions obtained from children tested in Rvachew and Jamieson (1989, Study 1). In order to participate in the study all of these children were required to demonstrate accurate identification of the words "seat" and "sheet" when presented with naturally produced live-voice stimuli. The children were then presented with a continuum of synthetic words that were constructed to be identical except for the centroid of the fricative portion of the word which was varied from a high frequency (for the "seat" endpoint at stimulus 1) to a much lower frequency (for the "sheet" endpoint at stimulus 7). Figure 7–5A shows identification functions obtained from 5 of the children who demonstrated categorical perception of this contrast based on spectral cues, allowing them to achieve perceptual performance that was similar to the

The small performance differences that are observed in speech discrimination tests involving natural speech stimuli occur because the child is not attending to or weighting appropriately the right set of cues for perceiving the contrast in question; this problem is magnified during more difficult tasks such as identification of synthetic speech in which the acoustic cues have been carefully controlled.

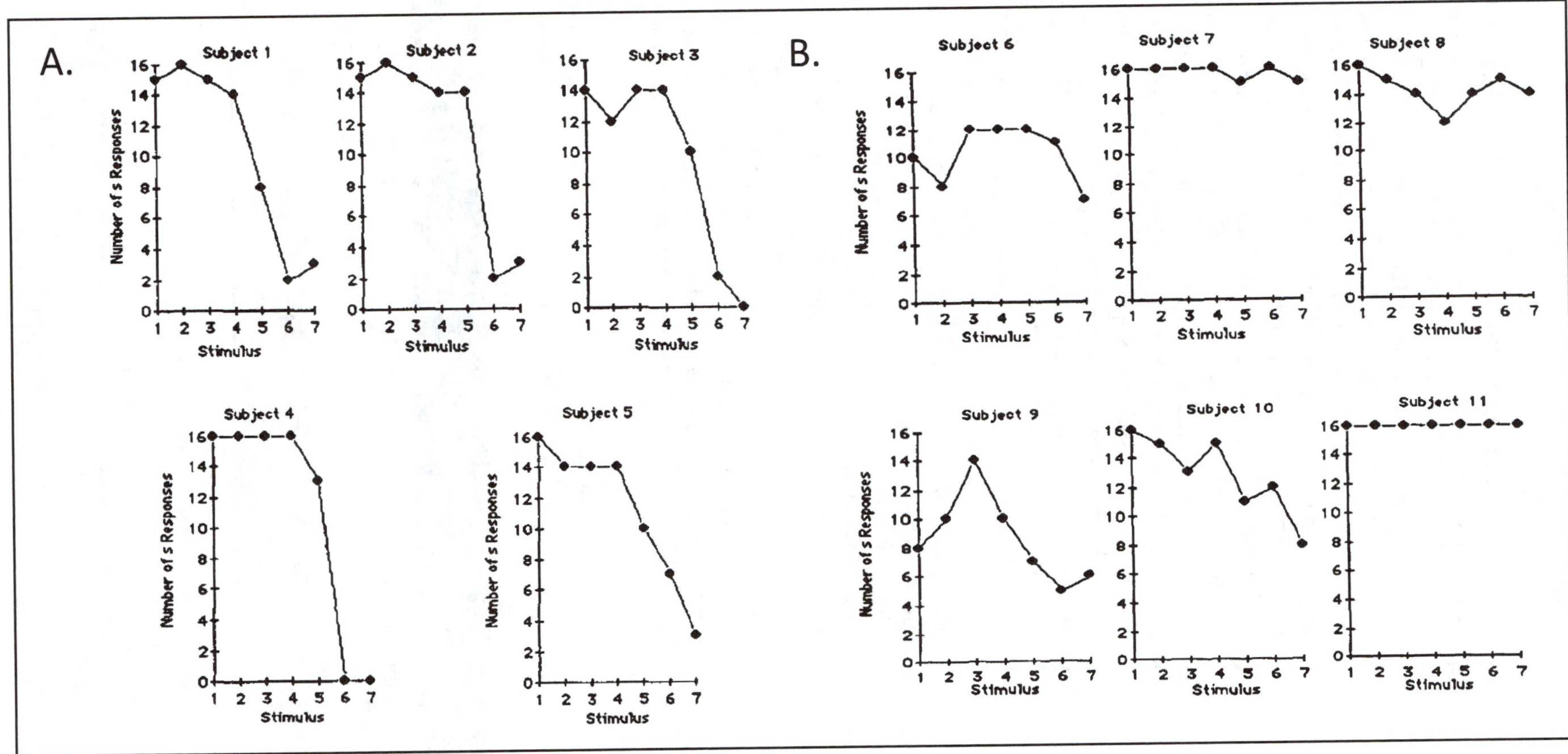

***Figure* 7–5.** *Mean number of "seat" responses to the stimuli in a 7-point seat-sheet synthetic speech continuum in which the centroid of the fricative was reduced in equal steps.* **A.** *Individual functions obtained from 5 children with DPD who responded similarly to children with normal speech.* **B.** *Individual functions obtained from 6 children with DPD who were unable to identify the stimuli as belonging to two discrete categories (the function of a 12th child who responded like Subject 6 is not shown due to space restrictions). Adapted from Rvachew and Jamieson (1989). Perception of voiceless fricatives by children with a functional articulation disorder.* Journal of Speech and Hearing Disorders, 54, *Study 1, Figure 3, p. 198 and Figure 4, p. 199. Adapted with permission of the American Speech-Hearing-Language Association.*

typically developing children and the adult subjects in this study, all of whom achieved categorical perception of this contrast. As can be seen in Figure 7–5B, the remaining children were completely unable to identify these stimuli as belonging to two discrete categories. It is likely that these children identified the live voice stimuli on the basis of the formant transition cues which allowed them to give the impression of having perceptual knowledge of this contrast when listening to natural speech. Failing to recognize the crucial importance of the spectral cue explains the children's perceptual performance during the synthetic speech task as well as their inability to learn the appropriate articulatory gestures for reproducing this acoustic-phonetic feature contrast in their own productions of these words.

Another reason for skepticism is the occasional failure to find a correlation between speech perception test scores and speech production accuracy (Aungst & Frick, 1964; Waldman, Singh, & Hayden, 1978). The primary reason for this finding is that speech perception deficits are very specific to the children's misarticulations (e.g., see Monnin & Huntington, 1974) and tests of speech perception often do not test contrasts that parallel the children's speech errors (Locke, 1980). Furthermore, good perceptual knowledge of a given contrast is a necessary but not sufficient condition for achievement of articulatory accuracy. Good perceptual performance does not guarantee that the child will demonstrate accurate production of the sound but does increase the likelihood that the child will learn to produce it soon. Consider the hierarchical multiple regression analyses shown in Table 7–8. These data are taken from a study in which 47 children received tests of speech perception (SAILS, a word identification/error detection task) and speech

Table 7–8. *Longitudinal Predictive Relationship Between Speech Perception Skills (SAILS) and Articulation Accuracy (GFTA-2) Measured Prior to Kindergarten Entry (preK) and at the End of the Kindergarten Year (K), as Determined by Hierarchical Multiple Regression Analysis*

	Dependent Variable	*Independent Variables*	R^2	ΔR^2	ΔF	p
A. Articulation (GFTA-2) does not predict growth in Speech Perception (SAILS)	SAILS K	SAILS PK	.207	.207	11.73	.001
		GFTA-2 PK	.254	.048	2.81	.101ns
B. Speech Perception (SAILS) predicts growth in Articulation (GFTA-2)	GFTA-2 K	GFTA-2 PK	.428	.428	33.64	.000
		SAILS PK	.503	.075	6.65	.013*

These analyses show that articulation skills prior to kindergarten did not predict unique variance in speech perception skills at the end of kindergarten, after controlling for prekindergarten speech perception skills, as shown by the nonsignificant (ns) result for change in variance explained in the second step of the analysis. On the other hand, speech perception skills prior to kindergarten predicted about 7.5% of variance in articulation skills at the end of kindergarten, after controlling for articulation skills prior to kindergarten, as shown by the significant (*) result for change in variance explained in the second step of the analysis. These results suggest that speech perception leads growth in articulation skills in developmental time.

Source: Adapted from Rvachew (2006). Longitudinal prediction of implicit phonological awareness skills. *American Journal of Speech-Language Pathology, 15*, Table 3 (p. 170). Used with permission of the American Speech-Language and Hearing Association.

production (GFTA-2) when they were 58 months old and again at the end of kindergarten when they were 70 months old. The concurrent correlation between speech perception test performance and number of errors on the GFTA-2 during the prekindergarten assessment was moderately large but not statistically significant; the longitudinal correlation between prekindergarten speech perception and articulation accuracy at the end of the kindergarten year was statistically significant, however ($r = -.47$). More importantly, the analysis shown in Table 7–8 shows that articulation accuracy prior to kindergarten did not explain growth in speech perception skills during the kindergarten year (Part A); on the other hand, speech perception skills prior to kindergarten entry did explain growth in articulation accuracy during the same year (Part B). The results of this analysis suggest that speech perception is causally related to the achievement of speech production accuracy, a causal relationship that has been confirmed in several intervention studies to be discussed in Chapter 9.

A third reason that there is skepticism about the role of speech perception in DPD is the confusion in the research about auditory processing as a causal factor in specific language impairment and dyslexia. The phonological processing deficits observed in children with speech, language, and reading disabilities have long been attributed to general auditory processing disorders with a hypothesized disorder in temporal processing (Tallal, 1980) being a specific version of this hypothesis that has generated a large body of research and a computer-based intervention (i.e., FastForWord; e.g., Merzenich et al., 1996). This literature is confusing because there is no consensus about the nature of the proposed auditory processing deficit (for alternatives to the temporal processing hypothesis, see Ahissar, 2007; Goswami et al., 2002) and because studies do not consistently demonstrate auditory processing difficulties among children with language and reading disabilities (for reviews, see Mody, 2003; Studdert-Kennedy, 2002). Furthermore, even when auditory processing deficits have been observed in these populations, nonsensory explanations cannot be ruled out (Halliday & Bishop, 2006) and causal relationships to the children's phonological processing deficits cannot be confirmed (Share, Jorm, MacLean, & Mathews, 2002). This degree of confusion leads readily to the conclusion that auditory processing difficulties are not an important causal factor in these disorders but this conclusion should not be generalized to the question of the causal role of speech perception deficits in DPD or indeed SLI or dyslexia.

Overall, it is now clear that speech perception deficits commonly occur in children who have concomitant language and reading impairments (Joanisse, Manis, Keating, & Seidenberg, 2000) and are associated with the phonological processing deficits that are causally related to the reading impairment (Stanovich & Siegel, 1994; Torgesen, Wagner, Rashotte, Burgess, & Hecht, 1997). Rather than the nonspeech auditory processing deficit causing speech

Animal models of neurological development suggest top-down mechanisms that explain why children with phonological processing deficits may or may not have deficits in more primary sensory domains.

perception difficulties, it appears that these problems may have a common cause. On the basis of animal models of neurological development, Ramus (2004) has proposed a mechanism by which ectopias (anomalies of cell migration during cortical development) lead to anatomical disruptions in thalamic nuclei that are important to sensory processing; interestingly, these top-down effects are quite heterogeneous with the specific outcomes dependent on the exact locations of the cortical ectopias and the mediating effects of hormonal conditions. Keeping in mind that the model is based on animal research, it provides a possible explanation for how some but not all children with a genetically based deficit in speech perception may or may not have concomitant difficulties with nonspeech sensory tasks. The model may also explain patterns of comorbidity among speech, language, and reading disability, a topic to which we return later in this chapter.

Ramus' neurobiological model of the etiology of dyslexia is consistent with brain imaging findings for children with Residual Speech Errors. Recall Preston et al.'s (2012) fMRI study in which brain activation patterns were significantly different for older children with speech errors while listening to speech relative to children without speech errors. The authors interpret their findings within the context of Hickok and Poeppel's (2007) model of speech processing (see Figure 2–12 and associated explanation in Chapter 2). Greater engagement of the superior temporal gyrus/supramarginal gyrus, precentral gyrus, and insula/putamen was interpreted as evidence that children with REs were relying on motor coding during perception, a strategy that only occurs when processing demands are high in normal listeners. Group differences in activation patterns in left temporal regions were interpreted as inefficient processing by the ventral stream that would explain impaired perception of novel phonological forms and deficient mapping of phonological to semantic representations.

The plausibility of this account does not rule out the possibility that some children suffer from an auditory processing disorder that causes speech perception and other phonological processing problems as in the "bottom-up" model of OME-related speech delay discussed earlier in this chapter. Furthermore, it must not be forgotten that speech perception is learned and the acquisition of appropriate cue-weighting strategies may be limited by lack of optimum input from the language environment. Nittrouer (2005) demonstrated that speech perception deficits can arise through multiple routes. Tests of speech perception and phonological awareness were administered to 5-year-old children representing 4 groups: those with chronic otitis media with effusion (OME), low socioeconomic status (low-SES), both conditions, or neither condition (control). The speech perception task involved identification of stimuli from a synthetic speech continuum in which the spectral characteristics of the fricative noise and the formant frequency transitions were varied. Many children with both chronic OME and low SES were

Speech perception deficits can arise through multiple routes with OME and poor environmental language inputs leading to similar difficulties with cue-weighting strategies.

unable to identify naturally produced words that began with the /s/ and /ʃ/ phonemes; therefore, synthetic speech identification data is shown for the remaining three groups only in Figure 7–6 (Chapter 1 explains how to interpret these figures as demonstrated in Figure 1–14; similar data for normally developing children are presented in Figure 2–9). The results clearly indicate less mature perceptual performance for all experimental groups compared to the control group as indicated by a greater reliance on the formant transition cue by the children with OME history or low SES versus greater reliance on the fricative spectrum cue by the children in the control group. These differences in speech perception performance were associated with differences in phonological awareness performance as well. The phonological awareness skills of children with DPD is discussed further in the next section as we move to studies that examine these children's underlying phonological knowledge.

Phonological Representations

In Chapter 4 we suggested that phonological knowledge emerges as the child stores increasing numbers of acoustic-phonetic representation for words in the lexicon, enriching the acoustic-phonetic detail within these representations, linking them to semantic representations and motor plans and organizing them to facilitate lexical access and higher levels of phonological processing. Many tasks tap the growing sophistication of the child's phonological knowledge as experience with language increases. We highlighted two specific classes of experimental task, phonological awareness and nonword repetition, as windows on the child's ability to abstract sublexical phonological units from the growing store of lexical representations. We begin with a review of the extensive literature on the phonological awareness skills of children with DPD.

Phonological awareness and nonword repetition tasks tap the growing sophistication of the child's phonological knowledge as experience with language increases.

Recall from Chapter 2 that phonological awareness (PA) refers to the child's awareness of sublexical units: syllables, onsets, rimes, and phonemes. The child may demonstrate implicit awareness in tasks such as matching words that share certain phonological elements or explicit awareness in tasks that require elision, segmentation, or blending of phonological units. Assessment tasks may require a nonverbal or a verbal response on the part of the child. These varying indexes of PA all tap a unitary construct despite these differences but the extent to which the task provides a sensitive measure of the child's phonological abilities varies with the difficulty level of the task relative to the child's age (Schatschneider, Francis, Foorman, Fletcher, & Mehta, 1999). Matching words on the basis of shared onsets for example provides good information about kindergarten age children's PA but elision tasks are better suited for older children and adults. Table 7–9 provides information about the PA abilities of children and adults with DPD relative to control groups with normally developing speech articulation abilities.

Phonological awareness refers to the child's awareness of sublexical units: syllables, onsets, rimes, and phonemes.

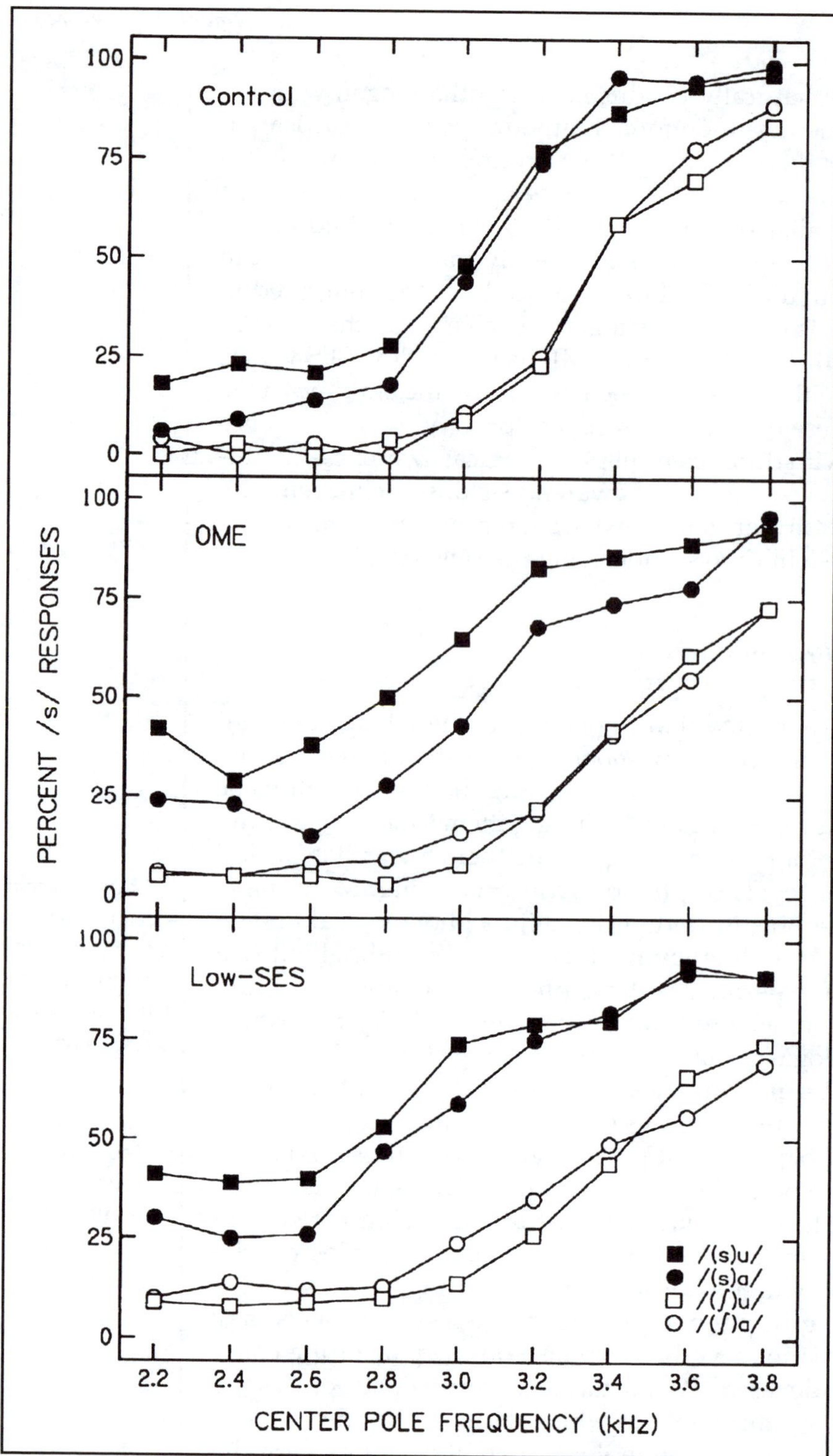

Figure 7–6. *Identification functions for a fricative-vowel speech perception task as performed by children with a history of chronic otitis media with effusion (OME), low socioeconomic status (low-SES), or neither risk factor (control). Sharper slopes indicate greater reliance on fricative centroid cues whereas greater separation between functions indicates greater reliance on formant transition cues (the less mature cue-weighting strategy). From* Nittrouer and Burton *(2005). The role of early language experience in the development of speech perception and phonological processing abilities: evidence from 5-year-olds with histories of otitis media with effusion and low socioeconomic status.* Journal of Communication Disorders *by Elsevier Inc., 38, Figure 1, p. 44. Reproduced with permission of Elsevier Inc. in the format Journal via Copyright Clearance Center.*

Table 7–9. Standardized Effect Sizes (Hedge's g) Representing Differences in Phonological Awareness Abilities of Clinical Samples Compared to Control Group Samples

Study	Sample	Age and/or Grade	Clinical N	Control N	Effect Size
Anthony et al. (2011): Explicit syllable, rime, and phoneme awareness	DPD	4;0 years	68	68	−1.03
Gillon (2000): Explicit syllable, rime, and phoneme awareness	DPD	6 years	23	30	−1.86
Gillon (2005): Phoneme matching	DPD	3;5 years	12	19	−0.77
Hesketh, Adams, Nightingale, & Hall (2000): Implicit and explicit rime and phoneme awareness	DPD	4 years	61	59	−0.47
Holm, Farrier, & Dodd (2007): Rime awareness	Delayed PD	5;6 years	14	15	−1.90
	Consistent Deviant	5;4 years	17	15	−1.80
	Inconsistent Deviant	5;4 years	15	15	−0.09
Larrivee & Catts (1999): Implicit and explicit syllable and phoneme awareness	DPD+LI	6 years/kindergarten	30	27	−1.46
Lewis et al. (2007): Explicit phoneme awareness with Pig Latin task	History DPD	Parents of children with DPD	24	111	−0.33
	History DPD+LI	Parents of children with DPD	12	111	−1.73
Lewis & Freebairn (1992): Explicit phoneme awareness with Pig Latin task	History DPD	Adults, 23 years	17	17	−0.78
Nathan, Stackhouse, Goulandris, & Snowling (2004): Rime awareness	DPD	5;8 years/kindergarten	19	19	−0.21
	DPD+LI	5;8 years/kindergarten	19	19	−0.78
Preston & Edwards (2007): Explicit phoneme awareness with spoonerism task	RE	12 years	13	14	−0.90
Raitano, Pennington, Tunick, Boada, & Shriberg (2004): Implicit and explicit rime and phoneme awareness	Normalized DPD, No LI	kindergarten	49	41	−0.78
	Persistent DPD, no LI	kindergarten	29	41	−1.02
	Persistent DPD, normalized LI	kindergarten	13	41	−1.68
	Normalized DPD Persistent LI	kindergarten	10	41	−2.30
Rvachew et al. (2003): Implicit awareness of onsets and rimes, nonverbal responses	DPD	4;8 months	13	13	−1.09

Samples are described as having a diagnosis of developmental phonological disorder (DPD) that was restricted to residual errors (RE) in one study and accompanied by language impairment (LI) in many but not all samples. See text for description of Dodd et al.'s subtype classifications.

For inclusion in this table full information about PA test performance, including mean scores and standard deviation for a clinical group and a control group (i.e., children with no current or past history of DPD), had to be available in the published article. Some valuable papers that have addressed this topic were excluded from this table because the test information was presented in visual form and thus the effect sizes could not be calculated (e.g., Bird, Bishop, & Freeman, 1995) or there was no control group (Hesketh, 2004; Lewis, Freebairn, & Taylor, 2000) or diagnosis of DPD for the clinical group could not be validated on the basis of standardized test scores (Webster, Plante, & Couvillion, 1997). Furthermore, when there were multiple measures in a single paper or multiple papers describing the same sample or overlapping samples of children, only one data point was included in the table so that all of the effect sizes reported are independent of each other.

Children with DPD consistently achieve lower scores on measures of phonological awareness in comparison to control groups.

Some generalizations about the PA abilities of children and adults with DPD are immediately apparent from Table 7–9. Every study yielded a negative effect size indicating that the group with DPD achieved lower scores on the measure of PA in comparison to the control group. This outcome confirms the strong relationship between speech production accuracy and phonological awareness that has been revealed by researchers using other methods, for example, studies comparing the speech accuracy of children with good versus poor PA or literacy skills (for review, see Preston, 2010). Second, the effect sizes are larger for groups with concomitant language impairment in comparison to the effect sizes for groups with isolated speech deficits. Nonetheless, the average effect sizes are large in each case: −0.92 for DPD alone versus −1.59 for combined DPD and language impairment. These effect sizes indicate that approximately half the participants with an isolated speech deficit scored lower than the control participants on the PA test whereas approximately three-quarters of the participants with combined speech and language deficits scored lower than the control participants on the PA test. Therefore, these data indicate that all children with DPD are at very high risk for PA deficits. Furthermore, these deficits persist even after resolution of the speech delay as can be seen by the large effect sizes observed for children with resolved DPD in Raitaino et al. (2004) and for adults with a history of DPD as preschoolers in Lewis and Freebairn (1992) and for parents of children with DPD in Lewis et al. (2007).

All children with DPD, even those without concomitant language impairment, are at very high risk for phonological awareness deficits.

In children with DPD, phonological awareness deficits can persist even after resolution of the speech delay.

Questions remain, however, that cannot be answered by the studies assembled in this review. The source of the children's PA deficit is not clear and various theoretical positions have been advanced. Some theorists have posited that phonological awareness emerges from language development in general (Dickinson, McCabe, Anastasopoulos, Peisner-Feinberg, & Poe, 2003) or lexical restructuring in particular (Metsala & Walley, 1998). Other theorists link PA more specifically to phonological development by suggesting that the child's awareness of sublexical units emerges from knowledge of articulatory gestures (Fowler, 1991; Ivry & Justus, 2001) or from improvements in speech perception skills that lead to better quality phonological representations (J. Zhang & McBride-Chang, 2010). In many of the studies summarized in Table 7–9 these variables were not well controlled so that the clinical and control groups differed from each other on these and other characteristics such as socioeconomic status and intelligence making it difficult to draw conclusions about why children with DPD are at risk or which specific children with DPD are most at risk for PA deficits (and consequently reading disability). Rvachew and colleagues explored these questions in a series of studies associated with a longitudinal follow-up of children with DPD first ascertained when they were 4 years of age.

In an initial small sample pilot study, 13 children with DPD were carefully matched to 13 children with normally developing speech on variables known to impact PA test performance, specifically chronological age, socioeconomic status, and receptive vocabulary ability. Speech perception was assessed using an error detection task (SAILS) in which the stimuli were natural speech recorded from children and adults, half of whom produced authentic misarticulations of the target phonemes, /k/, /l/, /s/, and /ɹ/. Phonological awareness was assessed with an implicit measure of onset and rime awareness that was developed by Bird, Bishop, and Freeman (1995) to ensure that the child's matching and segmentation abilities could be assessed via nonverbal responses. Figure 7–7 shows the children's percent correct responses on the measures of speech perception (SAILS) and phonological awareness (PAT). The

Children with DPD demonstrate deficits in speech perception and phonological awareness relative to control group children even when receptive vocabulary skills are controlled.

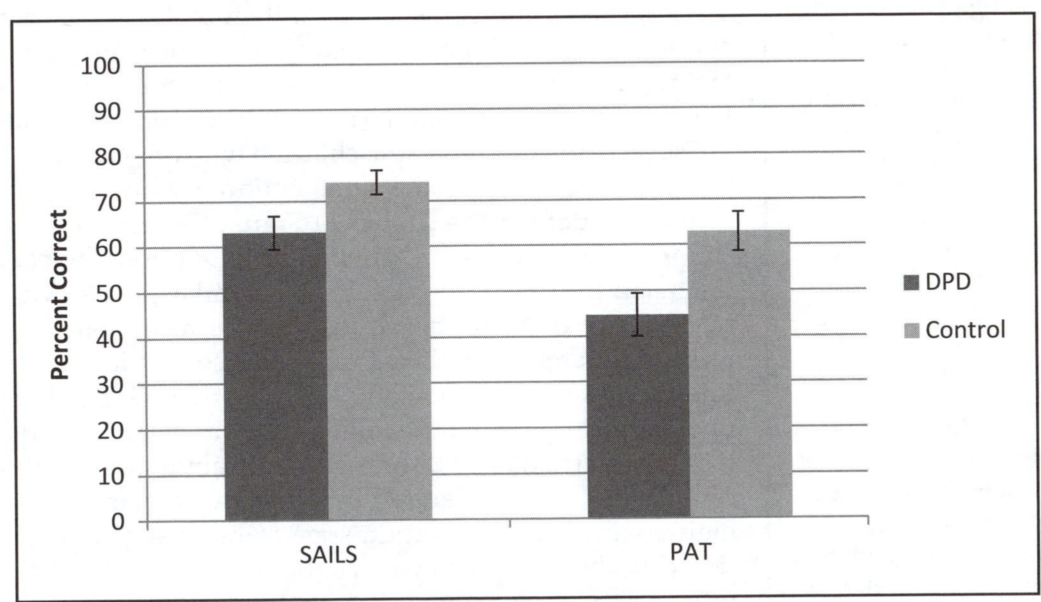

Figure 7–7. *Mean scores on tests of speech perception (SAILS) and phonological awareness (PAT) by children with developmental phonological disorders (DPD) and normally developing speech (control). Non-overlapping standard error bars reflect statistically significant differences in performance between groups for both measures. Adapted from Rvachew et al. (2003). Used with permission of the American Speech-Hearing-Language Association.*

children with DPD achieved significantly worse scores on both measures in comparison to the control group even though both groups had equally high scores on a test of receptive vocabulary skills (specifically, mean standard score of 108 for both groups on the Peabody Picture Vocabulary Test; Dunn & Dunn, 1997).

Eventually, this small sample grew to be 95 children with DPD which allowed us to use linear structural equation modeling to test hypotheses about the nature of the relationships among these variables (Rvachew & Grawburg, 2006). The best fitting model is shown in Figure 7–8. The model indicates that PA in 4-year-old children with DPD emerges from the joint impact of speech perception skills and vocabulary knowledge. After these variables were taken into account, articulation accuracy no longer explained significant unique variance in PA. As these children were followed through kindergarten and first grade these relationships were confirmed and the pathway towards the achievement of word reading skills was illuminated (Rvachew, 2006, 2007; Rvachew & Grawburg, 2008). The data revealed that speech perception skills and rime awareness prior to kindergarten explained onset awareness at the end of kindergarten; onset awareness and letter knowledge contributed to the emergence of the children's onset segmentation skills; at the end of first grade, onset segmentation ability was the primary predictor of nonword decoding skills whereas vocabulary knowledge was the primary predictor of sight word-reading skills.

A study of children with DPD revealed that phonological awareness emerged from the joint impact of speech perception and vocabulary skills with articulation accuracy contributing no unique variance.

The conclusion to be drawn from this longitudinal study is that children with DPD have phonological processing difficulties not because they misarticulate speech sounds but because they misperceive speech sounds. Inspection of Figure 7–5 suggests that not all children with DPD have difficulty with speech perception and in fact this longitudinal study revealed that about half of this population perceives speech similarly to children with normally developing speech. Furthermore, the children who do have difficulties with speech perception are the same children who have phonological awareness deficits, as shown in Figure 7–9. These two groups of children, those who have difficulties with phonological processing tasks and those who do not, have a similar profile with respect to the severity of their speech disorder as indicated by the nonsignificant differences in their PCC scores shown in Figure 7–9. These findings led Rvachew (2007) to suggest that the children with poor phonological processing skills formed a specific subtype of DPD that is at particular risk for reading disability although the degree of risk would be moderated by protective factors such as access to high quality language input, speech therapy, and reading instruction (Rvachew, 2007) as well as the presence of additional risk factors such as lower nonverbal intelligence (Peterson, Pennington, Shriberg, & Boada, 2009).

The research suggests that children with DPD have phonological processing difficulties not because they misarticulate speech sounds but because they misperceive speech sounds.

Children with poor phonological processing skills may form a specific subtype of DPD that is at particular risk for reading disability with the degree of risk moderated by protective factors as well as the presence of additional risk factors.

In summary, some children with DPD have significant difficulty with speech perception that results in poor quality acoustic-phonetic representations for words in the lexicon. These poor

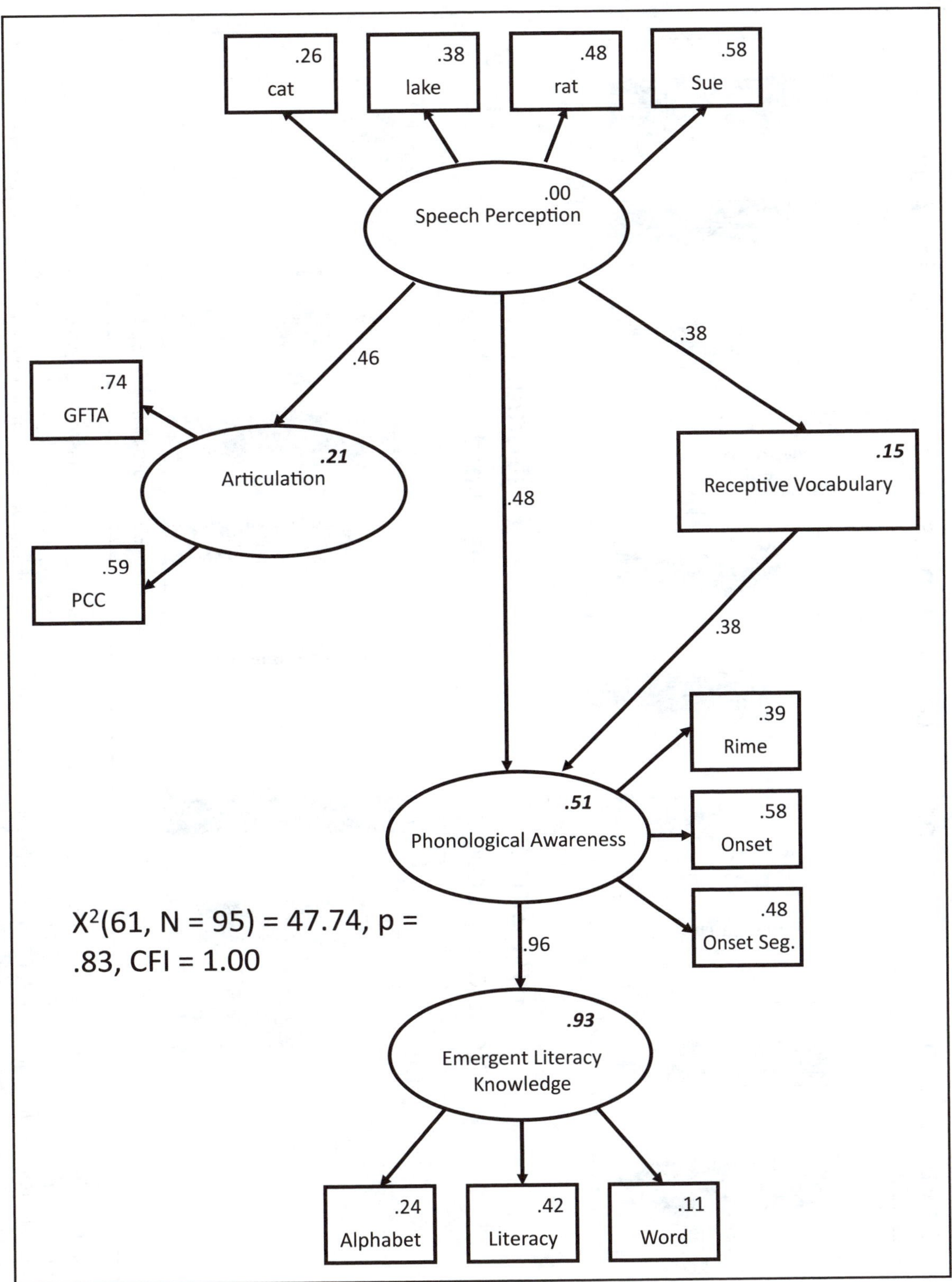

Figure 7–8. *Linear structure equation model of the relationships between the exogenous variable Perceptual Phonological Knowledge and the endogenous variables Articulation, Vocabulary Knowledge, Phonological Awareness, and Emergent Literacy Knowledge. Standardized regression weights are shown next to the path arrows and squared (multiple) correlations are shown within the markers for latent and observed variables. Adapted from Rvachew and Grawburg (2006). Correlates of phonological awareness in preschoolers with speech sound disorders.* Journal of Speech, Language, and Hearing Research, *49, Figure 1, p. 75. Used with permission of the American Speech-Hearing-Language Association.*

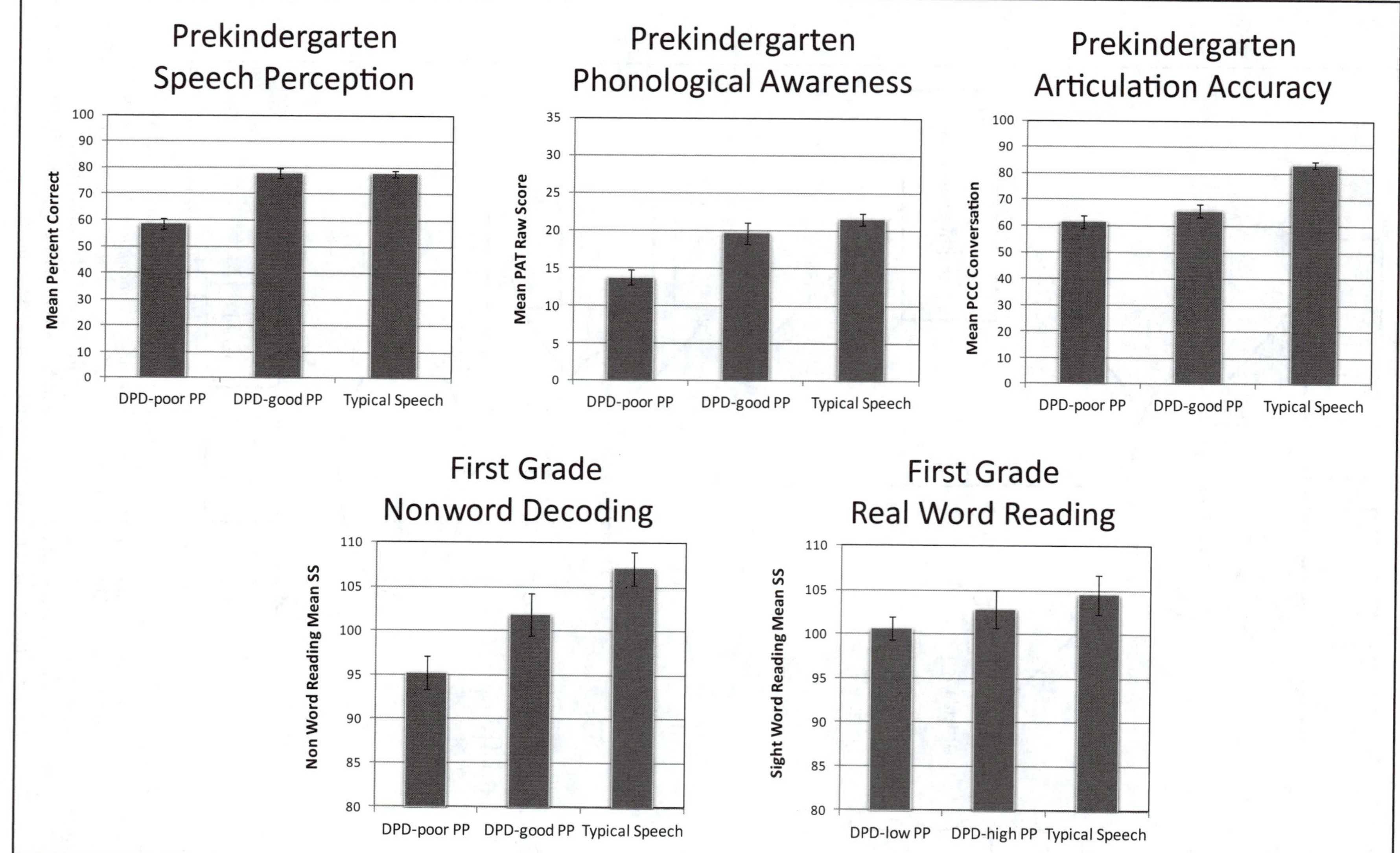

Figure 7–9. *Mean scores (with standard error bars) on prekindergarten predictors and first grade outcome variables for children with Development Phonological Disorders (DPD) and poor phonological processing skills (DPD low-PP,* n = 17*), children with DPD and good phonological processing skills (DPD hi-PP,* n = 16*), and children with normally developing speech (typical,* n = 35*). Note that the vertical axis for the reading variables ranges from* 80 *(lower limit of normal performance) to* 110 *(approximate mean receptive vocabulary score for all groups). Even the DPD low-PP group scores within normal limits for Nonword Decoding on average but this group scores well below expectations based on language functioning and significantly lower than the other two groups. Adapted from* Rvachew (2007). *Phonological processing and reading in children with speech sound disorders.* American Journal of Speech-Language Pathology, 16, *Table 2, p. 265 and Figure 1, p. 266.*

quality representations delay the children's achievement of speech production accuracy and hamper the development of the children's phonological awareness skills. Does this speech perception deficit impact other aspects of phonological knowledge that are abstracted from the lexicon? Munson and colleagues investigated children's phonotactic knowledge with a task in which they were required to repeat nonwords containing high or low probability phoneme sequences. The research design and the results for children with normally developing speech and language skills were presented in Chapter 4. Figure 4–17 shows that production accuracy improves with age and is always better for nonwords with high frequency phoneme sequences than for nonwords with low frequency phoneme sequences. Recall that Edwards, Beckman, and Munson (2004) concluded that large vocabulary sizes allowed the older children to abstract robust and generalized phonological knowledge at the phoneme level from their experience with specific words and syllables, thus explaining their superior performance with the repetition of novel sound sequences.

In a subsequent series of studies, similar data were obtained from children with DPD (Munson, Edwards, & Beckman, 2005b) or SLI (Munson, Kurtz, & Windsor, 2005). As would be expected, absolute accuracy of repetition varied between typical and clinical groups and was significantly correlated with speech perception and speech production accuracy. However, the difference in repetition accuracy between low- and high-frequency phoneme sequences was not at all correlated with speech perception or production performance for any group. Furthermore, children with DPD did not show a greater disadvantage when repeating low-frequency sequences than did typically developing children, relative to repetition accuracy for high-frequency sequences (Munson, Edwards, et al., 2005b). On the other hand, the performance difference across low- and high-frequency phoneme sequences was greater for children with SLI than for age-matched peers (Munson, Kurtz, et al., 2005). These findings, shown in Figure 7–10, suggest that difficulties with abstract phonological knowledge are not the source of the articulation errors that are observed in children with DPD. Rather, these children have difficulties constructing word representations in the more primary perceptual domain, an interpretation that is reinforced by other investigations involving a long-term repetition priming paradigm (Munson, Baylis, Krause, & Yim, 2006).

Nonword repetition accuracy is significantly correlated with speech perception and speech production accuracy in children with normal and delayed speech development.

Children with DPD respond to variations in **phonotactic probability** like control group children, suggesting that difficulties with abstract phonological knowledge are not the source of their articulation errors.

Thus far, the results of these studies are consistent with the model of phonological development that was presented in Plate 1. A child with speech perception difficulties develops poor quality acoustic-phonetic representations for words in the lexicon. The poor quality of these representations interacts with the size of the lexicon itself to determine the child's phonological awareness skills. Phonological knowledge that is abstracted across the lexicon as a whole, such as knowledge of language-specific phonotactic patterns, is also jointly determined by the number of lexical entries and the quality

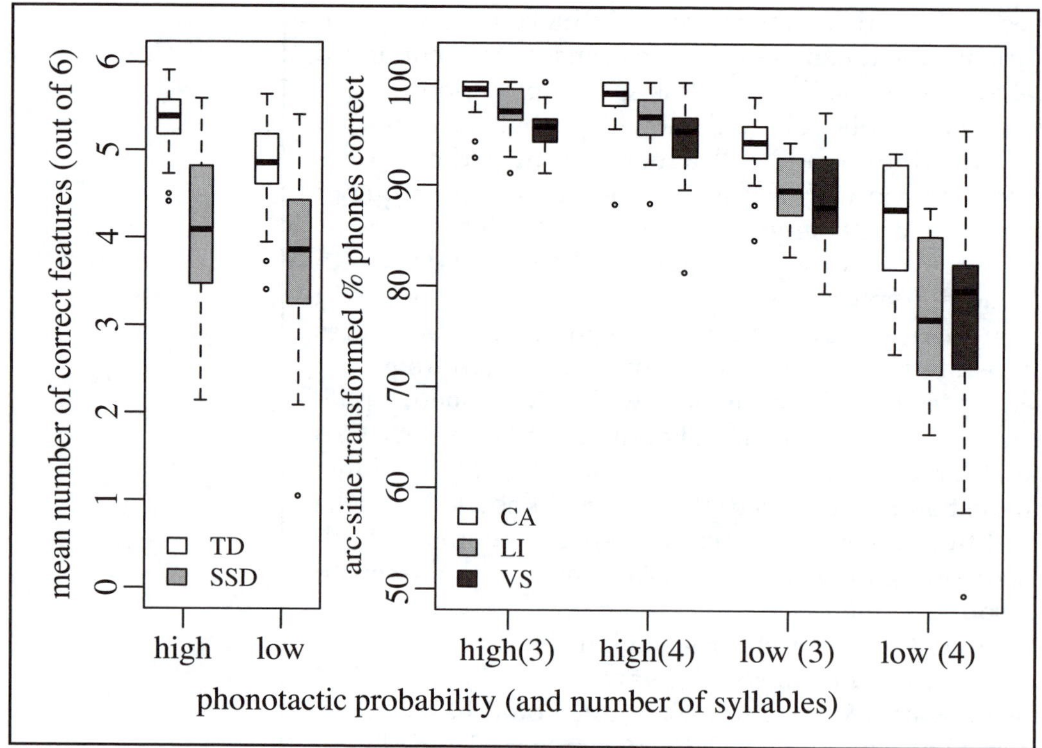

Figure 7–10. *Box plots show the medians and distributions of segmental accuracy scores for the repetition of biphone sequences with high versus low probability in nonwords, as a function of sequence type and group of participants (TD = typically development; SSD = speech sound disorder; LI = language impaired; CA = chronological age match to the LI sample; VS = receptive vocabulary age match to the LI sample). The chart on the left displays the number of correct features matched per sequence, summarized from Munson, Edwards, and Beckman (2005b), and shows that the difference in production accuracy between the two conditions is similar for the TD and SSD groups. The chart on the right displays the percentage of correctly produced phonemes per sequence, summarized from Munson, Kurtz, and Windsor (2005), and shows that the difference in production accuracy between the two conditions varies between groups and is associated with vocabulary knowledge.*

of the representations stored in the lexicon. Speech production accuracy is also limited by the quality of the acoustic-phonetic representations. We now turn to the quality of output, or articulatory, representations in children with DPD.

Output Representations

Throughout this book we have cautioned against making inferences about the child's ability to construct or execute a motor plan from phonetic transcriptions of the child's speech. In Chapter 4 we described a study in which segmental variability, as measured via phonetic transcription, was not always correlated with kinematic measures of movement variability (Goffman et al., 2007). We have introduced several instrumental methods of describing the child's speech output that provide a more adequate measure of the child's articulatory abilities including electropalatography (EPG), kinematic descriptions of tongue, lip, and jaw movements, and acoustic analysis of temporal and spectral characteristics of speech utterances. EPG studies of children with DPD have been particularly informative.

Traditionally, substitution errors (such as /k/ → [t] or /s/ → [θ]) in children's speech have been interpreted as reflecting deficiencies in the child's underlying phonological knowledge. Acoustic analysis can reveal covert contrasts in some children's speech indicating that the child has underlying knowledge of these contrasts but is articulating the distinction in a manner that it is not perceptible to the adult listener. EPG has proved to be a very important tool for revealing the articulatory gestures that children with DPD use when articulating these commonly misarticulated phonemes. As explained in Chapter 2, an artificial palate is used to record tongue contact and a "horse-shoe" shaped pattern of contacts between tongue and palate is expected during normal articulation of lingual phonemes such as /t/, /n/, and /s/. Observing changes in contact patterns over time allows the researcher or clinician to make inferences about the child's ability to independently control the tongue blade/tip, tongue dorsum, and lateral margins of the tongue during speech.

Lateral bracing of the tongue and independent control of the tongue blade is observed at least by age 6 years in children with normally developing speech (Gibbon, 1999). In contrast, Gibbon reviewed EPG studies indicating the presence of "undifferentiated lingual gestures" in 12 of 17 children with DPD (see Table 1, p. 388 of Gibbon, 1999). The children ranged in age from 5 to 12 years and their error patterns varied from residual speech errors (e.g., sibilant distortions) to multiple phonological processes. Undifferentiated lingual gestures (ULGs) are characterized by simultaneous anterior and posterior contact of the tongue across the palate during production of the lingual phonemes as illustrated in Figure 7–11A. One interesting characteristic of ULGs is that they can occur on misarticulated phonemes such as target /k/ produced perceptually as [t] but also on phonemes that sound perceptually correct such as target /d/ produced perceptually as [d]. Furthermore, this failure to manipulate the lingual gestures independently can underlie fricative distortions as well as stop substitution errors as shown in Figure 7–11B. Another characteristic is "articulatory drift" whereby placement of the gesture at onset is different from the placement at release of the undifferentiated gesture, resulting in variable perceptual outcomes for alveolar and velar targets, such that /t/ → [t, k] and /k/ → [t, k] (Gibbon & Wood, 2002). Gibbon (1999) demonstrated how a child can learn to control the release phase of the gesture to change a backing pattern to a more perceptually acceptable production of alveolar stops without fundamentally changing the ULG itself, as shown in Figure 7–12.

Electropalatography (EPG) has proved to be a very important tool for revealing the articulatory gestures that children with DPD use when articulating commonly misarticulated phonemes.

Changes in EPG contact patterns over time reveal the child's ability to independently control the tongue blade/tip, tongue dorsum, and lateral margins of the tongue during speech.

Lateral bracing of the tongue and independent control of the tongue blade is observed at least by age 6 years in children with normally developing speech.

Undifferentiated lingual gestures (ULGs) are characterized by simultaneous anterior and posterior contact of the tongue across the palate during production of the lingual phonemes.

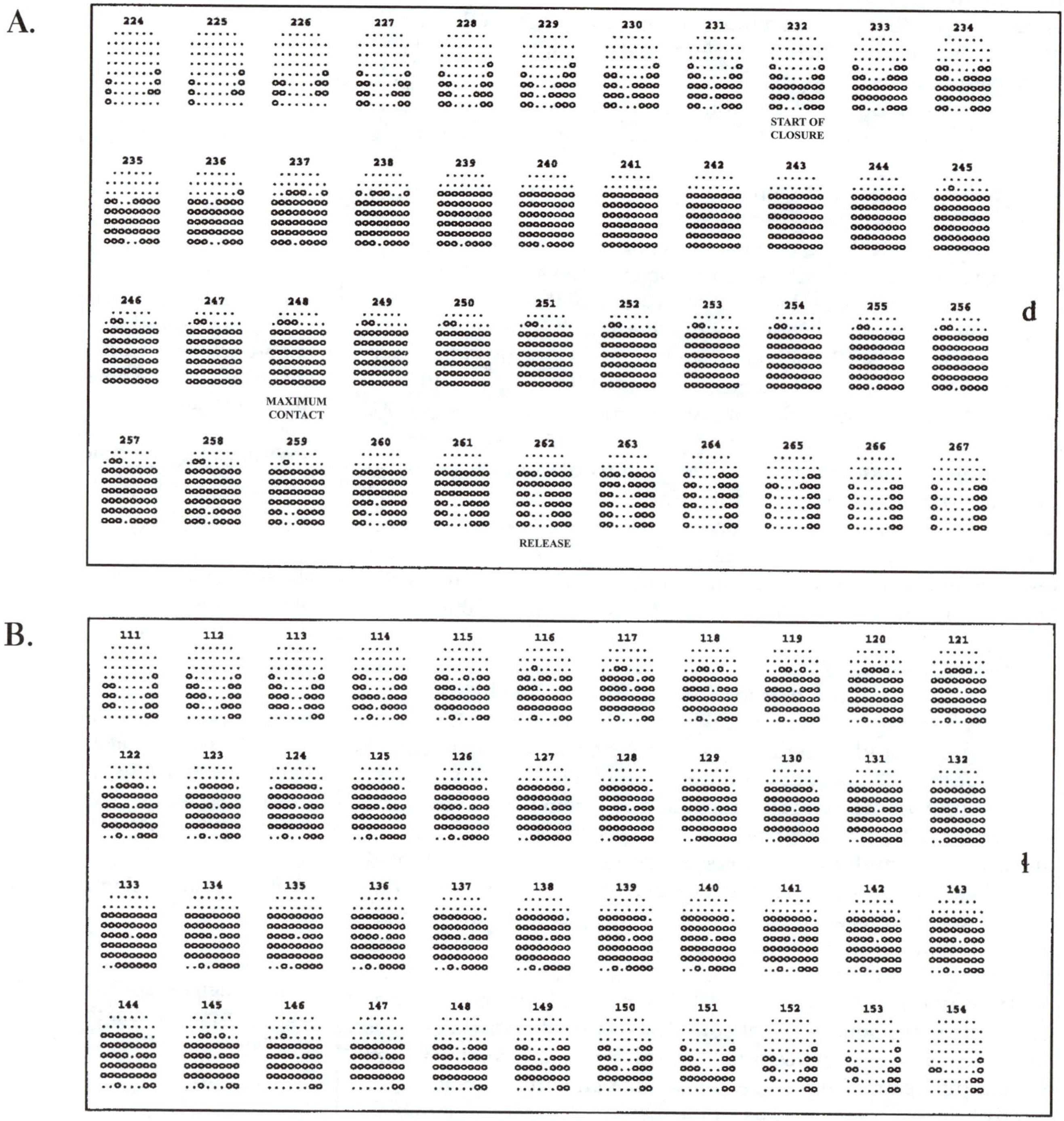

A.

START OF CLOSURE

MAXIMUM CONTACT

RELEASE

d

B.

ɬ

Figure 7–11. *Electropalatography recordings showing examples of undifferentiated lingual gestures.* **A**. *Printout from a child with DPD articulating the word "shed" with a perceptually correct target /d/.* **B**. *Printout from a child with DPD who lateralized the /s/ in the word "saw." Adapted from Gibbon (1999). Undifferentiated lingual gestures in children with articulation/phonological disorders.* Journal of Speech, Language, and Hearing Research, 42, *Figure 4, p.* 389 *and Figure 8, p.* 392. *Used with permission of the American Speech-Hearing-Language Association.*

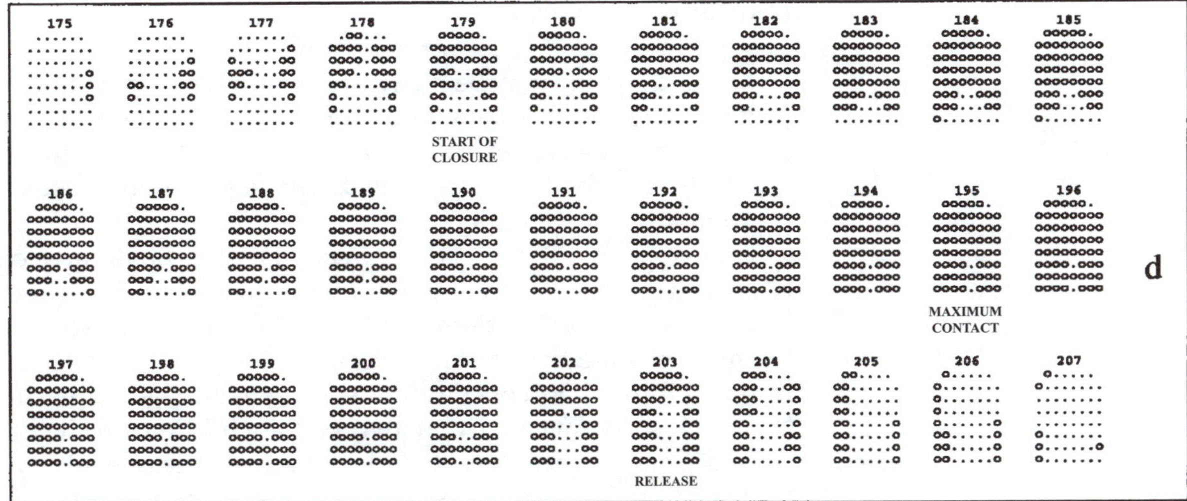

Figure 7–12. *Electropalatography recordings showing different outcomes of variable closure and release phases in undifferentiated lingual gestures.* ***A.*** *A child with DPD demonstrates underlying knowledge of the /d/-/g/ contrast by producing the target phones with different gestures although both targets are perceived as [g]. Target /d/ is produced with an undifferentiated lingual gesture with final release in the velar area. Target /g/ is produced with a discrete tongue dorsum contact in the posterior area of the artificial palate.* ***B.*** *This same child, after a period of speech therapy, is producing target /t/ so that it is perceived as [d] but the undifferentiated lingual gesture persists. The altered percept is accomplished by changing the topography of the gesture to ensure final release in the alveolar area. Adapted from Gibbon (1999). Undifferentiated lingual gestures in children with articulation/phonological disorders.* Journal of Speech, Language, and Hearing Research, 42, *Figure 5, 6 and 7, pp. 390–391. Used with permission of the American Speech-Hearing-Language Association.*

Gibbon (1999) argued that the articulatory patterns revealed by EPG reflect motor constraints in children with DPD for three reasons: first, the topography of the lingual gesture is reminiscent of the "everything moves at once" principle which is a known characteristic of immature oral motor control; second, the undifferentiated nature of the lingual gesture is pervasive in the children's speech, affecting both perceptually inaccurate phonemes such as lateralized sibilants and perceptually accurate sounds such as alveolar obstruents in the same child; and third, the presence of covert contrasts, even though the gestures used to produce them are immature, indicates that the child has appropriate underlying phonological knowledge. This review of EPG studies suggests that immature motor control may be a pervasive and potentially causal factor in DPD. However, this conclusion should be qualified by recognizing that the number of children studied with this technique remains small. Furthermore, children with ULGs appear to represent a very particular part of the population of children with DPD. Specifically, they are a relatively old group on average and thus the findings are characteristic of children with a trajectory of long-term normalization. Furthermore, atypical speech sound errors (including lateral lisps, backing of coronal obstruents and/or sibilants, and vowel errors) were reported for 15 of the 17 children. It is interesting to note that ULGs were not observed in the two children who had profiles of more typical errors (a 5-year-old with multiple phonological process errors and an 8-year-old with cluster reduction and dental distortion of sibilants).

The presence of **covert contrasts** in the EPG record, even though the gestures used to produce them are immature, indicates that the child has appropriate underlying phonological knowledge.

Children presenting with ULGs in research papers typically are older children with persistent atypical speech errors.

Goozée et al. (2007) provided more information about the kinds of children who may be likely to produce ULGs in a study in which kinematic measures of tongue control were gathered and an extensive clinical assessment of oral-motor abilities was conducted in addition to the EPG assessment. The description of the children's phonological patterns is abbreviated but lateral distortion of sibilants appeared to be a primary characteristic of all three children's speech. No measures of phonological processing were included in the test battery. No significant causal correlates were noted in the children's medical history except for OME for one child. Two of the children had concomitant specific language impairment. The EPG results revealed that two of the children produced lingual phonemes with differentiated lingual gestures despite the lateral distortion. The clinical assessment of these two children suggested dysarthria, confirmed by the finding of reduced tongue strength for these two children. The third child demonstrated ULGs during the EPG assessment and significant difficulties with the production of oral-motor sequences but no difficulties with tongue strength. The kinematic data derived from EMMA (see description in Chapter 1) indicated excessive tongue body movement during production of [t] and [s] and reduced acceleration of tongue body movement during [k] for this third child.

Some children with **lateral distortions** of sibilants have ULGs with normal tongue strength whereas others have differentiated tongue gestures and reduced tongue strength suggesting subclinical dysarthria.

These findings implicate reduced tongue strength as a correlate of DPD for at least some children, perhaps specifically in certain cases of lateral lisp. How common is reduced tongue strength in the DPD population? Unfortunately, it is difficult to be sure because the few studies that have examined tongue strength have involved cases of residual Speech Errors or CAS. Furthermore there are no large sample studies that have indicated the proportion of participants who have demonstrated low tongue strength. The six studies that have examined tongue strength in DPD to date, summarized in Table 7–10, have yielded mixed results suggesting that low tongue strength occurs in a minority of cases with severe or persistent speech disorder. Robin, Somodi, and Luschei (1991) point out that low tongue strength and endurance, detected in patients via instrumental assessment in their study, was missed upon standard clinical assessment and thus the prevalence of this problem with motor function is probably underestimated in the DPD population. A careful reading of these studies indicates that low tongue strength is associated with slow diadochokinetic rates (DKR) in every case, regardless of whether the stated diagnosis was SEs (Dworkin, 1980), CAS (Murdoch, Attarch, Ozanne, & Stokes, 1995), or suspected subclinical dysarthria (Goozée et al., 2007).

Studies that have examined **tongue strength** in DPD have yielded mixed results suggesting that low tongue strength occurs in a minority of cases with severe or persistent speech disorder.

When low tongue strength occurs, it is associated with slow **diadochokinetic rates**.

Table 7–10. *Summary of Studies Comparing Tongue Strength in a Group with Speech Errors to a Control Group with Normal Speech*

Study	*N*	*Age*	*Clinical Sample Characteristics*	*Findings Compared to Control Group*
Dworkin (1980)	5	8	Mild lispers (20% /s/ errors)	No difference in protrusive tongue force
	11	9	Moderate lispers (43% /s/ errors)	No difference in protrusive tongue force
	13	8	Marked lispers (66% /s/ errors)	No difference in protrusive tongue force
	16	8	Severe lispers (97% /s/ errors)	Significant difference in protrusive tongue force
Dworkin & Culatta (1980)	21	7–16	Frontal lispers with tongue thrust and open-bite malocclusion	No difference in protrusive tongue force
Fairbanks & Bebout (1950)	30	Adults	Residual errors, mostly sibilants	No difference in maximum tongue force
Goozée et al. (2007)	2	10	Lateral lispers with differentiated lingual gestures	Significantly reduced maximum pressure
	1	11	Lateral lisper, undifferentiated lingual gestures	Significantly higher maximum pressure
Murdoch et al. (1995)	6	5–11	Childhood apraxia of speech	Significantly reduced tongue strength and endurance
Robin et al. (1991)	5	8–10	Childhood apraxia of speech	Two CAS speakers' maximum strength was 3 times lower than the control children and 2 times lower than the other CAS children.

Reports of DKRs in children with DPD are rare, possibly because DPD implies normal DKR performance by definition. Several researchers have examined alternate motion rates (AMRs) in bi- or trisyllable repetition tasks, however. As reported in Table 7–5 a slow rate and/or an inability to repeat a trisyllable sequence is characteristic of CAS, whereas children with DPD achieve normal rates but may need extra trials to achieve an accurate production of /pataka/. McNutt (1977) reported significantly slower bisyllable repetition rates (AMRs) for older children with residual /ɹ/ errors but not for older children with residual /s/ errors. Preston and Edwards (2009) found that adolescents with residual errors repeated trisyllables at normal rates although accuracy was reduced relative to the control group.

Dodd and McIntosh (2008) described oral motor test results for 78 preschoolers with DPD and consistent speech errors in comparison to an age and sex matched control group. The children ranged in age from 36 to 66 months with a mean age of 4;5 years. Performance was scored according to a subjective scale reflecting accuracy and fluidity and no objective repetition rates are provided. They reported that 3.9% of the clinical sample performed below the normal range while repeating "pattacake." Bradford and Dodd (1996) administered the Robbins and Klee assessment (described in Chapter 5) to preschoolers diagnosed according to the subtypes Speech Delay (n = 22), Consistent Deviant (n = 15), Inconsistent Deviant (n = 9), and CAS (n = 5) in comparison to a Control group (n = 51). The percentage of children who made 2 or more errors on the multisyllable repetition task was reported to be 73, 53, 100, 80, and 37, respectively, for these groups but no data about repetition rates are provided. The errors were described as phonological process errors for the Speech Delay and Consistent Deviant groups and articulation errors, syllable structure errors, or phoneme sequencing errors for the Inconsistent Deviant and CAS groups.

In our lab we administered the Oral Speech Mechanism Screening Evaluation (Ruscello & St. Louis, 2000) to 57 French-speaking children with DPD with a mean age of 54 months. Repetition rates and the proportion of children meeting the minimum criteria for rate, accuracy and rhythm are shown for single and multiple syllable repetition tasks in Table 7–11. The rates were calculated from waveform displays of the digitized recordings of the children's responses to the tasks and rounding to the nearest tenth of a second. It can be seen that mean repetition rates per second fall at the lower end of the normal range in reference to the published literature for preschool-age children (e.g., Robbins & Klee, 1987). When considering the repetition rates specifically, approximately 15% demonstrated slow DKRs for at least one of the three single syllable tasks and approximately one-third of the sample demonstrated slow AMRs for at least one of the two multisyllable tasks. Half the children passed all five tasks, 10% failed 3 tasks, and 5% failed more than 3 tasks. Considering the DKR tasks specifically, only 7% failed

Table 7–11. *Performance of 57 Francophone Preschoolers with DPD on Single and Multiple Syllable Repetition Tasks*

	Repetitions/Sec				*Rate*	*Accuracy*	*Rhythm*
Task	*Minimum*	*Maximum*	*Mean*	*SD*	*Fail %*	*Fail %*	*Fail %*
[pa]	2.3	5.5	3.8	0.8	16	2	5
[ta]	2.6	6.5	4.0	0.9	0	4	4
[ka]	2.2	6.0	3.8	0.9	16	16	5
[pata]	0.7	4.0	1.9	0.6	28	34	30
[pataka]	<1	4.0	1.3	0.8	32	88	63

These tasks were administered using the procedures in the manual for the Oral Speech Mechanism Screening Evaluation (Ruscello & St. Louis, 2000). Many of the children were younger than the 5;0 year minimum for application of the norms. The outcomes showed that younger children were less likely to produce the required number of repetitions (16 for single syllables and 12 for [pataka]) but repetition rates in syllables/second were not correlated with age (i.e., 4-year-olds performed similarly to 5-year-olds, consistent with the findings of Williams & Stackhouse, 2000). Therefore, repetition times were converted to repetitions/second and the pass standard was prorated for the number of repetitions that the child accomplished. The resulting pass standards were 2.9, 2.3, 2.7, and .95 repetitions/second for [pa], [ta], [ka], and [pataka] repetitions, respectively. One child refused the [ka] and [pataka] tasks.

2 of the 3 and no child failed all 3 suggesting few cases of subclinical dysarthria in this sample. With respect to the AMR tasks, 25% failed one task and 18% failed both tasks. Children who achieved normal DKRs were identical to children who produced slower than average DKRs on all other assessments administered in this study (receptive vocabulary, nonverbal intelligence, articulation accuracy in single words and in conversation and phonological awareness). Children who achieved normal AMRs were also identical on average to children who produced slower than average AMRs except for significantly higher phonological awareness scores. This is interesting because the measure of phonological awareness used in this study is an adaptation of the Bird, Bishop, and Freeman (1995) task that requires no spoken responses from the children. Therefore, we suggest that multisyllable repetition tasks in young children tap phonological processing as well as motor planning skills. The children most likely to present with motor involvement over the long term are those who failed multiple DKR and AMR tasks, thus 5% of this sample. We hypothesize that the remaining quarter of the sample that had difficulty with AMR and phonological awareness tasks had difficulties that were at the levels of phonological processing and/or planning.

The proportion of preschool-age children with DPD who present with motor involvement as indicated by failing multiple DKR and AMR tasks is approximately 5%.

Slow multisyllable repetition rates in children with DPD may reflect difficulties with phonological processing and/or planning.

Although the findings of the studies cited thus far provide mixed outcomes, it appears that a small proportion of the DPD population presents with a motor impairment. The underlying cause of the motor impairment is not clear. Murdoch et al. (1995) suggest that, in the absence of documented evidence of neuropathology, symptoms such as poor tongue strength, slow rate, and sequencing difficulties should be attributed to a lack of volitional speech motor control. Terband et al. (2009) used the DIVA model to identify potential sources of deficits in the development of speech motor control. Revisiting Figure 3–15, it can be seen that auditory and somatosensory feedback are both critical to the learning of feedforward commands (i.e., motor plans). Recall that according to the DIVA model, the development of speech motor control takes place in two stages. During the "babbling stage" the model learns the mapping between auditory and somatosensory information and the corresponding feedforward commands. During the "imitation phase," the model learns to achieve the auditory targets that correspond to phonological units with the aid of auditory and somatosensory feedback. Over time, feed-forward control comes to dominate feedback control under normal speaking conditions (see Chapter 3 for a detailed discussion of feed-forward control). Terband et al. hypothesized that reduced or degraded oral sensitivity would force the learner to rely on feedback control. Subsequent modeling of this effect resulted in increased coarticulation, vowel distortion, and groping which they claim are core features of CAS. They noted that these speech outcomes occur as a consequence of hearing impairment as well, and that the DIVA model predicts that reductions in auditory feedback would also lead to an overreliance on feedback control.

Computer simulations lead to the prediction that reduced or degraded **oral sensitivity** will lead to an *overreliance on feedback control* and symptoms of CAS.

Is there evidence that children with DPD have degraded oral sensitivity as is predicted by these computer simulations? Surprisingly little research has addressed this question and most of the studies in this domain have been concerned with oral form discrimination (also called oral stereognosis). In these studies a pair of flat plastic forms is placed in the child's mouth, one form at a time in succession, and the child is asked to determine if the shape of the pair is the same or different. Results are reported separately for within-class and across-class form pairs (e.g., a square and a rectangle would be within-class but a square and a triangle are across-class). Ringel, House, Burk, Dolinsky, and Scott (1970) reported the number of errors in oral form discrimination for children and adults (167 research participants in all) divided into groups labeled normal, mild, moderate, and severe articulation disorder based on the number of sounds in error and the consistency of articulation errors per sound. The children ranged from first to fifth grade and had a mean age of 8 years. Children made many more errors than adults but in both age groups errors increased with the severity of the speech deficit. Poorer oral-form discrimination performance for children with articulation errors compared to children with normal speech was also reported by Sommers, Cox, and West (1972), McNutt (1977), and Speirs and Dean (1989) but contrary findings are reported by Lonegan (1974) and by Hetrick and Sommers (1988). Unfortunately, there are no studies on oral stereognosis that have adequate controls for potential confounds such as socioeconomic status, language skills, or verbal and performance I.Q. and thus this

Studies describing **oral-form discrimination** skills in children with DPD have yielded conflicting findings and lack controls for potential confounds.

literature is not as well advanced as the research on the speech perception abilities of children with DPD. Other tasks that have lower cognitive and linguistic load have been reported in the literature, specifically, two-point discrimination on the tongue (McNutt, 1977) and vibrotactile thresholds (Fucci, 1972; Lonegan, 1974), but insufficient research has been conducted and clear conclusions cannot be drawn.

Clinical Utility of the Psycholinguistic Approach

One of the cornerstones of the psycholinguistic approach is that each child is unique and thus there is no effort to fit each child into mutually exclusive categories. The SLP is expected to systematically investigate the child's underlying processing skills and target intervention at the child's specific point of breakdown. Numerous case studies have shown that children do demonstrate idiosyncratic profiles of strengths or weaknesses when assessed with a variety of tools targeting different areas of input processing, phonological knowledge, and output processing (e.g., see case study in Pascoe, Stackhouse, & Wells, 2005). In this review we have shown that difficulties with speech perception and phonological awareness are pervasive in this population. Concomitant language delay will intensify difficulties at the phonological level of representation. As a group, children with DPD tend to produce slow DKRs and AMRs but only approximately 5% of preschoolers with DPD show clear evidence of a motor speech disorder. Motor involvement is more frequent within samples of children with persistent speech delay. Issues with tongue strength and somatosensory feedback may occur in some children but the research literature is not clear on this point.

Systematic investigation of the child's strengths and weaknesses at all levels of processing can be an onerous task for the child and the clinician, not only because of the potential number of assessment procedures, but because normed and valid tests for all age groups are not readily available. Furthermore, careful attention to any of the models that underlie this approach should bring some skepticism about the possibility of isolating a single level of breakdown for any one child since a weakness at one level is bound to have repercussions throughout the system. The primary value of this approach and the research literature on the psycholinguistic functioning of children with DPD should be to remind us that speech development is a multifaceted endeavor that involves the gradual accrual of knowledge and skills at multiple levels of representation. It is not surprising therefore that, as a group, these children show weaknesses at all three levels relative to their normally developing peers. As we move forward to talk about effective treatment approaches it should not be a surprise to find that effective interventions also address input processing, output processing, and underlying phonological knowledge.

The research literature on the psycholinguistic functioning of children with DPD shows that speech development is a multifaceted endeavor that involves the gradual accrual of knowledge and skills at multiple levels of representation.

Prevalence, Comorbidity, and Long-Term Outcomes

7.4.1. Identify the best estimate of the prevalence of DPD among children aged approximately 5 years from among the studies reviewed.

7.4.2. Describe four possible outcomes with respect to reading ability according to the two-dimensional framework of oral language comprehension and word recognition skills.

7.4.3. Identify the factors that predict good versus poor literacy outcomes for children with DPD.

Prevalence

There is no consensus as to the correct estimate of the proportion of cases with speech delay in the population at any one time although the median **prevalence** estimate is approximately 6%.

Shriberg et al. (1999) reviewed over 100 studies of the prevalence of speech delay and concluded that there was no consensus as to the correct estimate of the proportion of cases with speech delay in the population at any one time. Law, Boyle, Harris, Harkness, and Nye (2000) confirm that the estimates vary widely, specifically from 2.3% to 24.6% for isolated speech disorder. Nonetheless, they report a median estimate of approximately 6% for speech impairment although it is not clear that this is a useful estimate given the extreme variation in the quality of the studies and the lack of consensus on the most appropriate procedure for identifying speech delay for any given age group. Here we report the details of three large-scale population-based studies in which it is possible to be absolutely sure of the definition of speech delay. Each of these studies reports the prevalence of speech delay in populations of children who are 5 or 6 years of age which means that children who had delayed speech at a younger age are obviously not taken into account.

Beitchman et al. (1986) estimated the prevalence of language-only, speech-only, and concomitant speech and language disorder among 5-year-old children in the Ottawa region of Canada using a two-stage process that began with the screening of a stratified random sample of one-third of all kindergarten children in the area. The screening consisted of a standardized citation form articulation test, two language screening tests and a checklist for voice and stuttering problems. Children scoring below the 30th percentile on the broad-based language screener or below the 10th percentile on the articulation test or failing the voice or fluency checklists progressed to the second phase of direct testing along with a random sample of 51 children who passed the screening tests. Notice that these criteria are likely to exclude children with normal language skills and residual distortion errors that place the child between the 10th and 16th percentile on the articulation test. At the second phase more extensive testing of language was conducted including the Test of Language Development (TOLD; Newcomer & Hammill, 1988) which includes subtests for word articulation and word discrimination. At the second phase of testing, failure of either of these subtests (i.e., scoring two or more standard deviations below the mean) or checklist scores indicating voice or fluency problems led to identification of speech disorder. After correcting for the observed rate of false negatives (which was quite high), the estimated prevalence of language-only, speech-only, and concomitant speech and language disorder was reported to be 8.04, 6.40, and 4.56, respectively. Therefore, the overall prevalence of communication disorders was estimated to be 19% and the estimated prevalence of speech disorders was estimated to be 11%. It is these children who provided the data about psychiatric outcomes at age 12.5 years shown in Table 7–2. A subsequent reanalysis of these data removed cases of secondary speech and language impairment yielding prevalence estimates of 10.5 for specific language impairment and 6.1 for specific speech impairment with no language component (Johnson et al., 1999).

Estimated prevalence of language-only, speech-only, and concomitant speech and language disorder was reported to be 8.04, 6.40, and 4.56, respectively among 5-year-olds in a Canadian study, providing a reliable estimate for the prevalence of speech impairments in the kindergarten population of 11%.

Shriberg et al. (1999) also used the word articulation subtest of the TOLD to estimate to prevalence of speech delay among English-speaking kindergarten-age children living in Iowa and Illinois in the United States. The initial screening phase of this study included selected items from the TOLD targeting language skills specifically. In the second phase of testing children who failed the screening completed a more extensive battery of language and cognitive tests that included the TOLD word articulation subtest. Shriberg et al. removed certain difficult words from consideration and ignored common distortion errors in order to yield a judgment of speech delay that would be consistent with the Speech Disorders Classification System. In other words, children with distortion errors were judged to have normal speech acquisition given their young age but children who had 2 or more "age-inappropriate" substitution and/or deletion errors were judged to have speech delay. Using these criteria, the prevalence of speech delay was estimated to be 3.9%. Both stages of this study, which was designed to identify language impairment, have design elements that clearly lead to an underestimate of the prevalence of speech delay. In the first stage, there is no screen for the presence of speech errors. In the second stage, distortion errors, even if they are unusually frequent or interfered with speech intelligibility, are discounted as a form of speech delay. Notwithstanding the difficulty of differentiating RE-A from RE-B and of predicting spontaneous resolution of distortion errors between 5 and 9 years of age, this decision appears to be unwarranted given the association between distortion errors and long-term persistence of speech delay, atypical neural imaging results, phonological processing impairments, and motor speech disorder, as reviewed above. The appendix to their report indicates that the sensitivity of the identification procedure was low and that the authors elected to not correct for false negatives; rather they report this prevalence estimate with the understanding that it is conservative. This very low estimate can be compared to the estimate of 18% reported by Roulstone et al. (2009) for the presence of speech errors (including both Speech Delay and Speech Error subtypes) among 8-year-old children in a large-scale population-based study conducted in the United Kingdom.

Among 8-year-olds in the United Kingdom, 18% have been found to present with speech delay or speech errors.

McLeod and Harrison (2009) used a combination of parent interview, teacher questionnaires, and direct assessment (of receptive vocabulary skills only) to assess 4983 Australian children aged 4;3 to 5;7 years using clustered random sampling to ensure a representative sample with proportional geographic distribution. One-quarter of parents expressed concern about how their child "talked and made speech sounds" with the most frequent concerns having to do with speech intelligibility: 12% of parents reported that their child's speech was not clear to others. Teacher ratings also indicated concern about expressive language competence for almost one-quarter of the children with high correspondence between teacher and parent expression of concern with respect to language output. These children form part of a national longitudinal study and thus it will be possible to determine how these functional measures of productive speech competence relate to future outcomes in multiple domains.

12% of parents of Australian 4- and 5-year-olds reported that their child's speech was not clear to others.

Comorbidity

Comorbidity with Specific Language Impairment

Shriberg et al. (1999) also reported comorbidity with specific language impairment (meaning language impairment in children with normal cognitive skills) to be 0.51% and comorbidity with language impairment in general to be 1.3%. The proportion of children with Speech Delay (defined as described above for the prevalence study) who also had language delay is illustrated in Figure 7–13. Notice that approximately one-third of the children identified with SD in this population based sample also had language impairment; this finding can be compared to the much higher rate of comorbid speech and language disorder described for a clinic-based sample in Table 7–1. Part of the discrepancy is undoubtedly due to differences in the ages of the children and the definition of speech delay employed. Most of the discrepancy is due to the known tendency for higher comorbidity of speech and language disorders on speech therapy caseloads however. It has been empirically established that parents are more likely to be aware of their child's language impairment if there is concomitant speech delay (Tomblin, Records, & Zhang, 1996) and a child with language impairment is more likely to receive treatment if he has articulation errors (Zhang & Tomblin, 2000).

Comorbidity of speech delay and language impairment is usually much higher in clinic samples than is observed in epidemiological studies involving samples drawn from the general population.

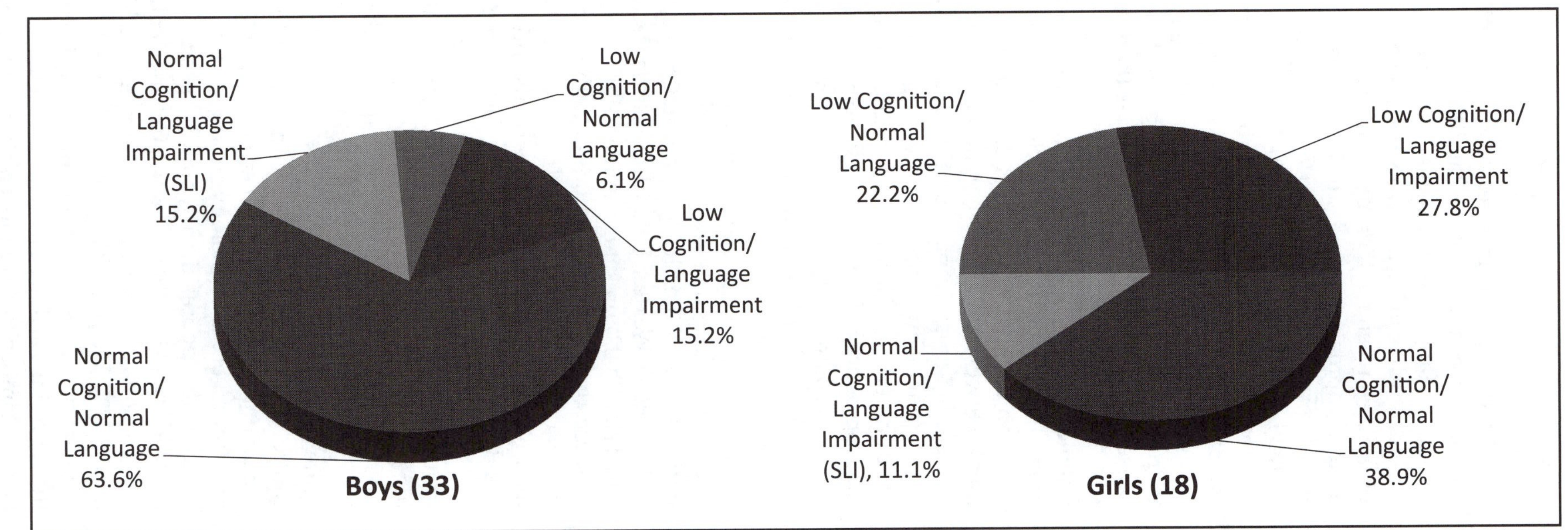

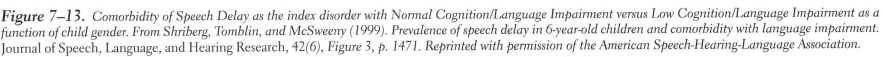

Figure 7–13. *Comorbidity of Speech Delay as the index disorder with Normal Cognition/Language Impairment versus Low Cognition/Language Impairment as a function of child gender. From Shriberg, Tomblin, and McSweeny (1999). Prevalence of speech delay in 6-year-old children and comorbidity with language impairment.* Journal of Speech, Language, and Hearing Research, 42(6), *Figure 3, p. 1471. Reprinted with permission of the American Speech-Hearing-Language Association.*

This difference in rates of comorbidity also accounts for an anomaly in estimates of heritability of language impairment. Heritability of language impairment has been reported to be high in several studies in which twins were selected from clinical samples of children receiving therapy for language impairment. However, in a large population-based study of twins in which language ability was determined at age 4 and 7 years, heritability was estimated to be negligible (Bishop & Hayiou-Thomas, 2008). On the other hand, the heritability estimate was high for this same twin sample when the phenotype was redefined to focus on aspects of speech production (i.e., Goldman-Fristoe Test of Articulation test scores and nonword repetition performance). The authors concluded that, "the presence of speech problems rather than language impairment is the phenotypic signature of a heritable disorder" (p. 370). This does not mean that there are not genetic influences on language development; they speculate that individual differences in language skills may be attributed to generalist genes that impact cognitive development. However, within the population of children diagnosed with specific language impairment, and thus having normal cognitive development by definition, the language problems appear to be environmental in origin whereas the concomitant speech production component of specific language impairment is highly heritable.

Articulation accuracy and nonword repetition performance were found to be the "phenotypic signature" of a heritable disorder in a large scale population study of twins followed prospectively between age 4 and 7 years.

Speech production problems may be directly associated with a very specific kind of language problem, however: a deficit in productive morphosyntax. Errors in the use of bound morphemes, and finite verb morphemes in particular, are considered to be a clinical marker for SLI and as such are typically explained by reference to impairments in the child's grammatical representations (Gopnik, 1997; Rice & Wexler, 1996; Rice, Wexler, & Cleave, 1995). Haskill and Tyler (2007) presented evidence that these kinds of errors may be more characteristic of children with DPD. They examined finite verb morphology use by children with DPD (grouped according to their use or nonuse of final consonants and consonant clusters) versus those with SLI. In this study the groups of children with DPD had concomitant phonological and language impairment. The SLI group had expressive language impairment with no accompanying phonological deficit. All children had borderline normal receptive language skills on average but normal nonverbal intelligence. Both groups of children with DPD achieved a significantly lower finite verb morphology composite than the normally developing control group whereas the group with SLI performed similarly to the control group on finite verb usage. Other studies have shown that finite verb morphology production in the DPD population is significantly poorer than would be predicted from their articulation accuracy (Rvachew, Gaines, Cloutier, & Blanchet, 2005) or their overall syntactic abilities (Mortimer & Rvachew, 2010; Paul & Shriberg, 1982). We find that these problems become more prominent than the speech deficit as the children get older. One implication of these findings is that many children with DPD as preschoolers may become similar to the children classified as SLI in the school-based

Difficulties with accurate production of **finite verb morphology** are associated with DPD.

prevalence studies discussed earlier. Strategies for treating morphosyntax while remediating speech production deficits are discussed in Chapter 9.

Comorbidity of DPD and Reading Disability

Although it is agreed that the ultimate goal of reading is to comprehend text, the acquisition of reading is a complex process that involves multiple components and thus there are many tests of "reading" that do not involve reading comprehension per se. To make sense of the literature on the comorbidity between DPD, SLI, and reading disability (RD) it is important to know what is being measured and why. It is also necessary to have some understanding of the debate about the appropriate definition of dyslexia.

According to the **simple view of reading**, a child's reading comprehension skills are determined by the product of his or her competence in decoding and oral language comprehension.

According to the simple view of reading (Gough & Tunmer, 1986), a child's reading comprehension skills (R) are determined by the product of his or her competence in decoding (D) and oral language comprehension (C), yielding the formula $R = D \times C$ such that competence in both decoding and oral language comprehension are required for average levels of achievement in reading comprehension. The best way to measure decoding depends on the child's developmental level (Tunmer & Greaney, 2010): at the beginning stages of reading the child should be asked to read (pronounce out loud) nonwords so that knowledge of sound-letter correspondences is tapped; after the child has received more reading instruction and practice, measures of context-free word identification should be included to assess knowledge of word-specific orthographic patterns; later, reading fluency should be assessed to capture automaticity in word recognition. Reading fluency is usually measured as the number of words read correctly per second, with a correction for lengthy hesitations or pauses, during the reading of meaningful passages. Appropriate measures of oral comprehension should also be developmentally constrained so that tests for younger children might focus more on vocabulary knowledge and simpler grammatical forms whereas tests for older children may require knowledge of more abstract vocabulary and complex syntactic forms and a higher level of inferencing and verbal reasoning ability. Decoding and oral language comprehension may not be completely independent of each other. Decoding skills emerge from the child's phonological awareness and letter knowledge and, as we indicated previously in this chapter, phonological awareness is jointly determined by speech perception skills and vocabulary development.

The Simple View of Reading predicts 4 classifications of reading comprehension ability, depicted in Figure 7–14. In each case, it is assumed that the children have received adequate literacy instruction and that they are otherwise normally developing. Normally developing readers will demonstrate average or better word recognition and oral language skills. Some children have good word recognition skills but poor oral language comprehension that causes a specific reading comprehension deficit. The largest category of

Good word recognition with poor oral language comprehension yields a **specific reading comprehension deficit.**

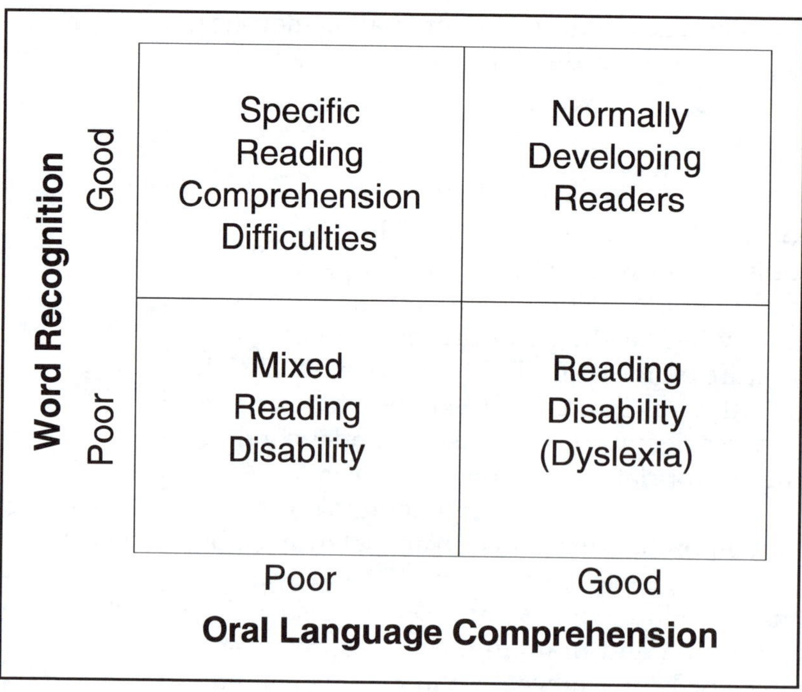

Figure 7–14. *Classification of different categories of reading disability. From Tunmer and Greaney (2010). Defining dyslexia.* Journal of Learning Disabilities *by Donald D. Hammill Foundation, 43, Figure 1, p. 233. Reproduced with permission of Pro-Ed Inc. in the format Journal via Copyright Clearance Center.*

Poor word recognition and poor oral language comprehension yields a **mixed deficit**.

Poor word recognition with relatively good oral language comprehension yields **dyslexia**.

A phonological processing deficit has been shown to be the core explanation for reading disability in children with otherwise good language and cognitive skills.

children with RD have poor word recognition and oral language skills and thus have a mixed deficit placing them in a category sometimes referred to as "garden variety poor readers." Finally, dyslexic children have much worse word recognition skills than would be predicted from their oral language comprehension skills. Although the children with DPD and phonological processing deficits represented in Figure 7–9 were not old enough for assessment of their reading comprehension skills, they appear to fall into this category by virtue of the large gap between their nonword decoding skills and their receptive vocabulary abilities. Indeed, a phonological processing deficit has been shown to be the core explanation for RD in children with otherwise good language and cognitive skills (Stanovich, 1988; Stanovich & Siegel, 1994; Torgesen et al., 1997). Following from this theoretical perspective and the research evidence, Tunmer and Greaney (2010) define dyslexia as "persistent literacy learning difficulties (especially difficulties in word recognition, spelling, and phonological recoding) in otherwise typically developing children . . . despite exposure to high quality, evidence-based literacy instruction and intervention, due to an impairment in the phonological processing skills required to learn to read and write" (p. 239). This definition differs from the commonly used discrepancy definition whereby the child's reading skills must be significantly lower than expectations based on nonverbal I.Q. However, many researchers have vigorously disputed the discrepancy definition (e.g., Siegel, 1992) on the grounds that poor readers with discrepant I.Q. profiles do not differ from poor readers with lower I.Q.s with respect to phonological processing skills, response to intervention, or long-term reading outcomes.

Several longitudinal population-based studies have determined the comorbidity of RD and language impairment. For example, using a discrepancy definition of dyslexia, Catts, Adlof, Hogan, and Weismer (2005) reported that 20% of children with SLI and 9% of children with normally developing language and cognitive skills were dyslexic in fourth grade. No such studies have been conducted with respect to speech disorders, but a recent study provided some data relating to speech disorders and reading fluency that is interesting because it included data for every child in Florida's Progress Monitoring and Reporting network for the years 2003 through 2006. From the total data base of students recorded for these years, 1991 reported to have "exceptionalities" in the speech or language area were compared to 8,833 children who had no primary "exceptionality." All of the children attended schools with a significant portion of children living in poverty. Speech Impairment was defined in relation to the number of speech sounds that were delayed by more than a year relative to age norms (see Appendix A of the paper for details and Chapter 8 for further discussion of these selection criteria) whereas Language Impairment (LI) was defined as scoring below a standard score of 77 on a standardized test of language functioning or having a large gap between receptive and expressive language functioning. The LI category included children who had concomitant SI and LI with no way to differentiate these children from a LI-only subgroup. These groups were further subdivided to reflect resolution of the impairment during first grade or persistence into second and third grade. Finally, subgroups were specified for those children whose diagnosis was changed from speech or language impairment to learning disability (defined as a large gap between I.Q. and school performance) during the first 3 years of school. Although the paper reports reading fluency outcomes for 4 timepoints over each of the first 3 grades, we have reproduced only the final timepoint here, in Table 7–12.

An initial observation from the table is that the risk of poor achievement in reading fluency was higher among children with LI (including those with concomitant SI, 78% at risk) than among children with SI alone (58% at risk), when summing across all risk groups. This finding is consistent with all studies of clinical samples that have examined speech-only versus speech-and-language impaired groups (Bird et al., 1995; Lewis et al., 2000). It should be pointed out however that children with DPD who go on to have reading disability often differ from those who do not on a variety of variables: not only are they more likely to have significantly worse

The risk of poor achievement in reading fluency was higher among children with language impairment (including those with concomitant speech impairment) than among children with speech impairment alone.

Table 7–12. *Percentage of Florida School Children Classified as At High Risk, Moderate Risk, or Achieving Bench Marks for Reading Fluency as a Function of Speech or Language Impairment Status at the End of Third Grade*

		Risk Level at End of Third Grade		
Subgroup	N	*High Risk*	*Moderate Risk*	*At or Above Grade Level*
SI-Resolved	278	17.3	34.0	48.7
LI-Resolved	65	16.1	33.9	50.0
SI-Persistent	1047	21.9	36.2	41.9
LI-Persistent	475	42.3	33.1	24.6
SI-Learning Disability	63	61.7	26.6	11.7
LI-Learning Disability	63	61.3	25.8	12.9
Local Reference group	8833	18.1	35.8	46.1

These samples were drawn from a data base of children attending Reading First schools in Florida which include significant numbers of children living in poverty. Risk status was determined from statewide benchmarks for reading fluency achievement. The sample includes all children in the database diagnosed with speech (SI) or language (LI) impairment and a reference sample who did not have a diagnosis of "primary exceptionality" in first, second, or third grade. LI category includes children with concomitant SI.

Source: Adapted from Puranik, Petcher, Al Otaiba, Catts, and Lonigan (2008). Development of oral reading fluency in children with speech or language impairments: A growth curve analysis. *Journal of Learning Disabilities, 41*, Table 1 (p. 548) and Table 5 (p. 555). Used with permission of Sage Publications.

language skills and more severe DPD than those who have good reading outcomes, they are likely to have lower nonverbal I.Q., to have poorer phonological awareness skills, and to have more disadvantaged social backgrounds (Larrivee & Catts, 1999; Peterson et al., 2009). In essence, the risk factors for reading disability among children with DPD are the same as the risk factors for reading disability in the general population but these risk factors tend to be associated with DPD thus elevating the risk of reading disability for this population overall.

A second observation is that the risk of reading fluency problems was no higher among children whose speech or language problem resolved during first grade than that observed in the reference group, confirming the "critical age hypothesis" advanced for SLI and DPD (Bishop & Adams, 1990; Nathan, Stackhouse, Goulandris, & Snowling, 2004). On the other hand, children with persistent SI had a 4% increased risk and children with persistent LI had a 21% increased risk relative to the reference group in this study. This finding highlights the crucial importance of treating speech and language problems prior to the onset of formal reading instruction.

Persistence of speech and/or language problems past the age of school entry elevates the risk of reading disability, highlighting the crucial importance of treating speech and language problems prior to the onset of formal reading instruction.

The risk of poor achievement in reading fluency was highest among children who were eventually diagnosed with learning disability: regardless of whether the original classification was SI or

LI, almost 90% of these children failed to achieve expectations. The chance of changing diagnosis to learning disability was twice as high for children with an original classification of LI compared to SI, however.

Puranik et al. (2008) also presented growth curve models for this sample showing that reading fluency performance and growth in first grade predicted the relative ranking of the groups throughout second and third grades. The finding that lags in phonological processing and reading in the early grades predict reading outcomes throughout the school years is commonly reported (e.g., see also Foster & Miller, 2007; Snowling, Bishop, & Stothard, 2000) and further highlights the urgency of providing appropriate early interventions for children with speech and language impairments in order to prevent school failure. Appropriate early interventions to address phonological processing are discussed in Chapters 9 and 11.

Medium and Long-Term Outcomes for Children with DPD

Outcomes have been documented for children with DPD in several domains including normalization of phonological functioning, literacy and academic achievement, social and psychiatric sequelae, and school and vocational success. As alluded to throughout this chapter, the results depend on the presence of concomitant language delay in most of these domains.

Another variable that impacts on long-term outcomes is speech and language status at school entry, in accordance with the "critical age hypothesis" mentioned above. Not many studies have reported short-term normalization rates for children who clearly had DPD at intake. Shriberg et al. (1994) studied short-term normalizing in a group of children who were 4 years old and had PCCs of approximately 63 at intake to the study. They reported that 18.5% of 54 children achieved short-term normalization when this goal was defined as normal speech acquisition within 2 years of identification or before 6 years of age. Rvachew et al. (2007) found that 26% of 58 children met this same criterion for short-term normalization in a study involving 4-year-old children who scored at the 5th percentile on the GFTA-2 on average at intake to the study. In contrast, Webster, Plante, and Couvillion reported that 66% of 45 children with an average age of 3 years at intake achieved normalized speech 3 years later. The Khan-Lewis Phonological Analysis was used to diagnose DPD in this study.

Baker and Cantwell (1987) reported long-term normalization rates for a sample of 300 children referred to a community speech clinic at a median age of 5 years. Ninety-three percent of the children presented with speech disorder (with or without accompanying language disorder) at the time of enrolment in the study. After a 5-year follow-up interval, only 30% of those children achieved normal speech even though 85% of the sample received at least 4 months of speech therapy.

Lewis et al. (2000) reported speech, language, and literacy outcomes for third graders who were treated for DPD as preschoolers. The children were recruited from speech therapy caseloads and admitted to this longitudinal study if they produced at least 3 phonological process-type errors on the Khan-Lewis Phonological Analysis. Results are reported separately for a group with phonological-only disorder (P group) and for a group with phonological and language disorder (PL group). It is very important to point out that the phonological-only group scored at the 30th percentile on the GFTA at the time of intake to this study. They also had higher nonverbal I.Q. and SES than the PL group. Intake characteristics and grade 3 outcomes for these two groups are shown in Table 7–13. The PL group had significantly worse decoding, sight word reading, reading comprehension and spelling scores than the P group in third grade. Thirty percent of the P group scored below normal limits for spelling despite their excellent language skills and otherwise good outcomes.

Children with a preschool history of DPD have an elevated risk of **spelling disorder** in school, even when there is no accompanying language impairment.

Similar findings have been reported for speech, language, and academic outcomes for young adults with a prior history of speech and/or language disorder. Johnson et al. (1999) reassessed the Ottawa sample when the participants were 19 years old, grouped according to diagnosis at age 5, that is, speech-only deficit or speech/

Table 7–13. *Group Characteristics at Time 1 and Percentage of Children with Communication Disorders in Third Grade*

Measure	*P Group*	*PL Group*
Sample size	28	24
Mean (SD) on Intake Variables at Time 1		
Age at intake (months)	5.0 (0.9)	5.1 (1.0)
Performance I.Q.	115.9 (13.1)	98.8 (13.0)
GFTA (percentile)	30.3 (20.4)	11.7 (12.4)
TOLD-P2 (standard score)	104.6 (10.8)	75.9 (7.3)
Number (Percentage) of Children with Communication Disorders in Third Grade		
Articulation disorder	1 (4%)	6 (22%)
Language disorder	4 (14%)	12 (60%)
Reading disorder	1 (4%)	11 (46%)
Spelling disorder	8 (30%)	14 (58%)

Time 1 test scores reflect performance at intake into the study and may reflect the impact of interventions received between the onset of treatment and the time of this assessment. The children were recruited from active speech therapy caseloads and may have obtained lower scores when first accepted for treatment.

Source: Adapted from Lewis, Freebairn, and Taylor (2000). Follow-up of children with early expressive phonology disorders. *Journal of Learning Disabilities*, 33(5), Tables 1–2 and Results text (pp. 436–438). Used with permission of Sage Publications.

language deficit compared to the control group (as described earlier in the section on psychiatric outcomes). Stability of the original classifications was high into young adulthood with 73% of the speech/language group continuing to show language impairment and 44% of the speech-only group continuing to show speech impairment. Overall, 56 of 114 individuals with speech or language diagnoses at age 5 produced speech errors as adults compared to 22/128 control participants. The majority of speech errors were liquid or sibilant distortions that did not impair intelligibility. The speech-only and control groups obtained similar scores on tests of cognitive function and academic achievement whereas the speech/language group scored significantly worse on all measures.

Other studies have shown that the sequelae of preschool speech disorders persist through the school years and into adulthood. Felsenfeld, Broen, and McGue (1994) described educational and occupational outcomes for two groups of adults drawn from a large study of children who had been assessed repeatedly from prekindergarten through fourth grade and again in high school (the Templin Longitudinal Study). Two subgroups of adults were selected from the data base to represent a group with moderately delayed development of articulation skills in the early school years (DPD group) and a comparison group with normal development of articulation skills (control group). Cognitive function was within normal limits for both groups but the DPD group had significantly lower verbal IQ than the control group. In comparison to the control group, adults with a history of childhood DPD performed significantly worse on tests of articulation accuracy, vocabulary knowledge, and language skills. They required more remedial help at school, achieved poorer grades, and completed fewer years of formal education. These adults were also more likely to hold unskilled or semiskilled occupations in comparison with the control group and their gender-matched siblings who were more likely to hold professional positions. The authors pointed out that even when educational outcomes were similar, individuals with a history of DPD were likely to choose occupations that required lower levels of reading and writing competency.

The sequelae of preschool speech disorders persist through the school years and into adulthood in many cases.

In comparison to the control group, adults with a history of childhood DPD performed significantly worse on tests of articulation accuracy, vocabulary knowledge, and language skills. They required more remedial help at school, achieved poorer grades, and completed fewer years of formal education.

In summary, approximately 11% of kindergarten-age children present with DPD with about a third of those children having concomitant language delay. The literature is lacking in good quality longitudinal studies for the preschool period. It is not known how many children have concomitant speech and language delay during the preschool period or what proportion might change diagnosis from language to speech delay or vice versa between age 3 and 6 years. Good estimates of recovery from speech delay during this period are also not available. It is clear that outcomes after the age of 5 years are strongly associated with persistence of the speech or language deficit and the presence of a concomitant language deficit. Essentially, the population of children with DPD appears to split into two divergent developmental trajectories. One group has difficulties that are primarily in the speech domain with relatively good language and cognitive skills and fewer social disadvantages; this group is likely to benefit from early intervention, achieving short-term normalization of speech competency and subsequently demonstrating good academic outcomes throughout the school years. However, it is also clear that these individuals will show traces of the underlying deficit into adulthood in the speech and phonological processing domains (see Tables 7–6 and 7–7; Johnson et al., 1999; Kenney, Barac-Cikoja, Finnegan, Jeffries, & Ludlow, 2006; Lewis et al., 2007; Lewis & Freebairn, 1992). One might speculate that achieving these good outcomes despite persistent underlying phonological processing deficits comes at a cost given the high rate of anxiety disorders that are observed in 12-year-olds who had speech or language delay at age 5 years (Beitchman et al., 1996). A second group has concomitant language impairment with relatively poorer nonverbal I.Q. and greater social disadvantages as well as greater persistence of the speech and language deficit. This group has a much greater probability of poor academic outcomes despite greater use of remedial services at school. Over the long term, psychiatric outcomes, school achievement and vocational accomplishments are significantly worse in comparison to adult peers with no history of speech and language impairment (Beitchman et al., 2001; Felsenfeld et al., 1994; Young et al., 2002). Unfortunately, none of these longitudinal studies examined the contribution of speech therapy to the outcomes experienced by these children over the short or long term. However, given the importance of speech and language status at school entry to academic and psychiatric outcomes throughout the school years and into adulthood, it is very likely that the effectiveness of early intervention for DPD is a critical protective factor in the lives of these children.

We turn now to the topic of treatment planning in Chapter 8, the final chapter of Part II. Having completed a thorough assessment of the child's phonological abilities at multiple levels of representation and interpreted the child's performance in relation to the scientific literature on the nature of DPD, a number of important decisions must be made before an intervention can be implemented. Most important among them is whether it is necessary to provide an intervention in order to ensure normalized speech acquisition. The selection of treatment goals, service delivery model, and approach to intervention are also important decisions that will flow directly from the results and interpretation of the assessment data.

References

Ahissar, M. (2007). Dyslexia and the anchoring-deficit hypothesis. *Trends in Cognitive Sciences*, *11*, 458–465.

American Speech-Language-Hearing Association. (2002). *Childhood apraxia of speech* [Technical report]. Available from http://www.asha.org/policy

Anthony, J. L., Aghara, R., Dunkelberger, M., Anthony, T. I., Williams, J. M., & Zhang, Z. (2011). What factors place children with speech sound disorders at risk for reading problems? *American Journal of Speech-Language Pathology, 20*, 146–160.

Aungst, L. F., & Frick, J. V. (1964). Auditory discrimination ability and consistency of articulation of /r/. *Journal of Speech and Hearing Disorders, 29*, 76–85.

Baker, L., & Cantwell, D. P. (1982). Developmental, social and behavioral characteristics of speech and language disordered children. *Child Psychiatry and Human Development, 12*, 195–206.

Baker, L. , & Cantwell, D. P. (1987a). A prospective psychiatric follow-up of children with speech/language disorders. *Journal of the American Academy of Child and Adolescent Psychiatry, 26*(4), 546–553.

Baker, L., & Cantwell, D. P. (1987b). Factors associated with the development of psychiatric illness in children with early speech/language problems. *Journal of Autism and Developmental Disorders, 17*(4), 499–510.

Beitchman, J. H., Brownlie, E. B., Inglis, A., Wild, J., Ferguson, B., Schachter, D., . . . Mathews, R. (1996). Seven-year follow-up of speech/language impaired and control children: Psychiatric outcome. *Journal of Child Psychology and Psychiatry, 37*(8), 961–970.

Beitchman, J. H., Nair, R., Clegg, M., Patel, P. G., Ferguson, B., Pressman, E., & Smith, A. (1986). Prevalence of speech and language disorders in 5-year-old kindergarten children in the Ottawa-Carleton region. *Journal of Speech and Hearing Disorders, 51*, 98–110.

Beitchman, J. H., Wilson, B., Johnson, C. J., Atkinson, L., Young, A. R., Adlaf, E., . . . Douglas, L. (2001). Fourteen-year follow-up of speech/language-impaired and control children: Psychiatric outcome. *Journal of the American Academy of Child and Adolescent Psychiatry, 40*(1), 75–82.

Bennett, K. E., & Haggard, M. P. (1999). Behavior and cognitive outcomes from middle ear disease. *Archives of Disorders in Children, 80*, 28–35.

Betz, S. K., & Stoel-Gammon, C. (2005). Measuring articulatory error consistency in children with developmental apraxia of speech. *Clinical Linguistics & Phonetics, 19*(1), 53–66.

Bird, J., Bishop, D. V. M., & Freeman, N. H. (1995). Phonological awareness and literacy development in children with expressive phonological impairments. *Journal of Speech and Hearing Research, 38*, 446–462.

Bishop, D. V. M. (2009). Genes, cognition, and communication: Insights from neurodevelopmental disorders. *Annals of the New York Academy of Sciences, 1156*, 1–18.

Bishop, D. V. M., & Adams, C. (1990). A prospective study of the relationship between specific language impairment, phonological disorders, and reading retardation. *Journal of Child Psychology and Psychiatry, 31*, 1027–1050.

Bishop, D. V. M., & Hayiou-Thomas, M. E. (2008). Heritability of specific language impairment depends on diagnostic criteria. *Genes, Brain, and Behavior, 7*, 365–372.

Bradford, A., & Dodd, B. (1996). Do all speech disordered children have motor deficits? *Clinical Linguistics & Phonetics, 10*, 77–101.

Broomfield, J., & Dodd, B. (2004). The nature of referred subtypes of primary speech disability. *Child Language and Teaching Therapy, 20*(2), 135–151.

Campbell, T. F., Dollaghan, C. A., Rockette, H. E., Paradise, J. L., Feldman, H. M., Shriberg, L. D., . . . Kurs-Lasky, M. (2003). Risk factors for speech delay of unknown origin in 3-year-old children. *Child Development, 74*, 346–357.

Canter, G. J., Trost, J. E., & Burns, M. S. (1985). Contrasting speech patterns in apraxia of speech and phonemic paraphasia. *Brain and Language, 24*, 204–222.

Cantwell, D. P., & Baker, E. (1987a). Comparison of well, emotionally disordered, and behaviorally disordered children with linguistic problems. *Journal of the American Academy of Child and Adolescent Psychiatry, 26*, 193–196.

Cantwell, D. P., & Baker, L. (1987b). Prevalence and type of psychiatric disorder and developmental disorders in three speech and language groups. *Journal of Communication Disorders, 20*(2), 151–160.

Carrell, J., & Pendergast, K. (1954). An experimental study of the possible relation between errors of speech and spelling. *Journal of Speech and Hearing Disorders, 19*, 327–334.

Catts, H. W., Adlof, S. M., Hogan, T. P., & Weismer, S. E. (2005). Are specific language impairment and dyslexia distinct disorders? *Journal of Speech, Language, and Hearing Research, 48*, 1378–1396.

Chiat, S. (2001). Mapping theories of developmental language impairment: Premises, predictions and evidence. *Language and Cognitive Processes, 16*, 113–142.

Cohen, N. J., Davine, M., Horodezky, N. B., Lipsett, L., & Isaacson, L. (1993). Unsuspected language impairment in psychiatrically disturbed children: Prevalence and language and behavioral characteristics. *Journal of the American Academy of Child and Adolescent Psychiatry, 32*, 595–603.

Cohen, N. J., Menna, R., Vallance, D. D., Barwick, M. A., Im, N., & Horodezky, N. B. (1998). Language, social cognitive processing, and behavioral characteristics of psychiatrically disturbed children with previously identified and unsuspected language impairments. *Journal of Child Psychology and Psychiatry, 39*(6), 853–864.

Conti-Ramsden, G., & Botting, N. (1999). Classification of children with specific language impairment: Longitudinal considerations. *Journal of Speech, Language, and Hearing Research, 42*(5), 1195–1204.

Dickinson, D. K., McCabe, A., Anastasopoulos, L., Peisner-Feinberg, E. S., & Poe, M. D. (2003). The comprehensive language approach to early literacy: The interrelationships among vocabulary, phonological sensitivity, and print knowledge among preschool-age children. *Journal of Educational Psychology, 95*(3), 465–481.

Dodd, B. (1995). Procedures for classification of subgroups of speech disorder. In B. Dodd (Ed.), *The differential diagnoses and treatment of children with speech disorder* (pp. 49–64). San Diego, CA: Singular.

Dodd, B. (2011). Differentiating speech delay from disorder: Does it matter? *Topics in Language Disorders, 31*, 96–111.

Dodd, B., Holm, A., Crosbie, S., & McCormack, P. (2005). Differential diagnosis of phonological disorders. In B. Dodd (Ed.), *Differential diagnosis and treatment of children with speech disorder* (pp. 71–82). London, UK: Whurr.

Dodd, B., & McIntosh, B. (2008). The input processing, cognitive linguistic and oro-motor skills of children with speech difficulty. *International Journal of Speech-Language Pathology, 10*, 169–178.

Dunn, L. M., & Dunn, L. M. (1997). *Peabody Picture Vocabulary Test* (3rd ed.). Circle Pines, MN: American Guidance Service.

Dworkin, J. P. (1980). Characteristics of frontal lispers clustered according to severity. *Journal of Speech and Hearing Disorders, 55,* 37–44.

Dworkin, J. P., & Culatta, R.A. (1980). Tongue strength: Its relationship to tongue thrusting, open-bite, and articulatory proficiency. *Journal of Speech and Hearing Disorders, 45*(2), 277–282.

Edwards, J., Beckman, M. E., & Munson, B. (2004). The interaction between vocabulary size and phonotactic probability effects on children's production accuracy and fluency in nonword repetition. *Journal of Speech, Language, and Hearing Research, 47,* 421–436.

Edwards, J., Fox, R. A., & Rogers, C. L. (2002). Final consonant discrimination in children: Effects of phonological disorder, vocabulary size, and articulatory accuracy. *Journal of Speech, Language, and Hearing Research, 45,* 231–242.

Fairbanks, G., & Bebout, B. (1950). A study of minor organic deviations in "functional" disorders of articulation: 3. The tongue. *Journal of Speech and Hearing Disorders, 15,* 348–352.

Felsenfeld, S., Broen, P. A., & McGue, M. (1994). A 28-year follow-up of adults with a history of moderate phonological disorder: Educational and occupational results. *Journal of Speech and Hearing Research, 37,* 1341–1353.

Fey, M. E. (1992). Articulation and phonology: Inextricable constructs in speech pathology. *Language, Speech, and Hearing Services in Schools, 32,* 225–232.

Foster, W. A., & Miller, M. (2007). Development of the literacy achievement gap: A longitudinal study of kindergarten through third grade. *Language, Speech, and Hearing Services in Schools, 38,* 173–181.

Fowler, A. E. (1991). How early phonological development might set the stage for phoneme awareness. *Haskins Laboratories Status Report on Speech Research, SR-105/106,* 53–64.

Fox, A. V., & Dodd, B. (2001). Phonologically disordered German-speaking children. *American Journal of Speech-Language Pathology, 10,* 291–307.

Fox, A. V., Dodd, B., & Howard, D. (2002). Risk factors for speech disorders in children. *International Journal of Language and Communication Disorders, 37,* 117–131.

Fria, T. J., Cantekin, E. I., & Eichler, J. A. (1985). Hearing acuity of children with otitis media with effusion. *Archives of Otolaryngology, 111,* 10–16.

Fucci, D. (1972). Oral vibrotactile sensation: An evaluation of normal and defective speakers. *Journal of Speech and Hearing Research, 15,* 179–184.

Gibbon, F., & Wood, S. E. (2002). Articulatory drift in the speech of children with articulation and phonological disorders. *Perceptual and Motor Skills, 95,* 295–307.

Gibbon, F. E. (1999). Undifferentiated lingual gestures in children with articulation/phonological disorders. *Journal of Speech, Language, and Hearing Research, 42,* 382–397.

Gierut, J. A. (1998). Treatment efficacy: Functional phonological disorders in children. *Journal of Speech, Language, and Hearing Research, 41,* S85–S100.

Gillon, G. T. (2000). The efficacy of phonological awareness intervention for children with spoken language impairment. *Language, Speech, and Hearing Services in Schools, 31,* 126–141.

Gillon, G. T. (2005). Facilitating phoneme awareness development in 3- and 4-year-old children with speech impairment. *Language, Speech, and Hearing Services in Schools, 36,* 308–324.

Goffman, L, Gerken, L, & Lucchesi, J. (2007). Relations between segmental and motor variability in prosodically complex nonword sequences. *Journal of Speech, Language, and Hearing Research, 50*, 444–458.

Goozée, J. V., Murdoch, B., Ozanne, A., Cheng, Y., Hill, A., & Gibbon, F. (2007). Lingual kinematics and coordination in speech-disordered children exhibiting differentiated versus undifferentiated lingual gestures. *International Journal of Language and Communication Disorders, 42*, 703–724.

Gopnik, M. (1997). Language deficits and genetic factors. *Trends in Cognitive Sciences, 1*(1), 5–9.

Goswami, U., Thomson, J., Richardson, U., Stainthorp, R., Hughes, D., Rosen, S., & Scott, S. K. (2002). Amplitude envelope onsets and developmental dyslexia: A new hypothesis. *Proceedings of the National Academy of Sciences, 99*, 10911–10916.

Gottesman, I. I., & Gould, T. D. (2003). The endophenotype concept in psychiatry: Etymology and strategic intentions. *American Journal of Psychiatry, 160*, 636–645.

Gottesman, I. I., & Hanson, D. R. (2005). Human development: Biological and genetic processes. *Annual Review of Psychology, 56*, 263–286.

Gough, P. B., & Tunmer, W. E. (1986). Decoding, reading, and reading disability. *Remedial and Special Education, 7*, 6–10.

Groenen, P., Maassen, B., & Crul, T. (1998). Formant transition duration and place perception in misarticulating children and adolescents. *Clinical Linguistics & Phonetics, 12*, 439–457.

Grunwell, P. (1981). *The nature of phonological disability in children*. London, UK: Academic Press.

Hallberg, U., Óskarsdóttir, S., & Klingberg, G. (2010). 22q11 deletion syndrome—the meaning of a diagnosis. A qualitative study on parental perspectives. *Child: Care, Health, and Development, 36*(5), 719–725.

Halliday, L. F., & Bishop, D. V. M. (2006). Auditory frequency discrimination in children with dyslexia. *Journal of Research in Reading, 29*(2), 213–228.

Harm, M. W., & Seidenberg, M. S. (1999). Phonology, reading acquisition, and dyslexia: Insights from connectionist models. *Psychological Review, 106*, 491–528.

Haskill, A. M., & Tyler, A. A. (2007). A comparison of linguistic profiles in subgroups of children with specific language impairment. *American Journal of Speech-Language Pathology, 16*, 209–221.

Hauner, K. K. Y., Shriberg, L. D., Kwiatkowski, J., & Allen, C. T. (2005). A subtype of speech delay associated with developmental psychosocial involvement. *Journal of Speech, Language, and Hearing Research, 48*, 635–650.

Hesketh, A. (2004). Early literacy achievement of children with a history of speech problems. *International Journal of Language and Communication Disorders, 39*(4), 453–468.

Hesketh, A., Adams, C., Nightingale, C., & Hall, R. (2000). Phonological awareness therapy and articulatory training approaches for children with phonological disorders: A comparative outcome study. *International Journal of Language and Communication Disorders, 35*(3), 337–354.

Hetrick, R. D., & Sommers, R. K. (1988). Unisensory and bisensory processing skills of children having misarticulations and normally speaking peers. *Journal of Speech and Hearing Research, 31*, 575–581.

Hewlett, N., Gibbon, F. E., & Cohen-McKenzie, W. (1998). When is a velar an alveolar? Evidence supporting a revised psycholinguistic model of speech production in children. *International Journal of Language and Communication Disorders, 33*, 161–176.

Hickok, G., & Poeppel, D. (2007). The cortical organization of speech processing. *Nature Reviews: Neuroscience, 8*, 393–402.

Hoff, E. (2003). The specificity of environmental influence: Socioeconomic status affects early vocabulary development via maternal speech. *Child Development, 74*(5), 1368–1378.

Hoffman, P. R., Daniloff, R. G., Bengoa, D., & Schuckers, G. (1985). Misarticulating and normally articulating children's identification and discrimination of synthetic [r] and [w]. *Journal of Speech and Hearing Disorders, 50*, 46–53.

Holm, A., Farrier, F., and Dodd, B. (2007). Phonological awareness, reading accuracy and spelling ability of children with inconsistent phonological disorder. *International Journal of Language and Communication Disorders, 43*, 300–322.

Ivry, R. B., & Justus, T. C. (2001). A neural instantiation of the motor theory of speech perception. *Trends in Neurosciences, 24*(9), 513–515.

Joanisse, M. F., Manis, F. R., Keating, P., & Seidenberg, M. S. (2000). Language deficits in dyslexic children: Speech perception, phonology, and morphology. *Journal of Experimental Child Psychology, 77*, 30–60.

Johnson, C. J., Beitchman, J. H., Esscobar, M., Atkinson, L., Wilson, B., Brownlee, E. B., . . . Wang, M. (1999). Fourteen-year follow-up of children with and without speech/language impairments: Speech/language stability and outcomes. *Journal of Speech, Language, and Hearing Research, 42*, 744–760.

Johnson, D. L., Swank, P. R., Owen, M. J., Baldwin, C. D., Howie, V. M., & McCormick, D. P. (2000). Effects of early middle ear effusion on child intelligence at three, five, and seven years of age. *Journal of Pediatric Psychology, 25*, 5–13.

Karlsson, H. B., Shriberg, L. D., Flipsen, P. Jr., & McSweeny, J. L. (2002). Acoustic phenotypes for speech-genetics studies: Toward an acoustic marker for residual /s/ distortions. *Clinical Linguistics & Phonetics, 16*(6), 403–424.

Karmiloff-Smith, A. (2006). The tortuous route from genes to behavior: A neuroconstructivist approach. *Cognitive, Affective, and Behavioral Neuroscience, 6*, 9–17.

Kenney, M. K., Barac-Cikoja, D., Finnegan, K., Jeffries, N., & Ludlow, C. L. (2006). Speech perception and short-term memory deficits in persistent developmental speech disorder. *Brain and Language, 96*(2), 178–190.

Klausen, O., Moller, P., Holmefjord, A., Reisaeter, S., & Asbjornsen, A. (2007). Lasting effects of otitis media with effusion on language skills and listening performance. *Acta Otolaryngologica, 543*, 73–76.

Kronvall, E. L., & Diehl, C. F. (1952). The relationship of auditory discrimination to articulatory defects of children with no known organic impairment. *Journal of Speech and Hearing Disorders, 19*, 335–338.

Larrivee, L. S., & Catts, H. W. (1999). Early reading achievement in children with expressive phonological disorders. *American Journal of Speech-Language Pathology, 8*, 118–128.

Law, J., Boyle, J., Harris, F., Harkness, A., & Nye, C. (2000). Prevalence and natural history of primary speech and language delay: Findings from a systematic review of the literature. *International Journal of Language and Communication Disorders, 35*(2), 165–188.

Lewis, B. A., Chen, X., Freebairn, L., Holland, S., & Tkach, J. (2010, November). *Neural correlates of speech production in speech sound disorders.* Poster presented at the annual convention of the American Speech-Language and Hearing Association, Philadelphia, PA.

Lewis, B. A., & Freebairn, L. (1992). Residual effects of preschool phonology disorders in grade school, adolescence, and adulthood. *Journal of Speech and Hearing Research, 35,* 819–831.

Lewis, B. A., Freebairn, L. A., Hansen, A. J., Iyengar, S. K., & Taylor, H. G. (2004). School-age follow-up of children with childhood apraxia of speech. *Language, Speech, and Hearing Services in Schools, 35,* 122–140.

Lewis, B. A., Freebairn, L. A., Hansen, A. J., Miscimarra, L., Iyengar, S. K., & Taylor, H. G. (2007). Speech and language skills of parents of children with speech sound disorders. *American Journal of Speech-Language Pathology, 16,* 108–118.

Lewis, B. A., Freebairn, L. A., Hansen, A. J., Taylor, H. G., Iyengar, S., & Shriberg, L. D. (2004). Family pedigrees of children with suspected childhool apraxia of speech. *Journal of Communication Disorders, 37,* 157–175.

Lewis, B. A., Freebairn, L. A., & Taylor, H. G. (2000). Follow-up of children with early expressive phonology disorders. *Journal of Learning Disabilities, 33*(5), 433–444.

Lewis, B. A., Shriberg, L. D., Freebairn, L. A., Hansen, A. J., Stein, C. M., Taylor, H. G., & Iyengar, S. K. (2006). The genetic bases of speech sound disorders: Evidence from spoken and written language. *Journal of Speech, Language, and Hearing Research, 49,* 1294–1312.

Locke, J. L. (1980). The inference of speech perception in the phonologically disordered child. Part I: A rationale, some criteria, the conventional tests. *Journal of Speech and Hearing Disorders, 45,* 431–444.

Lonegan, D. S. (1974). Vibrotactile thresholds and oral stereognosis in children. *Perceptual and Motor Skills, 38,* 11–14.

Maassen, B., Groenen, P., & Crul, T. (2003). Auditory and phonetic perception of vowels in children with apraxic speech disorders. *Clinical Linguistics & Phonetics, 17,* 447–467.

MacDermot, K. D., Bonora, E., Sykes, N., Coupe, A., Lai, C. S. L., Vernes, S. C., . . . Fisher, S. (2005). Identification of FOXP2 truncation as a novel cause of developmental speech and language deficits. *American Journal of Human Genetics, 76,* 1074–1080.

Makela, N. L., Birch, P. H., Friedman, J. M., & Marra, C. A. (2009). Parental perceived value of a diagnosis for intellectual disability (ID): A qualitative comparison of families with and without a diagnosis for their child's ID. *American Journal of Medical Genetics, Part A, 149,* 2393–2402.

Marquardt, T. P., & Saxman, J. H. (1972). Language comprehension and auditory discrimination in articulation deficient kindergarten children. *Journal of Speech and Hearing Research, 15,* 382–389.

McGrath, L. M., Pennington, B. F., Willcutt, E. G., Boada, R., Shriberg, L. D., & Smith, S. D. (2007). Gene x environment interactions in speech sound disorder predict language and preliteracy outcomes. *Development and Psychopathology, 19,* 1047–1072.

McLeod, S., & Harrison, L. J. (2009). Epidemiology of speech and language impairment in a nationally representative sample of 4- to 5-year-old children. *Journal of Speech, Language, and Hearing Research, 52,* 1213–1229.

McNeil, M. R. (2003). Clinical characteristics of apraxia of speech: Model/behavior coherence. In L. D. Shriberg & T. F. Campbell (Eds.), *Proceedings of the 2002 Childhood Apraxia of Speech Research Symposium*. The Hendrix Foundation.

McNutt, J. C. (1977). Oral sensory and motor behaviors of children with /s/ or /r/ misarticulations. *Journal of Speech and Hearing Research, 20*, 694–704.

McReynolds, L. V., Kohn, J., & Williams, G. C. (1975). Articulatory-defective children's discrimination of their production errors. *Journal of Speech and Hearing Disorders, 40*, 327–337.

Merzenich, M. M., Jenkins, W. M., Johnston, P., Schreiner, C., Miller, S. L., & Tallal, P. (1996). Temporal processing deficits of language-learning impaired children ameliorated by training. *Science, 271*(5245), 77–81.

Metsala, J. L., & Walley, A. C. (1998). Spoken vocabulary growth and the segmental restructuring of lexical representations: Precursors to phonemic awareness and early reading ability. In J. L. Metsala & L. C. Ehri (Eds.), *Word recognition in beginning literacy* (pp. 89–120). Mahwah, NJ: Erlbaum.

Mody, M. (2003). Phonological basis in reading disability: A review and analysis of the evidence. *Reading and Writing, 16*(1), 21–39.

Monnin, L. M., & Huntington, D. A. (1974). Relationship of articulatory defects to speech-sound identification. *Journal of Speech and Hearing Research, 17*, 352–366.

Morley, M. (1957). *The development and disorders of speech in childhood*. Edinburgh, UK: Churchill Livingstone.

Mortimer, J., & Rvachew, S. (2010). A longitudinal investigation of morphosyntax in children with speech sound disorders. *Journal of Communication Disorders, 43*, 61–76.

Mowrer, D. E. (1971). Transfer of training in articulation therapy. *Journal of Speech and Hearing Disorders, 36*, 427–446.

Munson, B., Baylis, A., Krause, M., & Yim, D.-S. (2006). *Representation and access in phonological impairment*. Paper presented at the 10th Conference on Laboratory Phonology, Paris, France, June 30–July 2.

Munson, B., Edwards, J., & Beckman, M. E. (2005a). Phonological knowledge in typical and atypical speech-sound development. *Topics in Language Disorders, 25*(3), 190–206.

Munson, B., Edwards, J., & Beckman, M. E. (2005b). Relationships between nonword repetition accuracy and other measures of linguistic development in children with phonological disorders. *Journal of Speech, Language, and Hearing Research, 48*, 61–78.

Munson, B., Kurtz, B. A., & Windsor, J. (2005). The influence of vocabulary size, phonotactic probability, and word likeness on nonword repetitions of children with and without specific language impairment. *Journal of Speech, Language, and Hearing Research, 48*(5), 1033–1047.

Murdoch, B. E., Attarch, M. D., Ozanne, A., & Stokes, P. D. (1995). Impaired tongue strength and endurance in developmental verbal dyspraxia: A physiological analysis. *European Journal of Disorders of Communication, 30*, 51–64.

Nathan, L., Stackhouse, J., Goulandris, N., & Snowling, M. J. (2004). The development of early literacy skills among children with speech difficulties: A test of the "critical age hypothesis." *Journal of Speech, Language, and Hearing Research, 47*, 377–391.

Newcomer, P., & Hammill, D. (1988). *Test of Language Development-2 Primary*. Austin, TX: Pro-Ed.

Nijland, L. (2009). Speech perception in children with speech output disorders. *Clinical Linguistics & Phonetics, 23*, 222–239.

Nittrouer, S. (1996). The relation between speech perception and phonemic awareness: Evidence from low-SES children and children with chronic otitis media. *Journal of Speech and Hearing Research, 39*, 1059–1070.

Nittrouer, S., & Burton, L. T. (2005). The role of early language experience in the development of speech perception and phonological processing abilities: Evidence from 5-year-olds with histories of otitis media with effusion and low socioeconomic status. *Journal of Communication Disorders, 38*, 29–63.

Osberger, M., & McGarr, N. S. ((1982)). Speech production characteristics of the hearing impaired. In N. J. Lass (Ed.), *Speech and language: Advances in basic research and practice* (pp. 221–283). New York, NY: Academic Press.

Ozanne, A. (1995). The search for developmental verbal dyspraxia. In B. Dodd (Ed.), *The differential diagnoses and treatment of children with speech disorder* (pp. 91–109). San Diego, CA: Singular.

Ozanne, A. (2005). Childhood apraxia of speech. In B. Dodd (Ed.), *Differential diagnosis and treatment of children with speech disorder* (pp. 71–82). London, UK: Whurr.

Paradise, J. L., Dollaghan, C. A., Campbell, T. F., Feldman, H. M., Bernard, B. S., Colborn, K.,. . . Smith, C. G. (2000). Language, speech sound production, and cognition in three-year-old children in relation to otitis media in their first three years of life. *Pediatrics, 105*(5), 1119–1130.

Paradise, J. L., Feldman, H. M., Campbell, T. F., Dollaghan, C. A., Colborn, D. K., Bernard, B. S., . . . Smith, C. G. (2001). Effect of early or delayed insertion of tympanostomy tubes for persistent otitis media on developmental outcomes at the age of three years. *New England Journal of Medicine, 344*(16), 1179–1187.

Paradise, J. L., Rockette, H. E., Colborn, D. K., Bernard, B. S., Smith, C. G., Kurs-Lasky, M., & Janosky, J. (1997). Otitis media in 2253 Pittsburgh-area infants: Prevalence and risk factors during the first two years of life. *Pediatrics, 99*(3), 318–333.

Pascoe, M., Stackhouse, J., & Wells, B. (2005). Phonological therapy within a psycholinguistic framework: Promoting change in a child with persisting speech difficulties. *International Journal of Language and Communication Disorders, 40*(2), 189–220.

Paul, R., & Shriberg, L. D. (1982). Associations between phonology and syntax in speech-delayed children. *Journal of Speech and Hearing Research, 25*, 536–547.

Peterson, R. L., Pennington, B. F., Shriberg, L. D., & Boada, R. (2009). What influences literacy outcome in children with speech sound disorder? *Journal of Speech, Language, and Hearing Research, 52*, 1175–1188.

Poehlmann, J., Clements, M., Abbeduto, L., Farsad, V., & Ferguson, D. (2005). Family experiences associatedwith a child's diagnosis of fragile X or Down syndrome: Evidence for disruption and resilience. *Mental Retardation, 43*(4), 255–267.

Polka, L., & Rvachew, S. (2005). The impact of otitis media with effusion on infant phonetic perception. *Infancy, 8*(2), 101–117.

Polka, L., Rvachew, S., & Molnar, M. (2008). Speech perception by 6- to 8-month-olds in the presence of distracting sounds. *Infancy, 13*, 421–439.

Popescu, M. V., & Polley, D. B. (2010). Monaural deprivation disrupts development of binaural selectivity in auditory midbrain and cortex. *Neuron, 65*, 718–731.

Preston, J. L. (2010). Speech and literacy: The connections and the relevance to clinical populations. In A. E. Harrison (Ed.), *Speech disorders: Causes, treatments and social effects* (pp. 43–73). Hauppauge, NY: Nova Science.

Preston, J. L., & Edwards, M. L. (2007). Phonological processing skills of adolescents with residual speech sound errors. *Language, Speech, and Hearing Services in Schools, 38*, 297–308.

Preston, J. L., & Edwards, M. L. (2009). Speed and accuracy of rapid speech output by adolescents with speech sound errors including rhotics. *Clinical Linguistics & Phonetics, 23*, 301–318.

Preston, J. L., & Edwards, M. L. (2010). Phonological awareness and types of sound errors in preschoolers with speech sound disorders. *Journal of Speech, Language, and Hearing Research, 53*(1), 44–60.

Preston, J. L., Felsenfeld, S., Frost, S. J., Mencl, W. E., Fulbright, R. K., Grigorenko, E. L., . . . Pugh, K. R. (2012). Functional brain activation differences in school-age children with speech sound errors: Speech and print processing. *Journal of Speech, Language, and Hearing Research, Papers in press* (January 9, 2012), doi:10.1044/1092-4388(2011/1011-0048).

Preston, J. L., & Koenig, L. L. (2011). Phonetic variability in residual speech sound disorders: Exploration of subtypes. *Topics in Language Disorders, 31*, 168–184.

Puranik, C. S., Petcher, Y., Al Otaiba, S., Catts, H. W., & Lonigan, C. J. (2008). Development of oral reading fluency in children with speech or language impairments: A growth curve analysis. *Journal of Learning Disabilities, 41*, 545–560.

Raitano, N. A., Pennington, B. F., Tunick, B. F., Boada, R., & Shriberg, L. D. (2004). Pre-literacy skills of subgroups of children with speech sound disorders. *Journal of Child Psychology and Psychiatry, 45*(4), 821–835.

Ramus, F. (2004). Neurobiology of dyslexia: a reinterpretation of the data. *Trends in Neurosciences, 27*, 720–726.

Raaymakers, E. M., & Crul, T. A. M. (1988). Perception and production of the final /s-ts/ contrast in Dutch by misarticulating children. *Journal of Speech and Hearing Disorders, 53*, 262–270.

Rice, M. L., Smith, S. D., & Gayán, J. (2009). Convergent genetic linkage and associations to language, speech and reading measures in families of probands with Specific Language Impairment. *Journal of Neurodevelopmental Disorders, 1*, 264–282.

Rice, M. L., & Wexler, K. (1996). Toward tense as a clinical marker of specific language impairment in English-speaking children. *Journal of Speech, Language, and Hearing Research, 39*(6), 1239–1257.

Rice, M. L., Wexler, K., & Cleave, P. L. (1995). Specific language impairment as a period of extended optional infinitive. *Journal of Speech, Language, and Hearing Research, 38*(4), 850–863.

Ringel, R. L., House, A. S., Burk, K. W., Dolinsky, J. P., & Scott, C. M. (1970). Some relations between orosensory discrimination and articulatory aspects of speech production. *Journal of Speech and Hearing Disorders, 35*, 3–11.

Robb, M. P., Hughes, M. C., & Frese, D. J. (1985). Oral diadochokinesis in hearing-impaired adolescents. *Journal of Communication Disorders, 18*, 79–89.

Robbins, J., & Klee, T. (1987). Clinical assessment of oropharyngeal motor development in young children. *Journal of Speech and Hearing Disorders, 52*, 271–277.

Roberts, J., Hunter, L., Gravel, J., Rosenfeld, R., Berman, S., Haggard, M., . . . Wallace, I. (2004). Otitis media, hearing loss, and language learning: Controversies and current research. *Journal of Developmental and Behavioral Pediatrics, 25*, 110–122.

Roberts, J. E., Rosenfeld, R. M., & Zeisel, S. A. (2004). Otitis media and speech and language: A meta-analysis of prospective studies. *Pediatrics, 113*(3), 238–248.

Robin, D. A., Somodi, C. B., & Luschei, E. S. (1991). Measurement of tongue strength and endurance in normal and articulation disordered subjects. In C. A. Moore, K. M. Yorkston, & D. R. Beukelman (Eds.), *Dysarthria and apraxia of speech: Perspectives on management*. Baltimore, MD: Paul H. Brookes.

Roulstone, S., Miller, L. L., Wren, Y., & Peters, T. J. (2009). The natural history of speech impairment of 8-year-old children in the Avon Longitudinal Study of parents and children: Error rates at 2 and 5 years. *International Journal of Speech-Language Pathology, 11*, 381–391.

Ruscello, D. M., & St. Louis, K. O. (2000). *Oral Speech Mechanism Screening Evaluation* (3rd ed.). Austin, TX: Pro-Ed.

Rvachew, S. (2006). Longitudinal prediction of implicit phonological awareness skills. *American Journal of Speech-Language Pathology, 15*, 165–176.

Rvachew, S. (2007). Phonological processing and reading in children with speech sound disorders. *American Journal of Speech-Language Pathology, 16*, 260–270.

Rvachew, S., Chiang, P., & Evans, N. (2007). Characteristics of speech errors produced by children with and without delayed phonological awareness skills. *Language, Speech, and Hearing Services in Schools, 38*, 60–71.

Rvachew, S., Gaines, B. R., Cloutier, G., & Blanchet, N. (2005). Productive morphology skills of children with speech delay. *Journal of Speech-Language Pathology and Audiology, 29*(2), 83–89.

Rvachew, S., & Grawburg, M. (2006). Correlates of phonological awareness in preschoolers with speech sound disorders. *Journal of Speech, Language, and Hearing Research, 49*, 74–87.

Rvachew, S., & Grawburg, M. (2008). Reflections on phonological working memory, letter knowledge and phonological awareness: A reply to Hartmann (2008). *Journal of Speech, Language, and Hearing Research, 51*, 1219–1226.

Rvachew, S., & Jamieson, D. G. (1989). Perception of voiceless fricatives by children with a functional articulation disorder. *Journal of Speech and Hearing Disorders, 54*, 193–208.

Rvachew, S., Ohberg, A., Grawburg, M., & Heyding, J. (2003). Phonological awareness and phonemic perception in 4-year-old children with delayed expressive phonology skills. *American Journal of Speech-Language Pathology, 12*, 463–471.

Rvachew, S., Slawinski, E. B., Williams, M., & Green, C. L. (1996). Formant frequencies of vowels produced by infants with and without early onset otitis media. *Canadian Acoustics, 24*, 19–28.

Rvachew, S., Slawinski, E. B., Williams, M., & Green, C. L. (1999). The impact of early onset otitis media on babbling and early language development. *Journal of the Acoustical Society of America, 105*, 467–475.

Schatschneider, C., Francis, D. J., Foorman, B. R., Fletcher, J. M., & Mehta, P. (1999). The dimensionality of phonological awareness: An application of item response theory. *Journal of Educational Psychology, 91*, 439–449.

Seymour, H. N., Baran, J., & Peaper, R. E. (1981). Auditory discrimination: Evaluation and intervention. In N. J. Lass (Ed.), *Speech and Language: Advances in Basic Research and Practice* (Vol. 6, pp. 1–56). New York, NY: Academic Press.

Share, D. L., Jorm, A. F., MacLean, R., & Mathews, R. (2002). Temporal processing and reading disability. *Reading and Writing: An Interdisciplinary Journal, 15*, 151–178.

Sherman, D., & Geith, A. (1967). Speech sound discrimination and articulation skill. *Journal of Speech and Hearing Research, 10*, 277–280.

Shriberg, L. D. (1993). Four new speech and prosody-voice measures for genetics research and other studies in developmental phonological disorders. *Journal of Speech and Hearing Research, 36*, 105–140.

Shriberg, L. D. (1994). Five subtypes of developmental phonological disorders. *Clinics in Communication Disorders, 4*, 38–53.

Shriberg, L. D. (1997). Developmental apraxia of speech: III. A subtype marked by inappropriate stress. *Journal of Speech, Language, and Hearing Research, 40*, 313–337.

Shriberg, L. D., Aram, D. M., & Kwiatkowski, J. (1997a). Developmental apraxia of speech: I. Descriptive and theoretical perspectives. *Journal of Speech, Language, and Hearing Research, 40*, 273–285.

Shriberg, L. D., Aram, D. M., & Kwiatkowski, J. (1997b). Developmental apraxia of speech: II. Toward a diagnostic marker. *Journal of Speech, Language, and Hearing Research, 40*, 286–312.

Shriberg, L. D., Austin, D., Lewis, B. A., McSweeny, J. L., & Wilson, D. L. (1997). The Speech Disorders Classification System (SDCS): Extensions and lifespan reference data. *Journal of Speech, Language, and Hearing Research, 40*(4), 723–740.

Shriberg, L. D., Ballard, K. J., Tomblin, J. B., Duffy, J. R., Odell, K. H., & Williams, C. A. (2006). Speech, prosody, and voice characteristics of a mother and daughter with a 7;13 translocation affecting FOXP2. *Journal of Speech, Language, and Hearing Research, 49*(3), 500–525.

Shriberg, L. D., Campbell, T. F., Karlsson, H. B., Brown, R. L., Mcsweeny, J. L., & Nadler, C. J. (2003). A diagnostic marker for childhood apraxia of speech: The lexical stress ratio. *Clinical Linguistics & Phonetics, 17*(7), 549–574.

Shriberg, L. D., Flipsen, P., Karlsson, H. B., & McSweeny, J. L. (2001). Acoustic phenotypes for speech-genetics studies: An acoustic marker for residual /ɝ/ distortions. *Clinical Linguistics & Phonetics, 15*, 631–650.

Shriberg, L. D., Flipsen, P., Kwiatkowski, J., & McSweeny, J. L. (2003). A diagnostic marker for speech delay associated with otitis media with effusion: The intelligibility-speech gap. *Clinical Linguistics & Phonetics, 17*, 507–528.

Shriberg, L. D., Fourakis, M., Hall, S. D., Karlsson, H. B., Lohmeier, H. L., McSweeny, J. L., . . . Wilson, D. L. (2010). Extensions to the Speech Disorders Classification System (SDSC). *Clinical Linguistics & Phonetics, 24*, 795–824.

Shriberg, L. D., Friel-Patti, S., Flipsen, P., & Brown, R. L. (2000). Otitis media, fluctuant hearing loss, and speech-language outcomes: A preliminary structural equation model. *Journal of Speech, Language, and Hearing Research, 43*, 100–120.

Shriberg, L. D., Green, J. R., Campbell, T. F., McSweeny, J. L., & Scheer, A. R. (2003). A diagnostic marker for childhood apraxia of speech: The coefficient of variation ratio. *Clinical Linguistics & Phonetics, 17*, 575–595.

Shriberg, L. D., Kwiatkowski, J., & Gruber, F. A. (1994). Developmental phonological disorders II: Short-term speech-sound normalization. *Journal of Speech, Language, and Hearing Research, 37*(5), 1127–1150.

Shriberg, L. D., Lewis, B. A., Tomblin, J. B., McSweeny, J. L., Karlsson, H. B., & Scheer, A. R. (2005). Toward diagnostic and phenotypic markers for genetically transmitted speech delay. *Journal of Speech, Language, and Hearing Research, 48*, 834–852.

Shriberg, L. D., Lohmeier, H. L., Strand, E. A., & Jakielski, K. J. (submitted). Encoding, memorial and transcoding deficits in childhood apraxia of speech.

Shriberg, L. D., Tomblin, J. B., & McSweeny, J. L. (1999). Prevalence of speech delay in 6-year-old children and comorbidity with language impairment. *Journal of Speech, Language, and Hearing Research, 42*(6), 1461–1481.

Shuster, L. I. (1998). The perception of correctly and incorrectly produced /r/. *Journal of Speech, Language, and Hearing Research, 41*, 941–950.

Siegel, L. S. (1992). An evaluation of the discrepancy definition of dyslexia. *Journal of Learning Disabilities, 25*(10), 618–629.

Silva, P. A., Justin, C., McGee, R., & Williams, S. M. (1984). Some developmental and behavioral characteristics of seven-year-old children with delayed speech development. *British Journal of Disorders of Communication, 19*, 147–154.

Smith, S. D., Pennington, B. F., Boada, R., & Shriberg, L. D. (2005). Linkage of speech sound disorder to reading disability loci. *Journal of Child Psychology and Psychiatry, 46*(10), 1057–1066.

Snowling, M. J., Bishop, D. V. M., & Stothard, S. E. (2000). Is preschool language impairment a risk factor for dyslexia in adolescence? *Journal of Child Psychology and Psychiatry, 41*(5), 587–600.

So, L. K. H., & Dodd, B. (1994). Phonologically disordered Cantonese-speaking children. *Clinical Linguistics & Phonetics, 18*, 235–255.

Sommers, R. K., Cox, S., & West, C. (1972). Articulatory effectiveness, stimulability, and children's performances on perceptual and memory tasks. *Journal of Speech and Hearing Research, 15*, 579–589.

Speirs, R. L., & Dean, P. M. (1989). Toffee clearance and lingual sensory and motor activities in normal children and children with articulation problems of speech. *Archives of Oral Biology, 34*, 637–644.

Stackhouse, J. (1992). Developmental verbal apraxia I: A review and critique. *European Journal of Disorders of Communication, 27*, 19–34.

Stackhouse, J., & Snowling, M. (1992). Developmental verbal dyspraxia II: A developmental perspective on two case studies. *European Journal of Disorders of Communication, 27*, 35–54.

Stackhouse, J., & Wells, B. (1993). Psycholinguistic assessment of developmental speech disorders. *European Journal of Disorders of Communication, 28*, 331–348.

Stanovich, K. E. (1988). Explaining the differences between the dyslexic and the garden-variety poor reader: The phonological-core variable-difference model. *Journal of Learning Disabilities, 21*(10), 590–612.

Stanovich, K. E., & Siegel, L.S. (1994). Phenotypic performance profile of children with reading disabilities: A regression-based test of the phonological-core variable-difference model. *Journal of Educational Psychology, 86*, 24–53.

Stein, C. M., Schick, J. H., Taylor, G., Shriberg, L. D., Millard, C., Kundtz-Kluge, A., . . . Iyengar, S. (2004). Pleiotropic effects of a chromosome 3 locus on speech-sound disorder and reading. *American Journal of Human Genetics, 74*, 283–297.

Studdert-Kennedy, M. (2002). Deficits in phoneme awareness do not arise from failures in rapid auditory processing. *Reading and Writing: An Interdisciplinary Journal, 15*, 5–14.

Tallal, P. (1980). Auditory temporal perception, phonics, and reading disabilities in children. *Brain and Language, 5*, 13–34.

Teele, D. W., Klein, J. O., Chase, C., Menyuk, P., Rosner, B. A., & Group, the Greater Boston Otitis Media Study (1984). Otitis media with effusion during the first three years of life and development of speech and language. *Pediatrics, 74*, 282–287.

Terband, H., Maassen, B., Guenther, F. H., & Brumberg, J. (2009). Computational neural modeling of speech motor control in childhood apraxia of speech (CAS). *Journal of Speech, Language, and Hearing Research, 52*, 1595–1609.

Thoonen, G., Maassen, B., Gabreels, F., & Schreuder, R. (1994). Feature analysis of singleton consonant errors in developmental verbal dyspraxia (DVD). *Journal of Speech and Hearing Research, 37*, 1424–1440.

Thoonen, G., Maassen, B., Gabreels, F., & Schreuder, R. (1999). Validity of maximum performance tasks to diagnose motor speech disorders in children. *Clinical Linguistics & Phonetics, 13*, 1–23.

Thoonen, G., Maassen, B., Wit, J., Gabreels, F. , & Schreuder, R. (1996). The integrated use of maximum performance tasks in differential diagnostic evaluations among children with motor speech disorders. *Clinical Linguistics & Phonetics, 10*, 311–336.

Tomblin, J. B., Records, N. L., & Zhang, J. (1996). A system for the diagnosis of specific language impairment in kindergarten children. *Journal of Speech and Hearing Research, 39*, 1284–1294.

Torgesen, J., Wagner, R. K., Rashotte, C. A., Burgess, S., & Hecht, S. (1997). Contributions of phonological awareness and rapid automatic naming ability to the growth of word-reading skills in second- to fifth-grade children. *Scientific Studies of Reading, 1*, 161–185.

Tunmer, W. E., & Greaney, K. (2010). Defining dyslexia. *Journal of Learning Disabilities, 43*, 229–243.

Vargha-Khadem, F., Gadian, D. G., Copp, A., & Mishkin, M. (2005). FOXP2 and the neuroanatomy of speech and language. *Neuroscience, 6*, 131–138.

Vargha-Khadem, F., Watkins, K., Alcock, K., Fletcher, P., & Passingham, R. (1995). Praxic and nonverbal cognitive deficits in a large family with a genetically transmitted speech and language disorder. *Proceedings of the National Academy of Sciences, 92*, 930–933.

Velleman, S. L., & Shriberg, L. D. (1999). Metrical analysis of the speech of children with suspected developmental apraxia of speech. *Journal of Speech, Language, and Hearing Research, 42*, 1444–1460.

Vernon-Feagans, L. (1999). Impact of otitis media on speech, language, cognition and behavior. In R. M. Rosenfeld & C. D. Bluestone (Eds.), *Evidence-based otitis media*. Hamilton, Ontario, Canada: Decker.

Waldman, F. R., Singh, S., & Hayden, M. E. (1978). A comparison of speech-sound production and discrimination in children with functional articulation disorders. *Language and Speech, 21*, 205–230.

Webster, P. E., Plante, A. S., & Couvillion, M. (1997). Phonologic impairment and prereading: Update on a longitudinal study. *Journal of Learning Disabilities, 30*(4), 365–376.

Wilkinson, R., & Marmot, M. (2003). *The social determinants of health: The solid facts* (2nd ed.). Copenhagen, Denmark: World Health Organization.

Wilkinson, R., & Pickett, K. (2010). *The spirit level: Why equality is better for everyone.* London, UK: Penguin.

Williams, N., & Chiat, S. (1993). Processing deficits in children with phonological disorder and delay: A comparison of responses to a series of output tasks. *Clinical Linguistics & Phonetics, 7*, 145–160.

Williams, R., Ingham, R. J., & Rosenthal, J. (1981). A further analysis for developmental apraxia of speech in children with defective articulation. *Journal of Speech and Hearing Research, 24*, 496–505.

Williams, P., & Stackhouse, J. (2000). Rate, accuracy and consistency: Diadochokinetic performance of young, normally developing children. *Clinical Linguistics & Phonetics, 14*, 267–293.

Winitz, H., & Darley, F. (1980). Speech production. In P. LaBenz & A. LaBenz (Eds.), *Early correlates of speech, language and hearing* (pp. 232–265). Littleton, MA: PSG.

Yont, K. M., Snow, C. E., & Vernon-Feagans, L. (2003). Is chronic otitis media associated with differences in parental input at 12 months of age? An analysis of joint attention and directives. *Applied Psycholinguistics, 24*, 581–602.

Yoss, K. A., & Darley, F. L. (1974). Developmental apraxia of speech in children with defective articulation. *Journal of Speech and Hearing Research, 17*, 399–416.

Young, A. R., Beitchman, J. H., Johnson, C., Douglas, L., Atkinson, L., Escobar, M., & Wilson, B. (2002). Young adult academic outcomes in a longitudinal sample of early identified language impaired and control children. *Journal of Child Psychology and Psychiatry, 43*(5), 635–645.

Zadeh, Z. Y., Im Bolter, N., & Cohen, N. J. (2007). Social cognition and externalizing psychopathology: An investigation of the mediating role of language. *Journal of Abnormal Child Psychology, 35*, 141–152.

Zhang, J., & McBride-Chang, C. (2010). Auditory sensitivity, speech perception, and reading development and impairment. *Educational Psychology Review, 22*(3), 323–338.

Zhang, X., & Tomblin, J. B. (2000). The association of intervention receipt with speech-language profiles and social-demographic variables. *American Journal of Speech-Language Pathology, 9*(4), 345–357.

Zhao, Y., Ma, H., Wang, Y., Gao, H., Xi, C., Hua, T., . . . Qiu, G. (2010). Association between FOXP2 gene and speech sound disorder in the Chinese population. *Psychiatry and Clinical Neurosciences, 64*(5), 565–573.

Chapter 8

Treatment Planning

In typical clinical practice, especially in publically funded settings, treatment planning decisions often occur in two phases and may even be made by different individuals at those two decision points. An initial assessment is conducted in accordance with the relevant standards as discussed in Chapter 5. The SLP will gather information about the child's functioning in a number of domains for the explicit purpose of making a diagnosis. An implicit purpose of this assessment is to determine whether the child needs a service and if so, what kind of service should be provided. There are many variations on the exact process that leads to this decision point—there may be a prior screening or triage step before the diagnostic assessment and there may be an opportunity for diagnostic therapy after but in every case there is a point at which someone decides what kind of service, if any, the child will receive (or be referred to receive). In a second phase, once the child is actually receiving treatment, an SLP will decide what the goals of the intervention will be and how best to help the child to achieve those goals. Comparatively speaking, there is a firm empirical basis for making decisions in the second phase of the process. Many books and articles have been written to help the clinician choose intervention goals and studies have been conducted to determine whether different approaches to this task have greater or lesser efficacy.

An implicit purpose of the diagnostic assessment is to determine whether the child needs a service and, if so, what kind of service should be provided.

In a second phase, once the child is actually receiving treatment, an SLP will decide what the goals of the intervention will be and how best to help the child to achieve those goals.

Almost nothing has been published in the scientific literature with respect to the first decision, however. Besides the fact that decades of debate about appropriate labels and diagnostic criteria have not yet yielded a consensus on these issues, a diagnosis and the decision about treatment options are not one and the same. Even if every SLP could agree that a given child should be diagnosed as

The diagnosis does not directly determine the treatment plan.

Treatment planning decisions include: (1) does the child require an intervention in order to achieve age-appropriate speech function? (2) if so, who should provide the intervention? (3) where should the intervention be provided? and (4) how frequently and with what intensity should the intervention be provided?

having a development phonological disorder, a series of decisions remain that do not follow directly from the diagnosis itself: (1) does the child require an intervention in order to achieve age-appropriate speech function? (2) if so, who should provide the intervention? (3) where should the intervention be provided? and (4) how frequently and with what intensity should the intervention be provided? Very few peer-reviewed systematic investigations have been published in the scientific literature that serve as an empirical basis for making these decisions. One reason for this gap may be that these decisions are so frequently made at an administrative level as they impact on the use of resources and relate directly to the specific mandate of the service provider. The administrative guidelines that are laid down, even when they are developed by front-line SLPs rather than administrators, typically are made in response to workload pressures and resource limitations rather than the needs of individual children. However, the harm that arises when these decisions are removed from treating clinicians is too great for our profession to be passive in the face of this empirical gap. We must ensure that these decisions are made for each child on the basis of the best available scientific evidence. We address this first level of planning in some depth in this chapter despite the absence of studies that specifically address best practice with respect to these questions. Before proceeding, we caution that the decisions made at these different time points (when the child is placed on a wait list for intervention and when the child actually receives the intervention) are not fully independent of each other even though they may be made by different individuals, sometimes months apart. If it is decided that a child with a severe DPD is eligible to receive a 6-week block of once-weekly group therapy, then the treating SLP will have to adjust the goals and choose a therapy approach that is compatible with those constraints. On the other hand, if the mandate of the service provider is to ensure that preschool-age children begin school with speech and language functioning within the average range, then the treating SLP should choose an intensity of service that will achieve that goal given the severity of the child's deficits and the amount of time that is available before school entry. We begin, however, with an even more fundamental question: Should the child receive an intervention?

Deciding Whether to Provide an Intervention

8.1.1. Describe three approaches to the process of deciding whether a child requires speech therapy for remediation of developmental phonological disorder.

8.1.2. Explain why selection criteria based on phoneme-specific norms should not be used to determine eligibility for speech therapy services.

8.1.3. Describe how to apply the predictive assessment protocol to monitor speech development in a school-age child with sibilant distortions.

8.1.4. Apply the flow chart shown in Figure 8–1 to assessment data gathered from preschool and school-age children and decide whether the children should be referred to receive speech therapy for remediation of DPD.

There are three basic perspectives on how to decide whether a child requires an intervention. The first is tied to the notion of a normative reference[1]: the child's performance is compared to that of a reference group that has similar age and demographic characteristics and treatment is prescribed if the child appears to be significantly delayed with respect to the mean of the group. The second is in the tradition of the medical approach to diagnosis and differentiates those with a speech disorder in contrast to a delay in phonological development.[2] The third, related to the ICF framework presented in the Introduction to Part II, would place a higher priority on treating impairments that impact on the child's activities and participation in specific contexts. Decision making from these three perspectives is discussed using case examples from a longitudinal follow-up study in which children were recruited from speech-language caseloads in pediatric hospitals and assessed annually for 3 years, at the end of junior kindergarten/preschool, kindergarten, and first grade. The measures that were used in this study are described in Rvachew and Grawburg (2006) and Rvachew (2007). The case study presentations include a list of phonemes that the child misarticulated in at least two of three word positions and clusters that were misarticulated at least twice on the Goldman-Fristoe Test of Articulation-2 (GFTA-2; Goldman & Fristoe, 2000), thus corresponding to the "customary production" criterion used in phoneme specific normative charts such as that shown in Figure 4–5.

There are three perspectives on determining **treatment eligibility**: (1) *norm-referenced approach*; (2) *medical approach*; and (3) *ICF framework*.

[1]Issues related to measurement theory and test construction are not covered in this book. It is assumed that the reader is familiar with the relevant concepts (e.g., Klee, 2008; McCauley & Swisher, 1984; Peña, Spaulding, & Plante, 2006). The SLP must choose a standardized instrument that is valid for the assessment purpose, normed on an appropriate reference sample, and proven to provide a reliable estimate of the child's performance on the construct of interest.

[2]We remind the reader that we do not believe that there is a fundamental distinction between phonological delay and phonological disorder as argued in the introduction to Part II and discussed in Chapter 7. Here we adopt terminology commonly used in criteria for qualifying children for service and demonstrate that these criteria will exclude children who are at significant risk of poor social and academic outcomes unless treatment is provided. Furthermore, the flow chart is not meant for the purpose of diagnosis; that is, children who score below the 10th percentile might be labeled with respect to any of the categories discussed in the Introduction to Part II and in Chapter 7, according to the child's psycholinguistic profile and developmental history of speech impairment, the SLP's preferred classification scheme, and the requirements of the local jurisdiction. In any case, scoring below the 10th percentile on a standardized test would indicate sufficient severity of speech impairment to warrant service provision.

Norm-Referenced Approach

The **norm-referenced approach** to determining eligibility for service is to compare the child's performance to a reference group based on a standardized test score and prescribe treatment if the child's score falls below a mandated minimum.

A common practice for determining eligibility for service is to compare the child's performance to a reference group based on a standardized test score and prescribe treatment if the child's score falls below a mandated minimum (Olswang & Bain, 1991; Spaulding, Plante, & Farinella, 2006). Normative based cutoff scores for recommending intervention are consistent with the "common disease/common variant" model of language and literacy disorders (Bishop, 2009; see also Chapter 7). In fact, Bishop points out that the use of the term "disease" is hardly appropriate by this view "because there are no clear dividing lines between normality and abnormality" (p. 14) given that common variants of many genes, each having a small effect, collectively account for continuous variations in verbal skills within the population. From this perspective, services are provided to children scoring at the low end of the distribution, not because of a qualitatively defined abnormality but because the magnitude of the discrepancy between the child's level of functioning and the population average is so great as to constitute a significant risk to the child or cost to society. One goal is to avoid wasting resources by providing services to children who will "catch up" to their peers, achieving intelligible speech by age 4;0 and error-free speech by age 9;0, without intervention. Even if there were unlimited resources for the provision of speech therapy services there are costs to providing the service unnecessarily (the risk of stigmatizing the child and depriving the child of the benefit of engaging in other activities) and thus over-treating is to be avoided. On the other hand, if the child's rate of progress is so slow that other risks are incurred along the way (failure to learn to read at the expected rate or bullying at school for example) then the benefit of preventing these outcomes is weighed against the cost of providing speech therapy to the child.

For the diagnosis of language impairment, it has been empirically established that a cutoff score of −1.25 standard deviations from the mean (i.e., 10th percentile or less) in two or more composite measures in five language domains provides good specificity and sensitivity in relation to clinician ratings of severity of speech and language functioning (Tomblin, Records, & Zhang, 1996). Despite the lack of similar empirical work for standardized tests in phonology, the 10th percentile cutoff used in the language domain seems to be a defensible cutoff score for determining eligibility for service on the basis of performance on a standardized test of articulation accuracy as well. This cutoff will result in samples that are roughly similar to those described in Chapter 7 that demonstrated elevated risk for significantly poor outcomes in the psychosocial, academic, and vocational domains. Some might argue that these outcomes were restricted to children with concomitant language impairments but a careful reading of Chapter 7 reveals that the "speech only" samples described in many studies as having good outcomes have scored considerably higher than the 10th percentile and/or presented with fluency or voice disorders rather than DPD. It is possible although unconfirmed that children with residual speech errors and no prior history of speech delay (i.e, RE-B) are not at risk for adverse academic and vocational outcomes. Children with a preschool history of moderate or severe DPD as determined by standardized measures of articulation accuracy are another population entirely: we believe that the incidence (if not the prevalence) of language impairment and/or phonological processing disorders is high among this group and thus the outcomes described for language impaired children may be reasonably predicted for these children as well. On these grounds, provision of intervention to young children who score at or below the 10th percentile on a standardized test of articulation accuracy is justified.

Provide intervention to young children who score at or below the 10th percentile on a standardized test of articulation accuracy in order to reduce risk of negative outcomes described in long-term follow-up studies for children who begin school with speech delay.

Case Study 8–1 provides an example of a child who received two years of speech and language therapy prior to entering kindergarten. At the age of 4;9 he scored at the 9th percentile on the GFTA-2 when assessed during the prekindergarten year. Phonemes subject to error in at least two out of three word positions are shown, indicating difficulties with interdental and postalveolar fricatives, affricates, and /ɹ/. Cluster reduction was pervasive. Receptive vocabulary skills were a strength and his expressive morphology and syntax abilities were generally age-appropriate although grammatical errors involving articles and the past-tense morpheme were apparent in the free speech sample. The child shows clear evidence of phonological processing difficulties with low scores for speech perception and phonological awareness. One year later his GFTA score had improved to the borderline normal range due to improved accuracy for /dʒ/ and l-clusters and his phonological awareness performance had improved to the average range. At the end of first grade gliding and distortion of /ɹ/ continued to be pervasive in his speech. Although his word reading scores were average overall, the large gap between his sight word reading and nonword reading score was worrying as was the gap between his word reading performance and his receptive vocabulary skills. This profile is consistent with dyslexia as discussed in Chapter 7. Despite the fact that his test scores are close to or within normal limits at this assessment point, there are a number of risk factors in the child's history that justify continued monitoring of his progress through the school years (specifically, he was a late talker and his mother received speech therapy as a child). Nonetheless, the speech and language intervention provided to him as a preschooler appeared to set him on a trajectory of reduced risk for poor outcomes given the normalized profile during the kindergarten assessment. Following from the outcomes reported in Stothard, Snowling, Bishop, Chipchase, and Kaplan (1998) for children who normalize speech and language functioning before school entry, we can expect that this child would have a good chance of maintaining grade-level reading achievement even though his poor phonological processing skills would likely persist throughout the school years.

Case Study 8–1

Case History: Child (PA211) was late talker; health history unremarkable; mom received speech therapy as a child; parents have postsecondary educations.

Preschool Test Scores (CA = 4;9)

SAILS	61%, $z = -2.53$
GFTA-2	9th percentile
PCC	70%, $z = -1.29$
PPVT	SS = 102
MLU	6.28
PAT	Raw score = 13, $z = -1.84$
Letters	Raw score = 10

Preschool Phoneme Errors

Target	Errors
ʃ	s
tʃ	t ts
ɹ	w null
dʒ	d
θ	f
ð	null v
l-clusters	reduced
r-clusters	reduced

Example Sentences from Preschool Speech Sample

Then the dog lying on the mat.

Then the baby lying on the mat too.

Then they go on elevator and go to bed on the mat

Then a baby very tired and need to go to bed.

Kindergarten Test Scores (CA = 5;8)

SAILS	80%, $z = -.34$
GFTA-2	16th percentile
PCC	85%, $z = -.24$
PPVT	SS = 108
MLU	6.55
PAT	Raw score = 28, $z = -.21$
Letters	Raw score = 11

Kindergarten Phoneme Errors

Target	Errors
ʃ	s
tʃ	ts
ɹ	w null
θ	f
ð	d v
r-clusters	reduced

Example Sentences from Kindergarten Speech Sample

And the (baby then the) baby hurt herself.

And then the dog got her up and taked her on the elevator.

And then they went to a bed department.

And then, the dog ate some of her food up.

And then he gave some to a baby.

First Grade Test Scores (CA = 6;9)

SAILS	87%, z = .43
GFTA-2	15th percentile
PCC	90%, z = −.21
PPVT	SS = 115
MLU	6.65
PAT	Raw score = 33, z = .43
TOWREsw	SS = 108
TOWREnw	SS = 87
TOWRE	SS = 97

First Grade Phoneme Errors

Target	Errors
ɹ	ɹʷ w null
ɹ-clusters	simplification

Example Sentences from First Grade Speech Sample

She's asking him to look after the baby.

Can I see the last page?

Then the baby sneaks out.

I know this story.

Then the dog's getting out of the room.

Then the baby comes with him.

Notes: SAILS = Speech Assessment and Interactive Learning System (measure of speech perception skills; see http://www.medicine.mcgill.ca/srvachew); GFTA-2 = Goldman Fristoe Test of Articulation-2 (Goldman & Fristoe, 2000); PCC = Percent Consonants Correct, assessed in conversation (see Chapters 4 and 5); PPVT = Peabody Picture Vocabulary Test (Dunn & Dunn, 1997); MLU = Mean Length of Utterance (in morphemes); PAT = Phonological Awareness Test (Bird, Bishop, & Freeman, 1995); Letters = number of letters named; TOWRE = Test of Word Reading Efficiency (Torgesen, Wagner, & Rashotte, 1999); TOWREsw = sight word reading subtest; TOWREns = nonword reading, that is, phonetic decoding subtest; SS = standard score where mean is 100 and standard deviation is 15.

A more common means of determining eligibility for speech therapy services is to compare the child's performance to phoneme specific norms. For example, the Appendix to Puranik, Petcher, Al Otaiba, Catts, and Lonigan (2008) provides the service eligibility criteria for Florida schools. The criteria for language services are relatively straightforward, being based on standard score cutoffs, but the first eligibility criterion to receive speech therapy involves a rather complicated formula for determining whether the frequency of incorrect sound production is "significant" in relation to normative data for phoneme acquisition: specifically, "three or more consonantal error sounds delayed by at least 1 year, two or more delayed by at least 2 years, one delayed by at least 3 years, or a pattern of five or more consonantal error sounds affecting overall intelligibility" (p. 557). We strongly recommend against the use of criteria based on age norms for individual phonemes, especially when the requirement is that the delay exceed the expected age of acquisition. Recall that the expected ages of acquisition, as indicated in most normative charts, are the ages at which 90% of children have achieved customary production of the phoneme in question. Presumably, the requirement that the child show a 2-year delay for two or more sounds reflects an expectation that the child might acquire the phonemes spontaneously during that two year period. However, for most phonemes there is no reason to think that a child is likely to show spontaneous acquisition of a phoneme once the expected age of acquisition has passed. Consider the pattern of errors presented in Case Study 8–2. This child, at the age of 4;7, has failed to achieve customary production for 10 phonemes and shows consistent simplification or reduction of word initial consonant clusters. All of the errors shown would be categorized as "typical developmental" except for the fronting of /k/ and /g/ as the expected age of acquisition for these phonemes is 4;0 according to Figure 4–5. Smit, Hand, Freilinger, Bernthal, and Bird (1990) found that these target phonemes are achieved by approximately 75% percent of children at age 3 years, approximately 90% of 4-year-olds and virtually all older children. The stability of the growth curves for these phonemes indicates clearly that there is no reason to wait beyond age 4;0 to intervene (especially when the child's overall test score indicates a DPD of moderate severity!) and yet this child would not clearly meet the criterion for two or more phonemes with a two year delay. Furthermore, this child has mild difficulties with morphosyntax and word finding and significant problems with speech perception and phonological awareness and thus fits the profile of children at significant risk for delayed acquisition of literacy skills (see PL group, Table 7–13 adapted from Lewis, Freebairn, & Taylor, 2000). One might argue that the child's language difficulties would qualify him for service but in fact, mild language difficulties are frequently missed unless an accompanying speech deficit results in referral to the SLP (Zhang & Tomblin, 2000), and thus it is important to not set the bar too high for the identification of speech or language impairments.

We strongly recommend against the use of criteria based on age norms for individual phonemes to determine eligibility for service.

There is no reason to think that a child is likely to show spontaneous acquisition of a phoneme once the expected age of acquisition has passed.

Mild language difficulties are frequently missed unless an accompanying speech deficit results in referral to the SLP, and thus it is important not to set the bar too high for the identification of speech or language impairments.

Case Study 8–2

Case History: Child (PA514); history unremarkable; no family history of speech, language or reading disorder; parents have university degrees.

Preschool Test Scores (CA = 4;7)

SAILS	47%, $z = -4.65$
GFTA-2	5th percentile
PCC	58%, $z = -2.8$
PPVT	SS = 95
MLU	3.41
PAT	Raw score = 8, $z = -2.92$
Letters	Raw score = 5

Preschool Phoneme Errors

Target	Error
k	t
g	d
ʃ	t
tʃ	ts
l	w null
dʒ	dz
ɹ	w null
θ	f t
s	t
z	d
r clusters	simplified
l clusters	simplified
s clusters	reduced

Example Sentences from Preschool Speech Sample

He biting her shirt.

Reading.

I don't know.

Playing.

She got a hat.

Kindergarten Test Scores (CA = 5;7)

SAILS	76%, $z = -1.00$
GFTA-2	43th percentile
PCC	77%, $z = -1.25$
PPVT	SS = 112
MLU	9.2
PAT	Raw score = 31, $z = .54$
Letters	Raw score = 12

Kindergarten Phoneme Errors

Target	Errors
θ	f

Example Sentences from Kindergarten Speech Sample

And then, the other picture, they're dressed up like stuff.

And then they went down to the attic in this picture.

Went downstairs into the attic.

And the baby down there, the dog went down there to get the baby.

They wrecked. . . (incomplete sentence).

First Grade Test Scores (CA = 6;7)

SAILS	77%, $z = -1.07$
GFTA-2	17th percentile
PCC	84%, $z = -1.40$
PPVT	SS = 100
MLU	6.04
PAT	Raw score = 31, $z = -.81$
TOWREsw	SS = 106
TOWREnw	SS = 89
TOWRE	SS = 97

First Grade Phoneme Errors

Target	Error
ɹ	ɹʷ w null
s	θ
ɹ-clusters	simplification

Example Sentences from First Grade Speech Sample

She's telling the dog to look after the baby.

Cause if he doesn't, (he might the) she might not give him a treat or something.

The baby's getting up and he went over there.

Climbing on him like a piggybank.

He's sorta smiling, the dog.

He's going into her mom's room and then the dog's on the bed.

Notes: SAILS = Speech Assessment and Interactive Learning System (measure of speech perception skills; see http://www.medicine.mcgill.ca/srvachew); GFTA-2 = Goldman Fristoe Test of Articulation-2 (Goldman & Fristoe, 2000); PCC = Percent Consonants Correct, assessed in conversation (see Chapters 4 and 5); PPVT = Peabody Picture Vocabulary Test (Dunn & Dunn, 1997); MLU = Mean Length of Utterance (in morphemes); PAT = Phonological Awareness Test (Bird et al., 1995); Letters = number of letters named; TOWRE = Test of Word Reading Efficiency (Torgesen et al., 1999); TOWREsw = sight word reading subtest; TOWREnw = nonword reading, that is, phonetic decoding subtest; SS = standard score where mean is 100 and standard deviation is 15.

The second reason to council against phoneme-based normative standards is that this kind of criterion does not take into account the type of error or the pattern of errors that occur in the child's speech. Neither of the children presented in Case Study 8–1 or 8–2 would qualify for service given the rule shown above and yet both children are using phonological processes that should be suppressed by the age of 3 years (fronting and stopping). It is true that standardized tests of articulation accuracy are based solely on the number of errors and therefore do not take the type of error into account either. However, phonological processes by definition apply to classes of phonemes and thus will typically result in a test score that falls at or below the 10th percentile as shown in Case Studies 8–1 and 8–2 because of the total number of errors involved. These two cases illustrate clearly that the use of phoneme-based age norms will deny service to children with significant phonological delay who are at risk for dyslexia, the very group of children that the school SLP is mandated to serve.

There is one exception in which the use of sound based norms might be reasonable: this is the case of children with Speech Errors (sometimes called questionable residual errors or QREs) especially of the RE-B type, as defined in Chapter 7. Recall that the growth curves for /s/and /z/ remain unstable between 6 and 9 years and Smit et al. (1990) had difficulty determining a clear age of acquisition for these phonemes. Relying on standardized test scores to determine service eligibility for children with QREs can lead to over and under identification of children who require service for remediation of sibilant distortions. Tests that contain many items targeting /s/-clusters may indicate a severe delay for a preschooler who has no errors except consistent dental distortion of sibilants. In other circumstances the child may obtain a test score within normal limits even though it is clear that the child will not achieve correct sibilant production spontaneously and the error is impacting on the child's speech intelligibility. Smit et al. recommended a course of predictive assessment in the case of RE-B type Speech Errors, as follows: (1) do not treat before age 7 unless the error is atypical (e.g., lateral distortion); (2) assess at age 7 years but delay treatment if any acceptable productions of /s/ and /z/ occur in the child's speech or if the child is stimulable or if the child's upper incisors have not erupted; (3) recheck at age 8 years and treat if there is no change over the past year or if there are participation restrictions that warrant initiating treatment at this time; otherwise (4) recheck at age 9 years and treat if clinically significant distortions remain in the child's speech.

Predictive assessment is recommended for children who present with *RE-B type speech errors* between the ages of 6 and 9 years.

We provide an example of a child with sibilant distortions in Case Study 8–3. This child is scoring within normal limits during the prekindergarten year despite interdental productions of sibilants, reduction of /s/-clusters and simplification of /ɹ/-clusters. We highlight this case because we sometimes find children such as this receiving treatment when we recruit research participants from speech therapy caseloads. When describing clinician reliability in the assignment of severity ratings during intake assessments,

Case Study 8–3

Case History: Child (APA005); health and developmental history unremarkable; no family history of speech, language or reading disorder; single parent family; mom has university degree.

Preschool Test Scores (CA = 4;6)

SAILS	80%, z = .35
GFTA-2	21st percentile
PCC	83%, z = .35
PPVT	SS = 119
MLU	5.85
PAT	Raw score = 22, z = .10
Letters	Raw score = 10

Preschool Phoneme Errors

Target	Errors
ʃ	θ
tʃ	tθ
dʒ	dð
s	θ
z	ð
r clusters	simplified
s clusters	reduced

Example Sentences from Preschool Speech Sample

Or it could be a escalator.

Hey, the dog's pressing the button to go up up up.

X X that's the up button and that could be the down button.

Up down down up.

They're playing in the toys.

Carl's putting the baby in X it the car the X way.

Kindergarten Test Scores (CA = 5;6)

SAILS	87%, $z = .80$
GFTA-2	22nd percentile
PCC	85%, $z = -.24$
PPVT	SS = 119
MLU	8.12
PAT	Raw score = 21, $z = -1.98$
Letters	Raw score = 12

Kindergarten Phoneme Errors

Target	Errors
ʃ	s θ
tʃ	ts θ
s	θ
r clusters	simplified
s clusters	reduced

Example Sentences from Kindergarten Speech Sample

The dog put the baby in the truck and pushed him to the toy.

And then it made a big mess and the baby took a toy.

And then they went to the library.

And then they looked at the books.

And then the baby (look) saw one and it, he liked it.

First Grade Test Scores (CA = 6;7)

SAILS	77%, $z = -1.07$
GFTA-2	26th percentile
PCC	93%, $z = .70$
PPVT	SS = 114
MLU	8.44
PAT	Raw score = 32, $z = .19$
TOWREsw	SS = 108
TOWREnw	SS = 107
TOWRE	SS = 109

First Grade Phoneme Errors

Target	Errors
s	θ

Example Sentences from First Grade Speech Sample

And then they were taking up clothes and the baby found a hat.

And uh, gloves.

And he put the gloves on the dog's nose.

And then they left.

Then they went (to s) to see them on TV

And then they started crying.

And then they went back downstairs and rolled in the rugs.

Notes: SAILS = Speech Assessment and Interactive Learning System (measure of speech perception skills; see http://www.medicine.mcgill.ca/srvachew); GFTA-2 = Goldman Fristoe Test of Articulation-2 (Goldman & Fristoe, 2000); PCC = Percent Consonants Correct, assessed in conversation (see Chapters 4 and 5); PPVT = Peabody Picture Vocabulary Test (Dunn & Dunn, 1997); MLU = Mean Length of Utterance (in morphemes); PAT = Phonological Awareness Test (Bird et al., 1995); Letters = number of letters named; TOWRE = Test of Word Reading Efficiency (Torgesen et al., 1999); TOWREsw = sight word reading subtest; TOWREnw = nonword reading, that is, phonetic decoding subtest; SS = standard score where mean is 100 and standard deviation is 15; X indicates unintelligible word in the free speech sample.

Rafaat, Rvachew, and Russell (1995) found that children with GFTA percentiles as high as 80 were deemed to have mild speech delay and children with GFTA percentiles as high as 20 were diagnosed with moderate DPD. In some cases these anomalies are justified because the standardized test scores do not capture the difference between typical and atypical error types. In other cases they are mistakes because the clinician has miscalculated the child's age or misinterpreted the phoneme-level normative charts (taking the left hand edge of the bars on Figure 4–5 to be the expected age of acquisition for example). In other cases the judgment reflects the use of tests based on phonological process norms which tend to inflate the severity rankings relative to norms based on a simple count of the number of errors. The child presented in Case Study 8–3 does produce an error pattern of concern relative to phonological process norms, specifically inconsistent cluster reduction. Given the ambiguity around the age at which cluster reduction is normally suppressed, a "wait and see" approach seems prudent. Indeed, no intervention was provided and he showed steady improvements throughout the 3-year period of monitoring. At the end of first grade, he does not meet the standards for initiating treatment according to Smit et al.'s protocol for predictive assessment because dentalization of /s/ and /z/ was quite inconsistent in conversation (e.g., [dɔgz noz̪]). Unlike Case Studies 8–1 and 8–2, there are no concerns about language or phonological processing skills and no evidence of discrepancies in the profile of reading acquisition in this case either. Furthermore, there is no family history of speech, language or reading disability. Overall, Case Study 8–3 illustrates a normal trajectory. What if we had assessed this child in a clinical rather than research context at the age of 4;6? We would have counseled the parents to provide focused stimulation (see Chapter 9) for the s-cluster errors and recommended that they contact a SLP if the distortions persisted past the age of 9 years and then discharged the child from further service.

Medical Approach

Another common approach is to reserve treatment for children who are diagnosed with a phonological disorder as differentiated from delayed phonological development. Presumably, the assumption is that children who are following the normal sequence of development but at a slower than expected rate will eventually achieve accurate speech production without intervention. By this view, children with a phonological disorder require treatment because their atypical speech patterns are an indication of impairment in some underlying process or mechanism. Stoel-Gammon and Dunn (1985) identified a number of characteristics of disordered trajectories of phonological development: (1) an early plateau reflecting

According to the **medical approach**, treatment is reserved for children who are diagnosed with a phonological disorder as differentiated from delayed phonological development.

persistence of phonological processes beyond the expected ages; (2) extreme variability in production rather than gradual improvement toward adult levels of consonant accuracy; (3) chronological mismatch with mastery of later developing sounds occurring alongside persistent misarticulation of early developing sounds; (4) idiosyncratic rules or processes not typically seen in normal development (at least not past the toddler period when we would argue that idiosyncratic productions are not atypical); and (5) restricted use of contrast.

Case Study 8–4 illustrates these characteristics in a boy who was aged 5;4 at the time of the first assessment. The plateau in development is reflected in the very minimal gains in an extraordinarily low PCC observed during the 3-year follow-up period. Variability in production is observed both within and between sampling intervals. Note for example, the alternative pronunciations of the words "elevator" and "pushing" during the assessment. Substitutions for specific targets were difficult to predict (for example, /f/ produced variously as [f], [p], or [t]). Variability over time was observed as well with the apparent mastery of the liquids in singleton contexts at the kindergarten assessment followed by the reappearance of gliding in the first grade assessment being one example. The kindergarten results give the appearance of chronological mismatch with the apparent mastery of later developing phonemes despite the fronting of velar stops. It is illusory, however, as errors on the later developing phonemes re-emerge at the first grade assessment. It is possible that the appearance of chronological mismatch in this case is a "therapy effect" that results from the targeting of phonemes in nondevelopmental order, a practice discussed later in this chapter. We have not conducted an in-depth analysis of the child's phonological system and thus cannot comment on the use of idiosyncratic rules or contrastive use of phones (as mentioned earlier, this step would typically occur after the decision to treat has been made and would require extensive sampling of the child's speech as described in Chapter 6). However, several atypical errors are readily apparent including affrication of /t/, the use of lateral fricatives, and substitution of a glide for /v/ during the preschool assessment as well as a mix of fronting and backing errors throughout the observation period. This child clearly meets the conventional criteria for phonological disorder and thus would qualify for service on these grounds. In fact, the child would be considered a high priority for treatment from any perspective given that he scored at or below the first percentile on the GFTA at each assessment, he showed at least a 2-year delay for two phonemes at each assessment, and his speech was unintelligible to unfamiliar listeners (without mentioning the expressive language delay).

The question is whether there is any rationale for denying intervention to the children shown in Case Studies 8–1 and 8–2 on the grounds that their phonological systems are delayed rather than disordered.

Case Study 8–4

Case History: Child (PA221) was a late talker but history is otherwise unremarkable; no family history of speech, language or reading disorder; both parents have advanced degrees; English is first and dominant language but there is some exposure to a second language in the home.

Preschool Test Scores (CA = 5;4)

SAILS	67%, $z = -1.62$
GFTA-2	1st percentile
PCC	45%, $z = -4.46$
PPVT	SS = 115
MLU	1.77
PAT	Raw score = 13, $z = -1.84$
Letters	Raw score = 11

Preschool Phoneme Errors

Target	Errors
f	p t
t	tʃ null
l	w null
dʒ	d null
θ	ɬ null t
v	w g f
s	ɬ t
z	s null
ð	d
l clusters	reduced
r clusters	reduced
s clusters	reduced

Example Sentences from Preschool Speech Sample

Baby is pulling (her her) his ear.
Elevator. [ɛdʒɛgeə]
Me don't know.
Pushing [pʊtɪŋ].
Pushing [pʊɬɪŋ] button.
With his paw.
Waiting.
Elevator [ɛgetə].

Kindergarten Test Scores (CA = 6;2)

SAILS	79%, – 51
GFTA-2	<1st percentile
PCC	50%, $z = -4.67$
PPVT	SS = 115
MLU	2.97
PAT	Raw score = 24, $z = -1.22$
Letters	Raw score = 12

Kindergarten Phoneme Errors

Target	Errors
g	d null
k	t g
dʒ	g null
θ	t null s
v	w null
z	s null
ð	s v
l clusters	reduced
r clusters	reduced
s clusters	reduced

Example Sentences from Kindergarten Speech Sample

Press the button.

No, up here.

Go up.

Elevator.

They play, they play, they play.

Play, play, play.

I know what you like.

I know there one bunny, you know that one.

One doggy.

First Grade Test Scores (CA = 6;7)

SAILS	70%, –2.11
GFTA-2	<1st percentile
PCC	53%, $z = -8.6$
PPVT	SS = 95
MLU	2.95
PAT	Raw score = 33, $z = .43$
TOWREsw	SS = 91
TOWREnw	SS = 81
TOWRE	SS = 83

First Grade Phoneme Errors

Target	Errors
g	null d
t	d k
ʃ	s null
tʃ	d t ts
l	j null
ɹ	w null
dʒ	g null
θ	f s
s	null
ð	v w
l clusters	Reduced
r clusters	Reduced

Example Sentences from First Grade Speech Sample

I can't read.

Hey, no pictures, no words.

What a good book.

The dog looking out the window.

They jump on the bed. (. . .)

Then the baby put make-up on the dog.

What is it?

Notes. SAILS = Speech Assessment and Interactive Learning System (measure of speech perception skills; see http://www.medicine.mcgill.ca/srvachew); GFTA-2 = Goldman Fristoe Test of Articulation-2 (Goldman & Fristoe, 2000); PCC = Percent Consonants Correct, assessed in conversation (see Chapters 4 and 5); PPVT = Peabody Picture Vocabulary Test (Dunn & Dunn, 1997); MLU = Mean Length of Utterance (in morphemes); PAT = Phonological Awareness Test (Bird et al., 1995); Letters = number of letters named; TOWRE = Test of Word Reading Efficiency (Torgesen et al., 1999); TOWREsw = sight word reading subtest; TOWREnw = nonword reading, that is, phonetic decoding subtest; SS = standard score where mean is 100 and standard deviation is 15; X indicates unintelligible word in the free speech sample.

Although it has been suggested that children with phonological delays are fundamentally different from children with phonological disorders, the research evidence has failed to confirm this hypothesis. For example, as reviewed in Chapter 7, a positive family history for speech-language disorder and difficulties with phonological awareness are characteristic of both the delayed and disordered subtypes. The frequency of atypical segment and syllable structure errors in children's speech reflects the age of the child and the severity of the child's speech deficit rather than fundamental differences in the cause or nature of the child's speech deficit (e.g., see Figure 7–1). This conclusion is reinforced by the similar profile of poor speech perception, phonological awareness skills, and nonword reading skills observed in Case Studies 8–1, 8–2, and 8–4. At the preschool observation interval, it would be our recommendation that all three children be referred for intervention on the basis of standardized test scores below the 10th percentile, making no distinction between the delay profiles illustrated in Case Studies 8–1 and 8–2 versus the disorder profile illustrated in Case Study 8–4. This does not mean that these children will respond equally well to the same approach to intervention. The issue of appropriate intervention approaches for children with these different error profiles is addressed in Chapters 9 through 11.

The hypothesis that children with phonological delays are fundamentally different from children whose error profile suggests a phonological disorder has not been empirically confirmed.

ICF Approach

A third approach privileges or at least takes into account the impact of the child's DPD on participation in everyday activities, those that are socially expected for the child as well as those that are personally valued by the child or the child's family, when deciding whether to provide an intervention. The importance of this perspective is highlighted by the finding that parental expectations for their preschooler's outcomes as a result of speech therapy reflect concerns about socialization and behavior in home, preschool, and community environments (Thomas-Stonell, Oddson, Robertson, & Rosenbaum, 2009). An extensive review of this topic will not be reproduced here as McCormack, McLeod, McAllister, and Harrison (2009) have published an excellent systematic review of the literature demonstrating restrictions on participation associated with speech delay across a broad range of ICF Activities and Participation Domains. Their review identified potential participation restrictions in domains related to: (1) learning and applying knowledge (reading, writing, calculating, thinking/attending, and speaking); (2) communication (writing messages and engaging in conversation); (3) mobility; (4) self-care; (5) interpersonal interactions and relationships; and (6) major life areas (e.g., educational and vocational outcomes). The likelihood that there will be participation restrictions in any of these domains depends on complex interactions between the nature of the speech impairment, the temperament, personality, and life goals of the child, the presence of

A third approach takes into account the impact of the child's DPD on participation in everyday activities using the **ICF-CY framework** as a guide.

Research shows that parental expectations for their preschooler's outcomes as a result of speech therapy reflect concerns about socialization and behavior in home, preschool, and community environments.

Speech impairments are associated with restrictions on participation across a broad range of **ICF Activities and Participation Domains**.

other impairments such as language disability or developmental coordination disorder, and environmental factors such as the attitudes and skills of teachers, parents, and peers. In other words, the presence of participation restrictions is not a linear function of the severity of the child's speech deficit but must be determined via direct assessment of these factors, using tools described in Chapter 5 (e.g., FOCUS; Thomas-Stonell, Oddson, Robertson, & Rosenbaum, 2009). Sometimes service providers who are specifically mandated to provide services based on participation considerations will use criteria that exclude children at high risk for participation restrictions in academic and social domains. For example, legislation in the United States mandates the provision of services for children with DPD if the impairment interferes with academic performance although social factors may also be considered in some school districts (Bernthal & Bankson, 2004). The qualifying criteria published for Florida (Puranik et al., 2008) that require the presence of a phonological disorder or a significant delay based on phoneme specific norms are presumably designed to ensure compliance with this mandate. However, as we have shown, application of the criteria will result in the exclusion of children who have significant risk factors for dyslexia. Even mild residual speech errors can have an impact on peer attitudes (Hall, 1991; Silverman, 1992); the possibility of significant psychosocial and academic sequelae cannot be predicted from standardized test scores alone. As discussed in detail in Chapter 5, the presence of participation restrictions must be explored directly for each child and given prominence in any decision to treat the child. By this view, the children described in Case Studies 8–1 and 8–2 might be recommended for services that serve to prevent reading or spelling disability even though their GFTA scores are borderline normal. Case Study 8–2 is an interesting case in this regard because his GFTA score at the kindergarten assessment is well within the average range but his PCC is below normal limits reflecting a high frequency of inconsistent omission and distortion errors in connected speech that did not occur during the single word naming test. These errors impacted his intelligibility and may have led to participation restrictions warranting treatment despite age-appropriate standardized test scores and apparent mastery of the phonemes that are expected given his age. Treatment of these children's residual speech errors would be justified if they were self-conscious about these misarticulations, they experienced negative reactions from peers, or the errors hindered their participation in desired activities.

The presence of **participation restrictions** is not a linear function of the severity of the child's speech deficit and therefore must be determined via direct assessment with appropriate measurement tools.

Even mild residual speech errors impact on **peer attitudes** and the possibility of significant psychosocial and academic sequelae cannot be predicted from standardized test scores alone.

Recommended Protocol for Deciding When to Treat

The **decision flow chart** begins with an intake assessment that includes a standardized assessment of the child's articulation accuracy.

In the spirit of the discussion thus far we have developed a flow chart to guide you through the decision making process that incorporates elements of these three perspectives. As shown in Figure 8–1,

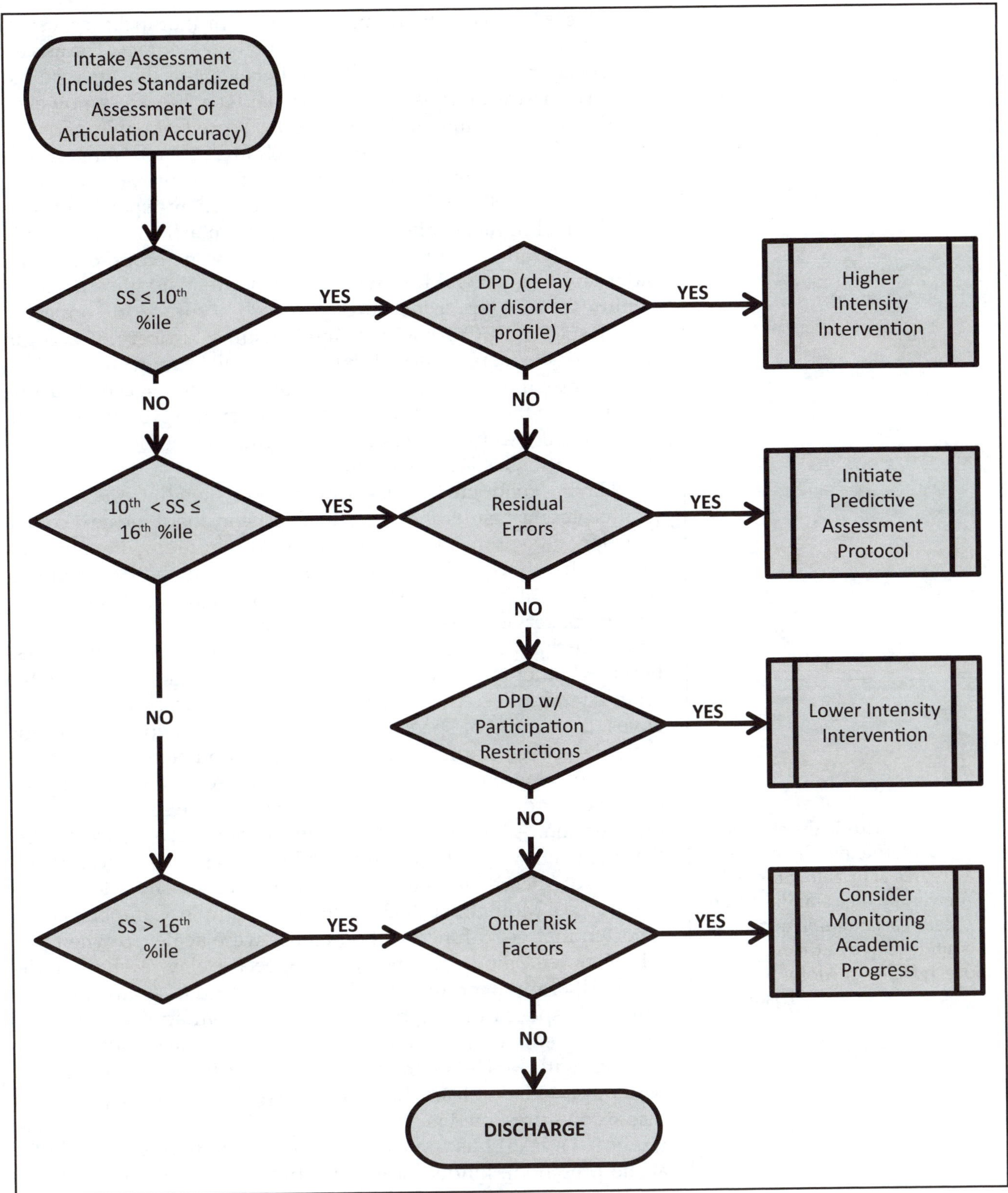

Figure 8–1. *Flow chart to facilitate treatment recommendations. SS = standard score (on a standardized measure of articulation accuracy); DPD = developmental phonological disorder. Predictive assessment protocol described in text and in Smit et al. (1990). See text for application guidelines with case examples.*

the process begins with an intake assessment that includes a standardized assessment of the child's articulation accuracy. The assessment, of course, must include all the other elements that are required in such an assessment, as outlined in Chapter 5. We stress, however, that the clinician must derive a standard score from at least one of the assessment tools that reflects the child's articulation accuracy relative to an appropriate normative reference group. It is essential not to omit this step in favor of relying on phoneme specific normative charts. For most children, a citation form articulation test will be perfectly adequate for this purpose. In some cases, especially older children, or children who demonstrate a significant intelligibility-speech gap, a measure of speech accuracy in connected speech such as PCC in conversation (Austin & Shriberg, 1997) or in sentences (Johnson, Weston, & Bain, 2004) will be more appropriate. In any case, the child's performance in connected speech must be compared to the appropriate normative reference group in order to determine if the child scores below the 10th percentile or 1.25 standard deviations below the mean.

Having conducted the assessment and scored the tests, it is time to interpret the results and arrive at a decision about the next course of action. Our protocol is focused on those children where the primary difficulty is in the area of phonology. Many of these children have concomitant disorders in the area of language; the child may qualify for service based on language test performance alone—this possibility has not been incorporated into Figure 8–1. The first question is whether the child has scored at or below the 10th percentile on the standardized measure of articulation accuracy. If the answer is yes, the profile of speech errors must be scanned to determine if child's speech errors are primarily distortion errors, placing the child in the Speech Error category. With the exception of these cases of Speech Errors, we recommend that the child be scheduled for an intervention. As discussed further in the next section, we predict that the need will be for a relatively high intensity intervention in the case of Speech Delay and an even higher intensity intervention in the case a Motor Speech Disorder. For example, Campbell (1999) reported that good functional outcomes were achieved when preschoolers with moderate and severe Speech Delay received twice-weekly therapy over a 90- to 120-day period (i.e., on average the children's speech intelligibility improved from approximately 50 to 75 % intelligible). On the other hand, equivalent outcomes in children with MSD-AOS required treatment for a 360- to 420-day period, provided at least three times a week. Considering the four case studies presented in this chapter, PA211 as a preschooler (Case Study 8–1), PA514 as a preschooler (Case Study 8–2), and PA221 at the preschool, kindergarten, and first grade time points (Case Study 8–4) were all eligible for a high intensity intervention.

Schedule the child for intervention if he or she scores at or below the 10th percentile on a standardized test of articulation accuracy and receives a diagnosis of Speech Delay or Motor Speech Disorder.

Another possibility is that a child scoring below the 10th percentile on a standardized measure of articulation accuracy presents primarily with residual distortion errors. For children in the Speech

Error category, it is recommended that the predictive assessment protocol be initiated (Smit et al., 1990), as described earlier in this chapter. The protocol ensures that these errors are less likely to be treated before the child is mature enough to achieve success or in cases where the child is capable of self-correction. On the other hand, the protocol recommends that these errors be targeted even before the age of 9 when it appears that the child is not likely to self-correct especially in cases where atypical errors are produced (in fact, atypical errors should be targeted prior to the age of 7). The predictive assessment protocol is also initiated when the child in the Speech Error category scores between the 10th and 16th percentile on a standardized test of articulation accuracy. Although Smit et al.'s predictive assessment protocol was directed specifically at sibilant distortions, /ɹ/-distortions are also vulnerable to a protracted and uncertain trajectory toward normalization. The risk of long-term normalization for children with /ɹ/-distortions may be especially high for those with slow diadochokinetic or alternate motion rates. Therefore, children such as PA211 at the first grade assessment (Case Study 8–1) would benefit from further monitoring and possible remediation of /ɹ/ misarticulations, especially given the lack of progress on this phoneme in the preceding three years (although note that this child qualifies for continued monitoring of his progress due to the presence of additional risk factors as discussed below).

For children in the Speech Error category, it is recommended that the predictive assessment protocol be initiated.

Atypical errors should be treated prior to the age of 7 years.

Other children scoring between the 10th and 16th percentile on a standardized measure of articulation accuracy, may present with mild Speech Delay rather than Speech Errors. In these cases, the SLP should consider whether there are participation restrictions that warrant providing a low intensity intervention that will facilitate participation in the relevant activities of daily life. Such interventions might include a short-term intensive intervention targeting specific needs, a home program, advice to the classroom teacher, or the services of a communication disorders assistant or integration aide to help ease the child's participation in difficult classroom situations or desired extracurricular activities. These kinds of interventions may be especially important for those children who have mild DPD with signs of motor involvement such as slow diadochokinetic and/or alternate motion rates, poor nonword repetition skills, low tongue strength, or evidence of poor somatosensory feedback. We recognize that many publically funded agencies may not be mandated to provide services to children who present with mild but persistent articulation impairments, especially if there is no concomitant language or literacy disorder. Nonetheless, children with "speech only" impairments are at risk for anxiety disorders and participation restrictions. In those cases where the agency mandate is based on the ICF perspective, these secondary impacts should be the primary concern and thus treatment could be recommended when these are objectively documented even if the DPD itself is mild. Furthermore, there would be no ethical reason for private practitioners

If the child presents with mild Speech Delay and participation restrictions, consider providing a low intensity intervention that will facilitate participation in the relevant activities of daily life.

to not provide services to such children scoring between the 10th and 16th percentile on standardized tests of articulation accuracy.

When risk factors associated with poor academic or psychosocial outcomes are present in a child who scores above the 10th percentile on a standardized measure of articulation accuracy, consider monitoring the child's progress.

A final reason for recommending a service is the presence of other risk factors (Olswang, Rodriguez, & Timler, 1998). Some children scoring above the 10th percentile, and in rare cases even above the 16th percentile, may raise concern due to the presence of risk factors associated with poor academic or psychosocial outcomes. Such factors include prior treatment for speech and language difficulties (especially language impairment), a family history of speech, language or reading disability, or a current history of the dyslexia profile that we described above. PA211 and PA514 at the kindergarten and first grade assessments (Case Studies 8–1 and 8–2) meet these criteria. When these additional risk factors co-occur with mild DPD or normalized speech proficiency, the SLP should consider monitoring the child's progress over time and implementing preventative interventions when necessary. Such monitoring may involve a formal schedule of periodic reassessment; alternatively, parents and teachers may be alerted to the potential risks for academic and psychosocial problems in the future and counseled to refer the child for additional services should the child appear to be struggling at school.

Finally, children who score above the 16th percentile and who do not have any concomitant risk factors or developmental disorders would be discharged as not requiring further service. APA005 (Case Study 8–3) meets this criterion. Although this child had distortion errors at every assessment, the frequency and consistency of the errors never resulted in the child receiving a GFTA score or PCC in conversation that was below normal limits. The only reason that this child was assessed repeatedly is that he was recruited into the control group of a longitudinal follow-up study. The repeated monitoring enabled us to confirm a normal trajectory with steady improvements in the production of the sibilants and clusters throughout the 3-year period of the study.

Service Delivery Options

8.2.1. Describe the required components of a service delivery model.

8.2.2. Explain why it is recommended that children with DPD receive a minimum of 12 to 20 hours of treatment in a given service year.

8.2.3. Imagine that two children with similar severity and profile of speech delay receive the same number of treatment sessions in a given school year (i.e., dose frequency is equal) but achieve very different outcomes.

Name and define at least three factors that might account for the variability in the outcomes.

8.2.4. Describe the conditions under which group therapy and parent administered therapy can be as effective as therapy provided by the SLP to a single child.

8.2.5. Apply the recommendations and research findings regarding service delivery models to Case Studies 8–1, 8–2, and 8–4 (prekindergarten assessment).

Cirrin et al. (2010) explain that a "service delivery model can be conceptualized as an organized configuration of resources aimed at achieving a particular educational [or therapeutic] goal. It must address questions of where service is to be delivered, by whom, and in what dosage" (p. 234). The case studies presented thus far, along with the decision flow chart shown in Figure 8–1, suggest that the service delivery model for a given child should be designed to vary treatment intensity as a function of the severity and nature of the child's speech deficit and the rate of the child's progress in speech therapy. Ideally, decisions about the appropriate service delivery model would be made dynamically over time in relation to the child's needs, and, consequently, issues related to the way in which intensity can be manipulated are discussed in later parts of this chapter (in relation to the selection of goals and goal attack strategies) and in later chapters of this book (in relation to the selection of treatment approaches and procedures). However, assignment of children to service delivery models are often made for administrative purposes and therefore we discuss some of the broader issues related to caseload management prior to turning to case-level decision making.

The **service delivery model** specifies who will deliver the intervention, where, and with what dosage to achieve the desired therapeutic goal for a given child.

Although the maximum recommended caseload size for a SLP is 40 individuals, school surveys indicate that the average is 25% higher and some caseloads are double the recommended maximum. Furthermore, the needs of the children on school caseloads have become more complex with a significant increase in the proportion of cases with severe secondary speech and language impairments in recent decades. Despite this increase in complex cases, the proportion of caseloads presenting with primary DPD in public health and school settings remains predominant (Broomfield & Dodd, 2004; Dowden et al., 2006; Joffe & Pring, 2008; Schooling, 2003). Clinicians and service providers respond to the resultant workload pressures with a variety of strategies that include: (1) rationing service to each child by providing standardized blocks of treatment of a predefined duration and intensity, (2) providing intervention to children in groups, and (3) providing the treatment through other agents, either parents or communication disorders assistants (CDAs). We attempt to derive some general principles about the conditions under which these practices are effective from the literature in the paragraphs

The maximum recommended **caseload size** for a SLP is 40 individuals.

In public health and school settings, a high proportion of the SLP caseload is composed of children with DPD.

to follow. We have in mind those children who score at or below the 10th percentile on a standardized measure of articulation accuracy and thus require a higher intensity service. This is a hazardous exercise because the efficacy of a given intervention can only be determined for a specific type of client receiving a specific type of intervention given with a specific intensity by a specific provider. Studies that have attempted to determine which service delivery models are effective or the conditions under which speech therapy can be effective have involved highly heterogeneous samples and undescribed treatments. As Pring (2004) pointed out, when you "ask a silly question" it is very difficult to get a helpful answer but we do our best to provide guidance with the evidence that is available.

How Much Intervention Is Enough?

The general rule about the **amount of intervention** to provide is that more is better but too much is a waste of resources.

The general rule about the amount of intervention to provide is that more is better but too much is a waste of resources. For example, Sommers et al. (1962) conducted a trial in which some children received weekly in-class "speech improvement work" for 16 weeks in first grade while others received the same intervention for 9 months. A third group received an additional 8 weeks of this intervention in second grade after having received it for 9 months in first grade. A control group received no intervention. The results revealed that greater improvements in articulation accuracy accrued to the group that received 9 months of intervention compared to 16 weeks in first grade but that there was no benefit to receiving an additional 8 weeks in second grade. The results suggested that the second grade plateau reflected two phenomena: children who had achieved age appropriate speech and did not need further intervention and children who required a different type or intensity of intervention to make further gains.

Sommers et al. do not provide an indication of how much intervention is required to achieve a reasonable outcome especially since the specific intervention provided (to be discussed further in Chapter 9) is not one that is currently in use. Jacoby, Levin, Lee, Creaghead, and Kummer (2002) reported information about the average amount of intervention that is associated with functional gains in communication skills, using the ASHA National Outcome Measurement System (NOMS) which includes a functional communication measure (FCM) for articulation that roughly reflects intelligibility of speech as rated by the child's SLP. The patients in the study were preschool-age children (3 to 6 years) receiving therapy for primary speech and language impairment in a pediatric hospital. Outcomes were expressed in terms of the number of levels of functional gain on the ASHA NOMS FCMs, with a change of 2 or more levels considered to be a reasonable amount of progress. For example, if a child began therapy with speech that was unintelligible to familiar listeners and progressed to producing speech that was occasionally intelligible to familiar listeners, this would represent 2 levels of improvement on the FCM. Amount of intervention duration was coded as the number of 15-minute units of intervention provided between the assignment of FCMs. FCM assessments occurred at intake, regularly schedule progress reports, and discharge. Three general conclusions were drawn from their data. First, it appeared that children who began therapy with more severe deficits (i.e., lower FCMs) required more units of therapy to achieve a functional gain but the trend was not statistically significant (this may be because the relationship is not linear: other researchers have found that children with moderate delays make the most progress in FCMs in a given amount of time relative to children with mild or severe delays; e.g., Thomas-Stonell, McConney-Ellis, Oddson, Robertson, & Rosenbaum, 2007). Second, younger children made a functional gain with fewer units of intervention than older children. Third, the amount of improvement observed was significantly correlated with the amount of service received. Specifically, an improvement of more than 2 levels on the FCM for articulation/phonology required receipt of at least 20 hours of therapy. The nationwide ASHA NOMS project also found a correlation between the number of levels of improvement observed and the amount of intervention received (Schooling, 2003). For preschoolers, the number of hours of service associated with no change, 1 level and 2 or more levels of change on the articulation FCM was approximately 11, 15, and 21 hours (American Speech-Language and Hearing Association, 2009b).

In general, children who begin therapy with more severe deficits require more units of therapy to achieve a functional gain, although this relationship is not strictly linear.

On average, younger children make a functional gain with fewer units of intervention than older children.

Amount of improvement observed was significantly correlated with the amount of service received.

The conclusion that 20 or more hours of treatment is required to obtain a clinically significant functional outcome is a "rule of thumb" that is highly dependent on interactions between the child, the family, the clinician, and the treatment program. We have shown one example of a child who failed to make a clinically significant improvement after 3 years even though the child was accessing a mix of public and private services throughout that time (see Case Study 8–4). We show other examples in later parts of this book of children achieving remarkable outcomes with less than 20 hours of intervention. It is difficult to say in advance, for any child, how long the intervention must be in order to achieve the desired goals. It is possible to predict on the basis of the ASHA NOMS project, however, that interventions lasting less than 10 hours are highly unlikely to effect a measurable change in speech intelligibility.

The conclusion that 20 or more hours of treatment is required to obtain a clinically significant functional outcome is a "rule of thumb" that is highly dependent on interactions between the child, the family, the clinician, and the treatment program.

Interventions lasting less than 10 hours are highly unlikely to effect a measurable change in speech intelligibility.

What happens when services are rationed to insufficient amounts of treatment? Glogowska, Roulstone, Enderby, and Peters (2000) randomly assigned preschoolers who were eligible to receive treatment for primary speech and/or language delay from community clinics in the U.K. to the treatment condition or a "watchful waiting" control condition. Outcomes were assessed after one year. During that time, the children in the treatment group received an average of 6 hours of intervention in 8 contacts that occurred approximately once per month. Measures of improvement in expressive language skills and phonology error rate revealed no significant differences between the two groups and 70% of all children continued to present with substantial deficits in these areas at the end of the trial. Follow-up assessments conducted when these children were 7 to 10 years of age revealed that one-third of the sample had ongoing language, literacy, and social difficulties at school (Glogowska, Roulstone, Peters, & Enderby, 2006).

Parents and clinicians often report that the child benefited from brief interventions even when the reported effects on communication and participation are not large enough to be detected by standardized tests or functional communication measures.

How is it that rationing of service to such brief amounts is routine in some jurisdictions when there is high quality evidence that 6 hours of intervention provides no more benefit than "watchful waiting"? One reason is that parents and clinicians overwhelmingly report that the child benefited from these brief interventions even though the reported effects on communication and participation are not large enough to be detected by standardized tests or functional communication measures (Thomas-Stonell et al., 2007). We have no doubt that parents and children derive tangible benefits from their interactions with SLPs but there is no evidence that these brief interventions, especially when they do not significantly reduce the severity of the child's impairment, serve to reduce the risk of academic failure and psychosocial sequelae that were reported in Chapter 7 for children who begin school with speech and language deficits. On the contrary, Glogowska et al. (2006) suggest that the risks remain substantial for children who receive insufficient treatment as preschoolers. Therefore, we conclude that there is no empirical justification for routine rationing of service to 10 or fewer hours of treatment in a one-year period. If the service provider prefers to organize service around standardized blocks of treatment to which each patient is entitled, the block should provide a minimum of 12 to 20 hours of service.

Intensity of the Treatment Schedule

Although the number of hours of treatment provided is one aspect of intensity, the way in which those hours are distributed over time is another variable that may impact on treatment outcomes. For example, in the randomized control trial conducted by Glogowska et al. (2000) in the United Kingdom, the children received 6 hours of intervention in approximately 8 monthly sessions. In the descriptive study reported by Thomas-Stonell et al. (2007) in Canada, children received approximately 8 weekly sessions. Very few studies have systematically explored the impact of varying treatment intensity on outcomes although there is some reason to believe that short periods of frequent treatment might be more effective than long periods of infrequent sessions (Allen, 2009; Barratt, Littlejohns, & Thompson, 1992).

Short periods of frequent treatment might be more effective than long periods of infrequent sessions.

Warren, Fey, and Yoder (2007) defined a number of variables that impact on treatment intensity and recommended that researchers focus attention on these issues when designing and testing interventions. These variables are listed in Table 8–1. Notice that

Table 8–1. *Variables That Impact on Treatment Intensity*

Variable	*Definition*
Treatment intensity	Quality and quantity of service provided in a given period of time
Dose	Number of properly implemented teaching episodes per session
Dose form	Task or activity within which the teaching episodes are delivered
Dose frequency	Number of sessions per unit of time (e.g., day/week/month)
Total intervention duration	Time period over which the intervention is provided (e.g., 5 days or 12 weeks or 9 months)
Cumulative intervention intensity	Dose × Dose Frequency × Total Intervention Duration

cumulative intervention intensity is not just the number of sessions provided (dose frequency) over a given period of time (total intervention duration)—a third variable, specifically, the number of teaching episodes per session (dose), is also entered into the equation. In our lab, we have found that speech-language pathology students increase session time devoted to direct teaching from one-third to one-half during the course of a 6-week phonology practicum (the remainder of the session is taken up by manipulation of therapy materials, documentation, off-task conversation with the child, and on- and off-task conversation with the parent). We presume that this increase in clinician efficiency will lead to greater effectiveness of the intervention but further research is required to determine optimum treatment intensity. At this time, it seems reasonable to assume that treatment intensity is an integral part of any treatment approach. In other words, in order to expect the same results that have been reported for any treatment that has been described in the research literature, it is necessary to provide it to similar patients at the same dose and dose frequency and for the same total duration. Furthermore, optimum dose and dose frequency can be expected to vary with the treatment goal and phase of the child's treatment program. Therefore, further discussion of these issues is reserved for later parts of this book where we discuss specific treatment approaches and procedures.

Cumulative intervention intensity is the number of sessions provided (*dose frequency*) over a given period of time (*total intervention duration*) times the number of teaching episodes per session (*dose*).

Group Therapy

Group therapy can have advantages and disadvantages. A potential advantage is that the presence of a group of peers provides authentic opportunities for communication and may facilitate carryover from the clinic to extra-clinic environments. For this reason, certain approaches to therapy (communication-based approaches)

In **group therapy**, the presence of peers provides authentic opportunities for communication and may facilitate carryover from the clinic to extra-clinic environments.

A group may reduce the active dose of therapy per unit of time for each child in the group relative to individual therapy.

require that the treatment be conducted in a group context (Creaghead, Newman, & Secord, 1989). On the other hand, a group may reduce the active dose of therapy per unit of time for each child in the group relative to individual therapy; therefore, if the child's needs or the effectiveness of the treatment approach that is being implemented require a high number of teaching episodes per session, group therapy may be a poor choice of service delivery model. Frequently, group therapy is implemented in response to caseload pressures and thus the extent to which this treatment model meets the child's particular needs may be accidental rather than planned (Dowden et al., 2006).

One particularly well-designed large sample randomized control trial of individual versus group therapy is often cited as an indication that group therapy is effective (Sommers et al., 1966). In the group therapy condition, children were treated in groups of 3 to 6 children who shared similar age, severity of impairment, and phase of treatment. A traditional approach to therapy was employed (described in Chapters 9 and 10) and games were kept to a minimum which presumably served to maintain dose and response frequency at high levels in both treatment conditions. Improvements were significantly greater for students with moderate impairment versus mild impairment but there were no differences as a function of service delivery model or grade level of the students. Furthermore, there was no interaction between severity of the child's speech deficit and the service delivery model. One very important methodological detail is typically omitted from reports of this study, however: individual sessions were 30 minutes long whereas group sessions were 45 minutes in duration. Therefore, an effort was made to narrow the gap in dose (and thus cumulative treatment intensity) by varying session duration between the two conditions. The authors felt that the most salient difference between the two modes of therapy was the interaction among the children. They point out that children with severe deficits were excluded from the study.

The finding from Sommers et al. (1966) that group therapy was as effective as individual therapy can be contrasted with data from the ASHA NOMS project that revealed a striking disadvantage to group therapy relative to individual therapy for preschoolers when the outcome was the articulation FCM (American Speech-Language-Hearing Association, 2009a). There are many differences between the studies including the superior validity of the research design in Sommers et al. and the age of the children. However, we think that the most likely explanation for the disparate findings is that SLPs in typical practice do not increase session length when implementing group therapy given that group therapy is used as a means of coping with excessively large caseloads. In fact, the ASHA NOMS data suggest that children receiving group therapy require more hours of therapy to obtain the same functional gain. Therefore, the important message to be drawn from these studies is that group therapy can be effective as long as dose per child is maintained at sufficiently high

Group therapy can be effective as long as dose per child is maintained at sufficiently high levels.

levels. The bottom line is that treatment outcomes are determined in large part by cumulative treatment intensity. Group therapy is more efficient only if it provides the same cumulative treatment intensity to each child as individual therapy for the same per session cost in SLP time and effort.

Parents as Intervention Agents

Involving parents in the rehabilitation program is one way to increase dose frequency and thus, if parents are effective in their role as therapists, they may serve to increase cumulative treatment intensity for a given amount of SLP input. A small number of excellent quality randomized control trials have investigated the effectiveness of parents as therapists in programs in which parents were trained as substitutes for SLP-provided intervention (Eiserman, Weber, & McCoun, 1992, 1995) and in programs in which parents were trained to act as adjuncts to SLP-provided intervention (Sommers, 1962; Sommers et al., 1964; Tufts & Holliday, 1959). In all of these studies the comparison condition was small group therapy provided directly to the children by a SLP. The time requirement for the SLP in the parent program varied from 50% to 100% of the time requirement to provide direct intervention to the children. In all studies, the interventions were relatively intensive in both the parent programs and the SLP provided interventions. Furthermore, the training provided to the parents was highly structured and standardized in all of these studies. The goal of the parent programs was to increase cumulative treatment intensity and to enhance parent involvement and satisfaction (as most parents prefer to be centrally involved in their child's treatment) rather than to reduce SLP input per child. Under these conditions parents were found to be effective intervention agents: when used as substitutes for SLP provided service, parents can be as effective as treatment provided directly to children by the SLP; when used as adjuncts to the SLP provided service, parents can significantly enhance the effectiveness of speech therapy. Two of these studies are described in more detail.

If parents are effective in their role as therapists, they may serve to increase cumulative treatment intensity for a given amount of SLP input when provided with a **structured home program**.

Eiserman et al. (1992) provided intervention to 40 3- and 4-year-old children with primary speech-language delay (specifically, moderately delayed phonological skills and mildly delayed expressive syntax abilities) and followed them over a 3-year period. Families were randomly assigned to receive direct intervention provided to groups of 2 children in the clinic on a weekly basis or to receive parent training provided in the home on a twice-monthly basis. The intervention programs in both conditions were described as including phonetic and phonological approaches to the remediation of the child's speech deficit with attention to language skills and other areas of development included as needed. The parent training component included specific training in the implementation of therapy techniques and data keeping. The training procedures included demonstrations and practice until the mother demonstrated mastery of the techniques targeted during the sessions. Mothers were also provided with materials to facilitate completion of home therapy activities. Mothers were encouraged to complete the activities daily or at least 4 times per week with their child. The intervention was provided for 7 months in each year until the child no longer met criteria to receive service. The numbers of children receiving service in each year by group was 20, 7, and 0 in the direct therapy (clinic based) group and 20, 5, and 0 in the parent therapy (home based) group. At the end of the second year, the two groups had improved their GFTA scores from the 4th to the 30th and 41st percentile for the clinic and home based conditions, respectively (the between group difference in year 2 was not statistically significant). Improvements in morphosyntax also showed a numerical advantage to the home-based intervention that was not statistically significant. At the end of the third year the two groups were similar on all measures (Eiserman et al., 1995).

Sommers (1962) examined the effect of training mothers to augment the impact of direct therapy provided to individuals or small groups of children aged 7 or 8 years of age with higher or lower intelligence quotients. Again, the mothers received very specific training in the implementation of speech therapy techniques, in sessions that occurred coincident with their child's speech therapy session and that included lectures, demonstrations, and observation of speech therapy provided by the SLP to their child. Parents who did not receive this training were offered the opportunity for brief interactions with SLPs after their child's session during which they could ask questions about their child's progress and receive homework assignments. The children in the study were randomly selected for participation and randomly assigned to conditions. Individual therapy was provided in 30-minute sessions once a day for 4 weeks. Group therapy was provided in 50-minute sessions to groups of approximately 4 children once a day for 4 weeks. The children in the study presented with "functional articulation disorders" and normal hearing and peripheral oral mechanism. However, half the group demonstrated average intelligence while the remainder achieved low-average I.Q. scores. The outcome measure was change in McDonald Deep Test scores for the production of 10 commonly misarticulated consonants from the pre- to the posttest assessment. These results are presented in Figure 8–2. It can be seen that for children with average intelligence, group and individual therapy was equally effective but training of the mothers enhanced the impact of the intervention considerably. For children with lower intelligence, the most effective condition was individual therapy augmented by support from mothers trained in speech therapy techniques. One interesting finding in this study was that mothers improved their own speech perception skills as a result of involvement in the parent training program and that there was a significant

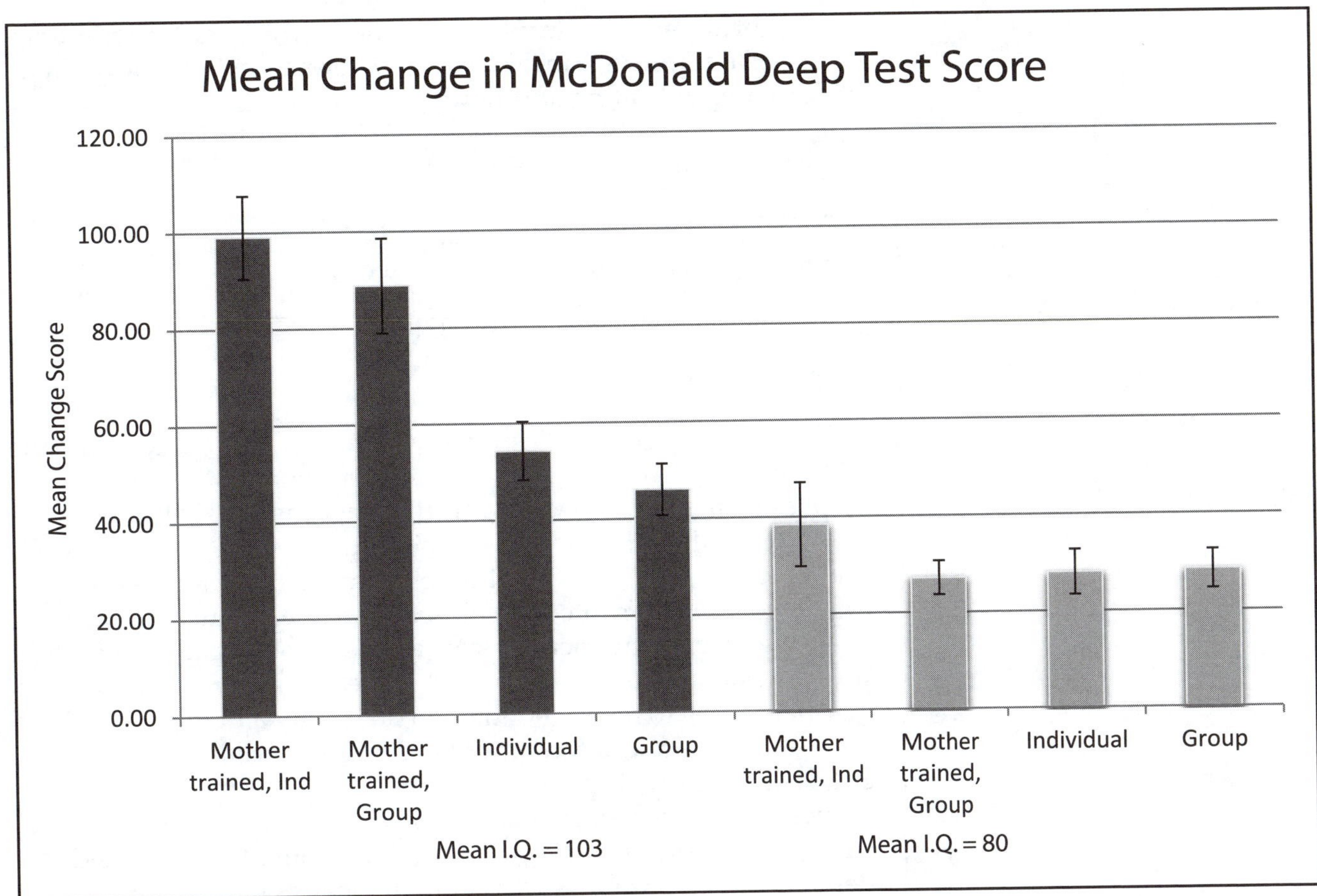

Figure 8–2. *Mean change in McDonald Deep Test Score after 20 speech therapy sessions as a function of service delivery model (group or individual therapy with or without a home program component in which mothers were trained to carry out the intervention at home). Ten children aged 7 or 8 years, with higher or lower intelligence quotients, were treated in each condition. Adapted from Sommers (1962), Table 2, p. 183. Factors in the effectiveness of mothers trained to aid in speech correction.* Journal of Speech and Hearing Disorders, 27, *Table 2, p. 183. Used with permission of the American Speech-Hearing-Language Association.*

correlation between maternal speech perception skills (posttreatment) and child outcomes.

What happens when parents are provided with home practice activities but are not trained in speech therapy techniques? Gardner's (2005) qualitative study of home practice interactions provides a picture of the confusion that can arise when the goal of "speech homework" is imperfectly apprehended by parent and child. The following short extract was selected for its brevity; the reader is referred to the original paper for longer examples that reveal a delightful earnestness on the part of parents and children in their approach to these exercises but a frightening lack of thought on the part of the SLPs who provided the stimuli and instructions! In this example, the goal of the activity was to practice the phone [z] in the context of the plural morpheme in the word "cars." The interaction selected from Gardner (2005, p. 63) proceeded as follows (with underscores indicating additional emphasis):

Child: [t^{h}ɑdz]

Mother: it's not tars it's cars, cars

Child: [t^{h}ɑz]

Mother: yes, but you're still saying [t^h], [k^h], its [k^{h}ɑzːd]

Child: tars:

The interaction is not especially helpful in terms of teaching the child the target because many aspects of the mother's input place emphasis on another phoneme ([k]) rather than the [z] that is supposed to be the target of the exercise; furthermore, the child does not receive a positive evaluation or reinforcement for correct production of the SLP's intended target phoneme. In our own research clinic we observe interactions such as this among children and their preprofessional student SLPs. Specific teaching is required to help clinicians learn to focus attention on one target and to provide both helpful models and informative feedback for children's responses. SLPs need to provide parents with specific instruction in these techniques before expecting them to carry them out at home. Gardner (2006) describes a pilot project for training parents, CDAs, and student SLPs to have more successful interactions with children in the context of speech therapy sessions.

Summary and Recommendations

Cumulative intervention intensity is a primary determinant of treatment outcomes.

This brief review reveals that cumulative intervention intensity is a primary determinant of treatment outcomes. It appears that 12 to 20 hours of intervention are required to effect a functional improvement in speech outcomes for the majority of children although there is considerable individual variability in the amount of treatment that is required to achieve program goals. Although the evidence is weak on this point, it is probable that short periods of intense intervention are more effective than scheduling infrequent sessions over a long period of time. When clinicians are unable to provide intervention on a frequent basis, parents can be taught to be effective treatment agents, and they are usually well positioned to increase dose frequency. Appropriately trained CDAs may also be effective although this has not been established for the remediation of speech errors. In fact, the only well-designed study to demonstrate CDA effectiveness specifically targeted vocabulary and excluded articulation therapy as being too specialized for CDAs to implement (Boyle, McCartney, Forbes, & O'Hare, 2007). Paraprofessionals, early childhood educators, and teachers have also been shown to be effective in the delivery of phonological awareness interventions (Ehri et al., 2001).

One way to put this information into practice might be to design a standardized intervention program that is likely to be beneficial to the average child while being feasible given your resources and total caseload size. We have had good success with such a model in our research clinic for 4- to 5-year-old children with moderate phonological disorders (Rvachew & Brosseau-Lapré, 2010). All children receive 12 weeks of intervention structured to provide 6 hours of individual therapy targeting remediation of speech errors and 6 hours of small group intervention targeting phonological awareness. Parents observe the individual sessions and then receive a 6-hour structured intervention designed to teach them to continue providing input at home for an additional 9 months. We have found that the success of this program is dependent on the exact nature of the treatment approach that is used as discussed further in Chapter 9.

Blakeley and Brockman (1995) describe an alternative approach, direct program management, implemented for children with craniofacial disorders. The implementation of this service delivery model resulted in a 93% success rate, defined as normalized speech, language, resonance, and hearing function by school age, even though a literature review revealed that the historical success rate with this population was approximately 50%. Although their project concerns a specific type of secondary phonological disorder, the basic principles that underlie this model are equally applicable for caseloads of children with primary phonological disorders. An important aspect of the model is the refocusing of program goals on the desired outcome (90% of children achieving normalization prior to school entry) rather than on process (providing most of the children with a standardized level of service). The key operational requirement was frequent monitoring of the child's progress starting at an early age. At each assessment, the parents were taught to provide appropriate interventions at home and the child's response to prior interventions was documented. If the child was not progressing at a rate that would ensure achievement of the goal, resources were mobilized to increase the intensity and/or change the configuration of the interventions as needed. Clinic staff worked to reduce barriers that prohibited the family's access to needed services and consulted with community clinicians to enhance their effectiveness. They provided direct treatment to children only when necessary to ensure the child's progress toward the goal of normalized function at school entry. The services received by each child varied greatly with approximately a third receiving no direct speech therapy, a third receiving speech therapy in the community, and a third receiving speech therapy from the craniofacial team. Dose frequency varied widely as did total intervention duration (ranging from 16 to 180 weeks of therapy). The provision of services by other professionals was also highly individualized, pointing to another key feature of this approach. In this project, the SLPs worked as part

Total program management is a service delivery model that focuses on achievement of the desired outcome for each child rather than on process goals for the clinic.

of an interprofessional team that collaborated with other human resources within the child's family and community to achieve the best possible outcome for each child. This is a very different view of the SLP role than that painted by Dowden et al. (2006) in which school SLPs struggled in isolation to provide services to their caseloads. The caveat is that collaborative approaches to service delivery work best when total caseload size is reasonable because collaboration exacerbates rather than alleviates the pressures of an overly large caseload (Katz, Maag, Fallon, Blenkarn, & Smith, 2010).

Response-to-Intervention (RTI) is a prevention model that features multiple tiers of interventions that are layered on children based on their individual needs.

Total program management shares elements with Response-to-Intervention (RTI), defined by Justice as "a prevention model that features multiple tiers of reading interventions that are layered on pupils based on their individual needs" (p. 285). The RTI model requires that SLPs work together with other school personnel to first ensure that the primary reading instruction environment is adequate. SLPs have an important role to play in this component as consultants and collaborators. The second component is the implementation of a program to identify those children who are not responding adequately to classroom-based instruction. Screening tools that are appropriate for young children were discussed in Chapter 5. The third component is the provision of supplementary instruction to small groups of children who require additional input to accelerate the children's progress. A variety of professionals and paraprofessionals may deliver these interventions but the SLP should be part of the team that determines the program goals, designs the instructional procedures, trains the interveners, and monitors the outcomes.

Two important elements of a successful service are frequent monitoring of a child's progress and effective teamwork to mobilize all possible resources to meet the child's needs in a dynamic fashion over time.

To sum up, the best service delivery model is obviously the configuration of resources that meets each child's individual needs. Providing an appropriate service is best achieved by focusing on the child's progress toward a well-defined goal and adjusting the provision of services as required to ensure that the child maintains a trajectory toward that goal. Two important elements of a successful service are frequent monitoring of a child's progress and effective teamwork to mobilize all possible resources to meet the child's needs in a dynamic fashion over time. Perhaps the most important element, however, is clear goal setting from the onset of the child's treatment program. We turn now to treatment planning at the level of the individual child.

Treatment Planning for the Individual Child

8.3.1. Define and distinguish basic, intermediate, and specific goals.

8.3.2. Define and distinguish vertical, horizontal, and cyclical goal attack strategies.

8.3.3. List six factors that should be considered when selecting treatment goals for a given child. Describe the conditions under which each of these factors predicts relatively rapid acquisition of a phoneme.

8.3.4. Compare the complexity approach to the traditional developmental approach to the selection of treatment goals with respect to underlying theory and hypothesized outcomes. Interpret Figures 8–4 and 8–5 to evaluate the actual outcomes when children receive treatment for the most complex targets first compared to the least complex targets first.

8.3.5. Given a sample of speech from a child with DPD, conduct a multilinear analysis, select three sets of intermediate and specific goals, and construct a treatment plan based on the principles shown in Table 8–4.

8.3.6. For the same child construct an alternate plan based on the goal ordering principles shown in Table 8–6.

8.3.7. For the same child, construct a progress monitoring plan.

Treatment planning requires detailed information about the child's phonological knowledge at multiple levels of representation, including an in-depth analysis of a representative sample of the child's speech as described in Chapters 5 and 6. Most of this section is devoted to the topic of goal selection including basic principles that guide the decision making process, a review of the research literature on this topic, a description of two published approaches to goal selection, and an example of recommended goals for a child whose sample was analyzed in depth in Chapter 6. The related topics of instructional objectives and discharge planning are also covered.

Goals and Goal Attack Strategies

An important aspect of treatment planning involves the selection of goals at three levels of specificity: basic goals, intermediate goals, and specific goals (Fey, 1992). For children with DPD, the basic goal is the achievement of intelligible speech. For children with residual speech errors, adultlike accuracy or social acceptability of the child's speech may be the basic goal. Preventing reading disability and other sequelae of the underlying phonological disorder might be goals of the treatment program as well. Building up and reorganizing the child's phonological knowledge at multiple levels of representation, necessary to the achievement intelligible and accurate speech at the surface level, are implicit basic level goals.

Intermediate goals are medium-term goals that have a superordinate hierarchical relationship to the specific goals of the treatment program. The nature of these goals and the way in which they

Treatment planning involves the **selection of goals** at three levels of specificity: *basic goals*, *intermediate goals*, and *specific goals*.

For children with DPD the **basic goal** is the achievement of intelligible speech.

Intermediate goals are medium term goals that are selected in accordance with the theoretical position taken by the SLP to relate in a hierarchical fashion to the specific goals.

Specific goals are the phonological units that are directly targeted in therapy.

Any level of the **phonological hierarchy** may be targeted when selecting intermediate and specific goals.

Three categories of **goal attack strategy** are available for addressing the goals over time: *vertical, horizontal, or cyclical.*

are related to the specific goals will reflect the theoretical position taken by the SLP. Specific goals are the phonological units that are directly targeted in therapy. Much of the discussion that follows in this chapter is focused on phonemes as potential therapy targets (simply because most research has focused on phoneme goals) but it must be remembered that any level of the phonological hierarchy may be targeted when selecting intermediate and specific goals. A second important point about specific goals is that these concern those phonological units that will be targeted in therapy with planned procedures and activities. It may be expected that other phonological units will change during the course of the treatment program, either as a result of maturation or as a result of generalization from a treated target, thus contributing to the achievement of the basic goal. These expected changes will be related to the basic and intermediate goals but do not constitute the specific goals of the treatment program. Specific goals may be selected to promote these kinds of changes, however. Some examples of hypothetical sets of basic, intermediate, and specific goals are provided in Table 8–2.

Once the intermediate and specific goals have been selected, a strategy for addressing the goals over time must also be selected. Fey (1992) identified three categories of goal attack strategy: vertical, horizontal, and cyclical. A vertical goal attack strategy is character-

Table 8–2. Examples of Hypothetical Basic, Intermediate, and Specific Treatment Goals

Basic Goal	*Intermediate Goals*	*Specific Goals*
Example 1		
Speech 75% intelligible to a stranger.	1. Word final codas 2. [+consonantal][+continuant]	1. C_2 = /k,g/ in CVC words 2. C_1 = /f,v/ in CV words
Example 2		
Adultlike accuracy and acceptability of speech articulation.	1. Mastery of /s/ 2. Mastery of /ɝ,ɚ/ 3. Mastery of /ɹ/-clusters	1. /s/ in complex codas 2. /ɝ/ in multisyllabic words 3. /kɹ,gɹ/ word onset clusters
Example 3		
Kindergarten level emergent literacy skills	1. Implicit awareness of subsyllabic units 2. Knowledge of letter sounds	1. Match CVC words with shared onsets or shared rimes 2. s, m, p, l, t, g, a, e
Example 4		
Improved quality of social interactions.	1. Improved use of question versus statement intonation contour.	1,2. I want the ______.
Improved speech intelligibility.	2. Increased PCC in multiword phrases.	1,2. Can I have the ______, please?

ized by two fundamental features: (a) one goal is targeted at a time; and (b) the targeted phonological unit is addressed in therapy until a predetermined level of production accuracy is achieved before a new goal is introduced. Traditionally, the child would be expected to master the target before switching to a new goal. However, as discussed later in this section, children will often make spontaneous gains toward mastery even if treatment is withdrawn prior to achievement of consistent production of a given phoneme. Therefore, the SLP could set a less stringent criterion for moving from one goal to the next (such as customary production). The criterion that is set may be determined by the child's abilities so that an approximation of the target may be considered to be a significant functional gain even if perfect production is not currently possible for a child with severe DPD. The choice of treatment approach also plays a role as some treatment approaches aim for perfect output whereas others accept approximations to the target, depending on the underlying theoretical basis for the intervention. These issues are discussed in greater depth in Part III. Referring to Table 8–2, Example 4, the SLP might practice the sentence "I want the ______." with different functional objects in the child's natural environment until consistent intelligible responses with an appropriate intonation contour are achieved before starting to practice the more difficult sentence, "Can I have the ______, please?" We can imagine that, in this case, the functional outcome of the child's verbal communications in social situations might be more important than absolute speech accuracy and thus the accuracy criterion might be set at a level lower than mastery for moving from one sentence to the next. Furthermore, the accuracy criterion for the intonation contour used during sentence production might be higher than the accuracy criterion for production of the phonetic content depending on the treatment goals and the way that these variables interact to determine communication effectiveness. However, Example 2 is focused on adultlike accuracy. In this case, when using a vertical strategy, the SLP might target /s/ until 90% accuracy in conversation is achieved before introducing the next goal /ɝ/.

When a **vertical goal attack strategy** is implemented a single goal is targeted until a predetermined level of production accuracy is achieved.

A horizontal goal attack strategy is different from the vertical strategy in that multiple goals are targeted at the same time. Several goals are addressed in therapy until predetermined criteria for discontinuing treatment on those goals are achieved. As with the vertical strategy, the SLP is free to choose more or less stringent criteria for deciding when to discontinue work with a particular target. The horizontal strategy allows the SLP to shift focus among the multiple goals as a function of changes in rate of progress during periods when the goal is being actively targeted in therapy and during periods when it is being monitored for spontaneous change. Revisiting Example 2 in Table 8–2, the SLP might initiate treatment for /s/, /ɝ/, and /gɹ/ at the same time, let's say in September. The criterion for discontinuing direct treatment on a goal might be set loosely at 40 to 75% correct production in conversation with an improving

A **horizontal goal attack strategy** involves targeting multiple goals at the same time.

trend. For example, if the performance in November is 25%, 50%, and 60% on the 3 goals, respectively, the SLP would shift focus to /s/ while monitoring performance on the other two goals. If in January conversational accuracy is 40%, 40%, and 75%, the SLP would continue to target /s/ while reintroducing /ɝ/ to stop the regression in performance for this phoneme. In April, improvements in accuracy to 75%, 80%, and 90% for the 3 goals would prompt the SLP to discontinue direct treatment but monitor progress at regular intervals thereafter.

A cyclical goal attack strategy is an integral component of Hodson's (2007) Cycles Phonological Remediation Approach. Detailed principles for selecting and ordering treatment goals according to this approach are presented later in this chapter. However, variants of the cyclical goal attack strategy have been implemented with other phonological approaches to remediation. This approach to targeting treatment goals is intended to facilitate gradual but broad-based change across the child's entire phonological system. Multiple intermediate goals are targeted during a given cycle but only one specific goal is targeted during any one treatment session. Specific goals are targeted for predetermined periods of time and then new goals are introduced in a fixed sequence regardless of the child's level of progress with prior goals. The sequence of intermediate goals is recycled with new specific goals until the targeted phonological patterns are observed in conversational speech. Referring to Example 1 in Table 8–2, the SLP could use a cyclical goal attack strategy to target these goals that were selected using a nonlinear phonological analysis of the child's speech. The SLP might target the first goal, word final codas, in the first 2 weeks of the intervention by working on words containing word-final /k/. In the second two weeks, words beginning with /f/ would be introduced as a means to facilitate emergence of the [+consonantal][+continuant] feature combination. In weeks 5 and 6, the voiced dorsal stop /g/ would be introduced, returning to the goal of encouraging word final codas. In weeks 7 and 8 the voiced labial continuant would reintroduce the [+consonantal][+continuant] feature combination. If codas and continuants were seen to be emerging in the child's spontaneous speech at this point, new intermediate goals would be selected for this child. If not, the intermediate goals would be recycled, either by returning to the specific goals already targeted or selecting new specific goals representing these intermediate targets.

When a **cyclical goal attack strategy** is implemented, specific goals are targeted for predetermined periods of time and then new goals are introduced in a fixed sequence regardless of the child's level of progress with prior goals.

Factors to Consider When Selecting Goals

One approach to goal selection seeks to accelerate the typical developmental processes that are presumed to be operating slowly in the child receiving treatment.

There are two basic approaches to goal selection in phonology therapy: one perspective seeks to accelerate the typical developmental processes which are presumed to be operating slowly in the child receiving treatment; the other seeks to dramatically alter the developmental course, triggering a sudden reorganization of the child's phonological system. These alternative approaches may result in very different choices of treatment goals for the same child. In either case, however, the same factors are taken into consideration when examining the potential goals that one might choose. These factors help the SLP answer the following questions about any potential intermediate or specific treatment goal: Is the child likely to achieve this goal without treatment? Is the child likely to achieve this goal at this time with treatment? Will the achievement of this goal effect substantial change toward the achievement of the basic goal(s)? Three of these factors reflect characteristics of the phonological units themselves without regard to the child's performance with the potential units that could be targeted in therapy: frequency and/or functional load of the units (usually phonemes) in the language, order of emergence of the units in normal development, and relative markedness of the phonological units. Two related factors directly reflect the child's performance with the phonological units in question at the surface level: stimulability and consistency of production. Finally, the child's phonological knowledge of the potential target at multiple levels of representation should be considered. These factors are discussed in turn.

An alternative approach to goal selection seeks to trigger a sudden and dramatic reorganization of the child's phonological system.

Recall from Chapter 4 that the roles of input frequency and functional load of a phoneme in explaining order of emergence and acquisition vary from one language to another based on the complexity of the language's phoneme inventory. Articulatory complexity plays a role in the time required to achieve mastery of a phoneme. Stokes and Suredran (2005) found that input frequency predicted age of emergence of phonemes in Cantonese but functional load was the best predictor for English. Therefore, /ð/ is a late developing phoneme in English despite extremely high frequency because very little information would be lost if this phoneme disappeared from the language. In contrast, /s/ has high frequency and high functional load but is frequently misarticulated, presumably due to the difficulty of the requisite articulatory gestures. Ensuring accurate articulation of this phoneme and appropriate phonological usage should have an important impact on the intelligibility of the child's speech. The phoneme /s/ also plays a role in the accurate production of important prosodic structures in English (complex onsets and codas) and in the production of frequently occurring grammatical morphemes (plural, possessive and third person singular morphemes). For all these reasons acquisition of this phoneme can have a broad impact on the child's communicative effectiveness and thus /s/ is a common treatment goal in speech therapy. Similar considerations can be applied to the choice of larger phonological units as treatment goals including complex onsets, rimes, syllables, and words, with the Child Corpus Calculator (Storkel & Hoover, 2010) providing useful information about potential treatment stimuli.

Input frequency and **functional load** of a phoneme are factors to consider when deciding whether a potential target will help the child achieve the basic goal.

Developmental order of emergence of potential phoneme targets is also a common consideration when selecting treatment goals.

Developmental order of emergence of potential phoneme targets is also a common consideration when selecting treatment goals. Unfortunately, there is no absolute consensus on the developmental order that should be used when selecting goals so this criterion does not lead to predictable targets. Not only is there variance between alternative sets of normative data (e.g., compare Figure 4–5 with Table 4–8) but there is considerable variance between the order of emergence and the order of mastery for phonemes and other phonological units and it is not clear which should take precedence (i.e., compare left and right edges of bars in Figure 4–5). Should the SLP introduce /s/ at age 3 years when 50% of children have achieved customary production of this phoneme or wait until age 8 years when 90% of children have achieved customary production of this phoneme? We have more to say on that question later in this chapter but, for now, the main point is that "earlier developing" phonemes are expected to be easier for the child to learn than "later developing" phonemes with or without treatment. There is plenty of ambiguity in the application of developmental norms to the choice of treatment goals, however, leading to anomalies such as Gierut, Morrisette, Hughes, and Rowlands (2001) classifying /ɹ/ as early developing in Study I and as late developing in Study II of the same paper on the role of developmental norms in the selection of treatment goals!

The **markedness** relationship between pairs of potential treatment goals can also be considered.

Another consideration based on characteristics of the potential phonological units themselves is the relative markedness of pairs of phonological units. For example, if a child's inventory was restricted to glides, nasals, and vowels one would have a choice of introducing either oral stops [+consonantal][−continuant], the unmarked option, or fricatives [+consonantal][+continuant], the marked option. The markedness relationship between these two options would lead you to predict that oral stops should be easier to teach; on the other hand, if the child learned to produce fricatives, oral stops should emerge spontaneously. You can see that this idea is related to the notion of the implicational hierarchy introduced in Chapter 4 (see Table 4–15 and associated discussion).

Stimulability refers to the child's ability to achieve a correct production of the potential target when provided with additional information intended to prompt a correct response.

Typically, stimulability is assessed by providing the child with a limited number of **audiovisual models**.

The next factor, stimulability, has been studied as a prognostic indicator in several large sample investigations. Stimulability refers to the child's ability to achieve a correct production of the potential target when provided with additional information intended to prompt a correct response. Techniques for assessing stimulability were described in Chapter 5 and range from brief unstructured procedures in which the SLP provides whatever cues necessary to induce a correct response for a specific sound to highly structured assessments in which the child is provided with a prescribed number of audiovisual models of many sounds to imitate and no additional information. In the former case, a successful result indicates that the child is physically capable of producing the articulatory gestures required for production of a given phoneme. The more structured procedures used in the studies that have examined the prognostic value of stimulability testing provide additional information about the child's phonological and learning abilities. For example, the Carter and Buck (1958) procedure involves asking the child to imitate multiple phones on repeated trials in nonsense syllables that vary syllable position and phonetic context. Greater numbers of accurate responses may indicate that the child has perceived the difference between his or her own attempts at the target and the examiner's model and is able to make spontaneous adjustments in articulatory gestures to achieve the correct targets. Thus, the task targets multiple domains relevant to success in treatment including speech perception skills, motor learning, attention, and motivation. Several studies have shown that children who achieve higher scores on such tests are more likely to master their error phonemes than lower-scoring children. This is true for children with normally developing speech and for children with DPD regardless of whether the child receives treatment (Carter & Buck, 1958; Miccio, Elbert, & Forrest, 1999; Sommers et al., 1967).

Children who achieve higher stimulability scores are more likely to master their error phonemes than lower-scoring children, regardless of whether the child receives treatment.

Sommers et al. (1967) found that treatment benefitted all children, those with low and high stimulability scores, but treatment benefits were greatest for children with low stimulability scores in a study in which treated children received traditional therapy weekly for 8 months. This conclusion is dependent on the nature and the intensity of the treatment provided however. Rvachew et al. (1999) observed no improvement for treated unstimulable phonemes in a 12-week group phonological intervention; within the same group of children, small improvements were observed for 53% of treated stimulable phonemes. This intervention involved a cycles goal attack strategy however so that the cumulative intervention intensity was limited for each specific goal. In this study, stimulability increased the probability of a good outcome but did not guarantee it. One reason for this outcome is that stimulability is independent of perceptual knowledge of a phoneme. Lof (1996) assessed children's stimulability for certain consonants and their perception of the same consonants using Locke's (1980) Speech Perception Production Task (as described in Chapter 5). Across a variety of commonly misarticulated phonemes, all possible combinations of performance for perception and stimulability were observed: successful perception and stimulability; successful perception without stimulability; misperception without stimulability; and stimulability despite misperception. The final combination occurred only in the case of the /f/-/θ/ contrast, however, reflecting the ease of imitating the articulatory gesture for /θ/ given visual input alone. Stimulability without perceptual knowledge was not observed for any other phonemes. In some cases, the children were misarticulating the phoneme in spontaneous speech despite having perceptual knowledge of the target and the ability to imitate the sound. In other cases, notably the majority of /ɹ/ misarticulators, the children were lacking both stimulability and perceptual knowledge. The majority of /k/ and /g/ misarticulators were unstimulable despite good

Stimulability is independent of perceptual knowledge of a phoneme.

The combination of good perceptual ability and stimulability predicts a good treatment outcome.

perceptual performance. Rvachew et al. (1999) found that the combination of good perceptual ability and stimulability was the best predictor of a good treatment outcome.

Inconsistency in the production of an error phoneme is traditionally viewed as a positive prognostic indicator but interactions with representational and motoric factors may prevent advancement toward mastery of an inconsistently produced phoneme.

Inconsistency in the production of an error phoneme is traditionally viewed as a positive prognostic indicator (e.g., Smit et al., 1990). It is not clear how the SLP is expected to operationalize the notion of consistency, however, and no research program has systematically explored the conditions under which consistency of production of phonemes and prosodic structures predict spontaneous improvement in children with DPD. One underlying assumption is that instability marks a phase transition in the child's phonological system and thus reorganization and stabilization at a higher level of function are imminent (e.g., see case studies in Grunwell, 1992). Another assumption is that occasional correct productions indicate a physical ability to produce the requisite articulatory gestures but inconsistency reflects immature speech motor control; increased consistency is expected to emerge with time and maturation. However, as discussed in Chapter 3, the relationship between segmental variability and motor stability is highly complex and interacts with representational factors (Goffman, Gerken, & Lucchesi, 2007). Even among children with speech and language deficits, systematic relationships between variability in the production of segments and kinematic measures of motor stability are not observed. Furthermore, occasional correct productions of a phoneme do not indicate that the child has adultlike underlying phonological knowledge of the phoneme in which case the child has no target to aim for and, thus, no basis for achieving progressive change toward mastery of the phoneme.

Perceptual phonological knowledge of a phoneme that the child misarticulates is a positive prognostic indicator.

Perceptual phonological knowledge of a phoneme that the child misarticulates is a positive prognostic indicator as we indicated earlier in reference to studies of stimulability. In Rvachew et al. (1999) improvements after 12 weeks of intervention were observed for 20% of targets that were misperceived prior to intervention and 64% of targets that were well perceived prior to treatment. In another study, we showed that speech perception skills predicted growth in articulation skills over the kindergarten year, a period when most of the sample of children with DPD were no longer receiving treatment (see Table 7–8; Rvachew, 2006).

Underlying phonological knowledge as indexed by a covert contrast predicts improvements in production accuracy.

Other researchers have shown that underlying phonological knowledge predicts changes in production accuracy. Tyler, Edwards, and Saxman (1990) observed changes in the phonological systems of four children, three of whom received treatment, focusing on the phonological processes of prevocalic voicing and velar fronting or backing depending on the pattern observed in the child's speech. Hypotheses about the status of the child's underlying phonological knowledge were derived from phonetic transcriptions and acoustic analysis. Initially, a phonological process analysis of the phonetic transcriptions was used to make predictions: obligatory application of a process was taken as an indicator of non-adultlike knowledge of the contrast whereas optional (i.e., inconsistent) application of a process was taken as an indicator of adultlike knowledge. The prediction that better progress would be observed in the case of optional versus obligatory process use was not supported. In a second analysis, acoustic measures were used to identify covert contrasts in the child's speech. In this case, a significant difference in the distribution of acoustic values between two categories (e.g., /t/ vs. /d/) even if it was not perceptible to the adult listener was taken as an indication of underlying knowledge of the contrast. On the other hand, overlapping distributions of the acoustic cue of interest indicated non-adultlike phonological knowledge of the contrast. The acoustic analysis revealed information about the children's underlying phonological knowledge that was predictive of faster improvements in speech accuracy for the 3 children who received treatment. The child who was not treated did not improve even though the acoustic analysis revealed underlying knowledge of the voicing contrast for this child.

Gierut, Elbert, and Dinnsen (1987) developed a tool for operationalizing productive phonological knowledge according to a continuum that reflects the child's knowledge of each consonant phoneme relative to the adult target. In their study, the ranking was derived from a single word production probe that targets consonants in initial, medial, and final word positions. We present data obtained from a child who completed this probe in Rvachew and Nowak (2001) in Case Study 8–5 and then show how her productive phonological knowledge for each phoneme would be coded in Table 8–3. You can see that the potential treatment goals should be taken from the lower half of Table 8–3, those phonemes at Type 4, 5, or 6 productive phonological knowledge. Although some errors were observed for /p,t,d/ these consisted of occasional errors that are commonly observed in children's speech (e.g., voicing errors, coda deletion) and thus are not impacting intelligibility. The absence of dorsals, liquids, affricates, and noncoronal supralaryngeal fricatives are all issues of significant concern, however. The question is, with so many potential phonemes to target in therapy, where does one start? Some SLPs might choose to facilitate mastery of /m/, /n/, or /s/. One might expect rapid success in speech therapy because this child is clearly stimulable for these phonemes and the nasals are very early developing phonemes. Furthermore, these phonemes have high functional load and thus early success with these sounds would have immediate impact on the child's speech intelligibility and communicative effectiveness. Another SLP might avoid these phonemes because they should improve without therapeutic intervention. Targeting a more difficult phoneme such as the complex and late developing /ɹ/, might trigger a broad-based reorganization of the child's phonological system. We discuss these opposing approaches to selecting treatment goals at length next.

Productive phonological knowledge can be ranked on a continuum that reflects the child's knowledge of each phoneme relative to the adult target.

Case Study 8–5
Pretreatment Results on Probe of Productive Phonological Knowledge

Participant TS30 from Rvachew and Nowak (2001)

pig	✓	big	✓	tub	✓	duck	✓	cup	t	gum	d
pie	✓	bite	✓	tear	✓	deer	✓	cob	t	gate	d
pants	✓	back	✓	toes	✓	done	✓	cut	t	girl	d
peach	✓	bus	✓	tail	✓	door	✓	coat	t	gun	d
paint	✓	boot	✓	tooth	✓	dog	✓	comb	t	goat	d
soupy	✓	tub-i	✓	eating	?	bed-i	✓	book-i	t	doggie	d
chip-i	✓	rubbing	✓	fatty	✓	reading	✓	duckie	d	froggie	d
soapy	✓	cob-i	✓	cutting	?	muddy	n	sock-i	t	piggie	d
cup-i	–	robe-i	✓	bootie	✓	riding	✓	rocky	d	baggie	d
sleeping	✓	web-i	✓	biting	✓	hiding	✓	back-i	t	hugging	d
soup	✓	tub	✓	eat	✓	bed	✓	book	t	dog	d
chip	✓	rub	✓	fat	✓	read	✓	duck	t	frog	–
soap	✓	cob	✓	cut	✓	mud	✓	sock	t	pig	d
cup	✓	robe	✓	boot	–	ride	✓	rock	t	bag	–
sleep	✓	web	✓	bite	✓	hide	✓	back	t	hug	d
# ✓ /p/	14	# ✓ /b/	15	# ✓ /t/	12	# ✓ /d/	14	# ✓ /k/	0	# ✓ /g/	0

mud	✓	knife	✓	fat	w	van	w	thumb	t	them	d
mouth	✓	nose	✓	face	w	vase	w	thunder	s͋	these	d
mother	✓	noise	✓	fire	w	vanilla	w͋	thankyou	s͋	there	d
mouse	✓	nail	✓	five	w	vacuum	w	thief	fw	theirs	d
moon	✓	nothing	✓	fish	w	valentine	w	thirsty	t	that	d
gum-i	b	raining	d	laughing	b	waving	b	toothy	t	feather	w
comb-i	b	running	d	coughing	b	shaving	b	bath-i	b	mother	d
thumb-i	b	moony	d	knife-i	P	glove-i	b	mouth-i	t	brother	d
swimming	b	van-i	d	leafy	b	driving	b	teeth-i	t	father	w
Tommy	b	sunny	d	roof-i	b	stove-i	b	wreath-i	p		
gum	–	rain	d	laugh	p	wave	b	tooth	t		
comb	✓	run	d	cough	p	shave	b	bath	b		
thumb	✓	moon	d	knife	p	glove	b	mouth	t		
swim	✓	van	d	leaf	p	drove	b	teeth	t		
Tom	✓	sun	~	roof	p	stove	w	wreath	p		
# ✓ /m/	9	# ✓ /n/	5	# ✓ /f/	0	# ✓ /v/	0	# ✓ /θ/	0	# ✓ /ð/	0

soup	~	zebra	~	shave	s	chip	t	juice	d	read	w
soap	~	zipper	✓	shoe	s	cheeze	t	jail	d	rock	w
sock	~	zoo	✓	shirt	~	chalk	t	jeep	d	rain	w
sun	s	zipping	✓	shovel	s	chair	t	jump	d	run	w
santa	s	ziggy	✓	shampoo	tz	chicken	t	jelly	d	ride	w
juicy	d	cheezy	d	fishing	d	peach-i	d	orange-y	d	starry	d
mouse-i	d	nosy	d	washing	d	catching	d	bridge-i	d	deer-i	j
icy	d	noisy	d	brushing	t	pinching	d	badge-i	d	door-i	w
bus-i	d	rosy	d	crashing	t	punching	d	cage-i	d	fire-i	w
dressy	d	buzzing	d	pushing	t	watching	d	page-i	d	chair-i	j
juice	t	cheese	d	fish	t	peach	t	orange	~	star	–
mouse	t	nose	~	wash	t	catch	t	bridge	d	deer	–
ice	t	noise	~	brush	t	pinch	t	badge	d	door	–
bus	~	rose	d	crash	t	punch	t	cage	d	fire	–
dress	t	buzz	d	push	t	watch	t	page	d	chair	–
# ✓ /s/:	2	# ✓ /z/	4	# ✓ /ʃ/	0	# ✓ /tʃ/	0	# ✓ /dʒ/	0	# ✓ /ɹ/	0

laugh	j	web	✓	yes	✓	hide	✓	sleep	j	**Comments**
leaf	j	watch	✓	yellow	✓	hug	✓	bluehouse	b	57 correct responses
light	j	wash	✓	you	✓	hill	✓	glove	g	
ladder	j	wave	✓	yawn	✓	hat	✓	blow	b	
leg	j	growing	✓	yard	✓	house	✓	snow	s	~ nasal emission
tail-i	j	sewing	✓	crayon	✓	treehouse	✓	star	t	
nail-i	j	blowing	✓	onion	–	grasshopper	✓	swim	w	
shovel-i	j	throwing	✓			beehouse	✓	stove	t	
calling	j	snowing	✓			forehead	✓	dress	d	
hilly	j	growing	✓			bluehouse	✓	brother	b	
tail	–	grow	✓					crash	t	
nail	–	sew	✓					treehouse	t	
shovel	–	throw	✓							
call	–	blow	✓							
hill	–	snow	✓							
# ✓ /l/	0	# ✓ /w/	15	# ✓ /j/	6	# ✓ /h/	10	# ✓	0	

Other Pretreatment Assessment Information:

Chronological Age: 51 months; Reynell Developmental Language Scale (Receptive) $z = 1.1$;

Structured Photographic Expressive Language Test-Preschool: 3rd percentile; Goldman-Fristoe Test of Articulation: below first percentile; Percent consonants correct in conversation: 67%;

Phonetic repertoire in conversation: [m n p b t d s h w j]; Syllable Structure Repertoire: V, CV, CVC, CVCV, CVCVC, CVCC (nasal clusters in coda),

Summary of Results from Assessments 1, 2, and 3

Number of matching productions on the PPPK by consonant and assessment time

Consonant	A1	A2	A3
p	14	12	12
b	15	12	15
t	12	15	12
d	14	14	15
k	0	0	0
g	0	0	0
m	9	15	6
n	5	13	9
f	0	6	6
v	0	3	0
θ	0	0	0
ð	0	1	1
s	2	2	2
z	4	2	2
ʃ	0	5	8
tʃ	0	4	2
dʒ	0	0	0
ɪ	0	9	9
l	0	12	15
w	15	15	15
j	6	7	7
h	10	10	10
Clusters	0	1	0
Total	106	158	146

Feature match ratios by assessment time

Node or Feature	A1	A2	A3
+Consonantal	0.81	0.90	0.96
+Sonorant	0.77	1.00	1.00
+nasal	0.54	0.93	0.50
+continuant	0.15	0.36	0.32
+branching continuant	0.00	0.13	0.07
+lateral	0.00	0.80	1.00
+voiced	0.94	0.95	0.97
+spread Glottis	0.76	0.77	0.90
Labial	0.90	0.97	1.00
+round	0.73	1.00	1.00
Coronal	0.81	0.91	0.93
−grooved	0.00	0.04	0.04
−anterior	0.09	0.37	0.39
Dorsal	0.00	0.00	0.00

Note: This case study has been adapted with permission from Rvachew and Bernhardt (2010) where she was referred to as ME30. PPPK = probe of productive phonological knowledge.

Table 8–3. *Example of Coding Productive Phonological Knowledge for Participant 30 Prior to Treatment in Rvachew and Nowak (2001)*

Type	*Description*	*Phonemes*
1	Never misarticulated. Correct in all morphemes and all positions.	b w h
2	Correct in all morphemes and positions except for certain position-specific alternations predictable by rule.	p t d
3	Correct in all morphemes and positions with the exception of some "fossilized" forms.	j
4	Consistently correct in at least one position but consistently incorrect in at least one other position.	m n
5	Consistently incorrect in one or more positions but occasional correct productions in one or more positions.	s z
6	Never produced correctly. Misarticulated in all morphemes and all positions.	k g f v θ ð ʃ tʃ dʒ l ɹ

Productive Phonological Knowledge Continuum adapted from Gierut et al. (1987, Table 2b, p. 466).

A Randomized Control Trial of Approaches to the Selection of Treatment Goals

The **complexity approach** to the selection of treatment goals invokes learnability theory as the justification for selecting the most complex potential treatment goals as the starting point for intervention.

Gierut (2007) promotes the selection of complex treatment goals by invoking "learnability theory," the notion that language is essentially unlearnable and thus the language acquisition process is constrained by a preexisting and universal system of unifying laws and hierarchically organized linguistic constituents. This is a version of an "inside-out" model of development as described in the Introduction to Part I of this book. According to Gierut, the child's earliest phonological system is constrained to be a restricted subset of the adult system, comprised primarily of simple (i.e., minimally complex, predictable, or unmarked) phonological elements. Over time, the child's system then unfolds to encompass all of the elements in the adult language as positive evidence from linguistic input sets parameters associated with increasingly complex or marked elements. The course of this developmental process is proposed to be governed by universal implicational laws that constrain the set of phonological elements that may exist in any child's underlying system. These constraints reflect markedness relationships between different classes of phonological elements. For example, it is stated that affricates are more complex (or marked) than fricatives according to an innately determined hierarchical relationship between these phoneme classes. From the perspective of learnability theory, there must be positive evidence in the ambient language of elements that are more marked than the fricatives if the child is to expand the complexity of a system that is, for example, at level C of the implicational hierarchy shown in Table 4–15.[3]

The clinical implications of learnability theory relate to the complexity of the treatment goals that speech-language patholo-

[3]Although the concept of the implicational hierarchy is invoked in the complexity approach, the hierarchy itself is not used in all studies as the definition of complexity. Note that affricates are not more complex than fricatives according to the implicational hierarchy shown in Table 4–15. This may be because this hierarchy reflects phonetic contrasts whereas it appears that phonemic contrasts are the source of the markedness relationships discussed in Gierut (2007). Notwithstanding a lack of consensus on so-called universal markedness relationships (Menn, Schmidt, & Nicholas, 2009), varying definitions of complexity from study to study are another challenge to any effort to provide empirical support for the efficacy of the complexity approach. In Gierut et al. (1987) the complexity of affricates relative to fricatives varied from child to child based on productive phonological knowledge; Dinnsen, Chin, Elbert, and Powell (1990) and Tyler and Figurski (1994) used the implicational hierarchy for phonetic feature classes, however, and thus affricates would have been classified as having equivalent complexity to fricatives; in Gierut et al. (2001) the affricate /tʃ/ would have been considered more complex than the fricative /ʃ/ according to the developmental norms used in Study I but these two phonemes would have been considered to be equally complex according to the developmental norms used in Study II. The basis for the claim in Gierut (2007) that affricates imply fricatives is not clear.

gists select for their clients. For example, a traditional approach to the treatment of TS30 (see Case Study 8–5) whose phonetic repertoire comprises the phones [m n p b t d s z h w j] might be first to increase the frequency of her accurate productions of the phoneme [s] and to then expand the fricative class to include, for example, [f v]. Gierut (2007) predicts that this strategy will enhance performance within the fricative class but will not facilitate any increase in the overall complexity of the child's system; therefore, spontaneous emergence of more complex phonetic elements such as affricates and liquids will not (indeed cannot) occur. She suggests that a more effective and efficient strategy would be to target "higher order categories to induce cascading effects on generalization learning" (p. 7). For example, targeting a complex onset such as /tw/ is expected to trigger spontaneous emergence of affricates because clusters are presumed to be a more marked syllable structure than affricates according to the universal implicational laws invoked by this theory.

The **traditional approach** to goal selection involves treating phonemes in developmental order from earlier to later developing while taking other factors into account such as stimulability and functional load.

Gierut (2007) points to a number of single subject studies (e.g., Gierut et al., 1987; Gierut et al., 2001) to support the recommendation that SLPs target complex phonological elements when treating children with DPD. These single case studies are viewed as support for treating complex targets, outside of the child's baseline system, if new elements are to emerge during therapy. These studies used a nonexperimental multiple probe design that lacks internal validity because it does not control for history or maturation effects (McReynolds & Kearns, 1983). The implementation of this design in these studies has been criticized for a number of faults, including the lack of stable baselines, the difficulty of determining the time intervals between probes, and the practice of comparing outcomes across rather than within children (Diedrich, 1989; Rvachew & Nowak, 2001, 2003). Careful study of these research outcomes reveals that changes in untreated phonemes that are considered to be generalization effects triggered by the treatment of complex phonemes are most likely maturation effects; in other words, changes in these less complex sounds would have occurred even if the children had not received intervention. In order to determine whether observed changes in children's speech are a true treatment effect, it is necessary to use a randomized controlled research design. We now describe the results of such a study in detail.

Single case studies have been used to support the hypothesis that treating complex targets facilitates across-class generalization.

Rvachew and Nowak (2001) contrasted the complexity approach to selecting treatment goals with a more traditional developmental approach. Forty-eight children with moderate or severe DPD received a pretreatment assessment (A1), a 6-week block of treatment targeting two consonant phonemes (block 1), a second assessment (A2), another 6-week block of treatment targeting two additional consonant phonemes (block 2), and a posttreatment assessment (A3). All assessments were conducted by a SLP who was blind to the child's group assignment and treatment targets.

Rvachew and Nowak (2001) contrasted the complexity approach to selecting treatment goals with a more traditional developmental approach using a randomized control between groups design.

The treatment approach during each block was focused on articulatory knowledge, with phonetic placement, shaping, and modeling techniques used to establish stimulability at the syllable level. Once stimulability in syllables was achieved the child was provided with opportunities for articulation practice in imitated words, spontaneous words, imitated patterned sentences, spontaneous patterned sentences, imitated sentences, and spontaneous sentences. All children began the treatment program at the stimulation phase and progressed from one treatment step to the next upon achieving 80% correct responding.

The phonemes that were targeted during the two treatment blocks depended on whether the child was assigned at random to the *most stimulable, early developing* (ME) group or the *least stimulable, late developing* (LL) group. At each of the three assessments the child was asked to imitate all items from the Productive Phonological Knowledge Profile and the child's responses were used to rank the child's unmastered phonemes according to type of Productive Phonological Knowledge as shown in Table 8–3. Potential treatment targets were those phonemes for which the child had Type 4, 5, or 6 productive phonological knowledge. These potential treatment targets were further ranked within each knowledge type according to the 90th percentile age of acquisition, using the normative data shown in Table 4–8. In each treatment block, children assigned to the ME group received treatment for the two sounds that were most stimulable and earliest developing, with the proviso that the two sounds not share the same manner class. Children assigned to the LL group received treatment for the two sounds that were least stimulable and latest developing, again with the constraint that the two sounds not share the same manner class. For example, participant TS30 (Case Study 8–5) was assigned to the ME group and received treatment for the phonemes /k/ and /s/ in the first treatment block. The criteria for choosing targets for children in the LL condition effectively ensured that this group would receive treatment for unstimulable sounds, at least during the first treatment block. For example, if Participant TS30 had been assigned to the LL group she would have received treatment for the phonemes /ɹ/ and /θ/, both late developing, unstimulable phonemes at different manners and places of articulation. The most frequently targeted sounds during the first treatment block for the ME group were /k/ and /f/. The most frequently targeted consonants during the first treatment block for the LL group were /s/ and /ɹ/.

Figure 8–3A shows the ME group's response accuracy for three sets of consonants from the Productive Phonological Knowledge Profile for the three assessments. The highest line on the chart (diamond-shaped markers) shows the change in percent correct responding for phonemes that were treated in the first block, both during the first block when these phonemes were targeted and during the second block when treatment was withdrawn for these

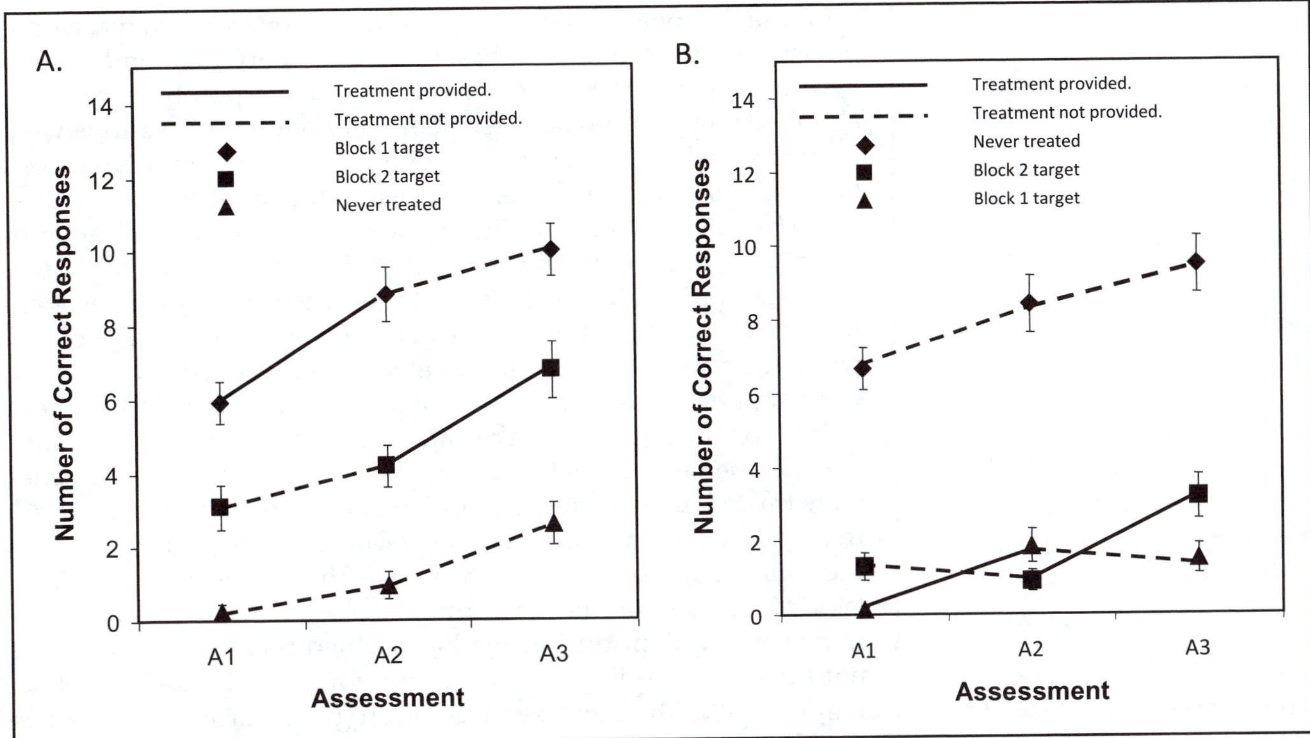

Figure 8–3. *Mean number of correct responses for certain consonants on the Productive Phonological Knowledge Profile, administered at three assessment points: prior to treatment (A1), after the first treatment block (A2), and after the second treatment block (A3).* **A.** *Results for children in the ME group.* **B.** *Results for the children in the LL group. From Rvachew (2005, Figure 2, p. 212) based on data reported in Rvachew and Nowak (2001). Reproduced with permission of American Speech-Language-Hearing Association in the format Textbook via Copyright Clearance Center.*

sounds. The middle line on the chart (square markers) shows the change in percent correct responding for the phonemes that were targeted during the second block, both during the first block before treatment was initiated for these consonants and during the second block when these phonemes were treated. The lowest line on the chart (triangular markers) shows change in percent correct responding for these children's least stimulable phonemes although these sounds were never targeted in treatment (i.e., these are the phonemes that would have been targeted in the first block *if* the child had been assigned to the LL group).

Figure 8–3B shows the LL group's response accuracy for three sets of consonants from the Productive Phonological Knowledge Profile for the three assessments. The lowest line on the chart (triangular markers) shows the change in percent correct responding for phonemes that were treated in the first block, both during the first block when these phonemes were targeted and during the second block when treatment was withdrawn for these sounds. The middle line on the chart (square markers) shows the change in percent correct responding for the phonemes that were targeted during the second block, both during the first block before treatment was initiated for these consonants and during the second block when these phonemes were treated. The highest line on the chart (diamond-shaped markers) shows change in percent correct responding for these children's most stimulable phonemes although these sounds were never treated (i.e., these are the phonemes that would have been targeted *if* the child had been assigned to the ME group).

The slopes of the lines in Figure 8–3 provide an indication of the rate of change during the first and second treatment blocks. First, the rate of change during blocks when the phonemes were treated was compared to the rate of change observed during blocks when the phonemes were not treated (all comparisons noted here were significant upon statistical analysis as reported in Rvachew, 2005). For the ME group, the rate of change for the most stimulable phonemes was higher during the block when these phonemes were treated, than during the block when these phonemes were not treated (see solid vs. dashed lines for block 1 and 2 targets in Figure 8–3A). For the LL group, the rate of change for the least stimulable phonemes was higher during the block when these phonemes were treated, than during the block when these phonemes were not treated (see solid vs. dashed lines for block 1 and 2 targets in Figure 8–3B). The increased rate of progress during blocks when the phoneme was targeted compared to blocks when the phoneme was not targeted is an important indicator of the effectiveness of speech therapy.

In Figure 8–3, the increased rate of progress during blocks when the phoneme was targeted compared to blocks when the phoneme was not targeted is an important indicator of the effectiveness of speech therapy.

The second analysis considered rate of change for treated phonemes when comparing the ME and LL groups. The rate of change in production accuracy from A1 to A3 for treated *stimulable* phonemes was greater than the rate of change for treated *unstimulable* phonemes (highest line in Figure 8–3A vs. lowest line on Figure 8–3B). In other words, the greatest amount of progress was observed for treated stimulable phonemes. Treatment progress was so poor for treated phonemes in the LL group that the children failed to achieve stimulability in isolation for 34% of these targets after 6 weeks of intervention. On average, the children in this group learned to produce the target in single words whereas the children in the ME group learned to produce their target phonemes in complete sentences during treatment sessions.

The randomized control trial showed that the greatest amount of progress was observed for treated stimulable phonemes with negligible progress observed for treated unstimulable phonemes.

The third analysis considered the relative rate of change for stimulable phonemes when comparing the ME and LL groups. From A1 to A3, the rate of change shown by the ME group for *treated* stimulable phonemes was numerically but not significantly greater than the rate of change shown by the LL group for *untreated* stimulable phonemes (highest line of Figure 8–3A vs. highest line on Figure 8–3B). The spontaneous gains for untreated stimulable (most knowledge) phonemes observed in the LL group, as shown in Figure 8–3B, provide support for the argument that it may not be efficient to target these phonemes in speech therapy.

The final analysis considered the rate of change for unstimulable phonemes across the ME and the LL groups. This is a crucial comparison because, from the perspective of the learnability argument, it is not possible to observe gains in these phonemes unless one adopts a complexity approach to selecting treatment goals. From A1 to A3, the rate of change shown by the ME group for *untreated* unstimulable phonemes was actually significantly *greater* than the rate of change shown by the LL group for *treated* unstimulable phonemes (lowest line on Figure 8–3A versus lowest line on Figure 8–3B). Overall, treatment progress was very poor for unstimulable phonemes but treating the stimulable phonemes first appeared to facilitate improvements for unstimulable phonemes in the ME group. This finding directly contradicts the predictions of the complexity approach and provides support for the practice of beginning treatment with less complex phonemes.

Overall, treatment progress was very poor for unstimulable phonemes but treating the stimulable phonemes first appeared to facilitate improvements for unstimulable phonemes.

Overall, in this study, children in the LL group made very poor gains regardless of their pretreatment performance on the probe of productive phonological knowledge for a given treatment target, as shown in Figure 8–4. The selection of new treatment targets in the second block of this study ensured that children in the LL group would move to somewhat easier targets but their poor outcomes in the first block seemed to inhibit their progress in the second half of the treatment program and had a measurable negative impact

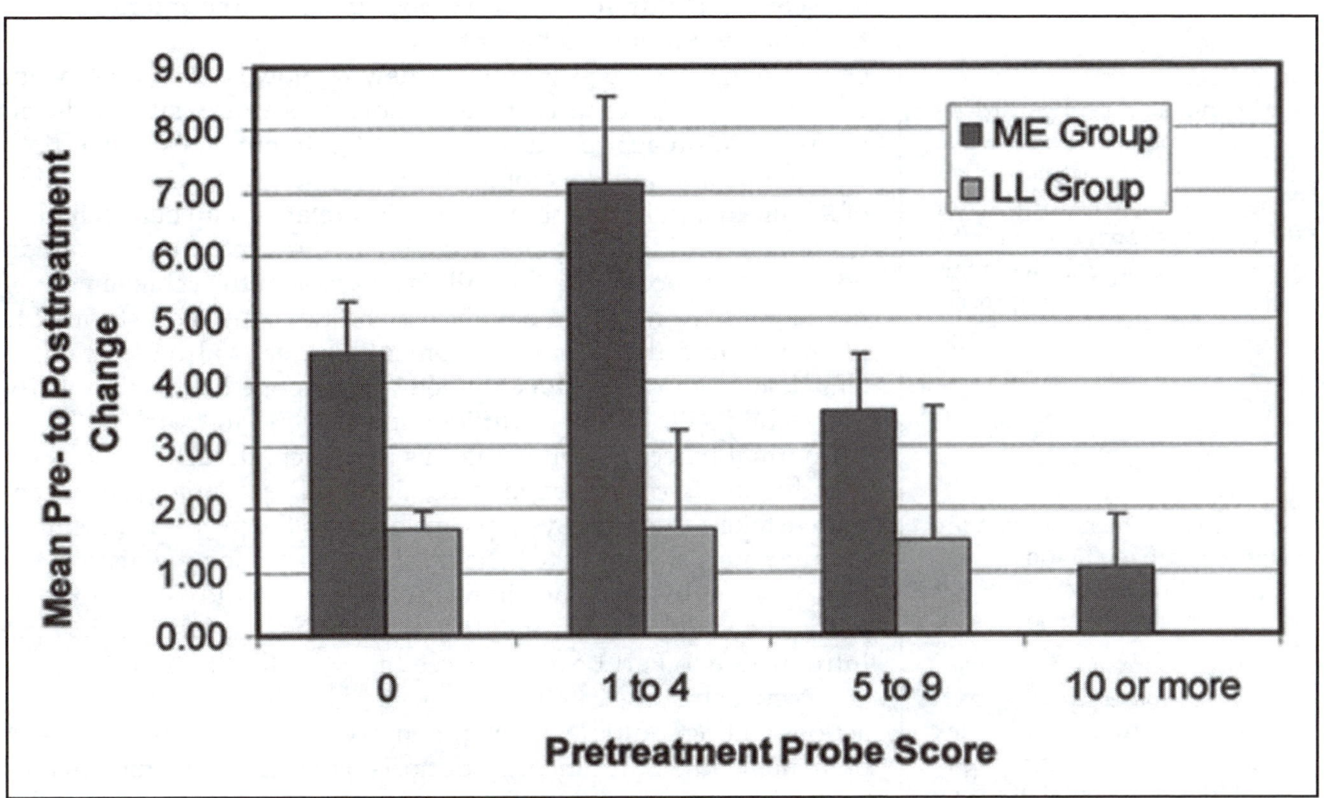

Figure 8–4. *Mean pre- and posttreatment gains in score on the probe of productive phonological knowledge as a function of pretreatment score category and treatment condition. From Rvachew and Nowak, 2003, Figure 2, p. 387. Reproduced with permission of American Speech-Language-Hearing Association in the format Textbook via Copyright Clearance Center.*

on their parents' satisfaction with their treatment outcomes. On the other hand, children in the ME group continued to enjoy good success even as they moved to more difficult phonemes in the second treatment block. The results shown in Figure 8–4 suggest that the greatest treatment benefits will be obtained when treatment is directed at phonemes for which the child has type 5 productive phonological knowledge (i.e., pretreatment probe scores of 1 to 4 points indicates some correct responses but less than mastery in any one word position). However, it may be premature to conclude that it is inefficient to begin the intervention with targets for which the child has most phonological knowledge because there is a strong suggestion that treating these phonemes first facilitated change in phonemes for which the child had less phonological knowledge.

The results shown in Figure 8–4 suggest that the greatest treatment benefits will be obtained when treatment is directed at phonemes for which the child has type 5 productive phonological knowledge (i.e., some correct responses but less than mastery in any one word position).

Dynamic Systems Perspective on the Selection of Treatment Goals

It should be clear that we strongly recommend against the complexity approach to the selection of treatment goals. We have demonstrated empirically that when the most complex treatment targets are selected children make very poor gains on those targets. Furthermore, we found no benefits in terms of reorganization of the child's phonological system (Rvachew & Nowak, 2001). We want to make it equally clear that we are not advocating a strictly developmental approach to the selection of treatment goals either. Both the complexity and developmental approaches invoke the notion of a built-in and immutable hierarchical relationship between phonemes. According to the developmental approach, the SLP can do no better than accelerate the child's progress in the achievement of the sequence. This approach, in which one focuses on stimulable phonemes introduced in developmental order, is also based on an "inside-out" model of development. Unless one begins very early in the child's life, it will be difficult for the child to "catch up" with the normal trajectory following this approach. In fact, we do want to induce a rapid reorganization of the child's phonological system but we take a dynamic systems approach to the process of facilitating the emergence of new behaviors. In this section we discuss the principles of this approach in relation to a case study first reported in Rvachew and Bernhardt (2010). It might be helpful to review the Introduction to Part I before proceeding with this section.

We strongly recommend against the complexity approach to the selection of treatment goals.

We are not advocating a strictly developmental approach to the selection of treatment goals because it will be difficult for the child to "catch up" with the normal trajectory following this approach.

We recommend a **dynamic systems approach** to the process of facilitating the emergence of new behaviors.

New behaviors can be seen to emerge from the complex interactions among multiple developmental domains coupled with task demands and environmental supports. From the dynamic systems perspective, it is not necessary to "set" a parameter in order to trigger the appearance of a new class of speech sounds. Rather, we begin by identifying the subcomponents that are necessary for the emergence of a new behavior paying particular attention to those

New behaviors can be seen to emerge from the complex interactions among multiple developmental domains coupled with task demands and environmental supports.

subcomponents that are not in place. As a consequence of the principle of nonlinearity, a therapy approach that induces gradual, linear changes in the appropriate subcomponents will lead to reorganization at the macroscopic level. The solution to the problem will be specific to each individual child because of individual variability in the developmental time tables for each of the components as well as the child's history of environmental input. If we consider TS30 (see Case Study 8–5), it is clear that the addition of new sound classes, specifically affricates and liquids, would be of significant benefit to this child. Figure 8–5 proposes exogenous and endogenous supports for the emergence of a new sound class in this child's system, focusing specifically on the affricates. A detailed description of TS30's progress in therapy during Block 1 will serve to illustrate how linear, incremental changes in these subcomponents led to the emergence of a new form, the palatoalveolar affricate /tʃ/, during this period, even though she never received intervention for this phoneme. As this child was assigned to the ME condition, the treatment goals were /m/(ambisyllabic) and /s/(codas) during the first block, representing type 4 phonological knowledge. In the second block, /l/(onsets) and /ʃ/(codas) were targeted, also representing type 4 productive phonological knowledge but introducing a new manner class and a new place of articulation relative to the block 1 goals.

As a consequence of the principle of **nonlinearity**, a therapy approach that induces gradual, linear changes in the appropriate subcomponents will lead to reorganization at the macroscopic level.

Figure 8–5 indicates that certain biological and environmental supports are the foundation for all aspects of language learning and are considered first. This child was very shy and reluctant to engage with the SLP for the first few sessions and actually reported that she had "no fun at all" during those sessions when responding to a pictograph-based questionnaire. Fortunately, the child was assigned the most experienced and effective SLP in the project who coached the mother to lead the speech therapy activities for the first few sessions and gradually built up rapport with the child to the extent that she was able to take over leading the activities by session 4 and the mother was able to leave the room briefly in session 5. The child reported having "lots of fun" for sessions 4 through 12 although sporadic refusals to engage in certain activities continued in the second therapy block. To further to the issue of environmental supports, the mother was very motivated to help the child improve her speech, engaging fully in all therapy sessions, completing all homework activities and asking for additional activities to target untreated sounds (e.g., /k/, although these materials were not provided until after the 12 week intervention was completed). The treatment program itself was essentially behaviorist in nature, providing many models of the target sounds, informative feedback about the child's attempts to produce those sounds, and both tangible and social reinforcement for correct responses. It is likely that these external motivational factors coupled with gradual improvements in the child's attitude toward speech therapy played a major role in her outcomes over the course of the intervention.

Certain biological and environmental supports are the foundation for all aspects of language learning and must be considered in treatment planning.

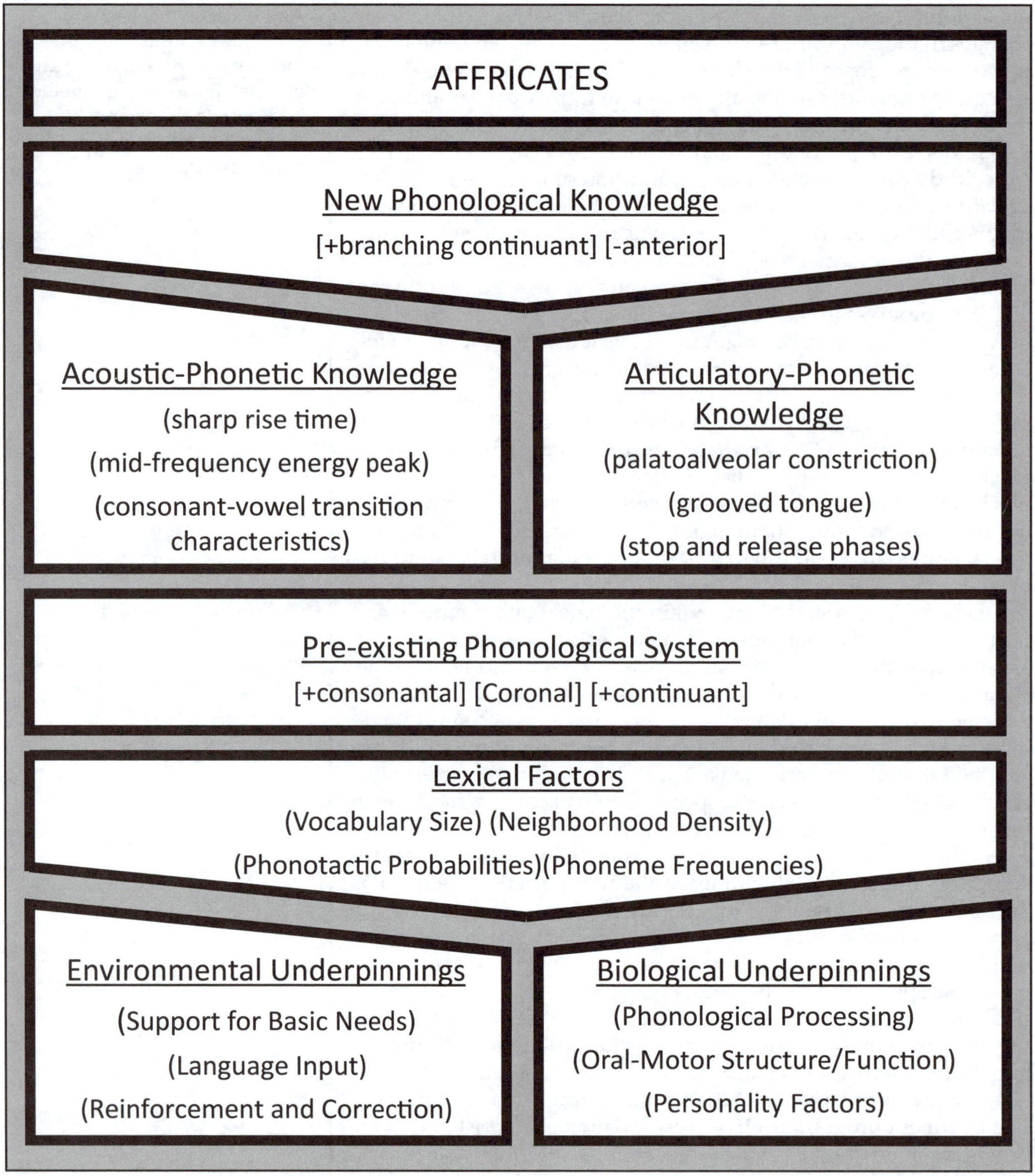

Figure 8–5. *Illustration of the endogenous and exogenous components that interact to explain the emergence of affricates in phonological development. From Rvachew and Bernhardt, 2010, Figure 1, p. 36. Reproduced with permission of American Speech-Language-Hearing Association in the format Textbook via Copyright Clearance Center.*

Turning to biological supports, there was no indication of oral-motor weaknesses as a cause of the child's difficulties. She passed an examination of oral structure and function and achieved stimulability for all target phonemes at the word level in 15 minutes or less. Unfortunately, no measures of speech perception or phonological processing were included as part of the assessment protocol for this study. However, there were some indications of possible difficulties with perceptual and/or phonological knowledge of phoneme contrasts. For example, even as she gradually reduced the frequency of stop substitutions for the interdental fricatives, she used [Labial] instead of [Coronal] substitutions, suggesting some perceptual confusion. Finally, in terms of basic supports, there were no obvious issues with lexical factors because her language comprehension skills were more than one standard deviation above average for her age.

Moving on to strengths and needs in her preexisting phonological system, the A1 assessment revealed that she did not have fully stable knowledge of the hypothesized prerequisite features for affricates: [+consonantal], [Coronal], or [+continuant]. Although [+consonantal] was consistently matched in stops, fricatives were frequently produced as glides in word onsets and stops elsewhere; although [+sonorant] was consistently matched in the glides, the liquids and the nasals were sometimes produced as stops and fricatives were sometimes produce with nasal emission. Altogether, there was a lack of consistent contrast between the [+consonantal] and [+sonorant] sound classes. Similarly, her knowledge of [Labial] versus [Coronal] place was almost but not fully stable: she matched those place features consistently in stops, nasals, and liquids, but used labials for interdental fricative targets. Her knowledge of [+continuant] was emerging with a match ratio of .15 reflecting mastery of [h] and very occasional use of [s] and [z], usually in word onsets. One goal for the first treatment block was to stabilize her knowledge of [+continuant] by targeting [s] in codas. In other words, the intervention involved promoting a linear (incremental) increase in the use of an emerging form ([+continuant]) rather than prompting a sudden, nonlinear change by introducing a new form ([+branching continuant]). Correct use of /m/ in the ambisyllabic position was also targeted during this block.

During the course of the treatment block a number of phonetic and phonological improvements occurred that laid the foundation for the emergence of the affricate. Overall, her knowledge of major manner classes improved; nasals were produced more accurately and fricatives were produced less often as glides. Further differentiation of the major manner classes occurred with a contrast between stops and fricatives (e.g., /p/ vs. /f/) within the obstruent class, and between glides and liquids (e.g., /j/ vs. /l/) within the sonorant class becoming reasonably well established during the first six weeks of intervention. Nasal emission was eliminated in her speech. With respect to the fricative treatment target, she quickly achieved stimulability for /s/, learning to produce the grooved tongue posture necessary for the sibilant acoustic output, and to coordinate the transition from the voiced vowel to the voiceless fricative. Subsequently, she made steady progress through the imitated and spontaneous phrase and sentence level activities. The match ratio for [+continuant] more than doubled between A1 and A2. Furthermore, she extended the use of the [+continuant] feature to target fricatives that were produced as stops or glides at A1 (specifically [f,v,θ,ð,ʃ]). Other changes in her phonological system also played a role. Her use of the feature [-anterior] was extended from [j] to [ɹ] and [ʃ], resulting in an increase in the match ratio from .09 to .39, and resulting in contrastive use of this feature within the fricative and liquid sound classes. These changes provided a firm foundation for the emergence of [+branching continuant] and subsequent integration with newly established features such as [−anterior] to form the affricate [tʃ].

It is clear that a hierarchical relationship among skills is invoked in this account of the child's phonological progress here. The hierarchy is not a preformed structure of abstract parameters that can be switched on all at once as if they were interlinked Christmas tree lights. Rather, the child's knowledge of increasingly complex sound classes emerges as a function of experience with the sensorimotor (phonetic) substrate of the phonological system. Green et al. (2000) identified two mechanisms of speech motor learning that allow for the emergence of new behaviors: differentiation (the modification of a preexisting behavior into more specialized ones) and integration (the integration of new behaviors with previously stabilized behaviors). In our description of TS30's progress above we have described the emergence of new sound classes as a kind of phonological differentiation, in which stabilization of the consonant-sonorant contrast allowed for the emergence of a stop-fricative contrast and stabilization of this contrast in turn led to the emergence of an affricate. In a further parallel between speech motor learning and phonological change, developmental regressions can occur in both domains. For example, Green et al. (2002) recount that reductions in jaw stability occurred as toddlers began the process of differentiating control of lip movements from jaw movements. We point out that TS30 demonstrated a regression in her acquisition of nasals when liquids were introduced in the second treatment block, perhaps reflecting the task of further differentiating the recently stabilized sonorant and obstruent sound classes into finer categories.

The emergence of new sound classes during therapy may be an example of **phonological differentiation**.

In a further parallel between speech motor learning and phonological change, developmental **regressions** can occur in both domains.

The second motor learning process, integration, can also be observed in TS30's phonological development. We have described the extension of features from one manner class to another, for example, [−anterior] from glides to liquids and then to fricatives (and affricates), as a form of integration that again requires some minimum degree of stabilization of use of the feature in one context before it is generalized to another. This is analogous to the pattern of development observed in Green et al. (2000), in which stabilization of lip control did not emerge until after a stable pattern of mandibular control was established. Note that Green et al.'s data

Integration also appears to play a role in phonological learning as the child extends the use of a feature from one manner class to another.

do not mean that lip control is impossible at earlier ages than those reported for stabilization of jaw control. In fact, young children do accomplish sophisticated lip movements during eating and drinking by providing themselves with external sources of support for the jaw through bite-stabilization on the spoon or cup. Nonetheless, in the early phases of learning to control the lips, external or internal stabilization of the jaw is necessary. Similarly, it seems unlikely that the palatoalveolar affricates could be successfully introduced into a system that was characterized by unstable knowledge of major manner and place contrasts such as stop-nasal and labial-coronal; indeed this pattern was not observed in any of the children enrolled in the Rvachew and Nowak (2001) trial.

These findings directly challenge Gierut's (2007) contention that, during speech therapy, "the child must be provided with crucial input about these more complex components [in order to learn] the remaining outlying structures of the target language" (p. 8). Although it is undeniably true that a child who receives no exposure to complex phonological structures will never acquire them, the data in this paper show that it is false to presume that phonological change in children with DPD requires that the SLP target only complex phonological structures. In the context of children receiving intervention for DPD, it is crucial to remember that the largest part of language input available to the child is provided outside of the clinic. The goal of the speech therapy program must be to position the child to benefit from that input.

Thus far, we have been focusing on phonemes as treatment targets. Selecting goals at the prosodic levels of the phonological hierarchy is necessary for the success of the treatment program however. In the next section we demonstrate the selection of treatment goals, using a multilinear analysis of the child's phonology.

Application of Multilinear Phonology to the Selection of Treatment Goals

Bernhardt and colleagues describe goal selection from the perspective of multilinear phonology in many publications (Bernhardt, 1992; Bernhardt & Gilbert, 1992; Bernhardt & Stemberger, 2000; Bernhardt, Stemberger, & Major, 2006; Bernhardt & Stoel-Gammon, 1994). Identification of the child's strengths and needs at multiple levels of the phonological hierarchy is combined with a description of strengths and needs in other developmental domains (perceptual, motoric, cognitive, psychosocial, semantic, syntactic, and pragmatic) to derive a treatment plan. We recommend the excellent case study by Bernhardt et al. (2006) that describes a comprehensive approach to treatment planning that considers every aspect of Jarrod's development, a case that is featured in a special issue of *Advances in Speech-Language Pathology* with extensive test data and video documentation (McLeod, 2006).

Identification of the child's **strengths and needs** at multiple levels of the phonological hierarchy is combined with a description of strengths and needs in other developmental domains to derive a treatment plan that is consistent with the principles of multilinear phonology.

General principles of goal selection from the perspective of multilinear perspective are listed in Table 8–4 and demonstrated for Amber whose speech data was presented in Chapter 6 (Case Study 6–2). This child, aged 4;8 when she started therapy, was a delightfully friendly little girl who enjoyed her speech therapy sessions. Unfortunately, however, she was experiencing significant upheavals in her home life so it was never certain who would be completing the assigned speech homework exercises and it often was not the individual who attended therapy sessions. It was important that these exercises be designed to minimize interpersonal conflict and maximize success. For this reason, treatment goals that serve to extend the use of stimulable phonemes and stabilize the use of emerging syllable structures are the most appropriate choices.

The multilinear analysis of Amber's speech, summarized in Table 6–7, suggests an overall strength in syllable marking. Delinking of the [+consonantal] feature from voiced obstruents and nasals in ambisyllabic contexts serves to weaken second syllables in trochees however. This is an unusual pattern that significantly impacts the intelligibility of Amber's speech. Therefore, encouraging inclusion of [+consonantal][+voiced] segments and [+consonantal][Nasal] segments in the ambisyllabic position of trochees is an important first goal. Given that [Labial] place is the only nondefault stimulable place of articulation, CVbV(C) and CVmV(C) words are the logical specific targets for the initial treatment sessions. After achieving success with these early developing phonemes, expanding her repertoire of phones in this position to include /v/ can be attempted; incorporating this trochaic structure into three and four syllable words will also serve to extend her emerging knowledge of this prosodic structure.

Table 8–4. *Principles of Goal Selection from the Multilinear Perspective*

1. Take into account all factors associated with the child's DPD (perceptual, motoric, cognitive, psychosocial, linguistic).
2. Determine strengths and needs at all levels of the phonological hierarchy (phrase, word, syllable structure, segment, feature, and associations between tiers).
3. Identify the child's default structures; be aware that these defaults may not correspond to the default/markedness relationships hypothesized for the adult system.
4. Use a horizontal or cycles goal attack strategy to alternate between prosodic and segmental goals within a given treatment block, starting with prosodic goals.
5. Strengths are used as supports for needs; that is, new syllable structures are targeted with established segments while new segments/features are introduced in the context of established word shapes/syllable structures.
6. With respect to segmental goals, marked features are targeted in emerging segments.
7. More complex and unstimulable segments may be introduced if the child is a "risk-taker" but avoided for children who need to experience immediate success.

With the exception of a single [ts] in word final position, complex onsets and codas are completely absent in Amber's speech although there is evidence that these elements are represented underlyingly. The high frequency of words with complex onsets and codas in English enhance the impact of this pattern on the intelligibility of Amber's speech and thus it is important to tackle this prosodic structure early. We can expect that she might have early success if the goal is to increase her use of stop + /s/ sequences in codas and then extend her use of complex codas to include nasal + stop sequences. The final prosodic mismatch, occasional resyllabification of words with nasals in the coda (e.g., CVm → CVmV), appears to be resolving spontaneously and need not be targeted in therapy.

Considering potential segmental targets, the analysis revealed good matching for [+consonantal][+continuant] segments in the coda to be a strength but [+continuant] was never matched in the context of supralaryngeal obstruents in the onset position. In other circumstances, we might like to target /ʃ/ as a means to discourage Amber's strong preference for [Labial] in onsets but given that she is not stimulable for this phoneme we opt for /f,v/ as the initial target, in this case avoiding the default [Coronal] place. The choice of /f/ or /v/ when the intermediate goal is [+consonantal][+continuant][Labial] may require a brief period of stimulability testing to determine which phone is easiest for the child to produce in CV syllables. Bernhardt and Stoel-Gammon (1994) recommend /v/ because [+continuant] is redundant with [+voice] and with the following vowel and thus should be a facilitating context for introducing [+consonantal][+continuant] into the onset position. However, word frequency plays a role in facilitating generalization of learning and /v/ has low frequency in English. Given that Amber has good knowledge of the voicing contrast in onsets, she may have success when both are targeted during the same treatment block.

In our experience, three goals in a given treatment block, whether using a horizontal or cycles goal attack strategy, is typically the most either the child or SLP can handle. Any more than three goals would reduce the cumulative intervention intensity per goal to unacceptable levels. In a 12-week treatment block this plan will have a marked effect on the intelligibility of Amber's speech by stabilizing her production of weak syllables in trochees, thus facilitating the emergence of complex codas and extending her use of the fricative sound class from the coda to the onset position of words. During a second 12-week treatment block, Amber will be well positioned to acquire /s/+stop and /s/+nasal clusters in the onset position. It will also be time to introduce a new place of articulation, either [−anterior] or [Dorsal] depending on the results of stimulability testing. Given a developmental approach, [Dorsal] consonants in the coda position would be the likely starting point, moving on to [Dorsal] in the onset as soon as possible. Increasing the use of these marked place features would result in a spontaneous reduction in the spreading of [Labial] from coda to onset that is so common in Amber's speech.

Finally, introducing the last major sound class to her system by targeting [+lateral] in the [+consonantal][+sonorant] segment /l/ would be a good third goal. We would begin with /l/ in the onset and then introduce the second liquid /ɹ/ later in the treatment block if she experiences early success with /l/. Given that /l/ in the coda is later developing than /l/ in the onset and that vowelization of liquids in this position does not have a severe impact on intelligibility, we would not see /l/ in the coda as a high priority goal for this treatment block.

The recommended intermediate and specific goals for the first and second treatment blocks are shown in Table 8–5. Alternative specific goals are shown in case Amber achieves good progress with the first specific goal before the end of the treatment block which is quite likely given 12-week treatment blocks. If she were treated in two 6-week blocks, the same treatment plan could be followed but the specific goals would be restricted to the primary goals.

We point out that the goals selected for Amber are consistent with neither the complexity approach nor a traditional approach based on developmental norms. Rather, the approach reflects our view of phonological development from a dynamic systems per-

Table 8–5. *Recommended Treatment Goals for Amber (Case Study 6–2) Using a Multilinear Phonological Analysis to Select Goals and a Horizontal Goal Attack Strategy over Two 12-Week Blocks*

Intermediate Goal	*Primary Specific Goal*	*Secondary Specific Goal*[a]
Treatment Block 1		
[+consonantal] in [+voice] or [Nasal] ambisyllabic segments (i.e., reduce weakening of second syllables in trochees)	1. 'CVbV(C), e.g., "rabbit" 2. 'CVmV(C) e.g., "tummy"	1. CV'CVCV(C), C_3 = voiced stop or nasal e.g., "pajama" 2. 'CVCV(C), C_2 = voiced fricative, e.g., "beaver"
Complex codas	1. CVCs or CVCVCs, e.g., "mops" (verb), "peanuts"	1. CVCC, C_2 = nasal, e.g., "jump," "dance"
[+consonantal][+continuant] in onsets	1. fVC(VC), e.g., "feet" 2. vVC(VC), e.g., "van"	1. ʃVC, e.g., "sheet" 2. ʃVv(VC), e.g., "shovel"
Treatment Block 2[b]		
Complex onsets	1. sCVC(VC), e.g., spot	1. ClCVC(VC), e.g., "plane"
[Dorsal]	1. CVk, e.g., "pack" 2. CVg, e.g., "mug"	1. kVC, e.g., "cake" 2. gVC, e.g., "game"
[+consonantal][+sonorant]	1. lVC(VC), e.g., "lamb"	2. ɹVC(VC), e.g., "rake"

[a]Secondary Specific Goal is introduced only if Amber reaches criterion level performance on the Primary Specific Goal and spontaneous achievement of the Secondary Specific Goal is not observed before the end of the treatment block.

[b]Treatment Block 2 begins after 12 weeks regardless of Amber's level of performance on the goals targeted in Treatment Block 1.

spective. Following Grunwell's (1992) advice, the first priority was to stabilize a highly variable structure because instability is a marker of "incipient change." The variable production of labial obstruents in the ambisyllabic position as [w j t s] is also devastating to the intelligibility of Amber's speech. We are expecting that the stabilization of /b, m/ in the ambisyllabic position will have a widespread impact on her phonological system, not only reducing the delinking of [+consonantal] in this position but also reducing the delinking and spreading of [Labial] from ambisyllabic and coda positions to the onset as well as the resyllabification of words with /m/ in the coda.

The first priority was to stabilize a highly variable structure because instability may be a marker of incipient change.

As was described for TS30 above, it is expected that facilitating gradual change in known features and structures by extending their use from one context to another will lay the groundwork for system expansion with the introduction of new features and phonemes. One first block goal will increase frequency of /s/-clusters in the coda and extend knowledge of complex codas to nasal clusters. Another first block target serves to extend Amber's knowledge of [+continuant] from the coda to the onset. She should experience rapid success with the stimulable targets /f,v/ in the onset at which time she will be ready to attempt /ʃ/. Given that she has underlying knowledge of /s/+clusters in the onset position, there is a chance that these might emerge spontaneously once [+continuant] in onsets is established. Success with [−anterior] in /ʃ/ may facilitate emergence of /tʃ/ and /ɹ/ especially after introduction of the liquid /l/.

Facilitating gradual change in known features and structures by extending their use from one context to another will lay the groundwork for system expansion.

Notice that we plan to introduce several new phonemes that are relatively late developing although the fricative /ʃ/ and the liquids /l/ and /ɹ/ are second rather than first choices for treatment goals. We are hoping that she will experience rapid success with the earlier developing targets allowing us to move to later developing phonemes before the end of the treatment blocks. The choice of phonemes as treatment goals is not constrained by the age of mastery for the phonemes relative to the child's age. In other words it is not necessary to wait until Amber is 5;0 to introduce /l/ or 5;6 to introduce /v/ or 6;0 to introduce /ʃ/. We approach the task like teaching a child to ride a bike: at 2 years parents provide a tricycle so that the child learns to pedal and steer; at age 3 parents often provide a bicycle but with training wheels so that the child learns to handle speed and braking without fear of falling over; at age 4 parents may provide a scooter which allows the child to learn to balance independently of the pedaling function; at age 5 the training wheels are removed but a parent provides physical support and verbal guidance as long as needed. With speech sounds we can introduce late developing phonemes at a young age as long as some basic foundational skills are in place and we offer sufficient support; we do not expect the child to achieve full mastery all at once; we know that we can reintroduce the phoneme again in the future with as much or as little support as the child needs until independence and consistency in the production of the phoneme is achieved. This is the philosophy that underlies the cycles approach, that is outlined next.

Finally we plan to introduce several new phonemes that are relatively late developing.

Cycles Remediation Approach

We discuss the Cycles Remediation Approach because speech sample analysis and goal selection based on phonological processes remains widespread and overall more accessible to SLPs than the multilinear approach. We feel that, for beginning clinicians, this highly structured approach can be a good choice when treating children who have moderate to severe DPD. The approach is well described in two books (Hodson, 2007; Hodson & Paden, 1983), target selection is based on an easy to use and interpret computerized-assessment tool (Hodson, 2004), and there is empirical evidence to support the efficacy of the intervention (Almost & Rosenbaum, 1998). However, the approach is designed to accelerate normal development and is meant to be implemented with high intensity over a long duration. Therefore, if your services are rationed to a fixed number of weeks of service per year, this may not be the most appropriate approach to use because very minimal gains are observed in the short term. Details about the treatment procedures are provided in Chapter 11. Here we discuss the selection of treatment goals and the cycles goal attack strategy.

The cycles approach is meant to be implemented with high intensity over a long duration.

Hodson (2007) defines a cycle as a period of time during which all of the selected target patterns for a given child are presented. Cycle duration is individualized for each child because it is determined by the number of pattern deficiencies that are identified for that child as potential intermediate targets and the number of stimulable phonemes that are available as potential specific targets. Phonological patterns are recycled during subsequent cycles while gradually increasing complexity, either by increasing the complexity of the phonetic environments in which a phoneme is targeted or by introducing more complex phoneme targets for a given pattern deficiency. Recycling of a target pattern is discontinued when generalization to conversation occurs, typically after 2 or 3 cycles. Each phoneme within a target pattern receives 60 minutes of treatment per cycle and each pattern is targeted for 2 or more hours per cycle.

A **cycle** is a period of time during which all selected target patterns for a given child are presented.

Phonological patterns are recycled during subsequent cycles while gradually increasing complexity.

Recycling of a target pattern is discontinued when generalization to conversation occurs, typically after 2 or 3 cycles.

Each phoneme within a target pattern receives 60 minutes of treatment per cycle and each pattern is targeted for 2 or more hours per cycle.

Specific guidelines for the selection and ordering of patterns are provided, as summarized in Table 8–6. Returning again to Amber's speech sample in Case Study 6–2, we can identify patterns that would be targeted according to this approach. We analyzed Amber's speech sample using the HAPP-3 (Hodson, 2004) and the following phonological patterns were identified as potential targets for intervention: Consonant Sequences, Prevocalic Liquids, Glides, Stridents, and Velars. As shown in Chapter 6, some of the major patterns in Amber's phonological system are missed by this analysis. However, the remaining patterns are clearly pervasive and deleterious to her speech intelligibility so there is no doubt that targeting issues such as consonant cluster reduction and velar fronting would have a beneficial effect on Amber's communicative effectiveness. A proposed treatment plan based on the cycles approach is shown in Table 8–7. The intermediate goals are Velars, Consonant Sequences,

Table 8–6. Cycles Remediation Approach: Target Patterns in Preferred Order of Selection

Pattern	Target
Primary Targets	
Word structures (omissions)	Stops, nasals, and glides in CV syllables compound words and 2 to 3 word phrases CVC (word final consonants) VCV (within word consonants)
Anterior-posterior contrasts	Fronting of velars, and/or Backing of alveolar or labial consonants
/s/ clusters	Stimulable word initial clusters Stimulable word-final clusters
Liquids	Word initial /l/ or /ɹ/ at the end of each cycle
Secondary Targets	
Palatals	/j, ʃ, tʃ, dʒ, ɝ, ɚ/
Other consonant sequences	Word internal sequences Glide clusters
Singleton stridents	/s/ or /f/
Voicing contrasts	
Assimilations	
Any remaining idiosyncratic patterns	

Source: Summarized from Hodson (2007), Hodson and Paden (1983), and Hodson (1989).

Table 8–7. Cycles Remediation Approach: Proposed Treatment Plan for Amber (First Four Cycles)

Cycle	Intermediate Goal	Specific Goal
I	Velars	/k/, word final, e.g., "make"
I	/s/ Clusters	/ts/, word final, e.g., "hats"
I	Liquids	/l/, word initial, e.g., "lime"
II	Velars	/g/, word initial, e.g., "go"
II	/s/ Clusters	/st/, word initial, e.g., "stop"
II	Liquids	/ɹ/, word intial, e.g., "read"
III	Velars	/g/, word final, e.g., "dog"
III	/s/ Clusters	/sp/, /sm/, word initial, e.g., "spoon"
III	Liquids	/pɹ/, /dɹ/, word initial, e.g., "drip"
IV	Velars	/gl/, /gɹ/, word initial, e.g., "glass"
IV	/s/ Clusters	/sk/, word final, e.g., "mask"
IV	Liquids	/ɹ/, word intial, e.g., "road"

and Liquids. Glides were omitted because improvements in the production of glides would have less impact on her intelligibility and the errors largely concerned consonant sequences. The issue with stridents is a "side effect" of stopping and is expected to resolve itself after working on /s/-clusters. Hodson recommends that a few minutes of each session be devoted to promoting stimulability of potential future phoneme targets and thus we assume that each target will be stimulable at the point that it is actually introduced in the therapy sequence. Notice that the work in each week is expected to facilitate the emergence of specific targets introduced in subsequent weeks. For example, the /ɹ/ clusters introduced in week 9 appears to be a difficult structure to target as a means of achieving Liquids as an intermediate goal but we have been targeting Liquids, Velars, and Clusters in previous weeks and clusters are a facilitative context for the emergence of /ɹ/ (Curtis & Hardy, 1959). The /sk/ cluster is only introduced when other /s/ clusters and the velar is well established. Practice with /ɹ/ in the context of rounded vowels is delayed until it is sure that the child can inhibit labialization of /ɹ/ in difficult words such as "road" and "rooster." The "plan" shown in Table 8–7 presumes very good progress with the proposed specific goals; in actual practice, specific goals would be determined from week to week on the basis of stimulability probes that occur at the end of each session and therefore long-term planning of intermediate goals is possible but the specific goals are entirely determined by the child's progress as the treatment program unfolds. If the child was struggling with the acquisition of the velar targets or if the child proved to be unstimulable for the velar clusters the specific targets would be very different. For example, the SLP could reprise the specific goal "/k/, word final" in Cycle III and repeat "/g/, word initial" in Cycle IV but expand from the word to the phrase level of production in each case.

Clusters are a facilitative context for the emergence of /ɹ/.

The recycling of these targets is discontinued when carry-over to conversation is observed. If the child is showing carryover of the targeted intermediate and specific goals to conversation by the end of Cycle IV, for example, a new set of secondary targets can be tackled in a new series of cycles. For Amber, these goals would be the palatals, any prevocalic stridents and clusters that did not emerge spontaneously, and resolution of the idiosyncratic pattern in the ambisyllabic position if this pattern was still present in her speech.

How is the cycles approach to goal selection different from the multilinear approach? Although the cycles approach is tied to the cycles goal attack strategy, this is not the unique feature of the remediation approach. The goals presented in Table 8–5 could be treated using any goal attack strategy and, in fact, Bernhardt (1992) describes an approach that is very similar to a cycles goal attack strategy. An obvious difference, of course, is the analysis itself, as discussed in Chapter 6. The multilinear analysis has led to a primary focus on interactions between the segmental and prosodic tiers in

Amber's speech, highlighting delinking rules that affect the production of the trochaic prosodic structure in particular and that serve to protect her preference for [Labial] in onsets and [Coronal] in non-onset syllable positions. These patterns will not be discovered by a computer-based phonological process analysis although an alert clinician might classify the mismatches in question as unusual patterns of fronting/backing or idiosyncratic phonological rules if a careful phonological process analysis were conducted by hand.

A second difference between the sets of goals shown in Tables 8–5 and 8–7 is that we opted to target singleton fricatives in the onset position and /s/-clusters and nasal clusters in the coda position before introducing complex onsets in the second treatment block when selecting goals from the multilinear analysis. In contrast, Hodson (2007) recommends that /s/-clusters be targeted very early in the treatment program. The rationale is that children who stop fricatives may find it easier to learn /s/-clusters than singleton /s/. The child will not have to inhibit the intervening stop between the strident and the vowel and Hodson claims that the /s/ is less likely to be distorted when taught in the cluster context.

Disregarding this difference in the ordering of the goals and given a 24-week treatment period both treatment plans would cover roughly the same intermediate treatment goals (velars, clusters, fricatives in singleton and/or cluster contexts, liquids, and palatals). The major difference is the focus on ambisyllabic obstruents and nasals, included in the multilinear plan but excluded from the cycles approach. It is difficult to predict the impact of missing a primary organizing characteristic of Amber's phonology at the prosodic level on the outcome of the treatment program.[4] Given this uncertainty we recommend multilinear analysis as providing the most complete description of a child's phonology and the soundest footing for the selection of treatment goals.

A **multilinear analysis** provides the most complete description of a child's phonology and the soundest footing for the selection of treatment goals.

[4]For those of you who are curious to know what actually happened with Amber, she made excellent progress when treated with a phonological process approach and a horizontal goal attack strategy. A phonological process analysis, carefully conducted by hand using procedures outlined by Ingram (1981), revealed the issue with ambisyllabic consonants as the priority. In the first 6 months, the goals were voiced obstruents and nasals in the ambisyllabic position and fricatives in the onset position. During the second 6 months, liquids in the onset position, velars in all word positions, and clusters in word initial and final positions were targeted. For each intermediate goal, all possible specific goals were targeted in a horizontal fashion. For example, focusing on the ambisyllabic consonant, we practiced words such as rabbit, table, poodle, pudding, tummy, banana, honey, beaver, heavy, feather, mother, fuzzy, puzzle, and treasure, more or less simultaneously during the first 6-month treatment period. After one year of therapy Amber achieved normalized speech accuracy with all phonemes mastered except /θ,ð,ɹ/ and no syllable structure errors remaining. Five years after she was discharged, Bernhardt and Stoel-Gammon's (1994) published their seminal paper introducing multilinear analysis to the SLP community. The relevance of the approach to this complex case led to its early adoption by the first author.

Instructional Objectives

Each session must also have goals, called **instructional objectives**, that are ordered in a logical fashion so as to achieve the intermediate and specific goals.

Each instructional objective has 3 components: (1) a **"do" statement**, (2) a **condition**, and (3) an **accuracy statement**.

Thus far, we have discussed treatment goals for relatively long time intervals with the basic goal covering the interval between the initiation of treatment and discharge from the treatment program and intermediate and specific goals being targeted repeatedly over the course of a given treatment block that may last from 6 to 24 weeks in duration, as we saw in our review of service delivery practices. Achievement of these goals requires that the SLP plan to implement procedures and activities during each session in a treatment block. Each session must also have goals that are ordered in a logical fashion so as to achieve the intermediate and specific goals. These session goals are called the instructional objectives and have a specific form (Mowrer, 1989). Each instructional objective has 3 components: (1) a "do" statement, (2) a condition, and (3) an accuracy statement. The "do" statement is an objective description of what the child will do during each trial of the activity. The condition statement describes the conditions under which the child will complete the task described in the "do" statement and must include at least the antecedent event. In addition to describing the event that precipitates the child's response on each trial, the SLP may also specify what will happen in the event of correct and incorrect responses on the part of the child. Finally, the level of accuracy that indicates achievement of the objective is stated so that the SLP knows when the objective has been reached. When the stated level of accuracy has been achieved it is time to introduce the next more complex instructional objective in the sequence; when the terminal objective in the sequence has been mastered a new specific goal can be introduced. The appropriate level of accuracy that should be required varies with the treatment approach, the overall goals of the treatment program, the specific goal, and the nature of the instructional objective itself as discussed further in Part III. In general, higher levels of accuracy are required when teaching phonetic skills whereas lower levels of accuracy are accepted when facilitating phonological change. Some examples of possible instructional objectives are shown in Table 8–8.

Monitoring Treatment Progress

Treatment planning is a dynamic process in which the selection and ordering of specific goals and instructional objectives undergoes continuous updating to adapt to the current status of the child's phonological knowledge.

The discussion thus far reveals that treatment planning is a dynamic rather than static process. An initial set of intermediate goals can be selected from the analysis of the child's speech at the onset of the treatment program but the selection and ordering of specific goals and instructional objectives will undergo continuous updating to adapt to the current status of the child's phonological knowledge. An effective intervention will result in rapid and sometimes dramatic changes in the child's phonological system and, thus, the treatment plan may need significant and frequent adjustments. Some children may not be responding to the treatment or may

Table 8–8. *Unpacking Instructional Objectives: Selected Hypothetical Examples for Treatment of [+consonantal][+continuant]*

Session	*Instructional Objective*
1	Amber will *identify correct productions of the word "feet"* when presented with recordings of correct and incorrect versions of the word (e.g., [fit], [pit], [sit], [θit] etc.) with **95% accuracy over 20 trials**.
2	Amber will *articulate /f/ in the words "feet," "fan," "face," "funny," and "fairy"* when shown pictures and asked, "What is this?" with **80% accuracy over 20 trials**.
3	Amber will *articulate /f/ in a phrase containing the word "feet" (e.g., "big feet," "small feet," "green feet," "two toed feet")* when asked, "What kind of feet should we draw on this monster?" with **80% accuracy over 5 trials**.
5	Amber will *correctly articulate /f/ in sentences* with **at least 45% accuracy** while talking about picture books **for 15 minutes**.
7	Amber will *imitate /v/ in the words "van," "vine," "vole," "village," and "Venus"* when presented with model sentences (e.g., "We went for a drive in the van.") with **80% accuracy over 20 trials**.
9	Amber will *round her lips when imitating* /ʃ/ presented in isolation on **5 consecutive trials.**

DO statement shown in italics; CONDITION is underlined; **ACCURACY statement shown in bold.**

respond slowly and the SLP will need to decide when to change treatment goals or procedures in order to prompt a more rapid rate of change in the child's phonology. Good clinical decision-making requires frequent monitoring of the child's progress. Olswang and Bain (1994) recommend that a program of quantitative and qualitative data collection be planned to address 3 questions: (1) Is the child responding to the treatment program? (2) Is significant and important change occurring? and (3) Is treatment responsible for the change?

Good clinical practice requires continuous adaptation to the child's changing status and thus it is essential to include a **progress monitoring plan** as part of the treatment planning process.

Determining whether the child is responding to the treatment program requires monitoring of the child's achievement of instructional objectives and specific goals. The adequacy of the data is entirely dependent on the quality of the instructional objectives as defined above: the objectives must identify a measurable behavior and the conditions under which the response is expected. The measure of progress includes both the accuracy of the child's responses and the amount of support that the child needs to achieve accurate responses. For example, the child who can produce 6 of 10 /f/ targets correctly while retelling a story has achieved a higher level of performance than a child who can imitate /f/ in words with 100% accuracy but consistently stops all fricatives while naming pictures spontaneously. Olswang and Bain (1994) pointed out that recording the accuracy of every response during therapy sessions interferes with the interaction between the child and SLP. Furthermore, performance during practice may not predict retention of the target

Recording the accuracy of every response during therapy sessions interferes with the interaction between the child and SLP.

Probe achievement of instructional objectives at *prespecified sampling intervals* to determine achievement of specific goals.

skills (Maas et al., 2008) and therefore specific probes scheduled to occur during prespecified sampling intervals will provide a better indication of learning. For example, if we consider the sequence of instructional objectives shown in Table 8–8, the SLP can estimate the child's achievement of the phrase level objective in session 4, indicating that a new instructional objective targeting longer sentences should be introduced. The terminal objective in the sequence for /f/ (correct productions while producing a narrative about pictures) would be a good time to record each response to be sure that the child has achieved the objective before introducing a new goal. Monitoring of progress during treatment may prompt a change in the intermediate goal when the child fails to change. An alternative scenario to the rapid progress hypothesized in Table 8–8 has the child failing to achieve stimulability for /f/ in syllables; for example, after 20 trials without success the SLP researches new procedures for stimulating production of /fV/ syllables; after 40 trials without change the SLP changes the specific goal to syllables that begin with /v/; after 60 trials without change, the SLP changes the intermediate goal to /s/-clusters. Barring these exceptional circumstances where unwise selection of goals or treatment approach leads to a complete lack of progress on the part of the child, the goal of monitoring treatment progress is to make decisions about the introduction of new instructional objectives toward the achievement of a given specific or intermediate goal.

The goal of monitoring treatment progress is to make decisions about the introduction of new instructional objectives toward the achievement of a given specific or intermediate goal.

Significant and important change is indexed by the amount of stimulus and response generalization that is observed.

Stimulus generalization occurs when the child transfers responses that were taught in therapy to new stimulus conditions (e.g., nontherapy contexts and to communication with individuals who are not the SLP).

Response generalization occurs when change occurs in items that are related to but not the same as the specific therapy targets.

Significant and important change is indexed by the amount of stimulus and response generalization that is observed. Stimulus generalization occurs when the child transfers items that were taught in therapy to nontherapy contexts and to communication with individuals who are not the SLP or other therapy agents. Response generalization occurs when change occurs in items that are related to but not the same as the specific therapy targets. Qualitative reports of stimulus and response generalization from family members, teachers, or other significant individuals in the child's life are valuable indicators of important change that should always be documented. In fact, the functional communication outcome measures discussed earlier in this chapter are dependent on this kind of data. Quantitative assessment of response generalization typically requires the development of a set of probe words with picture cards that can be administered at regular intervals. The words on the probe would be reserved for the probe and never targeted during therapy activities. The probe should take the specific and intermediate goal into account. Continuing with the example in which [+consonantal][+continuant] is the intermediate target and /f/ is the specific target, the probe would have 3 types of words: (1) words starting with /f/ that are never taught in therapy activities; (2) words starting with /v/ which is also a planned target for the treatment block; and (3) words starting with other [+consonantal][+continuant] phonemes that will not be targeted during treatment sessions. An example of a plan for monitoring treatment progress and stimulus and response generalization is shown in Table 8–9.

Table 8–9. *Progress Monitoring Plan for Amber: Treatment Block 1, [+consonantal][+continuant] Intermediate Goal*

Question	*Probe Type*	*Probe Items*	*Decision Rule*
1. Is Amber responding to the treatment program?	Treatment Probe (quantitative data estimated by SLP during drill-play activities in therapy sessions)	feet, fan, face, funny, fairy	Approximate minimum 80% to proceed to next instructional objective but less than 60% over 2 consecutive sessions triggers substep.
	Treatment Probe (quantitative data collected by SLP during narrative or conversation during every second therapy session)	/f/ onsets of words as they occur in the context of a narrative or conversation with the SLP about picture books or other concrete stimuli.	Minimum 45% correct to add /v/ specific goal.
2. Is significant and important change occurring?	Stimulus generalization reports (parent report data about use of therapy words at home with siblings, father, and grandparent and at daycare with teacher)	feet, fan, face, funny, fairy	Positive reports of spontaneous use of several words triggers switch to /v/ specific goal.
	Response generalization probe (quantitative data collected by SLP during spontaneous picture naming probe at end of alternate therapy sessions)	fire, finger, volley, vampire, sand, sippy-cup, Z, thimble, shelf, shampoo	40 to 74% over 2 probes to discontinue direct therapy on this intermediate goal.
3. Is treatment responsible for the change?	Control probe (quantitative data collected by SLP during spontaneous picture naming probe at end of alternate therapy sessions)	lid, laugh, ladder, jello, jar, rake, rice, berry, plan, prize	Faster rate of progress on response generalization probe relative to control probe indicates treatment effect.

Measures of stimulus and response generalization allow the SLP to decide when to discontinue therapy for selected intermediate goals and are essential for discharge planning. Several studies have shown that treatment can be discontinued for a goal when generalization probe performance is between approximately 40 and 75% accuracy (McKercher, McFarlane, & Schneider, 1995; Olswang & Bain, 1985). Most children will continue to make gains toward the achievement of a goal if this level of performance on the generalization probe is achieved and confidence in this prediction is enhanced if this level of probe performance is observed for 3 consecutive sessions. McKercher et al. further recommended that treatment be discontinued if generalization probe performance is at least 75% accurate for all goals. At this point, the child can be placed on a schedule of intermittent monitoring to ensure that there is no regression and that full mastery of developmentally appropriate speech sounds is achieved as expected.

Measures of stimulus and response generalization allow the SLP to decide when to discontinue therapy for selected intermediate goals and are essential for **discharge planning**.

Several studies have shown that treatment can be discontinued for a goal when generalization probe performance is between approximately 40 and 75% accuracy.

Monitoring performance on a control target shows that changes on treated targets were at least partly due to the treatment program if there is a difference in the rate of change on the two types of probe.

Olswang and Bain (1994) also recommend that the SLP monitor the child's performance on a control target; in other words, a phoneme or word structure that is not targeted in therapy and that is not expected to change as a result of the therapy program. The purpose of the control probe is to provide evidence that changes during therapy are at least partly due to the treatment program itself since we can expect that maturation and other events in the child's life will result in positive changes in phonological knowledge even if therapy was not provided. The choice of control probe target is not straightforward; as we demonstrated for TS30, untreated complex phonemes can emerge even when early developing and stimulable phonemes are targeted in therapy. However, as shown in Figure 8–3, the rate of change was greater for treated than untreated phonemes on average. Typically, phonemes from unrelated sound classes should serve as useful control targets on this probe. In Amber's case, it would be helpful to monitor her production of liquids during the first treatment block. The control probe will provide baseline data against which to compare her rate of change in the second block when these phonemes are treated. The control probe may also reveal emerging stimulability for one or the other phoneme, aiding in the selection of the first specific target when it comes time to target liquids in the second treatment block.

Summary

Treatment planning for the individual child begins with a thorough description of the child's phonological knowledge at multiple levels of the phonological hierarchy and multiple levels of representation, in the context of the whole child. Selection of intermediate goals should serve to stabilize highly variable aspects of the child's phonology, extend the child's phonological knowledge of features and prosodic structures from one context to another, and expand the child's system to encompass new features, segments, and prosodic structures. We feel that the research evidence supports the practice of aiming for early success, boosting the child's confidence and inducing rapid changes in the child's speech intelligibility as quickly as possible. This means choosing specific targets that are stimulable and have high functional load, always using strengths to support needs. However, with the appropriate ordering of instructional objectives and effective treatment procedures, new features, segments, and prosodic structures can be tackled quite early in the treatment program. As shown in Figure 8–4, the most dramatic gains are usually observed for targets that are just emerging in the child's phonological system. A horizontal or cycles goal attack strategy allows for work on multiple goals: while the child is enjoying rapid progress on some relatively easy targets, he or she may feel emboldened to persist with a more difficult target that will have long-term benefits to the complexity of the child's phonological system. It is important to remember that treatment planning is a dynamic process that takes place throughout the course of the child's treatment program. A plan for continuous monitoring of the child's progress must be put in place that reveals the child's response to the treatment program. The use of carefully designed generalization probes and information from the child's family will help guide the introduction of new instructional objectives, modifications to the planned treatment goals when necessary, and planning for eventual discharge of the child with fully intelligible speech.

References

Allen, M. M. (2009, November). *The impact of treatment intensity on a phonological intervention*. Paper presented at the annual convention of the American-Speech-Language and Hearing Association Conference in New Orleans, LA.

Almost, D., & Rosenbaum, P. (1998). Effectiveness of speech intervention for phonological disorders: A randomized controlled trial. *Developmental Medicine and Child Neurology, 40*, 319–325.

American Speech-Language and Hearing Association. (2009a). Prekindergarten NOMS Fact Sheet: Does service delivery model influence SLP outcomes in preschoolers? *NOMS National Data Reports and Fact Sheets*. Retrieved from http://www.asha.org/members/research/noms/noms_data.htm

American Speech-Language-Hearing Association. (2009b). Prekindergarten NOMS Fact Sheet: Does treatment time affect SLP outcomes in preschoolers? *NOMS National Data Reports and Fact Sheets*. Retrieved from http://www.asha.org/members/research/noms/noms_data.htm

Austin, D., & Shriberg, L. D. (1997). *Lifespan reference data for ten measures of articulation competence using the speech disorders classification system (SDSC)*. Waisman Center on Mental Retardation and Human Development, University of Wisconsin-Madison.

Barratt, J., Littlejohns, P., & Thompson, J (1992). Trial of intensive compared with weekly speech therapy in preschool children. *Archives of Disease in Childhood, 67*, 106–108.

Bernhardt, B. (1992). Application of nonlinear phonological theory to intervention with one phonologically disordered child. *Clinical Linguistics & Phonetics, 6*, 283–316.

Bernhardt, B., & Gilbert, J. (1992). Applying linguistic theory to speech-language pathology: The case for non-linear phonology. *Clinical Linguistics & Phonetics, 6*, 123–145.

Bernhardt, B., & Stemberger, J. P. (2000). *Workbook in nonlinear phonology for clinical application*. Austin, TX: Pro-Ed.

Bernhardt, B., Stemberger, J. P., & Major, E. M. (2006). General and nonlinear phonological intervention perspectives for a child with resistent phonological impairment. *Advances in Speech-Language Pathology, 8*, 190–206.

Bernhardt, B., & Stoel-Gammon, C. (1994). Nonlinear phonology: Introduction and clinical application. *Journal of Speech and Hearing Research, 37*, 123–143.

Bernthal, J. E., & Bankson, N. W. (2004). *Articulation and phonological disorders* (5th ed.). Boston, MA: Pearson Educational.

Bird, J., Bishop, D. V. M., & Freeman, N. H. (1995). Phonological awareness and literacy development in children with expressive phonological impairments. *Journal of Speech and Hearing Research, 38*, 446–462.

Bishop, D. V. M. (2009). Genes, cognition, and communication: Insights from neurodevelopmental disorders. *Annals of the New York Academy of Sciences, 1156*, 1–18.

Blakeley, R. W., & Brockman, J. H. (1995). Normal speech and hearing by age 5 as a goal for children with cleft palate: A demonstration project. *American Journal of Speech-Language Pathology, 4*(1), 25–32.

Boyle, J., McCartney, E., Forbes, J., & O'Hare, A. (2007). A randomised control trial and economic evaluation of direct versus indirect and individual versus group modes of speech and language therapy for children with primary language impairment. *Health Technology Assessment, 11*(25), iii–108. http://www.hta.ac.uk/1232

Broomfield, J., & Dodd, B. (2004). Children with speech and language disability: Caseload characteristics. *International Journal of Language and Communication Disorders, 39*(3), 303–324.

Campbell, T. F. (1999). Functional treatment outcomes in young children with motor speech disorders. In A. Caruso & E. A. Strand (Eds.), *Clinical management of motor speech disorders in children* (pp. 385–395). New York, NY: Thieme Medical.

Carter, E. T., & Buck, M. (1958). Prognostic testing for functional articulation disorders among children in the first grade. *Journal of Speech and Hearing Disorders, 23*, 124–133.

Cirrin, F. M., Schooling, T. L., Nelson, N. W., Diehl, S. F., Flynn, P. F., Staskowski, M., . . . Adamcyzk, D. F. (2010). Evidence-based systematic review: Effects of different service delivery models on communication outcomes for elementary school-age children. *Language, Speech, and Hearing Services in Schools, 41*(3), 233–264.

Creaghead, N. A., Newman, P. W., & Secord, W. A. (1989). *Assessment and remediation of articulatory and phonological disorders* (2nd ed.). New York, NY: Macmillan.

Curtis, J. F., & Hardy, J. C. (1959). A phonetic study of misarticulation of /r/. *Journal of Speech and Hearing Research, 2*(3), 244–257.

Diedrich, W. M. (1989). A response to Gierut, Elbert, and Dinnsen, "A functional analysis of phonological knowledge and generalization learning in misarticulating children." *Journal of Speech and Hearing Research, 32*, 219.

Dinnsen, D. A., Chin, S. B., Elbert, M., & Powell, T. W. (1990). Some constraints on functionally disordered phonologies: Phonetic inventories and phonotactics. *Journal of Speech and Hearing Research, 33*(1), 28–37.

Dowden, P., Alarcon, N., Vollan, T., Cumley, G. D., Kuehn, C. M., & Amtmann, D. (2006). Survey of SLP caseloads in Washington state schools: Implications and strategies for action. *Language, Speech, and Hearing Services in Schools, 37*, 104–117.

Dunn, L. M., & Dunn, L. M. (1997). *Peabody Picture Vocabulary Test* (3rd ed.). Circle Pines, MN: American Guidance Service.

Ehri, L. C., Nunes, S. R., Willows, D. M., Schuster, B. V., Yaghoub-Zadeh, Z., & Shanahan, T. (2001). Phonemic awareness instruction helps children learn to read: Evidence from the national reading panel's meta-analysis. *Reading Research Quarterly, 36*(3), 250–287.

Eiserman, W. D., Weber, C., & McCoun, M. (1992). Two alternative program models for serving speech-disordered preschoolers: A second year follow-up. *Journal of Communication Disorders, 25*(2–3), 77–106.

Eiserman, W. D., Weber, C., & McCoun, M. (1995). Parent and professional roles in early intervention: A longitudinal comparison of the effects of two intervention configurations. *Journal of Special Education, 28*, 20–44.

Fey, M. E. (1992). Articulation and phonology: An addendum. *Language, Speech, and Hearing Services in Schools, 23*, 277–282.

Gardner, H. (2005). A comparison of a mother and a therapist working on child speech. In K. Richards & P. Seedhouse (Eds.), *Applying conversation analysis*. Basingstoke, UK: Palgrave Macmillan.

Gardner, H. (2006). Training others in the art of therapy for speech sound disorders: an interactional approach. *Child Language and Teaching Therapy, 22*, 27–46.

Gierut, J. A. (2007). Phonological complexity and language learnability. *American Journal of Speech-Language Pathology, 16*, 6–17.

Gierut, J. A., Elbert, M., & Dinnsen, D. A. (1987). A functional analysis of phonological knowledge and generalization learning in misarticulating children. *Journal of Speech and Hearing Research, 30*, 462–479.

Gierut, J. A., Morrisette, M. L., Hughes, M. T., & Rowlands, S. (2001). Phonological treatment efficacy and developmental norms. *Language, Speech, and Hearing Services in Schools, 27*, 215–230.

Glogowska, M., Roulstone, S., Enderby, P., & Peters, T. J. (2000). Randomised controlled trial of community-based speech and language therapy in preschool children. *British Medical Journal, 321*, 923–928.

Glogowska, M., Roulstone, S., Peters, T. J., & Enderby, P. (2006). Early speech- and language-impaired children: linguistic, literacy, and social outcomes. *Developmental Medicine and Child Neurology, 48*, 489–494.

Goffman, L., Gerken, L., & Lucchesi, J. (2007). Relations between segmental and motor variability in prosodically complex nonword sequences. *Journal of Speech, Language, and Hearing Research, 50*, 444–458.

Goldman, R., & Fristoe, M. (2000). *Goldman-Fristoe Test of Articulation* (2nd ed.). Circle Pines, MN: American Guidance Service.

Green, J. R., Moore, C. A., Higashikawa, M., & Steeve, R. W. (2000). The physiological development of speech motor control: lip and jaw coordination. *Journal of Speech, Language, and Hearing Research, 43*, 239–255.

Grunwell, P. (1992). Processes of phonological change in developmental speech disorders. *Clinical Linguistics & Phonetics, 6*, 101–122.

Hall, B. J. C. (1991). Attitudes of fourth and sixth graders toward peers with mild articulation disorders. *Language, Speech, and Hearing Services in Schools, 22*, 334–340.

Hodson, B. W. (1989). Phonological remediaton: A cycles approach. In N. A. Creaghead, P. W. Newman, & W. A. Secord (Eds.), *Assessment and remediation of articulatory and phonological disorders* (2nd ed.). New York, NY: Macmillan.

Hodson, B. W. (2004). *Hodson Assessment of Phonological Patterns* (3rd ed.). Austin, TX: Pro-Ed.

Hodson, B. W. (2007). *Evaluating and enhancing children's phonological systems: Resarch & theory to practice*. Wichita, KS: Phonocomp.

Hodson, B. W., & Paden, E. P. (1983). *Targeting intelligible speech: A phonological approach to remediation*. Boston, MA: College-Hill.

Ingram, D. (1981). *Procedures for the phonological analysis of children's language*. Baltimore, MD: University Park Press.

Jacoby, G. P., Levin, L., Lee, L., Creaghead, N. A., & Kummer, A. W. (2002). The number of individual treatment units necessary to facilitate functional communication improvements in the speech and language of young children. *American Journal of Speech-Language Pathology, 11*, 370–390.

Joffe, V., & Pring, T. (2008). Children with phonological problems: A survey of clinical practice. *International Journal of Language and Communication Disorders, 43*, 154–164.

Johnson, C. A., Weston, A. D., & Bain, B. A. (2004). An objective and time efficient method for determining severity of childhood speech delay. *American Journal of Speech-Language Pathology, 13*, 55–65.

Katz, L. A., Maag, A., Fallon, K. A., Blenkarn, K., & Smith, M. K. (2010). What makes a caseload (un)manageable? School-based speech-language pathologists speak. *Language, Speech, and Hearing Services in Schools, 41*(2), 139–151.

Klee, T. (2008). Considerations for appraising diagnostic studies of communication disorders. *Evidence-Based Communication Assessment and Intervention, 2*(1), 34–45.

Lewis, B. A., Freebairn, L. A., & Taylor, H. G. (2000). Follow-up of children with early expressive phonology disorders. *Journal of Learning Disabilities, 33*(5), 433–444.

Locke, J. L. (1980). The inference of speech perception in the phonologically disordered child. Some clinically novel procedures, their use, some findings. *Journal of Speech and Hearing Disorders, 45*, 445–468.

Lof, G. L. (1996). Factors associated with speech-sound stimulability. *Journal of Communication Disorders, 29*, 255–278.

Maas, E., Robin, D. A., Austermann Hula, S. N., Freedman, S. E., Wulf, G., Ballard, K. J., & Schmidt, R. A. (2008). Principles of motor learning in treatment of motor speech disorders. *American Journal of Speech-Language Pathology, 17*, 277–298.

McCauley, R. J., & Swisher, L. (1984). Psychometric review of language and articulation tests for preschool children. *Journal of Speech and Hearing Disorders, 49*(1), 34–42.

McCormack, J., McLeod, S., McAllister, L., & Harrison, L. J. (2009). A systematic review of the association between childhood speech impairment and participation across the lifespan. *International Journal of Speech-Language Pathology, 11*, 155–170.

McKercher, M., McFarlane, L., & Schneider, P. (1995). Phonological treatment dismissal: Optimal criteria. *Journal of Speech-Language Pathology and Audiology, 19*, 115–123.

McLeod, S. (2006). Perspectives on a child with unintelligible speech. *Advances in Speech-Language Pathology, 8*, 153–155.

McReynolds, L. V., & Kearns, K. (1983). *Single-subject experimental designs in communicative disorders*. Austin, TX: Pro-Ed.

Menn, L., Schmidt, E., & Nicholas, B. (2009). Conspiracy and sabotage in the acquisition of phonology: dense data undermine existing theories, provide scaffolding for a new one. *Language Sciences, 31*(2–3), 285–304.

Miccio, A. W., Elbert, M., & Forrest, K. (1999). The relationship between stimulability and phonological acquisition in children with normally developing and disordered phonologies. *American Journal of Speech-Language Pathology, 8*, 347–363.

Mowrer, D. E. (1989). The behavioral approach to treatment. In N. A. Creaghead, P. W. Newman, & W. A. Secord (Eds.), *Assessment and remediation of articulatory and phonological disorders* (2nd ed., pp. 161–192). New York, NY: Macmillan.

Olswang, L. B., & Bain, B. (1985). Monitoring phoneme acquisition for making treatment withdrawal decisions. *Applied Psycholinguistics, 6*, 17–37.

Olswang, L. B., & Bain, B. (1994). Data collection: Monitoring children's treatment progress. *American Journal of Speech-Language Pathology, 3*, 55–66.

Olswang, L. B., & Bain, B. A. (1991). When to recommend intervention. *Language, Speech, and Hearing Services in Schools, 22*(4), 255–263.

Olswang, L. B., Rodriguez, B., & Timler, G. (1998). Recommending intervention for toddlers with specific language learning difficulties: We may not have all the answers, but we know a lot. *American Journal of Speech-Language Pathology, 7*(1), 23–32.

Peña, E. D., Spaulding, T. J., & Plante, E. (2006). The composition of normative groups and diagnostic decision making: Shooting ourselves in the foot. *American Journal of Speech-Language Pathology, 15*, 247–254.

Pring, T. (2004). Ask a silly question: Two decades of troublesome trials. *International Journal of Language and Communication Disorders, 39*(3), 285–302.

Puranik, C. S., Petcher, Y., Al Otaiba, S., Catts, H. W., & Lonigan, C. J. (2008). Development of oral reading fluency in children with speech or language impairments: A growth curve analysis. *Journal of Learning Disabilities, 41*, 545–560.

Rafaat, S., Rvachew, S., & Russell, R. S. C. (1995). Reliability of clinician judgments of severity of phonological impairment. *American Journal of Speech-Language Pathology, 4*(3), 39–46.

Rvachew, S. (2005). Stimulability and treatment success. *Topics in Language Disorders. Clinical Perspectives on Speech Sound Disorders, 25*(3), 207–219.

Rvachew, S. (2006). Longitudinal prediction of implicit phonological awareness skills. *American Journal of Speech-Language Pathology, 15*, 165–176.

Rvachew, S. (2007). Phonological processing and reading in children with speech sound disorders. *American Journal of Speech-Language Pathology, 16*, 260–270.

Rvachew, S., & Bernhardt, B. (2010). Clinical implications of the dynamic systems approach to phonological development. *American Journal of Speech-Language Pathology, 19*, 34–50.

Rvachew, S., & Brosseau-Lapré, F. (2010, November). *Improving phonological awareness in French-speaking children with speech delay*. Paper presented at the annual convention of the American Speech-Language and Hearing Association, Philadelphia, PA.

Rvachew, S., & Grawburg, M. (2006). Correlates of phonological awareness in preschoolers with speech sound disorders. *Journal of Speech, Language, and Hearing Research, 49*, 74–87.

Rvachew, S., & Nowak, M. (2001). The effect of target selection strategy on sound production learning. *Journal of Speech, Language, and Hearing Research, 44*, 610–623.

Rvachew, S., & Nowak, M. (2003). Clinical outcomes as a function of target selection strategy: A reply to Morrisette and Gierut. *Journal of Speech, Language, and Hearing Research, 46*(2), 386–389.

Rvachew, S., Rafaat, S., & Martin, M. (1999). Stimulability, speech perception and the treatment of phonological disorders. *American Journal of Speech-Language Pathology, 8*, 33–34.

Schooling, T. L. (2003). Lessons from the National Outcomes Measurement System (NOMS). *Seminars in Speech and Language, 24*(3), 245–256.

Silverman, F. H. (1992). Attitudes of teenagers toward peers who have a single articulation error. *Language, Speech, and Hearing Services in Schools, 23*, 187–188.

Smit, A. B., Hand, L., Freilinger, J. J., Bernthal, J. E., & Bird, A. (1990). The Iowa articulation norms project and its Nebraska replication. *Journal of Speech and Hearing Disorders, 55*, 779–798.

Sommers, R. K. (1962). Factors in the effectiveness of mothers trained to aid in speech correction. *Journal of Speech and Hearing Disorders, 27*, 178–186.

Sommers, R. K., Copetas, F. G., Bowser, D. C., Fichter, G. R., Furlong, A. K., Rhodes, F. E., & Saunders, Z. G. (1962). Effects of various durations of speech improvement upon articulation and reading. *Journal of Speech and Hearing Disorders, 27*, 54–61.

Sommers, R. K., Furlong, A. K., Rhodes, F. E., Fichter, G. R., Bowser, D. C., Copetas, F. G., & Saunders, Z. G. (1964). Effects of maternal attitudes upon improvements in articulation when mothers are trained to assist in speech correction. *Journal of Speech and Hearing Disorders, 29*, 126–132.

Sommers, R. K., Leiss, R. H., Delp, M., Gerber, A., Fundrella, D., Smith, R., . . . Haley, V. (1967). Factors relating to the effectiveness of articulation therapy for kindergarten, first, and second grade children. *Journal of Speech and Hearing Research, 13*, 428–437.

Sommers, R. K., Schaeffer, M. H., Leiss, R. H., Gerber, A., Bray, M. A., Fundrella, D., . . . Tomkins, E. R. (1966). The effectiveness of group and individual therapy. *Journal of Speech and Hearing Research, 9*, 219–225.

Spaulding, T. J., Plante, E., & Farinella, K. A. (2006). Eligibility criteria for language impairment: Is the low end of normal always appropriate? *Language, Speech and Hearing Services in Schools, 37*, 61–72.

Stoel-Gammon, C., & Dunn, C. (1985). *Normal and disordered phonology in children*. Baltimore, MD: University Park Press.

Stokes, S. F., & Suredran, D. (2005). Articulatory complexity, ambient frequency, and functional load as predictors of consonant development in children. *Journal of Speech, Language, and Hearing Research, 48*, 577–591.

Storkel, H. L., & Hoover, J. R. (2010). An online calculator to compute phonotactic probability and neighborhood density on the basis of child corpora or spoken American English. *Behavior Research Methods, 42*, 497–506.

Stothard, S. E., Snowling, M. J., Bishop, D. V. M., Chipchase, B. B., & Kaplan, C. A. (1998). Language-impaired preschoolers: A follow-up into adolescence. *Journal of Speech, Language, and Hearing Research, 41*, 407–418.

Thomas-Stonell, N., McConney-Ellis, S., Oddson, B., Robertson, B., & Rosenbaum, P. (2007). An evaluation of the responsiveness of the prekindergarten ASHA NOMS. *Canadian Journal of Speech-Language Pathology and Audiology, 31*(2), 74–82.

Thomas-Stonell, N. L., Oddson, B., Robertson, B., & Rosenbaum, P. L. (2009a). Development of the FOCUS (Focus on the Outcomes of Communication Under Six), a communication outcome measure for preschool children. *Developmental Medicine and Child Neurology, 52*(1), 47–53.

Thomas-Stonell, N., Oddson, B., Robertson, B., & Rosenbaum, P. (2009b). Predicted and observed outcomes in preschool children following speech and language treatment: Parent and clinician perspectives. *Journal of Communication Disorders, 42*(1), 29–42.

Tomblin, J. B., Records, N. L., & Zhang, J. (1996). A system for the diagnosis of Specific Language Impairment in kindergarten children. *Journal of Speech and Hearing Research, 39*, 1284–1294.

Torgesen, J., Wagner, R. K., & Rashotte, C. A. (1999). *Test of Word Reading Efficiency*. Austin, TX: Pro-Ed.

Tufts, L. C., & Holliday, A. R. (1959). Effectiveness of trained parents as speech therapists. *Journal of Speech and Hearing Disorders, 24*, 395–401.

Tyler, A. A., Edwards, M. L., & Saxman, J. H. (1990). Acoustic validation of phonological knowledge and its relationship to treatment. *Journal of Speech and Hearing Disorders, 55*, 251–261.

Tyler, A. A., & Figurski, G. R. (1994). Phonetic inventory changes after treating distinctions along an implicational hierarchy. *Clinical Linguistics & Phonetics, 8*, 91–107.

Warren, S. F., Fey, M. E., & Yoder, P. J. (2007). Differential treatment intensity research: A missing link to creating optimally effective communication interventions. *Mental Retardation and Developmental Disabilities Research Reviews, 13*, 70–77.

Zhang, X., & Tomblin, J. B.. (2000). The association of intervention receipt with speech-language profiles and social-demographic variables. *American Journal of Speech-Language Pathology, 9*(4), 345–357.

Part III

Intervention at Multiple Levels of Representation

In Part III we present principles of perceptual, motor, and phonological learning and describe input-oriented, output-oriented, and phonological procedures for teaching children skills in these domains. There are many effective procedures that can be applied in speech therapy and they have been combined to form a number of different packaged approaches (Williams, McLeod, & McCauley, 2010). Deciding which procedures to use with a given child is a difficult task that involves integrating clinical expertise, the child and family's needs and values, and the best research evidence (American Speech-Language-Hearing Association, 2004). A detailed discussion of evidence-based practice (EPB) is beyond the scope of this book but we provide a brief introduction to some concepts that underly the application of EPB in the clinic.

Deciding **which intervention procedures** to use with a given child involves integrating clinical expertise, the child and family's needs and values, and the best research evidence.

The first question to ask when considering the potential value of any treatment procedure for a given child is whether the practice is consistent with theory and basic research. The SLP needs to understand theory and research in the field of phonology in particular but also development more generally as well as learning in a therapeutic context. Every procedure that is used in therapy should be consistent with the SLP's theoretical perspective and the scientific literature (Bernstein Ratner, 2006). There must be a sensible reason for expecting the procedure to effect change in the child's phonological system and an understanding of the mechanisms that underly the effect. In other words, there must be answers to the questions *why* and *how* would this procedure work?

The first question to ask when considering the potential value of any treatment procedure for a given child is whether the practice is **consistent with theory and basic research**.

The second question to address is whether the procedure actually works. It is at this stage in the process that the SLP must evaluate

The second question to address is **whether the procedure actually works**.

The SLP must evaluate the **internal validity** of the *treatment efficacy studies* that are relevant to the procedure or approach in question.

Randomization of research participants to conditions is the only way to effectively control for variables other than the treatment that will contribute to changes in the child's phonology.

the internal validity of the treatment efficacy studies that are relevant to the procedure or approach in question. The American Speech-Language and Hearing Association (2004) has adapted the guidelines of the Scottish Intercollegiate Guideline Network for ranking studies in terms of validity and credibility, as shown in Table III–1. Randomized control trials (Level Ib) and meta-analyses of randomized control trials (Level Ia) have the highest level of credibility because randomization of research participants to conditions is the only way to effectively control for variables other than the treatment that will contribute to changes in the child's phonology and, thus, when well designed and carried out without bias, these studies provide the highest level of confidence that a given procedure or approach has a causal impact on phonological change. Clinicians are faced with three challenges in the task of evaluating the research evidence. The first is that the sheer weight of the scientific literature given time constraints in typical clinical practice is daunting and points to the need for increasing specialization in our profession. Fortunately the academic community is providing many venues for synthesis of this literature in accessible forms such as special forums in clinical journals. At the same time, some of these reviews, especially the cruder forms of meta-analysis, are not particularly informative as they reduce the question of "what works" to a single number (effect size) that hides the essential details about how the treatment works, with whom, and under what circumstances. There are no alternatives to reading the original treatment efficacy studies for any intervention that you are using.

The second challenge is related to the first: there are many studies suggesting that different procedures work and at first glance these disparate procedures appear to be theoretically incoherent leading some to the conclusion that all treatment approaches are essentially equivalent in terms of effectiveness (Kamhi, 2006). First

Table III–1. *Levels of Evidence for Studies of Treatment Efficacy*

Level	*Description*
Ia	Well-designed meta-analysis of >1 randomized control trial
Ib	Well-designed randomized control trial
IIa	Well-designed controlled study without randomization
IIb	Well-designed quasi-experimental study
III	Well-designed non-experimental study, i.e., correlational and case studies
IV	Expert committee report, consensus conference, clinical experience of respected authorities

Source: From Evidence-Based Practice in Communication Disorders: An Introduction [Technical report], by the American Speech-Language-Hearing Association, 2004. p. 2 (Table 1), http://www.asha.org/docs/html/TR2004-00001.html. Copyright 2004 by the American Speech-Language-Hearing Association. Reprinted with permission.

of all, it is not true that "everything works" and second, theoretical consistency in the treatment program is important to a good outcome (for further discussion, see Ingram, 2009; Weisz, Donenberg, Han, & Kauneckis, 1995). In the chapters to follow in Part III we try to link the procedures that we highlight to the theoretical perspective outlined in Chapter 4 and indicate how they apply at different points in the child's developmental trajectory.

Theoretical consistency in the treatment program is important to a good outcome.

The third challenge arises when a new (or more often old but forgotten) approach suddenly becomes popular, but there is no conventional treatment efficacy research demonstrating that the intervention is or is not effective. However, the absence of treatment efficacy data is a form of evidence that must be taken into account in the decision-making process. In order to obtain funds to conduct a randomized control trial a researcher must first demonstrate that there is a sound theoretical basis for a treatment and then collect preliminary evidence from quasi-experimental studies to show that the treatment is probably helpful and not harmful. If there are no randomized control trials to support the efficacy of a given procedure or approach, it is likely that the treatment has not passed the first two tests or that the preliminary studies were not successful (because it is difficult to publish negative evidence, the absence of negative evidence in published form does not mean that it does not exist). There are no procedures for which there is no evidence. Always begin by considering how and why the treatment might work given current theory and basic research. It is important not to be fooled by pseudoscience (Finn, Bothe, & Bramlett, 2005) which means having a deep understanding of the basic science that underlies your clinical specialty.

Finally, it is only the SLP who can decide whether a procedure that was effective on average in a given study might also be effective with a specific child in a given therapeutic context. The SLP must investigate very carefully the conditions under which a given practice was shown to work. How similar is the child you are treating to the children who were treated in the studies you reviewed? Can you provide the treatment in the same way and at the same intensity? Recall our conclusions in Chapter 8 about group therapy and home programming, practices that have been found to "work" in meta-analyses. In fact, child characteristics, cumulative intervention intensity and the structure of the support provided to parents makes a difference to the treatment effects observed (e.g., see Figure 8–2 and associated discussion). These kinds of important details can be obscured in meta-analyses and systematic reviews.

The SLP must investigate the **conditions under which** a given practice was shown to work. How similar is the child you are treating to the children who were treated in the studies you reviewed? Can you provide the treatment in the same way and at the same intensity?

Systematic monitoring of treatment progress, including the documentation of changes in performance on control probes is an important part of a treatment program because it is essential to the process of integrating clinical expertise with the scientific literature. Clinical experience and randomized control trials each provide essential but fundamentally different types of information. Randomized control trials increase confidence that a given procedure has an effect on children's phonological development, over

Systematic monitoring of treatment progress, including the documentation of changes in performance on control probes, is an important part of a treatment program because it is essential to the process of integrating clinical expertise with the scientific literature.

and above all other influences that serve to enhance the child's phonological knowledge. This is important because changes observed in the clinic arise from an amalgam of multiple influences; as discussed in Chapter 8, maturational change can be mistakenly attributed to treatment effects when the same change would be observed even if no treatment had been provided. When treatment effects are observed in a randomized control trial, these effects are reported as averages for groups of children that tend to be heterogeneous even when strict selection criteria are in place. Some children within the group will have responded to the treatment much more positively than others. It is only through careful monitoring in the clinic that the SLP can be sure that treatment is having the expected effect on an individual patient.

What does the SLP do when the current intervention research does not appear to be providing "the answer" for a particular child? In the following excerpt, the first author recalls an experience that makes the point that "evidence-based practice" is not all about the evidence. In the mid-1980s I was treating children in a wonderful program that provided half-day programming four days per week to children with multiple needs using a multidisciplinary approach. The 4-year-old child in question had an uneven cognitive profile, mild fine motor delays, and severe speech and language impairment (although no clear indications of motor speech disorder). When I first assessed him he produced the forms shown in Case Study III–1, indicating a highly restricted repertoire of vowels, consonants, and word shapes (70% of all words had the shape [CVs]); the consonant repertoire was restricted to [(m) p b k g h s]. The [s] was acquired from a previous therapist, who was using a phonological process approach and had some perverse success with "final consonant deletion" although it soon became clear that he had no underlying knowledge of codas to delete. I encouraged the program staff to use generalized language stimulation techniques to encour-

Case Study III–1
Representative Utterances from a 4-Year-Old Boy with Severe Developmental Phonological Disorder and Language Impairment

bath	[bæs]	duck	[gʌs]	phone	[hos]
bed	[bʌs]	doll	[gʌs]	fork	[hos]
boat	[bos]	drum	[gʌs]	flower	[hʌs]
ball	[bʌs]	cookie	[kes]	flag	[hæs]
blue	[bus]	squirrel	[kos]	Santa	[hæs]

age two word utterances while I attempted to add missing features and segments to his repertoire during individual speech therapy sessions; in particular, I focused on high vowels and coronal consonants in the syllable onset position. After a few months in the program he began to sequence words into multiword utterances, like this: "blue ball" → [bu bʌs]. You can see that the [s] was not properly integrated into his lexical representations! Other than this development I was having no success with his phonology—his system remained unchanged. His mother was becoming increasingly frantic because by Christmas break all the program staff (three child care workers, two physiotherapists, two occupational therapists, two SLPs, and one psychologist) were calling him "Gus" at least some of time, mimicking his own production of his name "Scott." I had been patiently explaining that because he could not say "bee" or "two" I was pretty sure I could not teach him to say his name, but finally I relented and changed the primary goal to focus on new functional words including, and most importantly, his name; subsequently, all the staff in the program devoted themselves to encouraging him to say his name correctly and by Easter he had mastered it. At which point everything changed: his word shape repertoire, vowel repertoire, and consonant repertoire suddenly opened up. Without being at all sure of the explanation, I can say that his rate of progress increased markedly. He was discharged to a lower intensity service at the end of the school year. I heard through the grapevine that the next SLP, who used the cycles approach with great success, thought that I was completely incompetent to have achieved so little with this child over the 9-month duration of the program.

Certainly I made some key mistakes in my handling of the case and I found those mistakes to be instructive as I moved forward in my clinical practice. A really big mistake was to forget that the research evidence must be integrated with the needs of the clients and their families. I certainly should have started working on his name in September! Another mistake was to not integrate the research evidence appropriately with clinical experience. At the time, the treatment techniques that I was using in my individual sessions were directed at his articulatory knowledge of phones that he did not produce and at his phonological knowledge of contrasts that were absent from his underlying phonological system. The approaches that I was using were consistent with theory and clinical research at the time. However, if I had been paying more attention I would have noticed that the most successful part of the intervention involved the "input-oriented techniques" (e.g., focused stimulation as discussed in Chapter 9) that the other staff and I were using to target language goals. I was very slow to pick up on the significance of difference in outcomes across the different goals and therapeutic techniques that were being used in "speech therapy" versus the general preschool program. Finally, when considering the evidence, I was far too focused on the speech-language pathology literature, searching for evidence of effective treatment approaches,

The **research evidence** must be integrated with the needs of the clients and their families.

when the answers lay in basic linguistic research that had been published 10 years earlier. I could be forgiven for not being aware of the core vocabulary approach, to be invented 20 years hence (see Chapter 10), but I was woefully unaware of Ferguson and Farwell's (1975) seminal paper on word-based phonologies even though this perspective held the key to understanding the essential problem that Scott had with acoustic-phonetic representations for words. It is very important to remember that the basic science forms a critical part of the evidence that must be considered when selecting and justifying the interventions we choose for our clients. Moving forward, new developments in genetics and the neurosciences may be as informative as randomized control trials when it comes to informing our practice with difficult cases.

In Part III we provide guidelines for the use of procedures for enhancing children's perceptual, articulatory, and phonological knowledge. In each chapter we begin with a review of the theory and basic science relevant to the principles of learning in each domain. We describe how the procedure should be applied in the clinical context given those principles. Then we consider the quality of the research evidence that supports (or does not support) procedures and approaches that are used to promote learning in each domain with careful attention to the conditions, if any, under which application of the procedure has been shown to be effective. Ultimately, however, the choice of treatment procedures will always be a trial and error process undertaken collaboratively with the child and the family. The SLP must plan a treatment that is informed by science but be prepared to adapt it quickly to the child's specific needs and response to therapy. An interesting economist (Harford, 2011) recently laid out "a recipe for successfully adapting. The three essential steps are: to try new things, in the expectation that some will fail; to make failure survivable, because it will be common; and to make sure that you know when you've failed" (p. 36). This sounds like a perfect recipe for continuous improvement in the practice of speech-language pathology.[1]

Ultimately, the choice of treatment procedures will always be a **trial and error process** undertaken collaboratively with the child and the family. The SLP must plan a treatment that is informed by science but be prepared to adapt it quickly to the child's specific needs and response to therapy.

References

American Speech-Language-Hearing Association. (2004). *Evidence-based practice in communication disorders: An introduction* [Technical report]. http://www.asha.org/docs/html/TR2004-00001.html

Bernstein Ratner, N. (2006). Evidence-based practice: An examination of its ramifications for the practice of speech-language pathology. *Language, Speech, and Hearing Services in Schools, 37*(4), 257–267.

[1]See also the TED Talk by Tim Harford, "Trial, Error and the God Complex," at http://www.ted.com/talks/tim_harford.html.

Ferguson, C., & Farwell, C. B. (1975). Words and sounds in early acquisition. *Language, 51*(2), 419–439.

Finn, P., Bothe, A. K., & Bramlett, R. E. (2005). Science and pseudoscience in communication disorders: Criteria and applications. *American Journal of Speech-Language Pathology, 14*, 172–186.

Harford, T. (2011). *Adapt: Why success always starts with failure*. Canada: Random House.

Ingram, D. (2009). The role of theory in SSD. In C. Bowen (Ed.), *Children's speech sound disorders* (pp. 23–26). Chicheser, UK: Wiley-Blackwell.

Kamhi, A. G. (2006). Treatment decisions for children with speech-sound disorders. *Language, Speech, and Hearing Services in Schools, 37*(4), 271–279.

Weisz, J. R., Donenberg, G. R., Han, S. S., & Kauneckis, D. (1995). Child and adolescent psychotherapy outcomes in experiments versus clinics: Why the disparity? *Journal of Abnormal Child Psychology, 23*, 83–106.

Williams, A. L., McLeod, S., & McCauley, R. J. (2010). *Interventions for speech sound disorders in children*. Baltimore, MD: Brookes.

Chapter 9

Input-Oriented Approaches to Intervention

The foundation of phonological development is the acquisition of acoustic-phonetic representations for words. As explained in Chapter 2, this process begins before birth and encompasses three types of knowledge that are largely although incompletely developed in the first few years of life. The child acquires knowledge of the acoustic-phonetic characteristics of the phonological units that are specific to the language or languages spoken in the ambient environment. The child learns how these units are used to contrast meaning and form meaningful words. The child also begins to develop an implicit awareness of the underlying structure of the sound system of the language by noticing similarities and differences among words. These milestones in the acquisition of acoustic-phonetic representations are illustrated in Plate 6.

The foundation of phonological development is the acquisition of **acoustic-phonetic representations for words**.

In Chapter 2 we outlined some of the learning mechanisms and environmental supports that contribute to normal speech perception development, summarized in Table 9–1. Particularly important in the early stages of speech perception development is the provision of speech input using an infant-directed register. Furthermore, the input must provide information about the distributional properties of acoustic cues for language specific phonetic categories. A powerful statistical learning mechanism allows the infant to extract phonetic categories from this variable input. This idea is represented in Plate 6 by varied colors for different speakers and varied placements of words along a voice-onset-time continuum with the modal frequency corresponding to the English category center for [b]. Research with human infants and computational modeling research shows that statistical learning leads to the grouping of

A powerful **statistical learning mechanism** allows the infant to extract phonetic categories from variable language input.

Table 9–1. Learning Mechanisms and Environmental Supports in the Natural Environment and Therapeutic Procedures for the Development of Speech Perception Skills in the Clinical Environment

Learning Mechanisms	Environmental Supports	Therapeutic Procedures	Expected Outcomes
1. Language Specific Phonetic Perception			
Attention to speech Statistical learning	Language input in infant-directed register Language input provided in a social context	Focused stimulation	Word segmentation skills Acoustic-phonetic representations for phones, words and prosodic patterns Increased size of lexicon Internal models to guide speech production
2. Phonemic Perception in Words			
Social learning mechanisms (e.g., detection of referential intent) Cognitive learning mechanisms (e.g., categorization skills) Phonological working memory Linkage of phonetic, phonological and semantic representations	Highly variable natural speech input from multiple talkers Engagement by the child with the input	"Ear training"	Phonemic perception skills Improved speech production accuracy for stimulable phones
3. Implicit Awareness of Onsets and Rimes			
Lexical restructuring triggered by growing size of lexicon and increasingly detailed acoustic-phonetic representations	Exposure to high quality language input Exposure to print materials Exposure to rime and alliteration	Dialogic reading	Continuing growth in the size of the lexicon and complexity of vocabulary knowledge Narrative skills Emerging phonological awareness skills

stimuli into "multidimensional islands" (McMurray & Aslin, 2005; McMurray, Aslin, & Toscano, 2009). In other words, infants do not learn distinctions between phonetic categories; rather they learn the distribution of exemplars that defines a given category independently of other categories. The developing phonetic categories also support the emergence of babbling skills and the development of an internal model that maps vocal tract configurations to speech output that corresponds to the language-specific acoustic-phonetic representations.

In the second year of life, phonemic perception emerges in concert with word learning abilities. Multiple cognitive and social learning mechanisms are involved but all interact with the amount and quality of the input provided. As described in Chapter 2, word learning skills are predicted by the size of the toddler's vocabulary which itself is determined by the maturity of the child's speech perception abilities in the first year of life and the cumulative number of words heard by the child in the context of social learning exchanges (Huttenlocher, 1998; Kuhl et al., 2008; Meltzoff, 2009; Mills et al., 2004; Werker & Curtin, 2005). As with phonetic perception in the first year of life, the shift to phonemic perception requires access to highly varied speech input with variation in talker characteristics being at least as important as variation in acoustic-phonetic characteristics within and between phonemic categories (Rost & McMurray, 2009). These developments also have an impact on the toddler's speech and language production skills.

Multiple cognitive and social learning mechanisms are involved but all interact with the amount and quality of the input provided to influence emergence of phonemic perception, word learning, and speech production skills in the second year of life.

Toward the end of the third year of life the child begins to develop an implicit awareness of the phonological units that make up words: syllables, onsets, and rimes. As shown in Figure 7–8, refinements in speech perception skills combined with a growing vocabulary size contribute to the development of implicit phonological awareness (Rvachew & Grawburg, 2006; Walley, Metsala, & Garlock, 2003). Emergent literacy skills are further enhanced by structured inputs from parents, especially exposure to print materials that highlight rhyme and alliteration and explicitly link the sound properties of the language to letter knowledge (Evans & Saint-Aubin, 2009; Senechal, LeFevre, Thomas, & Daley, 1998).

Toward the end of the third year of life, refinements in speech perception skills combined with a growing vocabulary size contribute to the development of **implicit phonological awareness.**

As reviewed in Chapter 7, a large proportion of children with DPD have significant difficulties with phonological processing that are manifested as poor speech perception and phonological awareness skills (see Figure 7–9), placing the children at risk for dyslexia even if the speech deficit is remediated. A minority may also have auditory processing difficulties (e.g., secondary to early onset and chronic otitis media with effusion) that also impact speech perception and phonological awareness skills. Poor language inputs are an additional risk factor that has a similar impact on phonological processing as shown in Figure 7–6. Not only are phonological processing deficits associated with speech impairment, linear structural equation modeling and longitudinal follow-up studies suggest that speech perception skills are causally related to the development of speech accuracy and phonological awareness skills (McBride-Chang, 1995; Rvachew, 2006; Rvachew & Grawburg, 2006). In this chapter we describe procedures for strengthening children's acoustic-phonetic representations for words, the foundation of good speech perception and phonological awareness skills. These procedures involve the provision of varied, concentrated, and focused speech input to the child. We also describe intervention studies that explore the hypothesized causal pathways and determine the conditions under which these procedures are effective.

Procedures for strengthening children's acoustic-phonetic representations for words involve the provision of **varied, concentrated, and focused speech input** to the child.

Our expectations about the kinds of procedures that might be effective in the remediation of speech perception and phonological processing deficits are drawn from our review of normal speech perception development, as shown in Table 9–1. In normal development, the learning processes that are engaged are on the implicit end of the continuum between conscious and unconscious processes, following Weinert's (2009) definition of "a passive, data-driven, nonconscious, and nonselective mode of learning that is based on parallel information processing and in which learning products are not necessarily accessible to metacognitive awareness" (p. 244). In the clinical context, children will be acquiring knowledge at older ages than in typical development. Although the therapeutic procedures that are proposed involve providing high quality input as in the normal learning environment, the adult may prompt specific responses from the child and provide informative feedback and thus the learning processes are somewhat more explicit than would be typical in normal development. Nonetheless, the procedures do not invoke the explicit metalinguistic abilities discussed in Chapter 11. Given that infants and young children are actually better implicit learners than adults and older children (e.g., Plante, Bahl, Vance, & Gerken, 2010), these procedures can be implemented at the earliest stages of language and phonological acquisition; there is no reason to reserve input-oriented procedures for older children as has sometimes been suggested (e.g., Bauman-Waengler, 2012).

We suggest teaching procedures that **engage implicit learning** processes that can be implemented at the earliest stages of language and phonological acquisition.

The three procedures that we cover in this chapter—focused stimulation, "ear training," and dialogic reading—all involve providing high quality varied input to the child. Depending on the developmental level of the child and the goals of the treatment program the input may be structured to highlight words, prosodic structures, syllables, subsyllabic units, phonemic contrasts, or morphophonemic structures. Collectively, these procedures are expected to impact the child's receptive vocabulary growth, speech perception skills, speech production accuracy, and phonological awareness by strengthening acoustic-phonetic representations for words and segments. We describe the correct application of these procedures and the research evidence relating to the efficacy of each procedure for the treatment of children with DPD.

Input-oriented intervention procedures may be structured to highlight words, prosodic structures, syllables, subsyllabic units, phonemic contrasts, or morphophonemic structures.

Focused Stimulation

9.1.1. List and provide examples of six techniques that can be used when implementing the focused stimulation procedure to enhance phonological knowledge of a given target.

9.1.2. List and describe five principles that underlay implementation of the focused stimulation procedure.

9.1.3 Demonstrate application of the focused stimulation procedure by designing two successive lesson plans that would be appropriate for a preschool-age child with DPD.

Focused stimulation is an intervention procedure in which the SLP applies a number of techniques in the context of an activity structured to provide the child with many exposures to a specific target form. Although the SLP structures the materials and the activity to ensure exposure to a preselected target, the child is a full partner in the exchange that ensues once the activity is initiated; the child has the freedom to direct the course of the activity and may or may not choose to produce the target structure. If the child produces the target, the SLP may imitate, recast, or expand the child's utterance so that the child can immediately compare his or her own production with the SLP's production of the target. However, no direct requests to produce or imitate the target are made, no instructions regarding accurate production are presented, and no specific corrective feedback, reinforcement, or punishment is provided contingent on the nature of the child's responses. These activities are referred to as hybrid intervention contexts because they include aspects of child-centered and clinician-directed contexts (Proctor-Williams, 2009). The techniques that may be used during these activities for the purpose of providing focused stimulation are listed and defined in Table 9–2. The effectiveness of these techniques singly and in combination have been systematically studied in the context of language interventions, especially for facilitating vocabulary growth and productive use of grammatical morphemes by children with cognitive impairments, children with SLI, and children with normally developing language skills. We have been adapting these techniques for the remediation of DPD and provide examples of these adaptations in Table 9–2. In the next section we will discuss the principles of focused stimulation as an intervention technique, as set out by Fey, Long, and Finestack (2003) for facilitating morphosyntax development in children with SLI, focusing on the research literature in this context. Subsequently, we provide demonstrations of focused stimulation applications for children with DPD. Finally, we review studies in which this technique has been used for the promotion of speech accuracy in children with DPD.

Focused stimulation is an intervention procedure in which the SLP applies a number of techniques in the context of an activity structured to provide the child with many exposures to a specific target form without explicitly requiring the child to imitate or otherwise produce the target.

Focused stimulation activities occur in **hybrid intervention contexts** because they include aspects of child-centered and clinician-directed contexts.

Focused stimulation techniques, adapted to enhance phonological knowledge, are described in Table 9–2.

Principles of Focused Stimulation

Focused stimulation is used as a procedure in a number of different approaches to language intervention that vary somewhat in their underlying theoretical orientation. In general, however, the procedure is compatible with any approach that posits some sort of limitation on the child's ability to process language input as a

Table 9–2. *Focused Stimulation Techniques Adapted to Enhance Phonological Knowledge with /ʃ/ as the Specific Goal in the Examples*

Technique	*Description*	*Example*
Time delay/slow rate	Slow pace of conversation and rate of presentation and wait longer than is typical for a desired child response.	SLP: Here is a black (pause) shoe. Here is a red (pause) shoe. Oh, look, here is the other black (pause) Child: [su]
Model	Present target form, often in contrast, without an opportunity for child production.	SLP: Look at Sherry. Sherry's shoe is too big. Look at Sue. Sue's shoe is too small. Oh no! Their shoes were switched.
Recast	Immediately respond to the child's utterance, repeating some of the child's words while correcting or modifying the target form.	Child: [dɪs hə su] SLP: It's her *shoe*.
Expansion	Immediately respond to the child's utterance, repeating some of the child's words while adding content that expands the child's meaning.	Child: [dɪs hə su] SLP: This shoe is the right size for Sherry.
Imitation/feedback	Immediately respond to the child's utterance by imitating the child's correct use of the target form.	Child: [dɪs hə ʃu] SLP: Yes, this is her shoe.
Question	Ask a question that may or may not include the target form in order to prompt production of the target from the child.	SLP: What will she do now? Child: Put on the red shoe.

Source: Adapted from "Dosage and Distribution in Morphosyntax Intervention: Current Evidence and Future Needs," by K. Proctor-Williams, 2009, *Topics in Language Disorders*, 29(4), Table 1, p. 297. Copyright 2009 by Lippincott Williams & Wilkins. Reprinted with permission.

primary causal factor in origin of the language deficit; furthermore, the nature of the language input in interaction with the social learning environment are seen as being important sources of variation in children's language outcomes in both normal and delayed language development. Therefore, the principles for application of focused stimulation serve to increase the frequency and salience of the target form in the input provided to the child so that the child can develop adultlike representations for forms that are incorrect, absent or inconsistently realized in the child's productive output. Fey et al. (2003) outlined the principles for implementing focused stimulation for facilitating productive grammar skills in children with SLI. We summarize five of these principles with adaptations to the DPD context in the paragraphs to follow.

The principles for application of focused stimulation serve to **increase the frequency and salience of the target form** in the input provided to the child so that the child can develop adultlike representations for forms that are incorrect, absent, or inconsistently realized in the child's productive output.

The first principle is that it is necessary for the SLP to plan the activity carefully to ensure that the goal of providing increased exposure to the target form is met. This means manipulating the physical, social, and linguistic environments to create opportunities for modeling and eliciting the target form. It goes without saying that the SLP must have a very clear notion of what the target form is when designing the activity. Our experience training SLPs to provide interventions in clinical trials has taught us that this is not always the case, especially in the context of these hybrid intervention contexts. The activities feel like unstructured play but the environment must be highly structured in advance to increase dose frequency during the treatment session. In the context of speech therapy for DPD, we recommend that dose frequency focus on the number of models provided per minute of therapy time in the early stages of the intervention. The goal is to strengthen the child's acoustic phonetic representation for the target form. A common strategy is to create narratives that have a repetitive structure with toys, flannel pieces, puppets, dramatic play materials, handmade books, and children's picture books that highlight the targeted phonological unit. Craft activities that require a large number of small parts (stickers, Popsicle sticks, puffballs, glue sticks, crayons of different colors, and so on) are another favorite. Free play with doll houses or barns that contain many small pieces also offer many opportunities for clinician input and child requests and vocalizations. Prompts for production, either in the form of pauses or questions, are used less frequently while the child is reluctant to attempt the form or is producing the form incorrectly. When the child begins to spontaneously offer correct productions of the form, the structure of the activity can be shifted to increase the frequency of prompts for production, increasing in turn the provision of recasts, imitations, or expansions of the child's production attempts by the SLP. Fey et al. recommend disrupting the physical environment or routines within the environment or the conversational flow as devices for prompting responses from the child. We believe that our advice to focus on modeling early in the treatment program and on eliciting spoken responses from the child later, when the child's representation for the target form is more stable, is consistent with the research evidence for language therapy (e.g., Hassink & Leonard, 2010; Proctor-Williams & Fey, 2007). We believe that it is also consistent with patterns of selection and avoidance in normal phonological development (Schwartz & Leonard, 1982). Unfortunately, however, there is no systematic research on the relative efficacy of these specific techniques in the DPD context.

The SLP must **plan the activity carefully** to create opportunities for frequent modeling and implicit elicitation of the target form.

We recommend that the SLP **focus on modeling target form** in the early stages of the intervention.

When the child begins to spontaneously offer correct productions of the form, **gradually increase the frequency of prompts for production**.

The next principle is to structure activities so that the children's needs in the areas of language and literacy are met in addition to focusing on the targeted phonological form. As stressed throughout Chapter 7 and demonstrated in the case studies in Chapter 8, the DPD population overlaps with dyslexia and SLI and they are at risk for delays in the development of literacy skills. Different textual genres provide authentic media for providing exposure to specific phonological targets that help prepare the child for the transition from oral to written language styles. Commercial speech therapy materials include "stories" that provide heavy exposure to certain phonemes but are often artificial in style and do not provide good

Structure activities so that the children's needs in the areas of language and literacy are met in addition to focusing on the targeted phonological form.

examples of common narrative styles that the child will experience in the classroom environment.

Increase salience of the target structure in *pragmatically felicitous contexts.*

The third principle is to make the target structure more salient in "pragmatically felicitous" contexts. The difficulty is in knowing how best to accomplish this goal. Researchers who are working to develop efficacious techniques for grammar facilitation have grappled with the problem of increasing the salience of grammatical morphemes while not distorting the metrical context in which these morphemes normally occur. For example, when teaching the present progressive morpheme "is," the SLP might say, "The boy IS running fast" in an effort to emphasize the target morpheme even though the resulting sentence will have a distorted metrical frame. An alternative way of emphasizing the target is to say, "The boy is running. He really IS." In language therapy it is thought that the second form is better than the first as this particular discourse modification provides a means of emphasizing the word "IS" in the phrase-final position where pitch changes and added duration are natural. Empirical evidence is lacking however in both the language and the speech therapy context. We share the concern that typical patterns of emphasis used in speech therapy serve to distort the normal cues to phoneme identity. For example, if the target form is /l/ and the SLP provides a model or recast with emphasis on this phoneme in the onset position, usually the static portion of the liquid will be prolonged, [lːʊk æt̚ ðə lːek], emphasizing acoustic elements that have more in common with the alveolar nasal than the dynamic transitional portion of the word that holds the acoustic cues that are most characteristic of the /l/ phoneme. The problem with manipulating cues for emphatic stress is that these techniques do effectively draw the listener's attention to specific parts of the speech input (Weismer & Hesketh, 1998) but with sometimes perverse effects when attention is drawn away from the actual target or when normally correlated cues become uncorrelated in the mind of the listener. Plante, Bahl, Vance, and Gerken (2010) demonstrated this in a study in which children learned novel stress assignment rules for an artificial language in an implicit learning paradigm. An interesting finding in this research program was that infants and preschool-age children are successful at this task whereas adults are not, highlighting the excellent implicit learning abilities of infants and young children. Follow-up studies revealed that adult ability to abstract the rules is somewhat improved by the addition of extra emphasis to stressed syllables in the input. On the other hand, the addition of additional amplitude to the stressed syllables interfered with children's learning of the stress assignment rules when testing children with normal and delayed language skills. Plante et al. concluded that the children interpreted the extra amplitude as an emphatic stress cue that drew their attention to specific syllables and away from the overall metrical pattern. Given that infants and young children use their knowledge of metrical patterns to abstract phonotactic cues and vice versa it may not be an efficacious practice to emphasize segments or syllables while distorting the metrical structure of the words and phrases in which those units occur. This may be true regardless of whether the target of the intervention is a metrical pattern (e.g., iambic stress pattern, CV'CVC), the segmental content of a given prosodic structure (e.g., [ɪŋ] in weak syllables) or a specific segment (e.g., [ɪ]). Once again, however, specific studies are required to determine the correct techniques to use when attempting to increase the salience of each of these kinds of target structures. In the absence of such evidence, our advice is to employ the technique that is used by mothers in the early stages of language development, specifically the use of an infant-directed speaking register as described in Chapter 2. In fact, one aspect of "motherese," a slower speaking rate, has been shown to impact word learning. Specifically, children with SLI learned to produce new words as well as normally developing children when the novel words were modeled in sentence frames at a slow speaking rate; their performance was significantly worse than that of the control group when the stimuli were presented at fast rates however (Weismer & Hesketh, 1996).

Do not distort the metrical structure of words and phrases by unnaturally emphasizing target structures within the language input.

Children with SLI learned to produce new words as well as normally developing children when the novel words were modeled in sentence frames at a **slow speaking rate**.

The fourth principle is to provide opportunities for the child to contrast his or her production with the correct production of the target. The technique used to meet this goal is to respond immediately to child attempts at the target with recasts of an incorrect production or imitations of a correct production. The nature of the interaction in which a recast is provided is expected to promote joint adult-child attention to the target form in the utterance produced by the child (known as the "platform") and the recast produced by the adult, thus increasing the saliency of the target form and the contrast to the platform utterance. As we indicated earlier, however, the effectiveness of recasts is variable, possibly greater for children with typical language than for children with SLI (Proctor-Williams & Fey, 2007) and enhanced in the later stages of therapy than the earlier stages when the child's representation of the target is unstable (Hassink & Leonard, 2010). This may be especially true when focused stimulation is used to facilitate phonological development. Even if the child perceives the difference between his or her own utterance and the clinician's utterance, the child may not perceive the difference in a way that supports a change in production. Consider the hypothetical exchange shown in Figure 9–1, which contains schematics of spectrograms of /ɹ/-initial words based on actual productions recorded during a treatment session conducted by the first author. In this case, the words "rock" and "walk" as produced by the adult are similar except for the starting frequencies of the second and third formants in the words: the third formant starts at a low frequency in the word "rock" and at a high frequency in the "walk"; the second formant starts at a medium frequency that is very close to the third in the word "rock" whereas it starts at a very low frequency that is far from the third in the word "walk." The child's productions of the words "rock" and "walk" also differ but in this case only the second formant is manipulated, a change that

Provide opportunities for the child to contrast his or her production with the correct production of the target.

The child's attempt to produce the target (**platform**) and the adult response containing a correct version of the child's utterance (**recast**) promotes joint attention to the target form.

Unless the child has a stable acoustic-phonetic representation for the target form, the child may not perceive the difference between the platform and the recast in a way that supports a change in production.

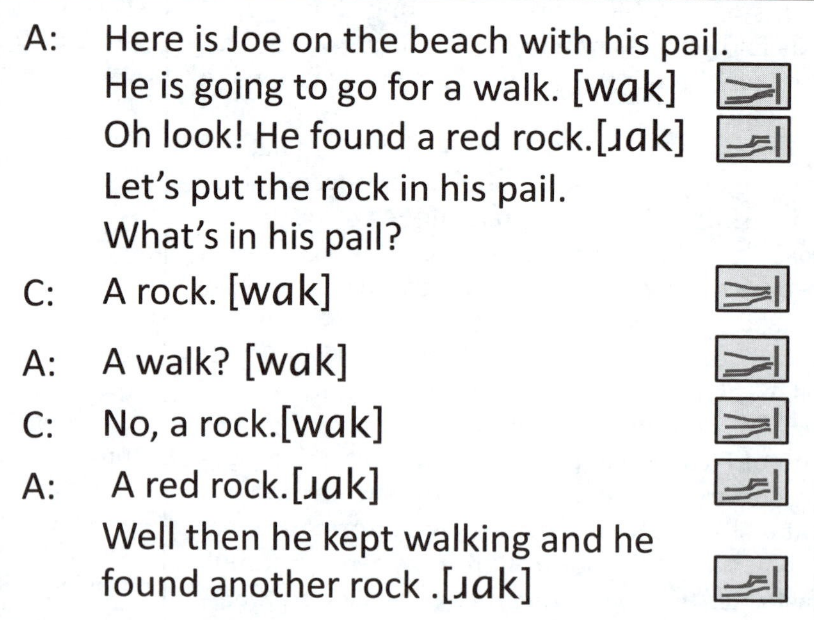

A: Here is Joe on the beach with his pail.
He is going to go for a walk. [wɑk]
Oh look! He found a red rock.[ɹɑk]
Let's put the rock in his pail.
What's in his pail?
C: A rock. [wɑk]
A: A walk? [wɑk]
C: No, a rock.[wɑk]
A: A red rock.[ɹɑk]
Well then he kept walking and he
found another rock .[ɹɑk]

Figure 9–1. *Hypothetical exchange between adult and child illustrating the possible ineffectiveness of recasts when the child's underlying representation of the target form is not adultlike. Schematics of the spectrograms for the words "walk" and "rock" are shown focusing on the first three formant transitions in the onset. Notice that the words "rock" and "walk" as produced by the adult are similar except for the starting frequencies of the second and third formants in the words: the third formant starts at a low frequency in the word "rock" and at a high frequency in the "walk"; the second formant starts at a medium frequency that is very close to the third in the word "rock" whereas it starts at a very low frequency which is far from the third in the word "walk." The child's productions of the words "rock" and "walk" also differ but in this case only the second formant is manipulated, a change that is not perceptible as a phonemic change to the adult listener: the third formant is high in both words but the second formant starts at a medium frequency in the word "rock" and at a low frequency in the word "walk."*

is not perceptible as a phonemic change to the adult listener: the third formant is high in both words but the second formant starts at a medium frequency in the word "rock" and at a low frequency in the word "walk." When the child says, "No, a rock [wɑk]" and the adult recasts and expands as "a red rock" the child may not attend to the difference in the third formant frequency; alternatively, the child may be aware of the acoustic difference in the words, but not be aware of the phonemic significance of the differences. In this case, concentrated exposure to highly variable but naturally produced models of the /ɹ/ phoneme may be required before recasting is an effective procedure for motivating change in the child's productions. Furthermore, activities that stimulate child productions at this stage (for the purpose of recasting them) have the perverse effect of strengthening the linkages between the child's inappropriate acoustic-phonetic and articulatory-phonetic representations for these /ɹ/-initial words.

To further the effective use of recasts, the recast must directly follow the child's platform utterance in a manner that is contingent upon the child's misarticulation of the target structure. Furthermore, the activity in which the recasts are embedded should not be designed to elicit productions that are far in advance of the child's abilities. For example, interrogative recasts ("Will you get it?") do not facilitate emergence of auxiliaries in children who do not produce auxiliary verbs in declarative sentences (Fey et al., 2003). Similarly, if a child were capable of producing [ʃ] in isolation but not syllables it might be appropriate to design an activity in which SH! is elicited in the context of putting dolls to bed; eliciting child production of doll names such as "Sherry" and "Shelly" during the same activity would be inappropriate although modeling of these names might be acceptable in the context of the activity. Activities designed to provide high quality input without eliciting spoken responses from the child are sometimes called "auditory bombardment" as we discuss later in this chapter.

The recast must directly follow the child's platform utterance in a manner that is **contingent** upon the child's misarticulation of the target structure.

Activities designed to provide high quality input without eliciting spoken responses from the child are sometimes called **auditory bombardment**.

Finally, users of focused stimulation are cautioned to avoid the use of telegraphic speech, a mandated form of modeling simplified utterances in some approaches to language therapy (for review, see van Kleeck et al., 2010). These kinds of utterances, in which content words are emphasized and grammatical parts of speech are omitted in an effort to simplify models for children (e.g., "baby go bed"), raise the same concerns about disrupting the normal relationships between prosody, phonology, semantics, and morphology that are so important to children's learning of word boundaries, phonotactics, semantic, and syntactic forms from the language input. Note however that sentence fragments that are otherwise grammatically correct are typical in normal conversation and acceptable in focused stimulation. For example, given the context and gestures that accompany the exchange, "The baby is going to bed" . . . "in the bed" . . . "all tucked in" . . . "night-night" . . . "oh! sleeping . . . finally" could be perfectly appropriate; on the other hand, "baby go bed," "baby in bed," "I tuck baby in," "baby go night-night," "baby sleep now" provide models of ungrammatical sentences that are stripped of important prosodic cues to word boundaries and grammatical classes.

When simplifying language models for children, avoid the use of **telegraphic speech**, in which content words are emphasized and grammatical parts of speech are omitted.

Demonstrations of Focused Stimulation to Remediate DPD

We provide some examples of applications of this procedure that are drawn from the published literature and our research transcripts with a view to demonstrating some of the ways in which focused stimulation can be applied for the remediation of DPD.

One of the peculiarities of research into focused stimulation is that the technique is expected to strengthen the child's representations for the targeted forms but the outcomes of the intervention are typically observed in the child's productive speech and language output. As the procedure includes a mix of techniques for providing speech input and eliciting speech output it is not completely assured that the impact of the approach on productive output is mediated by changes in the child's perceptual knowledge of the target forms. Nonetheless, in the examples to follow the intervention focus was heavily weighted toward providing models of the target; furthermore, any prompts for production attempts by the child were implicit rather than explicit; therefore, we assume that the treatments had their primary impacts at the level of acoustic-phonetic representations, with those representations in turn serving as a target for the development of motor plans once the child chose to practice speech production. We return to these questions when we review the research evidence in the section to follow.

In Demonstration 9–1, the student SLP is using a commercial picture book to present the child with many exposures to the target phoneme while engaging in a natural conversation about the story and the pictures and placing no pressure on the child to produce the target form. The child is enrolled in a randomized control trial of interventions that are being provided to French-speaking children with DPD. Half the children are receiving an input-focused intervention while the remainder received a traditional output-focused intervention. This child is in the input-focused condition which includes most of the procedures to be described in this chapter as well as some phonological therapy procedures to be described in Chapter 11. The original exchange, which occurred in French, targeted the phoneme /ʃ/ and involved the book *Michel, le mouton qui n'avait pas de chance* (Michel, the Sheep Who Had No Luck) by Sylvain Victor. The transcript has been altered to transmit the key characteristics of the exchange in English. For this purpose the target is /l/ and the imaginary book is *Lisa, the Unlucky Lamb*. In this project, every child is introduced to their target phoneme in the first treatment session: each phoneme is identified with a descriptive label and the auditory and articulatory characteristics of the target are demonstrated briefly. In this exchange the clinician begins by reminding the child that they are listening for the "tongue flipping" sound. Subsequently she does most of the talking although she answers his questions and asks questions about the story. She makes no effort to elicit productions of the target. The one time that he produces the target, incorrectly in this instance, she recasts by repeating the word with correct articulation. Although the actual activity lasted more than 10 minutes, only the first 90 seconds are reproduced here, a period during which the student SLP provided 30 presentations of the target and the child attempted the target once in 3 utterances. In most speech therapy activities (e.g., tradi-

Demonstration 9–1
Focused Stimulation Adapted to Increase Exposure to Target Phoneme /l/ in a Narrative and Conversational Context

Adult: Remember last week, I told you we would be listening for the tongue flipping sound [lə].

Child: (nods)

Adult: In this book the sound [lə] is hidden in the words.

Child: In the words?

Adult: Yes, the sound [lə] is hidden in the words. Listen.

Adult: (underlines title with finger) Lisa, the unlucky lamb.

Child: What means unlucky [ʌnwʌki]?

Adult: Unlucky? Unlucky means you have no luck. When you have luck good things happen. When you don't have luck—so sad, too bad. Things don't go so well. Let's read the book about Lisa the unlucky lamb. You will learn about being *unlucky*.

Adult: (turns to first page) Lisa loves raspberries. Here are some raspberries. But look, Lisa is not lucky! Why is she unlucky?

Child: She can't pass.

Adult: That's right. She can't pass through the hedge. She can't get the raspberries. Lisa is really unlucky.

Source: This exchange was adapted from a transcript of a therapy session conducted in French with participant 1110 in the Essai Clinique Randomisé sur les Interventions Phonologiques (ECRIP trial).

tional speech therapy as described in Chapter 10 or the dialogic reading procedure to be discussed later in this chapter) the unbalanced nature of the exchange would be a concern. Typically, one wants the child to contribute as least as much as the adult to the conversation. In contrast, the input focused procedures used in this research program were designed to encourage listening by the child and to ensure exposure to many exemplars of the target in a variety of words and phonetic contexts. Therefore, verbal and nonverbal responses were elicited only for the purpose of maintaining engagement of the child with the story and interaction between the child

Recasting phonological and syntactic information at the same time is not advisable because the child will not be able to process both kinds of changes to the platform utterance simultaneously.

and the adult. The most frequently used technique was modeling of correct /l/ phonemes in the context of the narrative. One corrective recast was offered (when the student SLP repeats the child utterance [ʌnwʌki] with corrected pronunciation. Notice that the recast is a pure "speech recast," adding information about the correct acoustic-phonetic realization of the /l/ but not adding semantic or syntactic complexity to the child's utterance. Yoder, Camarata, and Gardner (2005) explain that recasting phonological and syntactic information at the same time is not advisable because the child will not be able to process both kinds of changes to the platform utterance simultaneously. In this specific example, the student SLP could have provided a very complex recast such as, "What does unlucky mean?" but this recast may not have served to focus the child's attention on the misarticulated target phoneme because it also provides corrected syntactic information. If the treatment is intended to improve the child's speech intelligibility, the recast should be structured to provide information about the phonetic accuracy of the child's utterance. Later in the exchange reproduced in Demonstration 9–1, another technique was used when the child answered the question, "Why is Lisa unlucky." In this case the student SLP expanded the child's response to the question. The expansion provided more information but the target sound and word was not used in the question prompt or the expansion of the child's answer. Rather, it is a natural exchange that advances the narrative and maintains the child's engagement without placing any pressure on the child to produce the target.

The 58-month-old child highlighted in Demonstration 9–1 was a very good candidate for this treatment approach and responded really well with only 6 sessions of direct individual intervention targeting /ʃ/, /ʁ/-clusters, and /l/-clusters in each 45-minute session. Prior to treatment he obtained scores of 55% correct on a test of perception of /ʃ/ (indicating chance level performance) and 30% correct on a production probe for this target. This child also had very poor phonological awareness skills scoring 4 out of 34 points on the pretreatment test of implicit awareness of onsets and rimes. After 6 weeks of intervention in which focused stimulation and ear training were the primary intervention procedures the child demonstrated significant improvements with production probe performance doubling to 60% correct and phonological awareness test performance increasing to 14 points even though phonological awareness had not yet been addressed in the treatment program. The results of this trial are described at the end of this chapter.

Demonstration 9–2 provides an example of how powerful the technique can be even when applied by parents in the home environment. This case study was reported by Leonard and McGregor (1991).The child presented with an unusual phonological pattern that involved a preference for strident continuants in the coda position of syllables. The child was found upon assessment to have nor-

Demonstration 9–2
Changes in a Complex Phonological Pattern After 4 Months of Parent-Provided Focused Stimulation (Models and Recasts)

Productions of Words with Sibilant Onsets at Initial Assessment (Age 2;9)

[f]		[s]		[ʃ]	
fall	[af]	saw	[as]	sheep	[ips]
fine	[aɪnf]	school	[kus]	shines	[dains]
finger	[ɪŋges]	sink	[ɪŋks]	shirt	[ʌts]
five	[aɪf]	snake	[neks]	shoe	[us]
forks	[aks]	soap	[ops]	shoes	[us]

Changes in Productions of Words with Sibilant Onsets (Age 3;1)

Adultlike		Prolonged		Incorrect	
spoon	[spun]	seal	[s il]	fine	[ainf]
snake	[snek]	fish	[f ɪs]	school	[kus]
sock	[sɑk]	face	[s es]	snoopy	[nupis]
soup	[sup]			snowman	[nosmæn]
fork	[fɔk]			cereal	[iʊs]

Source: Selected from case study data presented in Leonard and McGregor (1991).

mal hearing and language skills. The mother's diary indicated that the child's first words, emerging at age 1;10, were "baby, bear, bed, blankie, bottle, bus, chair, daddy, Josh, mommie, pepsi, pizza, and truck" (p. 262). The first word to target a sibilant in the onset was "shoe," produced for the first time as [us] at the age of 2;0. At 2;9 she was observed to produce 12 phones representing stops, nasals, fricatives, and glides. Her syllable shape repertoire was also appropriate although clusters were produced only in the coda position. The unusual aspect of her phonology, demonstrated in selected words from the speech sample collected by Leonard and McGregor, was the delinking of strident continuants [f s z ʃ] from the onset position and their reappearance in the coda. The child's mother was taught to recast the child's mismatched productions, specifically, to repeat the child's word while prolonging the sibilant in the onset position. Two months later one can see movement toward resolution of the pattern as shown in the lower table in Demonstration 9–2. The authors report that other aspects of the child's phonology remained unchanged (i.e., stopping of affricates, omission of word-initial liquids, and reduction of word-initial liquid clusters continued as seen at the first assessment). This observation attests to the effectiveness and the specificity of the procedure in this case.

Empirical Evidence for the Efficacy of Focused Stimulation

Girolametto, Pearce, and Weitzman (1997) conducted a randomized controlled trial of focused stimulation in which mothers of late-talking toddlers were taught to provide their children with frequent exposure to specific target words. It was expected that the children's phonetic repertoire and syllable shape repertoire would expand along with the size of the lexicon given the "assumption that, at this early age, children learn words, not sounds" (p. 338). The children in the study, aged 23 to 35 months, had expressive and/or receptive language delays, restricted phonetic repertoires, low average to above average cognitive abilities and no known biological or social causal-correlates. Families were randomly assigned to receive immediate treatment or delayed treatment. The intervention consisted of 8 parent group sessions and 3 home visits that were used to teach parents a variety of parental input techniques, including: (a) child-oriented techniques to establish joint attention; (b) interaction promoting techniques to foster balanced turn-taking in nonverbal and verbal routines; (c) language modeling techniques applied incidentally in the natural environment to highlight relationships between language content, form, and use; and (d) focused stimulation techniques to teach 20 specific vocabulary items selected individually for each child. When examining change over a 4-month interval, large and significant differences were observed between groups on a variety of language and phonology outcomes including: (a) vocabulary size; (b) use of multiword utterances; (c) grammatical complexity of utterances; (d) complexity of syllable structures; (e) size of phonetic inventory in word-initial and final position; and (f) size of the phonetic inventory for early, middle, and late developing phones. Overall, articulation accuracy did not differ between groups (as measured by the PCC), highlighting the importance of using word-based measures of phonological development with young children as described in Chapter 4. The model of phonological development presented in Chapter 4 explains how exposure to good quality language input in a social learning context will have impacts on the child's representations at the acoustic-phonetic, semantic, articulatory, and phonological levels. The authors proposed that the opportunity to compare their own productions with the immediate recasts by the mothers was a key component of the intervention (although in fact this has not been established empirically). In addition, the expansion of the expressive lexicon

When parents were taught to use focused stimulation to increase vocabulary size in late-talking toddlers, improvements in many aspects of expressive phonology were observed.

itself forces a reorganization of the child's phonology in order to reduce homonymy and thus increase communicative effectiveness.

In contrast, Fey et al. (1994) did not find that focused stimulation targeting grammatical morphemes had a measurable impact on phonology. The 26 participants in this study, aged 44 to 70 months, had specific language impairment and concomitant delays in phonological development. After five months of intervention, children receiving either SLP or parent provided interventions had significantly higher Developmental Sentence Scores than the control group but there were no between-group differences in PCC. There was evidence that the children with milder phonological impairments experienced a significant reduction in the use of cluster reduction during the treatment period. Given that the morphosyntactic targets of the intervention often involved word final consonant sequences (i.e., as occur when producing third person singular or past tense morphemes), this finding suggests transfer of learning from the morphosyntactic targets to phonological forms. Therefore, this study suggests that focused stimulation, when applied with children who have progressed past the single word stage of language development, should target specific phonological goals to have an impact on phonological outcomes.

In contrast, focused stimulation targeting grammatical morphemes in older children did not have a measurable impact on phonology.

Camarata (2010) describes the application of "broad target recasts" within a focused stimulation approach designed to improve speech intelligibility in 3- to 4-year-old children with primary or secondary speech and language impairments. Camarata stresses that the goal of the intervention is to improve intelligibility of the child's speech, as in increase the number of utterances that can be understood by the listener, a goal distinguished from the more typical speech therapy goal of improving speech accuracy. With this approach the SLP decides on an utterance-by-utterance basis whether to recast the phonetic content of the child's platform utterance or, alternatively, to recast the grammar or expand the meaning of the child's utterance. Care was taken to not combine speech recasts with sentence recasts. Therefore, if a child said [dɪs din wɑən] the SLP might respond, "clean lion"; on the other hand, if the child produced a more intelligible but ungrammatical sentence such as [hɪm bæd dɑg] the SLP could respond, "He is a very bad dog." Yoder et al. (2005) describe the results of a randomized control trial to assess the efficacy of broad target recasts to improve speech intelligibility and sentence length in children aged 44 months with speech and language delays of unknown origin. Experimental group children received 3 half-hour treatment sessions per month for 6 months. Control group children were not treated as part of the project although children in both groups were free to seek additional interventions in the community. The primary outcome measures were proportion of fully intelligible utterances and MLU measured 10 and 14 months after study entry. No main effects of the intervention were revealed at either follow-up group

Broad target recasting, in which syntactic or phonological targets are recast on an utterance-by-utterance basis within the same session, does not appear to be effective as a treatment procedure for improving intelligibility globally in preschoolers with DPD.

There is evidence to suggest that phonological and morphological goals can be addressed effectively with focused stimulation in the same child using an **alternating goal attack strategy**.

for either outcome measure. The authors reported that the outcomes interacted with pretreatment status such that a treatment effect was observed for those children who showed the poorest pretreatment articulation accuracy. This effect was observed only at the 14-month follow-up assessment, however. The practical significance of the outcomes is difficult to judge because the outcome data as reported cannot be interpreted relative to age-level expectations for speech intelligibility or accuracy. Camarata's (2010) literature review does not provide strong and reliable evidence that broad target recasting is effective as a treatment procedure for targeting intelligibility globally in preschoolers with DPD.

Although the research evidence suggests that focused stimulation is more effective when applied to the correction of specific targets, there is evidence to suggest that phonological and morphological goals can be addressed effectively in the same child using an alternating goal attack strategy. Tyler, Lewis, Haskill, and Tolbert (2003) randomly assigned 47 preschoolers with co-occuring speech and language impairments to 4 different goal attack strategies implemented over a 24-week period: (1) 12-week phonology intervention followed by 12-week morphosyntax intervention; (2) 12-week morphosyntax intervention followed by 12-week phonology intervention; (3) phonology and morphosyntax interventions alternated weekly; and (4) phonology and morphosyntax goals addressed simultaneously in each session. Morphosyntax and phonology outcome data were collected from children in these 4 groups and from a wait-list control group that received no intervention. Treatment procedures when targeting phonology or morphosyntax included auditory awareness, focused stimulation, and elicited production procedures. The results revealed a clear advantage to the alternating goal attack strategy for improvements in morphosyntax. The authors speculate that the alternating strategy provided sustained attention to the children's morphosyntax difficulties over a long interval while replicating the normal learning process which is gradual in nature. They further speculate that the simultaneous condition was overwhelming for the children who had difficulties in both domains. With respect to phonological changes, equivalent outcomes were observed in all 4 treatment groups, with each group showing a large gain in productive phonology relative to the control group.

Summary: Focused Stimulation

Focused stimulation is a procedure that combines a series of techniques designed to provide children with frequent exposure to targeted linguistic forms without specifically requiring the child to imitate or otherwise produce the forms. The techniques are applied in the context of naturalistic, responsive interactions between adult and child after manipulating the environment to ensure frequent opportunities to produce the target in meaningful contexts. The research evidence indicates that the procedure is effective for promoting improvements in syntax when grammatical forms are targeted and vocabulary when words are targeted. The evidence for the use of the procedure to promote phonological development is mixed. One good quality randomized control trial indicates that facilitating expressive vocabulary development in late-talking toddlers has a corollary effect on the children's phonetic and syllable structure repertoires, an impact that makes sense given the strong relationship between phonological and lexical development in the early stages of language acquisition. Studies with older children have not yielded clear results with respect to carryover from language to phonological goals. One good quality randomized controlled trial has shown that the procedure can be used effectively to treat morphosyntax and phonological goals in the same children using an alternating goal attack strategy. Our interpretation of the findings thus far is that the procedure is most likely to be effective when specific target forms are selected and when the target is clear to both the clinician (and/or parent) and the child during any given activity. However, further research is required to test this hypothesis in the speech therapy context. It is also necessary to assess the relative impact of models versus recasts for children who have unstable acoustic-phonetic representations for the target forms. On a related point, further research involving a broader range of measures of phonological knowledge is required to determine whether the effect of focused stimulation techniques on children's productive output is moderated by improvements in the child's perceptual representations for the target forms, or by productive practice of those forms by the child. Laboratory research on novel word learning by normally developing children suggests the former process (see Richtsmeier, Goffman, & Hogan, 2009 as discussed in Chapter 4), but intervention research with the DPD population is required to clarify these issues. Finally, it is necessary to determine whether the procedure can be effective by itself or whether it needs to be combined with other procedures targeting knowledge at articulatory and phonological levels of representation. Currently, we recommend it as the best procedure for very young children, children at the early stages of language or phonological development and children who are reluctant to engage in traditional output-oriented approaches to articulation therapy. It also appears to be an effective component of interventions for older children with DPD (e.g., Tyler et al., 2003) but more comparative randomized controlled trials are required. As we will report later in this chapter we included it as one component of an intervention for 4- to 5-year-old children with DPD that was found to be effective in a randomized controlled trial but more research would be required to be sure that it was a necessary component of that intervention.

Ear Training

9.2.1. Describe and provide examples of four ear training techniques.

9.2.2. Demonstrate ability to construct discrimination (error detection) tasks to improve perception of specific phonological targets to be implemented by computer or in live-voice activities and at the single-word and sentence levels.

9.2.3. Evaluate the research evidence on "ear training" when provided live voice and with computer programs to identify the conditions under which it may be effective and predict the outcomes that are likely when it is used.

Charles Gage Van Riper (1905–1994) is the author of *Speech Correction: Principles and Methods*, reputed to be the first textbook in the field of speech pathology.

The **traditional approach** to speech therapy comprises two distinct stages, ear training followed by production training.

The purpose of the **ear training** stage is to help the child develop an internalized auditory model of the phoneme to serve as a target for the child's productions during the production training stage of the intervention.

The first ear training technique serves to **identify** the target for the child, highlighting the acoustic and articulatory characteristics of the phoneme.

The second technique—**isolation**—involves highlighting the contrast between the target and other phonemes.

The third technique—**stimulation** (also known as auditory bombardment)—involves providing concentrated exposure to the target.

Once the **internal model** is established the child is expected to use this model to make judgments about correct and incorrect productions of the sound as produced by the SLP in words.

Van Riper (1978), in a book first published in 1939, described a systematic approach to speech therapy comprising two distinct stages, ear training followed by production training (see also Hall Powers, 1957, a strong advocate of auditory training as an alternative to "oral gymnastics" and tongue excersises as the first phase of therapy). The purpose of the ear training stage is to help the child develop an internalized auditory model of the phoneme to serve as a target for the child's productions during the production training stage of the intervention. As defined in Table 9–3, four different techniques are employed that are somewhat more explicit and much more SLP-directed than those used during focused stimulation. The first technique serves to identify the target for the child, highlighting the acoustic and articulatory characteristics of the phoneme and naming it with a child-friendly label that can be used by the SLP and the child throughout the treatment program (e.g., [s] is the "snake" sound and [θ] is the "windmill" sound). The isolation technique involves highlighting the contrast between the target and other phonemes whereas stimulation (also known as auditory bombardment) involves providing concentrated exposure to the target. This is the primary technique for helping the child develop an internal acoustic model of the target sound. Once the internal model is established the child is expected to use this model to make judgments about correct and incorrect productions of the sound as produced by the SLP. During these activities the SLP attempts to simulate the child's error. Subsequently, the internal model of the sound would serve as a target for the speech production stage of the intervention and allow the child to make judgments about his or her own speech errors and provide a basis for self-correction once stimulability was established. Rather than providing step-by-step instructions with specific criteria for advancement from one step to the next, Van Riper described treatment sessions during which

Table 9–3. *Ear Training Techniques Summarized from Van Riper (1963)*

Technique	*Description*	*Example*
Identification	SLP identifies the target for the child by briefly demonstrating the auditory, visual and tactile-kinesthetic properties of the sound.	You are going to learn the "quiet sound," (finger in front of lips) [ʃ]. Watch and listen, [ʃ]. This is how I make the quiet sound: I round my lips and pull my tongue back in mouth like this—[ʃ].
Isolation	Child signals when he or she hears the target; SLP produces the target against a background of other speech sounds in isolation, words, phrases, and sentences.	(child is hiding behind door) When you hear me say the "quiet sound," jump out and scare me with a big BOO!: [fʌ], [si], [ʃe], [zɪ], [sʌ], [ʒu], [ʃɪ], [tʃe], [vʌ], [ʃoɪ] . . .
Stimulation	SLP presents the target to the child in a variety of different ways (also known as auditory bombardment).	Listen to this story: Sheep on a Ship, by Nancy E. Shaw. Sheep sail a ship on a deep-sea trip . . .
Discrimination[a]	SLP produces words with correct and incorrect articulations of the target, mimicking the child's error while the child identifies each word as correctly or incorrectly produced.	(Provide a set of colored markers and a series of faces drawn except for the mouth). Draw a smiley mouth when I say the [ʃ] sound correctly. Draw a frowny mouth when I say the [ʃ] sound incorrectly: [ʃip] , [sip], [θip], [sɪp], [ʃɪp], [θɪp] . . .

[a]Van Riper referred to this step in the program as "discrimination" but other terms such as "error detection" or "phoneme identification" would be more accurate labels because discrimination usually involves judging the similarity of pairs of stimuli rather than making judgments about individual stimuli presented one at a time.

ear training was implemented. These detailed descriptions reveal a number of defining characteristics of this procedure, the first being that the sessions should involve a variety of interactive and fun activities in which the child and SLP are equally engaged. Even stimulation (auditory bombardment) activities were designed to ensure full engagement and active responses by the child rather than passive listening. The second is that the SLP structured the environment and the activities to ensure that the child was not relying on visual cues when making judgments about the stimuli provided by the clinician. A third characteristic was a high degree of variability in the input: variation in utterance length from isolated sounds through syllables to words, phrases, and sentences as well as variations in loudness and intonation contours. Finally, for a single phoneme, the entire program of 4 techniques could be completed in a single 40-minute treatment session. In the examples given, children progressed to making perceptual judgments about their own speech and stimulability training in the second session. We stress this because ear training has been criticized as an unnecessary delay in the introduction of production training. Historically there appear to be two reasons that clinicians were engaging in long periods of unproductive ear training prior to the introduction of

Ear training sessions should involve a variety of interactive and fun activities in which the child and SLP are equally engaged.

Make sure the child is not relying on visual cues when making judgments about the verbal stimuli.

Provide a high degree of variability in the verbal input.

The entire program of 4 techniques can be completed in a single 40-minute treatment session before procedure to speech production practice in the second session.

production training even though the original intent was that these procedures last for a single session when introducing a new target. First, SLPs found that ear training could be conducted with large groups of children; furthermore, teachers and parents could be taught to implement them in place of the SLP (e.g., Chapman, 1942). Therefore, undue emphasis on ear training emerged as a caseload management technique rather than in response to the children's therapeutic needs. Second, the transformation of the procedures to conform to behaviorist teaching methods (i.e., "machine teaching techniques," Mowrer, 1971) stripped ear training of its key characteristics resulting in unsatisfactory outcomes even after long periods of training. We provide evidence below that an engaging form of "ear training" with variable stimuli can have dramatic effects with relatively brief exposures provided prior to or concurrently with production training.

Laboratory studies on second language speech perception have revealed that the most effective training paradigms involve the presentation of **highly variable natural speech input** for identification.

Van Riper (1963) claimed that this treatment approach would be valuable for children with speech problems and for individuals with foreign accent. Rvachew and Jamieson (1995) also suggested that there were commonalities in the learning challenge for children with DPD and adults learning a second language. Young first language learners of English and adult second language learners of English may misarticulate a given phoneme, for example, [θ], because of insufficient exposure to the phoneme in the input and inexperience with phonological contrasts involving this phoneme in their language use. Both groups may be unaware of the acoustic cues that differentiate [θ] from [f] or [t] even if they can readily produce the appropriate articulatory gestures associated with the phone. Many decades of laboratory studies on second language speech perception have revealed that the most effective training paradigms involve the presentation of highly variable natural speech input for identification. Van Riper's procedures call for considerable variation in utterance length and phonetic context in the presentation of correct exemplars of the target phoneme. However, carefully controlled variation in the acoustic cues that distinguish the target from neighboring phonemes is also important (Jamieson & Morosan, 1989) as is variation in nonphonetic aspects of speech such as that introduced by presenting tokens recorded from multiple talkers (Brosseau-Lapré, Rvachew, Clayards, & Dickson, in press; Lively, Logan, & Pisoni, 1993). Furthermore, research with children with DPD and with second language learners suggests that live-voice presentation of simulated errors may not be effective because it is difficult to exactly simulate errors that are based on inappropriate cue-weighting strategies rather than the substitution of one phoneme for another. For example, when remediating [ɹ] errors in children with DPD or Japanese learners of English, one might ask the learner to identify words such as "rock" and "walk." However, this activity does not lead directly to improved knowledge of the contrast in perception or production because these individuals are attending to the second formant frequency transition in these words rather than the third; in production, manipulation of this cue results in a phone that is midway between [w] and [ɹ], something that is difficult for an adult native speaker of English to produce (see Figure 9–1).

Rvachew (1994) developed a computer-based speech perception intervention called the Speech Assessment and Interactive Learning System (SAILS), designed to apply the research findings with second language learners to the clinical context. SAILS is a computer game in which the child listens to a series of recorded attempts to produce a particular word. The child's task is to indicate whether the stimulus presented on each trial constitutes the target word or not. The treatment levels of each SAILS model consist of natural recordings of the target word, half articulated correctly by various child or adult talkers with normal speech development and half misarticulated by various child talkers with DPD. Correct exemplars vary from highly prototypical versions of the target phoneme to versions that are less distinct members of the target phoneme class. The incorrect exemplars cover the full range of commonly occurring misarticulations of the target phoneme. The SAILS task is a two-alternative forced-choice identification procedure involving real words. Basic research has established clearly that an identification task is superior to a discrimination task (in which the listener makes same-different judgments about pairs of stimuli) for inducing categorical perception (Guenther, Husain, Cohen, & Shinn-Cunningham, 1999). We want the child to make a judgment about each word based on his or her own acoustic-phonetic representation for the target phoneme.

SAILS is a computer-based listening game in which children identify well-produced and misarticulated versions of words recorded from child and adult talkers that target commonly misarticulated consonants.

Although the program is designed to present variable natural speech input, the task itself is a departure from natural implicit category learning in that the child makes an explicit judgment about the category membership of each word and receives feedback about the accuracy of that judgment. McClelland, Fiez, and McCandliss (2002) demonstrated that Japanese-speaking adults learned to perceive the /ɹ/-/l/ contrast when the intervention involved identification of fixed blocks of training stimuli presented with feedback. This training condition was completely ineffective without feedback, however. Given that SAILS was developed for older children, aged 4 to 6, it was decided that they also would most likely benefit from explicit feedback about their responses (focused stimulation is probably the more appropriate procedure for younger children).

SAILS provides visual feedback for correct responses—specifically, a new item is added to a scene shown on the left side of the screen. Providing reinforcement without information can be counterproductive because in some circumstances, external reinforcers undermine the child's intrinsic interest in an activity (Cameron, Pierce, Basko, & Gear, 2005). For this reason, the visual feedback is intended to act more as a counting device that helps the child judge the passage of time. It is expected that informative feedback will be provided by the adult who is mediating the child's interaction with the program. Although the software is designed to allow independent play by the child, this feature was not used in any of the intervention studies conducted to date. Rather, an adult provided informative feedback if the child pointed to the wrong response alternative and did not allow the child to advance to the next trial until the missed trial was re-presented and the child selected the correct response alternative.

Demonstrations of Computer-Based and Live Voice Ear Training

Demonstration 9–3 illustrates game play for the Speech Assessment and Interactive Learning System. This program contains modules that target /k/, /f/, /s/, /ʃ/, /tʃ/, /θ/, /l/, and /ɹ/ in the initial position of single syllable words. The stimuli are natural recordings of speech produced by children and adults. There are two modules for each target phoneme. An important procedural point is that the child wears headphones when completing the SAILS activity. The use of good quality headphones allows for presentation of the stimuli at an amplitude that will be perceived as loud but not uncomfortable or distorted. Recall from Chapter 2 that children require much greater loudness in the input signal to achieve the same perceptual performance as an adult listener. The computer or laptop speakers cannot provide the necessary signal presentation level or protect against ambient noise—insist that the child wear headphones during the task. You will see from the demonstration that the SLP controls the mouse throughout the activity so that the child receives informative feedback and a second chance after each error response. Otherwise, feedback is kept to a minimum so that game play can progress rapidly. The SLP keeps track of the number of trials that required corrective feedback and repeats the SAILS activity at the beginning of each session until the child has mastered the modules for the target phoneme. An error detection task of this nature can be created by any SLP for these phonemes in other syllable positions (codas, complex onsets) or for other phonemes by recording pre- and posttreatment stimuli from clients using freely available digital recording software. Digital recordings can be presented along with clipart in Powerpoint slides so that children can decide whether the recorded words match the pictured target. The important features of the stimuli are the use of authentic errors and variability in the stimuli induced by recording the correct and incorrect exemplars from many different talkers.[1]

[1]For information about SAILS and how to obtain it, visit the first author's Web site: http://www.medicine.mcgill.ca/srvachew.

Demonstration 9–3
Use of the Speech Assessment and Interactive Learning System (SAILS) to Teach Perception of /ʃ/

SLP: Cooper, today we will begin with a computer game. When we play the game, we will listen for the word "shoe." The word "shoe" begins with the sound [ʃː]. When I say this word (points to picture of "shoe" on the monitor) the right way, it sounds like this: [ʃu]. Watch me and listen: [ʃu]. You will hear people trying to say the word "shoe." When you hear a person say the word "shoe" correctly, I want you to point to the picture of "shoe" here on the monitor. (Points to the shoe.) Sometimes a person will make a mistake. If the person says the word "shoe" the wrong way, I want you to point to the X on the computer screen. (Points to the X.) If you hear a word that is *not* shoe, point to the X, OK? Are you ready to listen?

Cooper: (Nods yes.)

SLP: I'll just put the headphones on. And now we're gonna start the game. (Puts headphones on Cooper and presents the first trial in the module.)

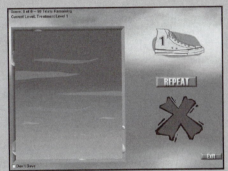

SAILS: [ʃu]

Cooper: (Points to shoe.)

SLP: Good listening Cooper! (Uses mouse to click the shoe.)

SAILS: (Adds frog and lily pad to pond.)

SAILS: [tʃu]

Cooper: (Points to shoe.)

SLP: Cooper, I didn't hear the [ʃː] sound. Watch me. It's not "shoe" unless you hear the [ʃː]. If it's *not* "shoe," point to the X. Let's listen to this one again. (Clicks the replay button.)

SAILS: [tʃu]

Cooper: (Points to shoe.)

SLP: Well, let's see what the computer thinks.

SAILS: (Presents error message: "That's not it!")

SLP: Oops, the computer didn't give you a frog. There was no [ʃː] sound in that word. Let's listen to another one.

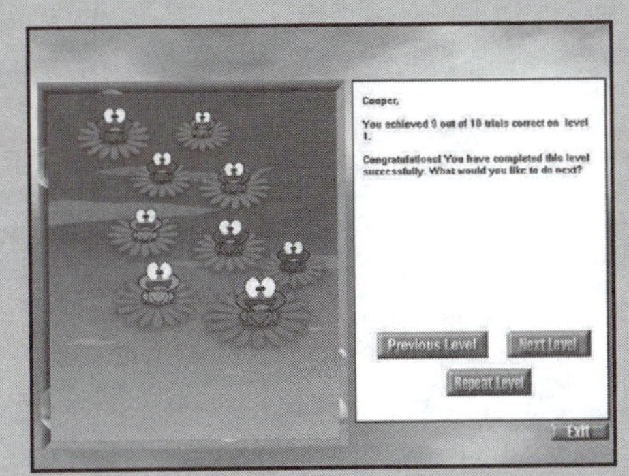

SAILS: [tu]

Cooper: (Points to X.)

SLP: Well done Cooper, there was no [ʃː] sound in that word. (Clicks the X.)

(Game play continues until ten trials are completed.)

Note: A video demonstration of the SAILS program in which author Brosseau-Lapré teaches a younger child, Shannon, to play the "feet" module, accompanies the book *Interventions of Speech Sound Disorders in Children*, by A. L. Williams, S. McLeod, & R. J. McCauley, 2010, pp. 159–177, Baltimore, MD: Brookes.

Live-voice error detection tasks allow the SLP to embed target stimuli in utterances with varying duration and complexity matched to the level of the child's language abilities.

We have also conducted live-voice error detection activities with children so that they can practice error detection when the stimuli are embedded in longer utterances. Demonstration 9–4 is an example of one such activity. The activity was conducted live-voice without amplification but ideally such activities would be conducted with a personal FM system, classroom sound-field system, or other technology that amplifies the SLP's and the child's voice. The exchange in the demonstration is an adaptation of an actual treatment session that was conducted in French, originally targeting /ʃ/ in the words "cheval" ([ʃəval]; "horse") and "vache" ([vaʃ]; "cow"). This 53-month-old child demonstrated chance level performance on a French version of the SAILS task prior to treatment as well as a complete inability to match words on the basis of shared onset or rime. He made rapid progress when taught to identify correct and incorrect productions of the /ʃ/ phoneme using the SAILS program, however. Spontaneous productions of the phoneme were beginning to emerge during focused stimulation and live-voice error detection tasks and therefore the student SLP was increasing the number of production prompts in the sessions. We have adapted the transcript to the English context so that the task is targeting velars in the English names of various farm animals. Otherwise, the exchange proceeds exactly as in the original video which is quite amusing to watch because the child has complete control of all the animals throughout the game. Although he is frustrated by the delay in being able to place the animal in the barn, he will not put it in until the student SLP says the name correctly and eventually is compelled to tell her exactly what to say! This child made good progress with respect to perceptual knowledge of the segmental and prosodic goals that were targeted during 6 weeks of individual sessions. Single word production probes for his three targets improved from 37 to 59% accuracy from the pretreatment assessment to the 6-week probe. Negligible change was observed in phonological awareness performance, however. The results of this trial are described in detail at the end of this chapter.

Empirical Evidence for the Efficacy of Ear Training

This review of treatment efficacy studies is divided into two sections, those concerned with the application of traditional live voice approaches to ear training and those testing the efficacy of the SAILS program, specifically. In these studies speech accuracy, speech perception, phonological awareness, and/or reading skills were the reported dependent variables.

Demonstration 9–4
Live-Voice Error Detection Task Combined with Production Prompts and Recasting.

Adult: OK, let's see what we have here. What is this? (hands cow to child)

Child: [tau]

Adult: A *c*ow. And this? (hands goat to child)

Child: [ʌ dot]

Adult: A *g*oat. And what about this one? (hands chick to child)

Child: [ʌ tjɪk]

Adult: Yes, a chi*ck*. And here's the last one. (hands duck to child)

Child: [dʌt]

Adult: A du*ck*. OK, you remember how we play this game? We can put the animals in the barn when I say the animal names the right way. Let's see, can we let in the [dit]?

Child: No.

Adult: No? Why not?

Child: You have to say it the right way!

Adult: Ok, can we let in the [dʌt]?

Child: No! If you say [dʌk], yes.

Adult: Oh! All right then. Can we let in the [dʌk]?

Child: Yes, it goes in this part here. (puts the duck in the barn)

Source: This exchange was adapted from a transcript of a therapy session conducted in French with participant 3101 in the Essai Clinique Randomisé sur les Interventions Phonologiques (ECRIP trial).

Efficacy of Live Voice Ear Training Procedures

The effectiveness of ear training was assessed in a large-scale trial in a school setting in which ear training was provided in some classrooms and some children with speech impairments received traditional speech therapy that included both ear training and speech production training.

Sommers et al. (1961) assessed the efficacy of Van Riper's treatment procedures in a large-scale study in which some children received "speech improvement" (ear training alone), others received speech therapy (ear training and production training) and others received neither intervention. Children who misarticulated one to five of the phonemes [v s ɹ l tʃ k ʃ f g θ] were in the "speech defective" group whereas children who articulated these phonemes correctly were placed in the "normal group." The speech improvement intervention was provided to both groups of children (because it was implemented in the classroom) but speech therapy was provided to the speech defective group only. Speech improvement was administered by speech therapists to first grade classrooms with the teacher present so that the teacher could observe and then repeat some activities from the weekly half-hour lesson for a few minutes each day. The lessons followed Van Riper's instructions for implementing identification, stimulation, isolation and discrimination techniques for the sounds [v s ɹ l tʃ k ʃ f g θ] with special emphasis on sounds that were misarticulated by any child in the classroom. No phonetic placement, choral speaking or other production activities were used in the speech improvement intervention. Homework assignments were not given in this condition. These activities were continued for 9 months in some classrooms, whereas other classes served as the controls and did not receive any intervention. Speech therapy was provided to small groups of 4 children with "defective speech," again following Van Riper's procedures, beginning with ear training and then proceeding to phonetic placement and other production practice techniques (to be discussed further in Chapter 10). Notebooks were used to provide homework activities for production practice in this condition. Some children received 9 months of weekly group speech therapy, others received 3 months of weekly group speech therapy, and others, assigned to the control group, received no intervention. Random assignment to treatment and control conditions occurred at the classroom level.

Pretreatment assessments revealed a good match for variables such as intelligence and socioeconomic status. Articulation outcomes were assessed via flashcards targeting the same 10 phonemes that were targeted in speech improvement and speech therapy. Scoring reliability was assessed by blind observers. Reading outcomes were also assessed at the end of the school year with a measure that targeted reading aptitude, auditory association, word recognition, and word attack. The results of the planned comparisons for the articulation and reading outcomes are shown in Table 9–4. With respect to outcomes for articulation accuracy, speech improvement classes were more effective than no treatment but 9 months of small group speech therapy was more effective than 9 months of classroom based speech improvement (ear training). Three months of speech therapy was not effective relative to the control condition and as effective as 9 months of speech improvement. The findings

For the improvement of articulation accuracy, traditional therapy that includes ear training and speech production training was more effective than no treatment or classroom-based ear training alone.

Table 9–4. Comparison of Speech Improvement Intervention (Ear Training) and Speech Therapy (Ear Training + Production Training) to Control Condition (No Intervention)

Groups	N	*Mean*[a]	SE[a]	*t*	*p*
Articulation Outcome Measure					
Speech improvement	402	3.31	0.338	3.28	0.01
Controls	245	2.20			
Speech improvement	402	3.31	0.427	2.88	0.01
Speech therapy (9 months)	69	4.54			
Speech improvement	402	3.31	0.488	.35	ns
Speech therapy (3 months)	36	3.14			
Speech therapy (3 months)	36	3.14	0.584	1.61	ns
Controls	245	2.20			
Speech therapy (9 months)	69	4.54	0.230	10.17	0.001
Controls	245	2.20			
Composite Reading Outcome Measure					
Speech improvement	402	36.56	1.81	2.61	0.01
Controls	245	31.83			
Speech improvement	402	36.56	1.69	2.98	0.01
Speech therapy (9 months)	69	31.53			
Speech improvement	402	36.56	1.97	2.51	0.01
Speech therapy (3 months)	36	31.62			
Speech therapy (3 months)	36	31.62	2.17		ns
Controls	245	31.83			
Speech therapy (9 months)	69	31.53	2.65		ns
Controls	245	31.83			

Note: Speech improvement intervention was provided by teachers at the classroom level. Duration of the intervention was approximately 9 months with some variation between classrooms. Speech therapy was provided by SLPs as a pull-out service to small groups of children with speech errors. Outcomes measures are reported here for children with speech errors only (i.e., data from children in the classrooms with age appropriate speech is excluded).

[a]Mean scores represent difference score on the post- versus pretreatment assessment and thus the SE is the standard error of the differences.

Source: From "Effects of Speech Therapy and Speech Improvement Upon Articulation and Reading," by R. K. Sommers, F. G. Copetas, D. C. Bowser, G. R. Fichter, A. K. Furlong, F. E. Rhodes, et al., 1962, *Journal of Speech and Hearing Disorders*, 26, p. 33 (Table 4) and p. 34 (Table 6). Copyright 1962 by the American Speech-Language and Hearing Association. Adapted with permission.

for reading were somewhat different in that changes in reading scores were greater for children in speech improvement classes in comparison to the control condition and in comparison to 3 and 9 months of speech therapy. Speech therapy did not lead to higher reading scores in comparison to the control condition. When examining outcomes for the children who did not misarticulate speech sounds, the speech improvement intervention also led to greater changes in reading scores compared to no intervention (37.58 vs. 34.83). To sum up, for children with mild and moderate speech problems, speech therapy that combines ear training with speech production training was shown to be effective for improving speech accuracy, in comparison to no treatment or speech improvement. The classroom-based speech improvement intervention, essentially ear training with no speech production component, proved to have a significant effect on the word reading abilities of children who had speech errors and children with normal speech.

This study also included 50 children who misarticulated 6 or more of the 10 phonemes on the pretreatment assessment, randomly assigned to one of two treatment conditions. One group was provided with the in-class speech improvement intervention and 9 months of weekly small group speech therapy. The other group received 9 months of speech improvement only. The outcomes for the group that received speech therapy and speech improvement, compared to the group that received speech improvement only, were very good for speech accuracy (mean change in articulation test scores being 7.82 vs. 3.05). Reading did not differ significantly between these groups (31.47 vs. 29.64).

Classroom-based ear training, by itself, was shown in this randomized controlled trial to be an inefficient and sometimes insufficient procedure for promoting speech accuracy although it was more effective than no intervention.

Ear training conducted in the classroom by the SLP and the teacher had a positive effect on single word reading, possibly as an early form of phonological awareness intervention.

Traditional speech therapy that included ear training did not have a significant effect on reading in this study although it did have a significant effect on speech accuracy compared to a no-treatment control condition.

Sommers and colleagues (Sommers et al., 1961; Sommers et al., 1962) demonstrated that classroom-based ear training, by itself, was an inefficient and sometimes insufficient procedure for promoting speech accuracy although it was more effective than no intervention. Speech improvement (ear training) conducted in the classroom by the SLP and the teacher did have a positive effect on single word reading, possibly as an early form of phonological awareness intervention. Speech therapy did not have a significant effect on reading in this study although it did have a significant effect on speech accuracy compared to no-treatment and compared to speech improvement classes.

Winitz and Bellerose (1967) demonstrated that a discrimination training task was clearly insufficient as the sole intervention in cases where the children were unstimulable for the target phoneme (in this study, the target was /ɹ/ and the 4 subjects were taught to discriminate pairs of stimuli contrasting /ɹ/-/w/ and /ɹ/-/ɹ^w/ using a same-different task). Shelton, Johnson, Ruscello, and Arndt (1978) questioned whether ear training was necessary at all when they conducted a study in which parents were provided with a home program for their preschoolers who failed an articulation screener. Unfortunately, the study does not provide an adequate test of the hypothesis that production training is effective without the addition of ear training procedures. The ear training was not implemented according to Van Riper's instructions. First, lessons were not individualized to the children's speech errors: 57 identical lessons targeting /s ɹ k f/ were provided regardless of the child's error phonemes. Second, nearly all of the training focused on isolated sounds and syllables with only 2 vowel contexts targeted so that the required stimulus variability was not provided. Treatment fidelity was unknown for most parents and poor in those cases where it was checked. The program provided approximately an hour of intervention per target phoneme which is sufficient but the distributed nature of the doses and the focus on child responses rather than parental inputs is not consistent with the principles of ear training. Parents received minimal training in the use of the prescribed booklets containing daily repetitive drill exercises that reportedly caused conflict between the parents and their children. The control group was 3 years old whereas the experimental group was 4 years old, but corrections for differences in pretreatment participant characteristics were not incorporated into the statistical analysis. Two-thirds of the sample dropped out of the study when the production therapy intervention (targeting /s/ or /ɹ/) was implemented so that, ultimately, it was not possible to compare outcomes for production treatment only to the combination of production treatment and ear training. Despite the flaws in this study it capped a decade of growing skepticism about the value of ear training and the emphasis shifted to perceptuomotor procedures in speech therapy (Mowrer, 1971; Seymour, Baran, & Peaper, 1981; Shelton & McReynolds, 1979). In general ear training fell into disuse with the exception of auditory bombardment, administered with amplification in some phonological process approaches to therapy (e.g., Hodson, 2007; Hodson & Paden, 1983).

SAILS: Computer-Based Speech Perception Training

The first randomized study involving SAILS (Rvachew, 1994) was designed to determine if speech perception training would facilitate children's response to production training for remediation of /ʃ/ misarticulations. Twenty-seven children aged 42 to 66 months with moderate DPD but normal language development participated. All of the children were unstimulable for the target phoneme (/ʃ/) during pretesting. The children were randomly assigned to three different treatment conditions. All of the children received 6 once-weekly treatment sessions. A research assistant administered 60 SAILS training trials at the beginning of each session. Subsequently, 20 minutes of articulation therapy, targeting the /ʃ/ phoneme, were provided by the first author who was blind to the child's speech perception training condition. The difference between treatment conditions lay solely with the nature of the stimuli presented during the speech perception training trials. Children in Group 1 listened to a variety of naturally produced exemplars of the word "shoe," half produced correctly and half produced incorrectly. Children in Group 2 listened to a single well-produced token of the word "shoe" and a single well-produced token of the word "moo," each token being presented 30 times. Group 3 children listened to the words "cat" and "Pete." Outcomes were assessed by an SLP who was blind to the child's group assignment.

This study showed that children do respond to prototypical stimuli produced by a single talker but that variable stimuli produced by multiple talkers results in a significantly larger effect on perception and production accuracy.

The outcomes assessed were perception of the words "sheet," acoustic measures of /ʃ/ quality, accuracy of /ʃ/ in the onsets of single words, and the highest level achieved in therapy (i.e., isolated sound, syllables, imitated words, etc.). Figure 9–2 shows pre- to posttreatment change on the speech perception test and a composite of the production outcome measures. Group 1 (shoe vs. Xshoe condition) demonstrated the greatest improvement in speech perception performance but Group 2 (shoe vs. moo condition) also showed significant gains in speech perception ability. Group 3 (cat vs. Pete condition) did not show any improvement in speech perception scores between the pre- and posttreatment assessments. With respect to improvements in speech production ability, all outcome measures indicated that Group 1 children made significantly more progress than Group 2 children who made significantly more progress than Group 3 children. In fact, only one child in Group 3 achieved stimulability for the target phoneme in isolation. On the other hand, 6 children in each of Groups 1 and 2 achieved stimulability in isolation and some children in Group 1 achieved mastery at the spontaneous sentence level. One explanation for the impact of the SAILS intervention in this study is that the children developed a strong internal representation for the /ʃ/ phoneme that allowed them to monitor the accuracy of their own productions and self-correct their errors. Although no homework exercises were assigned during this intervention, parents of children in Group 1 reported that their children engaged in self-practice when alone.

One explanation for the impact of the SAILS intervention in this study is that the children developed a strong internal representation for the /ʃ/ phoneme that allowed them to monitor the accuracy of their own productions and self-correct their errors.

The next study involving SAILS was a nonexperimental equivalent groups comparison of a modified cycles approach, with and without the inclusion of the SAILS intervention (Rvachew, Rafaat, & Martin, 1999). In the first year of this study, children received 12 weeks of small group therapy modeled after the cycles approach except that specific targets did not change as we cycled through 3 target processes during a 12-week treatment block (Hodson & Paden, 1983). Prior to the onset of the intervention the children's stimulability and perceptual knowledge of the target phonemes was assessed. Measurable improvements in production accuracy probes for these targets were observed if the child was stimulable for the sound and/or had good perceptual knowledge of the targeted phoneme category prior to treatment. When the child's speech perception performance for the target phoneme was poor or the child was unstimulable for the target, gains were unlikely to occur. Overall, measurable gains in production accuracy were observed for only 40% of the phonemes that were targeted during the 12 week intervention. In the second year of this study, children received the same small group intervention except that the first three group sessions

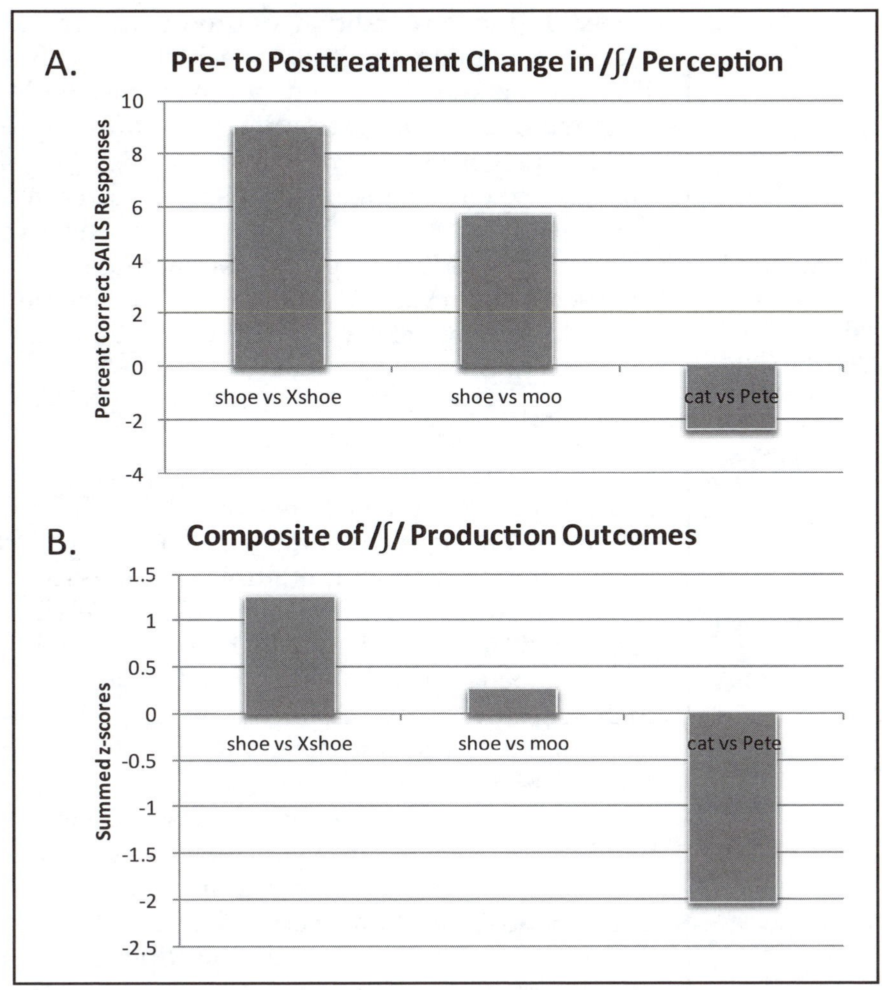

Figure 9–2. *Outcomes of a randomized control trial of the Speech Assessment and Interactive Learning System (SAILS) to remediate perception and production of /ʃ/ misarticulations in which 27 4-year-old children with DPD were assigned to one of three conditions: (1) the standard SAILS intervention involving varied stimuli recorded from multiple child and adult talkers (Group 1; shoe vs. Xshoe); (2) a word identification task with a maximal opposition in which the stimuli were produced by a single adult talker (Group 2; shoe vs. moo); or (3) a control condition in which the stimuli were unrelated to their speech errors (Group 3; cat vs. Pete).* **A.** *Change in percent correct on a measure of /ʃ/ perception (identifying correct and incorrect productions of the word "sheet").* **B.** *Composite measure (summed z scores) of post-treatment /ʃ/ production composed of an acoustic measure of /ʃ/ quality, correct production of /ʃ/ in the onsets of single words and highest level achieved in therapy.*

were replaced with brief individual therapy sessions during which phonetic placement was used to ensure stimulability of treatment targets, and SAILS was used to ensure good perceptual knowledge of the target phonemes. Posttreatment, improved performance was observed for 80% of all treatment targets, regardless of pretreatment level of speech perception skills and stimulability.

Wolfe, Presley, and Mesaris (2003) randomly assigned 9 children, aged 41 to 50 months, to receive either production training

Improvements in production accuracy were observed for twice as many target phonemes when a small group phonology intervention was modified to begin with a brief period of SAILS intervention coupled with stimulability training.

alone (Production condition) or production training combined with SAILS (Perception condition). Each child received between 9 and 17 treatment sessions targeting 3 phonemes with a horizontal goal attack strategy. Mean perception test scores improved from 6.58 to 9.03 for the Perception group and from 7.33 to 7.67 for the Production group. On average, target-specific production probe scores improved from .83 to 5.42 for the Perception group and from .40 to 3.80 for the Production group. Nonparametric statistical analyses revealed a significant advantage to the Perception condition when the child demonstrated poor perception of the target phoneme prior to intervention.

Statistical analyses revealed a significant advantage to group that received the SAILS intervention when the child demonstrated poor perception of the target phoneme prior to intervention.

The most recent study also involved preschool-age children with moderate or severe speech sound disorders (Rvachew, Nowak, & Cloutier, 2004). This study was designed to examine the effect of a SAILS intervention on more global aspects of speech performance as well as on the development of phonological awareness skills. Thirty-four children with multiple speech errors received 16 once-weekly treatment sessions lasting 45 minutes. These sessions were conducted by speech-language pathologists who were free to use any approach to speech therapy that they felt was appropriate. After each speech therapy session an undergraduate student research assistant helped the child's mother administer a 10- to 15-minute computer-based intervention. The experimental group received the SAILS intervention, targeting a different phoneme each week, in word-initial position during the first 8 weeks and in word final position during the last 8 weeks. The standard SAILS intervention task is a word identification or error detection task that corresponds to the ear training technique that Van Riper referred to as "discrimination" (see Table 9–3). For this study, new games were added to the intervention, one that involved matching isolated sounds to the target letter and another that involved matching words to the target letter (either on the basis of shared onset or shared rime/coda depending on the lesson). The stimuli for these identification tasks were recorded from multiple adult talkers. The control group listened to computerized books and answered questions about the pictures. The questions were provided to the mother in the form of a script based on standard dialogic reading techniques.

The speech-language pathologists who were responsible for the children's speech therapy programs were blind to the specific intervention that was provided during these sessions. Outcome measures included a test of speech perception skills, a test of implicit onset and rime awareness, the GFTA, and percent correct articulation of specific phonemes in conversation. Pre- and posttreatment assessments were conducted by a speech-language pathologist who was not involved in the child's speech therapy program and who was not aware of the whether the child was in the experimental or control group. The group that received the SAILS intervention showed large and significant improvements in speech perception skills relative to the control group whose perception performance remained unchanged over the 6-month interval between the two assessments. Improvements in production accuracy during picture naming and conversation were also significantly greater for the children who received the SAILS intervention in comparison with children who received the dialogic reading intervention (see Figure 9–3 for changes in consonant accuracy in conversation). In fact, the GFTA assessment indicated that the children who received the SAILS intervention made twice as much progress during the treatment period as the children in the control condition. Follow-up testing one year later when the children were in kindergarten revealed that 50% of the experimental group achieved normalized speech prior to first grade entry in comparison with 19% of the control group. Improvements in phonological awareness skills were equivalent in the two groups, however, both during the treatment period and during the follow-up interval. This finding is perhaps not surprising given the joint contributions of speech perception

The advantage to the group that received SAILS in addition to speech therapy was retained over a one-year follow-up interval when testing at the end of kindergarten revealed that 50% of the experimental group achieved normalized speech in comparison with 19% of the control group.

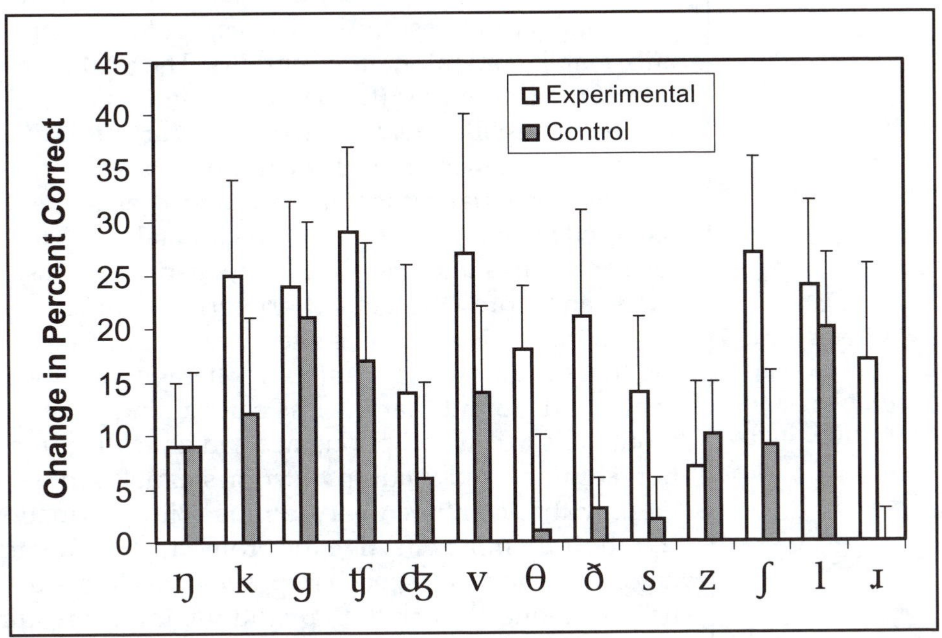

Figure 9–3. *Mean change in percentage of consonants correct in conversation for consonants that were not mastered by the majority of children prior to treatment (standard error bars are shown). Experimental group received the SAILS intervention targeting identification and discrimination of multiple phonemes in onset and coda position. Control group received a dialogic reading intervention. Experimental and control interventions were added to a 16-week course of weekly speech therapy in which the SLPs addressed speech production accuracy using the treatment approach that they felt was best suited to the child's needs.* Source: *From "Effect of Phonemic Perception Training on the Speech Production and Phonological Awareness Skills of Children with Expressive Phonological Delay," by S. Rvachew, M. Nowak, and G. Cloutier, 2004,* American Journal of Speech-Language Pathology, 13, *p. 257 (Figure 1). Copyright 2004 by the American Speech-Language-Hearing Association. Reprinted with permission.*

and vocabulary size to phonological awareness (see Figure 7–8) and the effectiveness of dialogic reading as a vocabulary intervention.

Other computer interventions have components that are similar to ear training but the research has been directed more explicitly at phonological awareness than speech perception skills and speech production outcomes per se: in the US, Daisy Quest (Lonigan, et al., 2003) and Earobics (Porkorni, Worthington, & Jamison, 2004), and in the UK, Phenomena (Moore, Rosenberg, & Coleman, 2005) and Phoneme Factory (Wren, Roulstone, & Williams, 2010).

Summary: Ear Training

Ear training includes a variety of techniques in which the child is made explicitly aware of the target phoneme, provided with concentrated exposure to the target phoneme in a variety of contexts, taught to identify the target in relation to contrasting phonemes and to identify correct productions versus incorrect productions of the phoneme. Van Riper (1963) instructed clinicians to provide plenty of variability in the stimuli with respect to phonetic contexts, utterance length, and intonation contours. The SAILS program replicates one of the techniques (termed a discrimination task by Van Riper) in which the child identifies words that are pronounced correctly or incorrectly. However, in this computer-based implementation, the stimuli are actual rather than simulated errors and the words are recorded from different adult and child talkers. The computer game format ensures that the child is engaged by the task and that many trials can be presented in a short period of time.

In this review we presented 4 randomized control trials showing that ear training is an effective therapeutic procedure.

In this review we presented 4 randomized control trials showing that ear training is an effective therapeutic procedure. Sommers et al. (1961) found that in-class ear training lessons targeting commonly misarticulated phonemes had a positive impact on articulation accuracy and reading outcomes. Small group pull-out speech therapy that combined ear training with production therapy was significantly more effective for promoting improvements in articulation accuracy than speech improvement classes that employed ear training alone. Speech therapy did not impact reading scores however. Randomized control trials with SAILS confirm that production therapy alone is less effective than production therapy combined with SAILS, an ear training procedure made more effective by the use of a computer game format and highly variable stimuli representing correct productions and authentic misarticulations of the target phonemes recorded from multiple child and adult talkers. Rvachew (1994) showed that children do respond to prototypical stimuli produced by a single talker but that variable stimuli produced by multiple talkers results in a significantly larger effect on perception and production accuracy.

One study did not find live voice ear training as implemented by parents to have a positive impact on articulation (Shelton et al.,

1978). It appears that the treatment was not implemented properly in this study since the home program did not present sufficient variability in the stimuli, the activities were not engaging for the children, the parents were not shown how to implement the tasks correctly, training was distributed over an excessive number of lessons and the program did not result in good perception outcomes either. This study shows that ear training can be ineffective if it is not implemented appropriately. Our research review highlights some of the key features of an effective implementation but not all issues have been fully explored.

Van Riper (1963) recommended that ear training be completed before any production therapy was attempted. This particular aspect of the traditional approach appears to have been a source of frustration for many SLPs who would prefer to launch into production training as early as possible (Kamhi, 2006). Vertical layering of the stages along with a vertical goal attack strategy in Van Riper's approach may be less efficient than parallel implementation of ear training and production training and a horizontal goal attack strategy. No systematic trials have determined whether it is better to ensure good perception prior to initiation of production therapy or if it is more efficient to target perception and production in parallel. At no time would we recommend persisting with speech perception training on a single phoneme for an entire semester (as described in Kamhi, 2006)! In our studies in which SAILS had a positive impact on speech perception and speech production learning, total exposure to the SAILS stimuli was between 30 and 60 minutes per phoneme. In each case, SAILS was implemented in parallel with stimulability or speech production training. With one exception, a horizontal goal attack strategy has been employed in our studies. In all of these studies the SAILS program was administered by parents or CDAs which improves the cost efficiency of the procedure. Overall, our reading of the literature suggests that the critical elements are stimulus variability and ensuring a match between the phoneme(s) targeted in perception training and the phoneme(s) targeted in production training.

No systematic trials have determined whether it is better to ensure good perception prior to initiation of production therapy or if it is more efficient to target perception and production in parallel.

The research suggests that the critical elements for successful ear training are stimulus variability and ensuring a match between the phoneme(s) targeted in perception training and the phoneme(s) targeted in production training.

Future research is required to determine how best to adapt SAILS and other live-voice or computer-based ear training approaches to target prosodic goals. As we indicated in Chapter 8, goal selection from the perspective of multilinear phonology will reveal weaknesses in the children's knowledge of prosodic structures and interactions between the segmental and prosodic tiers of the phonological hierarchy. Chapter 4 presents some information suggesting that perceptual factors may play a role in weak syllable deletion very early in normal development and our investigation of error types in children with and without phonological processing problems suggests that syllable structure errors may have a perceptual basis in DPD. However, no studies have assessed the efficacy of ear training procedures for the remediation of error patterns that are prosodic rather than segmental in nature. Despite this gap, a

The use of effective procedures to ensure that the child has good perceptual knowledge of the phonological units being targeted in therapy is an essential part of a speech therapy program.

number of good quality randomized control trials have now established that children's gains in production accuracy are significantly enhanced when computer-based ear training with variable stimuli is added to production training procedures. The use of effective procedures to ensure that the child has good perceptual knowledge of the phonological units being targeted in therapy is an essential part of a speech therapy program.

Dialogic Reading

9.3.1. Explain why children with DPD might benefit from parent-administered dialogic reading as a procedure to build vocabulary knowledge even when the primary focus of the direct intervention is on the child's speech intelligibility.

9.3.2. Define eight dialogic reading techniques and provide examples.

9.3.3. Describe the conditions under which parent-administered dialogic reading is most likely to be an effective technique for optimizing language and emergent literacy development in children with DPD.

Dialogic reading was developed as a means of improving the oral language skills of 2- to 3-year-old toddlers when employed by parents and subsequently adapted for use by preschool teachers with 4- to 5-year-old children.

Dialogic reading was developed by Whitehurst et al. (1988) as a means of improving the oral language skills of 2- to 3-year-old toddlers when employed by parents and subsequently adapted for use by preschool teachers with 4- to 5-year-old children (Lonigan & Whitehurst, 1998; Whitehurst et al., 1994; Whitehurst et al., 1999; Zevenbergen, Whitehurst, & Zevenbergen, 2003). Shared book reading may also be used as a means of facilitating emergent literacy skills such as awareness of print concepts or phonological units (Justice, McGinty, Piasta, Kaderavek, & Fan, 2010; Pile, Girolametto, Johnson, Chen, & Cleave, 2010). Programs for explicitly teaching phonological awareness are discussed in Chapter 11. In this chapter we focus on applications targeting oral language skills with incidental exposure to emergent literacy concepts in young children. Although the dialogic reading procedure does not target speech perception explicitly, there is a close relationship between vocabulary and speech perception development in infancy and in early childhood as discussed in Chapter 2 (Rvachew, 2006; Rvachew & Grawburg, 2006; Tsao, Huei-Mei, & Kuhl, 2004; Werker, Fennell, Corcoran, & Stager, 2002). Furthermore, shared book reading is another context in which adults can provide high quality language input to children. In fact, it has been shown that shared book reading is the context during which parents are most likely to provide a high density of sophisticated language input although they may need instruction in the use of techniques to support their child's learning of that vocabulary (Weizman & Snow, 2001). Given the cru-

Shared book reading is the context during which parents are most likely to provide a high density of sophisticated language input.

cial role of language input in language development, we feel that it is important to help parents of children with DPD learn to provide high quality language input to their child in a supportive context. Therefore, we include dialogic reading in this chapter as another input-oriented procedure that may strengthen young children's acoustic-phonetic representations for words and facilitate the mapping between acoustic-phonetic, semantic, articulatory, and phonological representations.

Vocabulary skills may be an area of relative strength for children with DPD and therefore it may seem unnecessary to teach their parents to use dialogic reading techniques to facilitate their child's vocabulary acquisition. If the child's speech is completely unintelligible, low average vocabulary skills are not likely to be the SLP's highest priority and with good reason! However, good vocabulary skills may be a protective factor for children with DPD with respect to literacy outcomes. Rvachew and Grawburg (2006) conducted a cluster analysis based on the speech perception, receptive vocabulary, and phonological awareness test scores of children with DPD. The results are shown graphically in Figure 9–4. In this figure,

Good vocabulary skills may be a **protective factor** for children with DPD with respect to literacy outcomes.

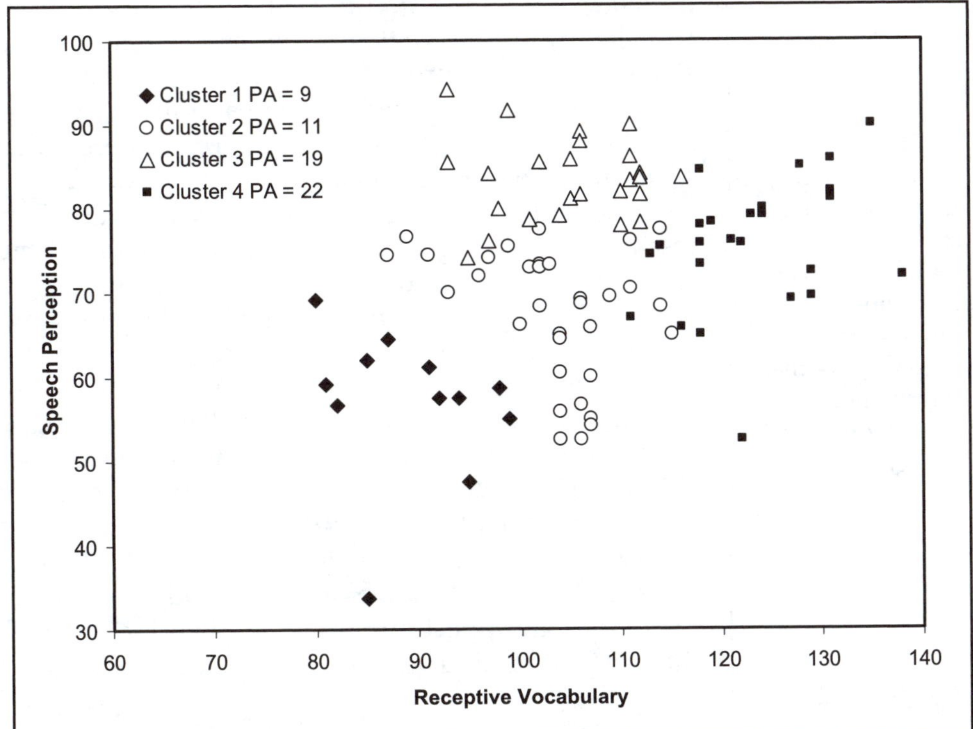

Figure 9–4. *Speech perception (percent correct) and receptive vocabulary (standard scores) performance for each of 95 children with DPD placed in four clusters by a* k-means *cluster analysis. Mean phonological awareness (PA) test scores are shown for each cluster in the legend.* Source: *From "Correlates of Phonological Awareness in Preschoolers with Speech Sound Disorders," by S. Rvachew and M. Grawburg, 2006,* Journal of Speech, Language, and Hearing Research, *49, p. 83 (Figure 2). Copyright 2006 by the American Speech-Language-Hearing Association. Reprinted with permission.*

receptive vocabulary (PPVT–III) standard scores are plotted against speech perception scores (SAILS; /k/, /s/, /l/, and /ɹ/ modules), with different markers for individual children in each cluster. The figure legend shows the mean phonological awareness (PA) test score for each cluster. The normal limits for PPVT performance are between 85 and 115. The lower limit of normal performance on the SAILS test is a score of approximately 70% correct. Clusters 3 and 4 achieved a mean PA test score within normal limits (i.e., a score higher than 15), whereas Clusters 1 and 2 scored below normal limits on average. The figure illustrates that the children who achieved the highest PA test scores had either exceptionally high vocabulary test scores or very good speech perception scores. The cluster with the lowest PPVT–III scores demonstrated the poorest speech perception and phonological awareness performance. These children can be predicted to have future literacy deficits on the basis of poor language skills alone (Peterson, Pennington, Shriberg, & Boada, 2009). The contrast between Clusters 2 and 3 shows that good speech perception performance is the best predictor of PA for children whose vocabulary scores are within the average range. All children with exceptionally high vocabulary skills achieved good PA scores, however, even those who scored below normal limits on the speech perception test. The mechanism for this outcome is revealed by studies that show an association between vocabulary size and language processing efficiency in 2-year-old children that in turn predicts language outcomes in multiple domains over the subsequent 6 years (Marchman & Fernald, 2008). Individual differences in processing efficiency may reflect endogenous variations in the functioning of underlying neural mechanisms in part; however, research with bilingual children shows that the primary influence is the amount of environmental language input. Greater exposure to language input in a given language "deepens language specific, as well as language-general, features of existing representations [leading to a] synergistic interaction between processing skills and vocabulary learning" (Marchman & Fernald, 2008, p. 835). From a public health perspective, teaching all parents to maximize their children's language development is part of the role of the SLP. For children with DPD it is especially important that parents not be so focused on "speech homework" that daily shared reading is set aside. SLPs can help the parents of children with DPD use shared reading as an opportunity to strengthen the child's language and literacy skills and provide opportunities for speech practice.

Individual differences in **processing efficiency** may reflect endogenous variations in the functioning of underlying neural mechanisms in part; however, research with bilingual children shows that the primary influence is the amount of environmental language input.

Dialogic Reading Techniques

Dialogic reading techniques are designed to gradually shift responsibility for storytelling from the parent to the child and thus active participation by the child is essential.

Dialogic reading techniques are designed to gradually shift responsibility for storytelling from the parent to the child. Active participation by the child is essential and the shift in story telling role from parent to child is a central characteristic of the procedure.

Parents are taught how to encourage active participation by evoking responses from their child and providing informative feedback in a manner that is responsive to their child's language abilities and familiarity with the story.

The kinds of prompts that parents might use are described using the CROWD acronym: completion, recall, open-ended, wh-questions, and distancing. Completion prompts involve producing a rhyme or phrase that reoccurs in the story to cue the end of the phrase or the next phrase that should occur. Recall prompts direct the child to retell parts of the story, either as just read or as read on a prior day. Open-ended prompts are questions that require relatively long answers, beyond yes/no or a single word ("Tell me what is happening here"). Wh-questions may require a simple labeling response in response to a "what" or "who" question or a more complex answer to a "when" or "why" question. Distancing prompts encourage the child to link story content to his or her own experiences. The complexity of the prompts should increase with rereading of a given book and with advancing age of the child. Van Kleeck, Vander Woude, and Hammett (2006), using a variation on the dialogic reading procedure, described the complexity of prompts in a shared book-reading intervention in terms of a literal-inferential continuum. We used the same framework to ensure a variety of prompts along the same continuum in our dialogic reading intervention in Rvachew et al. (2004). For example, on the first page of the electronic book *Grandma and Me* by Mercer Mayer, the prompts were: (1) Click the mailbox. (2) Where are Grandma and Little Critter going? (3) What do you think is in Grandma's basket? and (4) What might happen if Little Critter ran out on the road?

The kinds of **prompts** that parents might use to encourage active participation are described using the **CROWD** acronym: *completion, recall, open-ended, wh-questions*, and *distancing*.

Parents are also taught to provide informative feedback subsequent to the child's response to these prompts. Direct correction or expansions might be used to highlight the difference between what the child said and what the child might have said in response to the prompt. A follow-up question can be used to encourage the child to provide more information in response to the prompts. Parents should also encourage the child to repeat the expected response. The acronym PEER is used to structure these exchanges during the book reading interaction: Prompt, Evaluate, Expand, Repeat. Definitions of these techniques are provided in Table 9–5.

Parents are also taught to provide **informative feedback** subsequent to the child's response to these prompts.

The acronym **PEER** is used to structure parent-child exchanges during the book reading interaction: *Prompt, Evaluate, Expand, Repeat*.

Whitehurst et al. (1988) indicated that parental sensitivity to their child's language abilities is important to the success of this procedure. The parent is expected to gradually increase the complexity of the prompts and require greater participation by the child with repeated readings of a given book and as their child's language knowledge expands. It is not clear how parents are taught to implement this recommendation although the training program is structured to teach more concrete techniques first. In the first training session parents are taught to use completion, recall and wh-questions as prompts for object, function and attribute labels. Repeating the child's response, follow-up questions, and direct

Table 9–5. *Definitions of Dialogic Reading Techniques with Examples*

Technique	*Definition*	*Literal Example*	*Inferential Example*
Prompt	Evoke a response from the child.		
Completion		And the big bad wolf said . . .	What would you say if the wolf came to our house? You could say "Mr. Wolf . . ."
Recall		Do you remember how many pigs are in this story?	The wolf is going to go down the chimney. What will happen to him?
Open-ended		Tell me about this picture.	Oh-oh, I see the wolf coming. Tell me what happens next.
Wh-questions		What is this house made of?	Look at the expression on the pig's face here. What do you think he is he feeling right now?
Distancing		Do you remember when you made a house from blocks yesterday and it fell down? Tell me more about that.	Can you think of a time when you felt scared like this? Tell me more about that.
Evaluate	Provide feedback to indicate whether the response was correct or not.	No, not one.	I agree. The pig is scared.
Expand	Add information to the child's response.	Three, three little pigs.	In fact, I think he's terrified.
	Or, ask a question to get more information.	Yes, you see a wolf. What's the wolf doing?	What will happen to the house when he blows on it?
Repeat	Ask the child to repeat the correct response	Count with me. (pointing). One, two, three.	Say "terrified."
	or the new information.	Say "The wolf is hiding."	No, it *won't*. Say "The brick house *won't* fall down.

correction as forms of feedback are also introduced in the first training session along with following the child's lead. Open-ended questions and distancing prompts and expansions as feedback are introduced in a second training session. The parent training program is fairly brief, based on video recorded parent-child exchanges that model correct and incorrect use of the strategies. Each training session lasts no more than 90 minutes including discussion about the video-taped vignettes and role-play of dialogic reading techniques. The two sessions are separated by several weeks and the parents may be given books to use at home during the interval between the two sessions.

Demonstrations of Dialogic Reading

Demonstration 9–5 is a hypothetical exchange between a parent and a younger child reading "Thomas' Snowsuit" for the first time. The adult has to have a sense of humor to enjoy this irreverent take on a common problem but no child will fail to be delighted by a story in which the child refuses to wear his snowsuit, the teacher and the child end up in each other's clothes in one scene, the principal finds them both in their underwear in another, the principal is wearing the teacher's dress in a later scene (a problem ultimately solved by Thomas), and the book concludes with the principal retiring to Arizona where nobody wears snowsuits. For the younger child it provides an excellent introduction to story structure because there are multiple episodes of problem and resolution sequences involving the snowsuit. There are many opportunities to teach concrete vocabulary relating to the names, attributes, and functions of objects that occur in familiar home and school environments. Initially, participation by the child, when playing the role of Thomas, is undemanding (largely restricted to saying "no") but even very young children will enjoy taking on the adult roles which offer multiple opportunities to say, "Please put on your snowsuit."

In Demonstration 9–5, the interaction is somewhat unbalanced because the mother is reading the book for the first time and is producing most of the speech in the exchange. Furthermore, the imagined child is very young, between 2 and 3 years of age, and the adult does not have high expectations for the child's narrative abilities. She passes up some opportunities to prompt for child input as, for example, when she does not encourage the child to speculate on how the room shown on the front cover became wrecked. Clearly, however, this is not the typical "adult reads, child listens" book reading exchange. Conversational turns pass back and forth between adult and child as they discuss the story. The adult uses completion prompts to encourage the child to take the part of Thomas in the story, saying "no" at appropriate intervals. Wh-prompts are used to elicit color names and object labels. Open-ended prompts are used to evoke a description of the wrecked room and a prediction about upcoming events in the plot. A distancing prompt evokes a comment about the color of the child's own snowsuit. The PEER sequence is incorporated naturally into the exchange: "What color is the pocket?" (prompt); "No (evaluate), the snowsuit is brown but the pocket is yellow (expand). Say yellow (repeat)."

Demonstration 9–6 covers the same pages of this book but in this case an adult is reading the book to a somewhat older child, let's say almost 5 years old, who is very familiar with the story. The child takes on a larger role in the retelling of the story. The adult focuses more on teaching the child some difficult vocabulary related to the feelings of the characters as the plot progresses. The expressions on the characters' faces are drawn broadly in the illustrations and provide an excellent opportunity to discuss important but difficult concepts

Demonstration 9–5
Hypothetical Dialogic Reading Exchange Between Adult and Younger Child Reading *Thomas' Snowsuit* for the First Time

Adult	*Thomas' Snowsuit* by Robert Munsch. Oh my! Look at their house. Everything is wrecked.
Child	All messy.
Adult	Yes, it's messy. I wonder why? Let's find out how the house got messy.
Adult	*One day Thomas' mother bought him a nice new brown snowsuit.* Look at Thomas' mother—she is really happy about this new snowsuit. She must like this color. What color is this (pointing to the snowsuit)?
Child	Brown.
Adult	Brown, it's a brown snowsuit, with yellow pockets. Show me the yellow pockets.
Child	(Points to a yellow pocket).
Adult	Good for you! What color is the pocket?
Child	Brown.
Adult	No, the snowsuit is brown but the pocket is yellow. Say yellow.
Child	Yellow.
Adult	That's right, the pocket is yellow. What color is your snowsuit?
Child	Yellow.
Adult	Very good. Your snowsuit is a lovely yellow color. Thomas' new snowsuit is brown. The mother really likes this brown snowsuit. But look at Thomas' face!
Child	Yuck.
Adult	You got it, Thomas thinks it is yucky. *And when Thomas saw the snowsuit he said "That is the ugliest thing I have seen in my life! If you think that I am going to wear that ugly snowsuit you are crazy!" And his mother said "We will see about that."* (turns page)
Adult	*The next day, when it was time to go to school, the mother said "Thomas, please put on your snowsuit."* What do think Thomas said?
Child	No.

Adult	That's right; he said "no!" *His mother jumped up and down and said "Thomas, put on that snowsuit." And Thomas said . . .*
Child	No!
Adult	*So Thomas' mother picked up Thomas in one hand and she picked up the snowsuit in the other hand and she tried to stick them together. They had an enormous fight and when it was done, Thomas was in his snowsuit.* Now we know what happened to this room. Tell me about this picture.
Child	The chair tipped.
Adult	The chair is tipped over. They sure had a big fight to make such a mess. What else?
Child	Flowers everywhere.
Adult	Yes, the tulips were knocked over too. Do you know what this is? No? Say vase.
Child	Vase.
Adult	The vase fell over and the flowers fell out. I'll bet the water came out too and the carpet is wet now.
Child	(points at lamp) This broked.
Adult	That's a lamp. The lamp broke. Say "lamp."
Child	Lamp.
Adult	The lamp broke. (turns the page) Thomas went off to school and hung up his snowsuit. When it was time to go outside, all the other kids jumped into their snowsuits and ran out the door. Oh—but what about Thomas? (pause) What's gonna happen next? (pause) Will he put on his snowsuit?
Child	Him not put it on.

Source: Text of the book is shown in italics. A reading of *Thomas' Snowsuit* by Robert Munsch can be found at http://robertmunsch.com/.

such as disgust, frustration, anger, embarrassment, and satisfaction. Despite the absurdity of the specific events in the story, the nature of the conflict in the story is familiar to children and offers opportunities for discussing appropriate and inappropriate strategies for conflict resolution. In terms of the nature of this hypothetical interaction, the techniques used by the adult in Demonstration 9–6 are similar to those shown in Demonstration 9–5. The adult uses completion prompts to encourage the child to fill in repetitive parts of the

Demonstration 9–6
Hypothetical Dialogic Reading Exchange Between Adult and Older Child Reading *Thomas' Snowsuit*

Adult *Thomas' Snowsuit* by Robert Munsch. We haven't read this for a long time. It's such a fun book. Do you remember what happened to their house here?

Child They had a big fight about the snowsuit and wrecked the house.

Adult That's right, you do remember. Oh, look at this letter. That's the letter . . .

Child T, T is for Tyler.

Adult Yep, T makes the [t^{h}ə] sound. T is for Tyler and T is for Thomas. This word says "Thomas," *Thomas' Snowsuit*. Let's read the book together. You can help me.

Adult *One day Thomas' mother bought him a nice new brown snowsuit.* Look at Thomas' mother—how does she feel about this new snowsuit?

Child Happy.

Adult Why is she so happy?

Child Mom is happy because she really likes the snowsuit. (Points to Thomas' face). But he hates it—yuck.

Adult That's right. You see this look on his face. He is disgusted. Can you say disgusted?

Child Disgusted.

Adult Can you think of something that disgusts you? Something you really don't like?

Child Um, peas, I really don't like peas.

Adult Oh yeah, you won't eat peas. You think they are disgusting. But I like them a lot. Different strokes for different folks. Same thing with the snowsuit. Thomas' mother likes it but Thomas is disgusted. *When Thomas saw the snowsuit he said "That is the ugliest thing I have seen in my life! If you think that I am going to wear that ugly snowsuit you are . . .*

Child *Crazy*!

Adult And his mother said . . .

Child *"We'll see 'bout that."* (turns page)

Adult	The next day, when it was time to go to school, the mother said . . .
Child	"Thomas, please put on your snowsuit." And Thomas said "No."
Adult	That's right, he said "no!" *His mother jumped up and down and said . . .*
Child	"Thomas, put on your snowsuit." And Thomas said "No!"
Adult	And then what happened?
Child	The mum picked up Thomas and the snowsuit and tried to stick them together. Then they had a big fight and wrecked the room. And now Thomas is in the snowsuit.
Adult	That's right, *They had an enormous fight and when it was done, Thomas was in his snowsuit.* Look at Thomas' face now. How does he feel?
Child	He's unhappy.
Adult	Yeah, he's unhappy. I'd say disgruntled or grumpy. He's very grumpy in that snowsuit. And the mother?
Child	Her face is all red.
Adult	She's exhausted. The fight to get the snowsuit on wore her out. (turns the page) *Thomas went off to school and hung up his snowsuit. When it was time to go outside, all the other kids jumped into their snowsuits and ran out the door. But not Thomas. The teacher looked at Thomas and said . . .*
Child	Please put on your snowsuit but Thomas said "no" and then the teacher jumped up and down and said "put on your snowsuit!"
Adult	Look at Thomas' face here. What kind of expression is this?
Child	He's unhappy.
Adult	Yeah, he's not happy, that's for sure. I'd say he's defiant. He's not going to cooperate. He is defying the teacher's request. He's being defiant. Can you say defiant?
Child	Defiant.
Adult	And how do you think the teacher feels?
Child	Angry?
Adult	Maybe more like frustrated.

Source: Text of the book is shown in italics. A reading of *Thomas' Snowsuit* by Robert Munsch can be found at http://robertmunsch.com/.

story as well as recall and open-ended prompts to evoke descriptions of and predictions about story events. Wh-questions are used to elicit labels but in this case the labels are for abstract concepts rather than concrete objects with the exception of the letter name (T) on the front cover. A distancing prompt is used to connect Thomas' feeling about the snowsuit to the child's experience with feelings of disgust. The PEER sequence is apparent with liberal use of expansions. Follow-up questions to request more information, expansions and direct corrections are all used to provide feedback about the child's responses. Specific definitions of new words and direct requests to repeat difficult words are a key feature of this exchange with an older child. For example, "What kind of expression is this (prompt)? Yeah, he's not happy, that's for sure (evaluation). I'd say he's defiant. He's not going to cooperate. He is defying the teacher's request. He's being defiant (expansion and information). Can you say defiant (repeat)?"

Focused stimulation and dialogic reading procedures share several techniques in common but the adult's role is more directive in dialogic reading.

The focused stimulation and dialogic reading procedures share several techniques in common, in particular following the child's lead, prompts to elicit responses from the child and providing feedback to the child in the form of imitations and expansions of the child's response. Both procedures have the goal of encouraging active participation by the child in a turn-taking interaction with the adult. Although the child is intended to take over the story-telling role in dialogic reading, it is clear that the adult's teaching style is more directive in dialogic reading when compared to focused stimulation since new words are taught explicitly and the child is required to tell parts of the story, repeat corrected responses and imitate new vocabulary. The use of prompts in dialogic reading is also considerably more directive than in focused stimulation which relies more on environmental manipulations to stimulate certain responses from children. It appears that there may be more emphasis on recasting incorrect responses from children when implementing focused stimulation in contrast to a greater emphasis on modeling correct responses for children when implementing dialogic reading.

Another primary difference between the two procedures is the goal, given that focused stimulation was developed as a therapeutic procedure to focus on the form of children's utterances (e.g., morphosyntactic structures) whereas dialogic reading was developed for children who might be deprived of high quality inputs but are otherwise normally developing. The focus of dialogic reading is on the content and use of language: increasingly complex vocabulary knowledge, creation of narratives and extended discourse, and the use of decontextualized "meaning talk." Dialogic reading is seen as an ideal context for the joint construction of knowledge by adult and child. Focused stimulation is intended to provide opportunities for the child to notice disparities in the (mis)use of linguistic form by the child relative to adult utterances.

The focus of dialogic reading is on the content and use of language—increasingly complex vocabulary knowledge, creation of narratives and extended discourse, and the use of decontextualized "meaning talk."

Empirical Evidence for the Efficacy of Dialogic Reading

Two meta-analyses and a systematic review of randomized control trials that have assessed the efficacy of dialogic reading have concluded that this procedure has a significant effect on children's vocabulary development (Bus, Van Ijzendoorn, & Pellegrini, 1995; Mol, Bus, de Jong, & Smeeta, 2008; Reese & Cox, 1999), with a small effect size reported for receptive vocabulary and a moderate effect size reported for expressive vocabulary. The difference in outcomes for receptive versus expressive vocabulary may reflect the short observation intervals in most of these studies, often about 8 weeks; Whitehurst et al. (1994) found that effects on receptive vocabulary emerged over a 6-month follow-up interval when the intervention was implemented with high compliance at home and daycare. Mol et al. (2008) concluded that dialogic reading was most effective for toddlers and preschool-age children. Randomized control trials and observational studies suggest that children benefit from different reading strategies as a function of their level of language skills (Hindman, Connor, Jewkes, & Morrison, 2008; Reese & Cox, 1999). The "performance style" of reading, employed often by preschool teachers, involves discussions of the story before and after reading the book dramatically without interruptions (Dickinson & Tabors, 2001); this style has been shown to be beneficial to language development in kindergarten-age children.

Two meta-analyses and a systematic review of randomized control trials that have assessed the efficacy of dialogic reading have concluded that this procedure has a significant effect on children's vocabulary development.

Implementation of dialogic reading with language-impaired children by parents, teachers, and SLPs has had mixed results in randomized controlled trials. In a study that focused on inferential language use, language-impaired children, aged 3 to 5 years, received twice-weekly shared reading sessions from a research assistant in their daycare center over an 8-week period (van Kleeck, et al., 2006). In comparison to a no-treatment control condition, significant between-group differences were found on all standardized measures of language function, chosen to tap literal and inferential language skills, immediately posttreatment. Dale, Crain-Thoreson, Notari-Synverson, and Cole (1996) taught parents to implement one of two home-based language interventions, either dialogic reading or conversational language training (child-centered language stimulation techniques applied during every day activities, conversations and play). The participants, aged 3 to 6 years, had approximately 2-year delays in receptive and expressive language functioning. The dialogic reading intervention yielded superior results to the comparison intervention in number of different words used and mean length of utterance observed while playing with the mother. However, in a follow-up study in which the dialogic reading intervention was modified to teach parents to wait longer for child responses and the home-based parent intervention was compared to preschool-based dialogic reading, trends toward an effect did not reach statistical significance (Crain-Thoreson & Dale,

1999). Similarly, Pile et al. (2010) did not observe an effect of a joint SLP- and parent-implemented shared reading program on vocabulary diversity or mean length of utterance in a study that involved 4-year-old children with specific language impairment. One reason for these mixed outcomes for children with language impairments may be that it is necessary to have larger samples, longer intervention periods, and more sensitive outcome measures before changes in the language functioning of these children can be detected.

Kaderavek and Justice (2002) discuss child characteristics that may moderate response to dialogic reading. First, children with language impairments may be less likely than children with normally developing language skills to be engaged by books and stories, in which case parent-child interaction with toys and everyday activities might be better contexts for language teaching. This is an interesting hypothesis that highlights the importance of taking child temperament (and family culture) into account but it has not been established empirically. In fact, the dialogic reading procedure is designed to enhance engagement with books and shared book reading and the results of Dale et al. (1996) appear to directly counter the suggestion that play is a more effective context than story book reading for language facilitation with children whose language skills are deficient. Kaderavek and Justice further suggest that dialogic reading techniques may be too directive for children with low language competence. They note that parents tend to ask fewer questions and request less information when reading to children who have lower vocabulary knowledge and then gradually increase their expectations for child participation as their child's language knowledge expands. When children are reluctant to respond at all or have significant mismatches between their receptive and expressive language skills, it may be difficult to find the right level of prompts when using a directive teaching style. When children have unstable internal representations for words and phonemes they may need experience with greater amounts of input before they feel ready to produce new words "on demand." Dale et al. (1996) observed that parents frequently did not wait "long enough" for their child to respond in both the dialogic reading and conversation interaction conditions highlighting the transactional nature of shared book reading. The follow-up study in which parents were specifically taught to use waiting as a technique for prompting a response from their child did not have as good an outcome raising again the question of how directive parents should be when children have impaired language skills. It appears that parental sensitivity to child characteristics moderates the success of the intervention. The training program should enhance rather than inhibit the parents' intuitions as to appropriate expectations for their child's responses.

Dialogic reading techniques may be too directive for some children with low language competence.

Parental sensitivity to child characteristics may moderate the success of the intervention; the training program should enhance the parents' intuitions as to appropriate expectations for their child's responses.

We noticed another characteristic of shared book reading interventions with at-risk children that may contribute to disappointing results and that is the tendency to weigh the procedure down with multiple goals. Children with language impairments often have difficulties in several aspects of language functioning including semantics, syntax, pragmatics, phonology, and emergent literacy. Shared book reading is a potentially useful context for targeting therapeutic goals in all of these areas and it can be tempting to try to focus on multiple goals at once. We pointed out earlier in the chapter that focused stimulation works best when it is directed at a specific goal that is clear to the adult and child. The same may be true for dialogic reading. For example, Pile et al. (2010) combined an SLP-administered intervention with parent-administered dialogic reading but did not teach the dialogic reading techniques in the usual fashion. Parents were taught to teach print concepts, ask questions, and conduct phonological awareness activities in a single training session. Then the SLPs taught alphabet knowledge, literal and inferential language, and phonological awareness using book reading and targeted activities to the children in 9 weekly group sessions. Parents observed their child's treatment sessions and then received additional instructions for facilitating knowledge of print concepts and literal and inferential language during shared reading homework assignments. Significant improvements were noted in parental focus on print concepts (e.g., title and author of book) but other parental reading behaviors did not differ between the experimental and no-treatment control group. The lack of change in child language behaviors (the primary outcome measures being lexical diversity and mean length of utterance) is perhaps not surprising in this study that did not provide parents, SLPs, or children with a clear sense of the primary intervention goal.

No research has examined the specific effects of dialogic reading on outcomes for children with DPD but three studies shed some light on how this procedure might be useful with this population. Close examination of these studies suggests that dialogic reading, by itself, is unlikely to have a significant impact on children's speech accuracy. In the context of a randomized controlled trial, Whitehurst et al. (1991) provided an intervention to parents of language-delayed toddlers in 7 biweekly individual sessions, each lasting approximately 30 minutes. The children had normal receptive language skills but spoke very few words. Mothers were taught to use the prompting and feedback techniques during daily activities and during shared book reading. The children were followed from 28 to 65 months of age. Children in the treatment and control groups were free to seek other therapy services throughout the treatment and follow-up periods. At 34 months there was a significant advantage to the treatment group for receptive and expressive language ability. By the age of 44 months the control group had caught up to the experimental group on measures of language performance. Unfortunately there are no measures of phonological development at earlier ages but at 34 months both groups had significantly delayed articulation skills upon standardized testing. Delays in

Dialogic reading, by itself, is unlikely to have a significant impact on children's speech accuracy.

articulation skills persisted through 44 months; at 65 months both groups were scoring within normal limits on average although a quarter of the sample still had delayed articulation skills.

Rvachew et al. (2004) used parent-administered dialogic reading with computerized books as the control condition in contrast to a speech perception/phonological awareness intervention as described earlier in this chapter. Both interventions were combined with 16 weekly speech therapy sessions. The control group that received the dialogic reading intervention obtained significantly worse outcomes for articulation accuracy but showed similar improvements in phonological awareness in comparison with the group that received the speech perception intervention. As illustrated in the case studies in Rvachew and Brosseau-Lapré (2010) phonological awareness gains in the dialogic reading condition appeared to be associated with gains in vocabulary skills whereas phonological awareness gains in the speech perception condition were associated with gains in speech perception skills.

As a follow-up to this study, we conducted a randomized controlled trial of interventions for phonological disorders in French-speaking preschool-age children, with the results indicating that the impact of parent-administered dialogic reading depends upon the nature of the speech therapy program that the child receives (Rvachew & Brosseau-Lapré, 2011). The expectation was that a speech perception intervention, in combination with dialogic reading focused on vocabulary development, would facilitate children's response to a phonological awareness intervention, an outcome consistent with the model presented in Figure 7–8. The participants were 64 4- and 5-year-old children with mean percent consonant correct scores of 71% on a picture naming test. Receptive vocabulary skills were within normal limits as was nonverbal intelligence. All children received 6 one-hour sessions of individualized speech therapy provided once per week, each targeting three specific phonological goals using a horizontal goal attack strategy. Children were randomly assigned to receive an input-oriented or output-oriented approach to therapy (Table 9–6 presents details of the procedures employed). Production practice did occur in the input-oriented approach in the context of meaningful minimal contrast therapy (see Chapter 11 for description) but these activities were introduced when the child indicated readiness for production activities by initiating spontaneous productions of the target during focused stimulation activities. In contrast, children who were treated with the output-oriented approach engaged in speech production practice throughout all six treatment sessions. After the 6 weeks of individual therapy were completed the parents received 6 weeks of group training with random assignment to either a dialogic reading intervention or an articulation home program intervention. Although their parents were taught to implement dialogic reading or articulation therapy at home, the children all received a

Table 9–6. *Treatment Procedures Used in the Essai Clinique Randomisé sur les Interventions Phonologiques (Randomized Clinical Trial of Phonological Interventions; ECRIP Trial)*

Treatment Condition	*Procedure*	*Source*
Output Oriented	Stimulability training	Secord et al. (2007); Chapter 10
	Production training	Van Riper (1978); Chapter 10
	Articulation Home Program	Chapter 10
Input Oriented	Speech Perception training (SAILS adapted for French)	Rvachew & Brosseau-Lapré (2010); Chapter 9
	Ear Training	Van Riper (1978); Chapter 9
	Focused Stimulation	Fey et al. (2003); Chapter 9
	Meaningful Minimal Contrast Therapy	Weiner (1981); Chapter 11
	Dialogic Reading Home Program	Whitehurst (1988); Chapter 9
Phonological Awareness Groups	Sound Foundations (adapted for French)	Byrne & Fielding-Barnsley (1991); Chapter 11

phonological awareness intervention targeting implicit awareness of syllables, onsets, and rimes in small groups. These sessions lasted for one hour, offered weekly for 6 weeks.

In this study the primary outcome of interest was phonological awareness and the secondary outcome was improvements in speech production accuracy. Phonological awareness outcomes were assessed with a measure of explicit syllable and phoneme awareness with child and parent treatment conditions as the independent variables and pretreatment phonological awareness as the covariate. A significant interaction of individual treatment condition and parent group condition was observed: $F(1, 59) = 6.35$, $p = .01$. As shown in Figure 9–5, the best outcomes were observed for children who received the input-oriented approach to individual speech therapy when their parents received the dialogic reading intervention. Children who received standard output-oriented production therapy combined with an articulation home program provided by their parents also made gains in phonological awareness. The remaining two groups did not improve their explicit phonological awareness skills significantly. With respect to speech accuracy,

We found that an input oriented approach to individual speech therapy combined with a parent administered dialogic reading intervention produced good outcomes for speech accuracy and phonological awareness.

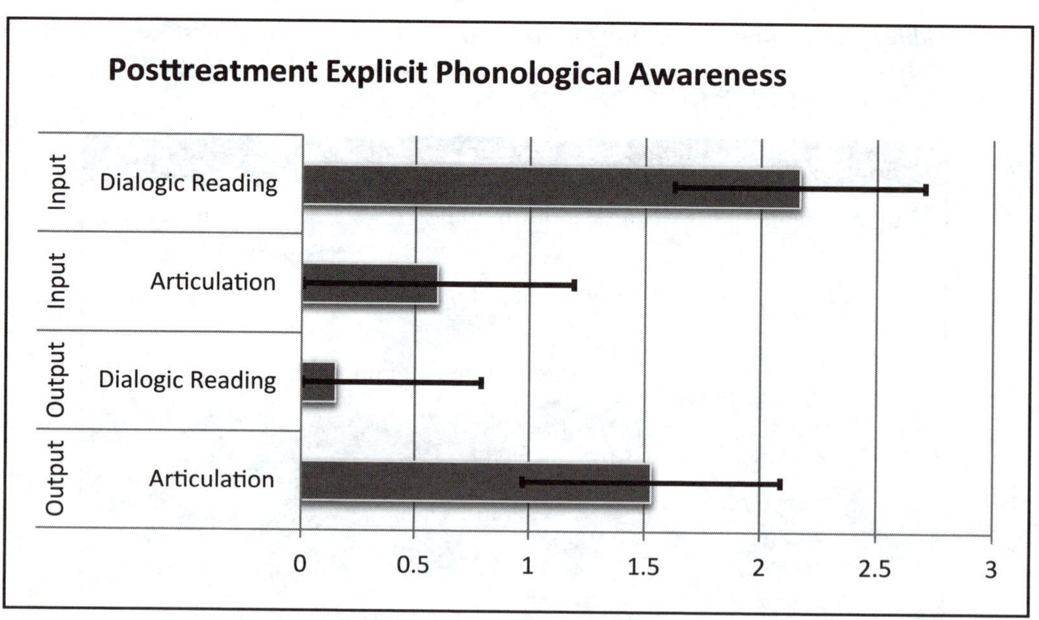

Figure 9–5. *Mean posttreatment performance on a measure of explicit phonological awareness by group in the ECRIP trial* (N = 64). *Two groups received output-oriented therapy in individual speech therapy sessions followed by either articulation home program or parent-administered dialogic reading; two groups received input-oriented therapy in individual speech therapy sessions followed by articulation home program or parent-administered dialogic reading. All groups received an implicit phonological awareness intervention in small groups. Standard error bars shown.*

all groups made a significant gain, averaging 7 percentage points, during the 12-week interval between the pre- and posttreatment assessments. The results are fully consistent with the model shown in Figure 7–8 in that a treatment approach that focused on strengthening children's speech perception skills combined with a home based intervention targeting vocabulary knowledge resulted in the best phonological awareness outcomes. The result is striking given that the outcomes represent generalization of implicit phonological awareness of large units (as taught during therapy) to explicit awareness of small units (as measured on a difficult deletion task posttreatment). Furthermore, the interventions for speech therapy, dialogic reading and phonological awareness were each quite brief lasting 6 hours over a 6-week period. We believe that the 6 individual therapy sessions that employed an input-oriented approach prepared the children to participate actively in and benefit from the dialogic reading program at home and helped the parents to implement the program more effectively once formal training in the techniques was initiated. Long-term follow-up of these children is underway in order to determine if the dialogic reading program will impact on the children's vocabulary skills over a 9-month period and if the gains in phonological awareness will be maintained.

Summary: Dialogic Reading

Dialogic reading is a procedure typically implemented by parents or early childhood educators with young children to create a context for the shared construction of knowledge around a topic of joint interest. The specific techniques that are used are designed to encourage a shift in story telling roles from the parent to the child and to facilitate development of the child's oral language skills. Randomized controlled trials have shown that the procedure has significant impacts on the vocabulary development of toddlers and preschool-age children. Not all applications with children with specific language impairment have been successful, however. It was suggested that children with delayed language skills may benefit from a less directive teaching style or that parents may have difficulty implementing dialogic reading in a fashion that is sufficiently responsive to the needs of children with language impairment. Alternatively, dialogic reading interventions that are implemented in the context of language therapy programs may suffer from a lack of focus with SLPs attempting to target too many language and literacy goals at once. For children with DPD, we have observed good phonological awareness outcomes in two studies in which parents were taught to implement dialogic reading techniques. In both studies, the focus of the parent training program was on prompting for literal and inferential language use with the provision of appropriate feedback for child responses. Although the curriculum in Rvachew and Brosseau-Lapré (2010) included a final session on the importance of phonological awareness and letter knowledge to school success, the parents were first taught to use dialogic reading to target language goals. Furthermore, the parents observed 6 weeks of individual speech therapy sessions during which student SLPs implemented focused stimulation and auditory bombardment procedures with their child. It is possible that improving these children's speech perception skills and teaching them to listen actively to speech input prepared them to benefit from the dialogic reading intervention. The parents may also have learned useful skills while observing the student SLPs work with their children during the 6 weeks of individual therapy prior to the implementation of the dialogic reading program (recall that we took a highly nondirective approach to focused stimulation in this study, placing the emphasis on modeling speech targets and demanding very little in the way of speech output). In any case, the particular combination of interventions in this study proved to be crucial, as the dialogic reading intervention was not effective when combined with 6-weeks of prior output-oriented speech therapy that focused on speech production practice.

Traditional output-oriented approaches to speech therapy are very directive in nature and the parent's participation in these sessions and the associated homework activities may have led them to take an overly directive approach to dialogic reading even though they received the same training program as the parents whose children received input-oriented speech therapy. We cannot confirm this hypothesis because we do not have measures of parent implementation of the program. However, this hypothesis is consistent with Kaderavek and Justice's (2002) speculation that dialogic reading can be too directive for some children. Firm conclusions about the use of dialogic reading with children who have DPD are difficult to draw at this time given the limited number of studies. It may be a useful adjunct to speech therapy but we believe that it should be implemented more or less as originally intended—in other words, the children should have a language age of between 2 and 4 years and their parents should be taught to implement the procedure for the purpose of facilitating their children's language development. At least two training sessions should occur that are structured to introduce the more concrete prompts and follow-up techniques first, leaving some time for parents to master these techniques and then introducing more difficult techniques at a later time. When the children have speech and language delays the implementation of an input-oriented approach to therapy with the child may help prepare the child to benefit from the shared book reading experience. Parents may need more support in order to learn to be maximally responsive to their child's needs, adjusting their demands appropriately to their child's receptive and expressive language skills and readiness to take on the story-telling role.

Conclusions and Recommendations

In Chapter 4 we cited Ferguson and Farwell's conclusion that the foundation of phonology is "a phonic core of remembered lexical items." Remembered lexical items emerge from the dynamic interplay of the child's attentional biases, perceptuomotor systems, and learning mechanisms with multiple sources of structured input from the social and physical environment. In normal development, experience is accrued at multiple levels of representation and woven tightly together so that the phonic core of individual words organizes itself into patterns that support generalization of learning in comprehension and production, allowing rapid increases in the complexity of linguistic knowledge. For children with DPD asynchronous developments in attentional, perceptuomotor or learning mechanisms mean that the multiple components do not come together in the right way at the right time. The phonic core is weakly constructed and the pattern is misshapen due to gaps in the fabric. The goal of these input-oriented procedures in the context of treatment for DPD is to provide a strong but flexible foundation for phonological development. Providing extra language input that targets these gaps is the only known means of strengthening the "phonic core of remembered lexical items" in children who are very likely to have difficulty processing phonological information from birth. It is important to remember that this foundation is built from words—infants do not learn speech sounds presented in isolation. The input must be plentiful and varied and meaningful.

Focused stimulation is a procedure that has a long and successful history in language therapy. When used to treat children with DPD we recommend that the initial focus be on providing high quality models of the target structure in varied contexts, shifting emphasis to eliciting productions from the child and providing recasts as the child indicates a willingness to attempt the new structure and an ability to approximate the target form. When treating very young children or children at the early stages of phonological development the target forms should be words.[2] Vocabulary items should be selected to satisfy semantic, pragmatic, and phonological needs. The clinical implications of patterns of selection and avoidance of phones and word shapes by young children in early development should be taken into account. In the early stages of treatment, new words should be selected to include phones and word shapes that match words that are in the child's productive repertoire. Subsequently, complexity should be increased by introducing words with new phones and word shapes. Words for young children or children with small vocabulary sizes should be selected to contrast the whole word rather than individual phonemes. For example, when treating the child introduced in Case Study 6–3, the first goal would be to expand her vocabulary by focusing on words that match her phone and syllable shape preferences. Focused stimulation activities that model words with a CV(V) structure such "no," "go," "bee," and "toy" would be consistent with this goal. Very quickly the complexity of the target words could be increased to include two syllable words that do not reduplicate the consonant (potty, puddle [pʌɾo], bottle [bɑɾo], pony, ducky, doggie, kitty, nappy, and napping [næpĩ]). Words that have a VC (e.g., egg, up, eat, in, on) or CVC structure are also important early targets (e.g., pop, beep, cake followed by bag, done, or other words with nonreduplicated consonants). When words with these structures begin to appear in her spontaneous speech, new phonemes could be introduced in the context of established word shapes, with "mummy" and "off" being excellent choices. Research has shown that phonological and lexical development is inextricably linked in early typical (e.g., McCune & Vihman, 2001) and atypical development (e.g., Girolametto et al.,

[2]In Chapters 10 and 11 we expand this concept of words to include nonsense words; in early language development we believe the focus should be on meaningful and functional language. In normal language development, the child's lexicon often includes items that would not be considered to be a "real word" by adult standards, that is, "phonetically consistent forms" or "protowords" and these may be included as therapy targets. In any case, the targets of focused stimulation activities would not normally be isolated speech sounds unless those sounds had conventional functions (e.g., "sh!").

1997). Our recommendation to use focused stimulation to target lexical items that expand the child's repertoire of phones and word shapes in graduated steps reflects these research findings and is further supported by good quality trials attesting to the efficacy of focused stimulation as a therapeutic procedure.

Older children with DPD present with speech error patterns that are organized at the level of prosodic structures, segments, or features and therefore therapy goals will be concerned with these levels of the phonological hierarchy. For these children ear training procedures are appropriate, especially when it is not clear that the child has good perceptual knowledge of the phoneme that is the specific goal of the therapy program. If we consider Case Study 6–2 for example, and the goals that were selected for her in Table 8–5, we see that the goals fall into two categories. There are specific goals that involve encouraging the use of known phonemes in syllable positions where they do not normally occur (i.e., prosodic goals) and there are specific goals that involve introducing segments that rarely or never occur in her inventory (segmental goals). The latter goals (specifically, /ʃ, k, l, ɹ/) are very good candidates for ear training, either as a prelude to production training or as an adjunct to the early phases of production training. There is no evidence that she has knowledge of these phonemes at any level of representation. Considering the model of speech motor control presented in Chapter 3, we can see that it is essential to ensure that she has good perceptual knowledge of an internally specified target phoneme so that the internal model can be tuned and an accurate match between the target input and the output of motor commands can be reliably achieved. Traditional ear training includes four techniques involving naturally produced speech presented by the clinician: identification, isolation, stimulation and discrimination. A large scale randomized controlled trial showed that, by itself, ear training has some impact on speech accuracy and even more impact on reading (Sommers et al., 1961). Ear training has more effect on speech accuracy when it is combined with production training. Randomized controlled trials have shown that the addition of computer-based word identification training considerably enhances the effectiveness of production training for phonemes that are absent from the phonetic repertoire (Rvachew, 1994, 2005). Furthermore, the use of multiple voices in the presentation of stimuli for word identification and error detection is more effective than training with a single voice. Additional studies are required to establish the effectiveness of ear training procedures to facilitate the acquisition of prosodic goals. However, given that prosodic errors such as weak syllable deletion are associated with the perceptual prominence of the syllable (see Chapter 4), it is probable that input-oriented approaches to the remediation of these errors will be effective as well. One thing to remember is that ear training should be fairly brief with 30 to 60 minutes of input per specific goal being sufficient in most cases and therefore there is no reason to omit a procedure that has been shown to dramatically enhance the effectiveness of speech therapy in well controlled studies. It is also important to understand that ear training is not expected to be effective without the addition of production practice. For Case Study 6-2 we would recommend beginning with a brief introduction to the new target, let's say /ʃ/, using identification techniques to point out the sibilant nature of the sound and the salient lip rounding during its production while providing a descriptive label, perhaps "the quiet sound," linking it to the familiar finger to lips gesture. We would follow this with the SAILS word identification task, providing informative feedback that references both the acoustic and articulatory characteristics of the stimuli if she identifies items such as [du], [tu], or [su] as being correct exemplars of the word "shoe." This procedure should last approximately 10 minutes and be followed with a stimulation (auditory bombardment) activity, preferably involving movement for a change of pace. For example, the child could search the office for "sheep" stickers while the SLP offers advice ("I think I hid a sheep on the top shelf") and running commentary ("You found two sheep on the bottom shelf") including recasts for any incorrect productions of the /ʃ/ phoneme offered by the child. Finally, the session would conclude with techniques to stimulate correct production of the phoneme in isolation, as will be described in the next chapter. The SAILS activities could be continued for one or two additional sessions and then proceed to live voice error detection tasks in which the SLP presents sentence level material. These ear training procedures would continue in parallel with production training activities; over time production activities would come to dominate the sessions and the child would assume an increasingly independent role with respect to self-monitoring and self-correction of speech errors.

The child presented in Case Study 6–2 is at risk for delayed acquisition of literacy skills simply by virtue of having DPD. Interventions that address phonological awareness and literacy skills are discussed in Chapter 11. However, it may be good practice to introduce all parents of young children with DPD to dialogic reading techniques as a means of maximizing oral language skills and ensuring exposure to enjoyable literacy experiences. It has been established that children with normally developing language skills benefit from dialogic reading when the outcome measure is growth in vocabulary size. The literature on the conditions under which dialogic reading is a useful tool for the treatment of speech and language disorders is not perfectly clear, however. Some studies have reported benefits for lexical diversity, utterance length, inferential language, or phonological awareness for 2- to 4-year-old children with speech and/or language delays. Other studies have failed to find an effect of dialogic reading on these children's language skills. We have tentatively suggested some reasons for disparate findings on the basis of our own experience with dialogic reading and our review of the literature. First, it is possible that parents of children with speech and language delays may need more intensive training in the application of these techniques in order to learn to be responsive to the particularities of their child's needs. Mismatches between their child's language comprehension, language expression, and speech production abilities may make it difficult for the parents to identify appropriate levels of prompts and responses to their children's answers. It has also been suggested that the traditional application of dialogic reading techniques may be too directive for children with speech and language delays. Our experience with dialogic reading may confirm this hypothesis. In our study, parent provided dialogic reading was associated with significantly higher phonological awareness skills when this intervention followed an input-oriented intervention provided by a student SLP weekly for 6 weeks. The dialogic reading intervention was not associated with improved phonological awareness performance when it followed an output-oriented intervention. The input-oriented intervention modeled a very nondirective style of interacting with their children that parents may have adopted as they applied the dialogic reading techniques with their child. Furthermore, the input-oriented intervention may have prepared the children to benefit from the intervention by improving their listening and speech processing skills. Both of these suggestions are highly speculative however. Finally, we suggested that dialogic reading is most likely to be effective when it has a relatively clear focus and parents are not asked to try to achieve too many goals at once. We continue to feel that maximizing oral language skills is an essential strategy for preventing literacy delays among children with DPD. Further research to determine the most effective and efficient strategies for children at different ages and levels of language skills is required.

References

Bauman-Waengler, J. (2012). *Articulatory and phonological impairments: A clinical focus* (4th ed.). Boston, MA: Allyn & Bacon.

Brosseau-Lapré, F., Rvachew, S, Clayards, M., & Dickson, D. (in press). Stimulus variability and perceptual learning of non-native vowel categories. *Applied Psycholinguistics*.

Bus, A. G., Van Ijzendoorn, Marinus H., & Pellegrini, A. D. (1995). Joint book reading makes for success in learning to read: A meta-analysis on intergenerational transmission of literacy. *Review of Educational Research, 65*, 1–21.

Byrne, B., & Fielding-Barnsley, R. (1991). Evaluation of a program to teach phonemic awareness to young children. *Journal of Educational Psychology, 83*(4), 451–455.

Camarata, S. M. (2010). Naturalistic intervention for speech intelligibility and speech accuracy. In A. L. Williams, S. McLeod, & R. J. McCauley (Eds.), *Interventions for speech sound disorders in children* (pp. 381–406). Baltimore, MD: Brookes.

Cameron, J., Pierce, W. D., Basko, K. M., & Gear, A. (2005). Achievement-based rewards and intrinsic motivation: A test of cognitive mediators. *Journal of Educational Psychology, 97*(4), 641–655.

Chapman, M. E. (1942). The speech clinician and the classroom teacher co-operate in a speech correction program. *Journal of Speech Disorders, 7*(1), 57–61.

Crain-Thoreson, C., & Dale, P. S. (1999). Enhancing linguistic performance: Parents and teachers as book reading partners for children with language delays. *Topics in Early Childhool Special Education, 19*, 28–39.

Dale, P. S., Crain-Thoreson, C., Notari-Synverson, A., & Cole, K. N. (1996). Parent-child book reading as an intervention technique for young children with language delays. *Topics in Early Childhool Special Education, 16*, 213–235.

Dickinson, D. K., & Tabors, P. O. (2001). *Beginning literacy with language: Young children learning at home and at school*. Baltimore, MD: Brookes.

Evans, M. A., & Saint-Aubin, J. (2009). Letter names and alphabet book reading by senior kindergartneners: An eye movement study. *Child Development, 80*, 1824–1841.

Fey, M. E., Cleave, P. L., Ravida, A. I., Long, S. H., Dejmal, A. E., & Easton, D. L. (1994). Effects of grammar facilitation on the phonological performance of children with speech and language impairments. *Journal of Speech and Hearing Research, 37*(3), 594–607.

Fey, M. E., Long, S. H., & Finestack, L. H. (2003). Ten principles of grammar facilitation for children with specific language impairments. *American Journal of Speech-Language Pathology, 12*(1), 3–15.

Girolametto, L., Pearce, P. S., & Weitzman, E. (1997). Effects of lexical intervention on the phonology of late talkers. *Journal of Speech, Language, and Hearing Research, 40*(2), 338–348.

Guenther, F. H., Husain, F. T., Cohen, M. A., & Shinn-Cunningham, B. G. (1999). Effects of categorization and discrimination training on auditory perceptual space. *Journal of the Acoustical Society of America, 106*, 2900–2912.

Hall Powers, M. (1957). Clinical and educational procedures in functional disorders of articulation. In L. E. Travis (Ed.), *Handbook of speech pathology* (pp. 769–804). New York, NY: Appleton-Century-Crofts.

Hassink, J. M., & Leonard, L. B. (2010). Within-treatment factors as predictors of outcomes following conversational recasting. *American Journal of Speech-Language Pathology, 19*, 213–224.

Hindman, A., Connor, C. M., Jewkes, A. M., & Morrison, F. J. (2008). Untangling the effects of shared book reading: Multiple factors and their associations with preschool literacy outcomes. *Early Childhood Research Quarterly, 23*, 330–350.

Hodson, B. (2007). *Evaluating and enhancing children's phonological systems: Research and theory to practice*. Wichita, KS: Phonocomp.

Hodson, B. W., & Paden, E. P. (1983). *Targeting intelligible speech: A phonological approach to remediation*. Boston, MA: College-Hill.

Huttenlocher, J. (1998). Language input and language growth. *Preventive Medicine, 27*, 195–199.

Jamieson, D. G., & Morosan, D. E. (1989). Training new, nonnative speech contrasts: A comparison of the prototype and perceptual fading techniques. *Canadian Journal of Psychology, 43*(1), 88–96.

Justice, L. M., McGinty, A. S., Piasta, S. B., Kaderavek, J. N., & Fan, X. (2010). Print-focused read-alouds in preschool classrooms: Intervention effectiveness and moderators of child outcomes. *Language, Speech, and Hearing Services in Schools, 41*, 504–520.

Kaderavek, J. N., & Justice, L. M. (2002). Shared storybook reading as an intervention context: Practices and potential pitfalls. *American Journal of Speech-Language Pathology, 11*, 395–406.

Kamhi, A. G. (2006). Treatment decisions for children with speech-sound disorders. *Language, Speech, and Hearing Services in Schools, 37*(4), 271–279.

Kuhl, P. K., Conboy, B. T., Coffey-Corina, S., Padden, D., Rivera-Gaxiola, M., & Nelson, T. (2008). Phonetic learning as a pathway to language: new data and native language magnet theory expanded (NLM-e). *Philosophical Transactions of the Royal Society, 363*, 979–1000.

Leonard, L., & McGregor, K. (1991). Unusual phonological patterns and their underlying representations: A case study. *Journal of Child Language, 18*, 261–271.

Lively, S. E., Logan, J. S., & Pisoni, D. (1993). Training Japanese listeners to identify English /r/ and /l/. II: The role of phonetic environment and talker variability in learning new perceptual categories. *Journal of the Acoustical Society of America, 94*(3), 1242–1255.

Lonigan, C. J., Driscoll, K., Phillips, B. M., Cantor, B. G., Anthony, J. L., & Goldstein, H. (2003). Evaluation of a computer-assisted instruction phonological sensitivity program with preschool children at-risk for reading problems. *Journal of Early Intervention, 25*, 248–262.

Lonigan, C. J., & Whitehurst, G. J. (1998). Relative efficacy of a parent teacher involvement in a shared-reading intervention for preschool children from low-income backgrounds. *Early Childhood Research Quarterly, 13*(2), 263–290.

Marchman, V. A., & Fernald, A. (2008). Speed of word recognition and vocabulary knowledge in infancy predict cognitive and language outcomes in later childhool. *Developmental Science, 11*, F9–F16.

McBride-Chang, C. (1995). What is phonological awareness? *Journal of Educational Psychology, 87*, 179–192.

McClelland, J. L., Fiez, J. A., & McCandliss, Bruce D. (2002). Teaching the /r/-/l/ discrimination to Japanese adults: Behavioral and neural aspects. *Physiology and Behavior, 77*, 657–662.

McCune, L., & Vihman, M. M. (2001). Early phonetic and lexical development: A productivity approach. *Journal of Speech, Language, and Hearing Research, 44*, 670–684.

McMurray, B., & Aslin, R. N. (2005). Infants are sensitive to within-category variation in speech perception. *Cognition, 95*, B15–B26.

McMurray, B., Aslin, R. N., & Toscano, J. C. (2009). Statistical learning of phonetic categories: Insights from a computational approach. *Developmental Science, 12*(3), 369–378.

Meltzoff, A. N. (2009). Foundations for a new science of learning. *Science, 284*, 284–288.

Mills, D. L., Prat, C., Zangl, R., Stager, C. L., Neville, H. J., & Werker, J. F. (2004). Language experience and the organization of brain activity to phonetically similar words: ERP evidence from 14- and 20-month-olds. *Journal of Cognitive Neuroscience, 16*, 1452–1464.

Mol, S. E., Bus, A. G., de Jong, M. T., & Smeeta, D. J. H. (2008). Added value of dialogic parent-child book readings: A meta-analysis. *Early Education and Development, 19*, 7–26.

Moore, D. R., Rosenberg, J. F., & Coleman, J. S. (2005). Discrimination training of phonemic contrasts enhances phonological processing in mainstream school children. *Brain and Language, 94*, 72–85.

Mowrer, D. E. (1971). Transfer of training in articulation therapy. *Journal of Speech and Hearing Disorders, 36*, 427–446.

Peterson, R. L., Pennington, B. F., Shriberg, L. D., & Boada, R. (2009). What influences literacy outcome in children with speech sound disorder? *Journal of Speech, Language, and Hearing Research, 52*, 1175–1188.

Pile, E. J. S., Girolametto, L., Johnson, C. J., Chen, X., & Cleave, P. L. (2010). Shared book reading intervention for children with language impairment: Using parents-as-aides in language intervention. *Canadian Journal of Speech-Language Pathology and Audiology, 34*, 96–109.

Plante, E., Bahl, M., Vance, R., & Gerken, L. (2010). Children with specific language impairment show rapid, implicit learning of stress assignment rules. *Journal of Communication Disorders, 43*(5), 397–406.

Porkorni, J. L., Worthington, C. K., & Jamison, P. J. (2004). Phonological awareness intervention: Comparison of Fast ForWord, Earobics, and LiPS. *Journal of Educational Research, 97*(3), 147–157.

Proctor-Williams, K. (2009). Dosage and distribution in morphosyntax intervention: Current evidence and future needs. *Topics in Language Disorders, 29*, 294–311.

Proctor-Williams, K., & Fey, M. E. (2007). Recast density and acquisition of novel irregular past tense verbs. *Journal of Speech, Language, and Hearing Research, 50*(4), 1029–1047.

Reese, E., & Cox, A. (1999). Quality of adult book reading affects children's emergent literacy. *Developmental Psychology, 35*(1), 20–28.

Richtsmeier, P. T., Gerken, L., Goffman, L., & Hogan, T. (2009). Statistical frequency in perception affects children's lexical production. *Cognition, 111*, 372–377.

Rost, G. C., & McMurray, B. (2009). Speaker variability augments phonological processing in early word learning. *Developmental Science, 12*, 339–349.

Rvachew, S. (1994). Speech perception training can facilitate sound production learning. *Journal of Speech and Hearing Research, 37*, 347–357.

Rvachew, S. (2005). Stimulability and treatment success. *Topics in Language Disorders. Clinical Perspectives on Speech Sound Disorders, 25*(3), 207–219.

Rvachew, S. (2006). Longitudinal prediction of implicit phonological awareness skills. *American Journal of Speech-Language Pathology, 15*, 165–176.

Rvachew, S., & Brosseau-Lapré, F. (2010). Speech perception intervention. In S. McLeod, L. Williams, & R. McCauley (Ed.), *Treatment of speech sound disorders in children*. Baltimore, MD: Brookes.

Rvachew, S., & Brosseau-Lapré, F. (2011). *A randomized trial of phonological interventions in French.* International Child Phonology Conference, June 17, 2011, York, UK.

Rvachew, S., & Grawburg, M. (2006). Correlates of phonological awareness in preschoolers with speech sound disorders. *Journal of Speech, Language, and Hearing Research, 49*, 74–87.

Rvachew, S., & Jamieson, D. G. (1995). Learning new speech contrasts: Evidence from learning a second language and children with speech disorders. In W. Strange (Ed.), *Speech perception and linguistic experience* (pp. 411–432). Timonium, MD: York Press.

Rvachew, S., Nowak, M., & Cloutier, G. (2004). Effect of phonemic perception training on the speech production and phonological awareness skills of children with expressive phonological delay. *American Journal of Speech-Language Pathology, 13*, 250–263.

Rvachew, S., Rafaat, S., & Martin, M. (1999). Stimulability, speech perception and the treatment of phonological disorders. *American Journal of Speech-Language Pathology, 8*, 33–34.

Schwartz, R., & Leonard, L. (1982). Do children pick and choose? An examination of selection and avoidance in early lexical acquisition. *Journal of Child Language, 9*, 319–336.

Secord, W. E., Boyce, S. E., Donahue, J. S., Fox, R. A.., & Shine, R. E. (2007). *Eliciting sounds: Techniques and strategies for clinicians* (2nd ed.). Florence, KY: Cengage Learning.

Senechal, M., LeFevre, J. , Thomas, E. M., & Daley, K. E. (1998). Differential effects of home literacy experiences on the development of oral and written language. *Reading Research Quarterly, 33*(1), 96–116.

Seymour, H. N., Baran, J., & Peaper, R. E. (1981). Auditory discrimination: Evaluation and intervention. In N. J. Lass (Ed.), *Speech and language: Advances in basic research and practice* (Vol. 6, pp. 1–56). New York, NY: Academic Press.

Shelton, R. L., Johnson, A. F., Ruscello, D. M., & Arndt, W. B. (1978). Assessment of parent-administered listening training for preschool children with articulation deficits. *Journal of Speech and Hearing Disorders, 43*(2), 242–254.

Shelton, R. L., & McReynolds, L. V. (1979). Functional articulation disorders: Preliminaries to treatment. In N. J. Lass (Ed.), *Speech and language: Advances in basic research and practice* (Vol. 2, pp. 2–112). New York, NY: Academic Press.

Sommers, R. K., Cockerille, C. E., Paul, C. D., Bowser, D. C., Fichter, G. R., Fenton, A. K., & Copetas, F. G. (1961). Effects of speech therapy and speech improvement upon articulation and reading. *Journal of Speech and Hearing Disorders, 26*(1), 27–38.

Sommers, R. K., Copetas, F. G., Bowser, D. C., Fichter, G. R., Furlong, A. K., Rhodes, F. E., & Saunders, Z. G. (1962). Effects of various durations of speech improvement upon articulation and reading. *Journal of Speech and Hearing Disorders, 27*, 54–61.

Tsao, F., Huei-Mei, L., & Kuhl, P. K. (2004). Speech perception in infancy predicts language development in the second year of life: A longitudinal study. *Child Development, 75*(4), 1067–1084.

Tyler, A. A., Lewis, K. E., Haskill, A., & Tolbert, L. C. (2003). Outcomes of different speech and language goal attack strategies. *Journal of Speech, Language, and Hearing Research, 46*, 1077–1094.

van Kleeck, A., Schwarz, A. L., Fey, M. E., Kaiser, A., Miller, J., & Weitzman, E. (2010). Should we use telegraphic or grammatical input in the early stages of language development with children who have language impairments? A meta-analysis of the research and expert opinion. *American Journal of Speech-Language Pathology, 19*, 3–21.

van Kleeck, A., Vander Woude, J., & Hammett, L. (2006). Fostering literal and inferential skills in Head Start preschoolers with language impairment using book-sharing discussions. *American Journal of Speech-Language Pathology, 15*, 85–95.

Van Riper, C. (1963). *Speech correction: Principles and methods*. Upper Saddle River, NJ: Prentice-Hall.

Van Riper, C. (1978). *Speech correction: Principles and methods*. Upper Saddle River, NJ: Prentice-Hall.

Walley, A. C., Metsala, J. L., & Garlock, V. M. (2003). Spoken vocabulary growth: Its role in the development of phoneme awareness and reading ability. *Reading and Writing: An Interdisciplinary Journal, 16*, 5–20.

Weiner, F. (1981). Treatment of phonological disability using the method of meaningful minimal contrasts: Two case studies. *Journal of Speech and Hearing Disorders, 46*, 97–103.

Weinert, S. (2009). Implicit and explicit modes of learning: Similarities and differences from a developmental perspective. *Linguistics, 47*, 241–271.

Weismer, S. E., & Hesketh, L. J. (1996). Lexical learning by children with specific language impairment: Effects of linguistic input presented at varying speaking rates. *Journal of Speech, Language, and Hearing Research, 39*, 177–190.

Weismer, S. E., & Hesketh, L. J. (1998). The impact of emphatic stress on novel word learning by children with specific language impairment. *Journal of Speech, Language, and Hearing Research, 41*(6), 1444–1458.

Weizman, Z.O., & Snow, C. E. (2001). Lexical input as related to children's vocabulary acquisition: Effects of sophisticated exposure and support for meaning. *Developmental Psychology, 37*(2), 265–279.

Werker, J. F., & Curtin, S. (2005). PRIMIR: A developmental framework of infant speech processing. *Language Learning and Development, 1*(2), 197–234.

Werker, J. F., Fennell, C. T., Corcoran, K. M., & Stager, C. L. (2002). Infants' ability to learn phonetically similar words: Effects of age and vocabulary size. *Infancy, 3*(1), 1–30.

Whitehurst, G. J., Epstein, J. N., Angell, A. L., Payne, A. C., Crone, D. A., & Fischel, J. E. (1994). A picture book reading intervention in day care and home for children from low-income families. *Developmental Psychology, 30*, 679–689.

Whitehurst, G. J., Falco, F., Lonigan, C. J., Fischel, J. E., DeBaryshe, B. D., Valdez-Menchaca, M. C., & Caulfield, M. (1988). Accelerating language development through picture book reading. *Developmental Psychology, 24*, 552–558.

Whitehurst, G. J., Fischel, J. E., Lonigan, C. J., Valdez-Menchaca, M. C., Arnold, D. S., & Smith, M. (1991). Treatment of early expressive language delay: If, when and how. *Topics in Language Disorders, 11*, 55–68.

Whitehurst, G. J., Zevenburger, A. A., Crone, D. A., Schultz, M. D., Velting, O. N., & Fischel, J. E. (1999). Outcomes of an emergent literacy intervention from Head Start through second grade. *Journal of Educational Psychology, 91*(2), 261–272.

Winitz, H., & Bellerose, B. (1967). Relation between sound discrimination and sound learning. *Journal of Communication Disorders, 1*, 215–235.

Wolfe, V., Presley, C., & Mesaris, J. (2003). The importance of sound identification training in phonological intervention. *American Journal of Speech-Language Pathology, 12*, 282–288.

Wren, Y., Roulstone, S., & Williams, A. L. (2010). Computer-based interventions. In A. L. Williams, S. McLeod, & R. J. McCauley (Eds.), *Interventions of speech sound disorders in children*. Baltimore, MD: Brookes.

Yoder, P. J., Camarata, S., & Gardner, E. (2005). Treatment effects on speech intelligibility and length of utterance in children with specific language and intelligibility impairments. *Journal of Early Intervention, 28*(1), 34–49.

Zevenbergen, A. A., Whitehurst, G. J., & Zevenbergen, J. A. (2003). Effects of a shared-reading intervention on the inclusion of evaluative devices in narratives of children from low-income families. *Applied Developmental Psychology, 24*, 1–15.

Chapter 10

Output-Oriented Approaches to Intervention

In Chapter 9 we described some input-oriented procedures that have the primary goal of strengthening children's acoustic-phonetic representations for words. We indicated that these procedures may also have a positive impact on speech accuracy by providing the child with clear targets for speech production, motivating speech production practice, and enhancing feedback about the match between the child's productions and the intended targets. Although input-oriented approaches alone play a role in the acquisition of internal models to guide speech movements, these approaches are not always sufficient. Children, whether exhibiting a normal or slow trajectory of phonological development, require years of practice to achieve adultlike speech accuracy and precision. In this chapter we describe procedures to maximize the effectiveness of speech practice to ensure normalized speech for children with DPD.

Children, whether exhibiting a normal or slow trajectory of phonological development, require years of **practice** to achieve adultlike speech accuracy and precision.

As outlined in Chapter 3, it would be a gross oversimplification to say that the development of speech motor control involves a succession of distinct stages characterized by unique learning challenges or mechanisms. Nonetheless, certain milestones stand out along the way from the infant's initial reflexive vocalizations to the achievement of adultlike speech. Furthermore, certain learning mechanisms appear to play a leading role in the acquisition of these milestones even though these mechanisms work in concert throughout development. Summarizing from Chapter 3 in Plate 7, we identify four key events in speech development. In the first few months an important foundation is laid as the infant explores the possibilities of the vocal production system and learns to produce a variety of protophones that contrast different forms of resonance, vocal tract closures at various places of articulation, and variable

Key milestones in normal speech acquisition form a roadmap for the selection of speech therapy goals.

phonatory and respiratory characteristics. The importance of the expansion stage in the laying of building blocks for later speech development is easy to forget when choosing goals for speech therapy, a topic to which we return shortly. Another important achievement during the infant period is the acquisition of canonical syllables when the child learns to control the variable parameters explored during the expansion stage, coordinating them to produce well-formed syllables in the context of babble, jargon, and early words. The repertoire of meaningful words is expanded through the reciprocal processes of selecting words to correspond to templates established in babble, adaptation of words to those well-practiced templates and gradual modification of existing templates so as to avoid homonymy in word production. Eventually, the templates become too limiting and greater flexibility is required to meet the child's growing language abilities. New phones, phonemes and words shapes are added to the repertoire, resulting in increased proximity of spoken words to their targets, culminating in fully intelligible speech by the age of 4 years for most children. Subsequently, consistency increases in a gradual fashion leading to adultlike accuracy by age 9 years and maximum precision for various speech parameters between 16 years and young adulthood.

Typical descriptions of speech acquisition focus on reductions in variability with age. Infants begin by producing words with high variability (see Figure 4–2) and converge on conventional and consistent productions of the appropriate sequence of phonemes. Kinematic studies reveal that stability upon repeated production of a phrase increases remarkably with age as shown in Figure 1–6. Standard studies of motor learning similarly focus on the conditions that result in a reduction in performance variability over time as shown in Figure 3–20. Therefore, it is not surprising that traditional speech therapy procedures are designed to enhance consistency and reduce variability in the production of phonemes with practice. However, variability is not always an impediment to speech learning and children with DPD often suffer from insufficient variability in their repertoire of speech behaviors. Performance variability can be viewed as facilitating, detrimental, or irrelevant to a successful outcome depending on the motor learning context (Vereijken, 2010). For example, the highly variable vocalizations of the expansion stage provide a complex foundation for the emergence of speech-like vocalizations at later stages. Infants who are described as being "quiet" during the first year of life lack sufficient variability for normal motor speech development. The normally developing infant harnesses rather than reduces this variability to coordinate the separate respiratory, phonatory, resonance, and articulatory components to produce babble in the next stage. Throughout the next 16 or so years there will be a continual interplay between adaptive variability to meet new challenges and increased stability to enhance precision. Some degree of variability is required to allow for continuous adaptations to changes in vocal tract structure and expansions in

Performance variability can be viewed as facilitating, detrimental, or irrelevant to a successful outcome depending on the motor learning context.

Throughout speech development there will be a continual interplay between **adaptive variability** to meet new challenges and increased stability to enhance precision.

linguistic complexity. During the same period, improvements in precision occur in a fashion that promotes stability in higher order goals despite shifting variability in underlying components. What this means is that the focus of speech therapy should be on the promotion of dynamic stability which is altogether different from a reduction in variability per se.

Speech therapy should focus on the promotion of **dynamic stability** rather than reducing variability.

How does the child achieve dynamic stability for speech? The foundation of dynamic stability is a set of well tuned internal models appropriate for a broad variety of speaking contexts, as described in Chapter 3 in relation to the DIVA model (see Figure 3–15, Guenther & Vladusich, 2009; Wolpert, Ghahramani, & Flanagan, 2001). In the speech context, the child must learn to predict the sensory consequences of motor commands that produce speech movements (internal forward dynamic models) and to select appropriate motor commands to achieve the desired vocal tract configuration given current inputs (internal inverse models). The kinematic mapping between vocal tract configurations and the speech sound outputs that correspond to the sound system of the language being learned by the infant must also be mastered during development. Wolpert et al. (2001) describe three learning mechanisms that play a role in the development of these models. Unsupervised learning occurs in a context in which the mapping between inputs to and outputs from the motor system is learned but the environment provides no specific target and no reinforcement or feedback as to the correctness of the behavioral responses. Essentially, the infant emits vocalizations, seemingly at random, and the correspondence between articulatory gestures and acoustic outcomes is linked in the internal model. Unsupervised learning can result in the extraction of representations from high dimensional inputs when linked to lower dimensional outputs as in the case of linking the many-to-one relationship between possible articulatory gestures and the acoustic outcomes associated a given phone (e.g., the variable gestures that produce the closely positioned F2 and F3 in [ɝ] as shown in Figure 1–3). Supervised learning occurs when the environment provides a specific target and the errors in the match between the target input and the output serve as a teaching signal. Supervised learning may involve an externally or internally provided target. Supervised learning plays a role in babbling during which the forward internal model can transform sensory errors into changes in the motor command to maintain repetition of syllables or syllable patterns during an utterance. Imitation learning is also a form of supervised learning but in this case the target is specified externally rather than internally. In reinforcement learning the environment provides information about the desirability of the behavior (rather than a model of the target behavior itself). In this case, especially when the endpoint behavior is complex, requiring the sequencing or superposition of many component parts, the information may not provide clear information about which motor commands to adjust in order to achieve the desired behavior.

The foundation of dynamic stability is a set of well-tuned **internal models** appropriate for a broad variety of speaking contexts.

Three **learning mechanisms** play a role in the development of internal models: *supervised learning, unsupervised learning, and reinforcement learning.*

Our expectations about the kinds of speech therapy procedures that might be effective for children with DPD are drawn from our review of normal speech development.

Our expectations about the kinds of speech therapy procedures that might be effective for children with DPD are drawn from our review of normal speech development as described in Chapter 3 and summarized in Table 10–1. For children who are at the earliest stage of speech development and who have restricted repertoires of speech elements we recommend procedures to encourage vocal play, primarily exploiting unsupervised learning mechanisms to promote variability in speech output but working in a social learning context to motivate free exploration of the vocal system. In the second section of this chapter, we focus on those children who appear capable of producing a base repertoire of segments and syllable structures but who evidence poor control of those elements. We describe some sensorimotor procedures designed to enhance control of this variability in the production of nonsense word sequences (essentially simulating babble) and in the production of first words selected to match and then gradually expand on those templates by building on the syllables that the child has mastered. In the third section, traditional speech therapy techniques to establish new phonemes and encourage practice of those phonemes in increasingly complex contexts are described. Finally, procedures to enhance and maintain precision during the transfer and maintenance phases of the speech therapy program are outlined in the fourth section. Each section is accompanied by detailed examples of the implementation of the procedures and a discussion of the research evidence to support the use of the procedures as described.

Explore Possibilities of the Vocal System

10.1.1. Describe the goal of procedures to encourage vocal play and distinguish this intervention from focused stimulation.

10.1.2. List and describe six techniques for encouraging vocal play in young children who are not readily imitating speech sounds.

Children who do not respond to traditional imitative approaches to speech therapy are commonly encountered in the clinic.

Dethorne, Johnson, Walder, and Mahurin-Smith (2009) point out that children who do not respond to traditional imitative approaches to speech therapy are commonly encountered in the clinic especially among children who are late-talking. Even among those children for whom the speech or language problem is primary (i.e., not secondary to cognitive delay, hearing impairment, autism, or some other primary condition), there will be children who have a limited repertoire of vocal forms and who are unwilling or unable to imitate new forms. In these cases, increasing variability is the specific target of intervention and the procedures used have the goal of supporting exploration of the vocal system: helping the child to

Table 10–1. Learning Mechanisms and Environmental Supports in the Natural Environment and Therapeutic Procedures for the Development of Speech Motor Control and Speech Production Accuracy in the Clinical Environment

Learning Mechanisms	*Environmental Supports*	*Therapeutic Procedures*	*Expected Outcomes*
1. Expansion Stage: Explore Possibilities of the Vocal System			
Practice Exploration Unsupervised learning	Self-produced speech inputs (auditory, somatosensory, proprioceptive feedback) Contingent speech input Contingent social input	Procedures to encourage vocal play (see text for details)	Increased variety of vocal outputs Learned inverse kinematic mappings between vocal tract configurations and articulator movements Expanded vowel space Improved coordination of phonation, resonance, and articulation to produce speechlike vowels and syllables
2. Babbling and Integrative Stage: Controlled Variability			
Practice Integration Selection Adaptation Supervised learning	Highly variable natural speech input from multiple talkers Self-produced speech inputs (auditory, somatosensory, proprioceptive feedback) Contingent speech input Contingent social input	Nonsense syllable practice Integral Stimulation Hierarchy Encourage functional word use based on established phonetic templates Encourage functional word use based on progressive variations in established phonetic templates	Tuning of internal models Linkage of vocal tract configurations to speech sounds Improved jaw stability Increased inter-articulator coupling (integration) Expansion of productive vocabulary through selection and adaptation to templates established in babbling repertoire
3. Early Speech Development: Expanding Repertoire of Phonemes and Word Shapes to Achieve Intelligible Speech			
Practice Differentiation Imitation Reinforcement Learning Social Learning	Self-produced speech inputs (auditory, somatosensory, proprioceptive feedback) Linguistic inputs in varied contexts Social inputs in varied contexts	Accurate speech models Phonetic placement Practice with knowledge of performance and results to establish new articulatory gestures and templates	Expanded repertoire of phones and phonemes Expanded repertoire of word shapes Improved proximity of words to targets Intelligible speech
4. Late Speech Development: Ongoing Refinements to Achieve Adultlike Speech Accuracy and Precision			
Practice Refinement Supervised Learning	Self-produced speech inputs (auditory, somatosensory, proprioceptive feedback) Social expectation for increasingly complex linguistic structure	Encourage practice with increasing variability and complexity Focus on authentic communication contexts and natural environment Provide knowledge of performance and results in accordance with principles of motor learning Focus on self-evaluation	Accurate production of all phonemes Consistent production of phonemes in varied contexts Speech planning for longer chunks of speech/language. Precise production of segmental and suprasegmental elements in varied contexts

The goal of the **vocal play** intervention is to encourage the child to explore the vocal system freely in order to experience the full range of auditory, somatosensory, proprioceptive, and even social effects that occur when different vocalizations are produced.

experience the full range of auditory, somatosensory, proprioceptive, and even social effects that occur when different vocalizations are produced. In this case, the SLP should have a range of experiences in mind but specific targets are not systematically provided or reinforced. Some of the techniques described are similar to those used for focused stimulation but there are subtle but important differences relating to the goals of the procedure. First, focused stimulation as e described in Chapter 9 has the goal of providing the child with multiple but varied exposures to a specific input form in order to strengthen acoustic-phonetic representations for the target form. The child may or may not choose to produce the form but a focus on many presentations of a specific target form is important to the success of the procedure. Recall that focused stimulation is a hybrid procedure with a balance of child and clinician direction. The vocal play procedures to be described here have a different goal. In this case we want to encourage the child to explore the vocal system freely. The activities are much more child-centered because self-exploration rather than the production of a given correct form is the goal. The SLP must provide a safe environment that permits this exploration with therapeutic guidance but without judgment. A 2-year-old with very limited vocalizations will need a secure environment in which it is socially appropriate to practice vocalizations more typical of a 4-month-old for a brief time. That same child will need emotional support to attempt vocalizing with an articulatory system over which he or she has not yet gained precise control. Techniques for providing therapeutic guidance in a child-centered context are described next.

Vocal play activities are much more **child-centered** than focus stimulation because self-exploration rather than the production of a given correct form is the goal.

Procedures to Encourage Vocal Play

Dethorne et al. (2009) reviewed evidence for five techniques for encouraging vocal play in young children who are not readily imitating speech sounds, specifically: (1) provide access to augmentative or alternative communication; (2) minimize pressure to speak; (3) imitate the child; (4) use an infant-direct speaking register (exaggerated pitch contours and slowed rate); (5) augment sensory and social feedback; and (6) avoid emphasis on nonspeech articulator movements (focus on function). We discuss these techniques in turn.

It is not uncommon for the parents of young children with severe speech delay to report that their child was a very quiet baby who nonetheless produced a few words at around the expected age and then simply stopped talking (Velleman & Strand, 1994). We know that this is a frustrating experience for the parents who will often attempt repeatedly to get the child to reproduce the seemingly forgotten words. We believe it is a frightening experience for the child who made an effort to speak and retreated to silence after finding speech to be an unreliable means of communicating. We cannot be sure of what is happening in the minds of children who stop talking after these early attempts but it is easy to imagine the internal reactions a child might have when experiencing different sensory and functional outcomes upon each attempt to say a word, despite having a clear sense of the word one wishes to say and the outcomes one is expecting to evoke. One reason to introduce an augmentative or alternative communication (AAC) system is to enhance the child's sense of self-efficacy, providing opportunities for successful communication in another modality and establishing a communicative framework onto which verbal communication can eventually be mapped. The optimum type of AAC system will depend on the child's communicative needs, cognitive capacity, and severity of speech deficit. If the child is very young with a small receptive vocabulary and you are expecting to establish verbal communication within a short time frame, it probably will be sufficient to encourage the use of relatively natural manual gestures or a small repertoire of conventional manual signs. For an older child who is making very slow progress a more formal AAC system will be required. In any case, it is wise to incorporate opportunities for the child to make choices into the treatment session, in keeping with the child-centered nature of this therapy approach. For a toddler this may mean simply offering multiple toys at the start of the session and encouraging the toddler to make a choice in the form of a pointing response. A small repertoire of manual signs could then be introduced, with signs such as "more" being useful, initially as a means of requesting repetition of an activity or interesting effect and later as a generative "pivot" when learning to sequence signs and words. A child whose motor delays preclude the learning of complex signs might use a picture booklet or formal AAC device to select and sequence activities within a therapy session. A well-designed randomized control trial involving toddlers with limited vocabulary size and cognitive delays found that AAC interventions facilitated the emergence of spoken words relative to an intervention that modeled and reinforced spoken language use (Romski et al., 2010). Although research evidence is scarce for children with less severe delays, there is no reason to believe that encouraging the use of manual language in late-talking children will inhibit the emergence of spoken language. In fact, all the evidence points to a strong positive relationship between gesture and oral language development (Goodwyn, Acredolo, & Brown, 2000; Rowe & Golden-Meadow, 2009) and thus we feel comfortable with the evidence base for this first technique.

The second technique is related to the first and that is to reduce pressure on the child to use speech as a means of communication. Some children require more language input before they are ready to attempt new words and, as reviewed in Chapter 9, focused stimulation is an effective procedure for these children when it comes time to focus on the evocation of specific linguistic forms (see also Kouri, 2005). However, the goal of the vocal play session is on free

One reason to introduce an **augmentative or alternative communication (AAC)** system is to enhance the child's sense of self-efficacy, providing opportunities for successful communication in another modality and establishing a communicative framework onto which verbal communication can eventually be mapped.

Incorporate opportunities for the child to make choices into the treatment session, in keeping with the child-centered nature of this therapy approach.

A randomized control trial found that AAC interventions facilitated the emergence of spoken words relative to an intervention that modeled and reinforced spoken language use.

All the evidence points to a strong positive relationship between gesture and oral language development.

Reduce pressure on the child to use speech as a means of communication.

exploration of the vocal system and therefore it is necessary to shift emphasis away from words, which will invite comparisons between output and the canonical form, to varied playful vocalizations. During vocal play there is no expectation that the child produce a specific form and thus less chance of distress because a given target is not achieved; rather, the goal is for the child to experience the sensory consequences of producing varied movements of the vocal system.

Provide the child with toys that invite playful vocalization and then **imitate** and expand those vocalizations as they occur.

Rather than eliciting specific vocal outputs from the child, the SLP should provide the child with toys that invite playful vocalization, imitate the child's nonverbal actions with the toys while waiting patiently for the child to vocalize, and then imitate the child's vocalizations when they occur. The technique mirrors the procedure used so effectively by Bloom to shift 3-month-old infants from quasiresonant to fully resonant vocalizations when speech input was provided contingent upon the infant's own vocalizations (Bloom, 1988). As the child becomes comfortable during therapy sessions and is vocalizing more frequently, direct imitations can become more playful: exaggerate variations in pitch, loudness, or resonance qualities to make the vocalization more interesting. Over time you can expand the child's vocalizations to introduce variation in vowel quality and eventually add consonantal closures produced in isolation or in combination with vocalic utterances. Throughout, use the fourth technique: the use of an infant-directed speaking register involving slowed rate of speech and exaggerations of pitch and prosodic contours as previously discussed in Chapters 2 and 9.

Use an **infant-directed speaking register** involving slowed rate of speech and exaggerations of pitch and prosodic contours.

Enhancing sensory feedback has the goal of helping the child establish the link between the motor commands used to produce movements of the articulators and the sensory consequences of those movements.

One reason for poor development of speech motor control might be deficiencies in **somatosensory feedback**.

The fifth technique—enhancing sensory feedback—has the goal of helping the child establish the link between the motor commands used to produce movements of the articulators and the sensory consequences of those movements. Recall from Chapter 8 that one reason for poor development of speech motor control might be deficiencies in somatosensory feedback (Terband, Maassen, Guenther, & Brumberg, 2009; Terband, Maassen, van Lieshout, & Nijland, 2011). Furthermore, there is some evidence that certain children with DPD have difficulties with oral sensory perception (Fucci, 1972; Fucci, Petrosino, Underwood, & Kendal, 1992; McNutt, 1977; Sommers, Cox, & West, 1972). Observation of infants in interaction with their caregivers reveals a correlation between oral-facial stimulation and sound making that may not be accidental. Raspberries and whooping noises just seem to go with face washing. Doll and puppet play provide opportunities for noisy kisses. The infant explores a delightful range of sound alternations while mouthing hands, toys, biscuits, or popsicles, possibly stimulated by the sensory characteristics of the objects or, alternatively, enabled by tongue and lip movements freed when the jaw is stabilized against the objects inserted into the mouth. There is no reason to not extend these activities that occur quite naturally with younger children into vocal play therapy sessions as they are not harmful and may motivate vocal practice on the part of the child. We must caution that,

Many natural forms of vocal play serendipitously involve elements that heighten oral sensory feedback.

although there are case studies describing the use of oral stimulation in speech therapy (e.g., see use of electric toothbrush by Lundeborg and McAllister, 2007), solid empirical evidence is lacking to support sensory stimulation as a therapeutic technique no matter how well justified on intuitive grounds. Even in the context of feeding interventions with premature infants, oral stimulation interventions have not yielded positive findings in controlled studies (Arvedson, Clarke, Lazarus, Schooling, & Frymark, 2010). Therefore we cannot recommend sustained attention to oral stimulation as a therapy technique based on current evidence. However, there is no harm in incorporating natural opportunities for sensory stimulation into vocal play routines.

Although there are case studies describing the use of **oral stimulation** in speech therapy, solid empirical evidence is lacking to support sensory stimulation as a therapeutic technique.

Furthermore, tuning of the internal models that link motor commands and their sensory outcomes requires practice on the part of the child and feedback provided by the SLP may play a role in motivating the child to initiate and repeat vocalizations. Recall from Chapter 3 that contingent social responses from mothers increased the quantity and improved the quality of infant vocalizations in a variety of studies. Although Goldstein, King, and West (2003) encouraged mothers to respond by smiling and touching their infants when they vocalized, social responses can be adapted for speech therapy to take into account the child's age, personality, and the specific play context. If the child crashes a car into a crowd of small dolls with an accompanying [p^h] sound, the socially appropriate and reinforcing response is to crash another car into the carnage with exaggerated movements and facial expression while uttering a loud "kapow." Resist the urge to suggest that crashing cars into people is not nice. After all, they are only dolls and you can now bring in the ambulances along with variations in vowel quality, pitch and loudness!

Notice in this example that the vocalizations are practiced in a functional context: crashing noises go with crashing actions and vowel sounds are practiced in the context of the speeding ambulance. The sixth vocal play technique is to focus on function; that is, do not practice nonspeech articulatory movements and do not isolate vocalizations from their playful context. Generally, if the therapy sessions are child-directed as intended there will be no opportunity for nonfunctional drills to occur.

Focus on **function**; that is, do not practice nonspeech articulatory movements and do not isolate vocalizations from their playful context.

Demonstration of Therapy to Encourage Vocal Play

Demonstration 10–1 describes the pre- and posttreatment phonetic and syllable structure repertoires for a toddler who received 12 weeks of intervention that focused primarily on the encouragement of vocal play. This child was a very quiet infant and toddler who had received heart surgery shortly after birth for correction of a congenital defect. His receptive language skills were within

Demonstration 10–1
Demonstration of Therapy to Encourage Vocal Play by a Late-Talking Toddler

Description of Child at 22 Months

Born with congenital heart defect requiring surgical correction.

Gross motor milestones met at expected ages but did not babble or say any words before 20 months of age.

Did not engage in vocal sound play except for occasional "car noises" while pushing cars.

Produced one spontaneous phonetically consistent form in a meaningful context: [ʌtʌ] or [ʌdʌ].

Pointed and grunted to indicate desired items.

Receptive language skills were age appropriate as were symbolic play skills.

Example of Therapy Activity Used During Weekly 45-Minute Sessions

SLP: Cory, what would you like to play with? Look, the barn or the playground?

Cory: (Points to playground).

SLP: (Arranges slide, swings, teeter-totter, park bench, pram, dog, and dolls on the table).

Cory: (Takes slide and boy doll. Manipulates doll up the slide steps) [ʌː↗] (and down slide). [ʌː↘]

SLP: (Takes girl doll). (Manipulates doll up the slide steps) [ʌp↗] [ʌp↗] [ʌp↗] (and down slide) [wiː↘].

Cory: (Takes baby doll). (Manipulates doll up the slide steps) [ʌʔ↗] [ʌʔ↗] [ʌʔ↗] (and down slide) [ʌː↘].

SLP: Oh no! The baby fell off the slide. She's crying!

Cory: [ʊʌː↗ ʊʌː↗].

SLP: [wʌːwʌː] She's crying. Will she feel better in the pram?

Cory: [ʊʌː↗ ʊʌː↗]. (Puts baby in the pram and gets the mother doll to push it).

SLP: (singing) Rockabye baby in the tree top . . . Is she still crying?

Cory: [ʊʌː↗ ʊʌː↗]. (pushes pram back and forth)

SLP: [wʌːwʌː] (singing) When the wind blows the cradle will rock . . .

Description of Child at 26 Months

Lots of vocal play in clinic and at home.

Spontaneous use of 12 meaningful words.

Vowel repertoire: [i ə ʌ u o].

Consonant repertoire: [m n p b t d k g ʃ].

Syllable structure repertoire: V, VV, CVC, CV, VCV, CVCV.

normal limits but he did not babble and produced only one phonetically consistent form and no conventional words. The demonstration contains an example of a therapy activity that motivated contrasts in pitch (rising while climbing the stairs and falling while descending the slide), contrasts in place of articulation, specifically for his preferred neutral vowel against the front vowel in "wee," gradations in lip aperture size from open through partially and fully closed ([ʌ], [wʌ], ([ʌp]) and contrasts in lip position from protruded to spread ([wi]). The first author encouraged nonverbal gestures as a means of communication and de-emphasized spoken language during the initial phase of the therapy program that focused instead on vocal play in functional contexts. Toys were selected to encourage natural vocalizations that could be generalized to other contexts such as the all purpose "wee" as an expression of excitement with speed on the playground. During the first few months of therapy, the primary therapy technique was to imitate and expand his utterances. The nature of the play, however, in which the SLP was fully engaged with the child and the activity, was meant to provide social reinforcement for the child's efforts to vocalize in a general sense. Notice that the singing was not intended as a target for the child to imitate but rather as contingent social feedback for the child's efforts to produce "crying noises" as well as being a social response that was well integrated into the "calming the crying baby" routine. By 26 months of age the child had built the foundation for continued speech therapy focusing on more specific syllabic and segmental targets whereas at intake his speech output was characterized by a lack of variability and complexity. In this case, the intervention targeting vocal play increased complexity and variability in his speech output, leading to improvements in his speech motor function, phonetic repertoire, and expressive language skills.

The intervention targeting vocal play increased complexity and variability in his speech output, leading to improvements in his speech motor function, phonetic repertoire, and expressive language skills.

Empirical Evidence for the Efficacy of Vocal Play Therapy

The therapy approach for encouraging vocal play that has been described here is motivated by the model of speech motor control presented in Chapter 3 and the basic science on early speech development presented in Chapters 3 and 4. No controlled studies have established the efficacy of the overall approach although the individual techniques have received some support in the scientific literature as reviewed by Dethorne et al. (2009) and summarized briefly above. The approach is consistent with the dynamic systems perspective that we have promoted throughout the book and is inspired by a new approach to physiotherapy that also focuses on enhancing self-exploration, increasing variability in movement patterns and guiding child discovery of multiple strategies for achieving postural control (Dusing & Harbourne, 2010). This approach to physiotherapy has been validated in a randomized controlled trial of approaches to intervention for premature infants that compared an approach based on schema theory to an approach based on dynamic systems theory, with a statistically significant advantage observed for the latter approach (Harbourne, Willett, Kyvelidou, Deffeyes, & Stergiou, 2010). We feel that this procedure is well suited for those children who present with an extremely limited repertoire of vocalizations, especially when they are reluctant to attempt to imitate new forms.

Controlled Variability in Babble and Early Words

10.2.1. Describe the purpose of nonsense syllable drills as implemented in the context of the sensorimotor approach.

10.2.2. Describe the principles of stimulus selection and ordering when implementing a sensorimotor approach to speech therapy.

10.2.3. Define the "challenge point" and describe three variables that determine the optimum challenge point on any given practice trial.

10.2.4. Given examples of different strategies for altering practice components to maintain practice at the optimum challenge point, identify the practice component that is modified. Distinguish strategies that are appropriate when the child's performance is too high versus too low.

10.2.5. Distinguish "knowledge of performance" and "knowledge of results" feedback.

10.2.6. Construct a lesson plan to implement the sensorimotor approach with a child who has been diagnosed with motor speech disorder—apraxia of speech.

During the late infant and toddler periods, **integration** plays an important role in the emergence of speechlike syllables and the development of dynamic stability in the production of these syllables in babble and early words.

In Chapter 3 we described the processes of integration, differentiation and refinement in the development of speech motor control (see Figure 3–6; Green, Moore, Higashikawa, & Steeve, 2000). During the late infant and toddler periods, integration plays an important role in the emergence of speechlike syllables and the development of dynamic stability in the production of these syllables in babble and early words. Free exploration of laryngeal states in squeals and growls and of articulatory closures in raspberries and nasals must now be controlled; integration of laryngeal and supralaryngeal events enables the production of stop + vowel syllables; lip movements are integrated into an increasingly stable jaw movement trajectory as the repertoire of disyllable words and multiword phrases expands. These developments require supervised learning in which the child practices the production of specific sounds, syllables, and words with the target specified internally or by the environment. During this stage, the child must practice selecting and then executing a feed-forward command (i.e., motor plan) to achieve a specific goal. Errors in the achievement of the goal are then transformed into corrective articulatory commands with a progressive reduction in errors and tuning of the inverse models (see Figure 3–15 and associated discussion).

These developments require **supervised learning** in which the child practices the production of specific targets that are specified internally or by the environment.

We are aware of two interventions that have the specific goal of practicing nonsense syllable sequences for the explicit purpose of tuning forward and inverse internal models: McDonald's sensorimotor approach (originally developed by and published in McDonald, 1964; described here from the summary in Shine, 1989) and Ling's approach to speech therapy for hearing-impaired children (Ling, 1976). The purpose of the nonsense syllable drills is to enhance "awareness of patterns of auditory, tactile, and proprioceptive/kinesthetic sensations associated with correct coarticulatory movements" (Shine, 1989, p. 345). In keeping with this goal, the speech practice materials involve phones that are reasonably well established or at least stimulable in the child's speech which means that the SLP must take care to explain the purpose of the activities to the child, caregivers, teachers, and other individuals involved in the child's intervention program in order to gain acceptance and compliance with the program. The SLP may also use other supportive techniques such as the integral stimulation hierarchy to facilitate accurate production of the syllable sequences and to promote independent motor programming as quickly as possible. Isolated sound practice is avoided. All practice materials are minimally targeted at the syllable level, with disyllables preferred, although for children with very restricted output, vowels and diphthongs may be the initial focus of therapy. Furthermore, variable contexts are stressed with combinations of consonants, vowels, and prosodic patterns systematically varied as the intervention progresses. Finally, principles of motor learning should be applied in a dynamic fashion to facilitate comparison of output with target and subsequent adjustment of articulatory commands as necessary.

An intervention developed by McDonald for children with speech delay and an intervention developed by Ling for hearing-impaired children have the specific goal of practicing **nonsense syllable sequences** for the explicit purpose of tuning forward and inverse internal models.

The purpose of the nonsense syllable drills is to enhance "awareness of patterns of auditory, tactile, and proprioceptive/kinesthetic sensations associated with correct coarticulatory movements."

Specific goals are syllables that include phones that are in the child's repertoire or at least stimulable.

All practice materials are minimally targeted at the syllable level, with disyllables preferred, although for children with very restricted output, vowels and diphthongs may be the initial focus of therapy.

As reviewed in Chapter 3, access to the auditory environment plays an important role in early speech development: perceptual knowledge of the target and auditory feedback of the outcome of the articulatory movements is essential for the achievement of canonical babbling. Therefore, the techniques that we describe to improve the child's control of articulatory movements can proceed in parallel with the procedures described in Chapter 9 to ensure the child's access to high quality verbal input and the development of acoustic-phonetic representations for language specific target forms, especially for those children who have difficulties with speech perception or a history of fluctuating or permanent hearing loss. Furthermore, therapeutic procedures may include techniques to enhance the child's access to sensory feedback (i.e., amplifica-

Perceptual knowledge of the targets and auditory feedback of the outcome of the articulatory movements is essential and thus these activities can proceed in parallel with appropriate input-oriented procedures.

tion and auditory bombardment; orosensory stimulation; mirrors, spectrographic displays, and other computer programs to provide visual feedback during speech practice).

Practice with nonsense syllables can be extended to meaningful word practice to be consistent with the notion of child selection and adaptation of words to match developing production templates as occurs in normal development.

In our description of these techniques we also describe an extension to meaningful word practice that is consistent with the notion of child selection and adaptation of words to match developing production templates in normal development as described in Chapter 4 (Vihman & Velleman, 2000). Velleman and Strand's (1994) recommended protocol for structuring therapy sessions to progress from syllable drills to meaningful speech is described and a lesson plan incorporating this protocol is presented along with a case study.

Sensorimotor Procedures to Enhance Dynamic Stability in the Production of Syllable Sequences

The first technique in the application of the sensorimotor approach involves the careful ordering of practice materials to ensure a gradual increase of complexity and a fine balance between repetition and variability so as to achieve dynamic stability in the production of syllable sequences.

The first technique in the application of the sensorimotor approach involves the careful ordering of practice materials to ensure a gradual increase of complexity and a fine balance between repetition and variability so as to achieve dynamic stability in the production of syllable sequences. Table 10–2 lists (with some modifications reflecting the authors' experience) the order of practice materials recommended by Ling (1976) followed by the order of practice materials recommended by Shine (1989). The first author has used the stimulus sequence in the first part of the table for over 30 years with very young children with severe DPD who have very restricted repertoires of phones and syllables shapes and suspected CAS (i.e., MSD-AOS). The child Cory as described at the 26-month point in Demonstration 10–1 represents a good candidate for this approach. The stimulus sequence in the second part of the table is recommended for children who have less restricted systems but nonetheless exhibit a large number of phoneme errors, high variability in error patterns, and/or poor speech motor control in maximum performance tests. The child PA221 presented in Case Study 8–4 might be a good candidate for the sensorimotor approach as described by Shine (1989). This child presented with a large phonetic repertoire but highly variable substitution patterns for any given phoneme and variable productions of individual words from one repetition to the next. At the same time, there was no change in his phonological status over a 3-year period with PCC remaining at approximately 50% and his delay remaining in the severe range despite receiving therapy continuously from public and private providers. An intervention that had the goal of helping him to achieve control over the production of syllables that were present in his repertoire while tuning internal models as the foundation for speech motor control may have been the key to helping him achieve intelligible speech. Certainly the standard procedures employed to introduce and stabilize production of new features and phonemes were not effective in his case.

Table 10–2. *Modified Sequence of Practice Materials Adapted from Ling (1976) and Shine (1989)*

Sequence of Practice Stimuli for Children with Restricted Phonetic Repertoires
1. Level 1: Corner vowels and vowel sequences (diphthongs).
a. V: [i], [u], [æ], [ɑ]
b. Vv: [ei], [ou], [ɑi], [ɑu], [oi]
2. Level 2: Labial consonants in increasingly complex syllable sequences
a. CV, CVv: C = [w], [m], [b], [f], e.g., [wi], [wu], [wæ], [wɑ] . . .
b. CVCV, CVvCVv: e.g., [bibi], [bubu], [bɑibɑi], [baubau] . . .
c. V(v)CV(v): e.g., [ɑwɑ], [iwi], [ouwou], [eiwei] . . .
d. $CV(v)_1CV(v)_2$: e.g., [mimu], [mɑmi], [mumɑi], [moimau] . . .
e. $C_1V(v)_1C_2V(v)_2$: e.g., [fimu], [woubi], [bɑfɑi], [mæwau] . . .
f. $C_1V(v)_1C_2V(v)_2$: vary intensity, pitch, stress patterns
3. Level 3: Coronal consonants in increasingly complex syllable sequences[a]
a–e Repeat sequence of syllables as for Level 2 but C = [j], [n], [d], [s], and [l]
Sequence of Practice Stimuli for Children with Larger Phonetic Repertoires
1. Reduplicated bisyllables: V= tense and lax vowels and diphthongs; C = consonants produced with "customary production" (correct more often than not)
a. CVCV: e.g., [titi], [tɑtɑ], [tɛtɛ], [tætæ] . . .
b. Repeat step 1a with another consonant and so on until C set is exhausted
2. Nonreduplicated disyllables
a. $C_1V_1C_2V_2$: [tisu], [lɑhi], [pɪfi], [tɑpou] . . .
b. ˈ$C_1V_1C_2V_2$ versus C_1V_1ˈC_2V_2 : [ˈpiku], [tɪˈsu] . . .
3. Nonreduplicated trisyllables
a. $C_1V_1C_2V_2\,C_3V_3$
b. ˈ$C_1V_1C_2V_2\,C_3V_3$ versus C_1V_1ˈ$C_2V_2\,C_3V_3$ versus $C_1V_1C_2V_2$ˈC_3V_3 : [lɑˈhidu] . . .
4. Abutting consonant sequences
a. VCCV, CVCCV, CVCCVC: [ɑtli] . . .
b. ˈVCCV, ˈCVCCV, ˈCVCCVC versus VCˈCV, CVCˈCV, CVCˈCVC: [ˈlænti], [ɛtˈlis]

[a]Ling (1976) includes additional levels for remaining places of articulation and, finally, voicing contrasts; however, in our experience the child has usually attained sufficient control and a large enough repertoire of phones and syllables shapes in spontaneous speech at this point that the SLP can proceed to phonological approaches as described in Chapter 11 after achieving this level. Alternatively, the SLP can continue with the levels suggested by Shine (1989), including these additional phonemes in the practice materials as long as they are produced at the level of customary production in the child's speech.

Table 10–2 reveals some common principles in stimulus selection and ordering for the two approaches, most notably the focus on syllables and syllable sequences. Although Ling recommends practice with the production and sequencing of vowels for those children with the most restricted phonetic repertoires (not surprising given the focus of his book on children with severe hearing impairment) both stimulus sets take the syllable as the primary unit of production and avoid practice with isolated consonants. The second common feature is the gradual increase in the complexity of the syllable sequences that are practiced. The sequences are somewhat simpler in the Ling approach, comprised of CV syllables sequenced to form VCV or CVCV disyllables. The McDonald sensorimotor approach takes the child through to more complex forms including trisyllables and sequences of VC and CVC forms that result in abutting consonant sequences within utterances. Careful attention to variations in prosodic contours is another important feature of this approach. The clinician should be attentive to the kinds of within-utterance coarticulatory sequences that are most problematic for the child and focus attention on these sequences; for example, some children may find it particularly difficult to shift from one articulator to another, e.g., [bikɑ]; or to change place of articulation within an articulator, e.g., [tɑkɑ]; others may have difficulty with large contrasts across the vowel space, e.g., [didu]; another may find it more difficult to sequence closely spaced vowels within an utterance, for example, [dɪdi]. The sequences that are difficult for the child can be introduced gradually, alternating between utterances before practicing difficult sound changes across syllables within the same utterance.

The **syllable** is the primary unit of production.

Along with a gradual increase in the complexity of the syllables practiced, careful attention to **variations in prosodic contours** is another important feature of this approach.

With respect to practice intensity, a distributed practice schedule with high treatment intensity over a relatively constrained total intervention duration is desirable. You do not want to be working on nonsense syllable drills for years and the child will not be able to tolerate long sessions of this activity. The practice schedule should provide for very frequent short sessions in the initial stages, hopefully allowing you to progress to more meaningful and conventional therapy approaches as soon as possible. Allen (2009) demonstrated that a multiple phoneme approach to intervention (to be described in Chapter 11) was not more effective than the 8-week control condition when implemented once weekly for 8 weeks or once weekly for 24 weeks. However, a significant improvement in articulation outcomes was observed when the treatment was implemented three times a week for 8 weeks. All multiple phoneme approaches including the sensorimotor approach described here involve a high degree of complexity in learning that benefits from greater treatment intensity. Supplementing with home practice in the form of focused syllable imitation drills one to three times daily is also desirable. These home practice sessions could last anywhere from one to ten minutes in duration depending on the child and the circumstances. However, as many practice trials as possible should occur during those brief sessions.

With respect to practice intensity, a **distributed practice schedule** with high treatment intensity over a relatively constrained total intervention duration is desirable.

Supplementing speech therapy sessions with **home practice** in the form of brief, focused syllable imitation drills one to three times daily is also desirable.

The conditions of practice within each therapy session are also critical to the amount of learning that will occur. It is important to define learning in this case as the skills that the child retains and generalizes from the nonsense syllable drills in the clinic to extra-clinic settings and to meaningful speech contexts. In other words, perfect performance during nonsense syllable practice is not the goal and would in fact be detrimental to learning. A large body of research has been devoted to identifying the practice conditions that will promote maximum retention and transfer of new motor skills (Maas et al., 2008). Most of these studies pertain to sports or laboratory perceptuo-motor tasks (e.g., see Figure 3–14) but some studies have been conducted in speech therapy contexts. Unfortunately, most of the studies have been conducted from the perspective of schema theory and have been concerned with differentiating principles of motor learning that promote acquisition of new generalized motor plans (GMP) versus transfer of learning across trained and novel parameterizations of a given GMP. For example, random practice of movements that constitute different parameterizations of a single GMP should promote learning, such as switching club lengths at random when practicing one's golf swing. On the other hand, blocked practice with your favorite club will result in good performance on the driving range but poor results on the course! However, as discussed in Chapter 3, there is no clear way to sort out which speech behaviors constitute a class of movements all belonging to the same GMP and thus we are not sure how to apply the principles to speech therapy. Furthermore, the research evidence suggests that all of the motor learning principles that have been suggested thus far interact with all of the other conditions of practice in a dynamic fashion, leading us to conclude that although the research studies yield valuable information the underlying theoretical perspective is lacking. We also worry that the principles as summarized in Maas et al. (2008) promote a rigid planning of practice conditions in advance of the treatment session based on the characteristics of the practice stimuli, as opposed to a dynamic adaptation of the conditions of practice during the speech therapy session in interaction with the child. One conceptual framework that helps to bring some order to the disparate findings emanating from this field of study is the notion of the "challenge point" as described by Guadagnoli and Lee (2004). This conceptual framework focuses attention on the information processing aspect of the acquisition of internal models for motor control. The framework is also consistent with dynamic systems theory because the optimum challenge point for learning emerges from the product of multiple interacting components of the practice situation linking the child, the task, and environmental inputs.

Guadagnoli and Lee (2004) define the challenge point as the intersection of functional task difficulty and practice performance when the learner is receiving the optimum amount of information to promote learning (defined as retention and transfer of the skill). When considering Figure 3–15, it is clear that the child must

Learning is defined as the skills that the child retains and generalizes from the nonsense syllable drills in the clinic to extraclinic settings and to meaningful speech contexts.

We promote dynamic adaptation of the conditions of practice during the speech therapy session in interaction with the child.

The **challenge point** conceptual framework focuses attention on the information processing aspect of the acquisition of internal models for motor control.

The optimum challenge point for learning emerges from the product of multiple interacting components of the practice situation linking the child, the task, and environmental inputs.

The challenge point is the intersection of functional task difficulty and practice performance when the learner is receiving the optimum amount of information to promote learning.

deal with many sources of information when practicing nonsense syllable imitation: the nature of the target, the status of the articulatory system prior to producing the utterance, the feed-forward command and predicted outcomes of executing the plan, actual auditory and somatosensory outcomes when executing the feed-forward command, auditory errors, and translation of errors in auditory coordinates to adjustments in articulatory coordinates. All of this information is useful when it comes in just the right amount. If functional task difficulty is too high and practice performance is very low, the child will be overloaded by all of the information and may not be able to interpret and use it effectively to develop flexible motor plans for future attempts. If functional task difficulty is too low and practice performance is too high the child is not receiving any error information and has no opportunity to experience the act of constructing new feed-forward commands or adjusting commands in response to unanticipated events and thus learning potential is diminished.

The **optimum challenge point** occurs when the child is experiencing a reasonably high level of performance during practice but even a small increase in functional task difficulty would result in a sharp decline in performance.

A number of interacting variables, involving the child, stimulus, task, and feedback, determine the optimum challenge point on any given practice trial.

Given that the optimum challenge point can be shifting from trial to trial within a therapy activity, the SLP must be alert to changes in the child's performance level and be prepared to alter one or more of these variables "on-line" in order to maintain the child at the optimum point.

The optimum challenge point occurs when the child is experiencing a reasonably high level of performance during practice but even a small increase in functional task difficulty would result in a sharp decline in performance. A number of interacting variables determine the optimum challenge point on any given practice trial: (a) the skill level of the child (determined in part by the severity of the child's deficit, the child's phonological knowledge of the target forms, the child's history of speech practice in prior therapy sessions and fluctuating state variables such as fatigue, mood and motivation); (b) the nominal difficulty of the task (in this case determined by the inherant difficulty of the phonemes in the syllables, the number of phonemes and syllables in the sequence, the coarticulatory challenge offered by the particular sequence, and the complexity of the context in which the task is embedded); (c) the support offered by the SLP in the manner of stimulus presentation (with multimodal models of the target providing more support than prompts for spontaneous production; see section on integral stimulation hierarchy below); (d) the structure of the practice schedule (with variable stimulus presentation from trial to trial increasing difficulty over blocked presentation of specific stimuli or stimulus classes); and (e) the nature of the feedback provided after the child's response (varying with respect to schedule and informativeness). Given that the optimum challenge point can be shifting from trial to trial within a therapy activity, the SLP must be alert to changes in the child's performance level and be prepared to alter one or more of these variables "on-line" in order to maintain the child at the optimum point. Table 10–3 lists some of the strategies that can be used if the child's performance is too high or too low to support optimum learning. We do not attempt to state a "rule" for the right amount of stimulus variability or the best feedback schedule: the application of these motor learning principles will vary not only across children but within a child as skill levels and task difficulty changes.

Table 10–3. Strategies for Altering Practice Conditions to Maintain Practice at the Optimum Challenge Point

Practice Component	*Practice Performance Is Too High*	*Practice Performance Is Too Low*
Child	Increase treatment intensity to induce fatigue, i.e., increase dose frequency or session duration.	Reduce treatment intensity to alleviate fatigue, i.e., reduce dose frequency, shorten session duration or take a break.
Nominal Task Difficulty	Increase task complexity, e.g., – stops → fricatives – bi → disyllables – di → trisyllables – trochaic → iambic – singletons → clusters	Decrease task complexity, e.g., – fricatives → stops – bi → single syllables – tri → disyllables – iambic → trochaic – clusters → singletons
Complexity of Context	Increase context complexity, e.g., – embed nonsense syllables in a functionally meaningful context and activity – practice the syllables in the context of a competing task (cutting out pictures, playing hopscotch, etc.)	Decrease context complexity, e.g., – decrease all distractions in the environment – reduce task to a simple stimulus-response-feedback routine – ensure that feedback is simple and fast and does not distract from the task
Practice Schedule	Increase variability of stimulus items from trial to trial (random practice schedule), e.g., ['fifi], ['bubu], [bɑ'bɑ], ['mæmæ], [wɑ'wɑ] . . .	Increase predictability of items from trial to trial (blocked practice schedule), e.g., ['bibi], ['bubu], ['bɑbɑ] . . . ['mimi], ['mumu],['mɑmɑ] . . .
Knowledge of Results	Provide summative information about response accuracy after sets of responses, e.g., SLP: OK, I want to hear a handful of funny words. Say ['fifi] Child: ['fifi] SLP: Say ['bubu] Child: ['bubu] SLP: Say [bɑ'bɑ] Child: [bɑ'bɑ] SLP: Say ['mæmæ] Child: [mɑ'mæ] SLP: Say [wɑ'wɑ] Child: [wɑ'wɑ] SLP: Pretty good but not quite the whole handful. You got 4 of them, (draws ring on the fingers of an outline of a hand drawn on a piece of paper with the syllables written on each finger that can be sent home for practice): ['fifi], ['bubu], [bɑ'bɑ], but not ['mæmæ], good work on [wɑ'wɑ]. See if you can get all of them with mum and then you'll get the ring for this finger.	Provide information about response accuracy immediately on each trial, e.g., SLP: Say ['bibi] Child: ['bibi] SLP: Good. Say ['bubu] Child: ['bubu] SLP: Another good one! Say ['bɑbɑ] Child: ['bubu] SLP: No, watch my lips and try again ['bɑbɑ]

continues

Table 10–3. continued

Practice Component	*Practice Performance Is Too High*	*Practice Performance Is Too Low*
Knowledge of Performance	Intermittently ask child for explicit evaluation of own performance, e.g., SLP: Say: [wifɑ] Child: [wiwɑ] SLP: Oops, what happened there? Child: points to lower lip and then bites it. SLP: That's right, you forgot to bite your lip on the second part.	Frequently, provide explicit information about movement parameters after correct responses and incorrect responses. SLP: Say [fifɑ] Child: [fifɑ] SLP: Excellent, you bit your lip for the [f] sound.
Stimulus Presentation	Move down the integral stimulation hierarchy (see Table 10–4). Cue access to internalized representation of the target, i.e., require spontaneous productions of the target forms	Move up the integral stimulation hierarchy (see Table 10–4) Provide a model of the target form with maximum multimodal information about its characteristics.

The ability to manage these practice conditions dynamically in interaction with the child is the mark of a skilled clinician.

A **random-blocked schedule** means that practice is repeated for a given parameter for a specified number of trials (e.g., 3) but new parameters are introduced at random with each new block of trials.

Among the practice conditions highlighted in Table 10–3, nominal task difficulty and practice schedule are of particular importance and indeed, attention to these issues is built into the stimulus orders suggested by Ling (1976) and by Shine (1989). The two treatment programs are designed to ensure that variability and complexity increases as the intervention progresses. Initially, reduplicated syllables are practiced, then vowels are varied within an utterance and finally consonants and vowels are varied. Research on motor learning in other domains suggests that a "random-blocked" schedule of trials within a session may be best, especially if the child is struggling with a particular step of the program (Pigott & Shapiro, 1984). A random-blocked schedule means that practice is repeated for a given parameter for a specified number of trials (e.g., 3) but new parameters are introduced at random with each new block of trials. For example, Level 2b of the Ling program might be practiced in blocked, random, or random-blocked schedule (in these examples the letter indicates an item involving that consonant): (1) blocked—all "b" items, all "m" items, all "w" items, all "f" items; (2) random—b, m, f, w, m, b, w, f, b, f, m, w; or (3) random-blocked—b, b, b, m, m, m, f, f, f, w, w, w. In fact, in keeping with the challenge point framework, the levels shown in Table 10–3 do not have to be rigidly applied; they can be adjusted for individual items in response to the child's performance levels. A young child practicing Level 2b of the Ling program might progress through the series of reduplicated syllables involving [b], [m], and [w] organized in random order with relative ease but struggle with items involving [f]. In this case it might be advisable to practice the set in mixed random and blocked-random order: in other words, practice the [f] item three times in succession before progressing to the next item, giving the child time to adjust and make corrections after producing an incorrect, slow or imprecise response. The amount of stimulation or support provided on each repeated trial could be gradually faded so that the child is encouraged to independently generate a motor plan and then evaluate (implicitly or explicitly) and correct his own responses from trial to trial, for example, [bibi], [bubu], [maimai], [maumau], [wiwi], [wuwu], [faifai], [faifai], [faifai], [baubau], [wiwi], [fufu], [fufu], [fufu], [maimai], [baubau], [fafa], [fufu], [fifi], [waba], . . . (notice that variability and nominal task difficulty is being adjusted as the task proceeds in response to imagined variations in the qualitative nature of the child's responses).

The way that stimuli are presented will depend on the age of the child, the nature of the stimuli (nonsense or meaningful words) and the amount of support that the child needs to achieve a correct response. The integral stimulation hierarchy is an ordered series of prompts that the SLP can choose from in order to stimulate a response from the child (Gildersleeve-Neumann, November 6, 2007; Rosenbek, Lemme, Ahern, Harris, & Wertz, 1973; Strand & Debertine, 2000; Strand & Skinder, 1999). The primary purpose of the prompt is to define the target that the child is expected to achieve, either providing a model from the environment for imitation or a cue that is designed to trigger access to an internally defined representation of the target response. The prompt may also provide support that helps the child select or construct a motor plan for achieving the target. On each trial the SLP can adjust the level of prompt up or down the hierarchy, providing more stimulation if the child is struggling and less when the child is producing the practice items with ease. Strand and Skinder (1999) provide detailed information on how to apply the hierarchy in a dynamic fashion based on the child's responding trial by trial during the treatment session. The integral stimulation hierarchy, adapted for a young child practicing nonsense word material, is shown with examples in Table 10–4.

The **integral stimulation hierarchy** is an ordered series of prompts that the SLP can choose from to stimulate a response from the child.

Finally, with respect to feedback our preference is to keep it to a minimum whenever possible so as to not interfere with the child's implicit mechanisms for detecting and responding to errors. Furthermore, elaborate systems for commenting on and rewarding the child's performance slows down the activity and may actually reduce the child's motivation to engage in nonsense syllable drills rather than motivate participation. There are three considerations when deciding on the frequency, timing, and nature of feedback to provide contingent upon the child's responses in any speech therapy task. The first consideration is the extent to which your feedback system will enhance or undermine the child's motivation to practice speech. Cognitive evaluation theory and the associated research indicates that tangible rewards undermine intrinsic motivation to participate in an activity when they are provided simply for engaging in an activity that is already intrinsically rewarding; under these conditions the controlling aspects of the reward system are paramount and the reward serves to undermine the child's

Keep **feedback** to a minimum whenever possible so as to not interfere with the child's implicit mechanisms for detecting and responding to errors.

Tangible rewards undermine intrinsic motivation to participate in an activity when they are provided simply for engaging in an activity that is already intrinsically rewarding.

Table 10–4. *Integral Stimulation Hierarchy Adapted for Children and Nonsense Word Stimuli*

Level	Prompts	Example
1.	Imitative prompt Coproduction	SLP: Watch me and listen. Let's say [moi]. SLP & Child together: [moi].
2.	Imitative prompt Mimed prompt	SLP: Watch me and listen. Let's say [boupai]. SLP: Mimes [boupai] while child says [boupai].
3.	Imitative prompt Repetition prompt (with or without delay)	SLP: Watch me and listen. When I raise my finger, say [boupai]. (raises 1 finger; immediately or with 1 to 3 second delay) Child: [boupai]. SLP: (raises next finger) Child: [boupai]. SLP: (raises next finger) Child: [boupai].
4.	Graphic cue Coproduction	SLP: Look at this picture (points to "bow") [bou]. And this one (points to "pie") [pai]. When we put them together we get a silly word. Let's say it together (pointing to pictures in sequence). SLP & child together: [boupai]
5.	Graphic cue (or other cue for spontaneous production such as printed text or a question)	SLP: Look at these pictures. Say the silly word. (pointing to pictures in sequence) Child: [boupai]

perceived autonomy (Cameron, Pierce, Basko, & Gear, 2005). On the other hand, tangible reinforcers can be motivating when they are provided to reward achievement of a specific level of performance because in this case the informational aspect of the reward is highlighted and the reward serves to enhance the child's perceived competence. In the context of the principles of motor learning (as opposed to operant conditioning), feedback is intended to provide information, specifically information about performance of the motor action or the results of the action, rather than control behavior. This brings us to the second consideration: the child's need for explicit extrinsic feedback about response accuracy relative to the target (i.e., knowledge of results). If the child has good acoustic-phonetic representations for the target forms that you are modeling, providing extrinsic feedback about results directly after every production may actually interfere with the child's self-evaluation of intrinsic feedback. On the other hand, in the early stages of therapy or in the case where the child does not have good internal representations of the acoustic-phonetic and/or articulatory target, the child may rely on extrinsic evaluative feedback about accuracy of each response. Finally, motor learning is also dependent on feedback about the actual performance of the motor act that results in the target form as perceived by the child. If the child has deficiencies in

The child's need for explicit extrinsic feedback about response accuracy relative to the target (i.e., **knowledge of results**) depends on the quality of his or her acoustic-phonetic representations for the target forms that you are modeling.

auditory or somatosensory perception it may be helpful to augment this intrinsic feedback with extrinsic verbal reports about performance or to provide biofeedback (e.g., visual feedback as discussed later in this chapter). In general it is recommended that knowledge of performance feedback be provided in a "prepractice" or "warm-up" activity that typically will involve a lower response frequency than the primary practice activity that is designed to maintain a high frequency of responding per unit of time. In order to maintain high dose frequency and to encourage self-evaluation by the child, we prefer to design simple feedback systems that provide summative information about response accuracy (with the size of the response set over which performance is evaluated determined by the child's performance level and personality). This kind of feedback system also serves as a "counter," allowing the child to predict the duration of the nonsense syllable drill activity. Every effort is made to maintain response frequency at a very high level so that treatment intensity can be maximized and total intervention duration minimized for this phase of therapy.

In general it is recommended that **knowledge of performance feedback** be provided in a "prepractice" or "warm-up" activity that typically will involve a lower response frequency than the primary practice activity that is designed to maintain a high frequency of responding per unit of time.

Summative feedback about response accuracy maintains high dose frequency and encourages self-evaluation by the child.

Demonstration of Sensorimotor Therapy to Enhance Controlled Variability in Babble and Early Words

Velleman and Strand (1994) suggest a lesson plan outline for the implementation of a sensorimotor approach with young children who have CAS that has four components: Warm-ups, Practicing the Scales, Practicing the Song, and Changing the Song. Warm-ups could be any number of activities designed to introduce the session activities and prepare the child to succeed at the tasks. These could include brief task instructions, a reminder of vocabulary used to refer to key articulators or target forms, a review of items covered in the previous session, or prepractice of new items to be introduced in the current session, with phonetic placement and "knowledge of performance" feedback provided as necessary. For children with secondary phonological disorders and primary motor impairments, warm-ups may include sensory stimulation to treat hypo- or hypersensitivity, the organization of specialized seating arrangements, and/or activities to normalize muscle tone or ensure trunk stability (Ernest, 2000). Practicing the Scales refers to the nonsense syllable drills implemented as described above. Subsequent to these drills, Practicing the Song involves meaningful play activities that focus on one or more words based on a template that matches the word shape and phonetic content practiced during the nonsense syllable drills. Changing the Song is the final activity in the session during which the target words are practiced in a more complex linguistic, prosodic, or pragmatic context.

A **sensorimotor lesson plan outline** for young children has four components: *Warm-Ups, Practicing the Scales, Practicing the Song*, and *Changing the Song*.

Demonstration 10–2 includes pre- and posttreatment data from a girl who received weekly individual therapy from the first author following the Ling program over a 6-month period. This case study information is accompanied by a lesson plan exemplifying the

Demonstration 10–2
Case Study and Example Lesson Plan Demonstrating the Sensorimotor Approach

Pretreatment Speech Sample (Age 2 years and 9 months)		Posttreatment Speech Sample (Age 3 years and 4 months)	
Consonant Repertoire	**Example Utterances**	**Consonant Repertoire**	**Example Utterances**
m n	[mi] "me"	m n	[dæ.i mʌmi di] "daddy mummy sleep"
b	[mʌ] "mom"	p b t d k g	[be.i kɑ] "baby crawl"
ʃ (isolation only)	[no] "no"	f θ s	[mɑi ko mʌmi] "my coat mummy"
	[be.i] "baby"	w h	[mɪtθ] "milk"
	[ɑ] "yes"		[bæk] "glasses"
	[ʃ], [un] "shoe"		[no dæ.i i] "no daddy read"
	[bi] "please"		[to.i] "turkey"
	[ɑ] "off"		[dʌ.i] "dirty"

Lesson Plan for Level 2d (Ling; see Table 10–2)

Task/Target	Stimulus Presentation	Practice Schedule	Feedback
1. **Warm-Ups**			
Produce [fə] on five consecutive trials when asked to make a "fishy sound" without prior model.	Demonstrate "fishy face" + "fishy sound" once in mirror, emphasizing light placement of upper teeth on lower lip with free flow of air over lip. Ask Brigit to make the "fishy sound." Repeat request to make "another fishy sound" until criterion is met.	Blocked practice.	100% knowledge of performance

Task/Target	Stimulus Presentation	Practice Schedule	Feedback
2. Practicing the Scales			
Produce $C_1V_1C_1V_2$ nonsense words with 80% accuracy where C = [b], [m], [w], [f].	Present imitative prompt on most trials. Increase stimulation for incorrect responses and then provide imitative prompt + repetition prompt to stimulate repetitions of difficult items.	Blocked practice (change to random if performance level is too high).	Summative feedback of results after every fourth trial. Repeat misarticulated items. Provide tangible reinforcement when 4 correct items are achieved.
3. Practicing the Song			
Produce "Mummy" and "Baby" spontaneously during doll play with 80% accuracy.	While playing with large doll house, using multiple baby and mummy dolls, ask questions: "Who's gonna sleep in this bed? Who's gonna sit in the high chair?" (etc.).	Random practice.	100% knowledge of results (give mummy or baby doll when question is answered with correctly pronounced response).
4. Changing the Song			
Produce "Mummy wants it" and "Baby wants it" while dressing dolls.	Ask "who wants the bib?" etc. and then provide co-production stimulus "baby wants it" or "mummy wants it" depending on the clothing item.	Random practice.	100% knowledge of results (give clothing when question is answered with correctly pronounced response; note that [bebi wa ʔɪ], [mʌmi wanɪ] and similar approximations are acceptable).

kinds of activities that were used in her treatment, organized according to Velleman and Strand's session plan outline. This child had a difficult start in life, suffering anoxia during birth due to the cord being wrapped around her neck during delivery. At age two and a half a neurologist noted abnormal tone in her legs and severe language delay and referred her for intervention. She also had a history of recurrent otitis media. At initial assessment her receptive language skills were within the average range but her primary expressive mode of communication was gestural. She did use a few words spontaneously as shown in the pretreatment case study information but had great difficulty imitating CV syllables even when they contained familiar phones; for example, although the phones [b] and [ʌ] were in her phonetic repertoire, she was unable to imitate the syllable [bʌ]. Therefore, treatment began at Level 1 of the Ling program as shown in Table 10–2 and progressed through to Level 3e. Follow through with the home practice program was excellent and she completed these levels within a 6-month period at which time her phonetic repertoire had expanded considerably, speech was her primary mode of communication, she was regularly communicating with short phrases although it was clear that her expressive language continued to be severely delayed. One of the most noticeable changes in her speech behavior was her ability to approximate a word with relative consistency during imitative and spontaneous speech contexts. During the early part of the treatment program groping and inconsistent productions were common even during imitation (e.g., "baby" being pronounced as [be.i], [bʌ], and [veis]). After 6 months of this intervention she had achieved sufficient stability to benefit from the reduced treatment intensity and more phonological approach employed by the therapist in her next placement (a multidisciplinary treatment program that provided speech, physio- and occupational therapy twice monthly in her daycare) although it was unfortunate that a high frequency of direct speech therapy could not be maintained. At age 4;6 standardized testing revealed borderline normal receptive language skills, severely delayed morphosyntax, and moderately delayed phonological skills characterized by cluster reduction, liquid gliding, and syllable deletions in complex multisyllabic words.

The demonstration also contains a lesson plan with four activities, the first two of which take place in front of a large mirror with the SLP seated directly behind the child but positioned so that both child and SLP faces are fully visible side by side in the mirror and so that the SLP is supporting the child in her chair. The warm-up consists of a review of the syllable [fə] because she had been struggling with these items during the previous session. During warm-ups phonetic placement may be provided and knowledge of performance feedback is provided with a high frequency. Proceeding quickly to the nonsense syllable drills, the SLP draws a beehive, an ocean, a mouse-hole, and a fishbowl on the mirror with a dry-erase pen taking care to not obscure the image of the child's face in the mirror. Reusable stickers depicting bees, whales, mice, and fish serve as tangible reinforcers and counters. The activity is finished when each item contains 5 stickers which are awarded for 4 correct productions of the items with the corresponding phoneme (i.e., correct production of the sequence [fifi], [fufu], [feifei], and [foufou] would yield a fish sticker to affix to the fishbowl picture). The activity will allow for 80 responses in a short space of time if task difficulty is adjusted appropriately through use of the integral stimulation hierarchy to ensure a high but not perfect level of responding. However, when proceeding to the activity involving meaningful (and whenever possible spontaneous) use of the words "baby" and "mummy" during doll play, feedback is provided on every trial and the response rate will be much slower. This activity allows for the provision of focused stimulation as well. Finally, the session ends with a fun but difficult task involving use of the words "mummy" and "baby" in a three-word phrase and thus coproduction is planned as the method of stimulation.

Overall, the lesson plan is designed to be consistent with the challenge point framework. There is no assumption that, as a general rule, random practice with arbitrarily defined "complex stimuli" is the most effective procedure for retention and transfer of learning. Rather, the starting point of therapy in the session was individualized to the profound severity of this child's speech deficit, selected to match her optimum challenge point (note that this idea is consistent with the discussion of complexity in the selection of treatment targets contained in Chapter 8). In her case, trial-to-trial variation in vowels while keeping the consonants constant within a set of practice stimuli was as much complexity as she could handle in the early weeks of the intervention program. If her skill level improved markedly during the session, a switch to randomized stimulus presentation across the [b], [m], and [w] sets could be implemented seamlessly within the context of the activity. Similarly, type of stimulus presentation and feedback schedule could be adjusted within the session dynamically in response to her performance level on a moment to moment basis.

Empirical Evidence for the Sensorimotor Approach

Pannbacker (1988) reviewed the evidence on the effectiveness of interventions for speech therapy interventions for the treatment of apraxia of speech. She identified 10 different approaches and concluded that there was research evidence supporting only two, one of which was systematic drill of movement sequences, including McDonald's sensorimotor approach as one example of this approach. This general approach is also recommended on the basis of the strength of the theoretical foundation as laid out in Chapter 3

A systematic review of the evidence on the effectiveness of speech therapy interventions for the treatment of apraxia of speech supports systematic drill of movement sequences.

and the empirical basis of the individual components. Research support for the motor learning principles is strong in non-speech domains and growing for speech therapy, as reviewed by Maas et al. (2008). The reinterpretation of the motor learning literature from the perspective of the challenge point framework is also well supported (see review by Guadagnoli & Lee, 2004). Recent randomized controlled trials in physiotherapy are validating applications that take a dynamic systems approach to the acquisition of dynamic stability rather than applying motor learning principles rigidly to achieve precision over repeated motor movements (e.g., Harbourne et al., 2010).

Clinical studies of the Nuffield Centre Dyspraxia Programme may appear to be another example of the approach espoused here that is backed by weak support. There are some similarities, in particular the explicit focus on motor programming as the treatment goal, systematic and gradual increases in the complexity of the utterances practiced, variable targets within sessions and the application of motor learning principles (for descriptions and literature review, see Williams, 2009; Williams & Stephens, 2010). However, there are some significant procedural differences that may lead to poor coarticulation and unusual prosody as unintended treatment effects. Differences include the use of meaningful stimuli (although practiced in nonmeaningful or nonfunctional contexts) and a focus on graphic stimuli to guide sequencing of elements within utterances. One concern with this program is an initial focus on nonspeech oral-motor exercises and the teaching of sounds in isolation (leading the authors to caution against "schwa insertion," which must be difficult to avoid with many phonemes). It is not clear that basic movement patterns with stimulable phonemes are established before more complex phonemes are introduced. This program also lacks systematic attention to variation in suprasegmental prosody. The published evidence in favor of this program is at the level of nonexperimental case studies. Experimental comparison to McDonald's sensorimotor approach would be informative with particular attention to measures of coarticulation, dynamic stability, and prosody as dependent variables.

The use of the integral stimulus hierarchy has received empirical support in the form of a few controlled single subject studies involving children with severe speech disorders (Strand & Debertine, 2000; Strand & Skinder, 1999). In these studies the practice materials are chosen for their functional importance to the patients who were treated but they are also ordered in a hierarchical fashion to increase in complexity. Nonsense syllable drills may also form part of the therapy program (see Lesson Plan structure in Demonstration 10–2). Integral stimulation as a procedure has a long history in SLP but the particular implementation described in these reports requires further assessment with larger samples.

Integral stimulation as a procedure has a long history in SLP and use of the hierarchy has received empirical support in the form of a few controlled single subject studies involving children with severe speech disorders.

Strand and Skinder (1999) summarized the rationale for the use of nonsense syllable stimuli with children who have apraxia of speech. Nonsense syllable drills are very common with these children because it is believed that they reduce the cognitive load and focus attention on the motor planning task that is the target of the intervention. The use of nonsense word stimuli in speech therapy for children with Speech Delay and Speech Errors has a very long and successful history as reviewed in Gierut, Morrisette, and Ziemer (2010). Furthermore, these authors provide a convincing demonstration of the efficacy of nonword stimuli even though the study was a retrospective nonexperimental comparison groups design. Their study involved 60 children with moderate or severe DPD and normal language skills who received conventional speech therapy targeting one phoneme that was absent from their phonemic repertoire. Half were treated with real words using picture naming tasks, whereas the remainder were treated with nonsense words, again using picture naming tasks since the words were associated with novel referents. Generalization probes were administered immediately posttreatment (an approximately 19-week interval) and 55 days posttreatment to assess transfer of training to untreated words involving all phonemes that were absent from the children's inventories at the pretreatment assessment. Immediately posttreatment, children in the nonsense words training condition showed superior transfer to words involving both the treated and untreated phonemes compared to children who were treated with real words. At follow-up, both groups achieved similar scores for the treated phonemes but the group that received training on nonsense words continued to show an advantage for untreated phonemes.

Nonsense syllable drills are recommended for the treatment of CAS because it is believed that they reduce the cognitive load and focus attention on the motor planning task that is the target of the intervention.

The use of nonsense words, paired with novel referents, has also been shown to promote transfer of learning when incorporated into phonology therapy.

Strong support for the sensorimotor approach described here is provided in a recent report of a prosody intervention that involved three school-age siblings with CAS who had received speech therapy for many years resulting in segmental accuracy but continued difficulties with prosody in conversational speech (Ballard, Robin, McCabe, & McDonald, 2010). The study employed a multiple baseline single subject design that provides good experimental control for history and maturation and other threats to internal validity and thus we can be reasonably sure that the changes in performance observed in the children's prosody were due to the intervention. Nonsense word stimuli were used to teach the children to produce trochaic and iambic patterns in the context of carrier sentences (e.g., "Can you find my BAguti?" or "He bought a taBUgi."). Principles of motor learning were carefully applied throughout the 12 session treatment program. Each session began with a prepractice period during which modeling, visual aids and detailed verbal performance feedback was provided to prepare the children for independent practice with the stimuli. Subsequently, printed text was used to stimulate high intensity practice of complex and varied stimuli while the SLP provided a declining and overall low frequency of feedback about accuracy of responding. Notice that all three-syllable strings involved readily pronounceable segments and thus the focus was clearly on the prosodic level of the phonological hierar-

The sensorimotor approach has been used to target prosody in children with CAS with some success.

chy. Probes targeting treated and untreated words were conducted during baseline, treatment and retention phases of the experiment with the children's ability to match the intended prosodic structure of the nonword measured using acoustic analysis to reveal changes in duration, vocal intensity, and F0. Some of the results reported for these children are reproduced in Figure 10–1 and indicate good transfer and retention for two of the three children. The third and youngest child shows poor retention of training for both trained and untrained words. The authors suggest that this child required more treatment sessions to achieve an optimum result because his prosodic difficulties were more severe than that of his older siblings. We have a different hypothesis, however. Observation of the within treatment results for these children shows that treatment session performance was roughly between 70 and 80% accurate for the older children with less severe prosodic disturbance. The younger child slowly improved from 30 to 80% accuracy over many sessions, however, suggesting that he was performing well below his challenge point for optimum learning for much of the treatment period. Perhaps the dynamic use of some of the strategies shown in Table 10–3 would have served to maintain treatment performance at an appropriate level and improved treatment efficiency. The rigid application of motor learning principles was effective for the children with a higher initial level of performance but the training task had a higher level of functional difficulty for the younger child and optimum learning potential was not achieved. Nonetheless, we feel that this study is a powerful indicator of the efficacy of the sensorimotor approach as applied with nonsense word stimuli for children with motor planning difficulties.

When the child performs well below the challenge point for optimum learning during practice sessions, retention and transfer of learning is less likely to occur.

Intelligible Speech

10.3.1. Describe five types of procedures for establishing correct articulation of a new phoneme.

10.3.2. Describe different strategies for ordering practice stimuli when implementing a traditional approach to speech therapy. If one word position is treated at a time, predict the likely outcomes with respect to generalization of learning based on the consistency of the child's pretreatment error pattern.

10.3.3. Evaluate the research evidence to identify elements of the traditional approach that are essential to its effectiveness.

Recall from Chapter 4 that speech intelligibility improves from 25% to 100% between 2 and 4 years of age in the normally developing child. The achievement of intelligible speech is associated with a

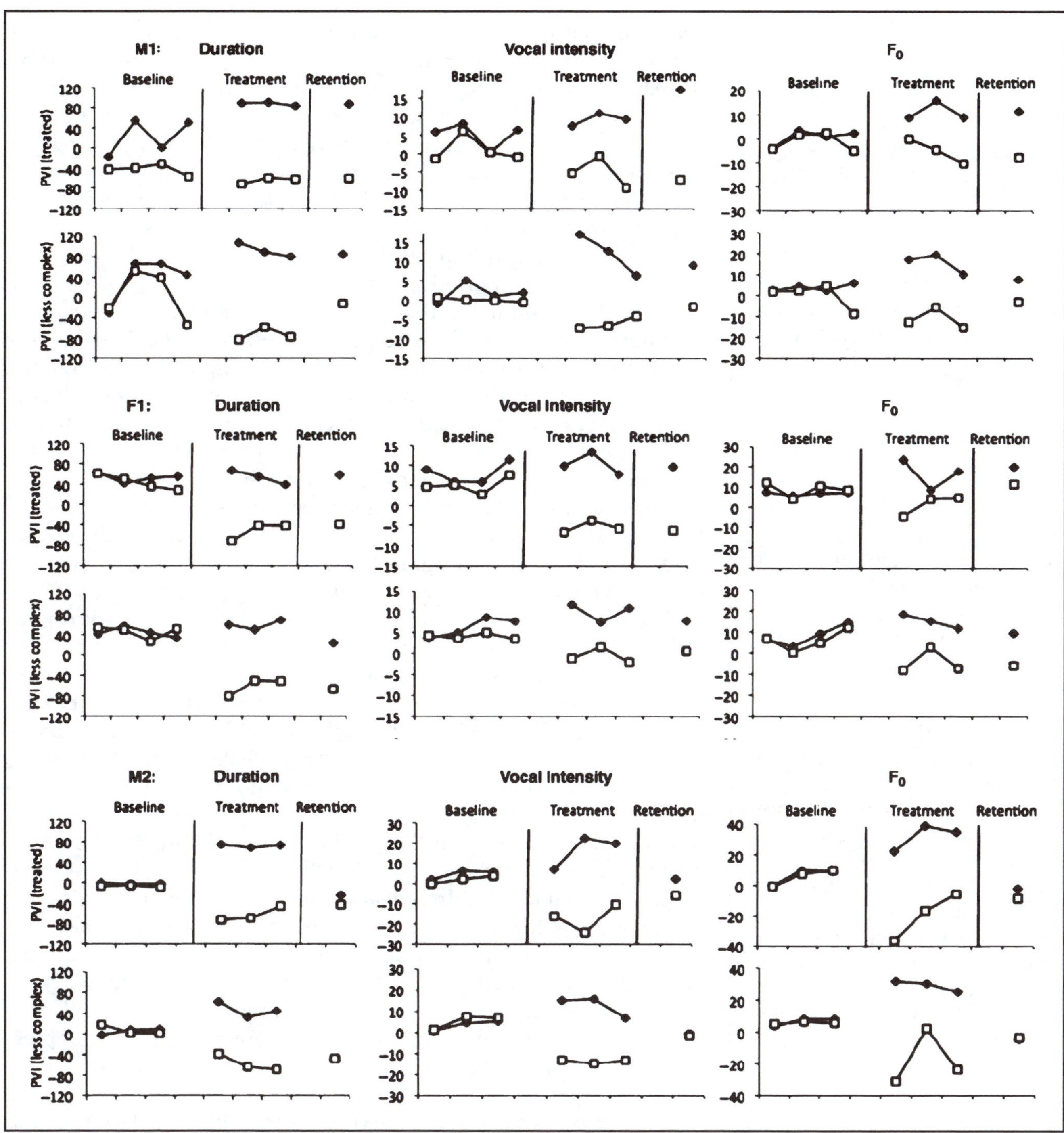

Figure 10–1. *Stress pattern data during baseline, treatment, and retention probes for three children* (M1, top; M2, middle; F1, bottom) *who received a sensorimotor intervention for the treatment of dysprosody. Outcomes are expressed as median pairwise variability indices (PVIs) for duration* (left panel), *intensity* (middle panel), *and* F_0 (right panel) *for generalization probes targeting the complex treated nonsense words in the first set of charts and less complex untreated nonsense words in the second set of charts for each child. A PVI of 0 indicates equal stress whereas a positive PVI indicates a SW stress pattern (expected for filled markers) and a negative PVI indicates a WS stress pattern (expected for open markers).* Source: *From "A Treatment for Dysprosody in Childhood Apraxia of Speech," by K. J. Ballard, D. A. Robin, and P. McCabe, 2010,* Journal of Speech and Hearing Disorders, 53, *selected panels of Figures 4, 5, and 6, pp. 1238–1240. Copyright 2010 by American Speech-Language-Hearing Association. Adapted with permission.*

sharp reduction in simplification processes in the child's speech, improved consistency in the use of emerging phonemes, and an increase in the percentage of correctly articulated consonants. In the previous section we discussed procedures to establish a foundation of basic word shapes with early developing phonemes across the spectrum of manner classes. Additional procedures may be required to help children with DPD establish later developing phonemes and prosodic structures. Reviewing Figure 3–6 and the associated text, we see that an important developmental process in speech motor control during this period is that of differentiation: lower lip is no longer tightly coupled to the jaw; upper and lower lip movements are now independent. The emergence of difficult phonemes such as /ʃ/, /dʒ/, and /ɹ/ requires independence of lips from jaw, tongue blade from tongue dorsum and differentiated control of the lateral margins of the tongue. The motor learning principles described in the previous section will continue to be important as the child will need to learn new motor plans specifying the spatiotemporal organization of articulator specific gestures for the production of each new sound. The child will also need to practice the production of these sounds in order to gain flexibility in the use of these plans in multiple contexts. For those children who are having difficulty acquiring new speech sounds, both supervised learning and reinforcement learning will be important means of acquiring the new articulatory gestures.

An important developmental process in speech motor control during the preschool period is that of **differentiation**.

For those children who are having difficulty acquiring new speech sounds, both **supervised learning** and **reinforcement learning** will be important means of acquiring the new articulatory gestures.

Traditional articulation therapy—procedures to establish a new phoneme followed by articulation practice to stabilize production of the phoneme in systematically more complex contexts—is the tried and true method for helping children acquire new phonemes in those cases when the absence of a phoneme can be traced to a lack of knowledge at the level of articulatory-phonetic representations. It is tempting to assume that these procedures are relevant only to those children deemed to have a "phonetic" disorder as defined in Chapter 7: a category that overlaps with an articulation disorder in Dodd's classification system and with the speech error category in Shriberg's SDCS (see Figure 7–3). However, this is not necessarily the case. Any child, even those whose overall profile appears to be more "phonemic" in nature may have incomplete or absent knowledge of the articulatory-phonetic characteristics of certain phonemes.

Traditional articulation therapy—procedures to establish a new phoneme followed by articulation practice to stabilize production of the phoneme in systematically more complex contexts—is the tried and true method for helping children acquire new phonemes in those cases when the absence of a phoneme can be traced to a lack of knowledge at the level of articulatory-phonetic representations.

The approach to be presented here has its historical roots in Van Riper's (1978) stimulation method. Intervention proceeds through a series of phases: ear training (sensory-perceptual training), sound establishment, sound stabilization, transfer and carryover, and maintenance. It is essential to not skip the ear training procedures or the computer based alternative that we described in detail in Chapter 9. Even if the child's primary difficulty appears to be at the level of articulatory-phonetic representations, you cannot assume that the child has good perceptual knowledge of the target phoneme. We have mentioned on several occasions Shuster's (1998) study of

Van Riper's stimulation intervention proceeds through a series of phases: ear training (sensory-perceptual training), sound establishment, sound stabilization, transfer and carryover, and maintenance.

school-age children who had failed to achieve /ɹ/ after 2 years of therapy: these children demonstrated an inability to identify correct and incorrect exemplars of the target phoneme in words — they lacked phonological knowledge of the critical acoustic-phonetic cue to the difference between /ɹ/ and their own distorted productions. Motor learning will not be successful unless the child has good perceptual knowledge of the target and can properly evaluate the sensory consequences of his or her own production attempts in relation to that target (see Figure 3–15 and the associated discussion of auditory feedback models of speech motor control).

Procedures to Establish Correct Articulation of a New Phoneme

When a child is not stimulable for a given speech sound, that child may simply lack the requisite "how-to" knowledge of the appropriate configuration of articulatory gestures; alternatively, the child may have specific underlying problems with the planning, programming, or execution of the requisite movements. In any case there are a variety of strategies that the SLP can bring to the task of helping the child achieve a correct production and then establish consistency in the execution of that production in syllables before proceeding to the sound stabilization phase of articulation therapy. The principles of motor learning as discussed in the previous section on sensorimotor approaches apply here but adapted to this context in which the child is learning a new and difficult configuration of articulatory gestures. In the previous section the emphasis was on dynamic stability: learning to achieve consistency across varied contexts in the production of stimulable phonemes. The essential ingredients of the sensorimotor treatment approach were a high degree of variability in stimuli from trial to trial and a moderately low frequency of "knowledge of results" feedback. When working to establish a new phoneme in the child's system, however, a move to blocked practice in brief periods of intense focus on the absent phoneme and the provision of "knowledge of performance" feedback on each trial is the rule. From the perspective of schema theory, different practice conditions are required for the learning of new GMPs versus different parameterizations of a given GMP (Shea & Wulf, 2005). However, the research findings on practice conditions across these two contexts can be unified within the challenge point framework (Guadagnoli & Lee, 2004). Teaching a child to produce an unstimulable phoneme can be one of the most difficult parts of the articulation therapy process — so difficult that one strategy is to simply avoid it (see discussion of goal selection strategies in Chapter 8). However, this is not always possible, often undesirable, and, given the many proven strategies for ensuring stimulability, not usually necessary. When a task presents a high level of functional difficulty for the child, the SLP will need to use the strategies shown in Table 10–3 to help the child practice

When a child is not **stimulable** for a given speech sound, that child may simply lack the requisite 'how to' knowledge of the appropriate configuration of articulatory gestures; alternatively, the child may have specific underlying problems with the planning, programming, or execution of the requisite movements.

When working to establish a new phoneme in the child's system, the appropriate practice schedule is blocked practice during brief periods of intense focus on the absent phoneme with "knowledge of performance" feedback provided on each trial.

at the challenge point; these strategies include reducing variability, which in this context means focusing on only one unstimulable phoneme at a time, and practicing in a simple context. That does not mean that variability is unimportant at this phase of therapy; unstimulability may be characterized by rigid performance by the child who perseverates on the usual response—creativity in motivating the child to attempt new ways of producing the phoneme is an important part of the therapeutic process. Furthermore, there are varied articulatory configurations and multiple contexts for the production of a given phoneme and the child may have to try many before finding the conditions that stimulate correct production. The procedures for establishing new phonemes to be discussed in this section also include providing multimodal stimulation in advance of the child's attempt and high quality feedback about performance and results subsequent to the child's response. The procedures to be covered here, in order, are: (1) stimulation, (2) contextual facilitation, (3) phonetic placement, (4) successive approximation, and (5) visual feedback.

Procedures for establishing new phonemes involve providing multimodal stimulation in advance of the child's attempt and high quality feedback about performance and results subsequent to the child's response.

Stimulation consists of providing the child with an auditory and visual model of the target phoneme and asking the child to imitate the model. The prompts suggested with respect to the integral stimulation hierarchy shown in Table 10–4 are stimulation techniques. Stimulation can be applied while seated face-to-face with the child or while seated at a mirror so that the child can see both the SLP's and his or her own face. Position the child so that your face is comfortably visible to the child; this might mean seating yourself in the child-sized chair and the child in the big chair (after providing appropriate supports for the child's feet and trunk). As with the sensorimotor approach, most phonemes are presented for imitation in the context of a syllable, that is, stops, glides, and liquids. Nasals and fricatives can be presented in isolation but should be put in a syllable context as soon as possible.

Stimulation consists of providing the child with an auditory and visual model of the target phoneme and asking the child to imitate the model.

If the child is not successful after a few attempts, use contextual facilitation techniques; this simply means searching for phonetic contexts that help the child achieve a correct production (although Kent, 1982, warns that facilitating contexts sometimes impact the listener's perception more than the child's production). Often, a facilitating context can be discovered by applying your knowledge of articulatory phonetics. For example, Stokes and Griffiths (2010) present an excellent case study in which back round vowels were used as a facilitative context to teach [ʃ] in word final position to a child with severe apraxia of speech. It has been suggested that [is] might be a facilitative context for stimulating [s] for certain children given that [s] is produced with the lips spread and the tongue blade in a high front position, articulatory gestures that are shared with the vowel [i] (see S-Pack as described in Mowrer, 1989). It makes sense to target fricatives in word final position because, as pointed out in Chapter 4, some children acquire fricatives in coda position before onsets. On the other hand, as noted in Chapter 8, Hodson (2007) recommends that /s/ be introduced in the [stV] con-

Contextual facilitation simply means searching for phonetic contexts that help the child achieve a correct production.

text initially, working with rather than against the tendency toward stopping in the onset position. Curtis and Hardy (1959) found that prevocalic clusters were a facilitative context for production of [ɹ]. They also found that [ɹɚ] stimulated a relatively high proportion of correct productions of the rhotic vowel that can subsequently be shaped to the prevocalic [ɹ]. Another strategy is to systematically probe the child's production in all possible phonetic contexts. The McDonald Deep Test (McDonald, 1964) was designed specifically for this purpose although a formal test is not required. Contextual facilitation is a key procedure in the implementation of the paired stimuli technique for establishing new phonemes. A simple reinforcement learning paradigm is used to promote generalization of production from the facilitative context to other contexts in which the child misarticulates the phoneme. Let us imagine, for example, that you have determined that the child is able to produce the word "hats" correctly; this word could be practiced along with 10 other words that the child produces with a distorted final /s/, for example, beets, cups, cakes, cats, mops, box, dance, mats, fox, nuts. Pictures of each item are interleaved with picture cards depicting 'hats' so that the trials alternate between the facilitative context and the more difficult words, for example, hats, beets, hats, cups, and so forth. The child is asked to name each picture so that the child's correct responses for "hats" serve as a model for correct production of the /s/ target on the subsequent trial. The SLP provides continuous reinforcement for correct /s/ responses on every trial including the word "hats." Irwin reported data for 388 children who were treated with this technique; an average of 83 minutes of intervention was required for the children to achieve at least 80% correct responding in a noncontingent single-word probe condition.

Contextual facilitation is a key procedure in the implementation of the **paired stimuli technique** for establishing new phonemes.

In the absence of a facilitating phonetic context, some additional information about the required articulatory gestures will be required. Phonetic placement involves a variety of techniques for helping the child correctly position and then move the articulators to produce the target phoneme or syllable. The techniques include verbal instructions, physical manipulation of the articulators, and amplified sensory feedback about the position of the articulators. A large number of tools and products have been applied in the process, ranging from everyday objects such as pencils (Shriberg, 1980) to dental tools such as flavored sponges (toothettes) to specially created tongue placement devices such as the Speech Buddies (http://www.speechbuddy.com). A comprehensive description of helpful techniques for each vowel and consonant in English is provided in Secord, Boyce, Donahue, Fox, and Shine (2007) and we recommend this source as an essential part of the SLP's toolkit rather than detailing any specific techniques here. However, we provide some cautionary guidelines about the application of these techniques. First, the techniques described in Secord et al. are meant to be practiced in a speech context. For example, when stimulating production of /ʃ/, two aspects of the articulatory gesture may be problematic: configuration of the tongue to produce a shallow groove in the center and

Phonetic placement involves a variety of techniques for helping the child correctly position and then move the articulators to produce the target phoneme or syllable.

Practicing isolated articulatory gestures in a nonspeech context will not generalize to the production of the target phoneme in a speech context.

Each new articulatory goal must be practiced in the context of the complete configuration of gestures that will lead to a successful production of the target phoneme or syllable.

Clinical trials show that exercises to improve articulator strength are not always successful and even when they are, increased strength by itself does not result in functional gains.

One special procedure that may be helpful for those rare cases who show signs of *subclinical dysarthria* is the use of a **bite-block** to stabilize the jaw while practicing independent movements of the tongue and lips.

stabilization of the lateral margins of the tongue against the upper bicuspids and molars. An infant spoon can be placed in the child's mouth to encourage fitting of the tongue around the bowl of the spoon and flavored sprays and tongue blades can be used to help the child locate the lateral margins of the tongue and place them along-side the inner molars. However, practicing these gestures in a non speech context is not likely to generalize to the production of [ʃ] (Forrest, 2002; Ruscello, 2009).

Once the child has achieved the correct tongue configuration or positioned the lateral margins of the tongue in the correct place, stimulate production of a fricative sound. Provide information about the child's articulatory performance relative to your expectations throughout the phonetic placement session, indicating the aspects of the gesture that are correct even if the sound is not quite right. You may need to establish individual parts of the articulatory configuration one at a time but those parts should not be abstracted from the whole in practice. In other words, you may need to shift attention sequentially from lip rounding, to the tongue groove, to the lateral margins of the tongue, to airflow characteristics, and to correct positioning of the blade of the tongue while establishing correct articulation of [ʃ]. Throughout the practice session, however, the child should be attempting to produce [ʃ] on each trial. Each new articulatory goal must be practiced in the context of the complete configuration of gestures that will lead to a successful production of the alveopalatal fricative. This is true even for children who have specific motor speech difficulties such as the children described by Goozée et al. (2007, see Chapter 7) who showed evidence of dysarthria in the form of reduced tongue strength and slow diadochokinetic rates in addition to lateral lisps and long-term normalization trajectories. Clinical trials show that exercises to improve articulator strength are not always successful and even when they are, increased strength by itself does not result in functional gains (Sjögreen, Màr, Kiliaridis, & Lohmander, 2010). One special procedure that may be helpful for those rare cases who show signs of subclinical dysarthria is the use of a bite-block to stabilize the jaw while practicing independent movements of the tongue and lips (Dworkin, 1978; Hodge, 2010; Netsell, 1985). Once again, however, actual speech is practiced while the bite block is in place. Furthermore, it is usually helpful to remain focused on the new articulatory gesture that you are trying to encourage at first and not worry too much about whether the resulting sound is perfectly correct: you want the child to feel comfortable experimenting with new articulatory postures and it is often easier to focus on one part of the new configuration at a time. If the child has a good internal model for the target sound he or she will know when the new gestures have been coordinated sufficiently well to produce a match or approximation to the target.

Finally, it is important to focus on changing those articulatory gestures that are truly essential to the production of the new phoneme. It is unfortunately fairly easy to establish bad articulatory habits or unusual distortions in the child's speech by providing incorrect advice. A common therapeutic error is to expend a lot of effort inhibiting lip rounding in children who substitute [w] for /ɹ/ even though a small amount of lip rounding is normal in /ɹ/ production. The gliding error reflects a failure to produce vocal tract constrictions with the tongue that lower the third formant and therefore it is these tongue gestures that should be the focus of therapy (more specifically, the therapeutic focus should be the acoustic result of producing constrictions in the pharyngeal and palatal areas). Hagiwara, Meyers Fosnot, and Alessi (2002) present an interesting case study in which the child's unusual distortion may have been learned during the course of speech therapy. Shriberg (1980) presents a systematic approach to the treatment of /ɹ/ distortions that takes into account the persistence of these learned habits while promoting active self-discovery of appropriate and varied tongue constrictions after stabilizing the jaw with a "bite stick" which is actually a clean pencil.

A useful adjunct to phonetic placement may be successive approximation or shaping to move the child from a known articulatory configuration to the new configuration in a sequence of small steps. Suggestions for shaping are also provided in Secord et al. (2007). Successful application of shaping procedures requires a careful "task analysis," in other words, good knowledge of the articulatory-phonetic characteristics of the target sound and the similar phone that is currently in the child's repertoire. Subsequently, a series of intermediate gestures from the known phone to the new phone can be taught in sequential order. Shaping from [t] to [s] by teaching the child to insert excessive aspiration after the [t] is very common for example. Shriberg (1975) provided detailed instructions for moving the child from sustained production of the liquid [l] to vocalic [ɝ]. Rather than reproduce the instructions here, we urge direct consultation with the original source because the paper contains a wealth of excellent advice for effective application of successive approximation techniques in general as well as a useful protocol for the evocation of [ɝ] in particular. Once having obtained a decent-sounding [ɝ] from the child through successive approximation, a related technique called chaining can be used to work the phone into syllables and words in varied syllable positions and contexts, for example: (1) prevocalic—[ɝ] - [ɝɹɛ] - [ɹɛ] - [ɹɛd] - [ɹid]; (2) postvocalic—[ɝ] - [iɝ] - [hiɝ] - [hɛɝ] - [pɛɝ]; and (3) intervocalic—[ɝ] - [ɝɹi] - [hɝɹi] - [hɛɹi] - [tʃɛɹi].

A useful adjunct to phonetic placement may be **successive approximation** or shaping to move the child from a known articulatory configuration to the new configuration in a sequence of small steps.

Once having obtained the new phone through successive approximation, a related technique called **chaining** can be used to work the phone into syllables and words in varied syllable positions and contexts.

Phonetic placement, successive approximation, and chaining all involve decomposing the task of producing a new phone or syllable into its constituent parts. Forrest (2002) reviewed the literature on the conditions under which task decomposition is helpful in motor learning. Segmentation is a form of task decomposition in which the task is broken up into spatially and/or temporally independent subcomponents. When a complex task is made up of sequentially ordered parts, each with a defined beginning and end, segmentation

Segmentation is a form of task decomposition in which the task is broken up into spatially and/or temporally independent subcomponents.

When a complex task is made up of sequentially ordered parts, each with a defined beginning and end, segmentation is an effective strategy for promoting learning of the parts and the whole.

is an effective strategy for promoting learning of the parts and the whole. In other words, motor learning research in multiple domains supports the use of chaining to help children master production of a phone in utterances of increasing length and complexity. The challenge point framework introduced in the previous section however should guide the SLP to maintain the task at the appropriate level of functional difficulty and move the child from the simplest part to the complex whole as quickly as is possible given the child's level of performance.

Fractionization involves decomposing the gestures associated with a phone into their individual subcomponents.

Fractionization involves decomposing the gestures associated with a phone into their individual subcomponents. We previously mentioned that production of [ʃ], even in isolation, involves rounded and slightly protruded lips, a shallow tongue groove, centrally directed airflow, anchoring of the lateral margins of the tongue against the upper bicuspids/molars, and positioning of the blade of the tongue behind the alveolar ridge. Notice that these articulatory gestures are not spatially and temporally independent; rather, they must overlap in time and space during production of [ʃ]. Theoretically, some of these parts could be practiced independently and in a manner that is abstracted from the speech context; for example, bubbles could be used to practice lip rounding or blow painting could be used to practice centrally directed airflow. This kind of fractionization of the parts of the [ʃ] task is known to be not only ineffective but detrimental to learning and we strongly advise against it. This is not the same as asking the child to repeatedly imitate [ʃ] while gradually shifting the focus of your performance feedback from one part of the articulatory gesture to another to ensure that the child is receiving the optimal amount of information during learning. We demonstrate that this latter practice can be effective later in this section but we repeat that using nonspeech exercises to practice parts of a speech movement outside of a speech context is ill-advised on theoretical and empirical grounds.

Fractionization is not only ineffective but detrimental to learning: using nonspeech exercises to practice parts of a speech movement outside of a speech context is ill advised on theoretical and empirical grounds.

In addition to providing verbal feedback about the child's performance ("Good, you rounded your lips!"), several technologies provide visual feedback about articulatory performance and may be helpful for those children who are having the most difficulty achieving production of a new phoneme. Some visual feedback devices are designed to provide reinforcement and knowledge of results without providing any external information about performance factors. For example, a device named Speech Viewer II was developed to provide interesting visual displays in response to the acoustic characteristics of the child's speech output. Pratt, Heintzelman, and Deming (1993) described the efficacy of the vowel accuracy module which showed a monkey advancing up a tree toward coconuts as the talker approximated a target vowel. They reported that the program did not sustain the attention of their preschool-age hearing-impaired clients. Additional modules designed to target contrasts between fricative phonemes did not provide accurate feedback. In general, we see no need for technology to replace the SLP or the child in the provision of "knowledge of results" feedback. Even in

Several technologies provide **visual feedback** about articulatory performance and may be helpful for those children who are having the most difficulty achieving production of a new phoneme.

the case of hearing-impaired talkers where such devices substitute for sensory feedback the talker may not be able to perceive, linking kinesthetic feedback of articulatory movements to functional feedback from the natural environment will be more useful for ensuring transfer and maintenance of the new skills to everyday communicative situations (see for example, minimal pairs therapy in Chapter 11).

In contrast, spectrograms can be used to provide more direct feedback about performance, with several software tools for speech analysis freely available as open source software. We caution that effective use of these tools does require some knowledge of acoustic phonetics and familiarity with the software controls for adjusting the analysis parameters for child speech (Kent & Read, 1992; Ladefoged, 1996). Case studies on the use of spectrographic feedback to stimulate [ɹ] production have been published (Masterson & Rvachew, 1999; Shuster, Ruscello, & Toth, 1995). Spectrographic, waveform, and pitch displays can also be used to target vowels, fricatives and prosodic structures. One of the primary advantages of spectrographic feedback is that it can be used to reinforce changes that are approaching the target even when they are not perceptible to the SLP or the child. Spectrographic feedback can also detect acoustic changes associated with articulatory gestures that are impossible to see (i.e., the lowering of the third formant in [ɝ] that occurs when a constriction is formed in the pharynx). A second advantage is that this therapeutic technique places the emphasis on producing a particular acoustic change (e.g., lowering the third formant) rather than producing a specific phoneme or SLP-defined articulatory gesture. The latter goals are often self-defeating when treating older children who have experienced long periods of failure in speech therapy. Asking the child to "say [ɝ]" may trigger the overlearned response that is associated with this phoneme or a defeated "I can't do that." Asking the child to try to make an orange line on the computer screen fall is quite a different challenge. Allowing the child to explore the possibilities of the vocal tract and discover the multiple articulatory configurations that bring the third formant down is fully consistent with our dynamic approach to therapy and much more productive.

One of the primary advantages of **spectrographic feedback** is that it can be used to reinforce changes that are approaching the target even when they are not perceptible to the SLP or the child.

Electropalatography (EPG) can be used to provide direct visual feedback of articulator placement and movement, although the performance feedback is restricted to information about contact of the tongue tip, blade, sides, and body with the alveolar ridge and palate (Morgan Barry, 1989). This approach requires that each client be custom-fitted with an artificial palate. The artificial palate contains sensors arranged in a grid pattern that provide feedback about tongue contact with the palate and teeth (see Figure 1–4). A target pattern of lingual-palatal contacts and the client's attempts are displayed on a computer monitor, either superimposed or adjacent to one another. Fletcher and Hasegawa (1983) described the use of this approach with a 3-year-old congenitally deaf girl who successfully acquired a high versus low vowel contrast in her productive speech. Dagenais, Critz-Crosby, and Adams (1994) presents two case studies in which EPG was used to treat lateral lisps in 8-year-old girls.

Electropalatography (EPG) can be used to provide direct visual feedback of articulator placement and movement, although the performance feedback is restricted to information about contact of the tongue tip, blade, sides, and body with the alveolar ridge and palate.

Good perceptual knowledge of /s/ was confirmed for both girls, using naturally recorded sentence length material, prior to the introduction of the EPG intervention. During therapy, contact patterns between tongue and artificial palate were presented to the child on a display that used different symbols to indicate sensors that should be contacted (prior to the attempt), and sensors that were appropriately contacted and sensors that were inappropriately contacted by the tongue during the attempt to produce the target utterance. Training began with lingual stops and progressed to the troublesome sibilants, first in CV and VC syllables and then working through words and phrases. In addition to EPG to teach correct tongue positioning, drinking straws were used to teach the correct tongue configuration, specifically, the central groove posture. The treatment was successful for one child who presented with undifferentiated lingual gestures prior to treatment and who achieved mastery of /s,z/ in sentences in 17 sessions over 7 weeks (although inconsistent lateralizations remained at the 6-month follow-up). The second child did not benefit from the intervention however. This second child did not produce the lateral lisp with an undifferentiated lingual gesture as her production was characterized by an appropriate tongue groove along with excessive lateral contact and inappropriate use of the tongue body. Interestingly the authors suggest that the first child was not an appropriate candidate for EPG because she could probably have been successfully treated without such an expensive procedure. The severity of the second child's speech disorder and the difficulty that she had in changing her articulatory pattern, in their opinion, made her a good candidate for EPG, although we note that she is not the only case in the published literature to not achieve normalization of /s/ even with the application of this extraordinary treatment. McAuliffe and Cornwell (2008) suggested that successful application of EPG requires incorporation of the principles of motor learning. In their case study they focused in particular on distributed practice, ensuring many short treatment sessions with a high dose frequency over a brief total intervention duration by scheduling in-clinic sessions trice weekly and providing the family with a portable unit for home practice and a structured home program requiring daily drill. After 4 weeks, tongue placement normalized for [t] but not [s]. Perceptual and acoustic measures revealed improved articulation of /s/, nonetheless.

Access to **portable ultrasound** units has made it possible to incorporate another method of visualizing the tongue into speech therapy sessions. In contrast to EPG, ultrasound provides information about the tongue configuration.

Access to portable ultrasound units has made it possible to incorporate another method of visualizing the tongue into speech therapy sessions. In contrast to EPG, ultrasound provides information about the tongue configuration and thus the presence of the groove so important to [s, z, ʃ, ʒ] can be revealed (Bernhardt, Gick, Bacsfalvi, & Adler-Bock, 2005). Furthermore, key tongue shape configurations for [ɹ] can be captured at multiple points of vocal tract constriction (Adler-Bock, Bernhardt, Bacsfalvi, & Gick, 2005). Figure 10–2 shows multiple ultrasound images of the tongue during production of retroflexed and bunched [ɹ] (Bernhardt, 2004). Adler-Bock,

A.

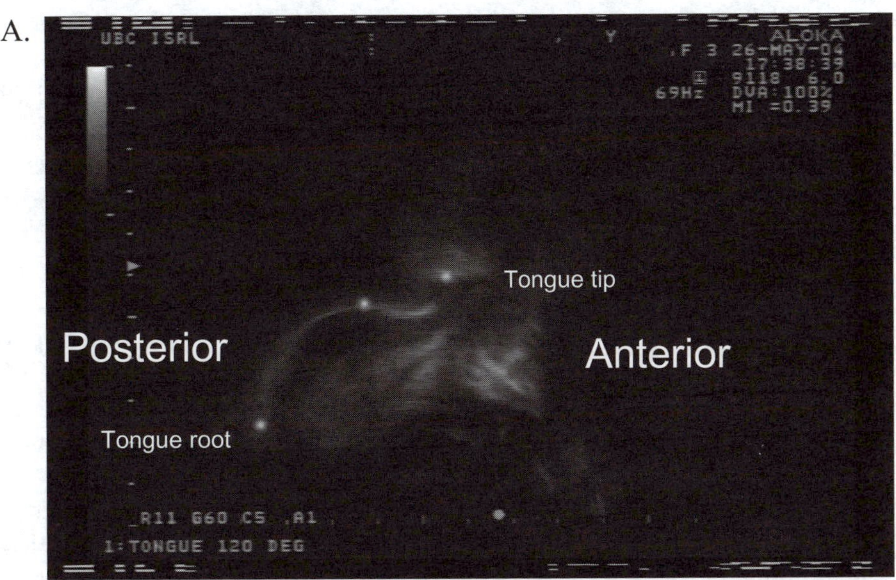

B.

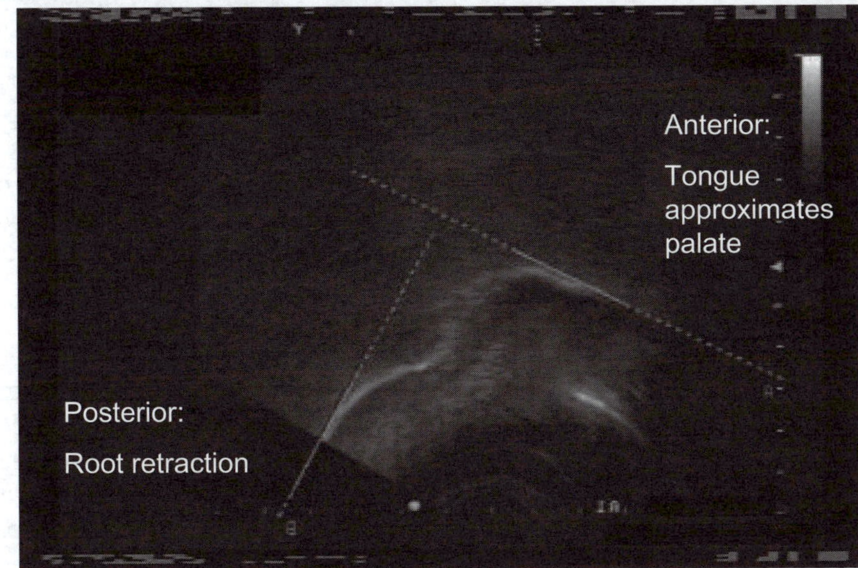

C.

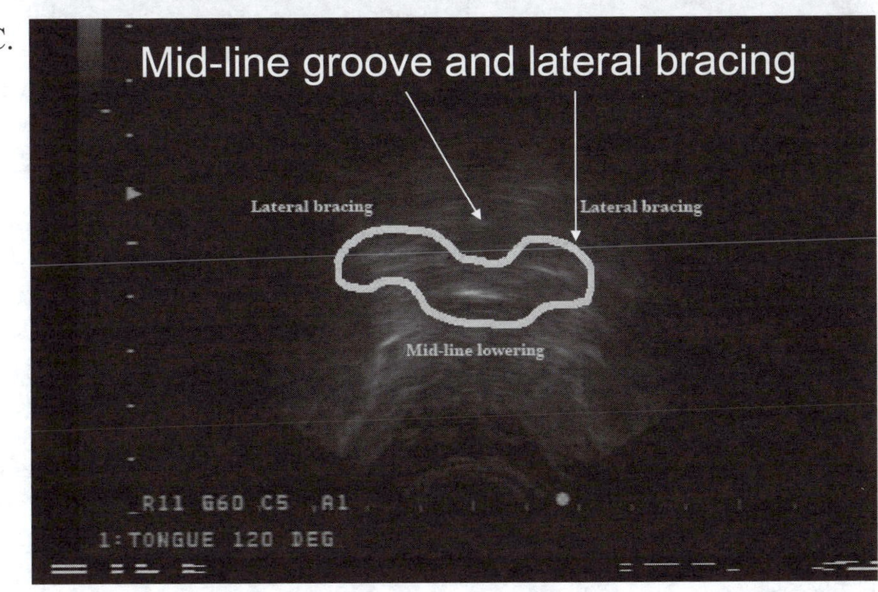

Figure 10–2. *Ultrasound images of (***A***) a sagittal view of the tongue during production of a "retroflexed" [ɹ]; (***B***) a sagittal view and (***C***) a coronal view of the tongue during production of a "bunched" [ɹ].* Source: *From* Evaluating Ultrasound as a Visual Feedback Tool in Speech Therapy, *by B. Bernhardt, 2004, paper presented at the American Speech-Language-Hearing Association, Philadelphia, PA. Reprinted with permission.*

Bernhardt, Gick, and Bacsfalvi (2007) describe two case studies in which 13 sessions of an ultrasound intervention led to positive changes in tongue shape, acoustic characteristics and perceptual accuracy in the adolescents' production of /ɹ/.

Demonstrations of Techniques to Establish New Phonemes

Demonstration 10–3 is a transcript of 10 minutes of a therapy session conducted by a McGill student SLP (Stephanie) who was treating a child enrolled in the ECRIP trial that we described in Chapter 9. In fact it is the first therapy session of the student's practicum and the first therapy experience for the child as well. The male child, Ben, was 4 years old and achieved a score of 73% consonants correct on the Test Francophone de Phonologie prior to the onset of therapy. His error productions for the /ʃ/ phoneme tended to be a fronted distortion, for example, /niʃ/ → [nis̪] ("niche" meaning "kennel"). However, this target was also vulnerable to spreading errors indicating that it was unmarked for place of articulation in his underlying system, for example, /ʃapo/ → [fapo] ("chapeau" meaning "hat"). The phonemes /ʃ/ and /ʒ/ were frequent targets in this trial because match ratios were poor for [+Coronal][−anterior] and the acquisition age for these high frequency phones is younger in French than in English. The treatment session commenced with a brief "identification" procedure designed to ensure that the child was aware of the target and understood the purpose of the therapy session (as described in Chapter 9). No ear training or other "input-oriented" procedures were provided because this child was randomly assigned to the "speech production" condition in which all therapy procedures focused on articulation practice. Subsequent to the identification procedure, Stephanie proceeded to an activity targeting [ʃ] in isolation. In preparation for the session, she created a number of paper dolls depicting babies dressed for sleep and color matched paper cribs that she laid out on the table next to a toy dog. She also brought a hand mirror to the session because the room was unfortunately not equipped with a wall mirror. Although the session was conducted in French, we provide an English translation of the session during which Stephanie guides the child toward a good [ʃ] production. Several aspects of the transcript are notable, some of which may not be fully transparent without access to the video. First, Ben is fully engaged with the activity; although he is amused by Stephanie's barking, he is anxious to silence the dog and place the baby in the crib. He has a remarkable level of motivation to achieve the goal (correct production of [ʃ]) and most of the time he is willing to wait until he has met Stephanie's performance standards before he puts the baby in the crib. She almost loses his attention at one point, however, because she has clearly allowed too many unsuccessful attempts to pass; a more experienced clinician would have introduced some other strategies to ensure the child had an opportunity to meet expectations and receive a baby before that point.

Demonstration 10–3
Student SLP (Stephanie) Uses of Stimulation to Elicit [ʃ] in Isolation from a 4-Year-Old Boy

Stephanie: I am going to start and then it's going to be your turn. (takes a paper baby and prepares to put him to sleep) So, I take the baby and I say: [ʃː] (places a finger in front of her lips when she pronounces the "quiet sound"). I make my lips nice and round and I say: [ʃ]. And then I place the baby in its crib (places the paper baby in the crib). Now, it's your turn.

"Woof, woof, woof, woof, woof, woof, woof" What are you going to say to the dog?

"Woof, woof, woof, woof, woof" Your baby won't be able to sleep! The dog keeps saying "woof, woof, woof"!

What do we say?

Ben: (smiles at the dog but does not respond)

We say: [ʃː]. Your turn!

Ben: (places a finger in front of his lips) [s̟]

Stephanie: Excellent! Ben, we are going to try again by making a nice circle with our lips, like this: [ʃ]

Ben: [s̟]

Ben: Oops, we're making round lips; you are showing me a big, beautiful smile! (Ben and Stephanie laugh) Because you are used to smiling, right? I am sure that is true.

But we are going to try to round our lips (Stephanie traces a circle on her lips with her finger). Can you make your lips round?

Can you make a nice circle? Come on, let's round our lips. (Stephanie demonstrates how the child should round his lips) [ʃ].

Ben: [s^y]

Stephanie: Oh, that was a little bit better, but we're going to keep practicing! I want to hear a [ʃ].

Ben: [s̟]

Stephanie: We have to bring the corners of our lips closer together. Just like this (Stephanie pushes the corners of her own lips in with her fingers to force rounded lips) [ʃ]. Shall we try? We take our lips and we bring them close together like a little fish.

It's exactly like a little fish (Stephanie and Ben laugh). It is funny, right? Try it, it's your turn. [ʃ].

Ben: (uses his fingers to make his lips round) [s̞ʲ]

Stephanie: Almost, we are going to keep practicing, ok? It's not exactly like that, but we are going to keep practicing. Good job, you are trying really hard! (Stephanie points to the crib to signal to the child that he may put his toy baby to sleep and the child places the toy baby in the crib) Excellent!

Stephanie: Shall we continue? Is it my turn or your turn?

Ben: It's my turn!

Stephanie: It's your turn again? (Stephanie laughs.) Ok, I'm going to let you choose another baby! You chose a pink baby; let's put the pink baby to sleep.

"Woof, woof, woof"

Ben: (looks at the dog and puts a finger in front of his lips) [fs̞]

Stephanie: Oops, let's try it again, Ben! Look, we're going to take our mirror (Stephanie takes a mirror and places it in front of herself and the child). We're making round lips.

Ben: [s̞]

Stephanie: [ʃ] (Stephanie takes the mirror and shows the child how to round his lips to pronounce the [ʃ] correctly). We are making a circle (Stephanie points toward the corners of her mouth to show how to round her lips). I see a big smile. And the big smiles, they make the sound [s]! They make the "snake sound." I don't want to hear the "snake sound." I want to hear the "quiet sound."

So, let's look in the mirror (Stephanie places the mirror in front of the child and shows him how to place his lips to make the "quiet sound"). [ʃ]

Ben: [s̞]

Stephanie: Oops, we have to make a circle, just like the one I'm making now! (Stephanie points toward the mirror, indicating her rounded lips.) We're making a circle with our lips. Can you make a circle with your lips?

(the child seems to have lost interest in the game and has stopped looking in the mirror) Ben, let's try this one more time and then you'll be able to put the baby to sleep.

Ben: [s̞]

Stephanie: (points toward her lips to show to the child that her lips are rounded) [ʃ]

Ben: (with rounded lips) [s̞]

Stephanie: Ok, I'm going to show you something. (Stephanie places the mirror in front of the child again) When you say [s], your tongue is here (she points toward the front of her mouth). Let's bring the tongue back a little (she points toward the back of her mouth). Let's send it more toward the back. [ʃ]

Ben: [ʃ]

Stephanie: Excellent! High-five! I heard [ʃ]; that was much better! Great job! (Stephanie takes two baby toys and gives them to the child.) I'm very happy, you can put two babies to sleep, because that was wonderful!

Shall we do another one? (The child nods.) It's my turn now!

(Stephanie takes a baby toy, while pointing to her own mouth.) So, I'm sending my tongue a little to the back of my mouth, Ben, and then I make a beautiful circle with my lips (she traces a circle on her lips with her finger): [ʃ].

Ben: [s̟ʃ]

Stephanie: (Pointing toward her tongue.) Send your tongue to the back of your mouth. [ʃ].

Ben: [s̟]

Stephanie: Your tongue is in front of your mouth! Can you send it toward the back of your mouth? (Points toward the back of her mouth, while keeping her mouth open while pronouncing the [ʃ], so that the child is able to see where the tongue is placed): [ʃ].

Ben: [h]

Stephanie: (Laughs.) We'll practice and we will have it. Let's continue. You're making great efforts, I'm very happy! It's your turn to pick a baby.

Ben: (Picks a baby and the dog starts to bark "woof woof.")

Stephanie: You won't be able to put your baby to sleep, the dog says "woof woof." (Stephanie places the mirror in front of the child.) Let's say it again. I'm sending my tongue to the back of my mouth (shows the child how she moves her tongue further back in her mouth); not to the front, this is too much to the front of the mouth, it is touching my teeth (shows the child how her tongue touches the front of her mouth). I'm sending my tongue toward the back. [ʃ]

Ben: [ʃ̟]

Stephanie: That's better, I didn't see a smile. That was great! And I saw that you tried to send your tongue to the back of your mouth. That was also excellent! (Points toward the crib.) So we can put the baby to sleep.

There are three left. Do we put them to sleep? Is it my turn or your turn?

Ben: My turn!

Stephanie: It's your turn? Ok! (Places the mirror in front of the child, while the child picks a baby toy.)

Ben: [s̘ʃ̙s̘]

Stephanie: Let's send the tongue to the back of the mouth! (Points toward the back of the mouth with her tongue and with her finger.)

Ben: [ʃ̙]

Stephanie: Excellent! You're trying very hard! We're making a beautiful circle with our lips, ok? I was seeing a nice smile (points toward her mouth in the mirror)!

Ben: [s̘ʃ̙s̘]

Stephanie: Oh! I hear some [sʃ], but it's great! You are in between the two! I think we're going to get it, what do you say? Do you think you'll get it? I certainly think so! Great job!

Shall we say it again? [ʃ].

Ben: (takes a deep breath and pronounces the sound at the same time as Stephanie does) [s̘ʃ̙ʃ]

Stephanie: Great job! That was perfect! That is exactly what I want, always! That was a beautiful "quiet sound"!

Mom, did you hear a nice "quiet sound"?

Mother: I'll say, Ben!

Stephanie: Wow, that was excellent! You can definitely do this, great job!

Oh, wait, there is another one! We don't have any babies in the yellow crib. We'll have to place a baby in our yellow crib. Ok, which one do you want? (The child chooses one of the toy babies and then puts it in the crib.) Ok?

Ben: [s s̘ʃ]

Stephanie: Excellent! Hey, I think, at the beginning, your tongue was in the front of the mouth, but then it went toward the back of the mouth. That is excellent! [ʃ].

Ben: [ʃ].

Note: Translated from the original French.

Fortunately, she is able to bring him back on task and he achieves lip rounding on the next trial. Overall, he is remarkably tolerant of not receiving the babies when he has not achieved her, and apparently his own, expectations. Clearly, the activity is not undermining his intrinsic motivation and the reinforcement he is receiving is serving to bolster his perceived competence. Second, Stephanie is providing a verbal description of his performance on every trial, remarking on aspects of the acoustic quality and the accuracy of his articulatory gestures (i.e., providing a high frequency of "knowledge of results" and "knowledge of performance" feedback). This feedback was generally clear and well matched to the characteristics of Ben's attempts to produce the sound. Occasionally, however, she provides "mixed signals" about the accuracy of Ben's response. In watching hours of treatment videos from this study we have found that the ability to manage these contingencies is a particularly difficult aspect of good clinical practice for student SLPs to master. Furthermore, it was an aspect of clinical practice that our student clinicians did not always change significantly during their practicum experience. Very good students such as Stephanie would improve, but students who provided erratic feedback at the beginning of their practicum tended to persist with this problem until the end as if their clinical educators were not quite aware of the problem. The ability to judge the accuracy of the child's response and provide helpful information about that response is an essential skill for the SLP. Third, Stephanie shifts the focus of her knowledge of performance feedback during the session: initially she provides information about lip-rounding; as soon as Ben produces this articulatory gesture, she shifts to providing information about tongue placement. However, on every trial she models and elicits these gestures in the context of the [ʃ] sound, never expecting Ben to produce them in isolation. In other words, she is using segmentation as a teaching strategy (by targeting the phone in isolation) but at no time does she fractionize [ʃ] into its component parts. It is possible that a more experienced clinician might have achieved the [ʃ] faster by using contextual facilitation or phonetic placement in addition to verbal instructions and audiovisual stimulation. On the other hand, we are sure that some experienced clinicians would not have persisted for the full 10 minutes thereby failing to achieve this successful outcome! Ben received a 6-week intervention using output-oriented procedures. During that time, 90 minutes was devoted to the intermediate goal [+coronal] [−anterior], targeting [ʃ] in the onset position specifically. Posttreatment, his match ratio for this feature had improved from .42 to .63 and he achieved 82% consonants correct on the Test Francophone de Phonologie. All round a job well done by child and clinician.

The ability to judge the accuracy of the child's response and provide helpful information about that response is an essential skill for the SLP.

Demonstration 10–4 illustrates the use of spectrographic feedback to establish production of the syllable "er" at the ends of words. The client was a 13-year-old boy who had received speech therapy since the age of two for severe apraxia of speech. As a teenager his speech was intelligible and generally accurate but some speech errors remained including consistent misarticulation of rhotic vowels.

Demonstration 10–4
Use of Spectrographic Feedback to Facilitate Acquisition of Word-Final /ɚ/

It is necessary to understand the acoustic theory of vowel production, the characteristics of correctly and incorrectly produced /ɹ,ɝ/ and the technical aspects of using spectral analysis software to produce good quality spectrograms from adult and child speech if you are going to use this technology effectively in speech therapy. The basic background knowledge can be obtained from other sources such as Kent and Read (1992) and Ladefoged (1996). Here we present some spectrograms illustrating the successful achievement of the rhotic vowel in word final syllabic contexts by a 13-year-old boy named Curt who had received speech therapy for apraxia of speech since he was two years of age. The demonstration begins with a description of the acoustic characteristics of /ɹ/ in word initial position before proceeding with the case study.

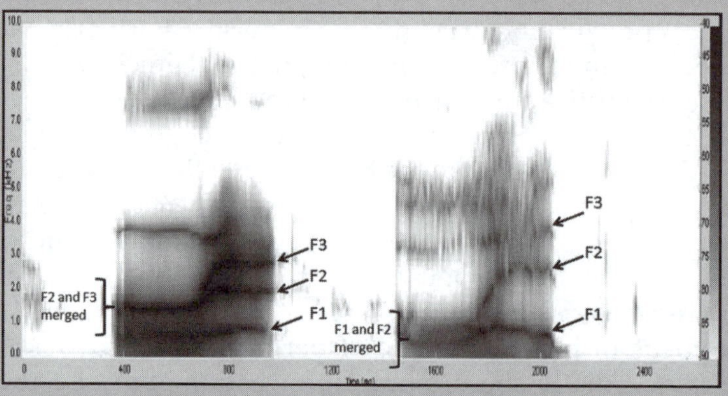

Adult-produced /ɹ/ (left); child-produced /ɹ/ distortion (right).

1. In this example the SLP produced the syllable /ɹʌ/ and the child (a 7-year-old girl) attempted to imitate the same syllable. Both talkers exaggerated the initial liquid, accounting for its excessive duration. The SLP production is characterized by the classic acoustic features of /ɹ/: the starting frequency of the third formant is so low that it has merged with the second formant; thereafter it rises sharply. In the child's production, the starting frequency of the second formant is so low that it has merged with the first formant. However, the third formant starts high and then rises only gently. This syllable is not perceived to be /ɹʌ/ or /wʌ/, rather it is a derhotacized distortion of the intended target. A word-final rhotic vowel would be roughly a mirror image of the spectrogram on the left.

2. The acoustic theory of vowel production leads to the prediction that constrictions at the pharynx, hard palate and lips will result in the lowering of the third formant as shown on the left, whereas constrictions at the velum and lips will result in lowering of the second formant as shown on the right in the figure shown above. You can imagine the difficulties inherent in attempting to shift the child's primary constriction from the velar area to the pharynx via verbal instructions and phonetic placement not to mention the impossibility of providing direct visual feedback! You will see with this demonstration that the technique is to allow the child to discover the combination of articulatory gestures and constriction degrees that result in the desired pattern of formant relationships and movements in the spectrogram through a process of trial and error as well as successive approximation.

3. This next spectrogram shows a model of the phrase "the writer" produced by the SLP for Curt in order to demonstrate the desired outcome of therapy and to introduce the parameters that he should attempt to manipulate during practice. The focus of treatment is the final syllable "er." T1 marker points to the highest value of the third formant (F3), just after release of the "t." The F3 falls in frequency, as expected for "er." The drop in frequency between the T1 and T2 markers is 781 Hz. Notice that the F2 is parallel to and very close in frequency to the F3. Both formants begin to fall immediately after release of the "t."

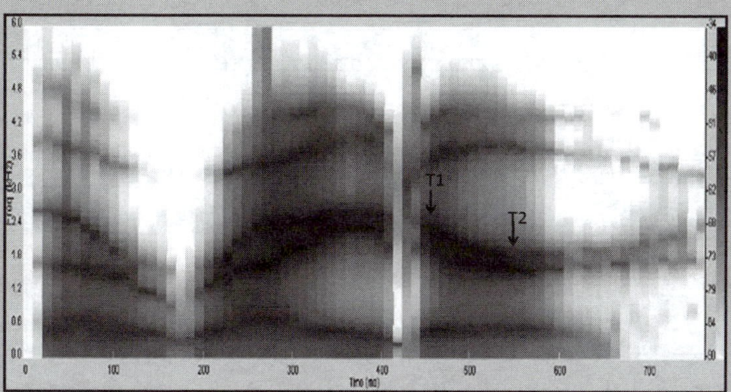

Spectogram of the clinician model of the phrase "the writer." T1 = 2465 Hz; T2 = 1684 Hz.

4. Curt's initial attempts at words with a word final "er" syllable are characterized by a relatively flat and high F3, not at all in proximity to the F2. In fact, there is even a slight rise in the measurable part of the third formant.

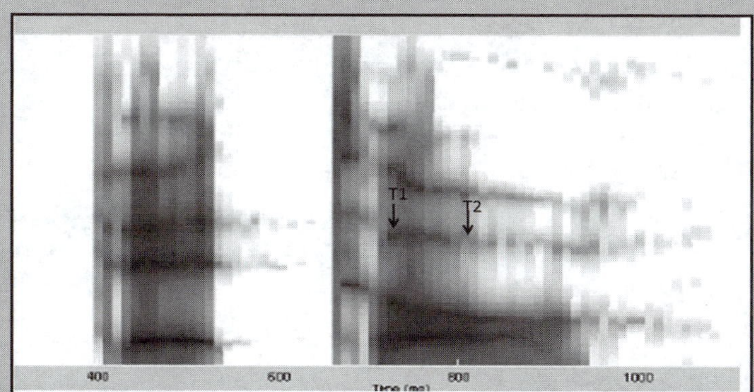

Curt's production of "pitter." (Note excessively long stop-gap for the ambisyllabic consonant followed by long duration of aspiration at release.) T1 = 2441 Hz; T2 = 2490 Hz.

5. Subsequently, Curt was encouraged to lower the frequency of the third formant between T1 and T2 in gradual steps, starting with small increments. The initial goal was to achieve a 50 Hz fall in the F3 between the highest point (T1) just after release of the consonant and the lowest measurable part of the F3 (T2). As the initial attempts involved a small rise even flat F3s were initially seen as improvement. No feedback regarding phonetic accuracy of the /ɚ/ was provided.

6. Curt gradually learned to reduce the F3 by progressively larger increments. By the end of the first session, he accomplished this 342 Hz change in F3 frequency near the end of the final syllable in the phrase "the writer." The syllable still does not sound correct, but the progress that could be observed in the spectrogram motivated Curt to continue trying. One of the advantages of spectral feedback is that it provides information about positive change toward the target that is not yet perceptible to the listener.

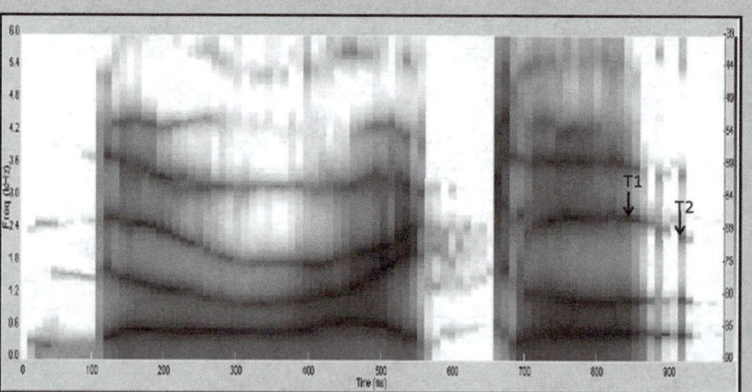

Although the F3 is flat throughout much of the syllable, Curt learned to produce progressively larger decrements in the formant at the end of the syllable. T1 = 2085 Hz; T2 = 2343 Hz.

7. After approximately 6 weeks of treatment, Curt was producing a consistent change in F3 frequency that corresponded to a perceptually correct "r." However, the fall in the F3 continued to be delayed, resulting in an "-or"-like percept at the end of the phrase "the writer." The F3 is more or less flat for 115 ms after release of the "t." Subsequent treatment focused on reducing the time interval between the release of the consonant and the descent of the formant.

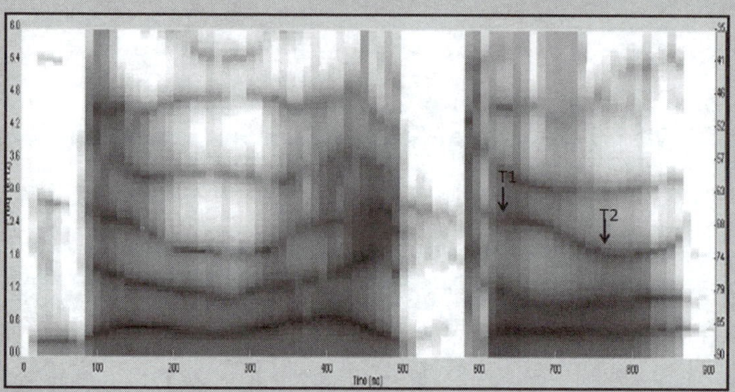

The F3 is flat for 115 ms and then it falls by 659 Hz, resulting in the syllable [ɔɚ]. T1 = 2563; T2 = 1904 Hz.

8. After Curt learned to lower his F3 sufficiently to produce a perceptable word final "er," attention shifted from the frequency characteristics to the temporal characteristics of F3 change. Future treatment focused on reducing the duration of this syllable and encouraging consistent use of word final "er" in conversational speech.

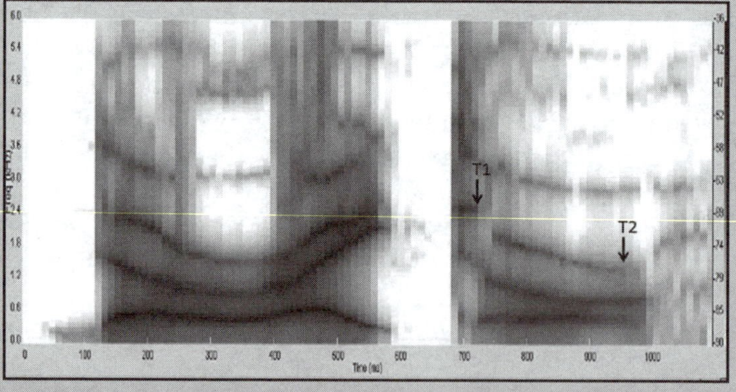

In this production, the F3 begins to fall 45 ms after the release of the [t]. T1 = 2563 Hz; T2 = 1489 Hz.

9. Audio files associated with these spectrograms can be accessed at http://www.medicine.mcgill/microp.

The phonemes /ɹ,ɝ,ɚ/ require close proximity of the first and second formants. Multiple articulatory configurations will produce this result but varying degrees of constriction are required in the pharyngeal and palatal areas (see Figures 10–2 and 1–3). The treating SLP (the first author) decided to focus on descent of the third formant as the goal. After he learned to produce these final syllables with a descending third formant as shown in the spectrograms taken from his treatment sessions, attention shifted to the temporal characteristics of the syllable (in fact, acoustic analysis revealed many unusual temporal characteristics in his speech including inappropriate syllable durations and unusually long stop gaps). Treatment sessions began with production of words and phrases with spectrographic feedback and ended with connected speech practice. Over time, the proportion of each session devoted to connected speech practice increased along with the length of the practice materials and the focus on self-monitoring. In Curt's case, many weeks of practice with spectrographic feedback were required before correct vocalic /ɚ,ɝ/ sounds were heard in his speech. More typically, clients will be younger with less severe impairments and one to three weeks of practice will be sufficient to establish these phones using this procedure. Spectrographic and waveform feedback can be used to practice vowel and fricative productions as well as aspects of prosody.

Treatment sessions began with production of words and phrases with spectrographic feedback and ended with connected speech practice in which self-monitoring was encouraged.

Stabilization of New Phonemes

After the child has learned to produce a new phoneme, therapy shifts to the goal of stabilizing production in utterances of increasing length and complexity. Following Van Riper (1978), a vertical goal attack strategy would be used to encourage practice of the target in syllables, words, phrases, and sentences. The child is expected to demonstrate automatic production at a high level of accuracy at each level of complexity before the next level is introduced. Within each level of complexity the SLP will usually begin with imitated productions and then proceed to spontaneous productions of the desired target structures. Principles of motor learning should be employed during practice sessions, being sure to maintain performance at the challenge point using the techniques listed in Table 10–3. Compared to the stimulation phase, the SLP will be shifting to less frequent knowledge of results feedback. Knowledge of performance feedback should not be required on a regular basis, perhaps only for a minute or two in prepractice activities as each new level is introduced.

The SLP will need to decide in advance how to introduce various word positions within the context of these levels. The traditional procedure is to systematically work through varied word positions early in the program, for example, if the target phoneme were /s/: (1) syllables, in order /sV/, /Vs/, /VsV/, /sVC/, /CVs/; (2) words,

After the child has learned to produce a new phoneme, therapy shifts to the goal of **stabilizing production** in utterances of increasing length and complexity.

A **vertical goal attack strategy** is traditionally used to encourage practice of the target in syllables, words, phrases, and sentences.

During the **stabilization phase**, the SLP should shift to less frequent knowledge of results feedback and knowledge of performance feedback should not be required on a regular basis.

The SLP will need to decide in advance the order in which to introduce various word positions.

prevocalic position, such as "soap," "sun"; (3) words, postvocalic position such as "mouse," "lace"; (4) words, intervocalic position such as "racing," "messy"; (5) phrases or patterned sentences such as "I like/don't like sardines/ice cream/salmon/sausage/lettuce//seaweed"; (6) complex words such as "necessary," "possible"; and (7) sentences such as "I bought 3 bars of soap at the pharmacy today" and "I like to eat ice cream sundaes with chocolate sauce." Some SLPs might even work the cluster contexts into this sequence, including /sCVC/ and CVCs/ syllables at the first level and introducing s-cluster words just prior to the patterned sentences level. An alternative to including all syllable positions in the sequence is to focus on a single word position from syllables through sentences with the expectation that learning at one position will spontaneously generalize to the untaught positions.

Generalization patterns across word positions is dependent on the child's pattern of substitution errors prior to treatment.

Forrest, Dinnsen, and Elbert (1997) observed that generalization patterns across word positions was dependent on the child's pattern of substitution errors prior to treatment. They described three patterns of consistency among 14 children with DPD. In some cases the child produced a consistent substitution for a given phoneme within and across word positions (CS group). Rvachew and Andrews (2002) found that this was a relatively rare pattern, occurring only 10% of the time. Examples of it in this book involve distortion errors such as that shown in Case Study 8–3 who produced /s/ → [θ] in all contexts (although note this child's speech accuracy was within normal limits overall). In a second pattern of error production, the child produced a predictable pattern that involved inconsistent substitutions across word positions (InAP group) that were consistent within word positions. This pattern is very common and is demonstrated in Case Study 6–2 (/v/ → [b] prevocalic, [w] intervocalic, and [s] postvocalic) and in Case Study 8–5 (/v/ → [w] prevocalic, [b] intervocalic and postvocalic). Some cases had no predictable substitutions within or across words positions (InWP). The child shown in Case Study 8–4 did not evidence consistent substitutions within word positions and could even be inconsistent within words ("pushing" → [pʊtɪŋ], [pʊɬɪŋ]). In a post hoc description of treatment outcomes for a study in which a minimal pairs approach was employed and in a prospective treatment study in which a traditional approach to intervention was implemented, different outcomes were observed depending on consistency of error pattern for the treated target (Forrest et al., 1997; Forrest, Elbert, & Dinnsen, 2000). Specifically, children in the CS group learned the treated sound (taught in a single word position) and generalized learning to untreated word positions. Children in the InAP group learned the treated sound in the treated word position but did not generalize to untreated word positions. Children in the InWP group did not learn the treated sound in treated or untreated word positions, echoing the very poor outcomes observed for PA221 over the 3 years of data shown in Case Study 8–4. These findings strongly suggest that different treatment approaches are required for these different groups of children (or targets).

First, those children that have a common error across all word positions and contexts (CS group) appear to be best suited to the traditional approach that is being described here, especially when the children present with residual speech errors on late developing phonemes such as /s/ →[s̪] or /θ/ → [f]. Given the excellent patterns of generalization across word positions described by Forrest and colleagues for these children it may not necessary however to systematically target the phoneme in all words positions. Rather, one could work through the levels—syllables, words, phrases, and sentences—at a single-word position and then probe to determine whether generalization was occurring to other syllable positions. If so, a treatment break with follow-up monitoring would be advisable. If generalization to the remaining syllable positions is not occurring there are two options. One repeats the sequence of levels, targeting the phoneme in a second syllable position. The other incorporates the other syllable positions into the sentence level without backtracking through all the simpler levels. The choice depends on the functional difficulty level of these alternative routes for the child. We are not aware of any randomized controlled trial evidence that establishes whether there is an efficiency or effectiveness advantage to these various options for ordering the practice stimuli. Theoretically, targeting all word positions at once (following Van Riper's original protocol) increases variability which is consistent with motor learning principles and may improve transfer of learning from the clinic to nonclinic situations. On the other hand, if the child is capable of phonological generalization from one word position to all the others there may be an efficiency advantage to focusing on one position at a time but this has not been established empirically.

The traditional approach that is described here appears to be best suited to phoneme targets that involve a consistent substitution or distortion error across all syllable/word positions.

Children in the InAP group, such as Amber, presented in Case Study 6–2, are not suitable candidates for the traditional approach because their error patterns are phonological in nature and usually involve multiple phonemes. For example, Amber delinked [+continuant] in prevocalic position, [Labial] in coda position, and [+consonantal] in the context of ambisyllabic voiced obstruents with some predictability. In cases such as this, multiphoneme approaches that target the interaction between feature and word position specifically are required. Procedures for treating children like Amber are presented in Chapter 11.

When the error patterns are inconsistent across syllable positions but consistent within syllable positions, multiphoneme approaches that target the interaction between feature and word position specifically are required.

Children in the InWP group appear to not benefit from traditional or phonological approaches, possibly because their underlying phonology is organized more at the level of the word than the phoneme or the problem is anchored in the more primary acoustic-phonetic and/or articulatory-phonetic domains. Some of these children may be diagnosed with apraxia of speech if they have significant difficulty with maximum performance tasks in addition to the extreme inconsistency in error patterns. Motor speech disorders are rare however and most children will not show clear evidence of motor speech disorder even though their AMR may be somewhat slow: in these cases the issue may be at a higher level of phonological

Children with highly inconsistent word productions appear to not benefit from traditional or phonological approaches, possibly because their underlying phonology is organized more at the level of the word than the phoneme or the problem is anchored in the more primary acoustic-phonetic and/or articulatory-phonetic domains.

planning and there may well be concomitant problems with phonological processing as described in Chapter 7. A multifaceted approach that targets acoustic-phonetic and articulatory-phonetic levels of representations is essential. The sensorimotor procedures to establish control of variability in nonsense syllable combinations as described earlier in this chapter may help to tune internal models. Focused stimulation procedures as described in Chapter 9 can be used to enhance acoustic-phonetic representations for words. Finally, a core vocabulary approach to encourage stability in the production of specific words is recommended (Crosbie, Holm, & Dodd, 2005; Iuzzini & Forrest, 2010). The core vocabulary approach is discussed further in Chapter 11.

Demonstration of Sound Stabilization Activities at the Patterned Sentence Level

Demonstration 10–5 shows alternative ways of implementing a stabilization activity at the patterned sentence level. In both cases the target is /f/ in the syllable onset but word internal position. In the first example, the activity is implemented as a drill activity in which the SLP writes sentences in the child's homework book and requests imitative responses from the child. Correct responses are rewarded with a token but tokens are removed when the child misarticulates the target. This kind of reinforcement system is referred to as a token economy because the tokens can be exchanged for something more interesting when sufficient tokens have been accumulated. The SLP reminds the child of the expected performance at the beginning of the session (good [f] with air blown across lip) but "knowledge of performance" feedback is not provided during the activity. The child is expected to monitor his own performance and make changes in response to the SLP's "knowledge of results" feedback. In fact this occurs as "redfish" is pronounced correctly without any extra stimulation after the incorrect response for "goldfish." The second demonstration implements a drill-play activity to achieve the same goal except that spontaneous rather than imitated responses are expected in this case. In this drill-play activity reinforcement for correct responses is built into the play context: the child keeps the fish when the sentences are produced correctly but are thrown back into the pond when the word "fish" is misarticulated. Again, the focus is on "knowledge of results" feedback. The SLP also takes every opportunity to provide repeated models of the target words in the course of natural conversation about the activity. In both examples, all speech errors not related to the target are ignored. Both activities involve the creation of a home practice activity. As discussed in Chapters 8 and 9, inclusion of the family in the treatment program is essential to a good outcome, especially when total intervention duration is rationed. However, the homework activities must complement the in-clinic goals and treatment approach and the parent must be well prepared to carry out the activities.

With a **token economy reinforcement** system the child earns tokens for correct responses (and may lose tokens for incorrect responses) and exchanges the tokens for something more interesting when sufficient tokens have been accumulated.

When implementing **drill-play** activities, natural reinforcement for correct responses is built into the play context.

During speech practice to stabilize new phonemes, all speech errors not related to the target are ignored.

Inclusion of the family in the treatment program is essential to a good outcome, especially when total intervention duration is rationed.

Homework activities must complement the in-clinic goals and treatment approach and the parent must be well prepared to carry out the activities.

Demonstration 10–5
Drill Versus Drill-Play Activity to Encourage Practice of Syllable-Initial, Within-Word /f/ at the Patterned Sentence Level

Patterned Sequence Activity Implemented as Drill

SLP: I am going to write some sentences in your homework book. After I read them, I want you to repeat the sentence. Each time I hear you say a good /f/ sound I am going to give you a token. But if you forget to blow the air across your lip I'm going to take a token back.

Child: What are the tokens for?

SLP: When we're done you can exchange them for baseball cards. You have to have 10 tokens to pick a card, OK?

Child: (nods)

SLP: (writes and reads) "I have a catfish."

Child: [ɑɪ hæbʌ kætfɪs]

SLP: That's it, here's a token. (writes and reads) "I have a goldfish."

Child: [ɑɪ hæbʌ goʊdbɪs]

SLP: Oops, that should be [goldfːɪs]. I'm taking this token back.

Child: Oh! That's not fair.

SLP: It's ok, I'll bet you can get it back with this one. (writes and reads) "I have a redfish."

Child: [ɑɪ hæbʌ wɛdfɪs]

SLP: Good one! You see, you earned it back. (gives token). (writes and reads) "Peter has a catfish."

Child: [pitə hæbʌ kætfɪs]

SLP: (gives token)

Child: That's two.

SLP: Yes, let's try the next one. (writes and reads) "Peter has a goldfish."

Patterned Sequence Activity Implemented as Drill-Play

SLP: You see the fish here in the sea. You get to catch them. If you can tell me what you have caught you can keep the fish. You can put them in this pail here. Later we will paste the fish in your homework book and you can tell your mom and dad what you caught. I want to hear you make a nice [fː] sound when you tell me what you have. Here is your fishing rod. Which one do you want to catch first?

Child: [ðæt kætfɪs]

SLP: Ok, see if you can get it.

Child: I caught it!

SLP: Ok, tell me what you caught, use a sentence, like this "I caught a . . ."

Child: [ɑɪ kɑɾə bɪg kætpɪs]

SLP: Oops, I didn't hear the nice [fː] sound. You have to throw him back.

Child: Oh no. But I'm gonna catch it again. Look.

SLP: Ok, what did you catch?

Child: [ɑɪ kɑɾə kætfɪs]

SLP: Excellent. Put it in the pail and then you can try to catch another fish. Which one this time?

Child: [ʌ wɛdfɪs]

SLP: I see you're trying to catch that redfish but it's trying to get away. You have to hold the fishing rod steady. Oh look, what did you do?

Child: [ɑɪ kɑɾə wɪdo wɛdfɪs]

SLP: Well said. Here's the fish pail. Now which one?

Child: [ə godfɪs]

SLP: OK, if you get it you will have three fish in your pail, a catfish, a redfish, and a goldfish.

In this example, the parent will need to understand that the goal is correct production of the /f/ and will need to be taught to ignore the errors that occur on the other phonemes. If this cannot be accomplished, stimulus items in the homework book will need to be structured to ensure that the child can produce the complete sentence correctly.

Empirical Support for the Traditional Approach to Sound Establishment and Stabilization

Empirical evidence that the traditional approach to speech therapy is effective, given sufficient cumulative intervention intensity, was presented in Chapter 9. Table 9–4 presents data from a randomized control trial in which small groups of children were treated with Van Riper's approach to speech therapy. Significantly higher speech accuracy for misarticulated phonemes on the McDonald Deep Test was observed for the treated children in comparison to outcomes for children who were not treated.

More recently, Günther and Hautvast (2010) demonstrated the effectiveness of the traditional approach in a non-experimental comparison groups study in which student SLPs provided therapy to three groups of 5-year-old German-speaking children with articulation disorder classified according to Dodd's assessment protocol (see Chapter 7). A wait-list control group received no intervention, a second group received the traditional intervention exactly as prescribed progressing through the ear training, stimulation, stabilization, and conversational speech stages, and a third group received a home program with contingency management in addition to the traditional therapy in the clinic. The children in the latter two groups received twice-weekly therapy for 8 weeks. The parents of the children in the third group were taught to use a token reinforcement system to reward homework completion: the children received stamps on special sheets such as a "reward snake" when they correctly articulated words during home practice sessions, which could be exchanged for mutually agreed upon rewards when the sheet was full. Study outcomes were measured as pre- to post-treatment change on probes of /s/ and /ʃ/ production accuracy in words and sentences with the results shown in Figure 10–3. It can be seen that the contingency management program to support home practice resulted in a higher mean score and reduced within-group variability in outcomes in comparison to the group that received the traditional approach in-clinic without the extra support for home practice. Both treated groups achieved significantly better outcomes than the wait-list comparison group. Between group differences in outcomes were also indicated by the percentage of children who were discharged from treatment after the 8-week intervention, specifically 40% in the second group versus 79% in the third group. Furthermore, outcomes were significantly correlated with minutes/week and frequency/week of reported homework completion in the treated groups.

Randomized control trials have established that the traditional approach to speech therapy is effective in comparison to a no-treatment control condition, with the effect enhanced by the addition of a structured home program.

The traditional approach comprises several elements and the DPD population is heterogeneous so it may be more useful to ask which specific elements of the approach are effective with which children? Specific elements of traditional speech therapy that may be considered independently are the procedures used during the ear training phase, the sound establishment phase, and stabilization phase as well as the vertical goal attack strategy that is a core feature of the traditional approach. Unfortunately, studies that examine these phases independently are rare and randomized control trials are rarer but some relevant research is reviewed here. Studies demonstrating that ear training is an essential element of the approach were reviewed in Chapter 9.

Ear training is an essential element of the traditional approach, as demonstrated in Chapter 9.

Procedures to establish a new sound in the child's repertoire are many and often the clinician will try several in an effort to elicit the target from the child. A few studies have examined the effectiveness

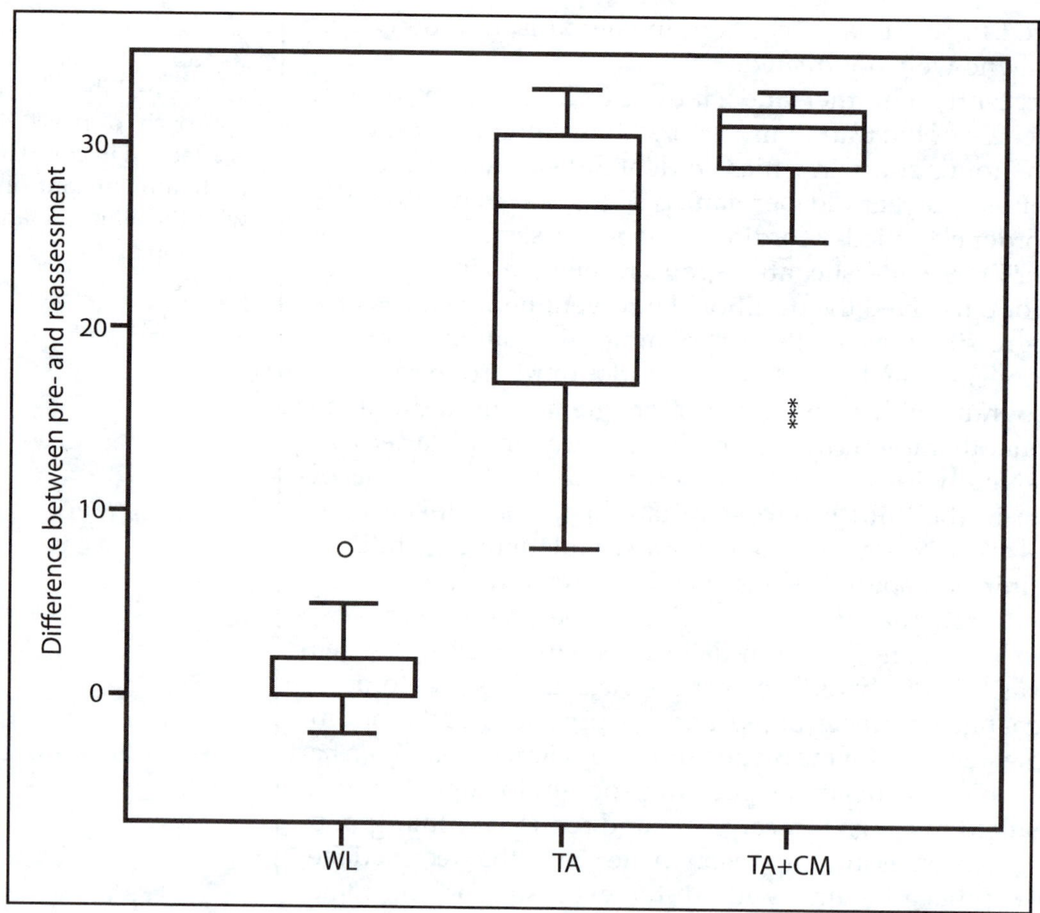

Figure 10–3. *Pre- to posttreatment improvement on target phoneme probes for the wait-list group (WL), the traditional articulation group (TA), and the contingency management group (TA+CM). The third group received traditional articulation therapy (TA) and used a token reinforcement system at home to reward performance during homework practice (CM), achieving the best outcome overall (see text for details).* Source: *From "Addition of Contingency Management to Increase Home Practice in Children with Speech Sound Disorder," by T. Günther and S. Hautvast, 2010,* International Journal of Language and Communication Disorders, *45(3), Figure 2, p. 350. Copyright 2010 by John Wiley & Sons, Inc. Reprinted with permission.*

In general, the research evidence supports the use of stimulation and phonetic placement techniques to establish new phones in the child's repertoire.

of including a phase of therapy where the SLP uses stimulation and phonetic placement in an uncontrolled fashion to elicit the target phonemes from the children, selecting procedures in response to the child's needs. Rvachew, Rafaat, and Martin (1999) examined the efficacy of ear training and stimulability training to enhance children's response to the cycles approach in a nonexperimental study. In the first year of the study, preschool-age children received 12 weeks of small group therapy modeled after the cycles approach (Hodson & Paden, 1983). Prior to the onset of the intervention the children's stimulability and perceptual knowledge of the target phonemes were assessed. Measurable improvements in production accuracy probes for these targets were observed if the child was stimulable for the sound and/or had good perceptual knowledge of the targeted phoneme category prior to treatment. When the child's speech perception performance for the target phoneme was poor or the child was unstimulable for the target, gains were unlikely to occur (forshadowing the findings of the randomized control trial conducted by Rvachew and Nowak, 2001, as described in Chapter 8). Overall, measurable gains in production accuracy were observed for only 40% of the phonemes that were targeted during the 12-week intervention. In the second year of this study, children received the same small group intervention except that the first three group sessions were replaced with individual therapy during which phonetic placement was used to ensure stimulability of treatment targets, and SAILS was used to ensure good perceptual knowledge of the target phonemes. Posttreatment, improved performance was observed for 80% of all treatment targets, regardless of pretreatment level of speech perception skills and stimulability.

More typically, research is focused on the implementation of specific procedures—those that are least likely to be used in the clinical setting! For example, Clark, Schwarz, and Blakeley (1993) describe a dental appliance that reshapes the maxillary arch so as to encourage a more posterior placement of the tongue during speech. Each appliance was constructed individually for each child in the study. They conducted a randomized controlled trial that demonstrated its usefulness in the establishment of /ɹ/. Although the procedure used in this study is not in common use in everyday clinical practice, the study is instructive. The device appears to have an effect that may be similar to certain more conventional phonetic placement techniques: it alters the sensory feedback that the child receives while talking, inhibits habitual tongue postures, and induces new patterns of articulation during production of /ɹ/. The participants in this study were school-age children who continued to misarticulate /ɹ/ after 6 months of traditional articulation therapy. The authors report that the children perceived the target but a natural voice discrimination task contrasting [ɹ]-[w] was used with only 85% correct responding required to demonstrate adequate perceptual knowledge of /ɹ/ and thus, given the inadequacy of the assessment method used, we would say that it is uncertain that the children's perceptual knowledge of the target was sufficient to support acquisition of [ɹ]. Four groups of children received two 15-minute treatment sessions per week for 6 weeks during which they practiced /ɹ/ in isolation, syllables, and words: two groups received the appliance, whereas two did not; in one of each of these groups, clinicians provided audiovisual stimulation by modeling expected responses during therapy; such models were not provided in the remaining two groups (in these latter groups the children were told to produce "the target" or printed stimuli were used to evoke the expected responses). The groups that practiced with the appliance made the best progress during therapy sessions, achieving correct production of the target within 30 minutes on average, regardless of whether they received audiovisual models of the target or not. However, carryover to conversation was only observed in the group that practiced with the appliance while receiving audiovisual models before each trial. The treatment protocol was carefully structured to ensure practice of /ɹ/ in a variety of vowel contexts and words positions and practice conditions were alternated so that the child mastered each step of the program with the appliance in place and then without the appliance before advancing to the next step. It seems that the children in this group were able to establish a new articulatory gesture that resulted in an acoustic output that matched the model provided by the clinician. Practice in varied contexts with appropriate feedback led to changes in internal models, allowing for generalization of learning from the drill tasks to conversational speech. The children in the two groups that did not receive the appliance did not learn to produce a good /ɹ/ or learned it too late to experience much practice with the new articulatory gesture. The children who did not receive clinician models prior to their own attempts at the target may have been lacking information essential for the effective operation of supervised learning mechanisms, in particular experience with the generation of corrective feedback commands in response to error signals that serve to tune the forward model. Overall, in spite of the unusual device applied in this study, the results validate standard techniques used during stimulability training, specifically, the provision of audiovisual models of the target and phonetic placement techniques to encourage new articulatory gestures in an effort to achieve the target sound. The authors also concluded that vocal exploration is a key factor in the learning of a new phoneme and the R-appliance is designed to encourage active discovery of new tongue postures and articulatory movements.

The conditions under which it is necessary to stabilize new phoneme production at a high level of accuracy in a hierarchical and sequential progression of steps organized according to word position and task complexity have not been empirically established.

The next element to consider is stabilization of the new phoneme in a hierarchical and sequential progression of steps organized according to word position and task complexity, with fairly high levels of performance expected at each step before moving from one level to the next. As discussed in Chapter 8, it is not clear that it is necessary to practice each phoneme until the child has achieved 90% accuracy in sentences or conversation over several sessions in order to ensure transfer and maintenance. First, studies have shown that children can transfer correct production of a new phoneme, taught in isolation or syllables, to untaught words, sentences, or even conversation (Clark et al., 1993; Mire & Montgomery, 2008; Powell & McReynolds, 1969). Furthermore, several studies have indicated that performance levels between 40 and 75% correct, even at the word level, are associated with further spontaneous gains on the part of the child. The proportion of older children with residual distortion errors who regress remains about 20% regardless of whether direct treatment is terminated when the children achieve 75% or 90% correct responding on single words or in conversation (Diedrich & Bangert, 1980). Altogether, these studies suggest that one might be able to provide a brief but intense intervention that establishes production of a new phoneme at the word level and then either introduce other phonemes that require intervention or place the child on treatment rest while monitoring to ensure further spontaneous gains toward the achievement of age-appropriate phonological competence. We caution, however, that children with certain subtypes of DPD will require continued practice in many linguistic contexts and speaking situations before mastery is achieved (e.g., children with lateral lisps or motor speech disorders).

The use of a **vertical goal attack strategy** is another element that may also be advisable for only some children—those children who present with a specific residual distortion error for example.

A **horizontal or cycles goal attack strategy** is likely to be more efficient with children who have multiple phoneme errors.

The use of a vertical goal attack strategy is another element that may also be advisable for only some children—those who present with a specific residual distortion error for example. A horizontal or cycles goal attack strategy is likely to be more efficient with children who have multiple phoneme errors. Klein (1996) conducted a retrospective chart review of outcomes for 4-year-old children with moderate or severe primary DPD. Outcomes were examined for the children who received traditional therapy compared to the children who were treated with phonological approach. The children in the two treatment conditions were matched for age and severity of their speech deficit at treatment onset. The traditional intervention included procedures such as ear training, phonetic placement, provision of models for imitation, and practice at increasing levels of complexity beginning with isolated sounds or syllables. The phonological intervention did not include ear training or phonetic placement; rather, multiple phonemes were taught at once and minimal pairs or imagery procedures were used to target phonological rules in the children's underlying phonology. Klein reported that children receiving phonological therapy achieved better speech outcomes after 13 months of therapy than children receiving traditional therapy for 22 months. This study is a nonexperimental design however and it is possible that the outcomes reflect differences in the children that led the clinicians to choose different approaches at the outset.

A more compelling demonstration of the efficiency advantage to the phonological approach was provided by Pamplona, Ysunza, and Espinoza (1999) who randomly assigned children with cleft palate to receive a traditional approach to therapy or a phonological approach to remediation of their compensatory articulation errors. The children received one-hour therapy sessions twice per week. Two examiners who were blind to treatment condition assessed each child in the study every three months until both agreed that the child's speech errors were completely resolved. A significant difference in time to resolution of the speech deficit was observed between groups: a median of 29 months for children receiving traditional therapy versus 13.5 months for children receiving phonological therapy.

To conclude, the specific procedures incorporated into the traditional approach have been shown to be effective and the approach as a whole is more effective than no treatment. For many children with multiple speech sound errors, however, a more efficient result will be obtained with a phonological approach (typically involving a horizontal or cycles goal attack strategy and a focus on phonological contrasts rather than individual phonemes).

Ongoing Refinements to Achieve Adultlike Speech Accuracy and Precision

10.4.1. List 13 strategies for promoting carryover.

10.4.2. Describe four strategies for promoting maintenance of precision and accuracy over the long-term for children with motor speech disorders.

The final stage of phonological development is characterized by a long period of gradual refinement.

Increased **consistency** with which certain phonemes are produced results in improved accuracy.

Increased **stability** in the achievement of speech motor goals results in improved precision.

Segmental consistency and motor stability do not always align.

The final stage of phonological development is characterized by a long period of gradual refinement that is marked by two progressive changes that promote enhanced speech intelligibility: (1) increased consistency with which certain phonemes are produced, resulting in improved accuracy and (2) increased stability in the achievement of speech motor goals, resulting in improved precision. We have previously pointed out that segmental consistency and motor stability do not always align, as shown in a study where children's production of prosodically complex utterances was described using phonetic transcription and kinematic measures (Goffman, Gerken, & Lucchesi, 2007). In this study, segment variability was vulnerable to complexity in the underlying hierarchical prosodic structure of the utterances, whereas motor stability was not influenced by these phonological variables. On the other hand, syllable prominence impacted segment variability and motor stability conjointly suggesting effects that were linked in the more primary phonetic domains. Therefore, we can consider segment variability and motor stability to be dissociable processes and discuss them separately.

Increased Segmental Consistency

As we discussed in Chapter 4, it is not clear to what extent the achievement of segmental consistency is a gradual process in normal speech development. Figures 4–6 and 4–7 illustrate cross-sectional data for the achievement of individual phonemes (/ʃ/ and /s/, respectively) and give the impression of very gradual increases in accuracy between 5 and 9 years of age. However, as we further indicated in Chapter 4, rare longitudinal investigations suggest that individual children acquire speech sounds quite rapidly (Hoffman, Schuckers, & Daniloff, 1980). The first author vividly remembers her daughter reading aloud a Dr. Seuss book in kindergarten and suddenly asking "Where is the 'f' in 'think'?" After explaining that there was no [f] in the word "think" because the first sound was in fact [θ], corresponding to the letters "th," her substitution of [f] for /θ/ resolved itself within the course of 48 hours. Although some of our clients struggle for months to achieve sound accuracy and to transfer new skills to connected speech (as in Demonstration 10–4), sudden mastery of new phonemes is quite common in clinical practice as well as normal phonological development. For example, Powell and McReynolds (1969) carefully monitored transfer of /s/ to untrained words at each step of a traditional therapy program provided to 4 children, aged 4 to 6 years, who evidenced no correct productions of this phoneme prior to treatment. Two of the four children generalized to words at or before the end of the nonsense syllable level of the sound establishment phase (in fact, one of these children was beginning to generalize after /s/ was established in isolation). These cases of rapid diffusion of a new phoneme throughout the child's system reflect generalization processes that are operating at the level of the child's underlying phonological knowledge. Rapid acquisition of a new phoneme will occur in many children when the treatment program addresses the children's absent or imperfect underlying representations for the segmental or prosodic structures at the acoustic-phonetic, articulatory-phonetic, and phonological levels. Most often, this will require the application of phonological approaches, to be discussed in Chapter 11, in combination with input- and output-oriented procedures.

Rapid diffusion of a new phoneme throughout the child's system reflects generalization processes that are operating at the level of the child's underlying phonological knowledge.

Given that some children transfer learning of a new phoneme from words to conversation and from clinic to home so readily, why is it that some clinicians find transfer of training to be such a struggle? Mowrer (1971) addressed this question when he reported that three-quarters of SLPs responding to large-sample surveys ranked carryover of a sound to spontaneous speech as their "most serious clinical problem." Unfortunately, the remedies proposed probably contributed more to the problem than the solution. At the time, researchers were promoting the transformation of traditional speech therapy, which Van Riper presented as a sensorimotor approach, into a behaviorist regimen via the application of programmed instruction techniques (Gray, 1974; Mowrer, 1989). From the perspective of phonological or motor learning, these programs had many elements that worked against the goal of ensuring carryover and thus a formal transfer and maintenance phase of the therapy program was required. The more efficient practice is to structure the establishment phase of the therapy program to promote spontaneous transfer and thus we discuss the more problematic aspects of the "machine learning" approach with the aim of deterring SLPs from adopting these counterproductive procedures.

At a time when behaviorist approaches to speech therapy were being promoted, three-quarters of SLPs responding to large-sample surveys ranked carryover of a sound to spontaneous speech as their "most serious clinical problem."

A key feature of behaviorist approaches is the structuring of the teaching sequence to ensure "errorless learning." Teaching steps are organized to lead the child in very small steps from the simplest skill toward the terminal goal (for example, practicing [i], [is], [s], [si] are each separate steps in a multistep sequence that eventually

A key feature of behaviorist approaches is the structuring of the teaching sequence to ensure "errorless learning."

terminates with [s] produced within complete sentences, according to a programmed learning program called the S-Pack. An associated requirement is that each "skill to be learned must be thoroughly mastered before the client can advance to the next task" (Mowrer, 1989, p. 179). For example, the Monterey Articulation Program requires 20 consecutive correct responses before the child can progress from one step to another (Gray, 1974). Notice how inconsistent this practice is with the notion of the challenge point in motor learning. The motor learning research shows clearly that a large amount of practice with one specific skill does indeed result in good performance during the practice session but very poor transfer of training to new movements and new contexts (Maas et al., 2008). We have recommended that task difficulty be set so that the child is essentially on the brink of failure: able to succeed but with approximately 20% error occurring so that experience with error correction allows for the tuning of forward models. When the task becomes too easy and the child is overpracticing a learned response, the complexity of the context or the task should be immediately increased as outlined in Table 10–3.

Behaviorist approaches also required overpractice of each step of the program before allowing the child to progress to the next step, a procedure that is inconsistent with the challenge point framework.

When the task becomes too easy and the child is overpracticing a learned response, the complexity of the context or the task should be immediately increased so that the child is practicing at the challenge point.

By definition a behavioral approach to therapy places control of the child's articulation accuracy in the hands of the SLP—"those who control the consequences of the behavior control the frequency of the behavior (p. 161)" is the succinct fashion in which Mowrer (1989) expressed this idea. As the behaviorists were explicitly opposed to "ear training" and the SLP was fully responsible for controlling the consequences of correct and incorrect productions of the target sound, the child was made dependent on the clinician for maintaining a high level of correct responding. The children were not provided with sufficient phonological knowledge of the target to spontaneously employ self-directed supervised learning mechanisms in the acquisition of the phoneme. And given that the SLP could not follow the child into all speaking situations, poor carryover and regressions after treatment dismissal were highly probable. It is no accident that SLPs using this approach were having difficulty with transfer of training. The motor learning approach espoused here does require the clinician to provide feedback after child responses; however, good acoustic-phonetic knowledge of the target should be established and the feedback should be delayed as in summative feedback or not provided on every trial. In other words the feedback schedule should give the child a chance to independently compare output to target and engage corrective mechanisms, empowering the child to take responsibility for learning and transfer.

By definition a behavioral approach to therapy places control of the child's articulation accuracy in the hands of the SLP.

Good acoustic-phonetic knowledge of the target should be established and the feedback schedule should give the child a chance to independently compare output to target and engage corrective mechanisms, empowering the child to take responsibility for learning and transfer.

Another characteristic of the behaviorist approach as implemented in the 1970s was a marked reduction in variability of the practice materials (relative to the therapy sessions described by Van Riper in his earlier appearing texts). A token economy and imitative drills were the order of the day. However, variability in form of the response (response length, phonetic context, prosodic contours, pragmatic function, etc.) is another essential component of an effective motor learning program. Some researchers are experimenting with the use of spinners and other devices to introduce variability in response form into the treatment session (Skelton, 2004). Drill-play activities offer the opportunity for the natural introduction of variability however as one can imagine for the activity shown in Demonstration 10–5. Both phrases and sentences are elicited in the course of the activity and there is the potential for different intonation patterns to emerge when the child is delighted to catch a fish or disappointed to lose one. The SLP can ask questions in different ways to encourage shifting prosodic contours (What did you do? I CAUGHT a redfish. Did you catch a goldfish? No, I caught a CATFISH! How many fish did you catch? I caught one, two, THREE fish.). Embedding speech practice in naturalistic or seminaturalistic contexts also meets one of the helpful behaviorist principles for promoting transfer and that is increasing similarity between the practice context and the transfer context. If one expects the child to say the word "soup" correctly during lunch, it makes sense to practice the word in the context of an activity that evokes the concept of a meal-time routine. However, the behaviorist notion that the response [sup] is conditioned by the stimulus cues for "eating soup" is a nightmare scenario for the SLP. It is not possible to practice all the "s" words in the contexts in which they will appear! Transfer of training is governed by processes internal to the child and linked to the quality of his or her acoustic-phonetic, articulatory-phonetic, and phonological representations.

Variability in form of the response (response length, phonetic context, prosodic contours, pragmatic function, etc.) is another essential component of an effective motor learning program.

Embedding speech practice in naturalistic or seminaturalistic contexts promotes transfer by increasing similarity between the practice context and the transfer context.

Transfer of training is governed by processes internal to the child and linked to the quality of his or her acoustic-phonetic, articulatory-phonetic, and phonological representations.

In the event that no transfer of learning from in-clinic drill to extraclinic conversation occurs, special procedures will need to be implemented to ensure carryover. One procedure that has been shown to be effective is teaching the child to monitor and record correct productions of the target in his or her own speech. Koegel, Koegel, and Ingham (1986) demonstrated that 6- to 10-year-old children with residual distortions of /s/ or /ɹ/ could learn to self-monitor within two treatment sessions. In this single-subject multiple baseline study, the children were first taught to produce the target phoneme(s) using a behaviorist approach in isolation, words, phrases, and sentences (imitatively, then spontaneously) to a criterion of 20 consecutive correct responses. This part of the treatment constituted the baseline phase and lasted between 1 month and 2 years depending on the child's rate of progress. At this point, the self-monitoring intervention was introduced for some children and phonemes but delayed for others in accordance with the multiple baseline across children design. In-clinic practice with the target continued at the conversational level in parallel with the self-monitoring intervention. The self-monitoring intervention consisted of teaching the child to mark a "+" on a recording sheet for each correct self-production of the target during conversation (ignoring

One procedure that promotes transfer of training is teaching the child to monitor and record correct productions of the target in his or her own speech.

incorrect productions). The child was expected to carry the recording sheets with them at home and school and record correct productions more-or-less continuously in conversational or narrative contexts. If the child brought the sheets to therapy sessions and the child's teacher and parent confirmed that the child was completing the task as instructed, the "+" marks could be exchanged for a promised event (e.g., pizza outing for 1,000 marks). The outcome measure was percentage of correct productions during conversation with a stranger; these generalization assessments occurred on a monthly basis throughout the study for each of 13 children. Figure 10–4 shows the results for one child but similar findings were reported for the remaining participants: no carryover was observed during the baseline (reinforcing the points we made above about the behaviorist approach) but rapid transfer was observed after self-monitoring was implemented. The authors describe the carryover period as being rapid but gradual because the children's initial efforts to produce the target in extraclinic conversations were "labored" but natural sounding speech was often achieved within

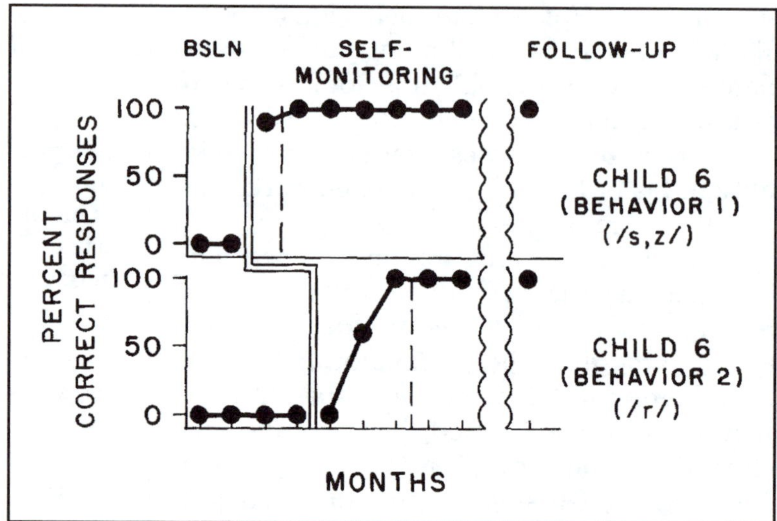

Figure 10–4. *Individual data on monthly generalization probes for a 7-year-old boy who received programmed speech therapy for two targets. Points represent percent correct production of the target during conversation with a stranger in the natural environment. Baseline covers the period during which the child was taught to produce the target in isolation, words, phrases and sentences by the SLP. Double-lines indicate initiation of self-monitoring of target production in conversational and reading-aloud contexts at home and school. Dashed lines indicate time when child stopped carrying the self-monitoring data sheets. Curly brackets indicate 3-month summer break.* Source: From *"Programming Rapid Generalization of Correct Articulation through Self-Monitoring Procedures," by L. K. Koegel, R. L. Koegel, and J. C. Ingham, 1986,* Journal of Speech and Hearing Disorders, 51, *Figure 3, p. 30. Copyright 1986 by American Speech-Language-Hearing Association. Reprinted with permission.*

a month. The authors note that subsequent to this experiment they implemented the procedure with wrist counters.

This procedure requires a certain amount of metalinguistic skill on the part of the child. With preschoolers we have had success teaching children to monitor the accuracy of specific words if the child is too young to grasp the notion of a speech sound. As discussed in Chapter 9, we teach children as young as 4;0 to make judgments about the accuracy of other's speech but this skill may not automatically carry over to self-monitoring. Spontaneous self-corrections on the part of the child should be reinforced and active self-monitoring may need to be taught. Van Riper (1978) actually recommended teaching self-monitoring directly upon completion of the ear training phase, in parallel with the early levels of sound establishment. It was only with the introduction of the programmed learning approach that self-monitoring was moved to the end of the treatment program, to occur in a defined "transfer" phase of the treatment program. We would agree, however, that asking the child to monitor conversation in the extraclinic environment should be introduced cautiously and only when the child is sure to achieve a reasonable level of success, both with correct production in connected speech and the self-monitoring task itself. We also prefer to limit self-monitoring to prescribed periods of time in the natural environment because we are not quite sure how continuous self-monitoring contributes to the goal of achieving automaticity in speech production. The parent and SLP need to think carefully about the appropriate time for this activity. On the one hand, it is best that the child not have the parent's full and undivided attention; the context should not be too much like regular speech practice time when the parent focused full attention on listening to and correcting the child's speech when completing homework exercises; rather the context should be more like regular conversation in the hurly-burly of everyday family life. On the other hand, the topic of the conversation should not be too important or emotionally laden; if, on the drive home from kindergarten each day, the child is likely to share information about exchanges with the class bully this would not be a good time for either party to be focusing on the form of the child's speech. Later, when mum is preparing the evening meal she could put a bowl of pennies on the kitchen counter so that the child can take one each time he hears himself produce a good /s/ sound. He can make a game of thinking of ways to work as many into the conversation as possible in a 10 minute period. We have included the promotion of self-monitoring on our list of tips for promoting carryover in Table 10–5.

Self-monitoring at the level of the phoneme requires a certain amount of metalinguistic skill on the part of the child and is best implemented with school-aged children.

With preschoolers we have had success teaching children to monitor the accuracy of specific words if the child is too young to grasp the notion of a speech sound.

Spontaneous self-corrections on the part of the child should be reinforced and active self-monitoring may need to be taught.

Van Riper recommended teaching self-monitoring directly upon completion of the ear training phase, in parallel with the early levels of sound establishment.

We prefer to limit self-monitoring to prescribed periods of time in the natural environment because we are not quite sure how continuous self-monitoring contributes to the goal of achieving automaticity in speech production.

Increased Motor Stability

The development of speech motor control continues well past the age at which the child achieves perceptually accurate speech sound

Table 10–5. *Tips to Promote Carryover*[a]

1. Ensure that the child has a good acoustic-phonetic representation for the target.
a. Use ear training procedures (see Chapter 9).
b. Provide auditory models of the target during the establishment phase.
2. Use a phonological approach to therapy when appropriate (see Chapter 11).
3. Apply principles of motor learning during the establishment phase.
a. Maintain performance level during practice at the "challenge point"(see Table 10–3).
b. Do not "overpractice." Practice with variable stimuli at multiple levels in a single session.
c. Provide knowledge of performance feedback during a prepractice "warm-up."
d. Provide intermittent, summative or delayed feedback of results during the practice activity.
4. Plan for stimulus generalization.
a. Reduce difference between treatment and natural environment.
b. Plan activities that provide naturalistic reinforcement for correct use of target.
c. Include family members and school personnel in the treatment program.
5. Empower the child to take responsibility for carryover.
a. Teach the child to self-monitor early in the treatment program (after "ear training").
b. Reinforce spontaneous self-corrections when they occur.
c. Prescribe brief but regular periods of self-monitoring in the extraclinic environment.

[a]Carryover is used here as a generic term referring to generalization of a taught phoneme from practiced contexts to unpracticed contexts (e.g., syllables to sentences, taught words to untaught words, prevocalic position to postvocalic position) as well as transfer of learning from the clinic to extraclinic settings (e.g., drill-play with SLP in the therapy room to conversation with Dad at home). Phonological generalization (from taught phonemes to other untaught phonemes) are discussed in Chapter 11.

production. Although the overall coordinative infrastructure for speech resembles the adult form in early childhood, children's articulatory movements are characterized by smaller displacements, longer durations, lower velocities, and greater variability than those observed in young adults. Gradual refinement toward adult values for displacement, duration, velocity, and variability continues past the age of 16 years. As we pointed out in Chapter 3, the higher levels of variability observed in lower order coordinative structures throughout childhood may provide flexibility to the system. Flexibility is required so that the child can adapt to ongoing developments in other domains including vocal tract structure, neurophysiological function, cognitive load, and linguistic knowledge. It is possible that children with DPD will have difficulty adapting to these future challenges however, perhaps accounting for regressions in speech accuracy. Therefore, monitoring children who have been discharged from direct intervention to ensure that they maintain the gains that they have achieved is an important step in the

Children with DPD may have difficulty adapting to future challenges such as developmental changes in vocal tract structure, neurophysiological function, cognitive load, and linguistic knowledge, accounting for regressions in speech accuracy after speech therapy is terminated.

speech therapy program. Children with the more severe disorders may need to return to speech therapy periodically if they need help maintaining speech accuracy in the face of increased expectations for language competence as they progress through school.

Callan, Kent, Guenther, and Vorperian (2000) developed a computational model based on DIVA (see Chapter 3 for description and discussion) to simulate maintenance of acoustic vowel targets despite developmental vocal tract restructuring between 3 and 45 months of age. The simulation demonstrated that the key to adapting to dramatic changes in vocal tract morphology was prior underlying knowledge of the acoustic-phonetic targets and practice with self-produced auditory feedback. The model shows that children will have to develop new motor plans as they grow older to achieve the same acoustic-phonetic targets. Slowness to adapt may result in the reappearance of distortion errors that were previously resolved although fluctuating frequencies of distortion errors with the child's age may also reflect variations in adult expectations for speech clarity (Munson, Edwards, Schellinger, Beckman, & Meyer, 2010). In any case, traditional therapy procedures implemented according to the principles of motor learning can be effective to help older children achieve precision in phoneme production. The practice materials must reflect the higher language production competence expected of the child, given his or her grade in school. Once again, it is critical to not omit the ear training step. In Chapter 9, ear training procedures and the SAILS error detection task focused at the single word level. When working with older children, complex sentence level material can be prepared for misarticulation judgments. If, for example, a group of Grade 5 children was working together to "tune up" their [ɹ], they could take turns recording complex sentences that the SLP has prepared to ensure appearance of the target in various prosodic positions ("The St. Louis Blues signed former New Jersey Devils star player, Jason Arnott, to a one-year contract yesterday." And "Arnott is a veteran forward who will be a valuable addition to our club said Blues General Manager Doug Armstrong."). The students can deliberately read them at different rates and levels of clarity. The following week the students can listen to them (presented in random order) and discuss the correctness of the [ɹ] targets in each sentence (guessing the talker will be part of the fun). It may be advisable to promote a "graded" scoring system in this case (Likert or visual analog scale) because many of the productions may not be clearly correct or incorrect. The process of listening for the targets, identifying them in running speech and discussing the quality of their production will be valuable in and of itself. Incorporating auditory models as well as self-monitoring into speech practice exercises is also important. Learning Fundamentals markets a product that allows self-practice of all commonly misarticulated consonants in English (e.g., Articulation IV: R, S, L, Th by LocuTour Multimedia on CD-ROM). The software presents a picture along with a printed and spoken sentence as the stimulus;

Traditional therapy procedures implemented according to the principles of motor learning can be effective to help older children achieve precision in phoneme production in the context of increasingly complex linguistic material.

Ear training and self-monitoring exercises are important components of the maintenance phase of the speech therapy program.

the client records their imitated response and then compares their own production to the model. The sentences are long enough to be appropriate for middle school children and usually contain multiple target forms (e.g., "The future looks bright for these students"). Progressing from these exercises to self-monitoring in longer passages of connected speech and then to the school environment, perhaps with group members supporting each other at this stage, is the final step.

Demonstration of a Plan to Promote Maintenance of Speech Accuracy

Children with apraxia of speech may need more comprehensive individualized attention as they progress through school given that they will have difficulty with language and reading in addition to speech accuracy. Let us image for example that you are monitoring a child who achieved age appropriate articulation test performance in third grade. In sixth grade he is concerned because half of his science grade is based on a term project requiring a model of a volcano, a written report, and an oral report at year-end. His individualized education plan allows him to type the report given his difficulties with handwriting and he has in-class support from an aide who will provide scaffolding for the development of the written report. He is very nervous about the oral presentation however. He knows that he will stumble over the difficult words in this context because he tends to omit weak syllables when he is nervous and speaking too quickly. Not only does the report involve words that are complex from the articulatory point of view, he sometimes mixes them up, saying "tectano" when he means "volcano" or "tectonic." Finally, he tends toward a monotone speaking style in class presentations that reduces his effectiveness. You could reinstitute individual therapy and reprise exercises targeting weak syllable deletion and prosody using the procedures described in Ballard et el. (2010, see Figure 10–1 in this chapter and associated discussion). We think it would be much more appropriate, however, to create a home or school program that focuses directly on the term project and student's specific concerns. We have presented some ideas for such a program in Demonstration 10–6.

Conclusions and Recommendations

There are a variety of procedures for helping children achieve improvements in the accuracy and precision of their speech but the common factor is the promotion of intense practice with feedback.

In this chapter we have presented a variety of procedures for helping children achieve improvements in the accuracy and precision of their speech. The common factor among all the procedures has been the promotion of intense practice with feedback: self-produced sensory feedback as well as feedback provided by the SLP according to motor learning principles. For children with very limited productive output, some procedures to encourage free vocal exploration across all speech parameters were provided. For children with

Demonstration 10–6
Proposed School Program to Prepare Student for Final Term Project: Oral Presentation on Plate Tectonics

1. **Word Level Articulation Practice with Flashcards**	
Instructional Objective:	Student will spontaneously produce vocabulary items with 100% segmental accuracy given variable cues.
Activity and therapy agent(s):	Student will create his own flash cards covering all of the difficult vocabulary to be covered in his report and producing three cards with different types of cues on each card, e.g., (1) Illustration: Photo of volcano; (2) Question: What is a landform where molten rock erupts through the surface of the planet? (3) Completion Prompt: The Mauna Loa is the world's largest active ______. (with 3 similar cards for each additional word—tectonic plate, magma, subduction, etc.). Student will shuffle the cards in random order and practice responding to the cards with his parents.
Feedback:	Student sorts cards into correct and incorrect piles with parental confirmation. Student tracks number in incorrect pile each day.

2. **Question and Answer to Vary Prosody**	
Instructional Objective:	Student will answer questions with 80% correct prosodic contours.
Activity and therapy agent(s):	CDA will ask questions that prompt vocabulary use in complete sentences with varying prosodic contours. e.g., Q: Does ice flow out of volcanoes? A: No, MAGMA flows out of volcanoes. Q: Do volcanoes form when continents collide? A. No, volcanoes form when TECTONIC PLATES collide. Does subduction cause a whirlpool? No, subduction causes a VOLCANO.
Feedback:	100% knowledge of performance feedback; use integral stimulation hierarchy to elicit repetition of each incorrect response with improved performance.

3. **Production of Difficult Vocabulary in Questions and Statements in Pragmatically Complex Context**	
Instructional Objective:	Student will respond quickly to prompts in competitive context with a correctly produced sentence or question (grammar, prosody, vocabulary, and articulation to be monitored).
Activity and therapy agent(s):	Classroom teacher will organize competitive team games among class members that include the target vocabulary and concepts. Suggested games include Jeopardy and Pantomime style competitions. CDA observes.
Feedback:	Summative feedback in private after the game has been completed. Compare CDA and student perspective on student's accuracy.

4. Accurate Production of Sentences in Oral Report	
Instructional Objective:	90% accurate production of segments and prosodic contours when producing sentences in the final oral report at varying speech rates.
Activity and therapy agent(s):	Student practices the sentences using Speech Analyzer with assistance from SLP. A spinner is used to determine if the sentence will be spoken at a slow, medium, or fast rate on each trial.
Feedback:	Student and SLP discuss performance after viewing spectrogram and wave form feedback of each sentence.
5. Accurate Production of Oral Report	
Instructional Objective:	90% accurate production of segments and prosodic contours when presenting the oral report to a selected audience.
Activity and therapy agent(s):	Student practices the oral report in front of pairs of listeners (e.g., parents, CDA and SLP, siblings, selected peers). Begin at slow rate and gradually increase to normal presentation style speaking rate.
Feedback:	Student identifies errors and rates performance from videotape of each practice effort. SLP offers advice as needed.

larger phonetic repertoires but limitations in the volitional control of speech output, an approach to the establishment of control in the production of nonsense syllable sequences and early words based on templates mirroring those sequences was presented. Techniques for eliciting new phonemes were described and the traditional approach to speech therapy was outlined. When implementing these procedures it was recommended that the SLP manipulate the conditions of practice, vary the stimuli, and control the feedback schedule in such a way as to ensure that the child is practicing new skills "at the challenge point." The challenge point can be determined by raising functional task difficulty so that the child's level of performance is high but even a small additional increase in task difficulty would result in a marked decline in performance.

It has been established that traditional therapy is more effective than no speech therapy at all.

Randomized controlled trials have established that ear training is effective and there is good reason to believe that stimulation and phonetic placement techniques are helpful in the establishment of new phonemes.

A vertical goal attack strategy and the systematic stabilization of sound production in syllables, words, phrases, and sentences is not the most efficient strategy in all cases.

In terms of the empirical foundation for these approaches to speech therapy, it has been established that traditional therapy is more effective than no speech therapy at all. The individual components of the traditional approach have also received research attention. Randomized controlled trials have established that ear training is effective and there is good reason to believe that stimulation and phonetic placement techniques are helpful in the establishment of new phonemes. A vertical goal attack strategy and the systematic stabilization of sound production in syllables, words, phrases, and sentences is not the most efficient strategy in all cases. As we discussed earlier the choice of treatment approach may depend on the nature of the child's error patterns. Typically, treatment approaches have been linked to apparent subtypes of children so that the traditional approach might be recommended for children with a "phonetic disorder," "articulation disorder," or a "speech error" diagnosis. However, taking a developmental approach, we would suggest that the intervention approach chosen depends on the nature of the child's error patterns and phase of the child's phonological disorder. Given that DPD changes in nature with age and severity, it is likely that multiple approaches will be appropriate with a single child over time. One can imagine a child in the "speech delay—genetic" category benefitting from focused stimulation as a toddler, requiring ear training procedures in combination with a phonological approach as a preschooler, and then returning to speech therapy in school when a traditional approach to remediate a lingering error on a late developing phoneme may well be the most appropriate choice. Similarly, a child in the "motor speech disorder—apraxia of speech" category may benefit from vocal play approaches as a toddler, the sensorimotor approach as a preschooler, a phonological approach in kindergarten, and the traditional approach as a school-age child depending on the way in which his or her speech error patterns change with development. There is no approach that is best for all children or even any one child. However, attention to underlying phonological representations will be required for any child presenting with multiple speech errors. We turn to phonological learning in the next and final chapter.

The choice of treatment approach may depend upon the nature of the child's error patterns and phase of the child's phonological disorder.

Given that DPD changes in nature with age and severity, it is likely that multiple approaches will be appropriate with a single child over time.

References

Adler-Bock, M., Bernhardt, B., Bacsfalvi, P., & Gick, B. (2005). Perceptual, acoustic, and tongue shape measures during /r/ production pre- and post-treatment using visual feedback from ultrasound: Case studies of two adolescents. *Journal of the Acoustical Society of America, 117*(4), 2605.

Adler-Bock, M., Bernhardt, B., Gick, B., & Bacsfalvi, P. (2007). The use of ultrasound in remediation of North American English /r/ in 2 adolescents. *American Journal of Speech-Language Pathology, 16*, 128–139.

Allen, M. M. (2009). *The impact of treatment intensity on a phonological intervention*. Paper presented at the American-Speech-Language and Hearing Association Conference in New Orleans, LA.

Arvedson, J., Clarke, H., Lazarus, C., Schooling, T.L., & Frymark, T. (2010). Evidence-based systematic review: Effects of oral motor interventions on feeding and swallowing in preterm infants. *American Journal of Speech-Language Pathology, 19*, 321–340.

Ballard, K. J., Robin, D. A., & McCabe, P. (2010). A treatment for dysprosody in childhood apraxia of speech. *Journal of Speech, Language, and Hearing Research, 53*, 1227–1245.

Bernhardt, B. (2004). *Evaluating ultrasound as a visual feedback tool in speech therapy.* Paper presented at the American Speech-Language-Hearing Association, Philadelphia, PA.

Bernhardt, B., Gick, B., Bacsfalvi, P., & Adler-Bock, M. (2005). Ultrasound in speech therapy with adolescents and adults. *Clinical Linguistics & Phonetics, 19*(6/7), 605–617.

Bloom, K (1988). Quality of adult vocalizations affects the quality of infant vocalizations. *Journal of Child Language, 15*(3), 469–480.

Callan, D. E., Kent, R. D., Guenther, F. H., & Vorperian, H. K. (2000). An auditory-feedback-based neural network model of speech production that is robust to developmental changes in the size and shape of the articulatory system. *Journal of Speech, Language, and Hearing Research, 43*, 721–738.

Cameron, J., Pierce, W. D., Basko, K. M., & Gear, A. (2005). Achievement-based rewards and intrinsic motivation: A test of cognitive mediators. *Journal of Educational Psychology, 97*(4), 641–655.

Clark, C. E., Schwarz, I. E., & Blakeley, R. W. (1993). The removable R-appliance as a practice device to facilitate correct production of /r/. *American Journal of Speech-Language Pathology, 2*, 84–92.

Crosbie, S., Holm, A., & Dodd, B. (2005). Intervention for children with severe speech disorder: A comparison of two approaches. *International Journal of Language and Communication Disorders, 40*(4), 467–491.

Curtis, J. F., & Hardy, J. C. (1959). A phonetic study of misarticulation of /r/. *Journal of Speech and Hearing Research, 2*(3), 244–257.

Dagenais, P. A., Critz-Crosby, P., & Adams, J. B. (1994). Defining and remediating persistent lateral lisps in children using electropalatography: Preliminary findings. *American Journal of Speech-Language Pathology, 3*(3), 67–76.

Dethorne, L. S., Johnson, C. J., Walder, L., & Mahurin-Smith, J. (2009). When "Simon Says" doesn't work: Alternatives to imitation for facilitating early speech development. *American Journal of Speech-Language Pathology, 18*, 133–145.

Diedrich, W. M., & Bangert, J. (1980). *Articulation learning*. Houston, TX: College-Hill Press.

Dusing, S. C., & Harbourne, R. T. (2010). Variability in postural control during infancy: Implications for development, assessment, and intervention. *Physical Therapy, 90*(12), 1838–1849.

Dworkin, J. P. (1978). A therapeutic technique for the improvement of lingua-alveolar valving abilities. *Language, Speech, and Hearing Services in Schools, 9*, 169–175.

Ernest, M. M. (2000). *Preschool motor speech evaluation and intervention*. Bisbee, AZ: Imaginart.

Forrest, K. (2002). Are oral-motor exercises useful in the treatment of phonological/articulatory disorders? *Seminars in Speech and Language, 23*(1), 15–25.

Forrest, K., Dinnsen, D. A., & Elbert, M. (1997). Impact of substitution patterns on phonological learning by misarticulating children. *Clinical Linguistics & Phonetics, 11*, 63–76.

Forrest, K., Elbert, M., & Dinnsen, D. A. (2000). The effect of substitution patterns on phonological treatment outcomes. *Clinical Linguistics & Phonetics, 14*, 519–531.

Fucci, D. (1972). Oral vibrotactile sensation: an evaluation of normal and defective speakers. *Journal of Speech and Hearing Research, 15*, 179–184.

Fucci, D., Petrosino, L., Underwood, G., & Kendal, C. (1992). Differences in lingual vibrotactile threshold shifts during magitude-estimation scaling between normal-speaking children and children with articulation problems. *Perceptual & Motor Skills, 75*, 495–504.

Gierut, J., Morrisette, M. L., & Ziemer, S. M. (2010). Nonwords and generalization in children with phonological disorders. *American Journal of Speech-Language Pathology, 19*, 167–177.

Gildersleeve-Neumann, C. E. (November 6, 2007). Treatment for childhood apraxia of speech. *ASHA Leader*. Retrieved from http://www.asha.org/Publications/leader/2007/071106/f071106a.htm

Goffman, L, Gerken, L, & Lucchesi, J. (2007). Relations between segmental and motor variability in prosodically complex nonword sequences. *Journal of Speech, Language, and Hearing Research, 50*, 444–458.

Goldstein, M. H., King, A. P., & West, M. J. (2003). Social interaction shapes babbling: Testing parallels between birdsong and speech. *Proceedings of the National Academy of Sciences, 100*(13), 8030–3035.

Goodwyn, S. W., Acredolo, L. P., & Brown, C. A. (2000). Impact of symbolic gesturing on early language development. *Journal of Nonverbal Behavior, 24*(2), 81–103.

Goozée, J. V., Murdoch, B., Ozanne, A., Cheng, Y., Hill, A., & Gibbon, F. (2007). Lingual kinematics and coordination in speech-disordered children exhibiting differentiated versus undifferentiated lingual gestures. *International Journal of Language and Communication Disorders, 42*, 703–724.

Gray, B. B. (1974). A field study on programmed articulation therapy. *Language, Speech, and Hearing Services in Schools, 5*, 119–131.

Green, J. R., Moore, C. A., Higashikawa, M., & Steeve, R. W. (2000). The physiologic development of speech motor control: Lip and jaw coordination. *Journal of Speech, Language, and Hearing Research, 43*(1), 239–255.

Guadagnoli, M. A., & Lee, T. D. (2004). Challenge point: A framework for conceptualizing the effects of various practice conditions in motor learning. *Journal of Motor Behavior, 36*, 212–224.

Guenther, F. H., & Vladusich, T. (2009). A neural theory of speech acquisition and production. *Journal of Neurolinguistics.* doi:10.1016/j.jneuroling.2009.08.006.

Günther, T., & Hautvast, S. (2010). Addition of contingency management to increase home practice in children with speech sound disorder. *International Journal of Language and Communication Disorders, 45*, 345–353.

Hagiwara, R., Meyers Fosnot, S., & Alessi, D. M. (2002). Acoustic phonetics in a clinical setting: case study of /r/-distortion therapy with surgical intervention. *Clinical Linguistics & Phonetics, 16*, 425–444.

Harbourne, R. T., Willett, S., Kyvelidou, A., Deffeyes, J., & Stergiou, N. (2010). A comparison of interventions for children with cerebral palsy to improve sitting postural control: A clinical trial. *Physical Therapy, 90*(12), 1881–1898.

Hodge, M. M. (2010). Developmental dysarthria intervention. In A. L. Williams, S. McLeod, & R. J. McCauley (Eds.), *Interventions for speech sound disorders in children* (pp. 557–578). Baltimore, MD: Brookes.

Hodson, B. W. (2007). *Evaluating and enhancing children's phonological systems: Research and theory to practice*. Wichita, KS: Phonocomp Publishers.

Hodson, B. W., & Paden, E. P. (1983). *Targeting intelligible speech: A phonological approach to remediation.* Boston, MA: College-Hill.

Hoffman, P. R., Schuckers, G. H., & Daniloff, R. G. (1980). Developmental trends in correct /r/ articulation as a function of allophone type. *Journal of Speech and Hearing Research, 23*, 746–756.

Iuzzini, J., & Forrest, K. (2010). Evaluation of a combined treatment approach for childhood apraxia of speech. *Clinical Linguistics & Phonetics, 24*, 335–345.

Kent, R. D. (1982). Contextual facilitation of correct sound production. *Language, Speech, and Hearing Services in Schools, 13*, 66–76.

Kent, R. D., & Read, C. (1992). *Introduction to the study of speech acoustics*. San Diego, CA: Singular.

Klein, E. S. (1996). Phonological/traditional approaches to articulation therapy: A retrospective group comparison. *Language, Speech, and Hearing Services in Schools, 27*(4), 314–323.

Koegel, L. K., Koegel, R. L., & Ingham, J. C. (1986). Programming rapid generalization of correct articulation through self-monitoring procedures. *Journal of Speech and Hearing Disorders, 51*(1), 24–32.

Kouri, T. A. (2005). Lexical training through modeling and elicitation procedures with late talkers who have specific language impairment and development delays. *Journal of Speech, Language, and Hearing Research, 48*, 157–171.

Ladefoged, P. (1996). *Elements of acoustic phonetics* (2nd ed.). Chicago, IL: University of Chicago Press.

Ling, D. (1976). *Speech and the hearing-impaired child: Theory and practice*. Washington, DC: Alexander Graham Bell Association for the Deaf.

Lundeborg, I., & McAllister, A. (2007). Treatment with a combination of intra-oral sensory stimulation and electropalatography in a child with severe developmental dyspraxia. *Logopedics Phoniatrics, 32*, 71–79.

Maas, E., Robin, D. A., Austermann Hula, S. N., Freedman, S. E., Wulf, G., Ballard, K. J., & Schmidt, R. A. (2008). Principles of motor learning in treatment of motor speech disorders. *American Journal of Speech-Language Pathology, 17*, 277–298.

Masterson, J. J., & Rvachew, S. (1999). Use of technology in phonology intervention. *Seminars in Speech and Language, 4*, 233–250.

McAuliffe, M. J., & Cornwell, P. L. (2008). Intervention for lateral /s/ using electropalatography (EPG) biofeedback and an intensive motor learning approach: A case report. *International Journal of Language and Communication Disorders, 43*(2), 219–229.

McDonald, E. T. (1964). *Deep Test of Articulation: Picture Form*. Pittsburgh, PA: Stanwix House.

McDonald, E. T. (1964). *Articulation testing and treatment: A sensory motor approach*. Pittsburgh, PA: Stanwix House.

McNutt, J. C. (1977). Oral sensory and motor behaviors of children with /s/ or /r/ misarticulations. *Journal of Speech and Hearing Research, 20*, 694–704.

Mire, S. P., & Montgomery, J. K. (2008). Early intervening for students with speech sound disorders: Lessons from a school district. *Communications Disorders Quarterly, 30*(3), 155–166.

Morgan Barry, R. A. (1989). EPG from square one: An overview of electropalatography as an aid to therapy. *Clinical Linguistics & Phonetics, 3*, 81–91.

Mowrer, D. E. (1971). Transfer of training in articulation therapy. *Journal of Speech and Hearing Disorders, 36*, 427–446.

Mowrer, D. E. (1989). The behavioral approach to treatment. In N. A. Creaghead, P. W. Newman, & W. A. Secord (Eds.), *Assessment and remediation of articulatory and phonological disorders* (2nd ed., pp. 161–192). New York, NY: Macmillan.

Munson, B., Edwards, J., Schellinger, S. K., Beckman, M. E., & Meyer, M. K. (2010). Deconstructing phonetic transcription: Covert contrast, perceptual bias, and an extraterrestrial view of Vox Humana. *Clinical Linguistics & Phonetics, 24*, 245–260.

Netsell, R. (1985). Construction and use of a bite-block for the evaluation and treatment of speech disorders. *Journal of Speech and Hearing Disorders, 50*(1), 103–106.

Pamplona, M. C., Ysunza, A., & Espinoza, J. (1999). A comparative trial of two modalities of speech intervention for compensatory articulation in cleft palate children: Phonological approach versus articulatory approach. *International Journal of Pediatric Otorhinolaryngology, 49*, 21–26.

Pannbacker, M. (1988). Management strategies for developmental apraxia of speech: A review of literature. *Journal of Communication Disorders, 21*(5), 363–371.

Pigott, R. E., & Shapiro, D. C. (1984). Motor schema: The structure of the variability session. *Research Quarterly for Exercise and Sport, 55*, 41–45.

Powell, J., & McReynolds, L. (1969). A procedure for testing position generalization from articulation training. *Journal of Speech and Hearing Research, 12*(3), 629–645.

Pratt, S. R., Heintzelman, A. T., & Deming, S. E. (1993). The efficacy of using the IBM Speech Viewer Vowel Accuracy Module to treat young children with hearing impairment. *Journal of Speech and Hearing Research, 36*, 1063–1074.

Romski, M. A., Sevcik, R. A., Adamson, L. B., Cheslock, M., Smith, A., Barker, R. M., & Bakeman, R. (2010). Randomized comparison of augmented and nonaugmented language interventions for toddlers with developmental delays and their parents. *Journal of Speech, Language, and Hearing Research, 53*(2), 350–364.

Rosenbek, J. C., Lemme, M. L., Ahern, M. B., Harris, E. H., & Wertz, R. T. (1973). A treatment for apraxia of speech in adults. *Journal of Speech and Hearing Disorders, 38*(4), 462–472.

Rowe, M. L., & Golden-Meadow, S. (2009). Early gesture selectively predicts later language learning. *Developmental Science, 12*, 182–187.

Ruscello, D. M. (2009). Nonspeech oral motor treatment issues related to children with developmental speech sound disorders. *Language, Speech, and Hearing Services in Schools, 39*, 380–391.

Rvachew, S., & Andrews, E. (2002). The influence of syllable position on children's production of consonants. *Clinical Linguistics & Phonetics, 16*(3), 183–198.

Rvachew, S., & Nowak, M. (2001). The effect of target selection strategy on sound production learning. *Journal of Speech, Language, and Hearing Research, 44*, 610–623.

Rvachew, S., Rafaat, S., & Martin, M. (1999). Stimulability, speech perception and the treatment of phonological disorders. *American Journal of Speech-Language Pathology, 8*, 33–34.

Secord, W. E., Boyce, S. E., Donahue, J. S., Fox, R. A., & Shine, R. E. (2007). *Eliciting sounds: Techniques and strategies for clinicians* (2nd ed.). Clifton Park, NY: Cengage Learning.

Shea, C. H., & Wulf, G. (2005). Schema theory: A critical appraisal and reevaluation. *Journal of Motor Behavior, 37*, 85–102.

Shine, R. E. (1989). Articulatory production training: A sensory motor approach. In N. A. Creaghead, P. W. Newman, & W. A. Secord (Eds.),

Assessment and remediation of articulatory and phonological disorders (2nd ed.). New York, NY: Macmillan.

Shriberg, L. D. (1975). A response evocation program for /r/. *Journal of Speech and Hearing Disorders, 40*, 92–105.

Shriberg, L. D. (1980). An intervention procedure for children with persistent /r/ errors. *Language, Speech, and Hearing Services in Schools, 11*, 102–110.

Shuster, L. I. (1998). The perception of correctly and incorrectly produced /r/. *Journal of Speech, Language, and Hearing Research, 41*, 941–950.

Shuster, L. I., Ruscello, D. M., & Toth, A. R. (1995). The use of visual feedback to elicit correct /r/. *American Journal of Speech-Language Pathology, 4*(2), 37–44.

Sjögreen, L., Màr, T., Kiliaridis, S., & Lohmander, A. (2010). The effect of lip strengthening exercises in children and adolescents with myotonic dystrophy type 1. *International Journal of Pediatric Otorhinolaryngology, 74*, 1126–1134.

Skelton, S. L. (2004). Concurrent task sequencing in single-phoneme phonologic treatment and generalization. *Journal of Communication Disorders, 37*(2), 131–155.

Sommers, R. K., Cox, S., & West, C. (1972). Articulatory effectiveness, stimulability, and children's performances on perceptual and memory tasks. *Journal of Speech and Hearing Research, 15*, 579–589.

Stokes, S. F., & Griffiths, R. (2010). The use of facilitative vowel contexts in the treatment of post-alveolar fronting: a case study. *International Journal of Language and Communication Disorders, 45*, 368–380.

Strand, E. A., & Debertine, P. (2000). The efficacy of integral stimulation intervention with developmental apraxia of speech. *Journal of Medical Speech-Language Pathology, 8*(4), 295–300.

Strand, E. A., & Skinder, A. (1999). Treatment of developmental apraxia of speech: Integral stimulation methods. In A. Caruso & E. A. Strand (Eds.), *Clinical management of motor speech disorders in children* (pp. 109–148). New York, NY: Thieme.

Terband, H., Maassen, B., Guenther, F. H., & Brumberg, J. (2009). Computational neural modeling of speech motor control in Childhood Apraxia of Speech (CAS). *Journal of Speech, Language, and Hearing Research, 52*, 1595–1609.

Terband, H., Maassen, B., van Lieshout, P., & Nijland, L. (2011). Stability and composition of functional synergies for speech movements in children with developmental speech disorders. *Journal of Communication Disorders, 44*, 59–74.

Van Riper, C. (1978). *Speech correction: Principles and methods*. Upper Saddle River, NJ: Prentice-Hall.

Velleman, S. L., & Strand, K. (1994). Developmental verbal apraxia. In J. Bernthal & N. W. Bankson (Eds.), *Child phonology: Characteristics, assessment, and intervention with special populations* (pp. 110–139). New York, NY: Thieme.

Vereijken, B. (2010). The complexity of childhood development: Variability in perspective. *Physical Therapy, 90*(12), 1850–1859.

Vihman, M. M., & Velleman, S. L. (2000). The construction of a first phonology. *Phonetica, 57*, 255–266.

Williams, P. (2009). The Nuffield Centre Dyspraxia Programme Third Edition (NDP3). In C. Bowen (Ed.), *Children's speech sound disorders* (pp. 269–275). Chichester, UK: Wiley-Blackwell.

Williams, P., & Stephens, H. (2010). The Nuffield Centre Dyspraxia Programme. In A. L. Williams, S. McLeod, & R. J. McCauley (Eds.), *Interventions for speech sound disorders in children* (pp. 159–177). Baltimore, MD: Brookes.

Wolpert, D. M., Ghahramani, Z., & Flanagan, J. R. (2001). Perspectives and problems in motor learning. *Trends in Cognitive Sciences, 5*(11), 487–494.

Chapter 11

Phonological Approaches to Intervention

In Chapter 10 we introduced the idea that the SLP may need to select and sequence different treatment approaches to correspond to the status of the child's knowledge across multiple levels of representation as the child progresses through intervention. By definition, a child with DPD will require an intervention that attends to their underlying knowledge of the phonological system of their language at some point in their developmental trajectory. Furthermore, as we indicated in Chapter 10, phonological approaches to intervention with these children are typically more efficient than the traditional approach to articulation therapy. As with traditional approaches, however, phonological approaches encompass a variety of procedures, and their application may be determined by the child's specific developmental needs.

By definition, a child with DPD will require an intervention that attends to their **underlying knowledge of the phonological system** of their language at some point in their developmental trajectory.

Phonological approaches to intervention are typically more **efficient** than the traditional approach to articulation therapy.

Phonological approaches encompass a variety of procedures, and their application may be determined by the child's specific developmental needs.

In Chapter 4 we traced the child's phonological development from first words through to the achievement of adultlike phonological knowledge. The earliest stage of phonological development is characterized by whole-word representations with the child's goal being to achieve a greater number of expressive word forms with closer proximity to adult targets while preserving lexical contrast so as to achieve maximum communicative effectiveness despite limitations at the level of the child's acoustic-phonetic and articulatory-phonetic representations for words. Ferguson and Farwell (1975) concluded their study of early phonological development by stating "that a phonic core of remembered lexical items and articulations which produce them is the foundation of an individual's phonology, and remains so throughout his entire linguistic lifetime" (p. 437). Therefore, there can be no sharp demarcation between a "whole-word" stage and a "phoneme-based" stage of phonological

The earliest stage of phonological development is characterized by **whole-word representations**.

As the child's vocabulary grows and the **lexicon self-organizes** to reflect the child's phonetic knowledge of the constituent word forms, phonological knowledge emerges at multiple levels of the phonological hierarchy.

During the school-age period, explicit **meta-phonological abilities** develop and permit acquisition of reading and spelling skills.

knowledge. However, as the child's vocabulary grows and the lexicon self-organizes to reflect the child's phonetic knowledge of the constituent word forms, phonological knowledge emerges at multiple levels of the phonological hierarchy. In keeping with the principles of dynamic systems theory (see Introduction to Part I), incremental changes in phonetic knowledge lead to an apparent discontinuity that reflects the emergence of this phonological knowledge. Shortly after the vocabulary spurt that occurs during infancy, the toddler's speech patterns become more predictable; subsequently, successive restructurings of phonological knowledge as new features and prosodic elements are mastered result in adultlike accuracy and intelligibility. During the school-age period, ongoing increases in vocabulary size, accumulations of phonetic and phonological knowledge and formal teaching allow the child explicit access to their phonological knowledge of these units; meta-phonological skills in turn permit the acquisition of reading and spelling skills. These three phases of phonological development, shown in Table 11–1 and illustrated in Plate 8, organize our discussion of procedures for facilitating phonological development in children with DPD.

Word-Based Phonology

11.1.1. Describe the characteristics of children who might benefit from the core vocabulary approach.

11.1.2. Identify the goal of the core vocabulary approach and describe the procedures that are used to achieve this goal.

Children with DPD are likely to be experiencing **heterochronous rates of development** so that the child might have quite a large lexicon and yet appear to be relying on word-based representations.

When the phonological system is organized for **lexical contrast**, the child may show excessive rigidity in speech patterns or excessively variable speech output.

In normal development, children whose phonological knowledge is limited to the level of lexical contrast will typically have very small vocabulary sizes and may produce emerging lexical forms with a great deal of variability as shown in Figures 4–1 and 4–2. Children with DPD however are likely to be experiencing heterochronous rates of development in semantic, acoustic-phonetic and articulatory-phonetic representations so that the child might have quite a large lexicon and yet appear to be relying on word-based representations. Some children at this stage may show excessive rigidity, for example, in the form of consonant-vowel co-occurrence patterns or preferred word templates that are highly resistant to change (e.g., see Case Study III–1). Other children at this stage may produce excessively variable speech output, with error patterns that are inconsistent within word positions, as described by Forrest, Dinnsen, and Elbert (1997, see Chapter 10).

Case Study 11–1 presents some data taken from a free speech sample provided by research subject PA214 who was assessed as part of a 3-year follow-up of English-speaking children receiving

Table 11–1. *Learning Mechanisms and Environmental Supports in the Natural Environment and Therapeutic Procedures for the Development of Phonological Knowledge in the Clinical Environment*

Learning Mechanisms	*Environmental Supports*	*Therapeutic Procedures*	*Expected Outcomes*
1. Word-Based Phonology and Emerging Phonological Structure			
Word-learning mechanisms Linkage of acoustic-phonetic, articulatory-phonetic, and semantic representations Selection and adaptation to templates	High quality language input provided in a social context Social supports for the child's use of spoken language	Core vocabulary	Increased proximity of spoken words to adult targets Increased phonetic repertoire Increased repertoire of word shapes Increased consistency in word production
2. Successive Reorganizations of Phonological Structure in Lexical Representations Lead to Mature System			
Social learning mechanisms Cognitive learning mechanisms Phonological working memory Linkage of phonetic, phonological, and semantic representations Linkage of lexical items with shared phonological structure	Support for lexical growth and complexity Support for increasingly complex language use	Target phonological classes Target phonological contrasts Meaningful minimal contrast procedure	Increased consistency in phonological patterns Decreased used of immature phonological patterns Emergence of new features and prosodic structures Increased match ratios for features and word shapes
3. Explicit Access to Phonological Structure			
Lexical restructuring triggered by growing size of lexicon and increasingly detailed acoustic-phonetic representations	Exposure to high quality language input Exposure to print materials Exposure to rime and alliteration Explicit teaching of print concepts Explicit teaching of prereading skills Explicit teaching of reading	Metaphonological procedures embedded in phonological therapy sessions Emergent literacy interventions Explicit interventions for phonological awareness, decoding, and spelling	Continuing growth in the size of lexicon and complexity of vocabulary knowledge Narrative skills Emerging phonological awareness skills Literacy skills

intervention for DPD. The words shown were selected from a sample recorded when he was 59 months old and presented with moderately impaired phonological skills. Highly inconsistent and often unusual patterns of phonological error are readily apparent in the sample. First, we show that he produces words inconsistently across repeated productions, even for words composed of simple syllable shapes and early developing phones such as "baby." He also produces a number of unusual syllable shape mismatches. Recall

Case Study 11–1
Selected Speech Sample Data Recorded from an Appropriate Candidate for the Core Vocabulary Approach (Research Participant PA214)

Prekindergarten Test Results (CA = 4;11)

SAILS (Phonemic Perception of /k/, /l/, /s/, /ɹ/)	61% (*z* = −2.53)
Goldman-Fristoe Test of Articulation-2	4th percentile
Percent Consonants Correct (in conversation)	58% (*z* = −2.81)
Peabody Picture Vocabulary Test	SS = 107
Mean Length of Utterance	2.76
Phonological Awareness Test	Raw score = 11 (*z* = −2.28)
Letter Name Knowledge	Raw score = 8

Selected Words from Prekindergarten Speech Sample

Inconsistent Within Word Productions	"baby" → [bebi], [ebi], [bevi]
	"glove" → [pɑt], [dʒʌdʒ]
	"dog"→ [dɑt], [dɑ], [dɑʊd] , [dɑn]
	"elevator"→ [eʊtedɚ], [vetɚ], [eʊgedɚ] , [eʊde]
Unusual Word Shape Mismatches	"going" → [bwoɪn]
	"riding" → [bɹaɪdɪŋ]
	"elevator"→ [ɛʊde]
	"picture"→ [pɪdʒ]
Manner Class Confusions	"wagon"→ [vædə]
	"telephone"→ [tɛvəfon]
	"pulling away"→ [pʌwɪŋ ʌve]
	"shovel"→ [fʌwə]
	"look"→ [hʊk]
	"balloons"→ [bɹunz]
	"doors"→ [dots]
	"running"→ [ɹʌvɪŋ]

Place Confusions		Vowel Errors	
	"cup"→ [tʌp]		"playing" → [pɛvi]
	"carrot"→ [tɛɹɪt]		"pulling" → [puwi]
	"taking"→ [tevi]		"reading" → [ɹaitɪŋ]
	"scissors" → [pvɪvə]		"trying" → [teɪvi]
	"quack" → [tʃæ]		

from Chapter 4 that certain syllable shape mismatches are common such as cluster reduction, final consonant deletion, and the deletion of unfooted weak syllables. These types of patterns do occur inconsistently in his speech alongside less common patterns such as deletion of weak syllables within a trochee and the addition of consonants to singleton onsets. With respect to consonant features, he has unstable knowledge of manner contrasts with confusions of approximants and obstruents in both directions. Further confusions within those classes are apparent with a clear differentiation between stops/fricatives/affricates not established, for example. Finally, place of articulation is frequently confused with an apparent preference for labial place of articulation. Two patterns are sometimes associated with apraxia of speech according to standard criteria (see Table 7–3): the inconsistency of errors for phonemes within words and the misarticulation of a phoneme in the target position of one word occurring alongside the inappropriate appearance of the same phone or phone combination in another word where it is not expected (e.g., "brush" → [ʌtʃ] despite "riding" → [bɹaɪdɪŋ]). However, the oral-peripheral examination revealed no clear indications of motor speech disorder in this case whereas evidence of phonological processing difficulties was unmistakable. During the prekindergarten assessment, he scored below normal limits for phonemic perception and implicit phonological awareness (his ability to identify misarticulated words or match words on the basis of shared rime or onset was no better than chance). When tested in first grade his nonword decoding score was 15 points (one standard deviation) lower than his sight word reading score. Therefore, his profile is more suggestive of Inconsistent Phonological Disorder as described by Dodd and outlined in Chapter 7. Crosbie, Holm, and Dodd (2005) attribute this subtype to difficulties at the level of phonological planning—selecting and ordering phonological units, as illustrated in Plate 5 (see level referred to as phonological encoding). They suggest that degraded motor programs for speech account for inconsistent speech output. We agree that these children have difficulty generating consistent feed-forward commands for speech but suggest that uncertain acoustic-phonetic targets for words and poor processing of auditory feedback during speech practice plays a key role in the genesis of the phonological encoding difficulties that some children experience.

Case Study 11-1 is an example of **inconsistent phonological disorder** and presents with a profile suggestive of *phonological planning difficulties.*

Crosbie et al. (2005) further recommend a unique form of intervention for this subtype relative to children with phonological delay or consistent phonological disorder. Standard phonological approaches would require targeting a feature (e.g., [Dorsal]) or phonological pattern (e.g., consonant sequences) but these goals assume a roughly adultlike structure to the child's underlying phonological knowledge. If the child's underlying phonological knowledge is organized at the whole word level such an approach would probably have a very poor outcome. The alternative intervention that is suggested for this subtype is the core vocabulary approach.

The **core vocabulary** approach is the recommended treatment for children with *inconsistent phonological disorder.*

Core Vocabulary Approach

We have previously demonstrated that lexical and phonological development are closely linked in early language development (e.g., Girolametto, Pearce, & Weitzman, 1997; see Chapter 9). When children have very small vocabularies, focused stimulation procedures can be used to increase the size of the child's lexicon and phonological structure will emerge as the child's store of linked acoustic-phonetic and articulatory-phonetic representations enlarges and the lexicon self-organizes. Here we have a different situation where the lexicon is already large but badly organized. You can imagine the disorder if your office contained a 10-year accumulation of patient files, labeled with a photo of the child, and arranged in stacks by hair color and gender because you had no knowledge of an alphabetic filing system. Someone could teach you the alphabet and how to file but you would not be able to put this information to good use until you had recovered the name of each child, clearly linked the names in your memory to each photo, and then written the names in alphabetic script on the outside of each file. Similarly, in the case of children with inconsistent phonological disorder, it is not helpful to try to teach them the phonological rules of the language without first stabilizing their phonetic knowledge of the individual items in their lexicon. For these children it is necessary to practice whole words and to focus on lexical rather than phonological contrast.

The core vocabulary approach is described as the targeting of consistency rather than accuracy in the production of a core set of functional vocabulary items chosen individually for the child.

The core vocabulary approach is described as the targeting of consistency rather than accuracy in the production of a core set of functional vocabulary items chosen individually for the child (Crosbie et al., 2005; Dodd & Bradford, 2000). The intervention begins with the parent selecting important vocabulary items for the child that will be used frequently in everyday communication. A set of approximately 50 words is recommended and we feel that it is wise to include multiple parts of speech beyond nouns on the list. The SLP then selects a small subset of the words as an initial starting point and determines a target pronunciation for each word based on the child's phonetic inventory and best pronunciation during practice trials. For example, acceptable pronunciations were listed as "grandma" → [gwænma], "banana" → [bænana], and "sandwich" → [sænwɪs] for a 3-year-old boy with a restricted phonetic repertoire. The SLP then drills production of the words in therapy sessions using segmentation and chaining techniques and cued articulation (linking elements of the word to letters, pictograms, or hand signs that are subsequently used to cue inclusion of all elements during production attempts). When consistent production is achieved at the word level, practice shifts to the phrase level and the child is expected to produce the word with consistent articulation in extraclinic environments. Parents and teachers are taught to continue practice of those words with daily drills and to reinforce consistent production of the words in everyday conversation. At that point, new words are introduced into in-clinic drills. When consistency is fully established, the word is withdrawn from practice and new words are introduced. One unique (and untested) aspect of the procedure is that imitation is avoided "since imitation provides a phonological plan that inconsistent children can use without having to generate their own plan for the word. Instead, the SLP provided information about the plan" (Crosbie et al., 2005, p. 481). We are somewhat uncomfortable with this aspect of the intervention on theoretical grounds, given the importance of auditory targets to the learning of feedforward commands (see DIVA model, Figure 3–15 and associated discussion) and on empirical grounds, given that treatment without models has been shown to be less effective than the use of models in a randomized control trial (Clark, Schwarz, & Blakeley, 1993; see discussion in Chapter 10). Given our sense that these children often lack sufficient detail in their acoustic-phonetic representations for the words, we would modify the approach to ensure a period of focused stimulation with the target words before requiring productive use in drill-play activities. Furthermore, we would be sure to produce a correct version of the word *after* the child's attempts at least some of the time (as is the typical procedure during focused stimulation), taking into account new research findings suggesting that postproduction stimulation by the adult can be more powerful than the provision of models for imitation as a teaching technique in both bird and infant vocal learning (Goldstein, Schwade, Menyhart, & DeVoogd, 2011). We have suggested some activities and provided an imagined therapeutic exchange based on this approach that would be helpful for PA214 in Demonstration 11–1.

Demonstration 11–1

Demonstration 11–1 suggests activities for implementing the core vocabulary approach that begin with the child's name. Let's imagine in this case that his name is Josh and his sister's name is Kelly. We can be sure (see Case Study 11–1) that these words will be difficult and inconsistently produced and yet they will be high priority items for him and his family to tackle first. The words are also convenient because the consonants comprise a range of manner classes: an affricate, a fricative, a stop, and a liquid. His responses to GFTA items indicate that he is stimulable for the constituent phonemes or at least has close equivalents: /dʒ/ in "pajama" → [dʒæmə], /s/ in "knife" → [naɪs], /g/ in "frog" → [pɹɔg], and /l/ in "ball" → [bɔl]. Therefore, the activity for the first few weeks will focus on these two names with /dʒɑs]/ and /kɛli/ being acceptable pronunciations. However, in our adaptation the first week will be devoted to providing auditory bombardment; focused stimulation and dialogic reading techniques will be used to elicit productions in subsequent weeks. The parents will need specific teaching to differentiate "listening" and "talking" phases of the intervention. During the first

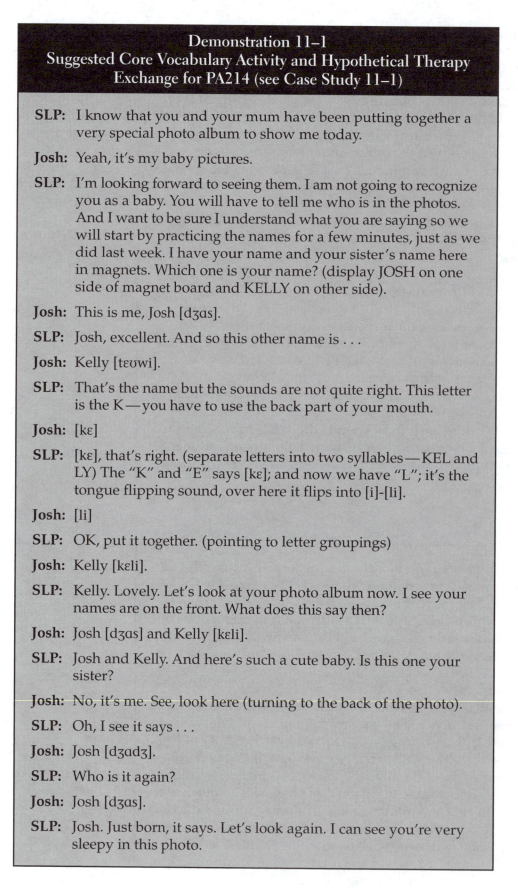

Demonstration 11–1
Suggested Core Vocabulary Activity and Hypothetical Therapy Exchange for PA214 (see Case Study 11–1)

SLP: I know that you and your mum have been putting together a very special photo album to show me today.

Josh: Yeah, it's my baby pictures.

SLP: I'm looking forward to seeing them. I am not going to recognize you as a baby. You will have to tell me who is in the photos. And I want to be sure I understand what you are saying so we will start by practicing the names for a few minutes, just as we did last week. I have your name and your sister's name here in magnets. Which one is your name? (display JOSH on one side of magnet board and KELLY on other side).

Josh: This is me, Josh [dʒɑs].

SLP: Josh, excellent. And so this other name is . . .

Josh: Kelly [tɛʊwi].

SLP: That's the name but the sounds are not quite right. This letter is the K—you have to use the back part of your mouth.

Josh: [kɛ]

SLP: [kɛ], that's right. (separate letters into two syllables—KEL and LY) The "K" and "E" says [kɛ]; and now we have "L"; it's the tongue flipping sound, over here it flips into [i]-[li].

Josh: [li]

SLP: OK, put it together. (pointing to letter groupings)

Josh: Kelly [kɛli].

SLP: Kelly. Lovely. Let's look at your photo album now. I see your names are on the front. What does this say then?

Josh: Josh [dʒɑs] and Kelly [kɛli].

SLP: Josh and Kelly. And here's such a cute baby. Is this one your sister?

Josh: No, it's me. See, look here (turning to the back of the photo).

SLP: Oh, I see it says . . .

Josh: Josh [dʒɑdʒ].

SLP: Who is it again?

Josh: Josh [dʒɑs].

SLP: Josh. Just born, it says. Let's look again. I can see you're very sleepy in this photo.

week the parents are asked to construct a photo album especially for therapy sessions, with Josh's collaboration. The album consists of baby photos of Josh and his sister, placed in transparent sleeves with the photo visible on the front side and the label on the back. The parents are asked to review the photo album with their children in the evening, using both siblings' names as frequently as possible to describe the photos and the events that occasioned the taking of the photograph. At the end of the week Josh brings the photo album to therapy. The SLP begins by practicing the names using magnetic letters as cues. Then they go through the photo album together while the SLP elicits the names Josh and Kelly using standard focused stimulation techniques such as time delay and questions to elicit responses and imitation and recasts after he has produced the target names (as described in Chapter 9; see Table 9–2). When the words have been mastered in-clinic, his parents are asked to encourage consistent use of the words at home. In preparation for targeting the next set of words, the parents are asked to make a second photo album which depicts a family picnic, scene by scene from preparations through the trip to the park and the picnic itself. The script is written to provide opportunities for use of the words "Uncle Radley," "hotdog," "taking," "putting," "chopping," and "minivan," as well as, of course, "Josh" and "Kelly." These words are functional and include a favorite relative, a favorite food and a mode of transportation in daily use so there will be frequent opportunities for practice in daily conversation when the structured practice part of the intervention is complete. Furthermore, they cover a range of manner and place contrasts and many words target the ambisyllabic word position which is particularly vulnerable to inconsistent errors. A few weeks are allowed for construction of the book and parental reading of the story so that Josh experiences multiple exposures to the words before he is expected to start retelling the story himself. The SLP begins active teaching of the pronunciation of the new words after the parents have completed the week of auditory bombardment (i.e., reading and rereading the story). As he begins to show stable production of individual core vocabulary words, Josh is encouraged to begin using them in a consistent fashion during the reading of the story (completion prompts and other dialogic reading techniques can be used to transfer responsibility for storytelling to Josh). Other activities can be devised to promote practice of the words in drill-play contexts and expectations for consistent use in the home environment will rise as the words are gradually mastered in words and phrases.

Empirical Basis for Core Vocabulary Approach

Crosbie et al. (2005) assessed the efficacy of the core vocabulary approach in a study in which treatment was provided to 18 4- to 6-year-old children with DPD. Following assessment, 10 were deemed to have inconsistent phonological disorder while the rest were found to have consistent phonological error patterns in their speech. The authors reported that a multiple baseline with alternating treatment design was implemented so that all children received 16 half-hour treatment sessions in each of two treatment approaches: core vocabulary and phonological contrast therapy (see meaningful minimal pairs procedure described later in this chapter). Order of treatment provision alternated based on the participants' order of referral to the project. In fact, most comparisons were made between groups of children depending upon type of DPD and treatment condition and therefore it would be more accurate to describe it as a nonexperimental between groups comparison. Significant interactions are reported for subtype and treatment type when observing changes in speech accuracy and consistency of speech production. Overall, the results strongly suggested that the phonological contrast intervention was most effective for children with consistent phonological disorder, whereas the core vocabulary intervention was most effective for children with inconsistent phonological disorder. Further studies with larger samples and randomized controlled design are required to confirm these findings.

Overall, the results strongly suggested that the phonological contrast intervention was most effective for children with consistent phonological disorder, whereas the core vocabulary intervention was most effective for children with inconsistent phonological disorder.

Despite these encouraging results we have some reservations about certain aspects of the treatment as indicated by our suggested modifications. First, we recommend a period of auditory bombardment in an authentic communicative context in order to provide the child with good quality exposure to auditory models of the target words. We want to establish stable acoustic-phonetic targets to guide the development of feed-forward commands during later speech practice. Secondly we suggest that the speech practice occur in two phases: (1) a prepractice warm-up during which "knowledge of performance" feedback and external cues are provided to aid production accuracy, according to the principles of motor learning as described in Chapter 10; and (2) a subsequent practice period using focused stimulation techniques that allow the clinician to repeat the child's productions subsequent to his attempts, providing further support for the process of comparing the child's output to the intended target. These modifications require systematic comparison to the standard procedure as described by Crosbie et al. (2005), in studies employing randomized controlled trial design.

We recommend a period of auditory bombardment to establish stable acoustic-phonetic targets to guide the development of *feed-forward commands* during later speech practice.

We suggest that the speech practice begin with a **prepractice warm-up** during which *knowledge of performance feedback* and external cues are provided to aid production accuracy, according to the principles of motor learning.

Subsequent speech practice could incorporate **focused stimulation techniques**.

Another issue that is open to empirical investigation is the selection of target words on purely functional grounds with little or no attention to their phonological characteristics. Children whose word productions are inconsistent at the segmental level may be consistent at the level of global word templates; indeed, the inconsistency may signal the child's efforts to break away from the constraints of those templates on lexical contrast. Adapting words to a limited number of templates is a common feature of early phonology (Vihman, 2006) that may persist in the speech of children with DPD, recognizable as the appearance of favorite phonemes especially in particular word positions. The child in Case Study 11–1 has

Children whose word productions are inconsistent at the segmental level may be consistent at the level of **global word templates**.

a preference for /v/ in ambisyllabic position and produces many words with the structure /CVvi/ or /CVvɪŋ/. Leonard and Brown (1984) present a case study of a child with specific language impairment who preferred /s/ in the coda (regardless of the target coda in the input and even in the case of null codas). Children who appear to be at this "templatic phonology" stage can demonstrate inconsistency and rigidity at the same time because multiple productions of the same word are allowed as long as the global template is preserved. For example, in Leonard and Brown's case study, the child's productions revealed systematicity in the form of lexical contrasts and preferred word templates despite within-word variability, for example, "Kathy" → [kækæs] or [kædəs] versus "Kelly" → [kebɪs] or [kəbəs]. A core vocabulary approach may also be recommended for a child in this stage of phonological development but it would seem appropriate to select words that deliberately challenge the preferred template and introduce new lexical contrasts in a principled fashion following a nonlinear analysis (Bernhardt & Stemberger, 2000) of the child's speech (see also Velleman, 2002 on "phonotactic therapy"). In fact, given an appropriate nonlinear analysis of the speech produced by children with apparently "inconsistent" errors, there may be less of a sharp demarcation between "inconsistent deviant" versus "phonological disorder" (see Case Study 11–1).

A child's productions may reveal systematicity in the form of lexical contrasts and preferred word templates despite within-word variability.

When using the core vocabulary approach, it would be appropriate to select words that deliberately challenge the preferred template and introduce new lexical contrasts in a principled fashion following a nonlinear analysis.

A final aspect of this procedure that is controversial is the teaching of "incorrect" word forms to children, given that the focus is on consistency rather than accuracy. Dodd and Bradford (2000) reported three case studies in which the children were treated with three different approaches including the core vocabulary approach. The two children who appeared to benefit from the core vocabulary approach had very large phonetic repertoires. Their gains during the core vocabulary treatment period were in the realm of consistency in the production of the target words and in improved production of prosodic structures (e.g., complex onsets, syllable codas). Similarly, PA214 in Case Study 11–1 has a reasonably complete phonetic repertoire and thus it would be possible to select words that he can say with fairly close if not perfect approximation to the adult model which increases comfort with the application of the approach. Further research, perhaps detailed longitudinal investigations of individual children, to determine the consequences of essentially teaching children to produce words incorrectly are required to validate this procedure.

Another aspect of the core vocabulary procedure that is controversial is the teaching of "incorrect" word forms to children, given that the focus is on consistency rather than accuracy.

In Dodd and Bradford (2000), the child who appeared to not benefit from the core vocabulary approach was described as having consistent disorder and thus not an appropriate candidate for the approach. It was suggested that this child was a more appropriate candidate for phonological contrast therapy. It also happens that this child had a very restricted repertoire of phones and syllable shapes and that his progress was slow overall regardless of treatment approach. Interestingly, consistency in the production of core vocabulary words actually declined during the core vocabulary treatment. Even if this child had presented with inconsistent productions within words prior to therapy, it is not clear that the core vocabulary approach would have been advisable. We would be uncomfortable applying the approach in such a case because it would entail teaching many word pronunciations that are markedly dissimilar from the adult target forms. On the other hand, the alternative choice of a phonological contrast approach would not have been appropriate unless it was clear that the child's phonology was organized at the level of phonemes and this is not always the case (consider again Case Study 11–1). We suggest that the choice of treatment approach cannot be made on the basis of the child's speech pattern alone in these cases; a full psycholinguistic assessment is in order. Given evidence of a motor speech disorder, the sensorimotor approach presented in Chapter 10 may be most appropriate; alternatively, if the issues are with speech perception or phonological processing, the input-oriented approach, as presented in Chapter 9, should probably precede application of a phonological approach. Validation of these hypotheses is another avenue for further research.

Emergence and Reorganization of Phonological Structure

11.2.1. Describe the basic goals of phonological approaches to therapy and the primary strategy used to achieve these goals.

11.2.2. Describe the rationale for implementing procedures to improve the child's phonetic knowledge of misarticulated phonemes when the basic goal is to reorganize phonological knowledge.

11.2.3. Describe 4 principles that underlie the treatment procedures used in the cycles approach to phonological therapy. Apply these principles in the development of lesson plans for commonly occurring targets.

11.2.4. Apply the procedures for implementation of the meaningful minimal pairs procedure for commonly occurring phonological targets.

More commonly, preschool-age children with DPD present with patterns that Forrest et al. (2000) described as "inconsistent across word position." For example, Amber (Case Study 6–2) produces an error pattern for /v/ that is variable but predictable: /v/ → [b] in syllable onsets, a glide in ambisyllabic position and [s] in the syllable coda position. In fact this pattern can be predicted by a small number of delinking rules that we demonstrated through nonlinear analysis: delinking of [+continuant] from consonants in the onset position, [+consonantal] from voiced obstruents in the ambisyllabic position and both [Labial] and [+voice] in the coda. The existence of these predictable patterns indicates that she has underlying knowledge of phonological units at multiple levels of the phonological hierarchy including the syllables, subsyllabic units, and features involved in the delinking rules that account for these error patterns. Phonological approaches to treatment take advantage of the child's phonological knowledge by planning for generalization from specific goals to untaught elements. Two aspects of the phonological treatment program are important: (1) the selection and ordering of treatment goals, and (2) the application of certain treatment procedures that are designed to heighten the child's awareness of the phonological contrast between the child's production and the adult target. We discuss these two aspects of phonological interventions in turn.

Phonological approaches to treatment take advantage of the child's phonological knowledge by planning for **generalization** from specific goals to untaught elements.

Two aspects of the **phonological treatment program** are important: (1) the selection and ordering of treatment goals, and (2) the application of treatment procedures to heighten the child's awareness of the phonological contrast between the child's production and the adult target.

Selecting Treatment Goals to Promote Phonological Generalization

Phonological generalization is the goal of a phonological intervention. If we teach Amber to produce words that begin with /v/, our expectation is that inclusion of [+consonantal][+continuant] will diffuse throughout her lexicon to affect not only the entire class of words that contain /v/ in the onset, but all words that contain this feature combination in the onset position and thus her production of /f/, /θ/, /ð/, /s/, /z/, and /ʃ/ should also be affected. In Chapter 8 we described multiple ways of organizing specific goals that are all potentially effective strategies for helping the child recognize the commonalities among phonemes, thus promoting generalization of learning across a sound class. A horizontal goal attack strategy would involve simultaneous targeting of all of the phonemes affected by the rule (e.g., delink [+continuant] from obstruents in the onset position), continuing until all the phonemes (e.g., /f, v, /θ/, /ð/, s, z, ʃ/) are produced at the level of customary production or better in generalization probes. In fact, this is the strategy that was actually used to treat Amber. Broen and Westman (1990) describe a successful application of this goal attack strategy in a parent-implemented phonological intervention with preschool-age children (see also Bountress & Bountress, 1985). Another strategy is to treat individual members of the class of phonemes under consideration in sequence for a preset period of time, rotating among the selected intermediate goals (cycles goal attack strategy). Two versions of this strategy were described in detail in Chapter 8. In Table 8–7, a plan consistent with the "cycles approach" (Hodson, 2007; Hodson & Paden, 1983) was mapped out so that a different intermediate goal (phonological pattern) would be targeted each week; each specific goal would receive one hour of intervention per week and each intermediate goal would receive 4 hours of interven-

Horizontal and cycles goal attack strategies organize specific goals to help the child recognize the commonalities among phonemes, thus promoting generalization of learning across a sound class.

tion per cycle. An alternative goal attack plan that involved cycling through intermediate goals selected according to a nonlinear analysis of Amber's speech was shown in Table 8–5. In this case, multiple specific targets for three intermediate goals would be treated in parallel for a full treatment block before new intermediate goals were selected, in a mixed horizontal-cycles goal attack strategy. Bernhardt and colleagues have described a number of case studies in which a similar strategy was implemented (Bernhardt, 1990, 1992; Bernhardt & Gilbert, 1992). Some researchers have implemented a vertical goal attack strategy, focusing on one phoneme (deliberately the most complex phoneme missing from the child's system) for many weeks even when there was no progress, hoping for generalization to other phonemes in the meantime (e.g., Cummings & Barlow, 2010). We do not recommend this strategy because the research evidence suggests that often there is no treatment effect and thus no generalization.

Another consideration when choosing specific treatment targets is the selection of the **target words** that will be practiced during therapy sessions.

The SLP chooses target words that can be used in **communicative contexts** during games in the clinic and in natural communicative exchanges in extraclinic settings.

The potential impact of the **lexical characteristics** of the target words may also be taken into account when selecting target words (e.g., *word frequency, neighborhood density*).

Another consideration when choosing specific treatment targets is the selection of the words that will be practiced during therapy sessions. Traditionally, the two primary considerations have been "picturability" and the functional value of the words to the child. The SLP wants words that can be used in communicative contexts during games in the clinic (thus the preference for words that can be depicted on picture cards) and in natural communicative exchanges in extraclinic settings (thus the preference for a core functional vocabulary). More recently, interest in the impact of the lexical characteristics of the target words has arisen. Currently, we take the view that rapid change in the child's system occurs not by changing a rule but by lexical diffusion. If Amber practices a small set of words that begin with /v/, changes at multiple levels of representations should occur for those words: her perceptual knowledge of /v/ will become more detailed and the category more defined relative to similar phonemes; the words will become linked to a new motor score that involves critical constriction degree at the lips; the underlying phonological representation will reorganize to mark [+continuant] in combination with [+consonantal] in the onset, and over time this feature combination should spread to other words that are linked to words such as "van" and "vine" and "vinegar" in the lexicon by virtue of shared onset characteristics. The individual words that are practiced will have certain lexical characteristics as we discussed in Chapter 4. For example, "van" is more frequently occurring than "vine" although they both reside in moderately dense neighborhoods. The word "vinegar" occurs almost as frequently as "vine" but has no neighbors. In contrast to any of these words, "feet" and "fire" will come up even more often in conversation and words starting with /f/ in general will have more neighbors. Theoretically, these differences in lexical characteristics may impact rate of diffusion of newly learned phonological pattern across the lexicon. It has been predicted that choosing high fre-

Theoretically, differences in lexical characteristics may impact rate of **diffusion** of newly learned phonological pattern across the lexicon.

quency words will enhance lexical diffusion because children and adults show an advantage in word recognition and word repetition studies when high frequency rather than low frequency words are the targets. The expectations with respect to neighborhood density are less clear because children do not react to manipulations in neighborhood density in a predictable fashion as do adults. Unfortunately, however, the studies that have examined these questions thus far have used single subject experimental designs that are ill suited to the research questions and the outcomes are very difficult to interpret; the specific findings may reflect differences in the developmental level of the phonemes targeted or individual differences in child response to therapy (Cummings & Barlow, 2010; Gierut, Morrisette, & Champion, 1999; Morrisette & Gierut, 2002). We cautiously suggest that high frequency target words may be conducive to the promotion of more rapid phonological reorganization of the lexicon.

We cautiously suggest that **high frequency target words** may be conducive to the promotion of more rapid phonological reorganization of the lexicon.

As we pointed out in Chapter 10, therapy can be conducted with nonwords, in the context of activities in which the "made-up word" is associated with a novel referent during therapy activities. Practice with nonwords can carry over to real-word targets and it is possible that generalization is more robust than when real words are targeted in therapy (Gierut, Morrisette, & Ziemer, 2010). One advantage of using nonword stimuli in therapy is that the phonological characteristics of the words can be very precisely controlled so that they match the problematic aspect of the child's system that is the specific therapy goal. Other characteristics such as phonotactic probability (as discussed in Chapter 4) can also be varied systematically. Some researchers are describing interesting relationships between word learning and lexical variables such as word frequency, neighborhood density, and phonotactic probability in studies that include young children who are developing speech and language at normal versus slower rates (Stokes, 2010; Storkel, Moskawa, & Hoover, 2010). Overall, the research findings are conflicting and the clinical implications are not clear (Stoel-Gammon, 2011) and not detailed here for that reason. One clear conclusion is that some of these effects reflect the way in which specific words are presented in the input (as opposed to the way that they are stored in the child's lexicon per se) and thus the message for the clinician should be to attend to the techniques that are used when teaching children new words, whether one's purpose is improving the child's lexical knowledge or phonological skills. We return to this issue in the next section when we discuss phonological intervention procedures.

Practice with **nonwords** can carry over to real word targets and it is possible that generalization is more robust than when real words are targeted in therapy.

Demonstration of Target Selection to Promote Phonological Reorganization

We demonstrated detailed analyses of a child's phonological system in Chapter 6 and discussed selection of treatment goals in depth in Chapter 8. However, the selection and ordering of treatment goals

Phonological interventions are equally concerned with the *prosodic* and *segmental levels* of the **phonological hierarchy**.

is so fundamental to the successful implementation of a phonological intervention that we provide one final example in Demonstration 11–2. This example has the further purpose of highlighting the point that phonological interventions are equally concerned with the prosodic and segmental levels of the phonological hierarchy. The sample shown in this demonstration was recorded from a 5-year-old child who had been receiving treatment for a year based on the cycles approach. The SLP had selected treatment goals that were largely concerned with segmental level phonological patterns. The child had made minimal gains and was becoming increasingly resistant in therapy sessions. His mother was especially distressed at his complete refusal to engage in practice activities at home. A consultation was requested from the first author as a prelude to recommending a "treatment rest." A subset of the speech sample that was recorded during the consultation is shown. The word list was constructed for a study of syllable position effects on consonant production (Rvachew & Andrews, 2002) and due to the complexity of the words, was elicited via imitation. The same patterns were observed in his conversational speech and during formal testing with an early version of the HAPP-3. The SLP had been working on patterns that are commonly observed in young children's speech

Demonstration 11–2
Selected Words from Speech Sample Recorded From 4-Year-Old Boy

abdomen	'æbɪnʔɑ	giraffe	'dʒaf	potato	'tedo
achieve	'tsiv	guitar	'tɑ	pumpkin	'pʌmtɪn
acknowledge	ʌ'nʌdʒɪn	judgment	'dʒʌdʒɪn	punishment	'pʌmptʃɪn
adventure	ʌ'vɛntʃʌ	Kellogg	'tɛnɪn	rabbit	'wæbnɪnt
alligator	'ægetə	kerchief	'tetʃɪn	recognize	'wɛtnɑɪz
although	æ'ʔo	magic	'mædʒɪn	rubbish	'wʌvɪnt
another	'nɛvə	mammoth	'mætʃɪn	sadly	'sædi
awake	'wet	observe	ʌ'zʌb	salad	'sæmɪnt
boastful	'bofɔ	pajamas	'dʒædʒɪnz	sausage	'sɑsɪnz
cabin	'tænɪn	parchment	'pɑtʃɪn	sherrif	'setɪn
cages	'tædʒɪn	piglet	'pinʌ	stomach	'sʌmɪnt
casino	tɪ'tʃino	pneumonia	'monʌ	toboggan	tə'bʌnɪn
crutches	'kɪʌtʃɪns	pocket	'pɑtɪn	uniform	'jufom
Edgar	'itʌ	popsicle	'pɑtʃo	wagon	'wɑnɪn

Graphic Summary of Mismatches in a 5-Year-Old's Phonological System Relative to Adult Targets

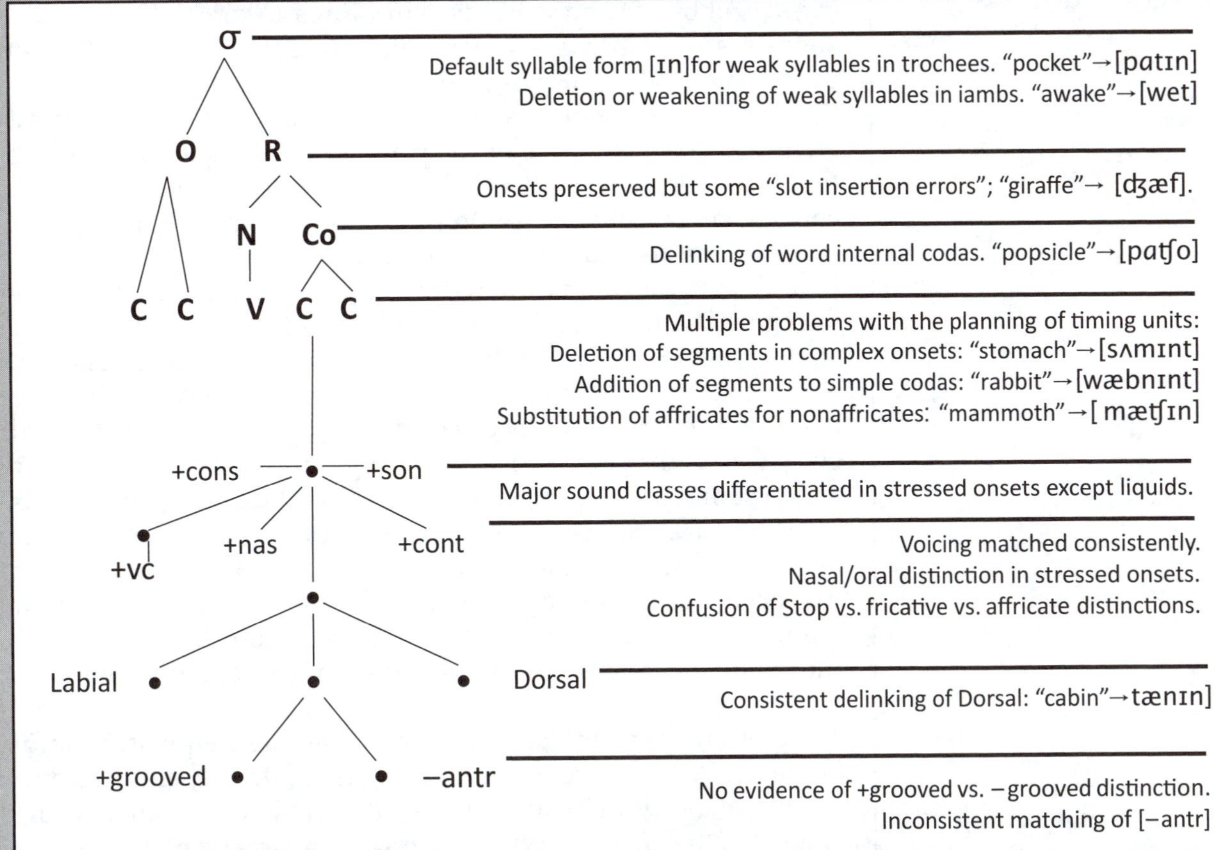

Suggested Treatment Goals

1. Intermediate Goal: Expand repertoire of weak syllables in trochaic contexts (eliminate default [ɪn]).
   a. Specific goal: 'CVCVC where all Cs are stimulable phones and C_3 is an obstruent.
   b. Suggested words: puppet, faucet, misses, famous, cages
2. Stabilize unfooted weak syllables in iambic contexts.
   a. Specific goal: V or CV shaped weak syllables in iambs within 2- and 3-syllable words.
   b. Suggested words: away, today, pajamas, bananas, potatoes, tomatoes
3. Establish coda in word internal contexts.
   a. Specific goal: Word internal codas in two syllable words with stimulable consonants.
   b. Suggested words: Poptart, passport, inchworm, halftime, hambone

and which do in fact occur in this child's sample although they are sometimes obscured by the larger issue: for example, consonant sequences (see cluster reduction in "stomach"); liquids (see gliding in "rubbish") and velars (see fronting in "kerchief"). Occasional successes were occurring with these targets (see "crutches") but overall his intelligibility remained markedly poor and his cooperation during treatment sessions was worsening. The computer-based analysis had missed one of the primary patterns in his speech and that was the use of a filler syllable for weak syllables in a trochaic context, specifically [ɪn] (with [ɪnt] and [ɪnz] as variants). A host of other errors also suggest severe difficulties at the level of phonological encoding including reduplication of segments and deletion of segments and syllables, especially those with low phonetic substance due to their prosodic position within the word. The vowel errors combined with age-appropriate performance on single- and disyllable repetition tasks also led to the impression that the difficulty was with phonological encoding rather than motor planning.

A summary of the primary patterns in the child speech is shown in Demonstration 11–2. At the prosodic level it can be seen that there are significant difficulties with the production of weak syllables in trochaic and iambic contexts and generalized difficulties with planning the timing units for word production. At the level of features, liquids are absent from the repertoire but [+consonantal] and [+sonorant] appear to be reasonably well differentiated otherwise. The stop/fricative/affricate sound classes are frequently confused however. With respect to place contrasts, [Dorsal] and [−grooved] are consistently delinked and [−anterior] is only matched in the context of the affricate. When the issues are organized hierarchically in this fashion it can be seen that the higher level prosodic issues should take precedence over cluster reduction, and the major sound class confusions should take precedence over velar fronting as treatment goals (in general the rule is work from the top to the bottom of the chart when selecting prosodic and feature level goals). Furthermore, given his growing resistance to therapy, a complete change in focus was called for. Therefore, it was recommended that the treatment targets be reconfigured to de-emphasize segments and focus on broad word-shapes that were problematic for this child. We have no data regarding his long-term outcome but it is known that the treatment rest did not occur and that his mother was very appreciative of her son's sudden cooperation with home practice exercises. We have suggested some word-shape targets as specific goals and some words that would be consistent with those goals in the demonstration. We have not suggested very many words for each goal because the expectation is that new patterns, once established, will generalize throughout the lexicon. We have this expectation because the existing patterns are consistent enough to form the basis for such generalization. For example, the consistency with which he inserts [ɪn] into weak syllable slots indicates that he has a specific representation for this structure in his lexical representations even though he is apparently uncertain of the phonetic content of those

We have not suggested very many words for each goal because, given the consistency of his phonological patterns, the expectation is that new patterns, once established, will generalize throughout the lexicon.

syllables. If he succeeds in learning alternative phonetic realizations for weak syllables within a trochee he should be able to generalize this new knowledge to other words having a similar prosodic structure. Normally, we would recommend targeting these prosodic goals in sequence but in parallel with attention to one or two segmental goals. In this special case, we recommend waiting until the child has experienced success toward the achievement of the word shape goals before reintroducing feature level goals.

Empirical Evidence for Phonological Generalization

The theoretical heart of phonological approaches to speech therapy is the notion of phonological generalization. The justification for taking the time to carefully analyze a child's phonological system is the promise that organizing treatment goals and stimuli so as to reorganize the child's underlying phonological knowledge will more efficiently lead to age-appropriate speech accuracy and intelligibility than traditional procedures that tackle the child's speech errors one phoneme at a time. Part of the empirical support for this argument resides in demonstrations of generalization of learning within sound classes, originating in studies of the distinctive feature approach to therapy.

The theoretical heart of phonological approaches to speech therapy is the notion of **phonological generalization**.

Organizing treatment goals and stimuli so as to reorganize the child's underlying phonological knowledge will more efficiently lead to age-appropriate speech accuracy and intelligibility than traditional procedures that tackle the child's speech errors one phoneme at a time.

Distinctive feature studies involved examination of treatment effects in single subjects, usually with a multiple baseline design, in which the internal validity rests upon three specific design elements. First, a stable baseline for the target phoneme followed by improved performance on the target when treatment was implemented suggests a treatment effect; second, lack of improvement (or significantly less improvement) on a control phoneme that has little feature overlap with the target confirms experimental control over the target, that is, indicates that improvements in the target are due to the treatment and not maturation or history effects or some other threat to the internal validity of the design; finally, stable baselines for the generalization phonemes that are related to the target, followed by improvements that are temporally related to change in the target, can be interpreted as a generalization effect. Not all studies included each of these design elements but most contained at least two and collectively these studies provide a reasonably convincing picture of within-class generalization. Randomized controlled trials would provide more confidence in the findings and are recommended given the fundamental importance of this topic from both a theoretical and clinical perspective. Notwithstanding some weaknesses in the research, a number of generalizations can be drawn from this literature as a whole.

Single subject studies that examined generalization patterns from the **distinctive feature** perspective have convincingly demonstrated within class generalization of learning in studies involving children with DPD.

First, and most importantly, it was established that generalization among preschoolers with multiple phoneme errors who were treated with phonological approaches occurred without any attention to a "transfer" stage of therapy. Elbert, Dinnsen, Swartzlander, and Chin (1990) demonstrated that when using a minimal pairs procedure at the word level, children would readily carry over learning

Treatment generalization among preschoolers with multiple phoneme errors who were treated with phonological approaches occurred without any attention to a "transfer" stage of therapy.

of new phonemes from trained words to new words in conversational speech. This was a significant achievement in view of the difficulties that clinicians were reporting with carryover when using behaviorist methods (although differences in client population may also have played a role). Subsequently, the researchers turned their attention to identifying the parameters that would predict the kinds of carryover that were likely to occur.

Studies of the distinctive feature approach established that "within-class" generalization was likely (although not certain) to occur when children learned the target phoneme.

Within-class generalization means that learning transferred from the taught phoneme to untaught phonemes with shared features.

Overall, studies of the distinctive feature approach established that within class generalization was likely (although not certain) to occur when children learned the target phoneme (Blache, Parsons, & Humphreys, 1981; Costello & Onstine, 1976; Elbert & McReynolds, 1985; McReynolds & Bennett, 1972). Within-class generalization means that learning transferred from the taught phoneme to untaught phonemes with shared features. For example, Costello and Onstine (1976) taught two children who stopped fricatives to produce /θ,s/ and observed varying amounts of transfer to words containing /ð,z,ʃ,tʃ,dʒ/ but no change in the control phoneme /ɹ/. Elbert and McReynolds (1985) taught a child who deleted both stops and fricatives from codas to produce (in successive phases of the treatment program) /b,t,g,s,z,f/ in the coda position of a nonsense syllable in contrast with the null onset. Transfer to real words with stop and fricative codas was probed repeatedly and increasing amounts of transfer to the generalization words was noted as treatment progressed (see data for Subject 1 in their report). Across-class generalization was not observed, however; teaching stops in the coda did not transfer to fricatives in this position. In another subject for whom the target order was reversed, teaching fricatives in the coda did not transfer to stops. Across these studies overall, patterns of generalization were idiosyncratic and linked to each individual child's sound system so that some children would generalize across word positions, whereas others would not; some children would generalize a feature across the complete sound class while others would restrict the new feature to certain feature combinations (for example, transfer of the feature +strident might be limited to −voice segments). Furthermore, children who did not learn the target phonemes were not observed to make gains on generalization probes.

Patterns of generalization were idiosyncratic and linked to each individual child's sound system.

After establishing that phonological relationships among phonemes based on shared features permitted within-class generalization, some researchers went further to hypothesize that across-class generalization would be possible on the basis of implicational relationships among phoneme classes.

After establishing that phonological relationships among phonemes based on shared features permitted within-class generalization, thus offering the hope of more efficient interventions for children with DPD, some researchers went further to hypothesize that across-class generalization would be possible on the basis of implicational relationships among phoneme classes (Elbert, Dinnsen, & Powell, 1984). Recall the notion of the implicational hierarchy as discussed in Chapter 4 (e.g., see Table 4–15) and in relation to the complexity approach to target selection in Chapter 8. Efforts to demonstrate across-class generalization continued to rely on single-subject research designs, either a multiple baseline or multiple-probe design, but in this case the logic of the research design is violated in that changes in what would ordinarily be considered to be a "control phoneme" were considered to be evidence of a treatment effect (transfer from the treatment target to unrelated phonemes) when such a change should be interpreted as a lack of experimental control over the dependent variables. Close examination of the data in these studies reveals that across-class generalization is more likely to reflect maturation or history than a true treatment effect, a conclusion reinforced by the outcomes of the randomized controlled trial described in detail in Chapter 8 (Rvachew & Nowak, 2001). We address this point one last time, however, because the false promise of across-class generalization leads to the persistence of some harmful treatment practices. As an example, we describe treatment outcomes for Subject 2 in Cummings and Barlow. This child received 19 treatment sessions during which she attempted to produce /ɹ/ in hundreds of practice trials and outcomes were plotted for this target across 23 production probes. Her score on these probes remained at 0 for the entire study. Generalization is reported as change in production performance between the pretreatment probe and a probe conducted two weeks posttreatment. These probes monitored production of multiple phonemes, specifically those that were produced with less than 50% accuracy prior to treatment. Subject 2 showed no change for the target /ɹ/ but changes were observed for other phonemes, for example, /v,tʃ,ŋ,d,k/. These changes were interpreted as "generalization" even though there was no treatment effect from which to generalize, and in the absence of a randomized control group, no way to know that the intervention played a role in these changes. In our lab, we conduct randomized control trials to assess the efficacy of varying treatment approaches and know that changes such as those reported can occur even when no treatment is provided. For example, in the study described in Chapter 9 (see Figure 9–5 and associated discussion) significant change overall was observed in articulation accuracy for treated children, whereas children in an untreated comparison group did not make significant improvements in PCC on average. However, patterns of change were observed in both treated and untreated children that were similar to those reported in Cummings and Barlow. For example, some children who received treatment for /ʃ/ and /ʁ/ made no gains on these phonemes but were observed to improve their production of other phonemes such as /f/ and /b/. We were able to find children in the untreated group with identical patterns of outcome, however: no gains in /ʃ/ and/ or /ʁ/ but significant gains in /f/ and/or /b/. It is clear that these changes in untreated early developing phonemes can occur even without treatment and constitute maturation rather than treatment effects. Therefore, it is important to choose treatment goals so as to plan for: (a) success on the treatment target(s), and (b) within-class generalization. Given that children with DPD so frequently present with multiple problematic phonological patterns, the prudent course of action is to target two or three patterns at once rather than targeting one phoneme and hoping for generalization to unrelated patterns.

It is important to choose treatment goals so as to plan for: (a) success on the treatment target(s), and (b) within-class generalization.

Enhancing and Integrating Knowledge of Phonetic Representations to Promote Phonological Reorganization

After the selection of intermediate and specific goals, the next step is to choose treatment procedures that will help the child learn the target words and generalize new knowledge.

After the selection of intermediate and specific goals, the next step is to choose treatment procedures that will help the child learn the target words and generalize new knowledge. In Chapter 7 we presented evidence that a large proportion of children with DPD have significant difficulty with the perception of sound contrasts corresponding to their misarticulated phonemes (see Tables 7–6 and 7–7). Furthermore, in Chapter 3 we described a model of speech motor control that explains how fuzzy knowledge of the acoustic-phonetic properties of phonemes and poor processing of acoustic feedback will interfere with the development of motor programs for speech production. In Chapter 4 we discussed how phonological knowledge emerges from linkages among these different types of phonetic knowledge in the lexicon. Mismatches in phonetic knowledge across different levels of representation can explain phonological patterns in children's speech. For example, fricatives and glides may be linked at the level of articulatory-phonetic representations because they are differentiated by only a small difference in constriction degree; large differences in the acoustic outcomes associated with this small difference in constriction degree should serve to distinguish the categories, however (Browman & Goldstein, 1989; Howard & Messum, 2011; Stevens & Keyser, 2009). If we consider Amber's difficulties with gliding voiced obstruents in the ambisyllabic position it is possible that she has incomplete knowledge of the acoustic-phonetic representations for these sound classes, possibly due to transient hearing problems at a younger age or an inherited problem with phonological processing. Furthermore, the pattern may be due to articulatory limitations because fricative production requires more differentiated control of tongue and jaw in the onset than coda syllable position (McAllister Byun, 2011). Finally, she may not have linked up her articulatory and acoustic knowledge of these sound categories properly, a process that is supported by feedback from caregivers according to some theories (Goldstein & Schwade, 2008; Howard & Messum, 2011; Kröger, Kopp, & Lowit, 2010). Given Amber's very difficult home situation insufficient social feedback is a possible contributor to her DPD. Therefore, the application of treatment procedures designed to improve phonetic representations of phonemes and to encourage internal linkages across multiple levels of representation is theoretically defensible even when the goal is to reorganize her phonological knowledge.

The application of treatment procedures designed to improve phonetic representations of phonemes and to encourage internal linkages across multiple levels of representation is theoretically defensible even when the goal is to reorganize phonological knowledge.

The cycles approach perfectly integrates attention to the child's acquisition of acoustic-phonetic, articulatory-phonetic, and phonological representations.

A treatment approach that perfectly exemplifies this principle is the cycles approach. Hodson (Hodson, 2011; Prezas & Hodson, 2010) recently explained the underlying principles of the treatment procedures that are used in this approach. First, the cycles goal attack strategy is justified on the grounds that it is more congruent with normal developmental processes in which children do not learn one phoneme to criterion before tackling the next one in line! At the same time, the organization of intermediate and specific goals within a cycle helps the child to link words that share the same phonological pattern. Second, auditory bombardment is an important procedure that is applied twice during each treatment session and during home practice because children learn speech "primarily by listening." Third, a large part of each session is devoted to production practice so that the children can associate kinesthetic and auditory feedback during the acquisition of new phonological patterns. This practice involves a small set of words carefully selected to maximize both phonetic context effects and phonological transfer. Finally, all techniques necessary are used to ensure that the child is experiencing the correct articulatory patterns while practicing the words; these techniques include choosing stimulable target phonemes, practicing words that maximize facilitative phonetic contexts and applying the principles of motor learning described in Chapter 10 with careful attention to the challenge point concept. Each session follows a standard outline that we demonstrate using the goals selected for Amber, based on her hypothetical treatment goals as laid out in Table 8–7.

Demonstration of a Treatment Session: Cycles Approach

Demonstration 11–3 outlines activities that would be appropriate to meet the first two goals proposed for Amber as laid out in Table 8–7. For the first session the intermediate goal would be Velars and the specific goal would be word final /k/. Given that this is the first session, a few minutes should be devoted to explaining the overall structure of the cycle and of each session to the parent as well as identifying the session target for the child and the mother. Introducing the homework booklet (containing the list of auditory bombardment stimuli) and ensuring that Amber is comfortable with the amplification equipment[1] will be necessary during this first session as well. The first activity is to read a list of approximately 20 words containing the session target to the child with slight amplification for about 30 seconds (the presentation level should be loud but not uncomfortable or distorted). Amber is expected to listen attentively but not repeat the words. Hodson (2007) cautions that it is important to say the words softly and naturally with amplification; do not present the words loudly without amplification which typically involves distorting the phonetic characteristics of the phonemes within the word.

During **auditory bombardment**, say the words softly and naturally with amplification; do not present the words loudly without amplification which typically involves distorting the phonetic characteristics of the phonemes within the word.

After this brief period of auditory bombardment, prepractice of the target words occurs with amplification. The target list is different from the auditory bombardment list in that it is shorter and the phonetic characteristics of the words have been carefully controlled.

[1]Many types of speech amplifiers are currently available for this purpose ranging from sophisticated FM systems to simple tube and funnel arrangements.

Demonstration 11–3
Suggested Lesson Plans for Amber (Case Study 6–2) Assuming Cycles Treatment and Goals Proposed in Table 8–7

Cycle I, Week 1, Session 1: Intermediate Goal VELARS

Goal	Activity	Stimuli	Expected Responses
Identify cycle and session targets.	Discussion with parent and child.	Homework book.	N/A
Establish acoustic-phonetic representation for target /k/(coda).	Auditory bombardment (SLP presents words to Amber with amplification).	make, back, cork, fork, rake, duck, knock, tack, walk, steak, snake, stomach, hammock, magic, paddock, backpack, pickpocket, picnic, kickback, checkmark.	Listen attentively.
Establish accurate production of the target words.	Imitate target words with amplification.	walk, back, park, mark, bake	Imitative single words, with chaining if necessary: [wɑː]-[k].
Practice accurate production of target words to establish new kinesthetic images ("integrative rehearsal").	Amber draws representations of the target words on index cards.	walk, back, park, mark, bake SLP Qs: What do you want to draw on this card, "walk" or "back"? What word do I write on this card? What did you draw on this card? Tell mum what you drew on this card.	Imitative → spontaneous single words.
Practice accurate production of target words to establish new kinesthetic images ("integrative rehearsal").	Amber mails the cards to her relatives after first stamping and addressing them.	walk, back, park, mark, bake SLP Qs: Which card goes to Grandma? What picture does Grandma get? Which picture gets the bird stamp? Which picture gets the yellow address label? Do you remember which one goes to Grandma? Which one will you mail first?	spontaneous single words → imitated phrases → spontaneous phrases.

Goal	Activity	Stimuli	Expected Responses
Probe stimulability of words for Session 2.	Word imitation task.	duck, tack, hammock, paddock, magic (use phonetic placement and successive approximation if necessary).	Imitative single word responses.
Reinforce acoustic-phonetic representation for target /k/(coda).	Repeat auditory bombardment and assign homework.	As above.	Listen attentively.

Cycle I, Week 2, Session 3: Intermediate Goal S-CLUSTERS

Goal	Activity	Stimuli	Expected Responses
Accurate production of /k/ (coda).	Review words from previous week.	Homework book (10 /k/ words from last week).	100% accuracy at spontaneous single word level.
Establish acoustic-phonetic representation for target /ts/(coda).	Auditory bombardment (SLP presents words to Amber with amplification).	Hits, pats, knots, meets, sits, cots, forts, mitts, pots, cats, rockets, puppets, lockets, hatchets, fidgets, sailboats, peanuts, golfcarts, snowsuits, tophats.	Listen attentively.
Establish accurate production of the target words.	Imitate target words with amplification.	hats, boats, bats, mats, beets	Imitative single words, with chaining if necessary: [hæt]-[s].
Practice accurate production of target words to establish new kinesthetic images ("integrative rehearsal").	Amber draws representations of the target words on index cards.	hats, boats, bats, mats, beets SLP Qs: What do you want to draw on this card, 'hats' or 'boats'? What word do I write on this card? What did you draw on this card? Did you draw 1 hat or 2 hats? How many cats did you draw on this card? Tell mum what you drew on this card.	Imitative → spontaneous single words.

Goal	Activity	Stimuli	Expected Responses
Practice accurate production of target words to establish new kinesthetic images ("integrative rehearsal").	SLP "hides" cards around office (in plain sight); Amber finds the cards and returns them to the SLP one at a time.	hats, boats, bats, mats, beets SLP Q: What did you find?	spontaneous single words → imitated phrases → spontaneous phrases.
Probe stimulability of words for Session 2.	Word imitation task.	walnuts, tophats, Poptarts, rabbits, puppets	Imitative single word responses.
Reinforce acoustic-phonetic representation for target /ts/(coda).	Repeat auditory bombardment and assign homework.	As above.	Listens attentively.

Target words are carefully selected to control for their phonetic characteristics and pre-practice of these words occurs with amplification.

In this case the 5 words have been selected to have a CVC structure with a labial in C_1 position and /k/ in C_2 position. Amber is stimulable for /k/ so it is expected that she will be able to imitate these words. However, any additional stimulation necessary can be applied as described in Chapter 10 to ensure correct production (e.g., integral stimulation, phonetic placement, chaining, and successive approximation); furthermore, knowledge of performance feedback can be provided as needed. When it is established that Amber can produce the words correctly, Amber removes the amplification equipment and creates a set of 5 pictures cards by drawing representations of the words onto index cards, each labeled by the SLP. These cards will serve as production practice materials at home and in the clinic.

Subsequently, a game, experiential play or craft activity serves as a foundation for practice of the target words.

Subsequently, a game, experiential play, or craft activity serves as a foundation for practice of the words at either the imitative or spontaneous level in words, phrases or sentences depending upon Amber's performance during the session. The notion of the challenge point applies here because the SLP should shift expectations from trial to trial to ensure practice at the highest possible level while maintaining correct responses. In contrast to the recommendation in Chapter 10 for a somewhat less than perfect response level, Hodson (2007) expects 100% correct responses on these carefully selected words, however. The activity is designed to provide seminatural reinforcement for correct responses. The planned activity should also ensure active participation on the part of the child in authentic interactions with the SLP; the nature of the exchanges between SLP and child are markedly different than those that occur in the context of the programmed learning approach (Gray, 1974; Mowrer, 1971) or even some phonological approaches that rely exclusively on a sequence of imitated followed by spontaneous picture naming (e.g., see Cummings & Barlow, 2010). In this case Amber will be "mailing" the cards to family members. She is asked to choose which card will be addressed to Mum, Dad, Grandma, and so forth. When the item on the card is said correctly, the SLP writes the name on the front of the card. Similarly, stamps and address labels are applied and the cards are placed in a letter-box made in advance of the session from construction paper. This activity also allows for the use of focused stimulation techniques by the SLP and for the natural occurrence of conversation during which transfer of learning can be monitored.

The second to last activity of each session is a few minutes of stimulability probing to confirm the specific goal and choose target words for the next session. If we presume that Amber is scheduled for two 30-minute sessions per week, the next session will continue with /k/ in the word-final position so this few minutes of probing will ensure that she is ready to progress to more complex words, for example, two syllable words and words containing coronal onsets. During the second session, stimulability probing will be conducted to identify /s/-cluster words that she can produce. The next sample lesson plan in Demonstration 11–3 is concerned with this third session that targets /ts/ in the word final position. The sequence of activities is the same except that the first activity is a review of the words from the previous session that targeted word final /k/.

The second to last activity of each session is a few minutes of stimulability probing to confirm the specific goal and choose target words for the next session.

Homework is a critical part of the treatment program. The treatment session itself allows for a limited amount of actual production practice (relative to what would be expected during a traditional speech therapy session). Home practice sessions need not be long but they should be frequent, at least daily, ensuring distributed rather than mass practice. We recommend that they have three components: first, reading of the auditory bombardment word list, which also contains a rhyme to facilitate rime awareness (e.g., for Session 1, "Jack and Jill); second, production practice with the 5 picture cards is essential (removing them from the letter-box, reviewing the intended recipients and remailing them will provide 20 practice trials in less than 2 minutes); and third, a phonological awareness activity can be provided to be completed once before the next session. In this case a rime matching activity would be a perfect complement to the Session 1 goal. Amber could sort and glue pictures to separate pages of the homework book, matching them to targets on the basis of shared rime: Jack—back, stack, pack, sack, tack; Jill—bill, pill, hill, till, fill. We also recommend that the clinic provide parent group education sessions so that parents are fully comfortable with the home practice procedures and have frequent opportunities to discuss issues that arise during home practice or with their child's progress in general. Recall from Chapter 8 research findings that a structured home program

Homework is a critical part of the treatment program.

Homework assignments should have three components: auditory bombardment, production practice, and phonological awareness.

benefits children's progress in therapy. Our own research shows that this effect is enhanced when the parents receive an intensive parent education program that is theoretically consistent with the treatment provided to their child (Rvachew & Brosseau-Lapré, 2010).

Children with the most severe DPD have been observed to achieve intelligible speech within 30 to 40 hours of intervention provided over 3 to 4 cycles.

An incremental rate of progress is not expected as in programmed learning approaches; rather the learning process is dynamic and nonlinear and very rapid increases in rate of change can occur in later cycles.

Hodson (2011) reported that over many decades of experience with this program, children with the most severe DPD have been observed to achieve intelligible speech within 30 to 40 hours of intervention provided over 3 to 4 cycles. Stoel-Gammon, Stone-Goldman, and Glaspey (2002) warn that progress may be slow during the first cycle; an incremental rate of progress is not expected as in programmed learning approaches; rather the learning process is dynamic and nonlinear and very rapid increases in rate of change can occur in later cycles. It is not recommended that the cycles intervention be applied with children who have milder deficits or that it be attempted in circumstances where children are rationed to brief therapy intervals. If a fixed block of intervention is mandated for the treatment of a child with severe DPD, the mixed horizontal-cycles goal attack strategy that is demonstrated in Table 8–5 is probably a better choice, combined with a structured home program.

Empirical Support for the Cycles Approach

The efficacy of the cycles approach has been validated in a well-designed randomized controlled trial.

The efficacy of the cycles approach has been validated in a well designed randomized controlled trial, conducted with 30 children, aged 33 to 61 months, who had severe DPD at intake to the study (Almost & Rosenbaum, 1998). A blinded randomization procedure was used to assign half the children to receive the intervention for 4 months followed by a 4-month break while the remainder received no treatment for the first 4 months and then received the treatment in the second 4-month block. Intervention was provided in twice weekly half-hour sessions and the target phonological process was changed every 4th session. Four to six patterns were selected as treatment goals for each child. In each group two children were lost to follow-up but the outcomes were assessed with an "intention-to-treat analysis." After the first 4-month treatment block, significant between group differences were observed on the Assessment of Phonological Processes—Revised, the Goldman-Fristoe Test of Articulation, and percent consonants correct (in conversation), in favor of the group that received treatment during that interval. After the second treatment block the group that received treatment in the first block continued to show superior speech accuracy in conversation relative to the group that received intervention in the second treatment block (no between-group differences were observed on the other measures). No significant between-group differences in mean length of utterance were observed at any point during the study. This study provides good quality evidence that the cycles approach is an effective intervention relative to a no-treatment control and further indicates that children who receive this intervention will continue to make gains after treatment is withdrawn.

Montgomery and Bonderman (1989) described a modification of the cycles program in which 9 children, aged between 3;0 and 4;10, with severe or profound DPD, received the intervention in a group from two SLPs. The intervention was provided in three 2-hour sessions each week for 17 weeks, followed by a 2-month break, and then again in a second 17-week cycle, during which time the children received three 2-hour sessions per week in the large group. The goal attack strategy and the treatment procedures were followed exactly as prescribed in Hodson and Paden (1983). A significant reduction in number of "phonological deviancies" was observed on the Assessment of Phonological Processes—Revised. They reported that the dismissal rate compared favorably with their prior experience with one-on-one therapy following a traditional approach but that the program was considerably more efficient in terms of the required number of treatment hours.

Tyler, Edwards, and Saxman (1987) described four case studies in which two children received a modified version of the cycles approach and two children received meaningful minimal pairs therapy. Patterns of generalization from taught phonemes and words to untaught phonemes and words were tracked over time. Generalization from taught to untaught words occurred and the children made significant gains for 7 different phonological processes over only 8 treatment sessions. Their application of the meaningful minimal pairs procedure also resulted in impressive gains, however.

Meaningful Minimal Pairs Procedures

Weiner (1981) presented the method of meaningful minimal pairs as a conceptual approach to phonological therapy that was theoretically consistent with the goal of changing the child's production of an entire sound class. Blache and Parsons (1980) also described this procedure as a uniquely linguistic approach to therapy in which words are used to teach distinctive features; more specifically, they posit that "teaching children the linguistic function of features is more important than the recognition or production of features or phonemes" (p. 203). The procedure has two key components: (1) teaching the child a pair of words that differs by a single phoneme, for example, "tea" /ti/ versus "key"/ki/; and (2) arranging the environment so that the child experiences a communication breakdown if both words are produced as a homophone, for example, "tea"→ [ti] and "key"→ [ti], thus motivating a change in production in order to avoid this situation. Phonological generalization is expected to other word pairs and phonemes that differ by the feature of interest (in this example, [Dorsal]). Generalization has been promoted in demonstrations of this procedure through the use of vertical or horizontal goal attack strategies as described below. The minimal pairs procedure has also been incorporated into the cycles approach by some researchers and clinicians.

The method of **meaningful minimal pairs** is a uniquely phonological approach to therapy in which children are taught the linguistic function of features.

A meaningful minimal pair is a pair of words that differs by a single phoneme, typically contrasting the feature that is the intermediate target of the intervention.

Arranging the environment so that the child experiences a communication breakdown if both words are produced as a homophone is a key component of the treatment procedure.

Application of the method of meaningful minimal pairs begins with a thorough linguistic analysis of the child's phonological system and the selection of a feature contrast as the therapy target.

Select 3 to 5 word pairs that differ only by the feature of interest in the selected syllable position.

In Step 1, ensure that the child knows the words and recognizes the pictures (or objects) that have been chosen to represent the word pairs.

Application of the method begins with a thorough linguistic analysis of the child's phonological system and the selection of a feature contrast as the therapy target. Most features of interest will impact a large number of phoneme pairs and thus a decision about which phoneme pairs to target and in which order must also be made. Blache and Parsons (1980) suggested tackling the affected phoneme pairs in developmental order. If the error pattern affects more than one word position, begin in word-initial position and then proceed to word-final if spontaneous generalization across word positions does not occur. Finally, in the treatment planning stage, select 3 to 5 word pairs that differ only by the feature of interest. The word pairs must be produced as homophones by the child. For example, Amber routinely devoiced obstruents in the coda; restricting the choice of word pairs to phonemes for which she is readily stimulable, p/b, t/d, f/v, and s/z are all potential candidates for this treatment procedure. Blache and Parsons (1980) would recommend beginning with p/b. Potential minimal pair words that differ only by these phonemes would be cap/cab, tap/tab, and cop/cob.

The meaningful minimal pairs procedure proceeds, for each word pair at a time, through a sequence of four steps, listed with the corresponding instructions in Table 11–2. First, it is necessary to ensure that the child knows the words and recognizes the pictures (or objects) that have been chosen to represent the word pairs; the

Table 11–2. *Steps in the Meaningful Minimal Pairs Procedure*

	Step	*Instructions (for example pair cap/cab)*
1	Test for Concepts	(Show the child the picture of the "cap" and the "cab" side by side) "This one is *cap*. This one is *cab*. Which one do you wear on your head? That's right we wear a cap on our head. Which one do we call when we need a ride to the airport? Yes, we call a cab when we need a ride."
2	Test for Discrimination	(Sit beside or behind the child. Show the child the picture of the "cap" and the "cab" side by side on the table.) "Touch *cab*. Touch *cap*." (Move pictures around, rearrange in random order between trials.) "Touch *cap*. Touch *cab*." (Repeat with random ordering of pictures and trials until child achieves 7 consecutive correct response pairs.)
3	Production Practice	(Place 4 pictures of "cap" and 5 pictures of "cab" in a haphazard arrangement on the table.) "Now it is your turn to be the teacher. Your job is to get me to pick up all the pictures on the table. When I have all the cards picked up, you can choose a sticker, OK? Start now, tell me what to pick up first."
4	Generalization	Repeat steps 1 to 3 as needed with new word pairs and phonemes until generalization has been achieved across the sound class at the word level. Then use traditional procedures to promote generalization to untrained words and to sentence level material and conversational speech as needed.

Note: Instructions adapted from Blache and Parsons (1980) and Weiner (1981).

child's understanding that the words have different meanings is an essential aspect of the intervention. Next, it is essential to ensure that the child has good perceptual knowledge of the phonemic contrast. We would try to complete this step by obscuring the child's access to visual feedback if possible (for example, by sitting beside or behind the child) when asking him or her to point to the cards when you name them. Blache and Parsons (1980) point out that 7 consecutive correct responses (to both members of the word pair) indicates that the child is responding above chance levels. When the child achieves this level of performance, proceed to production practice by reversing roles. Now it is the child's turn to talk: telling the SLP which cards to pick up or otherwise manipulate. It will be obvious by following the child's eye gaze which item is the intended target even if the child misarticulates the intended word. However, it is essential to the procedure that the SLP pick up the item that is indicated by the child's speech. If she says "Pick up the *cap*" when she meant "Pick up the *cab*," you must pick the cap. If there are no more caps on the table, indicate that you will not pick up a cab unless she says [kæb]. You can say something like this: I think you want me to pick up the ***cab*** but I keep hearing ***cap***; I will pick up the ***cab*** when you say [kæb] (with emphasis on the [b]). After two incorrect attempts, it is acceptable to offer verbal instructions or even phonetic placement in addition to the model to help the child achieve the intended articulation. The point is to ensure that the child learns the two categories by producing linguistically and functionally different responses in relation to the two items and experiencing different functional outcomes. This is quite different from the more artificial imitative learning scenario where the child produces a nonfunctional response and receives feedback about the accuracy of the response. Recent research in category learning in multiple domains indicates that the linking of motor responses to variable items within an auditory category with implicit feedback about category membership arising from functional experience with new categories is a more effective teaching strategy than traditional explicit training regimens (Liu & Holt, 2010).

In Step 2, ensure that the child has good perceptual knowledge of the phonemic contrast.

Step 3 is to ensure that the child learns the two categories by producing linguistically and functionally different responses in relation to the two items and experiencing different functional outcomes.

We have found that students in our clinic rarely set up or follow through with this procedure correctly without extra training and support. It is difficult to respond to what the child said rather than what she meant, especially if the child becomes distressed at the result of her miscommunication. However, it is exactly the opportunity for miscommunication that provides the "teachable moments" in the therapeutic exchange. Furthermore, the child's motivation to avoid these communication breakdowns is an important factor in the success of the procedure. Provided that you have matched the procedure to your client characteristics appropriately, there should not be any undue struggle in the elicitation of the appropriate word. In other words, if the child is unstimulable for the phoneme and the misarticulation has articulatory basis, a different approach to therapy is probably warranted or traditional procedures should be used

Step 4 is to ensure generalization to new word pairs and phonemes and conversation.

to ensure stimulability before the minimal pairs procedure is introduced (e.g., as in the implementation described in Tyler et al., 1987).

Blache and Parsons (1980) reported that it usually takes less than 10 minutes to repeat these steps with a single word pair. They would then probe for generalization to other word pairs and add additional word pairs representing the p/b contrast if generalization had not occurred. After 3 to 5 pairs, production will likely be stable enough to introduce the next phoneme pair, t/d, and so on. As an alternative to this vertical approach, Weiner (1981) described a horizontal approach where word pairs representing multiple phoneme contrasts are practiced at once. In other words, pairs of words representing voicing contrasts such as *cap/cab*, *pot/pod*, and *piece/peas* were all practiced in the same session.

Weiner also demonstrated the use of this procedure to target a word shape goal, specifically final consonant deletion. The use of the meaningful minimal pairs procedure to target consonant clusters can be tricky because the child's error usually involves more than one phoneme. For example, Amber tended to spread features within the complex onset resulting in coalescence (e.g., "smoke" → [pot]) as well as from the coda to complex onsets (e.g., "stove" → [pos]) resulting in cluster productions that were not good candidates for the meaningful minimal pairs procedure. Even when the child's error appears to be a simple deletion of one segment, application of the meaningful minimal pairs procedure can result in some confusing exchanges between child and SLP because the child's reduced version of the cluster may not result in an exact homophone. If we take a word pair such as "spin" and "pin" it is likely that the child's productions are differentiated by aspiration, that is, [pɪn] and [pʰɪn]. If the meaningful minimal word pairs procedure is to be applied in a case like this, it is important to implement it exactly as instructed, letting the child know that it is the functional effect of his pronunciation that is the problem. The problem is not that he is failing to produce a contrast (in fact, he is); the problem is that the contrast is not meaningful to you, the listener. The fact that [pɪn] means "spin" to him but "pin" to you is the communicative conflict that must be resolved by the addition of the key phoneme /s/ to the word "spin." Gardner (1997) observed therapy sessions in which the SLP incorrectly imitated the child's productions (not taking into account the child's phonetic implementation of the words), resulting in more confusion rather than clarification, as shown in this example in which the SLP is trying unsuccessfully to initiate a self-repair by the child:

- SLP: [sːpɑts] (spreads lips on /s/)
- CHILD: [pɑt] (looking at picture)
- SLP: [pʰɑts]?
- CHILD: [pɑts] (looking at SLP)
- SLP: Are they [pʰɑts]?
- CHILD: (shakes head no)

- SLP: Let's hear the Sammy snake sound at the beginning then, [sːpɑt].
- CHILD: [pʰɑt]

This brief example of a therapeutic exchange illustrates the kind of mismatch in phonological categories between talker and listener than can be resolved with the meaningful minimal pairs procedure. However, it is necessary to implement the procedure so as to focus on the linguistic function of the missing feature or segment from the listener's point of view. Many studies have been conducted in which minimal pair words (i.e., pairs of words differing by a single phoneme) have been presented to children for imitative or spontaneous production (e.g., as described in Barlow & Gierut, 2002). However, the procedures are implemented using behaviorist techniques rather than with a conceptual approach that focuses on the communicative breakdown that occurs when the child produces the pair as homophone. These studies are not discussed here because they are not examples of the meaningful minimal pairs procedure according to standard criteria.

Empirical Support for the Method of Meaningful Minimal Pairs

Baker (2011) conducted an extensive review of the scientific literature on the method of meaningful minimal pairs therapy and found 42 studies covering multiple levels of evidence including nonexperimental studies, quasi-experiments, single-subject experiments, and two randomized controlled trials. Taken together, these studies demonstrate that the procedure is effective and efficient. Baker (2011) suggested that the procedure is best suited to children who have mild or moderate DPD with a few consistent patterns of phonological error in their speech. The child should be stimulable for the phoneme pairs that are targeted in therapy. The research is characterized by a great deal of variability in the implementation of the procedure but certain elements are key to its effectiveness including ensuring that there is a production practice component with the provision of supports for accurate production attempts by the child. There should be parent involvement in the therapy and a structured home practice component. Some studies have revealed components of the intervention that are not essential to the success of the procedure. In particular, it may not be necessary to practice beyond the word level to achieve carryover to conversation and there is no need to practice many word pairs to achieve carryover either (Elbert et al., 1990; Elbert, Powell, & Swartzlander, 1991). In fact, many studies have shown that generalization can occur after practice with between 3 and 5 word pairs. In those cases where generalization did not occur after a small number of word pairs, the children involved were often shown to be inappropriate candidates for this intervention (they showed characteristics of motor speech disorder or inconsistent deviant phonological disorder). Other studies

The method of meaningful minimal pairs may be best suited to children who have mild or moderate DPD with a few consistent patterns of phonological error associated with stimulable phonemes.

The method of meaningful minimal pairs is more likely to be effective if the SLP ensures that there is a production practice component with the provision of supports for accurate production attempts by the child.

have shown clearly how not to implement the approach. For example, Saben and Costello Ingham (1991) achieved complete failure over a 10-month period with two children who were presented with multiple pairs of words contrasting a fricative with another phoneme. In this study a behaviorist intervention protocol was used to teach the children to imitate the words but reinforcement was given for responses that represented "suppression of the process" even if the response was a misarticulation of the target word. For example, one 4-year-old child with normal receptive language but a severe "phonological delay" (accompanied by soft neurological signs such as drooling) was treated in the study. He substituted glides for fricatives so a minimal pair such as "fight" and "white" might be a treatment target but "fight" → [sɑɪt] would be accepted as correct imitative or spontaneous response to the stimulus picture. The activities did not involve communicative exchanges with the SLP that invited ambiguity or uncertainty in message transmission and thus the child had no opportunity to learn how his misarticulations functioned in communication with a conversation partner. If the procedure had been implemented in the normal fashion perhaps the absurdity of picking up the "fight" card in response to [sɑɪt] would have been more apparent! Interestingly, the child did appear to make progress with /f/ initially but confusion ensued when /s/ and /θ/ were introduced and he reverted to 100% gliding of both treated and untreated target fricatives.

To emphasize the point that the procedure can be effective when implemented as intended, two studies are described in more detail here. Weiner (1981) applied the approach, using a single subject, multiple baseline across responses design, with two subjects who presented with multiple phonological patterns. Different phonological patterns were targeted in series but within each pattern, multiple phoneme pairs were targeted in parallel. Each child received intervention for deletion of final consonants (using the word pairs *bow-boat*, *bee-beed*, *pie-pipe*, *no-nose*, and *tea-teeth*), stopping of fricatives (using the word pairs *fin-pin*, *zip-dip*, and *sea-tea*) and velar fronting (using the word pairs *can-tan*, *key-tea*, *gum-dumb*, and *gate-date*). Treatment sessions occurred three times per week for one hour. Performance on treated words was tracked during therapy and generalization to untreated words was assessed once per treatment session throughout the experiment. Subject A mastered all three consonants within 6 sessions with generalization to untreated words being 50% or more, indicating an excellent probability that the child would acquire the phonemes without further treatment. Subject B required 14 sessions to achieve a similar result but nonetheless the number of phonemes affected and the degree of generalization observed (Figure 11–1) is remarkable in each case given the brevity of the treatment program (2 weeks in one case and 5 weeks in the other).

Dodd et al. (2008) compared two forms of choosing contrasts when implementing the meaningful minimal pairs procedure.

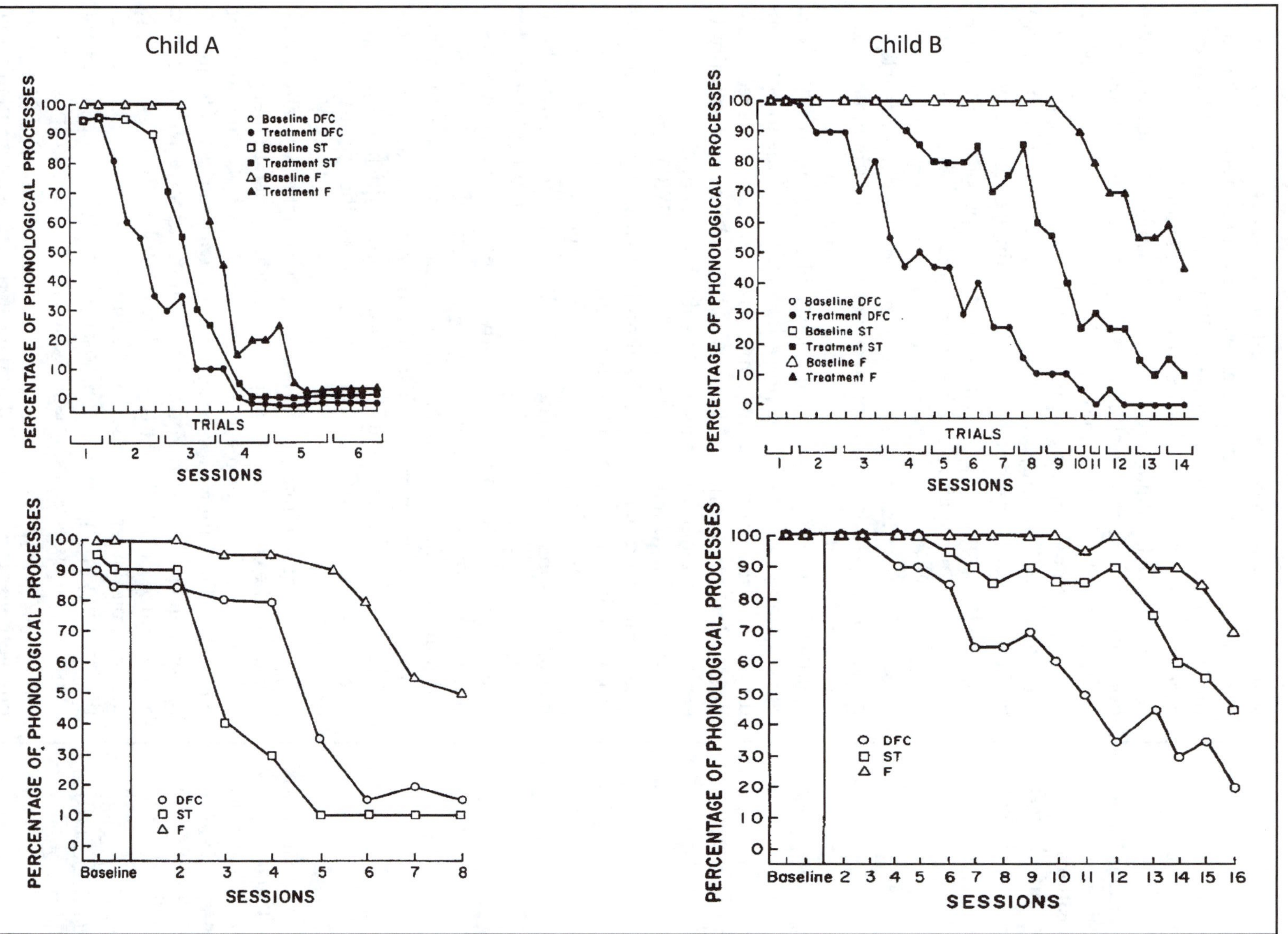

Figure 11–1. *Percent use of the phonological processes deletion of final consonants (DFC), stopping of fricatives (ST), and velar fronting (F) by two children who received a meaningful minimal pairs intervention. Performance during therapy is shown in the top charts and performance on generalization probes is shown in the bottom charts.* Source: *From "*Treatment of Phonological Disability Using the Method of Meaningful Minimal Contrast: Two Case Studies,*" by* F. Weiner,1981, Journal of Speech and Hearing Disorders, 46, *Figures 1 and 2, p. 100, and Figures 3 and 4, p. 101. Copyright 1981 by American Speech-Language-Hearing Association. Adapted with permission.*

The research participants were aged 3 to 5 years with moderate or severe DPD. They received 12 half-hour treatment sessions, scheduled once per week. Outcome assessments occurred at the end of the treatment block and again 8 to 10 weeks later. Children were randomly assigned to receive treatment with word pairs that represented either a minimal or a maximal opposition. Minimal oppositions involved a single feature change (e.g., "tea"→ [ti] and "key" → [ti] to target velar fronting) as in the standard application. Maximal oppositions contrasted phonemes that differed by many features (e.g., "me" → [mi] and "key" → [ti] to target velar fronting). In the case of cluster reduction, the contrasting conditions would be "top" → [tɑp] and "stop" → [stɑp] (minimal opposition) compared to "mop" → [mɑp] and "stop" → [stɑp] (maximal opposition). It is not completely clear how the procedure is implemented in the latter case; the report indicates that nonverbal and verbal feedback was provided for responses: the picture would or would not be picked up and information would be provided about the accuracy of the child's response ("You said that one well because I heard the 's' at the beginning"). Overtly, the procedure was the same in both conditions and the child had the opportunity to use the correct word productions in a functional context although the opportunity to experience listener uncertainty was subtly different in this application compared to that described in Weiner's (1981) report above. The comparison between minimal and maximal oppositions was motivated by the claim that the use of maximal oppositions leads to greater within- and across-class generalization than the use of minimal oppositions (Barlow & Gierut, 2002). However, this hypothesis was not confirmed in Dodd et al.'s (2008) randomized controlled trial. Both groups made statistically significant gains in percent consonants correct (with improvement from 58 to 74% overall). Measures of suppression of phonological processes and generalization to untreated phonemes also improved significantly over the 12-week treatment interval. There were no significant differences in any measured outcomes between groups either post-treatment or at follow-up.

Minimal oppositions involves a single feature change and **maximal oppositions** contrast phonemes that differ by many features.

Meaningful minimal pairs is a procedure that is typically implemented in the context of a comprehensive approach to therapy that includes other procedures and thus it is not always certain that the inclusion of the minimal pairs procedure was a critical element to the outcomes observed. For example, in Chapter 9 we described a randomized control trial in which we implemented meaningful minimal pairs along with focused stimulation and speech perception training. In the application described by Tyler et al. (1987), the minimal pairs procedure was preceded by speech perception training and speech production practice at the imitative and spontaneous word levels. Hodson (2007) suggested that meaningful minimal pairs could be incorporated into the cycles approach if the child had gained a high enough skill level to participate with success.

Meaningful minimal pairs is a procedure that is typically implemented in the context of a comprehensive approach to therapy that includes other procedures and thus it is not always certain that the inclusion of the minimal pairs procedure was a critical element to the outcomes observed.

Williams (2010) incorporates the procedure into the multiple oppositions approach along with a variety of other procedures including speech practice in a drill context and focused stimulation during interactive play activities. The focus of this approach is simultaneous practice with multiple word pairs that represent a "collapse" in the child's system to a single phone. For example, Williams (2010) describes a boy who produced all singleton obstruents and stop clusters as [g] word initially and all sonorants and fricative clusters as [w]. Beginning therapy with the collapse to [g], the intervention targeted multiple oppositions such as *gear*: *deer*, *fear*, *cheer*, *steer*. This is an interesting variation on the minimal pairs approach that was recently assessed with a randomized controlled trial (Allen, 2009). In this study, the multiple oppositions approach was only more effective than the control condition when provided 3 times a week for 8 weeks. The group that received the multiple oppositions intervention once a week did not achieve outcomes that were significantly better than the control group at 8 or 24 weeks.

As discussed briefly in Chapter 10, there is some research evidence suggesting that phonological approaches are more efficient than the traditional approach to speech therapy. However, these research applications involve high intensity interventions that may not be replicated in publically funded clinics. More randomized controlled trial studies are required to compare the relative effectiveness of different phonological approaches and to identify optimum intensities for each of these types of phonological intervention. When implementing these interventions it is important to remember that the outcomes reported in the research papers may not be achieved unless the service delivery models and treatment intensities applied in the research setting are carried over to the clinic.

More randomized controlled trial studies are required to compare the relative effectiveness of different phonological approaches and to identify optimum intensities for each of these types of phonological intervention.

Explicit Access to Phonological Structure

11.3.1. Distinguish three contexts in which the SLP may intervene to improve a child's metaphonological knowledge.

11.3.2. Distinguish procedures to improve speech perception skills versus procedures to improve phonological awareness skills.

11.3.3. Plan activities to teach awareness of syllables, onsets, rimes, phonemes, and features.

11.3.4. Describe five characteristics of effective phonological awareness interventions.

Some therapeutic procedures are designed to facilitate the child's explicit access to phonological structures at all levels of the phonological hierarchy. These activities improve the child's metaphonological knowledge of words, syllables, onsets and rimes, phonemes, and features. In some approaches the activities are integrated into speech therapy sessions and the goal is primarily to reorganize the

Some therapeutic procedures facilitate the child's explicit access to phonological structures thus improving the child's **metaphonological knowledge** of words, syllables, onsets and rimes, phonemes, and features.

child's phonological system and to improve speech intelligibility and accuracy with developments in phonological awareness being a fortunate side effect. However, given the risk of dyslexia among children with DPD, these children are prime targets for "response to intervention" or other programs that target emergent literacy skills as a means to prevent reading disability. Finally, speech-language pathologists are increasingly involved in the treatment of dyslexia and may intervene directly to improve children's decoding and spelling skills. The application of treatment procedures to improve metaphonology in each of these three contexts is discussed.

Metaphonological Approaches to Speech Therapy

Metaphonological or **"conceptual" approaches to speech therapy** have the goal of explicitly teaching the child about the phonological structure of speech as a means to reorganizing the child's phonological system and improving speech intelligibility and accuracy.

Metaphonological or "conceptual" approaches to speech therapy have the goal of explicitly teaching the child about the phonological structure of speech, especially structures that child misarticulates. As discussed in Chapter 3, these tasks will vary in terms of the unit that the child must focus on (with larger units generally being easier than smaller units) and the cognitive difficulty level of the task itself (with matching tasks being easier than explicit segmentation or deletion tasks for example). Some of the procedures are similar or even identical to the "input-oriented" procedures that we described in Chapter 9 but the goal is different. In Chapter 9 we were targeting the child's acoustic-phonetic representations for sounds and words. The procedures included providing focused and high quality exposure to specific targets (e.g., focused stimulation, auditory bombardment) and asking the child to make judgments about the quality of sounds or words presented (e.g., isolation, discrimination). When the child listens to many different exemplars of the word "sheet" and identifies the tokens that are produced correctly or incorrectly the child learns to focus on the acoustic cues that define the /ʃ/ category (recall from Chapter 1 that these cues are spread across the entire word). The procedures that we will describe here also involve presenting speech to the child and requiring explicit judgments about those speech inputs. However, the child is expected to learn about abstract phonological structures. For example, the child might learn that one class of consonants in English is characterized by long durations (the fricatives) compared to another class that is characterized by short durations (the stops). Another activity will teach the child that (at an abstract level) the word "sheet" is made up of three individual segments: /ʃ/, /i/, /t/. Notice that the child does not have to be explicitly or even implicitly aware of these individual segments to succeed at the mispronunciation task described above and thus speech perception tasks and phonological awareness tasks tap different levels of representation even though there are some superficial similarities in the nature of the activities. Table 11–3 contains a list of metaphonological activities that are routinely included in metaphonological treatment programs.

Conceptual approaches involve asking the child to make explicit judgments about speech inputs that are organized to help the child learn about abstract phonological structures.

Table 11–3. Examples of Metaphonological Activities at Multiple Levels of the Phonological Hierarchy and Three Levels of Difficulty

Syllables		
Matching: Place large caterpillar cutouts on the floor each with a head and either 1, 2, or 3 "body parts." Child selects from a selection of cards depicting foods (egg, melon, banana) and matches it to the appropriate caterpillar. After choosing the correct caterpillar the child jumps on each body part, pronouncing one syllable per part [e.g., ba (jump) – na (jump) – na (jump)] and then places food to be eaten on the caterpillar's mouth. (Omit 3 syllable words in the early stages of the intervention).	Identification: Present the child with a picture of a complex scene (a page from a Richard Scary book is a good example). The child picks a card that reveals either a 1 or a 2 and then proceeds to identify an item in the scene that represents either a one or two-syllable word.	Blending: Say one word with the syllables well segmented, to – ma – to. Child blends the syllables and produces the complete word. To make the task easier, especially for children with speech errors, provide four pictures as choices (e.g., potato, tomato, teapot, marmite). Child points to picture to identify the word. Practice production of the word when the correct picture has been identified. Reverse roles when the child masters the task.
Rimes		
Matching: Present two wizards named "Pat" and "Pete," each with a cauldron labeled with the wizard's name in large letters. Child sorts picture cards into their respective cauldrons based on match between word and wizard name (e.g., Pat—bat, hat; Pete—meat, feet, etc.) Do not label the word cards with text. When the cauldrons are full child says the magic word and the cauldron is removed to reveal a magic animal.	Rime generation with picture support: Create rimes and ask the child to fill in the blanks by choosing pictures from a selection, e.g., Mrs. Brown drove to the store, Where she noticed through the _____, Mr. Harper waving hi, Come with me and share my _____, I'd love to have your company, Let's sit here by this _____. (option cards: door, window, pie, cake, tree, bench).	Segmenting and matching: Give the child a puppet whose name is Snark. Snark only likes to eat things that rime with his name. The child must consider each picture card and decide if Snark will eat it or not. Options are bark, lark, park, shark, mark, snail, pear, car, cake, spear. (implicit rather than explicit segmenting)
Onsets and Phonemes		
Sorting: Label paper plates with letters or digraphs (e.g. P, CH, L). Child sorts pictures of food cut out of magazines onto the plates and then glues them on to make meals (porkchops, peas, potatoes; cheese, cherries, chicken; lettuce, leeks, lemons).	Segmenting: Provide a segmented template with 3 to 6 sections depending upon the length of the words that you will work with. Provide colored blocks. Say a word. Ask the child to produce the sounds of the word while pushing blocks, one sound at a time, into the sections of the template. Block colors should reflect similarities and differences in sounds, e.g., blue-red-green for "top" but green-red-green for "pop." Words can be built in chains: a - at - mat - sat - sit - pit - pot - pop - etc.	Deleting: Ask the child to "say '*beet*' without '*t*.'" If the child has some decoding skills progress to deletion within complex onsets and codas: "Say '*spit*' without the '*p*.'"

continues

Table 11–3. continued

Features		
Sorting by concept: Provide cut-outs of ears and tails and a sheet with drawings of bodies of different animals. Child selects the ears or tails, one at a time, at random from a container, and verbally indicates where it goes before gluing it to the appropriate animal, e.g., "These ears go on the front of the cow." Or "This tail goes on the back of the horse."	Matching sounds to concept: Provide child with model of the mouth or teath. Ask the child: Listen to this sound. Do I make it at the front where my teeth are, OR, at the back where I gargle? Produce /k/,/g/,/ŋ/,/t//d/,/n/ in random order.	Sorting words by feature: Provide stack of picture cards with word initial /k/ or /t/ and a large toy truck. Child puts the pictures of /k/ words in the back of the truck and pictures of /t/ words in the front of the truck. The child can be provided with an audiovisual stimulus ("Look at me. This is a cane.") or an auditory stimulus only (say "cane" while sitting behind the child) or no auditory stimulus (the child views the card silently and makes a decision). These cards should not contain the printed stimulus. The decision should be made on the basis of the child's internal representation of the sound of the presented word and not on the basis of a letter cue.

These treatment programs, when implemented with children who have DPD, may be general in nature, meaning that the phonemes targeted may not relate to the children's speech sound errors; alternatively, the intervention may be specifically targeted at the phonemes and syllable structures that the child has difficulty producing.

Metaphonological activities are often combined with phonological procedures such as the meaningful minimal pairs procedure. The metaphonological and production oriented activities may be targeted horizontally or they may be sequenced vertically so that the child is not required to practice speech production until after metaphonological knowledge of the phoneme target has been achieved. Dean and Howell (1986), in a description of their Metaphon approach, recommend that these phases be sequenced vertically. The metaphonological activities are designed to instill explicit awareness of the sound structure of the language, with a specific focus on those structures that the child has difficulty producing correctly. Subsequently, meaningful minimal pair and other phonological contrast activities are introduced to raise the child's awareness of his or her communicative effectiveness. They propose that metalinguistic awareness is essential to the development of the child's ability to implement repair strategies when there is a communicative breakdown and for this reason metaphonological skills are taught first. Subsequently, the child practices speech in contexts where communicative breakdowns may occur, triggering the use of repair strategies.

The **Metaphon** approach begins with activities to ensure metaphonological knowledge of target forms followed by procedures to raise awareness of communicative effectiveness.

Metaphonological skills are taught first in order to develop the child's ability to implement **repair strategies** when there is a communicative breakdown.

Demonstration of Metaphonological Approach

Demonstration 11–4 presents a series of activities, meant to be implemented in the sequence as presented, which could be implemented with Amber. Returning to the goals selected for Amber from the nonlinear analysis of her speech (see Table 8–5), one of the intermediate goals to be addressed in the first treatment block was [+consonantal][+continuant] in the onset position. Although Amber is stimulable for these segments (in fact she matches this feature combination in the coda position), she does not produce this feature combination in onsets. The specific goals to be targeted were /f/ and /v/, proceeding to /ʃ/ if progress permitted a third specific goal during the first block. When using a metaphonological approach the intervention would begin with activities to raise Amber's awareness of the feature [+continuant], using terms that are appropriate for a 4-year-old. It is suggested that the first activity ensure that she understands the concepts "long" and "short" and that she associate these words with objects of different lengths as well as whistle blasts of different durations. Once she has shown that she can make these associations it is a small step to associate the short and long objects with short and long speech sounds, specifically stops and fricatives produced in isolation. The activity as planned will largely involve the SLP producing speech sounds for Amber to respond to but if she proved to master the task quickly the roles could be reversed so that Amber could try producing short and long speech sounds for the SLP to respond to with appropriate sorting or matching responses. Even though only one-third of the first session would be devoted to this target, it is likely that these two activities could be completed in the time allowed.

The following week, the session could begin with a brief review of the short and long concepts and then the trains could be used for a new activity in which Amber points to the engine or the caboose to indicate whether she heard the "long" sound at the beginning or the end of the words presented by the SLP. This activity is recommended for Amber because she regularly produced "long sounds" in the coda but not in the onset. This conceptual activity will help her to focus attention on the onset position and provide some vocabulary for talking to Amber about her production of target words when it comes time to practice production of these phonemes. The next activity is a standard onset-matching activity—again focusing attention on the onset position but in this case the contrast between the specific target /f/ and /p/ is introduced along with the corresponding letters. The activity as planned provides opportunities for focused stimulation and some giggles especially if Amber and the SLP switch roles as the activity progresses. We recommend a role reversal if Amber begins to produce some of the target words spontaneously during the course of the activity. We also recommend homework activities that involve matching pictures to the letters "f" and "p" and "F" and "P."

Demonstration 11–4
Suggested Lesson Activities for Amber (Case Study 6–2) Assuming Non-linear Goals Proposed in Table 8–5 and Metaphonological Treatment Approach

Treatment Block 1: Intermediate Goal [+consonantal][+continuant] in onsets

Goal	Activity	Stimuli	Expected Responses
Multimodal comprehension of the concepts "short" and "long."	Load short and long toothpicks into short and long trains upon hearing short and long whistle blasts.	Provide toothpicks and a 2-car and 4-car train. Discuss the concepts "short" and "long" while sorting the toothpicks into piles by size. Blow long and short blasts of whistle in random order to trigger child's matching response until all toothpicks are loaded into appropriate railcars.	1. When long whistle is heard, pull long train into station and put long toothpick into rail car. 2. When short whistle is heard, pull short train into station and put short toothpick into rail car.
Associate concepts "long" and "short" with fricative and stop sounds.	Sort short and long toothpicks into short and long containers in homework book upon hearing short and long speech sounds. Reverse roles if Amber is capable.	Produce the sounds /p/, /t/, /b/, /d/, /f/, /v/, /s/, /ʃ/ in isolation and in random order. Paste short and long "pockets" into homework as containers for the toothpicks so that the activity can be repeated at home.	1. When a long sound (fricative) is heard, unload long toothpick from rail car and tuck into long pocket in homework booklet. 2. When a short sound (stop) is heard, unload short toothpick from rail car and tuck into short pocket in homework booklet. 3. Reverse roles so that Amber produces short and long sounds in isolation.
Raise awareness of fricatives in onset and coda positions of words.	Point to engine or caboose of train to indicate position of "long" sound in word.	Produce the words: Foot, purse, bush, van, fire, bath, toes, food, shoe, cash, sheet, calf.	Point to engine if the long sound is at the beginning of the word and to the caboose if the long sound is at the end of the word.

Goal	Activity	Stimuli	Expected Responses
Raise awareness of /f/ versus /p/ onsets.	Match actions to words based on onset sound, /f/ versus /p/.	Produce the words: feet, park, fire, fan, Pete, pan, pile, foal, fight, firetruck, football, potatoe (etc.).	While sitting on floor, Amber: (1) falls down slowly if a /f/ word is heard or (2) pops up quickly if a /p/ word is heard.
Produce /f/ and /p/ in appropriate meaningful context.	Meaningful minimal pairs procedure.	Provide multiple copies of picture cards depicting: feet-Pete; fan-pan; four-pour; fool-pool; fat-pat; file-pile.	Amber requests the cards or asks the SLP to carry out specific actions with the picture cards until there are none left on the table. Amber must produce the /f/ correctly in order to achieve the expected results with the /f/ picture cards.

Finally, the meaningful minimal pairs procedure shifts the focus of therapy to production practice. When implementing the meaningful minimal pairs procedure the SLP should use the language and concepts taught during the first phase to prompt repairs on the part of the child when miscommunications occur. For example, the SLP can say, "I am hearing a short sound but there are no words left on the table that begin with a short sound." Dean and Howell (1986) suggest an interesting variation on this procedure called the "secret messages" game. In this variation of the game, only one of each picture card in the target pair is shown face up on the table (e.g., "pan"—"fan"). The child has control of the remaining cards, in a randomized pile face down in front of her. She chooses a card, holding it so that the SLP cannot see it. Then she produces the name of the picture on her card and the SLP points to one of the cards on the table to indicate which word she heard. At this point the child reveals her card and discussion ensues if the card does not match the SLP's choice. If the card does match the SLP's choice the child gets to take a turn at a game she is playing with the SLP.

As with the standard meaningful minimal pairs approach, Amber would work through 3 to 5 pairs of words contrasting /f/ and /p/ until it was clear that generalization to untrained words was beginning to occur. Then words contrasting /v/ and /b/ could be introduced. Finally, words that contrast /ʃ/ versus /d/ could be practiced. This contrast will have to be planned carefully so that the initial pairs do not contain a labial phoneme elsewhere in the word. Words that contain /ʃ/ in the onset and a labial in the coda or ambisyllabic position may need to be practiced deliberately in Amber's case. There should be no need to practice /s/ and /z/ as these phonemes are unmarked for place and if [+continuant] is learned in the context of the nondefault labial and [–anterior] fricatives, the feature should generalize to the unmarked coronal obstruents spontaneously. The exception again is the difficulty with spreading of [Labial] from coda to onset position. If this pattern does not resolve itself spontaneously, practice with words containing a coronal fricative in the onset and a [Labial] fricative or stop in the coda will be necessary.

Amber produces other patterns that involve interactions between the segmental and prosodic levels of the phonological hierarchy, in particular the delinking of [+consonantal] in specific ambisyllabic contexts and cluster reduction complicated by spreading of features within the onset or from the coda to the onset. Bernhardt (1994) describes metaphonological activities for targeting prosodic goals that include raising awareness of target structures through the presentation of poems that have been specially constructed to contrast new structures with the child's preferred structure. Other techniques involve taking advantage of strengths to facilitate emergence of new structures. Teaching sound-letter combinations and working with nonsense words can be helpful with these exercises. For example, rapid sequencing of "IS-PE"(i.e., [aɪs↓pi], a nonsense sequence with two preferred structures ([Coronal] [+continuant] fricative in coda and [Labial] stop in onset), followed by movement of the break back by one segment yields "I-SPE" [aɪ↓spi]. In this way, metaphonological knowledge combined with letter knowledge can be used to facilitate emergence of a complex onset that can be practiced in words and generalized to many other /s/+consonant combinations.

Empirical Support for the Metaphonological Approach

A number of studies have reported outcomes for children with DPD who received metaphonological interventions. These studies reported good outcomes for phonological awareness and/or speech production accuracy in the short term (Gillon, 2000; Hesketh, Adams, Nightingale, & Hall, 2000; Hesketh, Dima, & Nelson, 2007; Major & Bernhardt, 1998) and for literacy outcomes in the longer term (Bernhardt & Major, 2005; Gillon, 2002). Most of these studies do not have randomized control groups, however, and therefore the outcomes are difficult to interpret. The two studies with the strongest research design are described here.

Hesketh et al. (2000) divided 61 3- to 5-year-old children with DPD into 4 groups: two groups with good phonological awareness skills, one treated with articulation therapy and the other with the metaphonological approach; and two groups with poor phonological awareness skills, one treated with articulation therapy and the other with the metaphonological approach. All children received 10 weekly individual therapy sessions. Articulation therapy followed the standard sequence of speech production practice from isolation through syllables, words, and sentences. The metaphonological intervention covered general metaphonological skills for the first four sessions; sessions 5 through 8 continued with metaphonological activities but focusing on the children's specific patterns of production error. Finally, in sessions 9 and 10 production practice was introduced in the context of meaningful minimal pair activities. Speech and phonological awareness outcomes were assessed immediately posttreatment and 3 months after cessation of treatment. The surprise result was that the two groups made roughly equivalent gains on all outcome measures. The authors point out that many traditional speech therapy procedures (i.e., identification of the target, segmentation, blending, chaining, etc.) may serve to improve the child's phonological awareness test performance. Although the children who received the articulation therapy appeared to make faster gains on target specific probes during the treatment interval, the differences were not statistically significant and the children who received the metaphonological intervention showed a faster rate of change during the follow-up interval than the children who received articulation therapy.

A metaphonological approach to speech therapy resulted in equivalent gains in speech accuracy in comparison to a traditional approach.

The results of Hesketh et al. (2000) are rather similar to the results we reported for our randomized control trial in Chapter 9 (Rvachew & Brosseau-Lapré, 2010). In our study the input-oriented and output-oriented approaches were equally effective but only when supported by a theoretically consistent home program. When the children received articulation therapy in the clinic but the parents were taught to provide dialogic reading at home the phonological awareness outcomes were significantly worse than when the parents supported the in-clinic therapy with an output-oriented home program. In both Hesketh et al. (2000) and Rvachew and Brosseau-Lapré (2010), the equivalent findings for speech production accuracy regardless of treatment approach are rather remarkable considering the small amount of speech production practice that was provided in the metaphonological intervention (in Hesketh et al., 2000) and in the input-oriented intervention (in Rvachew and Brosseau-Lapré, 2010) in comparison to the articulation therapy control groups. We suggest that the take home message from both studies is not that "anything works" but rather that treatment intensity is the key: the children must receive theoretically coherent interventions with sufficient intensity for the effects to stabilize in one domain and carry over to another. When children receive a properly implemented articulation therapy program that improves their articulatory-phonetic knowledge, perceptual and phonological knowledge will be impacted. The same is true for interventions that focus on perceptual knowledge or metaphonological knowledge but in either case the intensity of the intervention must be sufficient to effect substantive change in the targeted domain in order to achieve cross-domain effects. Further research is required to determine if one approach is more efficient than the other, especially when considering post-treatment generalization and maintenance.

Hesketh et al. (2007) carried out a randomized controlled trial to assess the efficacy of a more generalized phonological awareness intervention when conducted with 4-year-old children with DPD. In this case, the phonological awareness activities were not individualized to the children's speech errors and speech production practice was not provided. The control group received a language intervention focusing on vocabulary skills and print concepts. The interventions were provided over twenty 30-minute sessions two to three times per week. The group that received the phonological awareness intervention made significant gains in phonological awareness and surpassed the skills of the control group over the course of the intervention. Severity of the speech deficit was not significantly different between the groups before or after treatment, however.

A phonological awareness intervention that was not individualized to the children's speech errors resulted in significant improvements in phonological awareness but not articulation accuracy.

In conclusion, it appears that a metaphonological approach to speech therapy must focus on the child's specific error patterns in order to have a significant impact on speech accuracy as well as phonological awareness. Children with DPD clearly benefit from phonological awareness interventions although traditional speech therapy by itself may have a significant impact on children's metaphonological skills when it is provided with sufficient intensity. Further large sample randomized controlled trials with longer follow-up intervals are required to determine if a combination of metaphonological therapy and speech therapy protects children with DPD from the risk of dyslexia in the future. Further research is also required to determine if certain subsets of the DPD population are in particular need of a metaphonological approach.

Preventative Emergent Literacy Programs

Given the research evidence just reviewed on metaphonological approaches to speech therapy, what is the best way to prevent future academic problems for children like Amber who have severe DPD as preschoolers? We would argue that the first priority of the SLP who is responsible for providing individual therapy to Amber must be to ensure age-appropriate speech accuracy for this child before she begins formal schooling. The research that we reviewed in Chapter 7 indicates that persistence of the speech problem into kindergarten by itself would put her at risk for social, emotional, and academic difficulties over the long term. Furthermore, the SLP is the only professional with the training, skills and mandate to directly address her difficulties with productive phonology. Metaphonological activities may be a valuable part of the treatment program but they should be targeted at her phonological error patterns and have the primary goal of promoting speech intelligibility and speech accuracy. More generalized intervention for phonological awareness and emergent literacy can be provided by other individuals. The best practice would be for the SLP to ensure that the parents of their clients with DPD take advantage of education programs that teach parents to maximize their children's language development and emergent literacy skills. Every effort should be made to ensure that the children have access to high quality print materials and literacy experiences at home, daycare and school. From the public health perspective, the speech-language pathology profession as a whole has a large role to play in promoting public access to these kinds of programs for parents, child care workers, educators, and children. Randomized controlled trials have shown that vocabulary teaching and phonological awareness interventions can be implemented effectively by paraprofessionals and educators (Boyle, McCartney, Forbes, & O'Hare, 2007; Ehri et al., 2001; Wasik, Bond, & Hindman, 2006). The role of the SLP should be to work with community and school personnel to select or design evidence-based curricula and to educate parents, paraprofessionals and educators to implement effective teaching procedures in their homes and classrooms.

The role of the SLP should be to work with community and school personnel to select or design evidence-based curricula and to educate parents, paraprofessionals and educators to implement effective teaching procedures in their homes and classrooms.

An important first step for the SLP is to dispel some myths regarding best practice in the teaching of emergent literacy skills. Resistance to the development of such programs at the preschool level may come from those who believe phonological awareness and other emergent literacy skills are reading-related abilities that should be taught once the child begins first grade when the child is developmentally ready. In fact, the foundations of the reading skills that the child learns in school are laid during the preschool period starting at birth (Rvachew & Savage, 2006) with implicit phonological awareness skills emerging naturally from the child's growing experience with language. Children who do not experience a language rich environment in infancy and toddlerhood are at a disadvantage when they start school; the impact of the risk environment may be compounded by biological risk for dyslexia in some children (Noble, Farah, & McCandliss, 2006). The effects of social disadvantage on reading outcomes are entirely preventable with appropriate public inputs, however (Campbell, Ramey, Pugello, Sparling, & Miller-Johnson, 2002; Ramey, Campbell, & Ramey, 1999).

The foundations of the reading skills that the child learns in school are laid during the preschool period starting at birth.

The effects of social disadvantage on reading outcomes are preventable with appropriate public inputs.

The flip side of this myth is the idea that the prerequisite skills emerge naturally from being read to, and thus the popularity of programs that simply put books into the hands of parents (e.g., book bags for new mothers). First, as we indicated in Chapter 9, how one reads to the child is critical and thus the books need to be accompanied by education programs that teach developmentally appropriate techniques, dialogic reading for the parents of toddlers (Whitehurst et al., 1988), comprehensive language stimulation programs for preschool educators (Dickinson & Tabors, 2001; Wasik et al., 2006), and structured approaches to vocabulary teaching for grade school teachers (Biemiller & Boote, 2006; Graves, 2006). However, it must be recognized that children learn about language rather than reading while being read to. The research shows clearly that children do not even look at the text until after they have been explicitly taught to link knowledge of print concepts to their developing knowledge of phonological structure (Evans & Saint-Aubin, 2009; Senechal & LeFevre, 2002). Therefore, exposure to programs that provide explicit teaching of phonological awareness and letter knowledge during the preschool years and early school grades is essential, especially for those children who are disadvantaged due to poverty or a history of speech and language or other developmental delays.

Exposure to programs that provide explicit teaching of phonological awareness and letter knowledge during the preschool years and early school grades is essential, especially for those children who are disadvantaged due to poverty or a history of speech and language or other developmental delays.

Characteristics of Effective Phonological Awareness Interventions

A full review of the literature on family literacy and early intervention programs is well beyond the scope of this book but some basic principles are outlined and a few interventions that have proven efficacy and that should be of value for the DPD population are highlighted here. A large meta-analysis of good quality studies on phonological awareness interventions (Ehri, et al., 2001) concluded that the most effective programs are provided to small groups of preschool-age children, are relatively short (between 5 and 18 hours in total duration) and focus on a small number of skills that are taught to mastery (see summary of the conclusions of this national reading panel in Table 11–4). Perhaps the most important point in the summary is that phonological awareness interventions are most effective when they are provided early. Harm, McCandliss, and Seidenberg (2003) point out that several large scale meta-analyses have concluded that the impact of phonological awareness interventions on the acquisition of reading is considerably larger when the intervention occurs during the preschool period; even

Phonological awareness interventions are most effective when they are provided early.

Table 11–4. *Summary of the Conclusions of the National Reading Panel's Meta-Analysis of Scientific Investigations of Phonological Awareness (PA) Interventions*

1. PA instruction improves children's reading and spelling abilities.
2. PA instruction benefits low SES children as much as high SES children.
3. PA instructional benefits were especially large for preschool-age children.
4. Teachers can teach PA effectively.
5. Computer programs can be effective compared to no intervention but may be less effective than programs provided by teachers.
6. Effective programs taught one or two skills to mastery.
7. Effective programs lasted between 5 and 18 hours.
8. Effective programs made explicit links between PA skills and letter knowledge and/or reading.
9. Effective programs taught children in small groups.

waiting for kindergarten results in a marked reduction in the effect size. A related point is that the interventions are more effective when they are combined with instruction in letter-sound associations. Their computational modeling study served to confirm and explain why early exposure to phonological awareness and phonics instruction is essential to the acquisition of reading by supporting their mapping hypothesis: specifically, children who are at risk for dyslexia are likely to begin learning to read with noncomponential (i.e., whole-word) phonological representations in oral language which they subsequently map onto noncomponential orthographic representations in text. Phonological awareness instruction that is provided after the child has been taught to decode and after noncomponential orthographic representations have formed is of little benefit. When phonological awareness instruction is provided along with explicit teaching of sound-letter correspondence rules prior to formal reading instruction the child learns to map componential phonological representations to componential orthographic representations for words.

Phonological awareness interventions are more effective when they are combined with instruction in letter-sound associations.

Small groups are more efficient than interventions provided to a single child and more effective than interventions provided to the complete class. In the latter case there will be some children who do not understand the tasks and are unable to receive the extra support that they need to succeed. Programs that are provided at high intensity (for example, for 30 minutes per day each day of the school year) tend to focus on every possible phonological awareness task and to rush from one task to another which guarantees that a good proportion of the class will fail to master one skill before the next one is introduced. The meta-analysis showed that shorter duration programs with well-specified goals were more effective because all the children were more likely to master the constrained set of goals that were targeted by the activities. Finally, we point out that the meta-analysis showed that the programs were at least as effective when implemented by teachers in their classrooms as when implemented by researchers or other professionals in a "pull-out" fashion. One reason is that the phonological awareness skills should be linked to their functional applications and teachers are in a good position to ensure that these links are made in the classroom. For example, when children are learning to match words that share onsets or rimes, the teacher can reinforce the point that words have sounds as well as meanings during shared book reading sessions. The children's emerging segmentation skills can be linked to their efforts to spell words during journal writing and phoneme blending skills can be tapped as a strategy to improve decoding skills during reading. Similarly, if the SLP provides additional PA intervention to children with severe DPD, the child can be shown how to use these developing skills to support phonological planning and improve production accuracy for complex prosodic, segmental and morphological content (e.g., past tense and third person singular morphemes).

Small groups are more efficient than phonological awareness interventions provided to a single child and more effective than interventions provided to the complete class.

The meta-analysis showed that shorter duration programs with well-specified goals were more effective because all the children were more likely to master the constrained set of goals that were targeted by the activities.

Phonological awareness skills should be linked to their functional applications and teachers are in a good position to ensure that these links are made in the classroom.

Evidence-Based Phonological Awareness Interventions

One program that is particularly consistent with the recommendations of the National Reading Panel is Sound Foundations. Furthermore, this program was the subject of a randomized controlled trial that is an example of exceptional research design.[2] The program was implemented in 12 weekly half-hour sessions, administered to groups of 4 to 6 children, aged 4 years and attending preschool. The program focused on 7 consonants and 2 vowels: initial /s/, /ʃ/, /m/, /p/, /l/, /t/, /g/, final /s/, /m/, /p/, /t/, /l/, and the vowels /æ/ and /ɛ/. The first 11 lessons each focused on a single sound, with multiple activities for identifying words based on the target phoneme. Each lesson began with an appropriate song, rime or jingle that featured the target sound and letter. During the final lesson, card games and dominoes featuring /s/, /p/, /t/, and /l/ were introduced to teach matching and sorting words based on shared onset or coda. Children assigned to the control condition were also seen weekly in small groups and completed identical activities that focused on word meanings and semantic categories. The post-training results showed that the experimental group achieved significantly better phonological awareness performance in word initial and final position with generalization to untaught phonemes. Follow-up of these children revealed that nonword decoding was significantly better for children in the experimental group through fifth grade. Although significant differences were not observed for real word reading or reading comprehension, 16% of the experimental group compared to 28% of the control group scored below a standard score of 75 on one or more reading tests in fifth grade. Recently the intervention has been modified to include sensorimotor instruction of letter forms and dialogic reading to strengthen vocabulary skills (Hindson, Byrne, Fielding-Barnsley, Hine, & Shankweiler, 2005). Justice, Chow, Capellini, Flanigan, and Colton (2003) compared an explicit phoneme awareness intervention, similar to the Sound Foundations approach, to a shared reading/dialogic reading control condition. Growth in emergent literacy skills was significantly greater for children in the experimental intervention than for children in the control intervention.

Explicit teaching of phonological awareness skills has a greater impact on emergent literacy skills than a shared reading intervention.

[2]One aspect of the research design in Byrne and Fielding-Barnsley (1991) that is unique is the statistical treatment of the research groups. As is common in educational research the children were treated in small groups. In these circumstances the children's test scores are not independent of each other because the children in each group influence each other and the performance of all the children in the group is jointly influenced by the common teacher. Therefore, the statistical analysis must treat each group as if it were an individual subject. This study analyses the data appropriately in this respect whereas many if not most studies in which children were treated in groups inappropriately treat the tests scores from each child as individual data points which inflates the power of the study possibly leading to misleading results. Perversely, this aspect of the design (appropriately treating the group rather than the individual child as the unit of analysis) has led to the exclusion of this study from some meta-analyses for statistical reasons yielding inaccurate conclusions about the efficacy of this intervention.

For children who have speech and language impairments, impoverished access to language input, or who are English language learners, a combined approach that targets emergent literacy and oral language skills is essential. We recommend two curricula in particular for their comprehensive approach to language and literacy, both of which were designed for implementation by teachers with 4-year-old children in prekindergarten classrooms. The TELL curriculum was found to be effective in a randomized controlled trial when implemented specifically with children who had speech, language, and other developmental delays (Wilcox, Gray, Guimond, & Lafferty, 2011). Another effective program that provides a comprehensive array of elements targeting oral language and preliteracy skills is PAVEd for Success (Phonological Awareness and Vocabulary Enhancement). The program elements are briefly described in Table 11–5. Schwanenflugel et al. (2010) conducted a large-scale quasi-experimental study to investigate both the effectiveness and sustainability of the program in prekindergarten classrooms in low-income rural communities. Teachers in different schools were taught to implement different combinations of program elements so that, for example, some teachers implemented phonological awareness procedures, others vocabulary enhancement procedures, others both, and some neither. Outcomes were assessed at the end of the

For children who have speech and language impairments, impoverished access to language input, or who are English language learners, a combined approach that targets emergent literacy and oral language skills is essential.

Table 11–5. *PAVEd for Success: Program Elements*

Alphabet Knowledge[abcd]	Focus on a different letter each week within the context of developmentally appropriate activities, introducing letters in order from easiest to hardest.
Interactive Storybook Reading[abcd]	Ensure that each child experiences 5 whole group and 3 small group story book readings each week with teacher asking open-ended questions that probed competence, abstract knowledge, and relation to personal life.
Environmental Print[abcd]	Create a print-rich classroom.
Building Bridges[abcd]	Document 3 5-minute conversations per child each week, using techniques to encourage personal narratives and complex vocabulary and language.
Phonological Awareness[bd]	Provide phonological awareness lessons 3 times per week, spending 2 to 3 weeks on each of several developmentally appropriate skills (rime detection, syllable segmentation, onset detection, syllable and phoneme blending, sound-letter correspondence).
Explicit Vocabulary Practices[cd]	Design thematic units to teach 10 new vocabulary words per week using various strategies incorporated into the preschool routine and curriculum.

Note: One control school did not receive professional education in any of these techniques.

[a]Universal quality literacy practices (UQLP) were taught to all noncontrol schools including one group of schools that received education in only these base techniques.

[b]Phonological awareness techniques were taught in combination with UQLP in some schools.

[c]Explicit vocabulary practices were taught in combination with UQLP in some schools.

[d]The full PAVEd for Success program included all 6 program elements.

The most important finding with respect to child outcomes was that only the full PAVEd program (combining phonological awareness and vocabulary enhancement components) reduced the risk of reading disability for children shown to be at risk at study entry.

prekindergarten year (focusing on emergent literacy) and during the kindergarten year (focusing on prereading and reading skills). The most important finding with respect to child outcomes was that only the full PAVEd program reduced the risk of reading disability for children shown to be at risk at study entry. As we have discussed previously in Chapters 2 and 7, risk status for dyslexia is remarkably consistent. Children who present at school entry with phonological processing and decoding difficulties tend to demonstrate a stable profile throughout the school years. In this study, at-risk children who received the phonological awareness and vocabulary enhancement elements were significantly less likely to present with an at-risk profile in kindergarten. Children who received parts of the program learned from the program elements that were taught but risk status remained unchanged on average. Perhaps the more interesting findings in this study pertain to teacher response to the program. Classroom observations and teacher reports of fidelity to the program were observed during a 15-week implementation phase when teachers received support from the study staff and during a "sustainability phase" when this support was withdrawn. Teacher fidelity to the interactive reading and alphabet knowledge components of the program was high during the implementation and sustainability phases. Teachers were able to implement the phonological awareness program until the children mastered the skills they were taught to focus on and then they discontinued phonological awareness teaching, being uncertain about how to proceed. Fidelity to the language-related elements—building bridges and explicit vocabulary enhancement—was only moderate during the implementation phase and declined significantly during the sustainability phase of the study. The authors concluded that "teachers had much greater difficulty sustaining program features that had not been a previous emphasis in their classrooms" and that "when teachers have to learn skills not previously part of their training . . . long-term support likely will be needed" (p. 260). We feel that joining together with other school personnel to ensure that teachers receive this kind of support in their classrooms is an excellent role for the school SLP and the most efficient means of preventing reading disability among children who are exposed to multiple risk factors. Ehren and Ehren (2001) discuss strategies for expanding the SLP role to include collaborations with teachers in the provision of literacy programs. Schuele and Boudreau (2008) provide excellent guidance for school SLPs who are implementing phonological awareness interventions, either directly or through school personnel.

Direct Reading and Spelling Interventions

Even among children who are able to access speech therapy as preschoolers, a good proportion of children with DPD are likely to present with significant literacy delays in school, with the risk being especially high when the speech difficulties persist beyond the preschool period (Bird, Bishop, & Freeman, 1995; Glogowska, Roulstone, Peters, & Enderby, 2006; Lewis & Freebairn, 1992; Lewis, Freebairn, Hansen, Iyengar, & Taylor, 2004; Nathan, Stackhouse, Goulandris, & Snowling, 2004). As we indicated in Chapter 7, the risk of reading disability in third grade is almost 50% for children with a preschool history of speech and language disorder; the risk of spelling disorder in third grade is 30% for children with a preschool history of speech disorder and twice that for children with combined speech and language disorder as preschoolers (see Table 7–13). Children with childhood apraxia of speech are at particular risk and are very likely to require individual therapy during the school years for treatment of speech, language, and literacy problems. In the previous section we recommended standardized curricula implemented in the classroom as preventative programs for those children at risk for delayed acquisition of literacy skills. For those children who arrive in third grade with an identified reading or spelling disability, individual treatment, implemented by an SLP or paraprofessional working under the supervision of an SLP is required. The intervention should be carefully designed to specifically target gaps in the child's repertoire of language and literacy skills.

A good proportion of children with DPD are likely to present with significant literacy delays in school, with the risk being especially high when the speech difficulties persist beyond the preschool period.

An intervention for a child with an identified reading or spelling disorder should be carefully designed to specifically target gaps in the child's repertoire of language and literacy skills.

When children with DPD have difficulty with reading and spelling, there is likely to be a core deficit in phonological processing that manifests itself as a problem with decoding. Phonological awareness interventions alone will not be sufficient in the case of older children as we indicated earlier. Children older than age 6 or 7 years will require intensive phonics instruction that teaches them to apply their phonological awareness skills and knowledge of sound-symbol correspondence rules to the decoding of letters at all positions of the word, including words with complex structures such as three segment onsets. An intervention that has been shown to be effective with 7- to 10-year-old children with poor reading skills is the Word Building program (McCandliss, Beck, Sandak, & Perfetti, 2003). This program has the goal of improving the quality of the child's orthographic and phonological representations by forcing the child to attend to each letter in the printed word. The program consists of a series of progressively ordered lessons that build words from the CVC through the CCCVCC word shapes, with separate units for different word families (e.g., short vowels, long vowels, etc.). The child forms words with letter cards: inserting, deleting, and exchanging cards according to instructions provided by a tutor. Each new word is read by the child with support as needed from the tutor. Each lesson is preceded by a pretest: the lesson can be omitted if the child achieves a threshold of 90% pretest responding on the target words for the lesson. Advancement to the next lesson in the series requires achievement of the same threshold. An example of a typical lesson is shown in Figure 11–2. The structure of these lessons has many features in common with recommendations for promoting both motor and phonological planning as

Children older than age 6 or 7 years will require intensive **phonics instruction** that teaches them to apply their phonological awareness skills and knowledge of *sound-symbol correspondence rules* to the decoding of letters at all positions of the word.

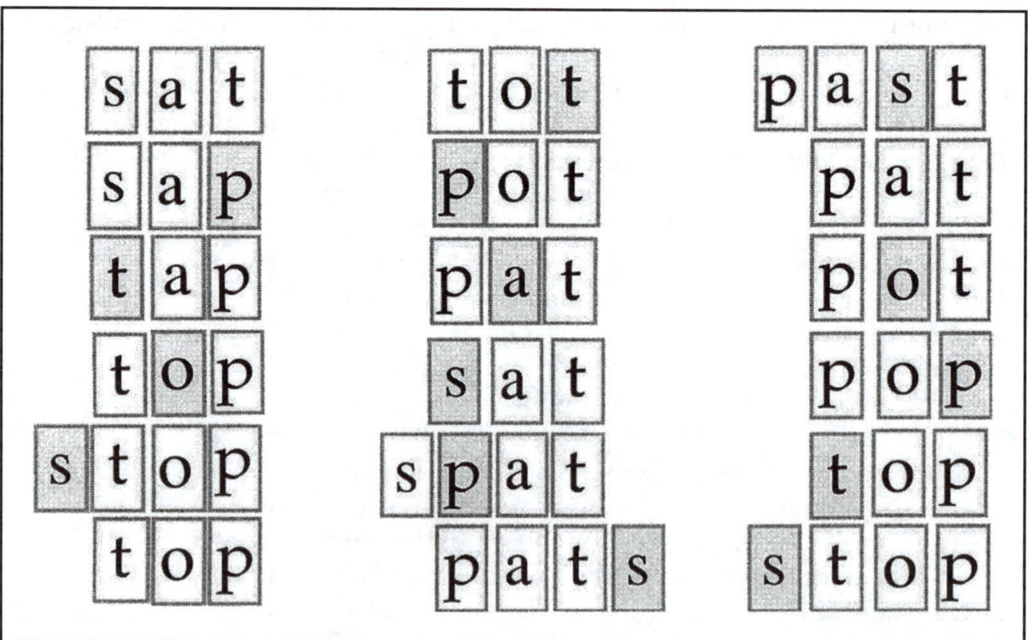

Figure 11–2. *Example of a word building lesson (see text for details).* Source: *From "Focusing Attention on Decoding for Children With Poor Reading Skills: Design and Preliminary Tests of the Word Building Intervention," by B. McCandliss, I. L. Beck, R. Sandak, and C. A. Perfetti,* 2003, Scientific Studies of Reading: The Official Journal of the Society for the Scientific Study of Reading, *7(1), Figure 1, p. 84. Copyright 2003 by Taylor & Francis Informa UK Ltd—Journals. Reprinted with permission.*

outlined in this chapter and Chapter 10 and therefore this appears to be a particularly promising program for children with concomitant DPD and reading disability. In a small sample randomized controlled trial, McCandliss et al. found that children demonstrated statistically and clinically significant gains in phonological awareness, nonword decoding, real word reading and reading comprehension, relative to a no-treatment control group, after 20 one hour lessons provided during the summer break from school. The outcomes were remarkable considering that phonological awareness and reading comprehension were not targeted by the intervention. Furthermore, the lessons were implemented by minimally trained undergraduate students.

For children with severe and persistent speech impairments, the Word Building approach could be supplemented with other programs that bring a more multisensory approach to the mapping of phonological and orthographic representations. The Lindamood Phoneme Sequencing Program has been shown to be effective for the promotion of phonological awareness in older children with reading impairments in randomized controlled trials (Porkorni, Worthington, & Jamison, 2004; Wise, Ring, & Olson, 1999). This program explicitly teaches awareness of the articulatory gestures

For children with severe and persistent speech impairments, the **Word Building approach** could be supplemented with other programs that bring a more multisensory approach to the mapping of phonological and orthographic representations.

associated with phonemes as well as relationships between phonemes in terms of place and manner of articulation. This knowledge is then incorporated into analytical exercises that target letter-sound relationships, manipulation of sounds within words, and spelling-sound patterns. Wise, Ring, and Olsen (1999) found that the articulatory awareness component of the program did not add to the effectiveness of the approach when implemented with children in second through fifth grade who were judged to be reading in the lowest decile in their classrooms. It is possible that this aspect of the program might be specifically helpful for the small minority of children with motor speech disorders but this has not been established empirically. Rvachew and Grawburg (2006) found that phonological awareness in children with DPD was associated with their speech perception skills rather than their speech production performance per se. There is some empirical evidence supporting the implementation of computer-based speech perception interventions as a means to facilitate the acquisition of phonological awareness in school age children although more randomized controlled trials with larger samples and longer follow-up intervals are required (in the UK, "Phenomena," Moore, Rosenberg, & Coleman, 2005; in the US, "Earobics," Porkorni et al., 2004).

With respect to spelling interventions we refer the reader to the excellent papers by Masterson and Crede (1999) and Scott (2000). Summarizing briefly, one of the most important principles of instruction for the SLP is to ensure that spelling instruction for clients with speech, language and learning disorders is fully individualized to the child's specific needs. Children with spelling difficulties will need more practice per word and more concentrated periods of study to learn new words than children who do not have learning disabilities. Therefore, it is essential to ensure that the child is not spending time practicing word lists that contain a high proportion of mastered words or spelling patterns. The activities used to teach children with spelling disorders are not different from those used in the classroom: memorization of word lists; analysis, identification, and sorting of words by common orthographic and morphological patterns; and integration of spelling practice with authentic reading and writing activities. The difference is that the child will require more support and individualized tutoring and concentrated study following a distributed practice schedule. Again, the tutoring will follow principles shown to be effective with all spellers: explicit, sequenced rule-based teaching of phoneme-grapheme correspondences, orthographic patterns, and morphological relationships (Wanzek et al., 2006). A variety of multisensory techniques can be implemented when studying difficult words including visualizing words with eyes closed before writing words, tracing words before writing from memory, and pronouncing words and spelling out loud before writing or typing the component letters. In closing this section, we point out a final and crucial principal and that is to work on words that will be used in the child's writing and to

Ensure that spelling instruction for clients with speech, language, and learning disorders is fully individualized to the child's specific needs.

The SLP should follow principles shown to be effective with all spellers: explicit, sequenced rule-based teaching of phoneme-grapheme correspondences, orthographic patterns, and morphological relationships.

A variety of multisensory techniques can be implemented when studying difficult words.

Plan for an appropriate mix of drill-practice and authentic writing activities in each session.

plan for an appropriate mix of drill-practice and authentic writing activities in each session. In Chapter 10 we presented a sample treatment plan for a child focused on an end of term project on plate tectonics (Demonstration 10–6). In this case the focus was speech intelligibility and accuracy. In a similar vein, we would suggest that individualized spelling instruction by the SLP be targeted at the specific challenges that the child is facing in the classroom and thus the details of the intervention will require collaboration with the classroom teacher and the involvement of the child in the selection of specific goals.

Conclusions and Recommendations

The phonological therapy program will be designed to promote generalization of learning from specific phonological structures taught in therapy to new words and new structures as efficiently as possible.

Phonological approaches all begin with a thorough analysis of the child's phonological knowledge at multiple levels of representation. The selection of basic, intermediate, and specific goals as outlined in Chapter 8 will focus on mismatches in the child's phonological knowledge relative to the adult system while taking advantage of strengths that can be used as a foundation for acquisition of new phonological knowledge. The phonological therapy program will be designed to promote generalization of learning from specific phonological structures taught in therapy to new words and new structures as efficiently as possible. A large part of the planning for generalization involves selecting and ordering treatment goals to promote diffusion of new knowledge through the lexicon on the basis of similar phonological characteristics. Practice words will typically be grouped to emphasize similarities at the level of overall word shape, syllable structure, segment composition, or features.

Procedures for strengthening acoustic-phonetic and articulatory-phonetic representations play an important role in laying the foundation for the emergence of phonological knowledge.

Metaphonological skills are taught, not only to promote speech intelligibility, but to facilitate the child's acquisition of reading and writing.

The choice of treatment procedures also plays a role in promoting generalization. First, procedures for strengthening acoustic-phonetic and articulatory-phonetic representations, as described in Chapters 9 and 10, play an important role in laying the foundation for the emergence of phonological knowledge. The cycles approach marries these procedures for strengthening phonetic knowledge together with a unique cycles goal attack strategy that raises awareness of phonological patterns and promotes gradual achievement of intelligible speech in accordance with developmental principles. Other procedures are metaphonological in nature, designed to instill explicit awareness of the sound structure of the language and to challenge the child with communicative breakdowns that trigger self-repairs when words are mispronounced. The success of these procedures requires a base level of phonological knowledge on the part of the child as well as perceptual awareness of the target phonological contrast and articulatory knowledge of the target phoneme. Finally, metaphonological skills are taught, not only to promote speech intelligibility, but to facilitate the child's acquisition of reading and writing. Provided a series of interventions, adapted to changing developmental needs and given with sufficient intensity, the child will meet this challenge too and be well positioned to achieve good social, emotional, and academic outcomes over the long term.

References

Allen, M. M. (2009, November). *The impact of treatment intensity on a phonological intervention*. Paper presented at the annual convention of the American-Speech-Language-Hearing Association, New Orleans, LA.

Almost, D., & Rosenbaum, P. (1998). Effectiveness of speech intervention for phonological disorders: A randomized controlled trial. *Developmental Medicine and Child Neurology, 40*, 319–325.

Baker, E. (2011). Minimal pair intervention. In A. L. Williams, S. McLeod, & R. J. McCauley (Eds.), *Interventions for speech sound disorders in children* (pp. 41–72). Baltimore, MD: Brookes.

Barlow, J. A., & Gierut, J. A. (2002). Minimal pair approaches to phonological remediation. *Seminars in Speech and Language, 23*(1), 57–67.

Bernhardt, B. (1990). *Application of nonlinear phonological theory to intervention with six phonologically disordered children.* University of British Columbia, Vancouver, Canada.

Bernhardt, B. (1992). Application of nonlinear phonological theory to intervention with one phonologically disordered child. *Clinical Linguistics & Phonetics, 6*, 283–316.

Bernhardt, B. (1994). Phonological intervention techniques for syllable and word structure development. *Clinics in Communication Disorders, 4*, 5–65.

Bernhardt, B., & Gilbert, J. (1992). Applying linguistic theory to speech-language pathology: The case for non-linear phonology. *Clinical Linguistics & Phonetics, 6*, 123–145.

Bernhardt, B., & Major, E. M. (2005). Speech, language and literacy skills three years later: A follow-up study of early phonological and metaphonological intervention. *International Journal of Language and Communication Disorders, 40*, 1–27.

Bernhardt, B., & Stemberger, J.P. (2000). *Workbook in nonlinear phonology for clinical application*. Austin, TX: Pro-Ed.

Biemiller, A., & Boote, C. (2006). An effective method for building meaning vocabulary in primary grades. *Journal of Educational Psychology, 98*(1), 44–62.

Bird, J., Bishop, D. V. M., & Freeman, N. H. (1995). Phonological awareness and literacy development in children with expressive phonological impairments. *Journal of Speech and Hearing Research, 38*, 446–462.

Blache, S. E., & Parsons, C. L. (1980). A linguistic approach to distinctive feature training. *Language, Speech, and Hearing Services in Schools, 11*, 203–207.

Blache, S. E., Parsons, C. L., & Humphreys, J. M. (1981). A minimal-word-pair model for teaching the linguistic significance of distinctive feature properties. *Journal of Speech and Hearing Disorders, 46*, 291–296.

Bountress, N. G., & Bountress, M. G. (1985). Modification of articulation error using a multiple-context, distinctive feature treatment program. *Perceptual and Motor Skills, 61*, 792–794.

Boyle, J., McCartney, E., Forbes, J., & O'Hare, A. (2007). A randomised control trial and economic evaluation of direct versus indirect and individual versus group modes of speech and language therapy for children with primary language impairment. *Health Technology Assessment, 11*(25), iii–108. Retrieved from http://www.hta.ac.uk/1232

Broen, P. A., & Westman, M. J. (1990). Project parent: A preschool speech program implemented through parents. *Journal of Speech and Hearing Disorders, 55*, 495–502.

Browman, C., & Goldstein, L. M. (1989). Articulatory gestures as phonological units. *Phonology, 6*, 201–251.

Byrne, B., & Fielding-Barnsley, R. (1991). Evaluation of a program to teach phonemic awareness to young children. *Journal of Educational Psychology, 83*(4), 451–455.

Campbell, F. A., Ramey, C. T., Pugello, E. P., Sparling, J., & Miller-Johnson, S. (2002). Early childhood education: Young adult outcomes from the Abecedarian Project. *Applied Developmental Science, 6*(3), 42–57.

Clark, C. E., Schwarz, I. E., & Blakeley, R. W. (1993). The removable R-appliance as a practice device to facilitate correct production of /r/. *American Journal of Speech-Language Pathology, 2*, 84–92.

Costello, J., & Onstine, J. M. (1976). The modification of multiple articulation errors based on distinctive feature theory. *Journal of Speech and Hearing Disorders, 41*(2), 199–215.

Crosbie, S., Holm, A., & Dodd, B. (2005). Intervention for children with severe speech disorder: A comparison of two approaches. *International Journal of Language and Communication Disorders, 40*(4), 467–491.

Cummings, A. E., & Barlow, J. A. (2010). A comparison of word lexicality in the treatment of speech sound disorders. *Clinical Linguistics & Phonetics, 25*, 265–286.

Dean, E., & Howell, J. (1986). Developing linguistic awareness: A theoretically based approach to phonological disorders. *British Journal of Disorders of Communication, 31*, 223–238.

Dickinson, D. K., & Tabors, P. O. (2001). *Beginning literacy with language: Young children learning at home and at school*. Baltimore, MD: Brookes.

Dodd, B., & Bradford, A. (2000). A comparison of three therapy methods for children with different types of developmental disorder. *International Journal of Language and Communication Disorders, 35*(2), 189–209.

Dodd, B., Crosbie, S., McIntosh, B., Holm, A., Harvey, C., Liddy, M., . . . Rigby, H. (2008). The impact of selecting different contrasts in phonological therapy. *International Journal of Speech-Language Pathology, 10*, 334–345.

Ehren, B. J., & Ehren, T. C. (2001). New or expanded literacy roles for speech-language pathologists: Making it happen in the schools. *Seminars in Speech and Language, 22*, 233–243.

Ehri, L. C, Nunes, S. R, Willows, D. M, Schuster, B. V., Yaghoub-Zadeh, Z., & Shanahan, T. (2001). Phonemic awareness instruction helps children learn to read: Evidence from the national reading panel's meta-analysis. *Reading Research Quarterly, 36*(3), 250–287.

Elbert, M., Dinnsen, D. A., & Powell, T. W. (1984). On the predition of phonological generalization learning patterns. *Journal of Speech and Hearing Disorders, 49*, 309–317.

Elbert, M., Dinnsen, D. A., Swartzlander, P., & Chin, S. B. (1990). Generalization to conversational speech. *Journal of Speech and Hearing Disorders, 55*, 694–699.

Elbert, M., & McReynolds, L. V. (1985). The generalization hypothesis: Final consonant deletion. *Language and Speech, 28*, 281–294.

Elbert, M., Powell, T. W., & Swartzlander, P. (1991). Toward a technology of generalization: How many exemplars are sufficient? *Journal of Speech and Hearing Research, 34*, 81–87.

Evans, M. A., & Saint-Aubin, J. (2009). Letter names and alphabet book reading by senior kindergartneners: An eye movement study. *Child Development, 80*, 1824–1841.

Ferguson, C., & Farwell, C. B. (1975). Words and sounds in early acquisition. *Language, 51*(2), 419–439.

Forrest, K., Dinnsen, D. A., & Elbert, M. (1997). Impact of substitution patterns on phonological learning by misarticulating children. *Clinical Linguistics & Phonetics, 11*, 63–76.

Forrest, K., Elbert, M., & Dinnsen, D. A. (2000). The effect of substitution patterns on phonological treatment outcomes. *Clinical Linguistics & Phonetics, 14*, 519–531.

Gardner, H. (1997). Are your minimal pairs too neat? The dangers of phonemicisation in phonology therapy. *European Journal of Disorders of Communication, 32*, 167–175.

Gierut, J., Morrisette, M. L., & Ziemer, S. M. (2010). Nonwords and generalization in children with phonological disorders. *American Journal of Speech-Language Pathology, 19*, 167–177.

Gierut, J. A., Morrisette, M. L., & Champion, A. H. (1999). Lexical constraints in phonological acquisition. *Journal of Child Language, 26*, 261–294.

Gillon, G. T. (2000). The efficacy of phonological awareness intervention for children with spoken language impairment. *Language, Speech, and Hearing Services in Schools, 31*, 126–141.

Gillon, G. T. (2002). Follow-up study investigating benefits of phonological awareness intervention for children with spoken language impairment. *International Journal of Language and Communication Disorders, 37*, 381–400.

Girolametto, L., Pearce, P. S., & Weitzman, E. (1997). Effects of lexical intervention on the phonology of late talkers. *Journal of Speech, Language, and Hearing Research, 40*(2), 338–348.

Glogowska, M., Roulstone, S., Peters, T. J., & Enderby, P. (2006). Early speech- and language-impaired children: Linguistic, literacy, and social outcomes. *Developmental Medicine and Child Neurology, 48*, 489–494.

Goldstein, M. H., & Schwade, J. A. (2008). Social feedback to infants' babbling facilitates rapid phonological learning. *Psychological Science, 19*(5), 515–523.

Goldstein, M. H., Schwade, J. H., Menyhart, O., & DeVoogd, T. J. (2011). *From birds to words: Social interactions at small timescales yield big effects on the development of vocal communication*. Paper presented at the 2011 biennial meeting of the Society for Research in Child Development, Montréal, Québec, Canada.

Graves, M. (2006). *The vocabulary book: Learning and instruction*. New York: NY: Teachers College Press.

Gray, B. B. (1974). A field study on programmed articulation therapy. *Language, Speech, and Hearing Services in Schools, 5*, 119–131.

Harm, M. W., McCandliss, B. D., & Seidenberg, M. S. (2003). Modeling the successes and failures of interventions for disabled readers. *Scientific Studies of Reading, 7*(2), 155–182.

Hesketh, A., Adams, C., Nightingale, C., & Hall, R. (2000). Phonological awareness therapy and articulatory training approaches for children with phonological disorders: a comparative outcome study. *International Journal of Language and Communication Disorders, 35*(3), 337–354.

Hesketh, A., Dima, E., & Nelson, V. (2007). Teaching phoneme awareness to pre-literate children with speech disorder: a randomized controlled trial. *International Journal of Language and Communication Disorders, 42*(3), 251–271.

Hindson, B., Byrne, B., Fielding-Barnsley, R., Hine, D. W., & Shankweiler, D. (2005). Assessment and early instruction of preschool children at risk for reading disability. *Journal of Educational Psychology, 97*(4), 687–704.

Hodson, B. (2007). *Evaluating and enhancing children's phonological systems: Research and theory to practice.* Wichita, KS: Phonocomp.

Hodson, B. W. (2011, April 5). Enhancing phonological patterns of young children with highly unintelligible speech. *ASHA Leader.*

Hodson, B. W., & Paden, E. P. (1983). *Targeting intelligible speech: A phonological approach to remediation.* Boston, MA: College Hill.

Howard, I. S., & Messum, P. (2011). Modeling the development of pronunciation in infant speech acquisition. *Motor Control, 15*, 85–117.

Justice, L. M., Chow, S., Capellini, C., Flanigan, K., & Colton, S. (2003). Emergent literacy intervention for vulnerable preschoolers: Relative effects of two approaches. *American Journal of Speech-Language Pathology, 12*, 320–332.

Kröger, B. J., Kopp, S., & Lowit, A. (2010). A model for production, perception, and acquisition of actions in face-to-face communication. *Cognitive Processing, 11*, 187–205. doi: 10.1007/s10339-009-0351-2

Leonard, L. B., & Brown, B. L. (1984). Nature and boundaries of phonological categories: A case study of an unusual phonologic pattern in a language-impaired child. *Journal of Speech and Hearing Disorders, 49*, 419–428.

Lewis, B. A., & Freebairn, L. (1992). Residual effects of preschool phonology disorders in grade school, adolescence, and adulthood. *Journal of Speech and Hearing Research, 35*, 819–831.

Lewis, B. A., Freebairn, L. A., Hansen, A. J., Iyengar, S. K., & Taylor, H. G. (2004). School-age follow-up children with childhood apraxia of speech. *Language, Speech, and Hearing Services in Schools, 35*, 122–140.

Liu, R., & Holt, L. L. (2010). Neural changes associated with nonspeech auditory category learning parallel those of speech category acquisition. *Journal of Cognitive Neuroscience, 23*(3), 683–698.

Major, E. M., & Bernhardt, B. (1998). Metaphonological skills of children with phonological disorders before and after phonological and metaphonological intervention. *International Journal of Language and Communication Disorders, 33*, 413–444.

Masterson, J., & Crede, L. A. (1999). Learning to spell: Implications for assessment and intervention. *Language, Speech, and Hearing Services in Schools, 30*, 243–254.

McAllister Byun, T. (2011). A gestural account of a child-specific neutralisation in strong position. *Phonology, 28*, 371–412. doi:10.1017/S0952675711000297

McCandliss, B., Beck, I. L., Sandak, R., & Perfetti, C. A. (2003). Focusing attention on decoding for children with poor reading skills: Design and preliminary tests of the word building intervention. *Scientific Studies of Reading, 7*(1), 75–104.

McReynolds, L. V., & Bennett, S. (1972). Distinctive feature generalization in articulation training. *Journal of Speech and Hearing Disorders, 37*, 462–470.

Montgomery, J. K., & Bonderman, I. R. (1989). Serving preschool children with severe phonological disorders. *Language, Speech, and Hearing Services in Schools, 20*(1), 76–84.

Moore, D. R., Rosenberg, J. F., & Coleman, J. S. (2005). Discrimination training of phonemic contrasts enhances phonological processing in mainstream school children. *Brain and Language, 94*, 72–85.

Morrisette, M. L., & Gierut, J. A. (2002). Lexical organization and phonological change in treatment. *Journal of Speech, Language, and Hearing Research, 45*, 143–159.

Mowrer, D. E. (1971). Transfer of training in articulation therapy. *Journal of Speech and Hearing Disorders, 36*, 427–446.

Nathan, L., Stackhouse, J., Goulandris, N., & Snowling, M. J. (2004). Educational consequences of developmental speech disorder: Key Stage I national curriculum assessment results in English and mathematics. *British Journal of Educational Psychology, 74*, 173–186.

Noble, K. G., Farah, M. J., & McCandliss, B. (2006). Socioeconomic background modulates cognition-achievement relationships in reading. *Cognitive Development, 21*, 349–368.

Porkorni, J. L., Worthington, C. K., & Jamison, P. J. (2004). Phonological awareness intervention: Comparison of Fast ForWord, Earobics, and LiPS. *Journal of Educational Research, 97*(3), 147–157.

Prezas, R. F., & Hodson, B. W. (2010). The cycles phonological remediation approach. In A. L. Williams, S. McLeod, & R. J. McCauley (Eds.), *Interventions for speech sound disorders in children* (pp. 137–158). Baltimore, MD: Brookes.

Ramey, C. T., Campbell, F. A., & Ramey, S. L. (1999). Early intervention: Succesful pathways to improving intellectual development. *Developmental Neuropsychology, 16*(3), 385–392.

Rvachew, S., & Andrews, E. (2002). The influence of syllable position on children's production of consonants. *Clinical Linguistics & Phonetics, 16*(3), 183–198.

Rvachew, S, & Brosseau-Lapré, F. (2010, November). *Improving phonological awareness in French-speaking children with speech delay*. Paper presented at the annual convention of the American Speech-Language-Hearing Association, Philadelphia, PA.

Rvachew, S., & Grawburg, M. (2006). Correlates of phonological awareness in preschoolers with speech sound disorders. *Journal of Speech, Language, and Hearing Research, 49*, 74–87.

Rvachew, S., & Nowak, M. (2001). The effect of target selection strategy on sound production learning. *Journal of Speech, Language, and Hearing Research, 44*, 610–623.

Rvachew, S., & Savage, R. (2006). Preschool foundations of early reading acquisition. *Pediatrics and Child Health, 11*, 589–593.

Saben, C. B., & Costello Ingham, J. (1991). The effects of a minimal pairs treatment on the speech-sound production of two children with phonologic disorders. *Journal of Speech and Hearing Research, 34*, 1023–1040.

Schuele, C. M., & Boudreau, D. (2008). Phonological awareness intervention: Beyond the basics. *Language, Speech, and Hearing Services in Schools, 39*, 3–20.

Schwanenflugel, P. J., Hamilton, A., Neuharth-Pritchett, S., Restrepo, M. A., Bradley, B. A., & Webb, M. (2010). PAVEd for Success: An evaluation of a comprehensive program for four-year-old children. *Journal of Literacy Research, 42*, 227–275.

Scott, C. M. (2000). Principles and methods of spelling instruction: Applications for poor spellers. *Topics in Language Disorders, 20*, 66–82.

Senechal, M., & LeFevre, J. (2002). Parental involvement in the development of children's reading: A five-year longitudinal study. *Child Development, 73*(2), 445–460.

Stevens, K. N., & Keyser, S. J. (2009). Quantal theory, enhancement and overlap. *Journal of Phonetics*. doi:10.1016/ j.wocn.2008.1010.1004

Stoel-Gammon, C. (2011). Relationship between lexical and phonological development in young children. *Journal of Child Language, 38*, 1–34.

Stoel-Gammon, C., Stone-Goldman, J., & Glaspey, A. (2002). Pattern based approaches to phonological therapy. *Seminars in Speech and Language, 23*, 3–13.

Stokes, S. F. (2010). Neighborhood density and word frequency predict vocabulary size in toddlers. *Journal of Speech, Language, and Hearing Research, 53*, 670–683.

Storkel, H. L., Moskawa, J., & Hoover, J. R. (2010). Differentiating the effects of phonotactic probability and neighborhood density on vocabulary comprehension and production: A comparison of preschool children with versus without phonological delays. *Journal of Speech, Language, and Hearing Research, 53*, 933–949.

Tyler, A. A., Edwards, M. L., & Saxman, J. H. (1987). Clinical application of two phonologically based treatment procedures. *Journal of Speech and Hearing Research, 52*, 393–409.

Velleman, S. L. (2002). Phonotactic therapy. *Seminars in Speech and Language, 23*, 43–55.

Vihman, M. M. (2006, June). *Phonological templates in early words: A cross-linguistic study.* Paper presented at the 10th Conference on Laboratory Phonology, Paris, France.

Wanzek, J., Vaughn, S., Wexler, J., Swenson, E. A., Edmonds, M., & Kim A. (2006). A synthesis of spelling and reading inerventions and their effects on the spelling outcomes of students with LD. *Journal of Learning Disabilities, 39*, 528–543.

Wasik, B. A., Bond, M. A., & Hindman, A. (2006). The effects of a language and literacy intervention on Head Start children and teachers. *Journal of Educational Psychology, 98*(1), 63–74.

Weiner, F. (1981). Treatment of phonological disability using the method of meaningful minimal contrasts: Two case studies. *Journal of Speech and Hearing Disorders, 46*, 97–103.

Whitehurst, G. J., Falco, F., Lonigan, C. J., Fischel, J. E., DeBaryshe, B. D., Valdez-Menchaca, M. C., & Caulfield, M. (1988). Accelerating language development through picture book reading. *Developmental Psychology, 24*, 552–558.

Wilcox, M. J., Gray, S. L., Guimond, A. B., & Lafferty, A. E. (2011). Efficacy of the TELL language and literacy curriculum for preschoolers with developmental speech and/or language impairments. *Early Childhood Research Quarterly, 26*, 278–294.

Williams, A. L. (2010). Multiple oppositions intervention. In A. L. Williams, S. McLeod, & R. J. McCauley (Eds.), *Interventions for speech sound disorders in children* (pp. 73–93). Baltimore, MD: Brookes.

Wise, B. W., Ring, J., & Olson, R. K. (1999). Training phonological awareness with and without explicit attention to articulation. *Journal of Experimental Child Psychology, 72*, 271–304.

Index

Note: Page numbers in **bold** indicate nontext material.

D

H

I

J

K

L

M

N

O

P

Q

R

S

T

U

V

W

Z